Nuclear Medicine and PET/CT

Technology and Techniques

NUCLEAR MEDICINE AND PET/CT
Technology and Techniques

Seventh Edition

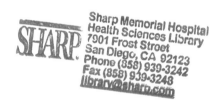

Paul E. Christian, BS, CNMT, FSNMTS, PET
Associate Director, Molecular Imaging Program
Director, Cyclotron Radiochemistry Laboratory
Huntsman Cancer Institute
University of Utah
Salt Lake City, Utah

Kristen M. Waterstram-Rich, MS, CNMT, FSNMTS
Professor
Director, Premedical Studies
Biomedical Sciences Program Director
Rochester Institute of Technology
Rochester, New York

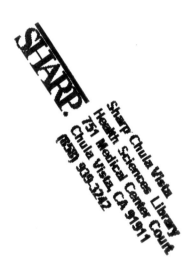

ELSEVIER
MOSBY

3251 Riverport Lane
St. Louis, Missouri 63043

NUCLEAR MEDICINE AND PET/CT TECHNOLOGY AND TECHNIQUES, SEVENTH EDITION

ISBN: 978-0-323-07192-5

ISBN: 978-0-323-07192-5

Acquisitions Editor: Jeanne Olson
Developmental Editor: Luke Held
Publishing Services Manager: Julie Eddy
Senior Project Manager: Laura Loveall
Design Direction: Margaret Reid

Printed in the United States

Last digit is the print number: 9 8 7 6 5 4 3 2 1

Carolyn J. Anderson, PhD
Professor
Radiology, Biochemistry &
    Molecular Biophysics and
    Chemistry Department
Washington University
St. Louis, Missouri

Crystal Botkin, MPH, CNMT, PET
NMT Clinical Coordinator
Saint Louis University
Doisy College of Health Sciences
Department of Medical Imaging
    and Radiation Therapeutics
St. Louis, Missouri

Paul H. Brown, PhD
Associate Professor of
    Radiology
Oregon Health Sciences University
Portland, Oregon

**Paul E. Christian, BS, CNMT,
FSNMTS, PET**
Associate Director, Molecular
    Imaging Program
Director, Cyclotron Radiochemistry
    Laboratory
Huntsman Cancer Institute
University of Utah
Salt Lake City, Utah

**Gary L. Dillehay, MD, FACNP,
FACR**
Professor of Radiology
Department of Nuclear Medicine
Northwestern Memorial Hospital
Chicago, Illinois

Kevin Donohoe, MD
Staff Physician, Division of Nuclear
    Medicine
Beth Israel Deaconess Medical
    Center
Assistant Professor of
    Radiology
Harvard Medical School
Boston, Massachusetts

**Helen H. Drew, MT(ASCP),
CNMT(NMTCB)**
Technical Specialist, Core Special
    Chemistry Laboratories
Department of Pathology
Johns Hopkins Hospital
Baltimore, Maryland

Tracy L. Faber, PhD
Professor of Radiology
Emory University
Atlanta, Georgia

James R. Galt, PhD
Assistant Professor, Emory
    University
Nuclear Medicine, Emory
    University Hospital
Atlanta, Georgia

**David Gilmore, MS, CNMT, NCT,
RT(R)(N)**
Program Director, School of
    Nuclear Medicine
    Technology
Beth Israel Deaconess Medical
    Center, a Harvard Medical
    School Affiliate
Boston, Massachusetts

Stanley J. Goldsmith, BA, MD
Director, Nuclear Medicine &
    Molecular Imaging
Professor of Radiology and
    Medicine
Weill Medical College of Cornell
    University
New York-Presbyterian Hospital/
    Weill Cornell Medical
    Center
New York, New York

Ravinder K. Grewal, MD
Assistant Attending Physician
Nuclear Medicine Service
Memorial Sloan Kettering Cancer
    Center
New York, New York

**William Hubble, MA, CNMT,
RT(R)(N)(CT), FSNMTS**
Academic Chair/NMT Program
    Director
Associate Professor
Saint Louis University
Doisy College of Health Sciences
Department of Medical Imaging
    and Radiation Therapeutics
St. Louis, Missouri

Kathy Thompson Hunt, MS, CNMT
Program Chair, Nuclear Medicine
    Technology
Baptist College of Health Sciences
Memphis, Tennessee

Peter Jenkins, MS, CHP
Medical Physicist
University of Utah Hospitals and
    Clinics
Salt Lake City, Utah

Karen S. Langley, MS
Radiation Safety Officer, Director
Radiological Health Department
University of Utah
Salt Lake City, Utah

Janice Leggett, RTNM
Supervisor, Division of Nuclear
    Medicine
British Columbia Children's Hospital
Radiology Department
Vancouver, British Columbia
Canada

**Mark T. Madsen, PhD, FAAPM,
FACR**
Professor of Radiology
University of Iowa
Iowa City, Iowa

Leon S. Malmud, MD
Dean Emeritus, Temple University
    School of Medicine
Temple University Hospital
Philadelphia, Pennsylvania

Donna C. Mars, MEd, CNMT, NCT
Assistant Professor, Allied Health
  Division
Baptist College of Health Sciences
Memphis, Tennessee

Derek McGuire, RTNM, CDT
Nuclear Medicine Technologist
British Columbia Children's
  Hospital
Radiology Department
Vancouver, British Columbia
Canada

Denise A. Merlino, CPC, CNMT, MBA
President, Merlino Healthcare
  Consulting Corp.
Magnolia, Massachusetts

Frances L. Neagley, CNMT, FSNMTS
Editor, Journal of Nuclear Medicine
  Technology
Society of Nuclear Medicine
Reston, Virginia

Neeta Pandit-Taskar, MD
Associate Attending Physician
Nuclear Medicine Service
Memorial Sloan Kettering Cancer
  Center
New York, New York

Henry Royal, MD
Professor, Radiology
Associate Director, Division of
  Nuclear Medicine
Mallinckrodt Institute of Radiology
Washington University School of
  Medicine
St. Louis, Missouri

Sally Schwarz, RPh, MS
Washington University School of
  Medicine
Department of Radiology/Division
  of Nuclear Medicine
St. Louis, Missouri

Akash Sharma, MD
Instructor in Radiology
Division of Nuclear Medicine
Mallinckrodt Institute of Radiology
Washington University School of
  Medicine
St. Louis, Missouri

H. William Strauss, MD
Attending Physician
Nuclear Medicine Service
Memorial Sloan Kettering Cancer
  Center
New York, New York

Nancy M. Swanston, CNMT, PET, RT(N)
Manager, Diagnostic Imaging
Section of Positron Emission
  Tomography
Division of Diagnostic Imaging
The University of Texas MD
  Anderson Cancer Center
Houston, Texas

Kathy Thomas, MHA, CNMT, PET
Applications/Technical Support
Capintec, Inc.
Battle Ground, Washington

Jean-Luc Urbain, MD
St. Joseph Hospital
London, Ontario
Canada

Mark Wallenmeyer, MBA, CNMT, FSNMTS
Assistant Professor of Nuclear
  Medicine Imaging Sciences
University of Arkansas for Medical
  Sciences
Little Rock, Arkansas

Kristen M. Waterstram-Rich, MS, CNMT, FSNMTS
Professor
Director, Premedical Studies
Biomedical Sciences Program
  Director
Rochester Institute of Technology
Rochester, New York

Katherine Zukotynski, BASc, MD, FRCP(C)
Staff Radiologist, Dana-Farber
  Cancer Institute
Associate Radiologist, Brigham and
  Women's Hospital
Instructor in Radiology, Harvard
  Medical School
Boston, Massachusetts

The production of a textbook is a labor of love. To have reached the status of a seventh edition shows a level of dedication amongst the authors and editors that is unusual. For almost three decades, this book has provided a mainstay in the education of nuclear medicine technologists. When one looks back, nuclear medicine was much simpler when the first edition of this book was published. Without significant change from either the first or the sixth edition, this book would not be of much use. A look at the book today, now in its seventh edition, shows it to be current and demonstrates a blending of old and new while also addressing future developments. The changes to the current edition make it ideal for the education of the nuclear medicine technologist. (It is also a great source of information for anyone in the first who wants an eminently readable text.)

Today's seventh edition is as up-to-date as a book can be. A completely new chapter on instrumentation by Mark Madsen brings into focus all of the current devices and is filled with excellent illustrations and descriptive material that is current and understandable. In the sixth edition, a new chapter was added on CT physics. Now a new addition to this text is a chapter on the physics and principles of MRI. At first glance, this would seem to be a somewhat unusual addition to a nuclear medicine text; however, it shows how the editors and authors are preparing the reader to deal with future clinical developments in imaging. A completely new chapter on brain imaging from the Boston group with so much experience in this area is another example of the forward-looking nature of this text. In the group of new and updated chapters is a complete revision of the chapter on cardiac imaging that incorporates imaging guidelines for clinical appropriateness. The nuclear medicine technologist is going to find himself/herself right in the middle of implementation of appropriateness criteria, and this is a wonderful starting place to get accustomed to the terminology and implementation of such guidelines.

The chapter on computer science has undergone a major revision with the focus shifting more to computer applications and practical digital imaging. The reader of this chapter will also be introduced to basics of PACS, networking, and image co-registration (fusion) of digital images. The chapter on radiochemistry and radiopharmacology has been updated with increased focus on the operation of the ^{99}Mo-^{99m}Tc generator and more information on PET radiopharmaceuticals. Further, the reader is introduced to some of the new regulatory changes, including USP Chapter <797>. Other chapters have had facelifts as appropriate to keep them current.

A feature that I particularly like is the outline at the beginning of chapters and the list of learning objectives and key terms for the chapter. Preceding the objectives is a standard outline of the chapter that is directed at those looking for a quick reference on a given topic. For educators, this structure is particularly useful. The quality of illustrations is excellent, and they have been chosen to drive home or illustrate principles in the text. The illustrations and captions are clear and understandable.

One of the interesting features of this text is its integration with the Evolve website. This integration allows the instructor to enrich their own materials with images from the textbook. Downloadable examination questions permit the use of the most current thinking to assess the student's comprehension of the presented material. Although this text is directed primarily at the nuclear medicine technology student, its organization and quality make it a text useable by radiology and nuclear medicine residents as well an absolute necessity on everyone's reference shelf.

Robert E Henkin, MD, FACNM, FACR
Professor Emeritus of Radiology
Loyola University Stritch School of Medicine
Maywood, Illinois

CONTENT

Writing a book is definitely a labor of love and a testament to patience. The process takes over two years, and the work waxes and wanes throughout the time period; but it is not until the very end that one gets a glimpse of how the book will look in print.

This book, now in its seventh edition, has stood the test of time. It continues to keep pace with the changes in the field of nuclear medicine and healthcare as it expands and evolves to meet the needs of the professionals facing the challenges of changing technology and medical practice. Through all of the revisions, it has stayed true to its focus of providing information that covers all aspects of nuclear medicine, thereby serving as a comprehensive introductory text for nuclear medicine professionals to enter practice in this field. This book is intended for use by technologists and student technologists, and it is also intended as a reference guide for physicians and scientists entering nuclear medicine. It is used by many nuclear medicine technologist educational programs and as a resource in many nuclear medicine departments worldwide.

The textbook remains divided into two main sections: the basic science chapters and the clinical applications. The knowledge base formed from the basic science chapters (e.g., mathematics, physics, instrumentation, patient care, and radiation safety) provide the foundation on which the clinical chapters build. In the clinical chapters, the science is expanded to include anatomy and physiology, and it is in the clinical chapters where you can see the complexity of the field of nuclear medicine and how the interconnectedness of physics, chemistry, anatomy, and physiology result in diagnostic images, or are used in clinical and therapeutic applications. The clinical chapters essentially start at the head and work their way down the body. The last two chapters, "Inflammatory/Tumor/Oncology Imaging and Therapy" and "Pediatric Imaging," include topics that span all body systems. This coherent framework for the knowledge base of the book provides an efficient and logical approach to studying the field of nuclear medicine that allows for students to see a unifying theme or connectedness of the information. An appendix of radiopharmaceuticals, which summarizes many of the radionuclide properties, radiopharmaceutical names, and clinical applications, is also included as an easy reference.

NEW TO THIS EDITION

Each revised edition captures the changes that have occurred since the previous edition and gives a glimpse into changes and advancements that are under investigation. The many expert contributors of the chapters have reviewed and updated the information in this edition to bring the materials and figures to the current level of clinical practice. There are several chapters that have undergone notable revisions. Chapter 3, "Instrumentation," has been replaced with a new chapter by a new contributing author in an effort to make this topic more easily understood and comprehensive and to provide an uptake to changes in this expanding area and new device configurations. Chapter 12, "Principles of Magnetic Resonance Imaging," is a completely new chapter. Chapter 12 has been added to provide the reader with a familiarity of magnetic resonance and magnetic resonance imaging, and it is not intended to be a comprehensive study of MRI. Chapter 14, "Central Nervous System," was revised by a new group of contributing authors from Boston who have provided a major revision to the chapter. There are also new co-authors in Chapters 15, 19, 21, and 23. Chapter 22 has a new title "Inflammatory/Tumor/Oncology Imaging and Therapy." As described by its title, the chapter has expanded to include the growing area of nuclear medicine therapy in oncology. Lastly, each chapter has protocols separated from the text for easy reference.

LEARNING ENHANCEMENTS

Each chapter begins with an outline, learning objectives, and key terms. The key terms appear in the front of each chapter to aid students in identifying terms with which they should become familiar. Each term will appear in boldface the first time that it used in the chapter. The key terms are also defined in the Glossary at the end of the book. There are also summaries at the end of each chapter to highlight a few of the important concepts in each chapter. The full-color PET/CT and cardiac scan insert has been expanded to provide additional examples of realistic scans found in practice.

Chapter 1, "Mathematics and Statistics," gives the reader opportunities to practice the basic math skills necessary to function as a nuclear medicine technologist. The answers for these questions are provided at the end of the book so that the reader can assess their knowledge before proceeding to the next chapter.

Boxes and tables are used throughout the book to call attention to important information. The information and writing style are targeted toward readers new to nuclear medicine. The fundamentals are addressed first, and then topics build to become more complex.

INSTRUCTOR ANCILLARIES

The Evolve website is a secure and interactive learning environment designed to work in coordination with *Nuclear Medicine and PET/CT Technology and Techniques,* seventh edition. The instructor materials available on Evolve will assist the educator in preparing exams and presenting material. The following assets are included on Evolve:

- A test bank with multiple choice questions in Exam-View and Word formats, including rationales for correct answers and references to the coordinating page number in the textbook

- An electronic image collection with all of the images from the textbook in .jpeg and PowerPoint formats

Instructors may use Evolve to provide an Internet-based course component that reinforces and expands the concepts presented in class. Evolve may be used to publish the class syllabus, outlines, and lecture notes; set up "virtual office hours" and email communication; share important dates and information through the online class calendar; and encourage student participation through chat rooms and discussion boards. Evolve also allows instructors to post exams and manage their grade books online. For more information, visit http://evolve.elsevier.com/Christian/nuclear/ or contact an Elsevier sales representative.

ACKNOWLEDGMENTS

We would like to thank the hard work and extraordinary efforts of the contributing authors of this text. Without their dedication and commitment to the project, it would not have been possible. It is also their talent in presenting information that allows the reader to transform this information into a knowledge base through which they can practice nuclear medicine.

We would also like to thank and recognize the co-workers, families, and loved ones of all of those involved in the book whose names do not appear in writing but endured the time commitment made by the authors to ensure the delivery of quality material.

Lastly, we would like to thank and extend our appreciation to our editors at Elsevier/Mosby, as well as the production and design team, whose support, guidance, patience, and diligent work have made this project a success.

Paul E. Christian
Kristen M. Waterstram-Rich

CONTENTS

6   Radiochemistry and Radiopharmacology, 151

Sally W. Schwarz, Reiko Oyama, Carolyn J. Anderson

7   Radiation Safety in Nuclear Medicine, 184

Peter A. Jenkins, Karen S. Langley

8   Patient Care and Quality Improvement, 219

Kathy Thompson Hunt, Donna C. Mars, Denise A. Merlino

Mathematics and Statistics

Paul H. Brown

OUTLINE

OBJECTIVES

After completing this chapter, the reader will be able to:
- Use scientific notation in performing algebraic operations.
- Use the inverse square law to calculate the intensity of a radiation field at various distances.
- Perform radioactive dilution calculations.
- Define the units of radioactivity, radiation exposure, radiation absorbed dose, and radiation dose equivalent.
- Perform calculations with logarithms and exponents using a calculator.
- Discuss numeric accuracy, significant digits, and rounding.
- Calculate quantities of radioactivity using the general form of the decay equation and decay factors.
- Use tables of decay factors to calculate remaining radioactivity.
- Calculate concentration and volume and radioactivity for patient doses.
- Compute the concentration of ^{99}Mo in ^{99m}Tc.
- Compute effective half-life and biological half-life.
- Calculate intensity with half-value layers.
- Diagram various types of graphs and graphing techniques.
- Discuss curve-fitting techniques.
- Define mean, standard deviation, and coefficient of variation.
- Discuss Gaussian and Poisson distributions.
- State the formula for standard deviation, and perform calculations in the presence of background.
- Explain the function of the chi-square test and interpretation of results.
- Interpret the results of a chi-square test using a probability table.
- Discuss the use and interpretation of *t*-tests.
- Describe the interpretation of sensitivity, specificity, prevalence, and accuracy.

KEY TERMS

accuracy
biological half-life
chi-square test
coefficient of variation (CV)
decay constant
decay factor
effective half-life
Euler's number

exponent
half-value layer (HVL)
inverse square law
least squares curve fit
linear attenuation coefficient
logarithm
mean
natural logarithm

physical half-life
Poisson distribution
proportional
scientific notation
sensitivity
significant figures
specificity
standard deviation (SD)

Nuclear medicine technology occupies a unique position in the allied health sciences because of its strong dependence on quantitative, or mathematical, results. This chapter attempts to provide a sound basis for performing calculations that are typically required of nuclear medicine technologists. The emphasis here is on practical use, not on theoretical principles. Practical examples are provided, and each type of calculation includes a discussion on the use of pocket calculators and rudimentary instructions for the use of Microsoft Excel. This chapter reviews elementary algebra, graphing techniques, and statistical principles, always with an emphasis on practical applications. It is presumed that readers have a working knowledge of high school–level mathematics. The more advanced reader may wish to skip to the Practical Applications section of this chapter. The reader who requires a more basic review of algebra may wish to consult another mathematics text.[1]

FUNDAMENTALS

Scientific Notation

Numbers in scientific calculations are often very small, such as 0.0015, or very large, such as 23,000. **Scientific notation** allows these numbers to be presented in a more convenient notation without cumbersome commas and zeros: 1.5×10^{-3} and $2.3E \times 10^4$. The **exponent** on the 10 specifies how many places the decimal point in the number is to be shifted to the left (for negative exponents) or shifted to the right (for positive exponents). Sometimes these numbers are alternatively represented as 1.5E–3 and 2.3E+4, a form found on pocket calculators or in printed tabular data (e.g., in calculations of internal radiation dosimetry), where the superscript is cumbersome to print. Pocket calculators typically have an "EE" key (for "enter exponent"), which allows easy entry of data in scientific notation. For example, if it is desired to calculate:

$$(1.5 \times 10^{-3}) \div (2.3 \times 10^4)$$

the procedure on the calculator would be as follows (Figure 1-1):

1.5   enter value for numerator
EE   *enter exponent* key
+/–   *change sign* key to make the exponent negative
3   enter the value of the exponent
÷   *divide* key
2.3   enter the value for denominator
EE   *enter exponent* key
4   enter the value of the exponent
=   (see result of 6.5217391E–8 in display)

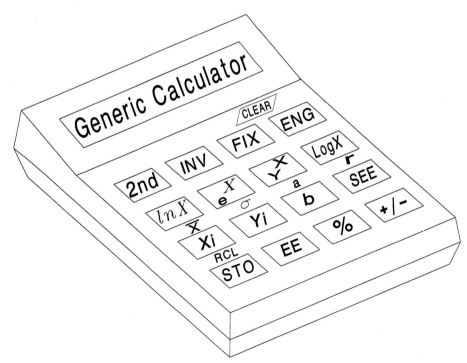

FIGURE 1-1 Generic scientific calculator demonstrating keys useful in nuclear medicine. The *2nd* key produces the function above the key (e.g., *2nd*) and $\overline{X}_i$ produces the mean of X_i values. The *INV* key produces the functional inverse of the key. *INV* and *lnX* are e^x functions. Most calculators do not have an e^x key if they offer *INV* and *lnX* keys. The *FIX* key sets the number of decimal places to be displaced (e.g., *FIX* and *3* will display only three decimal places for all subsequent calculations). The *ENG* key causes the calculator to display results in scientific notation. The X_i key is used to enter x values to calculate the mean and standard deviation σ. The X_i and Y_i keys are used to enter x and y values for least squares curve fit (linear regression) to produce a straight line with intercept a, slope b, correlation r, and standard error of estimate *SEE*. The +/– key changes the sign of a number.

TABLE 1-1	Numeric Prefixes	
Abbreviation	**Prefix**	**Numeric Value**
A	atto-	10^{-18}, one quintillionth
F	femto-	10^{-15}, one quadrillionth
P	pico-	10^{-12}, one trillionth
N	nano-	10^{-9}, one billionth
μ	micro-	10^{-6}, one millionth
M	milli-	10^{-3}, one thousandth
C	centi-	10^{-2}, one hundredth
D	deci-	10^{-1}, one tenth
Da	deka-	10^{1}, ten
K	kilo-	10^{3}, thousand
M	mega-	10^{6}, million
G	giga-	10^{9}, billion
T	tera-	10^{12}, trillion
P	peta-	10^{15}, quadrillion

This is precisely the same result as would be obtained by dividing 0.0015 by 23,000 on the calculator.

It is often desirable to use numeric prefixes to represent very small or large numbers (Table 1-1). The value 6.52×10^{-8} grams (g), or 6.52E–8 g, can be more conveniently represented by converting the exponent to one of the exponent values shown in Table 1-1, which are usually exponents divisible by 3 (such as 3, 6, 9, and so on). Thus 6.52×10^{-8} g can be represented as 65.2×10^{-9} g, or in convenient shorthand form as 65.2 nanograms (ng), where *nano* stands for 10^{-9}. Notice that the decimal point in the number 6.52×10^{-8} can be shifted to the right by making the exponent smaller by 1 for each right shift of the decimal (e.g., $6.52 \times 10^{-8} = 65.2 \times 10^{-9}$), the object being to have an exponent that is divisible by 3 so that the numeric prefixes in Table 1-1 can be used. Similarly, a number like 2.3×10^{4} counts (ct) can be expressed as 23.0×10^{3} ct, or 23 kct, with the k denoting *kilo*, or thousand.

This type of notation is often used for units of radioactivity, which is measured in becquerels (Bq). A patient might be injected with 7.4×10^{8} Bq of radioactivity, which can be written 0.74×10^{9} Bq (the decimal point can be shifted *left* if the exponent is *increased* by 1 for each left shift). So the injected radioactivity could be represented as 0.74 GBq. Alternately, the value 7.4×10^{8} Bq could be written 740.0×10^{6} Bq = 740 MBq (the decimal was shifted two places to the right, so the exponent is decreased by 2). Choosing between the two forms is simply a matter of preference. Note that pocket calculators often have an *engineering notation* key, which controls the scientific notation exponents in the calculator display to always be a power of 3. For example, 7.4×10^{8} Bq is displayed as 740E6 on the calculator, which the user understands to be the same as 740 MBq.

Fractions and Percentages

Fractions, such as $\frac{1}{3}$, consist of a numerator (1) that is to be divided by a denominator (3). The value of a fraction may also be expressed decimally, such as $\frac{3}{4} = 0.750$ (a fraction that terminates in a zero digit), or $\frac{4}{3} = 1.3333 \ldots$ (a fraction that never terminates in a zero digit). The mathematical manipulation of fractions requires care as to the number of digits and placement of the decimal point. The safest way to handle the mathematical manipulation of fractions is to simply use the power of the pocket calculator to perform calculations such as $\frac{1}{3} + \frac{3}{4}$ by first converting the fractions to decimals and then carrying out the other arithmetic:

$$\frac{1}{3} = 0.333$$
$$\frac{3}{4} = 2.250$$
$$\text{sum} = 2.583$$

As a general rule the arithmetic should maintain at least one more digit in each fraction than is necessary in the final result. For example, if it is desired to describe the area of a rectangle (area = width × length) to the nearest centimeter, then measurements of the width and length of the rectangle should be made to the nearest tenth of a centimeter. Use of the pocket calculator generally produces at least eight digits of accuracy, which is more than enough for nuclear medicine calculations.

Percentages are values expressed as a fraction of some whole, entire value: 75% of some number is the same as 0.75 multiplied by that number. This is exemplified in the following:

$$75\% \text{ of } 5\,ml = 0.75 \times 5\,ml = 3.75\,ml$$

Many pocket calculators have a % key, which makes it unnecessary to first convert the percentage to a decimal:

75	enter percent value
%	*percent* key
×	*multiply* key
5	enter 5
=	(see result of 3.75 in display)

Percentages are often used to express percentage change between two values. For example, a patient may have had a kidney function test last month that showed a kidney clearance rate of 42 milliliters per minute (ml/min). The patient returns today and has a kidney clearance rate of 58 ml/min. The patient's kidney function has improved by 38% based on the following:

$$\% \text{ change} = [(\text{new value} - \text{old value})/\text{old value}] \times 100$$
$$= [(58 - 42)/42] \times 100$$
$$= (16/42) \times 100$$
$$= 0.38 \times 100 = 38\%$$

Algebraic Equations and Ratios

Calculations in nuclear medicine often involve expressing a mathematical concept as a ratio. For example, an intensity setting of 240 on a display screen may produce a suitable image for a bar phantom with 500,000 ct in the acquisition. Now it is desired to acquire an image to 300,000 ct. The intensity on the screen is known to change linearly with the intensity control setting. What intensity setting should be used for the new 300,000 ct image? This translates mathematically into the following:

$$\frac{x}{300\,kct} = \frac{240\,intensity}{500\,kct}$$

This is typical of numeric equations in nuclear medicine. First, it is necessary to translate a mathematical concept, expressed in words, into an algebraic equation. The equation generally contains several numbers and one unknown value; here the new intensity setting is the unknown value (x). The object is to solve for the unknown value by rearranging the terms in the equation. In this example the unknown intensity x can be isolated on one side of the equation by multiplying both sides of the equation by 300 kct. Remember, any math operation can always be done to both sides of an equation without changing the equality. Many students may have learned this technique as cross-multiplying to solve a proportion.

$$300\,kct \times \left[\frac{x}{300\,kct}\right] = 300\,kct \times \left[\frac{240\,intensity}{500\,kct}\right]$$

The 300 kct cancels in the left numerator and denominator, so

$$x = 300\,kct \times \frac{240\,intensity}{500\,kct} = 144\,intensity$$

Another frequently encountered problem relates to radioactivity concentrations in patient doses. For example, the morning elution of the ^{99}Mo-^{99m}Tc generator yields 943 millicuries (mCi) of ^{99m}Tc radioactivity in 20 ml of saline eluate. What volume should be withdrawn from the eluate vial into a patient syringe to perform a 20 mCi patient scan (assume that no decay correction is needed)?

$$\frac{x}{20\,mCi} = \frac{20\,ml}{940\,mCi}$$
$$x = 20\,mCi \times \frac{20\,ml}{943\,mCi} = 0.42\,ml$$

Inverse Square Law

The radiation exposure from a radioactive point source is governed by a mathematical relationship called the **inverse square law**. This states that the radiation exposure or intensity (I) at a distance (d) from a radioactive source is proportional to the inverse square of the distance. This law holds for a point source (a source that is very small compared with the distance from the source) that emits radiation not absorbed while traveling over the distances involved. Syringe source γ-rays at a distance of 1 meter (m) or more in air would qualify as a point source. Air is a weak absorber of x-rays or γ-rays in the energy ranges typically encountered in nuclear medicine. A syringe source for exposure to the hands does not obey the inverse square law because the distance from the syringe to the hands is not large compared with the syringe dimensions. Similarly, the exposure from standing near patients does not follow the simple inverse square law. Mathematically the inverse square law states:

$$I \alpha \frac{k}{d^2}$$

where k is a proportionality constant that depends on the type of radioactive source and its activity. The symbol ∝ means "is **proportional** to." The inverse square law results in the radiation intensity quadrupling if the distance from the source is halved, or the radiation intensity decreasing to one fourth of its value if the distance is doubled. Changing the distance by a factor of 3 results in a factor of 9 change in intensity (nine times more intensity for one third the distance, or one ninth the intensity for three times the distance). This is usually stated in a form relating the old intensity (I_2) at some old distance (d_2) to a new intensity (I_1) at some new distance (d_1):

$$I_1(d_1)^2 = I_2(d_2)^2$$

The intensity of radiation is usually measured in units of roentgens (R) or milliroentgens (mR) per hour (hr). For example, suppose a technologist working 2 m from a small vial of radioactivity results in an intensity or exposure level of 2.5 mR/hr at 2 m. If the technologist moves to a distance of 3 m from the source, what is the new radiation intensity?

$$I_1 \times (3\,m)^2 = (2.5\,mR/hr) \times (2\,m)^2$$

or

$$I_1 = (2.5\,mR/hr) \times (2\,m)^2 / (3\,m)^2$$
$$I_1 = (2.5\,mR/hr) \times (4/9) = 1.1\,mR/hr$$

The technologist's radiation exposure is more than halved by moving 1 m further from the source. Note that pocket calculators generally have an x^2 key, which facilitates the calculation:

2.5	enter intensity value
×	*multiply* key
2	enter old distance value
x^2	*squaring* key
÷	*divide* key
3	enter new distance value
x^2	*squaring* key
=	(see result of 1.1 in display)

In another example, a technologist is working 4 feet (ft) from a point source that results in an intensity of 0.62 mR/hr. Concerns for radiation safety suggest that the intensity should be maintained at no more than 0.25 mR/hr for a safe working environment. To what distance from the source should the technologist move to achieve an exposure level of 0.25 mR/hr?

$$0.25\,mR/hr \times (d_1)^2 = 0.62\,mR/hr \times (4\,ft)^2$$

$$(d_1)^2 = \frac{(0.62\,mR/hr) \times (4\,ft)^2}{0.25\,mR/hr}$$

$$(d_1)^2 = \frac{(0.62\,mR/hr) \times 16\,ft^2}{0.25\,mR/hr}$$

$$(d_1)^2 = 39.7\,ft^2$$

$$\sqrt{(d_1)^2} = \sqrt{39.7\,ft^2}$$

$$d_1 = 6.3\,ft^2$$

Again, pocket calculators generally have a *square root* key ($\sqrt{\ }$), which facilitates calculation:

0.62   enter old intensity value
×   *multiply* key
4   enter old distance value
x^2 *squaring* key
÷   *divide* key
0.25   enter new intensity value
=   results of division
$\sqrt{\ }$ *square root* key (see result of 6.3 in display)

Notice that in solving this problem the left side of the equation contained $(d_1)^2$, but because the object was to solve for d_1, the square root of both sides of the equation was taken. The squaring function and the square root function canceled on the left side of the equation because $x^2 = x$. Functions that have this property are called *inverse functions*. The squaring function $(x)^2$ and the square root function ($\sqrt{\ }$) are inverse functions.

For example, a dilute standard solution is made by diluting a 1-ml volume of some standard source of radioactivity up to a 500-ml volume. This dilute standard, which has a low enough radioactivity to be accurately counted in a well counter, is then counted, and 2 ml of the diluted standard yields 15,346 ct. How many counts were in the original 1 ml of the standard?

$$C_1 V_1 = C_2 V_2$$

$$C_1 \times 1\,ml = \left(\frac{15,346\,ct}{2\,ml} \right) \times 500\,ml$$

$$C_1 = 3,836,500\,ct/ml$$

Notice how the units are carefully included with each number.

The dilution principle can also be used to measure an unknown volume. For example, suppose a 2-ml sample of a standard solution produces 647,530 ct per minute (cpm) in a well counter. This standard sample is then injected intravenously into a patient, and a 2-ml sample of the patient's blood yields 2600 ct in 10 minutes (or 260 cpm). What is the patient's blood volume?

$$C_1 V_1 = C_2 V_2$$

$$\left(\frac{260\,cpm}{2\,ml} \right) \times V_1 = \left(\frac{647,530\,cpm}{2\,ml} \right) \times 2\,ml$$

$$V_1 = 4981\,ml$$

Often it is necessary to inject a patient with a more concentrated solution than can be accurately counted in a well counter to ensure an adequate concentration of counts in the patient blood, without undue statistical counting noise. In the previous example, for instance, the patient blood counts yielded only 260 cpm/2 ml, which would be subject to a large statistical uncertainty (as discussed in the following section). It would therefore be necessary to obtain more blood counts. This requires increasing the activity in the standard source, which then becomes too concentrated to be accurately counted in the well counter. The problem is either that the standard is too strong or the patient sample is too weak because of the large count dilution in the patient blood volume. The answer to the problem is to dilute a portion of the standard and count this diluted standard while the full-strength undiluted standard can be injected into the patient. The standard can be diluted by adding 1 ml of it to a flask, which is then filled to 500 ml. The dilution factor is then 500. For example, a 2-ml sample of the 1:500 diluted standard in a well counter might yield 26,835 cpm. Then 5 ml of the undiluted standard is injected into the patient, producing blood plasma counts of 26,500 cpm in 2 ml of plasma. What is the plasma volume?

$$C_1 V_1 = C_2 V_2$$

$$\left(\frac{26,500\,cpm}{2\,ml} \right) \times V_1 = \left(500 \times \frac{26,835\,cpm}{2\,ml} \right) \times 5\,ml$$

$$V_1 = 2530\,ml$$

Notice here that the standard counts had to be multiplied by the dilution factor of 500 to obtain the true standard concentration, which was injected into the patient.

Units

When manipulating numbers, it is critical to always consider the units of the numbers involved. Forgetting to specify whether a patient was injected with 5 μCi or 5 mCi of iodine-131 (^{131}I) radioactivity can have disastrous consequences. It is best to develop a habit of writing down the units for all the numbers in any calculation.

Units are agreed-upon, standard quantities of measurement. They are often composed of some combination of the three fundamental properties of mass, length, and time. These are the properties that can be measured in the physical or biological world. From these fundamental units other units can be derived, such as speed in

TABLE 1-2	Units		
Measured Property	**Old Unit**	**SI Unit**	**Conversion Factor**
Radioactivity	curie (Ci) = 3.7×10^{10} dps	becquerel (Bq) = 1 dps	1 Ci = 3.7×10^{10} Bq 1 Bq = 2.7×10^{-11} Ci
Radiation exposure C/kg	roentgen (R) = 2.58×10^{-4} C/kg	coulomb/kg (C/kg)	1 R = 2.58×10^{-4} C/kg 1 C/kg = 3.88×10^{3} R
Radiation absorbed dose	rad = 100 erg/g	gray (Gy) = 1 joule/kg	1 rad = 0.01 Gy 1 rad = 10 mGy 1 Gy = 100 rad
Radiation dose equivalent	rem = QF × rad	sievert (Sv) = QF × Gy	1 rem = 0.01 Sv 1 rem = 10 mSv 1 Sv = 100 rem

QF, Quality factor; *SI,* Système Internationale.

meters per second (m/sec), centimeters per second (cm/sec), or ft/sec. These three units of speed are derived from three different measurement systems that arose many years ago: the meter-kilogram-second (mks) system of units; the centimeter-gram-second (cgs) system of units; and the foot-pound-second system of units. Also commonly encountered are energy units of 1 joule (1 kg × m^2/sec^2) in the mks system and 1 erg (1 kg × cm^2/sec^2) in the cgs system. Table 1-2 lists units often encountered in nuclear medicine. In 1977 the three existing unit systems were modified when the "worldwide" Système International d'Unités (SI) was developed. Although the intent of SI units was simplification, both the old units and SI units continue to be in use in the United States. In SI, each unit is named after a person, and numeric factors are not present in the definition of the SI unit. For example, the old temperature scale of centigrade was renamed *Celsius,* and the old unit of radioactivity, the curie (3.7×10^{10} disintegrations per second [dps]), was replaced in SI units by the Bq (1 dps), which has no complicating numeric factor in the definition. The reader should be familiar with both the old units and the SI units shown in Table 1-2. It is often necessary to convert between various systems for consistency in applying mathematical equations. Most common is the necessity to convert between the old units and SI units for radioactivity, radiation exposure, absorbed dose, and dose equivalent. For example, how many Bq are equivalent to 20 mCi of a radionuclide? This can be calculated from the conversion factor in Table 1-2 as follows:

$$\text{Activity in Bq} = 20\,\text{mCi} \times \left(10^{-3}\,\frac{\text{Ci}}{\text{mCi}}\right) \times \left(3.7 \times 10^{10}\,\frac{\text{Bq}}{\text{Ci}}\right)$$
$$= 20 \times 10^{-3} \times 3.7 \times 10^{10}\,\text{Bq}$$
$$= 7.4 \times 10^{8}\,\text{Bq} = 740 \times 10^{6}\,\text{Bq}$$
$$= 740\,\text{MBq (or 0.74 GBq)}$$

So 20 mCi is the same activity as 740 MBq. Notice how all the units except Bq canceled between numerator and denominator in the conversion. Use of the *enter exponent* key for scientific notation on the pocket calculator facilitates such calculations.

In radiation safety calculations, it is common to encounter measurements of radiation expressed either in older historical units (commonly used in the United States), or in the newer internationally standardized SI units. For example, radiation absorbed dose can be specified in units of rad (the old unit), or in SI units of Gray (Gy). The conversion of radiation absorbed dose from old to SI units is defined by 1 Gy = 100 rad. So, to convert a measurement of 5 rad in the old units into SI units:

$$\text{Absorbed dose} = 5\,\text{rad} \times \frac{1\,\text{Gy}}{100\,\text{rad}} = 0.05\,\text{Gy}$$
$$= 5\,\text{centigrays (cGy)}$$

So 5 rad (old units) is the same absorbed dose as 5 cGy (new SI units).

Similarly, in radiation safety considerations it is common to encounter measurement of dose equivalent, either in old units of rem or in new SI units of Sievert (Sv). The conversion factor is defined by 1 Sv = 100 rem. So to convert 1 cSv of dose equivalent in the new SI unit of cSv to the old unit of rem:

$$\text{Dose equivalent} = 1\,\text{cSv} \times 10^{-2}\,\frac{\text{Sv}}{\text{cSv}} \times \frac{100\,\text{rem}}{\text{Sv}}$$
$$= 1\,\text{rem}$$

So 1 cSv (in SI units) is the same dose equivalent as 1 rem (in old units). Again, notice that all the units except the final desired value cancel in numerator and denominator.

Use of the radioactive decay equations discussed in the following section often requires converting between different time units. Suppose it is necessary to convert the time difference between 10:45 AM and 1:20 PM to units of days. The time difference is 155 minutes, which can be converted to days:

$$155\,\text{min} \times \frac{1\,\text{hr}}{60\,\text{min}} \times \frac{1\,\text{day}}{24\,\text{hr}} = 0.108\,\text{days}$$

The process of converting such units consists of repeatedly multiplying by a conversion factor of 1 (expressed as a fraction, such as 1 hr/60 min) until the desired final unit result is obtained. For example, to convert the speed of light (3×10^{10} cm/sec) to a speed measured in furlongs (⅛ mile [mi]) per fortnight (14 days):

$$\frac{3 \times 10^{10} \text{ cm}}{\text{sec}} \times \frac{\left(\dfrac{1 \text{ in}}{2.54 \text{ cm}}\right) \times \left(\dfrac{1 \text{ ft}}{12 \text{ in}}\right) \times \left(\dfrac{1 \text{ mi}}{5280 \text{ ft}}\right) \times \left(\dfrac{8 \text{ furlong}}{\text{mi}}\right)}{\left(\dfrac{1 \text{ min}}{60 \text{ sec}}\right) \times \left(\dfrac{1 \text{ hr}}{60 \text{ min}}\right) \times \left(\dfrac{1 \text{ day}}{24 \text{ hr}}\right) \times \left(\dfrac{1 \text{ fortnight}}{14 \text{ days}}\right)}$$

$$= \frac{(3 \times 10^{10}) \times \left(\dfrac{1}{2.54}\right) \times \left(\dfrac{1}{12}\right) \times \left(\dfrac{1}{5280}\right) \times (8) \text{ furlong}}{\left(\dfrac{1}{60}\right) \times \left(\dfrac{1}{60}\right) \times \left(\dfrac{1}{24}\right) \times \left(\dfrac{1}{14}\right) \text{ fortnight}}$$

$$= \frac{1.49 \times 10^{6} \text{ furlong}}{8.27 \times 10^{-7} \text{ fortnight}}$$

$$= 1.8 \times 10^{12} \text{ furlong/fortnight}$$

The conversion factors in the numerator convert centimeters to furlongs, and the conversion factors in the denominator convert seconds to fortnights. Completion of this otherwise silly problem on the calculator provides useful practice in unit conversion and calculator manipulation. Notice how the units in juxtaposed conversion factors always cancel between numerator and denominator until only the final desired units remain.

Lengthy calculations such as this one may best be handled on the calculator by first calculating the numerical value of the numerator and denominator separately. Calculate for the numerator with the following progression of keys:

3
EE
10
÷
2.54
÷
12
÷
5280
×
8
=   (see result 1.4912909E6 for numerator in display)

Calculate for the denominator with the following progression of keys:

1
÷
60
÷
60
÷
24
÷
14
=   (see result of 0.0000008 in display)
EE   put calculator in scientific notation (see result of 8.2671958E−7 in display)

Notice that the calculator had to be placed in scientific notation mode for the denominator to observe more than one significant figure in the display. Calculators from various manufacturers might function differently. The calculation is then completed by dividing the numerator by the denominator to obtain the final answer of 1.8×10^{12} furlongs/fortnight. Most scientific calculators have memory locations where the numerator result can be stored temporarily in one memory location, with the denominator result stored in another. Then the memory locations can easily be recalled to divide numerator by denominator without having to enter the intermediate results by hand.

Exponent Laws and Logarithms

This section expands the algebra of exponents and logarithms. In general, exponent notation is set up as follows:

$$\text{base}^{\text{exponent}} = \text{number}$$

For example,

$$10^4 = 10,000$$

The exponent notation of 10^4 means the same as 10 multiplied four times:

$$10^4 = 10 \times 10 \times 10 \times 10 = 10,000$$

Generally one is confronted with exponential calculations involving raising a base of 10, 2, or e to some power. Base 2 problems often arise in computer considerations where it might be required to calculate

$$2^8 = 2 \times 2 \times 2 \times 2 \times 2 \times 2 \times 2 \times 2 = 256$$

Scientific pocket calculators generally have a Y^X key, meaning raise the base Y to the power x, which facilitates this type of calculation. To find 2^8 using the calculator,

2   enter base value Y
Y^X *exponentiation* key
8   enter exponent value x
=   (see result of 256 in display)

A special case arises when the exponent is zero. By mathematics definition any number (except zero) raised to the zero power is equal to 1:

$$e^0 = 1$$
$$10^0 = 1$$
$$2^0 = 1$$

Negative exponents provide a convenient form for representing small numbers:

$$10^{-4} = \frac{1}{10^4} = 0.0001$$

Notice that this shows how a number in exponent notation can be moved from numerator to denominator simply by changing the sign of the exponent:

$$2^8 = \frac{1}{2^{-8}} = 256$$

The algebra of exponents in equations follows certain rules.

Multiplication: add the exponents.

$$B^x \times B^y = B^{x+y}$$
$$10^2 \times 10^3 = 10^5$$
$$10^4 \times 10^{-5} = 10^{-1}$$

To find the area of a rectangle, multiply width times height:

$$\text{area} = 20\,\text{cm} \times 30\,\text{cm} = 600\,\text{cm}^2$$

Notice how this follows the rule for multiplying exponents:

$$\text{cm}^1 \times \text{cm}^1 = \text{cm}^2$$

Division: subtract the exponents.

$$\frac{B^x}{B^y} = B^{x-y}$$
$$\frac{10^2}{10^3} = 10^{2-3} = 10^{-1}$$
$$\frac{10^4}{10^{-5}} = 10^{4-(-5)} = 10^9$$
$$\frac{2^3}{2^3} = 2^0 = 1$$

A practical problem might involve calculation of the *mass* attenuation coefficient μ_m, which is defined by the quotient of the **linear attenuation coefficient** μ (in units of cm^{-1} or 1/cm) divided by the density ρ (in units of g/cm^3) for some substances such as human soft tissues. For example,

$$\text{if } \mu = 0.121/\text{cm, and } \rho = 3.4\,\text{g/cm}^3, \text{ then}$$
$$\mu_m = \frac{0.121/\text{cm}}{3.4\,\text{g/cm}^3}$$

The difficulty here is how to evaluate the units. First eliminate denominator units within each term of the equation—that is, write 1/cm as cm^{-1} and g/cm^3 as $\text{g} \times \text{cm}^{-3}$, using the rule discussed previously for moving from denominator to numerator by changing the sign of the exponent. Then,

$$\mu_m = \frac{0.12\,\text{cm}^{-1}}{3.4\,\text{g/cm}^{-3}}$$

Now follow the previous rule for division of exponents with cm dimensions:

$$\mu_m = \frac{0.12\,\text{cm}^{-1-(-3)}}{3.4\,\text{g}} = \frac{0.12\,\text{cm}^2}{3.4\,\text{g}} = 0.035\frac{\text{cm}^2}{\text{g}}$$

Alternatively, the units of μ_m might be written as:

$$\mu_m = 0.035\,\text{cm}^2 \times \text{g}^{-1}$$

Another example is hertz (Hz), the measure of frequency expressed as the number of waves or cycles per second. For example, if three waves pass by a certain point in space in 1 second, then the frequency (*v*) is given by:

$$v = 3/\text{sec, or } 3\,\text{sec}^{-1}, \text{or } 3\,\text{Hz}$$

Taking the root of a number is the inverse of raising to a power. A special case is the square root ($\sqrt{\ }$) of a positive number x, which is defined by:

$$\sqrt{x} \times \sqrt{x} = x$$
$$\text{e.g., } \sqrt{9} \times \sqrt{9} = 3 \times 3 = 9$$

Note that finding the square root is the same as raising a number to the half power: $\sqrt{x} = x^{1/2}$ As mentioned previously, the square root and squaring operation are inverses of each other because

$$\sqrt{(x^2)} = x$$
$$\text{and} \left(\sqrt{x}\right)^2 = x$$

Whether the squaring or the square root is performed first, the inverse function always cancels the other operation and simply returns the number x. Other roots can be calculated as the *n*th root of a number, which is written as $\sqrt[n]{x}$ For example, $\sqrt[3]{64} = 4$, because $4 \times 4 \times 4 = 64$. Some pocket calculators have a *root* key such as $\sqrt[x]{y}$, or the calculator might have an *inverse* (INV) key (see Figure 1-1), which is pressed before pressing another function to get the inverse of that function. For example, to calculate $\sqrt[3]{64}$ on the calculator:

64	enter value y to find cube root:
INV and Y^x	or *root* key $\sqrt[x]{y}$, which is same as INV – Y^x
3	enter root value x
=	(see display of result, 4)

The base e (= 2.718 …) is an irrational number called **Euler's number,** named after Swiss mathematician and physicist Leonhard Euler (1707-1783). Calculations involving e pervade the mathematical, physical, and biological world: radioactive decay, absorption of radiation, growth of bacteria, and radiation damage to cells. Scientific pocket calculators often have a special e^x key that is used for calculations. Some calculators require the user to invoke the e^x function by virtue of the fact that the e^x function and the natural logarithm function (ln x) are inverses of each other. This means that $\ln(e^x) = x$, and $e^{(\ln x)} = x$. For example, a radioactive decay problem might require the following calculation:

$$e^{-0.693} \times 4.5/6.0 = e^{-0.51975} = 0.59$$

This can be performed on the pocket calculator as follows:

0.693	enter value
+/−	*change sign* key
×	*multiply* key
4.5	enter value
÷	*divide* key
6	enter value

= (see result of division)

INV and ln x or e^x key (see result of 0.59 in display)

Logarithms provide another convenient system of notation that can make mathematical problems easier to solve. In nuclear medicine, logarithms can be used to linearize certain graphs (change a curved line into a straight line), solve problems in radioactive decay or radiation absorption, or provide a graphic axis scale capable of accommodating a wide range of numeric values. The pocket calculator quickly computes logarithms, so the reader only needs to become familiar with their algebraic properties. The logarithm ($\log_b x$) of a number (x) is the value to which the base (b) must be raised to equal the number:

$$x = b^{\log_b^x}$$

For example, for base 10 logarithms the $\log_{10} 1000 = 3$, because $1000 = 10^3$. Note that the expression $\log_{10} 1000$ is read as *the base 10 log of 1000*. Some examples follow:

$$\log_{10} 0.01 = -2$$
$$\log_{10} 0.1 = -1$$
$$\log_{10} 10 = 1$$
$$\log_{10} 100 = 2$$
$$\log_{10} 10^n = n$$

If a $\log_b x$ is written without any value specified for the base (as $\log x$), then base 10 is understood.

The blackness of a nuclear medicine image on a piece of photographic film is measured by the optical density (OD) of the film, which is defined by shining a beam of light through the film:

$$OD = \log(100\% / \% \text{ transmitted through film})$$

The human eye can generally distinguish optical densities in the 0.25 to 2.25 range; below 0.25 is too dim to be seen, and above 2.25 is too black. The OD corresponds to the percentage of light transmitted through the film.

% Light Transmitted through Film	OD
100	log 100/100 = 0
10	log 100/10 = 1
1	log 100/1 = 2
0.1	log 100/0.1 = 3

Logarithms have certain algebraic properties that can simplify mathematical calculations.

Multiplication: $\log xy = \log x + \log y$
Division: $\log x/y = \log x - \log y$
Exponents: $\log x^n = n \times \log x$

The other frequently encountered base for logarithms is the base e, or the **natural logarithm,** which is denoted by the special symbol *ln:*

$$\ln x = \log_e x$$

Pocket calculators usually have an ln x key, which allows easy calculation. The major use of natural logarithms in nuclear medicine is to solve problems in radioactive decay and radiation absorption, such as the time of decay *(t)* in the following equation:

$$0.25 = e^{-0.693 \times t / 6 \, hr}$$

The difficulty here is to solve for *t* by removing it from within the exponent. To eliminate a function (like e^x), the natural logarithm of both sides of the equation can be taken:

$$\ln(0.25) = \ln\left(e^{-0.693 \times t / 6 \, hr}\right)$$

Using the rule for log of exponents,

$$\ln 0.25 = \left(\frac{-0.693 \times t}{6 \, hr}\right) \times \ln e$$

And now using ln $e = 1$:

$$\ln 0.25 = \frac{-0.693 \times t}{6 \, hr}$$

Notice that the minus sign and units are carefully retained. Simply rearranging algebraically to solve for *t* then results in:

$$t = \frac{-6 \, hr \times \ln 0.25}{0.693}$$
$$= \frac{-6 \, hr \times (-1.386)}{0.693} = +12 \, hr$$

The minus from the original equation times the negative value of ln 0.25 results in a + sign.

Numeric Accuracy: Significance and Rounding

The **accuracy** of mathematical calculations is governed by three concepts: significant figures, rounding, and significant decimal places. **Significant figures** refers to the number of digits required to preserve the mathematical accuracy in a number.

Numeric accuracy rule 1. For a number with no leading or trailing zeros, the number of significant figures is the number of digits.

Number	Number of Significant Figures
3	1
3.45	3

Numeric accuracy rule 2. For a number with leading zeros, the leading zeros are not significant.

Number	Number of Significant Figures
0.0015	2
0.0463	3

Notice that expressing a number like 0.0015 in scientific notation as 1.5×10^{-3} eliminates the leading zeros and therefore eliminates the need for rule 2.

Numeric accuracy rule 3. Trailing zeros in a number should be retained only if they are significant, which depends on the context of the problem. Thus a problem may state that a drug costs $37; the cost has two significant figures. Or the problem may state that the drug costs $37.00, which is interpreted as being accurate in both dollars and cents; it has four significant figures. A length expressed as 4 cm has one significant figure; the length was measured to the nearest centimeter. But a length expressed as 4.0 cm has two significant figures; the length was measured more accurately to the nearest millimeter.

Numeric accuracy rule 4. The accuracy of the result in multiplication or division is such that the product or quotient has the number of significant figures equal to that of the term with the smaller number of significant figures.

For example, $2 \times 2.54 = 5$; the correct answer has only one significant figure because the 2 in the calculation has only one significant figure. But $2.00 \times 2.54 = 5.08$; the result has three significant figures because it is presumed that the trailing zeros in the 2.00 are significant. In another example,

$$\frac{0.061}{12.34} = 0.0049$$

or

$$\frac{6.1 \times 10^{-2}}{12.34} = 4.9 \times 10^{-3}$$

The result has only two significant figures. Note that a calculator display might show 0.0049433 or 4.9432739E-3, but the proper answer to record as a result is 0.0049 or 4.9E-3, with only two significant figures.

It is necessary to properly round off the result from the calculator before recording the result. For example,

$$\frac{0.061}{1.233} = 0.0494728 = 0.049$$

whereas

$$\frac{0.061}{1.232} = 0.0495130 = 0.050$$

Both answers have two significant figures, but the results are different because of rounding. The mechanics of rounding off a number consist of carrying the mathematical calculations to several more digits than are needed in the final answer. Then the final result is rounded off by the following rules.

Numeric accuracy rule 5. If the rightmost digits, beyond the significant figures in the final result, are less than 5000, then simply drop the rightmost digits. As an example, consider $0.061/1.233 = 0.0494728$, which must be rounded to two significant figures (because 0.061 has two significant figures). The rightmost digits are 4728, which is less than 5000, so the 0.049 is the correct rounded-off final answer.

Numeric accuracy rule 6. If the rightmost digits beyond the significant figures are greater than 5000, then increase the least significant figure by 1. As an example, consider $0.061/1.232 = 0.0495130$, which again must be rounded to two significant figures (because of the 0.061). The rightmost digits are 5130, which is greater than 5000, so the final answer needs to be rounded up by one least significant digit $(0.049 + 0.001)$. The final answer is 0.050, rounded off correctly to two significant figures.

Numeric accuracy rule 7. It may sometimes be necessary to round off a number when the rightmost digit is exactly 5. The rule here is to round down the number if the digit to the left of the 5 is even, and round up the number if the digit to the left of the 5 is odd. For example 2.45 is 2.4, rounded to two significant figures; 1.5 is 2, rounded to one significant figure. This rounding scheme for numbers that end in 5 is arbitrary and results in averaging out rounding errors when a large number of calculations are performed.

Numeric accuracy rule 8. For addition and subtraction the final result has the same number of significant decimal places (rather than significant figures) as the number in the problem with the least number of significant decimal places. For example,

$$0.123 + 3.42 = 3.54 \, (\text{two significant decimal places})$$
$$0.1 + 3.42 = 3.5 \, (\text{one significant decimal place})$$
$$1 + 3.42 = 4 \, (0 \text{ significant decimal places})$$

Sometimes addition and rounding must be employed simultaneously, as in $0.125 + 3.42 = 3.547$, which should properly be rounded to 3.55 with only two significant decimal places because the 3.42 has only two significant decimal places.

Scientific pocket calculators often have a key for fixing the number of decimal places to be used in a calculation. The calculator also does the rounding off, simplifying such calculations.

Calculators and Personal Computers

Examples throughout this chapter have emphasized the use of the pocket scientific calculator. These scientific calculators are available from many manufacturers and should offer, as a minimum, the $\ln x$ and e^x functions. On some calculators, these options may be presented through a combination of $\ln x$ and inverse keys, as discussed in the previous examples. Figure 1-1 shows a typical calculator keyboard that would be useful in nuclear medicine. Generally, a scientific calculator also offers other useful statistical functions such as mean, standard deviation, and linear regression (or **least squares curve fit**). Mastering the pocket calculator will greatly speed the results of many common nuclear medicine tests. Calculation of the variability in a nuclear counting system through a chi-square test, for example, can be conveniently derived from the standard deviation function on the pocket calculator.

A programmable calculator allows the user to store the instructions for frequently performed functions in the calculator memory or on a magnetic media program card of some sort that is inserted into the calculator. This would allow the user to program a function such as

$$GFR = a\left[1 - e^{-b(c-d)}\right]$$

into the calculator. Simply entering *a, b, c,* and *d* would produce the answer for glomerular filtration rate (GFR). Other options for calculating such results include using a programming language such as BASIC, FORTRAN, or C, which is sometimes available on imaging computers or on PC-type computers within the nuclear medicine department. Whether using a pocket calculator or other computers, the user must master some software to extend the range of user-defined calculations.

Several spreadsheet programs such as Microsoft Excel are now available for personal computers and greatly increase the number of mathematical calculations available to the user. In Excel, for instance, the user could simply enter numeric data values for *a, b, c,* and *d* in the previous equation for GFR into four data cells (e.g., A1, A2, A3, A4) and then enter the GFR formula in another cell, B1, by clicking on cell B1 and typing in the following:

$$= A1*(1 - \exp(-A2*(A3 - A4)))$$

Excel would calculate the GFR and place the answer in cell B1. Note that the symbol *exp* is a particular language that Excel understands to mean e^x, and the = sign in the previous equation is something that Excel interprets as *evaluate the numerical value of this equation, and place the result in cell B1.* The use of PC software, instead of the scientific calculator, also offers several operation advantages: the ability to easily save the data, the ability to easily edit the data, and the ability to create hard-copy printouts and graphing.

PRACTICAL APPLICATIONS

Radioactive Decay

Nuclei that have an unstable balance of neutrons and protons spontaneously undergo radioactive decay to achieve a more stable nuclear configuration. The number of radioactive nuclei that decay per unit time defines the radioactivity, which is measured in Ci or Bq (see Table 1-2). A radioactivity level is computed as follows:

$$1\,mCi = \left(1 \times 10^{-3}\,\frac{Ci}{mCi}\right) \times \left(3.7 \times 10^{10}\,\frac{dps}{Ci}\right)$$

$$= 3.7 \times 10^7\,dps$$

meaning that 3.7×10^7 dps occur in the sample of radioactive material. The equation that defines the decay of the activity *(A)* over time *(t)* arises from a differential equation, which states that the number of atoms decaying per second is proportional to the number of atoms present. If the number of atoms in a sample of radioactive material is doubled, then the number of atoms decaying per second is also doubled. Solving the differential equation yields the radioactive decay law:

$$A = A_0 e^{-\lambda t}$$

where

$$A = \text{activity at time } t$$
$$A_0 = \text{activity at starting time}$$
$$\lambda = \text{decay constant}$$
$$t = \text{time since starting time}$$

The **decay constant** λ is the fraction of atoms that decay per (small) time interval, and it has units of 1 over time (e.g., 1/hr) or inverse time (hr^{-1}). The decay constant for ^{99m}Tc, for example, is 0.115 hr^{-1}, which means that *about* 0.115 (or 11.5%) of the ^{99m}Tc atoms decay per hour.

Note carefully that the verbal *interpretation* of the decay constant λ as the fraction that decays per some time interval is an *approximation* that holds only when the period being considered leads to a very small fractional decay. It is incorrect, for example, to conclude that $\lambda = 0.115\ hr^{-1}$ means that in 6 hours a fraction of 6×0.115 or 69% of the atoms decay (it is really 50%). Even saying 11.5% decay per hour is only approximate (it is really 10.9%). It is advisable to simply use λ for the exact mathematical calculations using the radioactive decay equation and to avoid using the inaccurate verbal interpretation as fractional decay.

The typical radioactive decay calculation required in nuclear medicine specifies three of the four variables *(A, A_0, λ, t)* in the decay equation, requiring that the fourth unknown variable be solved for. For example, a radiopharmacy delivers a 20.0-mCi dose of ^{99m}Tc ($\lambda = 0.115\ hr^{-1}$) to the nuclear medicine department at 8 AM. What amount of radioactivity would remain to be injected into the patient for an 11 AM nuclear medicine scan?

$$A_0 = 20.0\,mCi,\ \lambda = 0.115\,hr^{-1},\ \text{and}\ t = 3.00\,hr$$
$$A = A_0 e^{-\lambda t}$$
$$A = 20.0\,mCi \times e^{-(0.115\,hr-1) \times (3.00\,hr)}$$
$$A = 20.0\,mCi \times e^{-0.345}$$
$$A = 14.2\,mCi$$

To solve this problem on the pocket calculator, it is best to first evaluate the exponential expression and then multiply by 20.

0.115	enter λ value
+/−	*change sign* key to make negative
×	*multiply* key
3	enter *t* value

=   do the multiplication
INV − ln x or e^x key
×   *multiply* key
20   enter A_0 value
=   (see result of 14.2 in display)

The radioactive decay law is often expressed in an algebraic form involving the half-life ($t_{1/2}$), rather than the decay constant 2. The $t_{1/2}$, which depends on the radioactive material involved, is that time at which the activity is decreased to half its original value. The radioactive decay law may alternatively be expressed as:

$$A = A_0 e^{-0.693 \times (t/t_{1/2})}$$

The factor 0.693 is actually ln 2, which is commonly written with three significant figures. Each half-life of radioactive decay causes the activity level to drop by 50%. Following is a timeline for radioactivity remaining:

$$\text{Activity remaining} = 100\% \rightarrow 50\% \rightarrow 25\% \rightarrow 12.5\% \ldots$$
$$\text{At time} = 0 \rightarrow t_{1/2} \rightarrow 2t_{1/2} \rightarrow 3t_{1/2} \ldots$$

(See Figure 1-3 for a graph of the radioactive decay law as a function of time for ^{99m}Tc with $t_{1/2}$ = 6 hours.)

Because both forms of the radioactive decay law are valid, it can be written as:

$$A = A_0 e^{-\lambda t} = A_0 e^{-(0.693) \times (t/t_{1/2})} = A_0 e^{-(0.693/t_{1/2}) \times t}$$

Because the expressions in the exponent e in these equations are equal, it can be seen that a relationship between λ and $t_{1/2}$ is given by:

$$\lambda = \frac{0.693}{t_{1/2}}$$

The λ and $t_{1/2}$ are inversely proportional to each other: a large λ means a small $t_{1/2}$ and vice versa. Whether to use one form of the radioactive decay law or the other is simply a matter of convenience. Given λ, $t_{1/2}$ can be calculated easily (and vice versa). For example, given that the decay constant λ for ^{99m}Tc is 0.1153 hr^{-1}, what is the $t_{1/2}$?

$$t_{1/2} = \frac{0.693}{\lambda} = \frac{0.693}{0.1153 \, \text{hr}^{-1}} = 6.01 \, \text{hr}$$

Careful attention to the units is necessary to avoid errors. To make the units clearer, this might be restated as:

$$t_{1/2} = \frac{0.693}{0.1153 \dfrac{1}{\text{hr}}}$$

To get the units of 1/hr out of the denominator, multiply both numerator and denominator by units of hours (essentially multiply by 1):

$$t_{1/2} = \frac{0.693}{0.1153 \dfrac{1}{\text{hr}}} \frac{\text{hr}}{\text{hr}}$$

The 1/hr and the hr cancel in the denominator, leaving:

$$t_{1/2} = \frac{0.693}{0.1153} \text{hr}$$

The common radioactivity problem is to solve for one of the four variables (A, A_0, t, $t_{1/2}$) when the problem specifies three of them.

For example, on Monday at 8 AM, a sample of ^{131}I ($t_{1/2}$ = 8.04 days) is calibrated for an activity of 10 µCi. What amount of radioactivity will be given to the patient if the dose is administered on the following Friday at 2 PM?

Given: $A_0 = 10 \, \mu\text{Ci}$, t = Mon 8 am → Fri 2 pm,
$$t_{1/2} = 8.04 \text{ days}$$
Solve for: $A = A_0 e^{-(0.693) \times (t/t_{1/2})}$

Here, a digression to discuss units is necessary. Remember the good practice of always writing down the units associated with every number. Any problem involving the e^x function must have a dimensionless number for the value of x, so it is absolutely necessary that identical units be used for both t and $t_{1/2}$. Then the units cancel in the numerator and denominator of $t/t_{1/2}$, making the calculation independent of the units chosen to measure time. In this problem the time of decay (Mon 8 AM → Fri 2 PM) is 102 hours, but $t_{1/2}$ has already been given in days. It would be correct to express the time of decay t as 4.25 days (rather than 102 hours) with the $t_{1/2}$ also in days, or it would be correct to express the $t_{1/2}$ as 193 hours (rather than 8.04 days) with the t also in hours.

$$A = 10 \, \mu\text{Ci} \times e^{-0.693} \times (4.25 \text{ days}/8.04 \text{ days})$$

or

$$A = 10 \, \mu\text{Ci} \times e^{-0.693 \times (102 \, \text{hr}/193 \, \text{hr})}$$
$$A = 10 \, \mu\text{Ci} \times e^{-0.366} = 6.93 \, \mu\text{Ci}$$

A quick check of the results of the calculator's answer is also useful, based on the 100% → 50% → 25% → ... timeline for each half-life. In this example the decay time of 4.25 days is less than one $t_{1/2}$ (8.04 days), so the answer should be between 100% and 50% of the initial 10-µCi activity. The calculator result of 6.93 µCi agrees with the mental check. Inadvertent calculator usage errors can be prevented with these mental checks.

A radionuclide is often calibrated for some activity level on a Friday, but it might have been administered to the patient on the previous Monday. This type of radioactivity problem can be solved using negative time values for times that precede the time of A_0 calibration. For example, a radionuclide with a 2-day half-life is calibrated for Friday at noon to be 3 mCi. What activity level was present on the preceding Monday at noon?

Given: $A_0 = 3 \, \text{mCi}$
$$t = -96 \text{ hr (4 days)}, t_{1/2} = 2 \text{ days}$$
Find: $A = A_0 e^{0.693 \times (t/t_{1/2})}$
$$A = 3 \, \text{mCi} \times e^{-0.693 \times (-4 \text{ days}/2 \text{ days})}$$

$A = 3\,mCi \times e^{+1.386}$ (notice $[-]$ times $[-]$ is $[+]$)
$A = 12\,mCi$

This result is easy to check mentally since the time difference is exactly 2 half-lives; the answer should be that Monday noon has four times the activity of Friday noon, in agreement with the calculator result.

Sometimes a problem concerns only the fraction of remaining radioactivity (A/A_0), rather than the actual remaining activity in mCi. For example, what fraction of radioactivity is left at a time equal to 3 half-lives? Here, $t = 3t_{1/2}$ is given and the object is to find A/A_0. The radioactive decay law can be algebraically rearranged (dividing both sides of the decay equation by A_0) as:

$$A/A_0 = e^{-0.693 \times (t/t_{1/2})}$$
$$A/A_0 = e^{-0.693 \times (3t_{1/2}/t_{1/2})}$$
$$A/A_0 = e^{-0.693 \times 3}$$
$$A/A_0 = e^{-2.079}$$
$$A/A_0 = 0.125$$

A quick mental check confirms the result: in 3 half-lives the radioactivity should decay 100% → 50% → 25% → 12.5%.

Remember that the radioactive decay equation always refers to the *remaining activity*, which is the same as 100% minus the decayed activity. It is important to determine whether the problem is stating the amount of radioactivity remaining, which the decay equation predicts, or the radioactivity that has decayed away. For example, the previous problem showed that only 12.5% of the original radioactivity remains after 3 half-lives. This problem could also state that 87.5% of the radioactivity decays away in 3 half-lives.

Radioactive decay problems can also require the t or $t_{1/2}$ value to be solved for in the radioactive decay law. These values are contained in the decay law as part of the exponent function, so the exponent must be removed. An example might be to calculate the time necessary for 99.9% of a sample of ^{99m}Tc to decay away. Remember that the decay law works with the remaining radioactivity.

Given: $A/A_0 = 0.1\% = 0.001$
$t_{1/2} = 6.01\,hr$
Solve for $t_{1/2}$ *in*: $A/A_0 = e^{-(0.693) \times (t/t_{1/2})}$
$$0.001 = e^{-0.693 \times (t/6.01\,hr)}$$

Taking the natural logarithm of both sides and using $\ln(e^x) = x$ yields:

$$\ln(0.001) = -0.693 \times t/6.01\,hr$$

Now the t value is out of the exponent and the equation can be simply rearranged algebraically:

$$t = -6.01\,hr \times \ln(0.001)/0.693$$

Notice how the minus sign and the units are carried correctly. Now using $\ln(0.001) = -6.908$ yields:

$$t = -6.01\,hr \times (-6.908/0.693) = 59.9\,hr$$

The two minus signs are multiplied and cancel each other. About 60 hours (or about 10 half-lives) is necessary for the radioactivity of ^{99m}Tc to decay to $\frac{1}{1000}$ of its original value. For a radionuclide such as ^{131}I, it is still true that 10 half-lives cause decay to about $\frac{1}{1000}$ of the original activity, but for ^{131}I, 10 half-lives is 10×8.04 days = 80.4 days.

As another example, an experiment finds that a sample of radioactivity decays to 30% of its original value in 5 hours. What is the $t_{1/2}$?

$$A/A_0 = e^{-0.693 \times (t/t_{1/2})}$$
$$0.30 = e^{-0.693 \times (5\,hr/t_{1/2})}$$
$$\ln(0.30) = -0.693 \times (5\,hr/t_{1/2})$$
$$-1.204 = -0.693 \times (5\,hr/t_{1/2})$$

so

$$t_{1/2} = -0.693 \times \frac{5\,hr}{-1.204} = 2.9\,hr$$

Do the mental check. Does this seem a reasonable answer? If 2.9 hours is the correct $t_{1/2}$, then a decay time of 5 hours is not quite 2 half-lives. So the expected answer is that 5 hours of decay with a 2.9-hour $t_{1/2}$ should leave slightly more than 25% of the radioactivity remaining. The problem has sensible results: 30% remaining at time just less than 2 half-lives.

Decay Factor Tables for Radioactive Decay

Tables of radioactive decay factors provide an alternative methodology for doing calculation of radioactive decay problems, instead of using a calculator or spreadsheet. The **decay factor** is the fraction of radioactivity remaining at some time after the calibration time. Refer to Table 1-3, a decay factor table for ^{99m}Tc.

Example 1. Using Table 1-3, what is the decay factor, the fraction of ^{99m}Tc activity remaining, at 3 hours past

TABLE 1-3	Radioactive Decay Factors for ^{99m}Tc
^{99m}Tc Decay Time (hr)	Decay Factor (Fraction of Activity Remaining)
0	1.00
1	0.89
2	0.80
3	0.71
4	0.63
5	0.56
6	0.50
7	0.45
8	0.40
9	0.36
10	0.32
11	0.28
12	0.25

calibration time? Entering the row of the first column of Table 1-3 for a decay time of 3 hours, Table 1-3 yields a decay factor of 0.71. If there was for example 5 mCi present at the calibration time = 0, then 3 hours later the remaining activity is 0.71 × 5 = 3.6 mCi.

Example 2. Using Table 1-3, what is the decay factor, the fraction of ^{99m}Tc activity remaining, at 9.5 hours past calibration time? Since this decay time is not a time found exactly in any of rows of the first column of Table 1-3, the best that can be said from Table 1-3 (using the rows of the first column of the table for 9 and 10 hours) is that the fraction remaining, the decay factor, is less than 0.36 but more than 0.32. If for example there was 7 mCi present at the calibration time = 0, then 9.5 hrs later the remaining activity is less than 0.36 × 7 = 2.5 mCi, but more than 0.32 × 7 = 2.2 mCi. Interpolation between two adjacent rows of Table 1-3 would be necessary to produce a more specific decay factor. Of course use of a calculator to do the exact equations would produce an exact number for the remaining activity without the need for any interpolating between rows of a decay factor table.

Since there is a wide range of the half-lives for radionuclides that are commonly used in nuclear medicine, it is impossible to have a decay factor table for every common radionuclide. However, Appendix A offers radioactive decay tables for ^{18}F, ^{67}Ga, ^{123}I, ^{131}I, ^{111}In, ^{99m}Tc, ^{201}Tl, and ^{133}Xe. Alternatively, instead of using a decay factor table specific to any one radionuclide as in Appendix A, Table 1-4 presents a "universally applicable decay factor table" that can be used with *any* radionuclide. Extreme care however must be exercised to insure that the time since calibration and the half-life used with Table 1-4 are both expressed in the same units of time.

Example 1. Using Table 1-4, what fraction of ^{111}In ($t_{1/2}$ = 2.81 days) activity is remaining at 11 AM on Tuesday, given that the calibration time was the day before, Monday at 8 AM? In this case the decay time is 27 hours, which much be expressed in days (to be in same units as is $t_{1/2}$) before entering Table 1-4. Since 27 hours is 1.12 days, the (decay time/$t_{1/2}$) to use for the first column in Table 1-4 is:

$$(\text{decay time}/t_{1/2}) = 1.12 \text{ days}/2.81 \text{ days} = 0.40$$

Entering Table 1-4 for the value 0.4 in the first column, the fraction of activity remaining, the decay factor, is 0.76 at 11 AM Tuesday. If for example the calibration activity was 3 mCi at 8 AM Monday, then the activity remaining is 0.76 × 3 = 2.3 mCi at 11 AM, Tuesday.

Example 2. Using Table 1-4, what fraction of ^{18}F ($t_{1/2}$ = 109 minutes) activity is remaining at 11 AM, given that the calibration time was at 8 AM? In this case the decay time is 3 hrs, which much be expressed in minutes (to be in same units as is $t_{1/2}$) before entering Table 1-4. Since 3 hrs is 180 minutes, the (decay time/$t_{1/2}$) to use for the first column in Table 1-4 is:

TABLE 1-4	Radioactive Decay Factors, Universally Applicable for any Radionuclide
(Decay Time)/($t_{1/2}$)*	**Decay Factor (Fraction of Activity Remaining)**
0.0	1.00
0.1	0.93
0.2	0.87
0.3	0.81
0.4	0.76
0.5	0.71
0.6	0.66
0.7	0.62
0.8	0.57
0.9	0.54
1.0	0.50
1.1	0.47
1.2	0.44
1.3	0.41
1.4	0.38
1.5	0.35
1.6	0.33
1.7	0.31
1.8	0.29
1.9	0.27
2.0	0.25

*Decay time and $t_{1/2}$ must be expressed in same units of time.

$$(\text{decay time}/t_{1/2}) = 180 \text{ minutes}/109 \text{ minutes} = 1.65$$

Since this is not a number found exactly in the first column of Table 1-4, the best that can be said from Table 1-4, using the rows of the first column in the table for (decay time/$t_{1/2}$) of 1.6 and 1.7, is that at 11 AM the decay factor is between 0.33 and 0.31. If for example the calibration time activity was 15 mCi, then 3 hours later the remaining activity is less than 0.33 × 15 = 5.0 mCi but more than 0.31 × 15 = 4.7 mCi. Interpolation between two adjacent rows of Table 1-4 would be necessary to produce a more specific decay factor.

Concentration-Volume Calculations

The majority of nuclear medicine isotopes are administered to a patient in liquid form. When a radiopharmacy prepares nuclear medicine isotopes, pharmaceutical activity is provided in a concentration of liquid. The concentration, that is the activity, (typically in mCi) per volume (typically in ml), holds essential information for identifying the exact amount of nuclear isotope in a volume.

When a clinic receives a vial containing 30 mCi of an isotope but only needs to inject a patient with 20 mCi, concentration information becomes essential to knowing how much volume to draw out of the vial for proper patient dosing. In this example, 20 mCi represents ⅔ of a 30 mCi vial, so the technologist would need to draw

⅔ of the liquid from that vial. But how much volume do you draw? You need some more information to make this calculation. The radiopharmacy should provide you with the concentration, amount of activity, and volume in the vial. While all that information is useful, if the radiopharmacy provides you with any two of those variables, the third one is simple to figure out. The basic formula to use is:

$$Activity = Concentration \times Volume$$

which can be solved for any one of the three variables. Here are some examples.

Example 1. The vial is labeled: concentration 10 mCi/ml, volume 3 ml. How much activity is in the vial? Using the formula:

$$Activity = Concentration \times Volume$$
$$Activity = (10\,mCi/ml) \times (3\,ml)$$
$$Activity = 30\,mCi$$

Example 2. The vial is labeled: activity 30 mCi, concentration 10 mCi/ml. How many milliliters is the volume in this vial?

$$Volume = Activity/Concentration$$
$$Volume = 30\,mCi/(10\,mCi/ml)$$
$$Volume = 3\,ml$$

Example 3. The vial is labeled: activity 30 mCi, volume 3 ml, concentration 10 mCi/ml. How much volume do you draw out of the vial if you need to inject 20 mCi?

$$Volume = Activity/Concentration$$
$$Volume = 20\,mCi/(10\,mCi/ml)$$
$$Volume = 2\,ml$$

The technologist will need to draw 2 ml from the vial to get a 20-mCi dose.

There are many important calculations to make in a clinic when a dose needs to be adjusted to give a patient a specified activity. Although many nuclear medicine clinics today receive unit doses, technologists still need to have the skill of adjusting the patient dose. In a day-to-day operation of a nuclear medicine clinic, a variety of factors require dose adjustment including but not limited to patients coming to their appointment early/late, weight, pediatric, or change in prescription.

Along with drawing a certain volume for a specific activity amount, technologists are also asked to dilute doses. Diluting a dose is done to increase the volume of a dose, decrease concentration, or both. Dilution requires an addition of a liquid, usually saline, which always increases volume and decreases concentration (inverse relationship). To calculate the necessary volume needed for proper dilution, use the following formula:

$$Volume\,(to\,add\,to\,vial) = Volume\,(final) - Volume\,(initial)$$

Example 4. A radiologist orders a heart shunt study with 20 mCi ^{99m}Tc-pertechnetate, to be injected as an

0.5-ml bolus. The ^{99m}Tc-pertechnetate vial from the radiopharmacy is labeled: activity 20 mCi, volume 0.2 ml, concentration 100 mCi/ml.

How much saline should be added to the vial, and what will the concentration be once it is diluted? Using the following formula:

$$Volume\,(to\,add\,to\,vial) = Volume\,(final) - Volume\,(initial)$$
$$Volume\,(to\,add\,to\,vial) = 0.5 - 0.2 = 0.3\,ml$$

The technologist should add 0.3 ml of saline to the vial.

What is the concentration in the new 0.5 ml volume?

$$Concentration = Activity/Volume$$
$$Concentration = 20\,mCi/0.5\,ml = 40\,mCi/ml$$

Often it is necessary to combine radioactive decay calculations with concentration-volume problems. The nuclear medicine department may obtain its radioactivity from a ^{99}Mo-^{99m}Tc generator through an early-morning elution of the generator. This eluate decays throughout the day, resulting in a changing concentration (in mCi/ml). For example, a generator is eluted at 7 AM, yielding 900 mCi in 20 ml of eluate solution. What volume should be withdrawn from the eluate vial into a syringe to yield 15 mCi for a scan at 2 PM? First calculate the radioactivity remaining in the eluate vial at 2 PM:

$$A = 900\,mCi \times e^{-0.693 \times (7\,hr/6.01\,hr)} = 402\,mCi$$

(A quick mental check confirms the reasonableness of this answer: slightly less than 50% remaining at a time slightly greater than $t_{1/2}$.) The concentration (radioactivity per volume) in the eluate vial is then (402 mCi/20 ml) at 2 PM. The volume needed to be withdrawn into the syringe for a 15-μCi dose at 2 PM can be calculated from the equation: activity = concentration × volume.

$$A = C \times V$$
$$15\,mCi = \left(\frac{402\,mCi}{20\,ml}\right) \times V$$
$$15\,mCi = \left(\frac{20.1\,mCi}{ml}\right) \times V$$

so

$$V = \frac{15\,mCi}{\left(20.1\frac{mCi}{ml}\right)} = 0.75\,ml$$

^{99}Mo-^{99m}Tc Radionuclide Generators

Another common problem for radioactive decay is to calculate the ratio of ^{99}Mo ($t_{1/2} = 65.9$ hours) activity to ^{99m}Tc activity in generator eluate. The problem is that some ^{99}Mo is also eluted out along with the ^{99m}Tc in the morning elution. The ^{99}Mo is a radionuclidic impurity that is limited by regulatory agencies to be less than 0.15 μCi ^{99}Mo per mCi ^{99m}Tc at the time of injection into a patient. Consider a generator that is eluted at 7 AM and yields an eluate vial containing 30 μCi ^{99}Mo along with 250 mCi ^{99m}Tc. Can this eluate be used for a brain scan at the elution time of 7 AM? Calculate the ratio of ^{99}Mo to ^{99m}Tc activity at 7 AM as:

$$\frac{^{99}\text{Mo}}{^{99m}\text{Tc}} = \frac{30\,\mu\text{Ci}^{99}\text{Mo}}{250\,\text{mCi}^{99m}\text{Tc}} = 0.12\frac{\mu\text{Ci}^{99}\text{Mo}}{\text{mCi}^{99m}\text{Tc}}$$

This eluate is less than the regulatory limit (0.15) and may be used.

Could this same eluate be used 6 hours later to prepare a lung scan? Now the ratio of activities at 1 PM is

$$\frac{^{99}\text{Mo}}{^{99m}\text{Tc}} = \frac{30\,\mu\text{Ci}\times e^{-0.693\times(6\,\text{hr}/65.9\,\text{hr})}}{250\,\text{mCi}\times e^{-(0.693)\times(6\,\text{hr}/6.01\,\text{hr})}}$$

$$= \frac{30\,\mu\text{Ci}\times 0.939}{250\,\text{mCi}\times 0.500} = \frac{28.17\,\text{Ci}^{99}\text{Mo}}{125\,\text{mCi}^{99m}\text{Tc}}$$

$$= 0.23\frac{\mu\text{Ci}^{99}\text{Mo}}{\text{mCi}^{99m}\text{Tc}}$$

This eluate cannot be used, since the ^{99}Mo/^{99m}Tc ratio is greater than the 0.15 regulatory limit. The ^{99}Mo has not changed very much in the 6 hours since generator elution, but the ^{99m}Tc activity has halved, resulting in a large increase in the ^{99}Mo/^{99m}Tc ratio.

The mathematics of this type of radionuclide generator are governed by the laws of radioactivity,[2] relating radionuclides denoted as a parent-daughter-granddaughter (and so on) decay chain. The parent radionuclide ^{99}Mo decays to the daughter ^{99m}Tc, which in turn decays to the granddaughter ^{99}Tc, and the decay chain continues. Without dealing with the exponential algebra for this type of decay, it is possible to easily calculate the ^{99m}Tc radioactivity expected to be eluted from the generator by knowing three values:

1. The activity of ^{99}Mo in the generator, which is given by the manufacturer's calibration date and the decay law for ^{99}Mo ($t_{1/2} = 65.9$ hours)
2. The time since the last elution of the generator, which is commonly 24 hours for daily elutions
3. The ratio of ^{99m}Tc to ^{99}Mo in the generator, which depends on the time since the last elution (^{99m}Tc to ^{99}Mo ratios are shown in Table 1-5 as a function of the time since last elution)

For example, a generator is delivered on Saturday and calibrated by the manufacturer for the following Monday at 6 PM to contain 2 Ci of ^{99}Mo. The generator is eluted daily (Monday-Friday) at 7 AM. What activity of ^{99m}Tc is available in the generator at 7 AM on Tuesday? The required data are as follows:

1. ^{99}Mo activity Tuesday 7 AM, 13 hours after calibration time.

$$A = 2\,\text{Ci}\times e^{-0.693\times(13\,\text{hr}/65.9\,\text{hr})}$$

$$A = 1744\,\text{mCi of }^{99}\text{Mo in the generator, Tuesday 7 am}$$

TABLE 1-5	Generator ^{99m}Tc/^{99}Mo Activity Ratio
Time Since Last Elution (hr)	**^{99m}Tc/^{99}Mo Activity Ratio**
1	0.094
2	0.18
3	0.25
4	0.32
5	0.39
6	0.44
7	0.49
8	0.54
10	0.61
12	0.68
14	0.73
16	0.78
18	0.80
20	0.83
22	0.85
24	0.87
26	0.88
30	0.91
∞	0.95

2. Time since last elution is 24 hours, since the generator is eluted daily.
3. From Table 1-5, the ^{99m}Tc/^{99}Mo ratio is 0.87 for 24 hours since last elution, so:

$$\text{Activity }^{99m}\text{Tc} = 0.87\times \text{Activity }^{99}\text{Mo}$$

$$= 0.87\times 1744\,\text{mCi}$$

$$= 1518\,\text{mCi}$$

Depending on the quality of the generator, only a percentage of this 1518 mCi of ^{99m}Tc will appear in the eluate. This is known as the *elution efficiency of the generator*. If the elution efficiency is 95%, then the ^{99m}Tc found in the Tuesday morning eluate would be calculated as 0.95 × 1518 mCi = 1442 mCi. This is available for patient studies.

Half-Life: Biological, Physical, and Effective

In most clinical applications the nuclear medicine gamma camera measures the radioactive counts over an organ of interest in the patient's body. Typically the patient's organ excretes the radiopharmaceutical with some biological half-life t_B while the radioactivity also decays physically with a **physical half-life** that is denoted as t_P. The **biological half-life** is an indicator of the physiological fate of the radiopharmaceutical, t_B. The counts observed by the gamma camera follow an exponential decay law based on the **effective half-life** t_E, where:

$$\frac{1}{t_E} = \frac{1}{t_P} + \frac{1}{t_B}$$

or, in a format that is much easier for calculation purposes,

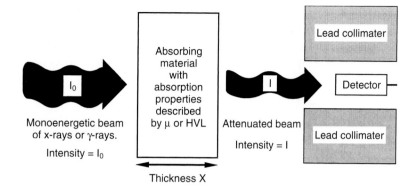

$$I = I_0 e^{-\mu X} = I_0 e^{-0.693(X/HVL)}$$

FIGURE 1-2 Attenuation of radiation in an absorbing medium.

$$t_E = \frac{t_P \times t_B}{(t_P + t_B)}$$

For example, if the liver excretes a ^{99m}Tc radiopharmaceutical with t_B = 3 hours, then the gamma camera over the liver would observe an effective half-life of

$$t_E = \frac{6\,hr \times 3\,hr}{(6\,hr + 3\,hr)} = 2\,hr$$

The effective half-life is always less than or equal to the smaller of t_P or t_B.

Attenuation of Radiation

The calculation of the intensity (I) of x-ray or γ-ray photons transmitted through some thickness (x) of absorbing material follows exactly the same algebra as the equations for radioactive decay. Figure 1-2 shows a beam of monoenergetic x-ray or γ-ray photons striking a thickness of absorbing material. Monoenergetic means that the photons all have the same energy, such as a beam of photons from a ^{99m}Tc radionuclide source that emits photons with an energy of 140 keV. The electron volt (eV) is a common unit for specifying energy. In nuclear medicine the energy of photons is commonly expressed in units of thousands of electron volts, abbreviated keV. The initial intensity (number of photons per second) entering the absorbing material is called I_0. The material attenuates, or absorbs, some fraction of the photons, and the photon beam emerges with a transmitted (i.e., not absorbed) intensity I. The intensity of the transmitted radiation is given by:

$$I = I_0 e^{-\mu x}$$

where μ is the linear attenuation coefficient, or the fraction of the beam absorbed in some (very small) thickness x. The linear attenuation coefficient μ is the analog of the decay constant λ in radioactive decay. The linear attenuation coefficient μ depends on the type of absorbing material and the energy of the photons. A large μ value means a strongly absorbing material. For ^{99m}Tc

γ-rays the μ value in lead is about 23 cm^{-1}, whereas the μ in water is only 0.15 cm^{-1}. Lead is a material that absorbs much more strongly than water.

A typical calculation deals with the fraction I/I_0 transmitted through a thickness x. For example, what percentage of 140-keV photons are transmitted through 10 cm of water (μ = 0.15 cm^{-1})?

$$I/I_0 = e^{-\mu x}$$
$$I/I_0 = e^{-0.15\,cm^{-1} \times 10\,cm}$$
$$I/I_0 = e^{-1.5} = 0.22, \text{ or } 22\%$$

Because 22% are transmitted, it can also be said that 78% are absorbed in 10 cm of water.

Consider a problem that asks what fraction of ^{131}I photons at energy 364 keV is transmitted through a half inch of lead (μ = 2.2 cm^{-1} at 364 keV). An initial inclination might be to calculate as follows:

$$I/I_0 = e^{-\mu x}$$

but

$$I/I_0 \neq e^{-2.2\,cm^{-1} \times 0.5\,in}$$

The calculation is incorrect because the units in the exponent do not cancel each other. A dimensionless number must be in the exponent to make the result independent of the units used to describe μ and x. Any units can be used as long as the units of μ and x are inverse of each other. It is easiest to look up the μ values, from published tables, and then convert the thickness x to the corresponding units, rather than convert the units of μ to correspond with those of x. For this problem, convert x = 0.5 inch to 1.27 cm to obtain

$$I/I_0 = e^{-2.2\,cm^{-1} \times 1.27\,cm} = 0.061$$

So 0.5 inch of lead transmits only 6.1% of a beam of 364-keV photons from ^{131}I. This also means that the lead absorbs 93.9% of the photons. The linear attenuation coefficient suffers from the same problem as λ; it is difficult to conceptualize. It is therefore common to follow the method used in radioactive decay and define a **half-value layer** (HVL) as that thickness of material that absorbs 50% of the photons. The HVL is the analog of $t_{1/2}$ in radioactive decay. One HVL transmits 50% of the photons, two HVLs transmit 25% of the original beam, and so on. The absorption line looks like the following:

$$\text{Photon intensity} = \rightarrow 100\% \rightarrow 50\% \rightarrow 25\% \rightarrow 12.5\% \dots$$

$$\text{Thickness} = \rightarrow 0 \rightarrow 1\,\text{HVL} \rightarrow 2\,\text{HVL} \rightarrow 3\,\text{HVL} \dots$$

The equation of photon attenuation then can be expressed as

$$I = I_0 e^{-\mu x} = I_0 e^{-0.693 \times (x/\text{HVL})}$$

and a relationship exists between μ and HVL, given by $\mu = 0.693/\text{HVL}$. If the HVL or μ value is known, it is a straightforward calculation to find the other and use whichever attenuation equation is most convenient.

As an example, what percentage of 140-keV photons from ^{99m}Tc are attenuated by 10 cm of water? The HVL for 140 photons in water is 4.6 cm.

$$I/I_0 = e^{-0.693 \times (x/\text{HVL})}$$

$$I/I_0 = e^{-0.693 \times (10\,\text{cm}/4.6\,\text{cm})}$$

$$I/I_0 = 0.22, \text{ or } 22\%$$

Remember the units of x and HVL must be the same, and remember that this equation calculates the *transmitted* intensity. A fraction (0.22) of the photons is transmitted. This is precisely the same result that was obtained previously in this section using the attenuation equation with μ. The problem, however, asks what fraction is *attenuated* by the water, so $1 - 0.22 = 0.78$ is the attenuated fraction; 10 cm of water absorbs 78% of the photons emitted by ^{99m}Tc. This type of calculation can be carried out easily on the pocket scientific calculator.

0.693	enter value
+/–	*change sign* key
×	*multiply* key
10	enter thickness value
÷	*divide* key
4.6	enter HVL value
=	(see result of division)
INV and ln x	or e^x key
	(see result of 0.22 in display)

A quick mental check of the calculator result is useful. The thickness here (10 cm) is slightly more than 2 HVLs (since HVL = 4.6 cm), so the attenuation answer should be slightly less than 25%.

Another problem might require solving the attenuation equation for either x or the HVL, both of which are contained in the exponent in the attenuation equation. Just as in radioactive decay (where t or $t_{1/2}$ needed to be solved for), the exponent with the natural logarithm can be eliminated as the inverse function of e^x.

$$I/I_0 = e^{-\mu x} - e^{-0.693 \times (x/\text{HVL})}$$

or

$$\ln(I/I_0) = -\mu x = -0.693 \times (x/\text{HVL})$$

For example, if 10 cm is known to transmit 22% of the photon beam, what is the HVL?

$$\ln(0.22) = -0.693 \times (10\,\text{cm}/\text{HVL}),$$

so

$$\text{HVL} = \frac{-0.693 \times 10\,\text{cm}}{\ln(0.22)}$$

$$= \frac{-0.693 \times 10\,\text{cm}}{-1.51} = 4.6\,\text{cm}$$

Note how the minus signs cancel and how the units are carefully carried. To calculate the HVL on the pocket calculator, perform the following steps:

0.693	enter value
+/–	change sign key
×	multiply key
10	enter x value
÷	divide key
0.22	enter fraction value
ln x	natural logarithm key
=	(see result of 4.6 cm in display)

One further nuance occurs for attenuation of photons. The μ value, or the corresponding HVL value, for any material also depends on the physical density ρ (g/cm^3); the HVL in water vapor is different from the HVL in liquid water, which is also different from the HVL in ice, and so on. This makes calculations using the μ or HVL values somewhat difficult because the μ values are usually tabulated only for the common physical state of the material in question (e.g., for liquid water). To circumvent this problem, a new parameter is defined as the *mass attenuation coefficient* μ_m (cm^2/g) = μ/ρ. The mass attenuation coefficient is *independent* of the physical density of the absorber and is therefore easily tabulated. The transmission of photons can then be expressed in one of three equivalent forms:

$$I/I_0 = e^{-\mu x}$$

$$I/I_0 = e^{-0.693 \times (x/\text{HVL})}$$

$$I/I_0 = e^{-\rho \mu_m x}$$

Calculation of a result using the more easily tabulated value of mass attenuation coefficient also requires looking up the density *(ρ)* of the absorbing material.

It should also be noted that these equations for the transmitted fraction of photons apply only to a situation known as *good geometry*, or *narrow-beam geometry*, meaning that a very thin, pencil-like beam of photons enters the absorber and is detected by a small collimated detector. Scattered photons (photons not traveling in a straight line between the origin of the photon and the detector) are excluded by the good geometry. In most practical applications, such as photons arising in the patient's heart and being detected by a gamma camera, the geometry is broad-beam. The photons can leave the

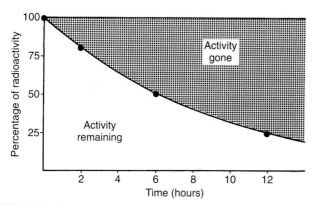

FIGURE 1-3 Linear plot of radioactive decay for $t_{1/2}$ = 6 hours.

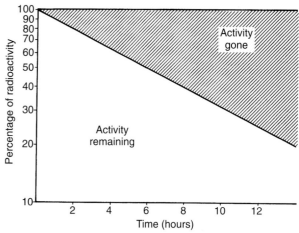

FIGURE 1-4 Semilog plot of radioactivity for $t_{1/2}$ = 6 hours. The y-axis is logarithmic.

patient's heart and move toward the thyroid, for example, and then scatter in the thyroid and travel toward the gamma camera to be detected as a photon apparently arising from the thyroid. The scattered photons increase the apparent transmission through the patient's body, and the equation is typically modified by a multiplicative buildup factor B, with $B \geq 1$. Buildup factors are dependent on the absorbing material, energy of the photon, and geometry. A large patient has a buildup factor greater than that of a thin patient, so in broad-beam geometry:

$$I/I_0 = Be^{-\mu x}$$

Specification of the buildup factor, or some other correction for scatter, such as arbitrarily using a smaller μ value, may be necessary for accurate quantification of photons originating inside a patient.

Graphs

In the modern technological world, people are inundated with data. Graphs provide a practical, highly visual way to convey large amounts of information. They can also be used to predict one variable based on another. The most common type of graph uses a linear set of x and y axes in the familiar Cartesian coordinate system. Figure 1-3 shows a graph or plot of the remaining radioactivity level versus time from a sample of radioactive material with $t_{1/2}$ = 6 hours. The x-axis (or abscissa) shows the time of each data point (for 0, 2, 6, and 12 hours), and the y-axis (or ordinate) shows the activity in millicurie for each data point. One variable is often considered to depend on another independent variable. The independent variable is generally plotted on the x-axis, with the dependent variable on the y-axis. In Figure 1-3, time is considered the independent variable on the x-axis, and activity level is considered the dependent variable on the y-axis.

Mathematically, activity (y) is a function of time, or $y = f(t)$. The data points in Figure 1-3 are called *discrete data points* because a measurement of activity was taken

at four discrete, individual data points (0, 2, 6, and 12 hours). Graphs of discrete data points may or may not, at the user's discretion, show the data points joined by smooth curves or a connect-the-dots type of straight line. Knowledge of the decay process suggests a smooth curve should best represent radioactive decay. On the other hand, a graph of the number of monthly kidney scans might be graphed as discrete data points joined in a connect-the-dots fashion because no reason implies a smoother curve.

Figure 1-3 shows a continuous curve of activity versus time for the radioactive decay equation:

$$A = A_0 e^{-\lambda t}$$

The $t_{1/2}$ for the data in Figure 1-3 is 6 hours because the radioactivity drops 100%, 50%, and 25% in 0, 6, and 12 hours, respectively. If the natural logarithm is taken on both sides of the equation, the curve in Figure 1-3 will simplify into the straight line shown in Figure 1-4 because:

$$\ln A = \ln\left(A_0 e^{-\lambda t}\right)$$
$$\ln A = \ln A_0 + \ln\left(e^{-\lambda t}\right)$$
$$\ln A = \ln A_0 - \lambda t$$

or

$$y = a + bt$$

This is the equation of a straight line with y-intercept $a = \ln A_0$, and slope $b = -\lambda$. This is an important practical result: the logarithm of radioactive decay data plotted versus time is a straight-line graph with negative slope equal to the decay constant. Note that the logarithmic plot of activity still shows the activity dropping by 50% every 6 hours.

A brief review of the graphic interpretation of straight-line data seems pertinent. A straight-line graph of y versus x is represented by the general formula:

$$y = a + bx$$

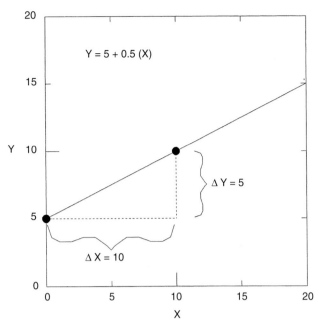

FIGURE 1-5 Straight-line graph with slope = 0.5 and intercept = 5.

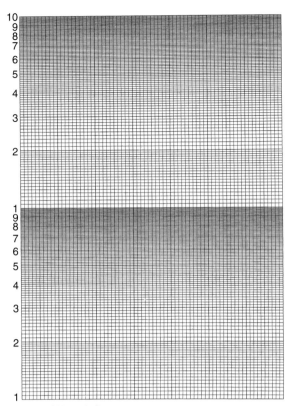

FIGURE 1-6 Two-cycle semilog graph paper.

The y-intercept, which is the value of y at $x = 0$, is represented by a. The slope, which represents the steepness of the line, is represented by b. Figure 1-5 shows a straight-line graph with $b = 0.5$ as the slope. The slope is calculated from any two arbitrary points on the line as:

$$\text{Slope} = \frac{\Delta y}{\Delta x} = \frac{(y_2 - y_1)}{(x_2 - x_1)}$$

In Figure 1-5 the slope is calculated from the points $(x_1, y_1) = (0, 5)$ and $(x_2, y_2) = (10, 10)$.

$$\text{Slope} = \frac{(10 - 5)}{(10 - 0)} = 0.5$$

For a straight-line graph, it does not matter which two points on the line are chosen to calculate the slope; the same answer is obtained. In Figure 1-5 the y-intercept $a = 5$ because the value of y is 5 at $x = 0$. Hence the equation of the straight line in Figure 1-5 is given by:

$$y = 5 + 0.5x$$

Given any x value, the equation can be used to calculate the y value. The sign of the slope merely reflects whether the curve slopes upward (a positive slope) or downward (a negative slope). Straight-line curves are generally used in nuclear medicine to prove a direct or linear relationship between two variables or to predict some y variable based on the value of the x variable.

Mathematical relationships or curves that are nonlinear, such as radioactivity versus time, are often transformed by a mathematical operation to make the graph a straight line. For exponential curves such as radioactive decay, taking the natural logarithm of the activity transforms the data into a straight line. The straight-line form might be preferred because subsequent interpretations or calculations are simplified. The use of logarithms as a process to transform curvilinear data into straight lines is so common that a special type of graph paper is often used to simplify the process (Figure 1-6). Semilogarithmic graph paper has axes with divisions that are proportional to the logarithm of the y-axis, so the y values are simply plotted at the appropriate point without the necessity of calculating the logarithm of the y-axis data. Semilogarithmic graph paper is available with a varying number of cycles, or powers of 10, on the y-axis. Figure 1-6 shows two-cycle graph paper, which can accommodate y values that span a range of no more than 10^2. The user simply relabels the numeric values on the y-axis to correspond to the range of the data involved. For example, the y values could range from 0.23 to 7.9, with the y-axis labeled with 0.1 at the bottom, 1.0 in the middle, and 10.0 at the top. Alternatively, the data might fall into the range of 200 to 8000, with the cycles labeled from 100 through 1000 to 10,000.

Measurement of Effective Half-Life

A typical procedure with nuclear medicine data is to calculate the effective $t_{1/2}$ of excretion from some organ in the body. As an example, consider a patient who is given a meal of radioactive food to determine the $t_{1/2}$ of the emptying of the stomach. The radioactivity counts

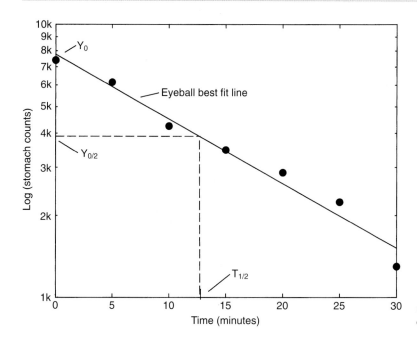

FIGURE 1-7 Measurement of effective $t_{1/2}$ = 12.5 minutes in the stomach by visual estimate of best-fit line on semilog plot.

emanating from the stomach are plotted on semilogarithmic graph paper (Figure 1-7). The $t_{1/2}$ of excretion can be determined by drawing a freehand visual-estimate straight line through the data points. Each data point is contaminated with statistical and systematic noise, or uncertainty, in the actual y value, so the straight line will probably not pass exactly through all, if any, of the data points. Use of this method to determine $t_{1/2}$ relies on the data points being reasonably well represented as a straight line on a semilogarithmic plot. Often the data appear more and more like a straight line at later time values, so these values are used to estimate the straight-line fit. After the straight line is drawn, the $t_{1/2}$ can be determined as the interval needed for the straight line to decrease by a factor of $\frac{1}{2}$. Just pick any convenient starting value for y, then read from off the graph the time needed to reach $\frac{y}{2}$. In Figure 1-7 the visual-estimate best-fit straight line has a y-intercept (or y_0) of 7800 ct, and the line falls to 3900 ct ($\frac{y_0}{2}$) in 12.5 minutes, so $t_{1/2}$ = 12.5 minutes by the visual-estimate best-fit line.

In some cases the data never decrease by a factor of $\frac{1}{2}$ over the time of the experiment, but it is still desired to calculate the $t_{1/2}$. In this case the proper calculation (remembering radioactive decay follows the equation ln y = ln $y_0 - \lambda t$) is to find the slope, which is equal to $-\lambda$, and the negative decay constant, which is based on the counts (y) and time (t) of any two points on the straight line.

$$-\lambda = \frac{[\ln(y_2) - \ln(y_1)]}{[t_2 - t_1]}$$

Then the $t_{1/2}$ is calculated from the $t_{1/2} = 0.693/\lambda$. Note that the equation for the decay constant slope requires calculation of the natural logarithm of the count values in the numerator. The logarithm need not be calculated

to *plot* the data (because of the convenience of semilogarithmic graph paper), but calculation of the slope λ *does* require calculation of the logarithm of any two arbitrary points on the straight line. Suppose that the data were acquired through only 10 minutes and that it was desired to still calculate $t_{1/2}$, although the data do not decrease to $\frac{y_0}{2}$ in only 10 minutes. Using two points on the estimated best-fit straight line—(0, 7800) and (10, 4400)—the decay constant is calculated as follows:

$$-\lambda = \frac{[\ln(4400) - \ln(7800)]}{[10\,\text{min} - 0\,\text{min}]} = \frac{-0.573}{10\,\text{min}}$$

so

$$\lambda = 0.0573\,\text{min}^{-1}$$

Then $t_{1/2} = 0.693/\lambda$ is calculated as 12.1 minutes, in close agreement with the graphic method, which estimated $t_{1/2}$ = 12.5 minutes.

Note that many nuclear medicine procedures yield graphs of counts versus time that do not follow a simple straight line on semilogarithmic plots. Several half-lives or several organs might be excreting a radiopharmaceutical from the body. It is then not correct to calculate a single $t_{1/2}$ from any data that do not appear to follow a straight line. Analysis of multiple half-life data requires other methods, such as curve stripping and nonlinear least squares.

Least Squares Curve Fitting

The technique of visually estimating the best-fit straight line is fraught with inaccuracy and imprecision because each observer's visual estimate line is unique. This could result in different values for the $t_{1/2}$, which is based on the straight line, or in different values for predicting a y

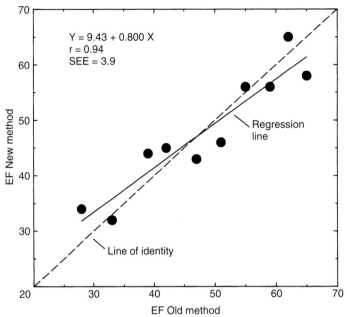

FIGURE 1-8 Regression analysis or least squares best-fit curve to compare old and new methods for calculating ejection fraction (EF).

value at any x value using the straight-line fit to the data. A more mathematically precise method to fit the straight line to the data is the method of least squares, or linear regression.[1] In this technique a set of n data values at the points (x_i, y_i), where $i = 1 \rightarrow n$, is graphed and fitted with a mathematically exact technique. No imprecision occurs; every observer who uses this method obtains exactly same answer. This type of calculation is generally performed to show a linear relationship between two variables or to predict some y variable based on measurement of some x variable.

Figure 1-8 shows data for x, y values from an experiment involving measurement of cardiac ejection fraction (EF) by two different techniques: a previously used method and the new method, which involves some change in experimental technique. Do these data show that the old method and the new method yield identical results? Or, given some value for EF by the old method (an x value), what would be the predicted results for EF by the new method (a y value)? The least squares method, or linear regression, calculates the best-fit values for y-intercept (a) and slope (b) in the best-fit straight line: $y = a + bx$. The intercept and slope parameters define a straight line, as discussed previously. The least squares method calculates the a and b that minimize the sum of the square of the distance in the y direction between the best-fit straight line and the data points. Use of a scientific pocket calculator can greatly speed calculations. Typically, a calculator requires the user to enter the first x value and press some key (e.g., X_i in Figure 1-1), telling the calculator this is x_1; to enter the corresponding first y value and tell the calculator this is y_1 (with the Y_i key; see Figure 1-1); and to enter x_2, y_2, and so on, until all n data points have been entered. Then the calculator displays the intercept and slope. Use of a computer is

TABLE 1-6	Linear Regression: Comparison of Two Methods for Calculation of Ejection Fraction*
Old Method: x (%)	**New Method: y (%)**
47	43
62	65
39	44
33	32
55	56
42	45
59	56
65	58
28	34
51	46

*$y = 9.43 + 0.800x$; $r = 0.94$; standard error of the estimate (SEE) = 3.9.

even simpler; the user enters x, y values in a spreadsheet format and instructs the computer to plot the data and the regression line. Almost all popular spreadsheet and graphics software packages offer linear regression (e.g., a personal computer [PC] spreadsheet program calculates and plots the best-fit line).

Calculation of the regression line by hand is tedious but not really complicated. The first step is the calculation of four sums based on the x, y data values. Then some simple multiplication and division produce the intercept and slope as follows. First calculate the four required sums, using the data for Figure 1-8, as shown in Table 1-6:

$$\Sigma x = x_1 + x_2 \cdots + x_n$$
$$= 47 + 62 + \cdots + 51 = 481$$
$$\Sigma y = y_1 + y_2 + \cdots + y_n$$
$$= 43 + 65 + \cdots + 46 = 479$$

$$\Sigma xy = x_1 y_1 + x_2 y_2 + \cdots + x_n y_n$$
$$= 47(43) + 62(65) + \cdots + 51(46) = 24{,}165$$

$$\Sigma x^2 = x_1^2 + x_2^2 + \cdots + x_n^2$$
$$= 47^2 + 62^2 + \cdots + 51^2 = 24{,}543$$

Then the intercept and slope are calculated as:

$$a = \frac{\left[\Sigma x^2 (\Sigma y) - \Sigma x (\Sigma y)\right]}{\left[n(\Sigma x^2) - \Sigma x (\Sigma x)\right]}$$

$$a = \frac{\left[24543(479) - 481(24165)\right]}{\left[10(24543) - 481(481)\right]} = 9.43$$

and

$$b = \frac{\left[n(\Sigma xy) - \Sigma x (\Sigma y)\right]}{\left[n(\Sigma x^2) - \Sigma x (\Sigma x)\right]}$$

$$b = \frac{\left[10(24165) - 481(479)\right]}{\left[10(24543) - 481(481)\right]} = 0.800$$

The best-fit line is then given by:

$$y = 9.43 + 0.80(x)$$

This line is drawn onto the graph of y versus x by calculating two points at the endpoints of the regression line and then joining these points with a straight line. At $x = 20$ the best-fit line value of y is $9.43 + 0.80(20) = 25$, and at $x = 70$ the best-fit line value of y is $9.43 + 0.8(70) = 65$. The regression line has been drawn in Figure 1-8. Also shown in Figure 1-8 is the line of identity, which is the line with a y-intercept of 0 and a slope equal to 1, defined by $y = x$. The line of identity is often drawn on regression graphs when the *same* parameter, here the EF, is being plotted on both the x- and y-axes. The line of identity facilitates an evaluation of whether the two methods (the x- and y-axes) are predicting the same result for the EF. If the two methods produce the same value for the EF, then the regression line should be the same as the line of identity. The line of identity is not a useful concept if the particular experiment being considered does not have identical parameters on the x- and y-axes. A regression of blood pressure versus age, for example, would not use the line of identity.

So what does the regression equation predict in Figure 1-8? The old and new methods do not predict exactly the same EF since the predicted regression line does not coincide exactly with the line of identity. For any given old method result (the x value), the regression equation or graph can be used to predict what the new method would yield for an EF result. This prediction of a y value, based on some measured x value, is the goal of regression analysis. Figure 1-8 shows that the new method produces results greater than the old method for EFs below about 47 by the old method because the regression line is above the line of identity. The new method underestimates the EF, compared with the old method, for EFs greater than 47 by the old method.

Figure 1-8 also lists the value of goodness of fit parameters, which help determine whether it is reasonable that the data points are truly represented by a straight line. The linear correlation coefficient r is calculated from the sums used to find the intercept and slope, along with one additional sum from the data points (Σy^2):

$$r = \frac{n(\Sigma xy) - \Sigma x (\Sigma y)}{\left[n(\Sigma x^2) - \Sigma x (\Sigma x)\right]^{1/2} \left[n(\Sigma y^2) - \Sigma y (\Sigma y)\right]^{1/2}}$$

The sign of the correlation coefficient is merely the same as the sign of the slope. A correlation $r = 1$ is a perfect fit, with the straight line passing exactly through each data point. The closer r is to 1, the more highly correlated are the x and y data. A chance, or probability (P), always exists that data that are truly not linearly related to each other will randomly appear in a fairly linear fashion. The statistical significance of correlation values less than 1 must be evaluated from statistical tables of probability (Table 1-7). If the correlation value for the n data points shows a P value of less than 0.05 from the statistical tables, then the data are said to be linearly correlated. Figure 1-8 shows $r = 0.94$ for $n = 10$ data points, which from Table 1-7 has $P < 0.001$, so the data are highly linearly correlated. If the r value was 0.632 or less (the $P = 0.05$ value for $n = 10$ from Table 1-7), then the data are not shown to be linearly correlated and it would not be prudent to apply a best-fit straight line to the data. A statistically significant correlation (meaning an r value with $P < 0.05$) merely implies a linear relationship between the x and y variables. This linear correlation or relationship does not necessarily suggest that x causes y. A graph, for instance, of the number of human babies (y) versus the number of stork nests (x) would probably show a high correlation, but this does not mean storks bring babies. More likely, both x and y depend on some other variable, such as the number of people in the house: people have babies, people live in houses, storks build nests on these houses.

TABLE 1-7	Linear Correlation Coefficient r at a Probability of P				
Number of Data Points	**Probability (P)**				
	0.100	**0.050***	**0.010**	**0.005**	**0.001**
5	0.805	0.878	0.959	0.974	0.991
10	0.549	0.632	0.765	0.805	0.872
15	0.441	0.514	0.641	0.683	0.760
20	0.378	0.444	0.561	0.602	0.679
30	0.306	0.361	0.463	0.499	0.570

*Minimum value of correlation coefficient for significant correlation is in this column. Larger r values are more highly correlated.

The use of Microsoft Excel for linear regression is quite straightforward. If 10 pairs of x, y data are known, as in Table 1-6, enter these data into a new Excel spreadsheet with x values entered into column A, and y values entered into column B. Then click on cell C1 and type in the following:

$$= SLOPE(B1:B10,A1:A10)$$

Click on cell C2 and type in

$$= INTERCEPT(B1:B10,A1:A10)$$

Click on cell C3 and type in

$$= CORREL(B1:B10,A1:A10)$$

Note that Excel then calculates slope, intercept, and correlation coefficient into cells C1, C2, and C3. The results can now be printed, the *x, y* data can be changed, and so on. If the *x, y* data values change, note that the values for slope and other items will also change. The user can also quickly ask Excel to plot the data: highlight the block of cells containing the *x, y* data by painting a box around them by holding down the left mouse button. Then click on the *Chart Wizard* icon near the top of the desktop and select *XY-Scatter* for the type of plot. After the plot appears, ask Excel to add the linear regression line to the graph by doing the following: click on the center of the graph, click the word *Chart* at the top of the display, and then choose *Add Trendline*. The least squares line will be added to the graph.

The other goodness of fit parameter shown in Figure 1-8 is the standard error of the estimate (SEE), sometimes denoted S_{yx}, which is defined as follows:

$$SEE = \left[\Sigma(y - a - bx)^2 / (n - 2) \right]^{1/2}$$

The *SEE* is the root mean square average deviation in the *y* direction of a data point from the regression line—that is, how far away the average data point is from the regression line in the *y* direction. In Figure 1-8, *SEE* = 3.9 so the average data point is about 4 units on the *y*-axis from the regression line. Another interpretation of *SEE* might be that the old and new EF methods disagree by 4, on average. A line that passes exactly through each data point produces *r* = 1 and *SEE* = 0 for a perfect fit. The *SEE* grows larger as the data points fall farther from the regression line. There is no easy way to state a *P* value for whether the *SEE* is small enough or not small enough to say the fit is statistically acceptable.

Least squares curve fitting could also be used to improve the precision of measurement of effective $t_{1/2}$ of data such as that shown in Figure 1-7. The calculation merely requires using the time as *x* values and the ln (counts) as the *y* values in the regression equations. The best-fit line has a slope that is the decay constant λ, and the half-life is then $t_{1/2} = 0.693/\lambda$. This least squares fit eliminates the imprecision of visual-estimate best-fit lines.

Several other caveats are known regarding least squares curve fitting. The linear correlation coefficient *r* describes only the degree of *linear* relationship between *x* and *y*. Some exact *nonlinear* relationship may in fact exist between *x* and *y* that yields a nonsignificant linear correlation. Data generated from the relationship $y = x^2$

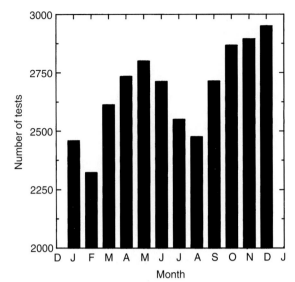

FIGURE 1-9 Histogram showing monthly variation in number of tests.

(x = −2, −1, 0, 1, 2 with corresponding y = 4, 1, 0, 1, 4) would produce the straight-line fit $y = 0.0 + 2 \times x$, with $r = 0$. An exact relationship in fact exists between x and y, but it is not linear.

The least squares best-fit line intercept and slope values have ± standard error uncertainties, according to formulas available in statistics texts.[3] This results in a range of possible best-fit lines. A statistical uncertainty is actually in the predicted y value for any x value. These uncertainties in the predicted line can be used, for example, to ascertain whether the predicted regression line is really different from the line of identity, or the x and y values can be tested for difference using t-tests, as discussed in the following section.

Other Graphs

Another graph useful in nuclear medicine is a histogram, which is used to display a single list of numbers such as the number of tests per month (Figure 1-9). Note that the *y*-axis is displayed with a minimum value of 2000 rather than 0 to accentuate month-to-month differences. Another type of graph is the pie chart, which is typically used to present some whole object broken down into its component parts. The width of each slice of the pie is proportional to each component's percentage share.

STATISTICS

Mean and Standard Deviation

Statistical analysis in nuclear medicine allows for consideration of such things as the level of confidence in the accuracy of some measurement or the level of confidence in a patient's test value differing from a normal result. Two concepts that often emerge in statistical considerations are *precision* and *accuracy*. *Precision* refers to the spread, or range, of data values obtained when some parameter is measured many times or in many patients. A small precision means that little variation exists in the data values. Accuracy, on the other hand, refers to how close the results are to the true, or "gold standard," result. Suppose that the length of a 96-inch–long board is measured twice, obtaining results of 94 inches and 98 inches. These data could be called accurate because the average (or **mean**) value of the two yields the correct answer of 96 inches. The average (or mean) of a group of measurements is simply the sum of all the measurements divided by the number of separate measurements that were made. The large range of the data (94 to 98 inches), however, would be considered not nearly precise enough for any practical construction measurements. Another person might measure the length of the board and obtain 96.25 and 96.50 inches. These results are more precise (smaller range of data) but less accurate (the average is 96.37 inches) than the previous measurement. A good measurement is both accurate and precise, but no necessarily fixed relationship exists between accuracy and precision in any experiment. Statistical parameters, such as the mean and standard deviation, allow quantification of the concepts of accuracy and precision.

Suppose that some parameter x is measured n times. Then the mean (or average) of the n values of the parameters x is defined by the symbol:

$$\bar{x} = \frac{\Sigma x}{n}$$

The symbol Σx means the sum of all the measurements of x.

As an example, a patient has four measurements of serum thyroxine (T_4, a thyroid hormone) given by 9.5, 9.0, 9.2, and 8.7 µg/dl. The mean value x is calculated as follows:

$$\bar{x} = \frac{(9.5 + 9.0 + 9.2 + 8.7)}{4} = 9.1 \mu g/dl$$

If the true answer for the serum T_4 was known, then the mean value $x = 9.1$ µg/dl could be compared with the true value to discuss the accuracy of the test. The **standard deviation**, a measure of the precision of the data, is given by the symbol σ, defined as

$$\sigma = \left[\Sigma (x - \bar{x})^2 / (n-1) \right]^{1/2}$$

Recall that an exponent of $\frac{1}{2}$ means the same as the square root ($\sqrt{\ }$). The standard deviation is a measure of the deviation or spread of the data points from the mean value. For the thyroid T_4 data:

$$\sigma = \left\{ \left[(9.5 - 9.1)^2 + (9.0 - 9.1)^2 + (9.2 - 9.1)^2 + (8.7 - 9.1)^2 \right] / [4-1] \right\}^{1/2}$$
$$\sigma = [(0.16 + 0.01 + 0.01 + 0.16)/3]^{1/2}$$

$$\sigma = (0.34/3)^{1/2} = 0.1133^{1/2} = 0.3366$$
$\sigma = 0.3\,\mu g/dl$, correctly rounded to one significant decimal place

The standard deviation is often expressed in a format of the mean value $\pm\sigma$, so this patient has a T_4 test result of 9.1 ± 0.3 µg/dl. A large σ value indicates data with a large range and therefore poor precision.

Sometimes it is more useful to express standard deviation as a percentage of the mean value, which is frequently called the *percent standard deviation,* or **coefficient of variation (CV)**:

$$CV = \left(\frac{\sigma}{\bar{x}} \right) \times 100$$

For the thyroid T_4 data presented earlier,

$$CV = \left(\frac{0.3367}{9.10} \right) \times 100 = 3.7\%$$

The *CV* merely shows how large the standard deviation is when compared with the mean value. For example, consider two separate experimental measurements of the length of an object. Both experiments produce the same standard deviation of 2 cm, but the two objects have different mean lengths of 2 m and 2 km. So one experiment has a CV of (2 cm/200 cm) × 100, or 1%, whereas the other experiment has a CV of (2 cm/200,000 cm) × 100, or 0.001%. The standard deviations of the two experiments are the same, but the CVs are vastly different, showing a much better precision in the second experiment (CV = 0.001%) than in the first experiment (CV = 1%).

Microsoft Excel can be used to calculate statistical parameters. As an example, for the four values of T_4, enter these data values in cells A1, A2, A3, and A4 in a new Excel spreadsheet. Then, in cell B1, type:

$$= AVERAGE(A1:A4)$$

In cell B2, type:

$$= STDEV(A1:A4)$$

In cell B3, type:

$$= B2/B1$$

Note the coefficient of variation is calculated in cell B3 as 0.036995, and the user must realize that this is 3.6995%, properly rounded to 3.7%.

As another example, consider two different blueberry farms. Suppose Farm A has blueberries of diameter 6 ± 7 mm and Farm B has blueberries of diameter 9 ± 2 mm. Which farm has the more desirable blueberries? It depends on what the buyer wants. Farm A has a wider range of blueberry diameters. Indeed, some Farm A blueberries must be quite small or large to produce such a significant 7-mm standard deviation, but the average blueberry is only 6 mm at Farm A. Farm B has blueberries that are bigger (9 mm) on the average, but the standard deviation for Farm B is smaller, so few really big (or small) blueberries are at Farm B.

The scientific pocket calculator generally has keys for calculation of mean and standard deviation. The user enters the first data value and then pushes the key (e.g., X_i) that tells the calculator this is x_1. Then the second data value is entered and the X_i key is pushed again, telling the calculator this is x_2, and so on up to x_n. Then press the key to display the mean and σ (sometimes denoted on calculators as σ_{n-1}).

Further calculations with statistics require consideration of the *theoretical distribution* of the data values. The user may know that a sample of blueberries produces diameters of 9 ± 2 mm, but suppose the user wants to know how many blueberries have diameters greater than 11 mm or what the probability is of getting a blueberry bigger than 13 mm. The theoretical distribution refers to a theoretical measurement of *all* the blueberries of Farm A, or of the T_4 values in *all* patients, and so on. The distribution is a theoretical graph of how many blueberries there are with which diameters or of how many patients there are with a certain value of T_4. What is usually measured in an experiment is not the theoretical distribution but rather a *sample* of data values (say 20 blueberries or 10 patients) that is part of the whole theoretical distribution. Two types of theoretical distributions of data values are important in nuclear medicine: the *Gaussian distribution* and the **Poisson distribution.** Many measurable quantities can be described by a Gaussian distribution, whereas the only thing of interest to nuclear medicine that follows a Poisson distribution is counting statistics.

Gaussian Distributions

The Gaussian distribution is also called the *bell-shaped distribution* or the *normal distribution.*[3] In general, measurements of some parameter might be expected to follow a Gaussian distribution if a reasonably large sample is taken from a very large distribution, where the parameter being measured is expected to vary randomly. For example, the diameters of blueberries in a 1-gallon sample would be expected to follow a Gaussian distribution. The measurement of the decay counts of a sample of several thousand radioactive atoms (sampled from the distribution of about 10^{23} atoms in a small sample of radioactive material) would also be expected to follow a Gaussian distribution. Student scores on an examination might follow a Gaussian distribution. Saying that something follows a Gaussian distribution means that if the number of times a certain value occurs is plotted on the y-axis versus the measured numeric value (e.g., blueberry diameter or number of counts) on the x-axis, then a graph such as Figure 1-10 is obtained. Analysis reveals that a Gaussian distribution has 68% of all results within the range $\bar{x} \pm 1\sigma$, 95% of all results within $\bar{x} \pm 2\sigma$, and

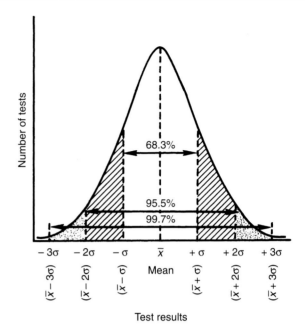

FIGURE 1-10 Gaussian distribution for test results can be expected to show the results in large population where test value is expected to vary randomly. Note that 68% of all test results are within the mean ±1 standard deviation (±1σ), 95% of all test results are in the range of ±2σ, and so on.

99% within $\bar{x} \pm 3\sigma$. Figure 1-10 shows this distribution. Hence returning to the sample of blueberries, if = 9 mm and $\sigma = 2$ mm, then if all the blueberries in the bucket are examined, the following would be expected:

68% within 7 to 11 mm $(\bar{x} \pm 1\sigma)$
95% within 5 to 13 mm $(\bar{x} \pm 2\sigma)$
99% within 3 to 15 mm $(\bar{x} \pm 3\sigma)$

The chance of getting a blueberry less than 5 mm, or greater than 13 mm, is only 5%. This is called *the area in the tails* (the ends) of the distribution. Because 95% are within $\bar{x} \pm 2\sigma$, it must be that only 5% are beyond the range $\bar{x} \pm 2\sigma$.

The properties of the Gaussian distribution are often used in quality control procedures and to determine normal ranges A quality control procedure might measure some daily parameter to determine whether an instrument is working properly. If today's value is beyond the $\bar{x} \pm 2\sigma$ value (based on previous measurements), then the instrument might be considered to be operating improperly because the probability of getting a result beyond $\bar{x} \pm 2\sigma$ is only 5%. This type of quality control, or normal value range determination, uses the 95% confidence interval (the $\bar{x} \pm 2\sigma$ range) as a conventionally accepted range. This means that a 1 in 20 (or 5%) chance exists that an acceptable quality control test will be incorrectly rejected, or a 5% chance exists that a normal subject would be incorrectly called *abnormal.* The preponderance of results, 19 out of 20 (95%), will be correctly classified.

Poisson Distributions and Counting Statistics

Counting statistics, meaning the number of counts expected from a sample, follow the Poisson distribution. In the Poisson distribution the standard deviation (σ_C) for any number of counts *(C)* is fixed at the square root of *C*:

$$\sigma_C = \sqrt{C}$$

This fixed definition of standard deviation does not exist in Gaussian distributions; essentially only counting statistics are Poisson. One farm could have a Gaussian distribution of blueberries of diameter 9 ± 2 mm (i.e., mean ± σ), and another farm could have blueberries of diameter 9 ± 4 mm. Neither farm has $\sigma = \sqrt{9}$. Any combination of a mean value and a standard deviation is possible in Gaussian data, whereas Poisson counting statistics always have the standard deviation of the counts from a sample equal to the square root of the counts.

Example:
What is the standard deviation of a sample that produced 10,000 ct?

$$\sigma_C = \sqrt{10,000} = 100 \text{ counts}$$

Example:
What is the coefficient of variation of 10,000 ct?

$$CV = \left(\frac{\sigma_C}{C}\right) \times 100 = \left(\frac{100}{10,000}\right) \times 100\% = 1\%$$

Example:
What are the σ_C and CV for 100 ct?

$$\sigma_C = \sqrt{100} = 10 \text{ counts}$$
$$CV = \left(\frac{\sqrt{100}}{100}\right) \times 100\% = 10\%$$

These examples show that as the number of counts increases from 100 to 10,000, the absolute magnitude of the standard deviation goes up (from 10 to 100 ct), but the percent standard deviation or CV goes down (from 10% to 1%). Less relative variability occurs in large count values.

Counting statistics, besides being Poisson, are also described by a Gaussian distribution as long as the number of counts is greater than about 30. Hence given some number of counts C, the standard deviation is automatically known. It is known that 68% of repeat measures of the sample fall within $C \pm \sqrt{C}$ and 95% of repeat measures of the sample fall within $C \pm 2\sqrt{C}$, and so on.

Example:
What is the 95% confidence interval for a sample with 10,000 ct?

$$\begin{aligned} 95\% \text{ confidence} &= C \pm 2\sigma_C = C \pm 2\sqrt{C} \\ &= 10,000 \pm 2\sqrt{10,000} \\ &= 10,000 \pm 200 \text{ counts} \end{aligned}$$

The 95% confidence interval is then from 9800 to 10,200 ct. If this represents a sample of the counts actually emanating from radioactive material, it can be said they are 95% sure that the true counts from this radioactive material are in the 9800 to 10,200 range (it is expected that 95% of repeat measurements would be in the range 9800 to 10,200 ct). The number of counts actually emitted by a radioactive source varies from time to time, in a random fashion, according to both Poisson and Gaussian distributions. The variation in the number of counts is often referred to as *counting noise*.

Sometimes this type of problem is expressed by saying that 10,000 ct are needed to be 95% confident that the true count is within 2% of the measured value. The presence of two different percentage values can seem confusing. The 95% confidence interval on 10,000 ct is ±200 ct, and this figure of 200 ct represents 2% of 10,000 ct. The general formula expressing the number of counts needed to be $n\sigma$ sure that the true answer is within some percent *(p)* of the measured counts is given by:

$$C = \left[\frac{n}{\left(\frac{P}{100\%}\right)}\right]^2$$

In this formula, *n* is replaced with a 1 for 68% confidence, a 2 for 95% confidence, and a 3 for 99% confidence.

Example:
How many counts are needed to be 95% sure that the true answer is within 1% of the measured value? Here *n* = 2 and *p* = 1%.

$$C = \left[\frac{2}{\left(\frac{1\%}{100\%}\right)}\right]^2 = \left[\frac{2}{.01}\right]^2 = 40,000 \text{ counts}$$

If this sample were recounted, then 95% of repeat measurements would be in the range $40,000 \pm 2\sqrt{40,000}$ or 40,000 ± 400, which represents a 1% uncertainty (because 400 is 1% of 40,000). Some radiation counters may have a preset count dial labeled as the percent error at the 95% confidence level, rather than a preset count dial actually labeled in number of counts. Setting such a preset count dial at 1% error would be the same as collecting 40,000 ct. Setting such a preset count dial at 5% would mean collecting 1600 ct, since

$$1600 = \left(\frac{2}{0.05}\right)^2$$

Some problems may deal with the count rate R that is obtained by counting a number of counts C in time T:

$$R = \frac{C}{T}$$

The standard deviation in the count rate is σ_R:

$$\sigma_R = \left(\frac{\sqrt{C}}{T}\right)$$

This presumes that no error occurs in measurement of the time T. By using $C = RT$, the σ_R can be alternatively written as the following:

$$\sigma_R = \frac{\sqrt{(RT)}}{T} = \sqrt{\left(\frac{R}{T}\right)}$$

Example:
A sample shows 43,627 ct in 5 minutes. What are the count rate and standard deviation in the count rate?

$$R = \frac{43,627 \text{ counts}}{5 \text{ min}}$$

$$R = \frac{8725 \text{ counts}}{\text{min}} = 8725 \text{ cpm}$$

$$\sigma_R = \frac{\sqrt{43,627}}{5} = 42 \text{ cpm}$$

Hence the count rate would be expressed as 8725 ± 42 cpm.

Example:
The count rate is 8765 cpm for a 2-minute count. What range of count rates would be predicted to occur in 68% of repeat measurements? This is simply asking what is the value of σ_R because 1 σ_R is the 68% confidence interval.

$$\sigma_R = \sqrt{(R/T)} = \sqrt{8765/2} = \sqrt{4382.5} = 66 \text{ cpm}$$

If the experiment were then repeated, it would be predicted that 68% of the repeat measurements would be in the range 8765 ± 66 cpm.

Background counts are a problem in most measurements of counts from a radioactive sample. Background arises from natural terrestrial and cosmic sources of radioactivity or from other nearby sources of radioactive material. The sample is usually counted in the presence of some background radiation, yielding a gross count for sample plus background, denoted by the letter C. Then the sample is removed from the counter and the background B is counted. The net, or true, counts,

which represent the sample only, is denoted by N and given by:

$$N = C - B$$

The standard deviation of the net counts is given by:

$$\sigma_N = \sqrt{(C + B)}$$

This is an example of the rules for combinations of errors,[1] which state that for addition or subtraction, errors add in quadrature within the square root:

$$\sigma_N = \sqrt{(\sigma_C^2 + \sigma_B^2)}$$

Additionally, since $\sigma_C = \sqrt{C}$ and $\sigma_B = \sqrt{B}$, one obtains $\sigma_N = \sqrt{(C + B)}$.

Example:
A sample is counted in the presence of background yielding $C = 1600$ ct. Then the background is counted alone, producing 900 ct. What are the true or net counts and standard deviation?

$$N = C - B = 1600 - 900 = 700 \text{ counts}$$

$$\sigma_N = \sqrt{(1600 + 900)} = \sqrt{2500} = 50 \text{ counts}$$

Hence the net counts can be expressed as 700 ± 50 ct. Note that the presence of background has increased the statistical uncertainty in the results. If there were *no* background, the sample in this example would have produced $N = 700 \pm \sqrt{700} = 700 \pm 26$ counts.

Similar considerations can yield the rules for the net count *rate*:

$$R_N = R_C - R_B = C/T_C - B/T_B$$

$$\sigma_{RN} = \sqrt{(\sigma^2 R_C + \sigma^2 R_B)}$$

$$\sigma_{RN} = \sqrt{(C/T_C^2 + B/T_B^2)}$$

or

$$\sigma_{RN} = \sqrt{(R_C/T_C + R_B/T_B)}$$

Chi-Square Tests

Suppose the wish is to test the reliability of the operation of some counting instrument, as a quality control test, by confirming that the instrument consistently produces the same counts in a reliable fashion. How can this be done when it is now known that the number of counts recorded will vary from measurement to measurement because of the statistical nature of radioactive decay? The answer is to count a sample a reasonable number of times (typically 10 repeat measurements are used) and then determine if the 10 different values show an acceptable or reasonable amount of variation. Too little or too much variation in the repeat measurements indicates a counter that may not be functioning properly. The **chi-square test** (χ^2) is used to determine an acceptable range of variability in the repeat measurements. The mean $\bar{C}$

of the 10 measurements is determined ($\bar{C} = \Sigma C/n$), and χ^2 is calculated as:

$$x^2 = \frac{\left[\Sigma(C-\bar{C})^2\right]}{\bar{C}}$$

Table 1-8 shows the calculation of χ^2 for some counter, which yielded a value of 24.7 for χ^2. Is this an acceptable amount of variation between the 10 measurements? The definition of acceptable χ^2 is given by looking up the probability *(P)* of this χ^2 value for the *n* (here 10) repeated measures in Table 1-9. Too little variation is shown by a χ^2 smaller than the $P = 0.9$ value; an amount of variation exactly as expected from the statistical nature of the decay process would yield $P = 0.50$; and an unacceptably large χ^2 would yield a P value greater than 0.10:

If $0.90 > (P \text{ of } \chi^2) > 0.10$, detector is OK.
If $(P \text{ of } \chi^2) > 0.90$, the detector shows too little variation.
If $(P \text{ of } \chi^2) < 0.10$, the detector exhibits too much variation.

For the data in Table 1-8, χ^2 was calculated = 24.7. In Table 1-9, this $n = 10$ measurement has a P value < 0.01, so this detector is *not* operating properly; if the χ^2 is too large, the detector is showing too much variation in counts. The detector probably needs to be repaired. An acceptable χ^2 for 10 measurements would be in the range $4.17 < \chi^2 < 14.7$ because the table of values reveals that this is the $0.90 > P > 0.10$ range. It is only common convention that fixes the $P = 0.90 - 0.10$ range as acceptable. Some laboratories might be willing to accept more variation, or they may be willing to use $0.95 - 0.05$ as the acceptable P range for χ^2.

Notice the similarities in statistical approach for calculating the linear correlation coefficient r and χ^2. Both are calculated from the data based on some equation, and then the P value of the r or χ^2 is determined to assess the significance of the result. This is typical of most statistical tests: calculate a parameter and then look up the probability of this result.

Does the result for the data in Table 1-8 seem sensible, that the detector is showing too much variation? Consider that a properly operating detector should have 68% (about 7 out of 10) of repeat measurements within the mean count $\pm\sqrt{(\text{mean count})}$. So the deviation $C-\bar{C}$ in Table 1-8 should be less than 1σ, less than $\pm\sqrt{10179.3}$ counts, in 7 out of 10 measurements. Examination of Table 1-8 shows that only four of the measurements (instead of the expected seven) have deviations from the mean within $\pm1\sigma$, or within ±101 ct. Too many measurement values are beyond $\pm1\sigma$. The detector is not working properly by this crude visual check, in agreement with the excessively large χ^2 value. Similar visual checks can be made to assess that only one out of 20 measurements should have deviations from the mean of more than $\pm2 \times 101$ ct. In fact, Table 1-8 shows that one measure is a deviation of -333 ct (about 3σ) and another is almost 2σ (actually -193 ct), so about 2 out of 10 are beyond $\pm2\sigma$ in contrast with the predicted 1 out of 20 measurements with this much variation. The calculated P value of χ^2 will always agree with such commonsense data checks.

Lastly, a word about calculating χ^2: most scientific pocket calculators do not have a calculation function for χ^2, but most calculators can calculate the standard

TABLE 1-8	Calculation of Chi-Square		
Observation	Counts (C)	Deviation (C − C̄)	Square (C − C̄)²
1	10,324	144.7	20,938.1
2	10,285	105.7	11,172.5
3	9,847	−332.3	110,423.3
4	10,168	−11.3	127.7
5	10,352	172.7	29,825.3
6	10,234	54.7	2,992.1
7	9,986	−193.3	37,364.9
8	10,139	−40.3	1,624.1
9	10,356	176.7	31,222.9
10	10,102	−77.3	5,975.3
	$\Sigma = 101,793$	$\Sigma = 0$	$\Sigma = 251,666$

$\bar{C} = 10,179.3$
$x^2 = \Sigma(C-\bar{C})^2/\bar{C}$
$x^2 = \dfrac{251,666}{10,179.3} = 24.7$
$SD = \left[\Sigma(C-\bar{C})\right]^2/(n-1)^{1/2}$
$SD = (251,666/9)^{1/2} = 167.2$

TABLE 1-9	Chi-Square Value at Probability P						
Number of Sample Measurements	Probability (P)						
	0.99	0.95	0.90*	0.50	0.10†	0.05	0.01
5	0.30	0.71	1.06	3.36	7.78	9.49	13.3
10	2.09	3.33	4.17	8.34	14.7	16.9	21.2
15	4.66	6.57	7.79	13.3	21.1	23.7	29.1
20	7.63	10.1	11.7	18.3	27.2	30.1	36.2

*Smallest acceptable χ^2 is in this column.
†Largest acceptable χ^2 is in this column.

deviation of the repeat count measurements, denoted here as *SD*:

$$SD = \left[\frac{\Sigma(C - \bar{C})^2}{(n-1)} \right]^{1/2}$$

This can be algebraically solved for $\Sigma(C - \bar{C})^2$:

$$\Sigma(C - \bar{C})^2 = (n-1) \times (SD)^2$$

This is simply the numerator of the definition of χ^2, so the equation for χ^2 can be written in terms of the mean and SD as the following:

$$\chi^2 = (n-1) \times \frac{(SD)^2}{\bar{C}}$$

To calculate χ^2, therefore, the pocket calculator (or the PC computer spreadsheet program) is used as described previously to calculate the SD and the mean, which are then used in the above equation for χ^2. The data in Table 1-8 show $SD = 167.2$ with a mean $\bar{C} = 10179.3$, so

$$\chi^2 = \frac{(10-1) \times (167.2)^2}{10179.3} = 24.7$$

exactly as obtained previously in Table 1-8.

To use Microsoft Excel to calculate χ^2, using the data of Table 1-8, just enter the data into cells A1 through A10 in a new Excel spreadsheet. In cell B1, type the number 10, or the number of data points. In cell C1, type

$$= (B1 - 1) * STDEV(A1:A10) \wedge 2 / AVERAGE(A1:A10)$$

Excel then places the value of χ^2 in cell C1.

The χ^2 statistic, in other algebraic definitions, has other uses besides a test for stability of counters in nuclear medicine. Chi-squared is commonly used in 2×2 contingency tables,[3] which could consider, for example, the number of persons who are well or ill, tabulated according to being male or female. Alternatively, a categorization could be made of the number of persons with positive or negative imaging tests using gamma cameras from two different manufacturers. A χ^2 calculation would show whether the two gamma cameras find different or same numbers of positive/negative test results.

t-Tests

The *t*-test is used to test for differences between *mean* values.[3] This test is also commonly referred to as the *Student* t-test because the original proposal for this test was published by an author using the pseudonym *Student*. The two forms of the *t*-test are for *independent* samples and *paired* samples.

For independent *t*-tests, two independent groups of data are used. For example, some test result is measured in a group of n_1 ill patients and a group of n_2 well patients. The two groups are completely independent.

No relationship or correlation exists between the two groups, typically because the groups represent different patients. The two groups have mean and standard deviations denoted by $\bar{x}_1$, SD_1, $\bar{x}_2$, and SD_2.

The *t*-test is a test of a null hypothesis that the mean values in the two groups are equal. The hypothesis being tested can be abbreviated $H_0 := \bar{x}_1 = \bar{x}_2$. The null hypothesis is statistical nomenclature, meaning that no difference is found. This test is called a *two-tailed test* because either group could be equally expected to have the larger mean value. The calculation of the *t*-test requires no new algebraic details from the data; the *t*-test result is simply calculated from the means and standard deviations in the two groups as follows:

$$t = (\bar{x}_1 - \bar{x}_2) \bigg/ \left\{ \frac{\left[(n_1 - 1) \times SD_1^2 + (n_2 - 1) \times SD_2^2 \right] \times \left(\frac{1}{n_1} \times \frac{1}{n_2} \right)}{n_1 + n_2 - 2} \right\}^{1/2}$$

The calculated t is then compared with tabulated values of the critical *t*-test (Table 1-10) with $n_1 + n_2 - 2$ degrees of freedom *(v)* at the $P = 0.05$ level:

If $t \le t_{n_1 + n_2 - 2, 0.05}$, then the study does not reject $H_0 := \bar{x}_1 = \bar{x}_2$, and no statistically significant difference is shown between the two groups.

If $t > t_{n_1 + n_2 - 2, 0.05}$, then the hypothesis $H_0 := \bar{x}_1 = \bar{x}_2$ is rejected, and the difference between the two groups is said to be statistically significant.

Example:
One group of $n_1 = 6$ patients is given a drug, and their thyroid T_4 levels (8.8, 8.7, 9.2, 8.6, 8.5, 9.0) have $\bar{x}_1 = 8.80$ and $SD_1 = 0.26$. A second group of $n_2 = 5$ patients is given a placebo, and their T_4 results (8.3, 8.5, 8.2, 8.1, 8.4) have $\bar{x}_2 = 8.3$ and $SD_2 = 0.16$. Is there a difference in T_4 levels between the two groups? Did the drug affect T_4 level?

$$t = (8.80 - 8.30) \bigg/ \left\{ \frac{\left[(6-1) \times (0.26)^2 + (5-1) \times (0.16)^2 \right] \times \left(\frac{1}{6} + \frac{1}{5} \right)}{(6 + 5 - 2)} \right\}^{1/2}$$

$$t = \frac{0.50}{\left\{ \frac{[0.4404] \times (0.3667)}{9} \right\}^{1/2}}$$

$$t = \frac{0.50}{(0.01794)^{1/2}} = 3.73$$

From Table 1-10 the critical t value at the 5% or 0.05 level with $n_1 + n_2 - 2 = 9$ degrees of freedom is $t_{9, 0.05} = 2.26$. Because calculated t is greater than critical t, it can be concluded that a statistically significant difference exists between the drug and placebo groups. The drug *did* make a statistically significant difference. In fact, the statistical tables show the critical t statistic at the 1% level $t_{9, 0.01} = 3.25$, thus demonstrating more than 99% confidence that a difference exists between the drug group and the placebo group because calculated t is greater than $t_{9, 0.01}$. It can also be said that less than

TABLE 1-10	*t*-Test Value at Probability *P*			
Degrees of Freedom (*v*)	Probability (*P*)			
	0.10	0.05*	0.01	0.001
4	2.13	2.78	4.60	8.61
5	2.01	2.57	4.03	6.87
6	1.94	2.45	3.71	5.96
7	1.89	2.36	3.50	5.41
8	1.86	2.31	3.36	5.04
9	1.83	2.26	3.25	4.78
10	1.81	2.23	3.17	4.59
15	1.75	2.13	2.95	4.07
20	1.72	2.09	2.84	3.85
30	1.70	2.04	2.75	3.65
60	1.67	2.00	2.66	3.46
∞	1.64	1.96	2.58	3.29

*Minimum value of *t*-test for significant difference is in this column. Larger *t* values imply a more significant difference.

a 1% likelihood exists that the difference between the drug and placebo groups is the result of a chance occurrence rather than because of the drug.

Most PC-type computer software packages (spreadsheets, statistics software) offer calculation capabilities of *t*-tests for which the user simply enters two columns of data values and selects an independent or paired *t*-test. The PC calculates the *t*-test result and the associated probability, sparing the user from any tedious calculations. In using such software it can be helpful to enter some test data, such as from the examples given here, to ensure that the software produces the same *t*-test and probability values as in the examples given here. Alternatively, the *t*-test can be performed as in the example here, after first using the pocket calculator to calculate the means and standard deviations of the two groups as discussed previously. To use Microsoft Excel for an independent *t*-test, for the T_4 data example, enter the first group's set of data values in column A (cells A1, A2, ..., A6), enter the number of data points for the first group in cell B1 (i.e., for the T_4 example data, enter the number 6 in cell B1), enter the data values for the second group in cells C1 through C5, and enter the number 5 in cell D1 (representing the number of data values in the second group). Then click on cell E1 and type in:

= TINV(E2,B1+D1-2)

Click on cell E2 and type in:

= TTEST(A1:A6,C1:C5,2,2)

In the Excel equation above for TTEST, the numbers 2, 2 are telling Excel to do an independent two-tailed *t*-test. Excel then places the *t*-statistic (3.73) in cell E1, and the probability *P* (0.00466) for this *t*-statistic in cell E2. If $P \leq 0.05$, then H_0 is rejected and a statistically significant difference becomes evident between the two groups. If $P > 0.05$, then H_0 cannot be rejected; a statistically significant difference between the two groups was

not found. In this example, the *P* value of 0.00466 is <0.01, so H_0 can be rejected even more stringently at the 1% level, while being more than 99% sure that the differences between the two groups are not caused by chance, just as concluded by the hand calculations for the *P* value being <0.01.

A special term, *standard error (SE)*, is used when referring to the variability in *mean* values. The SE governs the variability of repeated measurements of the *mean* value, whereas the standard deviation *(SD)* governs the variability of any one *individual* patient measurement. The result of an experiment to measure a mean value usually is expressed as $\bar{x} \pm SE$, rather than $\bar{x} \pm SD$, although this is not universal practice and confusion occurs if the specification of SE or SD is not made clear. The SE is given by:

$$SE = SD/\sqrt{n}$$

The data in the *t*-test example above would most commonly be specified as mean ± SE:

Drug group mean $= 8.80 \pm 0.11\,\mu g/dl$
Placebo group mean $= 8.30 \pm 0.07\,\mu g/dl$

Stating the data in this manner helps compare the means in the two groups. A graphic representation often shows the individual data values as dots on the graph, with a separate symbol for the mean. The mean symbol on the graph often includes ±SE bars, drawn as vertical lines of length equal to 1 SE above and below the mean value. The *t*-test is essentially a measure of how far apart the mean values are, measured in terms of their standard errors.

A paired *t*-test is used for testing differences between two mean values when the data are from the *same* patient. For example, a group of *n* patients could have their ventricular EF measured before (x_1) and after (x_2) taking some drug. The EFs before and after drug administration are correlated; a patient with a large EF before drug administration could also be expected to have a large EF after drug administration. What matters in paired data is the difference $d = x_1 - x_2$ between any two values. The difference between the first and second measurement is tabulated in each patient to calculate the mean difference $\bar{d}$:

$$\bar{d} = \frac{\Sigma(x_1 - x_2)}{n}$$

The standard deviation of the difference (SDD) is defined in the following manner:

$$SDD = \left\{ \frac{\Sigma(d - \bar{d})^2}{(n-1)} \right\}^{1/2}$$

Note that the algebraic sign, either + or −, of the difference *(d)* in each patient must be carefully used in calculating $\bar{d}$ and SDD. Then the paired *t*-test tests the null hypothesis that no mean difference exists

TABLE 1-11	Paired *t*-Test Data			
EF Old Method	EF New Method	Difference (d = Old – New)	$d - \bar{d}$	$(d - \bar{d})^2$
47	43	4	3.8	14.44
62	65	–3	–3.2	10.24
39	44	–5	–5.2	27.04
33	32	1	0.8	0.64
55	56	–1	–1.2	1.44
42	45	–3	–3.2	10.24
59	56	3	2.8	7.84
65	58	7	6.8	46.24
28	34	–6	38.44	–6.2
51	46	<5	4.8	23.04
			$\bar{d} = 0.2$	Sum = 179.60

$$SDD = \left[\Sigma(d - \bar{d})^2 / (n-1)^{1/2} \right]$$

$$= \left[179.6 / (10-1)^{1/2} \right]$$

$$= [19.96]^{1/2} = 4.47$$

$$t_9 = \bar{d} / (SDD / \sqrt{n})$$

$$= 0.2 / (4.47 / \sqrt{10}) = 0.14$$

between the first and second measurements, $H_0 : \bar{d} = 0$, by comparing the calculated *t*-statistic, $t = \bar{d} / (SDD / \sqrt{n})$, to the critical *t* value at the 0.05 level with $n - 1$ degrees of freedom ($= t_{n-1, 0.05}$). If $t > t_{n-1, 0.05}$, no difference is shown between the two measurements. If $t > t_{n-1, 0.05}$, a statistically significant difference exists between the first and second measurements. If the calculated *t* is just greater than the critical *t* with $n - 1$ degrees of freedom at the *P* confidence level (e.g., $P = 0.05, 0.01, 0.005, 0.001$, and so on), then it can be said that a difference is shown between the two measurements at the *P* confidence level.

Table 1-11 shows calculation of $\bar{d}$ and *SDD* for the old versus new EF data from Table 1-6. Note carefully how the algebraic sign (+ or –) of d and $d - \bar{d}$ is considered in Table 1-11. The null hypothesis being tested is H_0: old *EF* = new *EF*. The calculated $t = 0.14$ is much less than the critical *t* value ($t_{9, 0.05} = 2.26$) from Table 1-10, so the conclusion is that no statistically significant difference exists between the old and new *EF* values; H_0 cannot be rejected. This is another way of saying that the linear regression line in Figure 1-8 is not statistically different from the line of identity.

To use Microsoft Excel for a paired *t*-test, proceed to enter the data values exactly as described above for using Excel for an independent *t*-test. For the example data of Table 1-10, there would be 10 data values in column A and 10 data values in column C. Cells B1 and D1 would both be entered as 10, but now enter the Excel formulas as follows:

Click on cell E1 and enter:

$$= TINV(E2, B1-1)$$

Click on cell E2 and enter:

$$= TTEST(A1:A10, C1:C10, 2, 1)$$

The *2, 1* in the Excel TTEST equation here is telling Excel to do a two-tailed, paired *t*-test. Excel places the *t*-statistic (0.14) in cell E1 and the *P* value (0.89) in cell E2. Because *P* is >0.05, the null hypothesis cannot be rejected; no difference between the two EF methods was found, which is exactly as concluded by the hand calculation method previously.

Note that a *t*-test (for either independent or paired data) either fails to show a statistically significant difference ($t \geq t$-critical) or does show a statistically significant difference ($t < t$-critical). A *t*-test that fails to show a difference does *not* prove that the two mean values are equal[3]; it merely indicates that the data are inadequate to prove a difference exists. A semantic nuance that may be encountered is that independent *t*-tests consider the difference between the means, whereas a paired *t*-test considers the mean of the differences.

If more than two mean values are involved, the simple *t*-test is not appropriate. For example, one might wish to know whether a difference exists between the means of a test value in four independent groups of patients. The null hypothesis is $(H_0 : \bar{x}_1 = \bar{x}_2 = \bar{x}_3 = \bar{x}_4)$. This test requires a method called *analysis of variance (ANOVA)*— the most powerful way to find differences between the four groups. ANOVA also offers various methods for testing not just for whether all the means are the same but also for differences between pairs of the mean value. Alternatively to ANOVA, but less powerful for finding differences, the data can be tested for all pairs of differences with a *t*-test using the Bonferroni method, which requires lowering the significant *P* value from 0.05 to $0.05/n$, where *n* is the number of possible tests. For four groups of patients there are six possible *t*-tests: group 1 versus 2, 3, and 4; group 2 versus 3 and 4; group 3 versus 4. All six *t*-tests can be done and with a significant difference claimed only between pairs of mean values with a *t* value larger than the critical *t* value at the $0.05/6 = 0.0083$ *P* value.

Medical Decision Making

Medical decision making would not be necessary if medical tests always produced a result that correctly identified the patient as either ill or well. Unfortunately, because of the diversity of biological response, possible statistical noise in data, and other technological deficiencies, many medical tests can often produce identical results for ill and well patients. Therefore by a somewhat arbitrary method, a normal test result range is established for well people and then results outside this normal range are said to indicate illness. For example, suppose T_4 thyroid hormone is measured in a group of well people, and it is found that the mean ±2 *SD* normal range is from 4 to 12 µg/dl. Any subsequent patient test would be defined as normal or euthyroid for $4 \geq T_4 \geq 12$ and hyperthyroid for $T_4 \geq 12$. However, isn't using an absolute upper limit of 12 to define an abnormally high T_4 value a bit dogmatic? A patient with $T_4 = 11.9$ is labeled *well*, whereas a patient with $T_4 = 12.1$ is labeled *ill*, even though the difference in the two values may be within the limit of accuracy of the experimental technique. This is because most test values indicate a continuum of results, not a yes or no answer, as in pregnancy. What about a patient image test that produces an image that looks suspicious, that is, not quite clearly normal but not extremely abnormal? The image test can be called either *positive* (yes, it shows a defect) or *negative* (no defect is shown). What are the consequences of being a lax image reader (i.e., one who calls lots of positive studies) versus a strict image reader (i.e., one who requires very strong abnormal image characteristics before calling an image positive)? These are some of the questions that medical decision making can consider.

A test that finds a result for which the test was performed is called a *positive test*. A positive test for hyperthyroidism would be a $T_4 > 12$ µg/dl. A positive myocardial perfusion imaging test would be a patient image with a cold defect in the heart. A positive ^{99m}Tc bone scan would be a patient image with a hot spot in the bone. The test result might be low, high, cold, or hot, but it is positive for the condition for which it is being tested.

A test that does not show the tested-for result is called a *negative test*. A T_4 result in the euthyroid (normal) range would be a negative test for hyperthyroidism. A myocardial perfusion scan with no defects in the heart image would be a negative scan for coronary artery disease. Note carefully that the positive or negative value refers to the *test* result; positive or negative is not defined by the patient's clinical condition.

The patient's condition can be similarly categorized as either well or ill. This categorization must be obtained from some test *other than* the one being considered as the nuclear medicine test with positive or negative results. The patient condition is usually established as well or ill through some other medical test called the *gold standard test*. A patient, for example, could have either a positive or a negative myocardial perfusion imaging test, and the true state of the patient, as being well or ill, is usually established using some other clinical test such as coronary angiography. An imaging phantom study could have an image result that is called either *positive* or *negative*, and the true gold standard result is the known fact about whether the phantom contains an imaging abnormality or defect. Some presentations of this subject material might use the terms *normal* and *abnormal* in lieu of *well* and *ill*.

Given these definitions, all of the following material relates to placing each patient's test result into one of four categories:

1. *True positive (TP):* persons with a positive test result who are truly ill
2. *False positive (FP):* persons with a positive test result who are not ill
3. *True negative (TN):* persons with a negative test result who are truly well
4. *False negative (FN):* persons with a negative test result who are not well

A woman with a positive pregnancy test who is actually pregnant is called a *TP result*. If the pregnancy test result was negative but the woman is actually pregnant, then the result is an *FN result*. More typically, in nuclear medicine a decision is made to call an image test positive if the image shows some agreed-on defect. Then patients are categorized as TP, FP, TN, or FN by combining their nuclear medicine image test result with that of some other gold standard clinical test. A patient with a negative myocardial perfusion imaging test (no abnormal defects on the image study) who is known to have coronary artery disease would be called an *FN result*. A phantom study that calls the image *positive* in an area of the phantom where a lesion definitely exists would be a TP result.

Now consider the following test results. A study of imaging tests in 1000 patients produced the following data:

	Test Result	
	(–)	**(+)**
Well	836 = TN	44 = FP
Ill	26 = FN	94 = TP

Several other parameters that define the usefulness of the test can be derived from these categorized data.

The **sensitivity,** or *true positive fraction (TPF)*, is the percentage or fraction of ill patients who have a positive test:

$$\text{Sensitivity} = \text{TPF} = \frac{\text{TP}}{(\text{TP} + \text{FN})}$$

For the above data,

$$\text{Sensitivity} = \frac{94}{(94 + 26)} = 78\%$$

meaning that the study found a positive test result in 78% of the ill people. Note the distinction between similarly appearing symbols, TP and TPF.

The **specificity,** or *true negative fraction (TNF)*, is the percentage or fraction of well patients who have a negative test:

$$\text{Specificity} = \text{TNF} = \left(\frac{\text{TN}}{\text{TN} + \text{FP}}\right)$$

For the above data,

$$\text{Specificity} = \frac{836}{(836 + 44)} = 95\%$$

meaning that the study found a negative test result in 95% of the well people. Again, note the distinction between similarly appearing symbols, TN and TNF. (The decision on whether to use the term *sensitivity* or *TPF* and *specificity* or *TNF* is purely arbitrary.) The above data show a sensitivity of 78%, which is less than the specificity of 95%, meaning that this test does a better job at correctly diagnosing well people than it does at correctly diagnosing ill people.

The ideal medical test would have sensitivity and specificity both equal 100%. Unfortunately, medical data usually appear as in Figure 1-11, with an overlap between the test results for the well and ill patient populations. Which is more important, high sensitivity (i.e., correctly finding ill people) or high specificity (i.e., correctly finding well people)? The answer to this question is complex and often depends on the medical, economic, and social consequences of the test. If the imaging test is intended to detect brain tumors that are known always to be fatal, but for which a simple medical cure with no side effects can be found even in well people, then a high sensitivity might be preferred. The consequences of misdiagnosing an ill person would be death, whereas the consequences of misdiagnosing a well person would be a harmless drug regimen. On the other hand, suppose the consequence of finding a positive result in an imaging scan was immediate total frontal lobotomy, which would prolong the patient's life by only a few months. Given the dire consequences of treatment, a high specificity would be preferred to avoid misdiagnosing well patients.

Another factor that affects the most desirable sensitivity and specificity of a test is the prevalence of disease. The *prevalence* is the fraction or percentage of ill persons in the study population:

$$\text{Prevalence} = \frac{(TP + FN)}{(TP + FN + TN + FP)}$$

The preceding test result data had a prevalence of:

$$\frac{(26 + 94)}{(26 + 94 + 839 + 44)} = 12\%$$

meaning that 12% of the study subjects were ill.

The prevalence is characteristic of the patient population; prevalence is not a characteristic of the test itself. Prevalence is shown graphically in Figure 1-11 by the area under the ill curve compared with the area under both the ill and well curves. The relative heights of the ill and well curves show the prevalence, which can vary from one hospital to another. If the prevalence is high, many sick people are present, and the optimum test may be one that gives priority to a high sensitivity at the expense of lowered specificity (i.e., a few FP errors are more easily afforded in the small number of well people). To the contrary, a screening test for some rare disease operates in a patient population with a low prevalence, where the optimum test may be one that gives priority to a high specificity at the expense of lowered sensitivity

to avoid a large number of FP results in the preponderance of well people.

A parameter that specifies the total number of correct answers, regardless of being ill or well, is the *accuracy* of the test.

$$\begin{aligned} \text{Accuracy} &= \frac{(\text{Total number correct})}{(\text{Total number of persons})} \\ &= \frac{(TN + TP)}{(TN + TP + FP + FN)} \end{aligned}$$

The test result data show an accuracy of:

$$\frac{(836 + 94)}{(836 + 94 + 44 + 26)} = 93\%$$

meaning that the test correctly diagnosed 93% of all patients as ill or well. One problem is that the accuracy of a test depends strongly on the prevalence of disease for the same sensitivity and specificity of a test. This means that the accuracy between two hospitals can be very different for the same test because the prevalence at the two hospitals can be very different. Accuracy can be written specifically in terms of sensitivity, specificity, and prevalence as:

$$\text{Accuracy} = (\text{Sensitivity} \times \text{Prevalence}) + \text{Specificity} \times (1 - \text{Prevalence})$$

where prevalence is expressed as a fraction and not a percent.

Using these parameters for defining the goodness of a test, consider the following situation. A patient has a positive test result on some nuclear medicine study. Hence this must be either a TP result in a truly ill person or an FP result in a truly well person. The referring physician simply wants to know the probability of disease, given the positive test result. The referring physician can be provided a wealth of parameters about the goodness of the *test*: sensitivity = 78%, specificity = 95%, prevalence = 12%, accuracy = 93%. However, these parameters do not answer the clinical question at hand: what is the chance that this patient, who had a positive test result, is truly ill? A parameter is needed that deals with the clinical usefulness of the test, not just goodness-of-the-test parameters such as sensitivity.

The *positive predictive value* or *predictive value of a positive test* P(D+ : T+) can be read as the conditional probability of having disease (D+), given a positive test result (T+). This is merely the fraction of persons with positive test results who are truly ill:

$$P(D+:T+) = \frac{TP}{(TP + FP)}$$

For the test result data,

$$P(D+:T+) = \frac{94}{(94 + 44)} = 68\%$$

meaning that the answer to the referring physician's question is that only a 68% chance exists that the patient with the positive test result is truly ill. Of course this means that a 32% chance exists that the patient with this positive nuclear medicine test result is not ill. These considerations are a reflection of a mathematical concept called Bayes' theorem, after Thomas Bayes (1702-1761), an English mathematician and theologian. It allows recalculation of the probability of illness based on the new information of a positive test result. Before the nuclear medicine test, the chance that the patient had disease was simply the prevalence (often referred to as the *pretest probability of disease*) of 12%. After a positive test, however, the probability of disease has jumped to a posttest probability of 68%.

Conversely, the *negative predictive value* or *predictive value of a negative test* $P(D- : T-)$ is the probability P of not having disease (D–), given a negative test result (T–), or the fraction of all persons with a negative test who are truly well:

$$P(D-:T-) = \frac{TN}{(TN+FN)}$$

For the test result data, $P(D- : T-) = 836/(836 + 26) = 97\%$, meaning that a patient with a negative nuclear medicine test result has a 97% chance of being truly well. Note Bayes' theorem at work here. Before the nuclear medicine test, the patient had a (1-prevalence), or 88% chance of being well (i.e., the pretest probability of wellness was 88%). After a negative nuclear medicine test, the posttest probability that the patient is truly well jumped to 97%.

The discussion so far has not touched on how the patient's true condition, well or ill, is determined from some gold standard test. Calculation of all the parameters (such as TN, FP, sensitivity, specificity, or accuracy) requires that it is known from some other test, who is truly ill or well. Hence when evaluating the goodness of test results such as sensitivity, it is always necessary to ask what was used for the gold standard to define illness. Two hospitals may have vastly different parameters for sensitivity and specificity, not because of any difference in the nuclear medicine test result, but rather because the two hospitals define illness in different terms. For example, an invasive procedure such as coronary angiography is often used as a gold standard to calculate the sensitivity and other parameters of nuclear medicine myocardial perfusion imaging, but there may be no commonly agreed-on definition of illness in the gold standard test. One hospital might say that the test must show coronary arteries narrowed by only 40% for a diagnosis of illness, but a second hospital might say that a patient is not ill until the gold standard coronary angiography test shows more than 70% narrowing of the coronary arteries. This difference in the gold standard combines with the characteristics of the nuclear medicine test to produce different sensitivities and other parameters at the two hospitals.

When calculating sensitivity, for example, it is necessary to carefully define the test criterion level that characterizes a positive test. One hospital may say a positive test for hyperthyroidism is any $T_4 > 10.5$ µg/dl, whereas another hospital may say $T_4 > 12.5$ µg/dl is a positive test result. Different sensitivity values result. In fact, when information from the diagnostic test is received, any criterion level can be chosen to define a positive test. A lax criterion level (e.g., calling a nuclear medicine study positive with just a hint of abnormality in the image) leads to high sensitivity and low specificity. If a high sensitivity is desired, all tests can be called *positive*, resulting in a sensitivity of 100%. Of course, there would then be no TN tests, so the specificity would be zero. If a high specificity is desired, all tests can be called *negative*, resulting in a specificity of 100% (but unfortunately, the sensitivity would be zero).

As the criterion level that defines a negative or positive test result is moved left or right in Figure 1-11, the sensitivity and specificity change accordingly. Sensitivity and specificity then are not parameters fixed as constants in nature by some inherent property of a test or by an image reader's skill level. Rather, sensitivity and specificity depend on the gold standard used to define illness *and* on the criterion level that defines a positive test. In Figure 1-11, if the criterion level is slid to the right so that it is stricter in calling a positive test result, the sensitivity decreases while specificity increases. Slide the criterion level to the left so that it becomes more lax in defining a positive test, and the sensitivity improves while specificity worsens. For further guidance when thinking about these matters, a *receiver operating characteristic (ROC) curve* can be plotted, which shows sensitivity and specificity as a function of the criterion level used to call a test positive.

An ROC curve is shown in Figure 1-12. The *y*-axis is the sensitivity, and the *x*-axis is the specificity. Note that the *x*-axis is inverted in the sense that it *decreases* left to right from 100% to 0% specificity. (An alternate labeling for the axes of an ROC curve will have true positive fraction [TPF] from 0 to 1 on the *y*-axis, and false positive fraction [FPF] from 0 to 1 on the *x*-axis.) The ideal point for a test result would be the upper left corner of the ROC curve in Figure 1-12, with sensitivity = 100% and specificity = 100%.

An ROC curve is a graphic representation of the effect of changing the criterion level, just as the criterion level was moved left or right in Figure 1-11. A wealth of information can be gleaned from an ROC curve concerning which sensitivity/specificity is the optimum operating point, that is, the optimum criterion level that should be used to call a test positive. No definitive answers may be available, but the ROC curve clearly shows the available options. The ROC curve is still dependent on prevalence and the gold standard test to define illness. Suppose that a planar imaging study is reported in the literature with specificity = 61% and sensitivity = 86%. Another study in the literature reports a tomographic study with specificity = 82% and

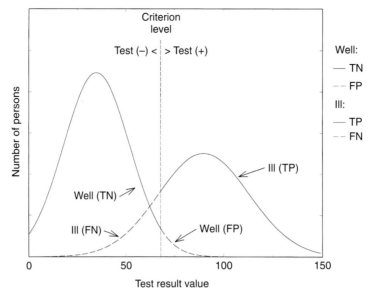

FIGURE 1-11 Distribution of test results for two groups: well (D−) and ill (D+). Test result is called *negative* (T−) or *positive* (T+) depending on whether it is below or above criterion level. Note that the well and ill populations overlap, creating well persons who are either TN or FP, and ill persons who are either TP or FN.

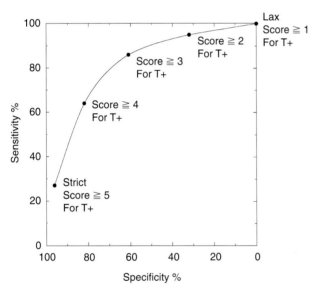

FIGURE 1-12 Receiver operating characteristic (ROC) curve showing sensitivity and specificity as a function of the minimum image score needed to call an image *positive*. Note that the x-axis for specificity reads left-to-right, from 100 to 0. A lax reader might call any image with a score ≥2 positive, with high sensitivity and low specificity. A strict reader would require a high score to call the image positive, resulting in low sensitivity and high specificity. The best overall test operates near the upper left corner of the ROC curve.

sensitivity = 64%. Which is the better test: planar or tomographic?

The question of which test is better cannot be answered unless *both* sensitivity and specificity are improved in one of the tests. In fact, these data could represent the same test results; the difference could simply be from a

changed criterion level for calling a test result positive. The hospital with the planar data could be calling a test result positive with a lower degree of image abnormality, leading to improved sensitivity but worsened specificity. It cannot be clearly determined which test is better without seeing the entire ROC curve for both the planar and tomographic data.

To form an ROC curve from any data, simply tabulate the TP, FN, TN, and FP results to calculate sensitivity and specificity for each criterion level that defines a positive test. For an in vitro T_4 blood test, just calculate sensitivity and specificity using different criterion levels for a positive test (e.g., calculate sensitivity and specificity for T+ defined as $T_4 \geq 0$, as $T_4 \geq 1$, as $T_4 \geq 2$, and so on). Then a plot of sensitivity versus specificity at the various criterion levels yields the ROC curve. Image data are somewhat different because a quantifiable, numeric result for imaging studies is not always available. Hence a rating scale is typically employed to score an image from 1 to 5 as follows:

Image Score	Meaning
1	Definitely normal image
2	Probably normal image
3	Possibly abnormal image
4	Probably abnormal image
5	Definitely abnormal image

Suppose an imaging study with 50 patients is conducted. From some other gold standard test, it is known which patients are truly ill or well: 28 are well, and 22 are ill. A reader scores each image as above. The sensitivity and specificity can be calculated from the TN, FP, FN, and TP results for each criterion level as follows:

Positive Test = Score ≥	TN	FP	FN	TP	Specificity (%)	Sensitivity (%)
1 (lax)	0	28	0	22	0	100
2	9	19	1	21	32	86
3	17	11	3	19	61	86
4	23	5	8	14	82	64
5 (strict)	27	1	16	6	96	27

Figure 1-12 is an ROC curve for these data. The planar and tomographic results above could represent just two different operating points on this single ROC curve. The planar test could have been called *abnormal* for an image score ≥3, whereas the tomographic data may have been called a *positive test* only for a stricter image score ≥4. Alternatively, a difference in ROC curves could be noted for the planar and tomographic results, but this could be ascertained only from seeing the entire ROC curve for both studies.

A medical test cannot be judged solely on sensitivity and specificity because these parameters are a strong function of the definition of the test criterion level used to call a test positive. The ideal operating point on the ROC curve could be at the upper left corner, with sensitivity equaling 100% and specificity equaling 100%. In general, the test that is closest to this ideal is the better test, so the best operating point (at what score to call a test positive) may be the one that results in an operating point closest to the upper left corner of the ROC curve. Alternatively, as discussed previously, considerations of prevalence of disease and consequences of diagnosis may suggest favoring sensitivity over specificity, or vice versa. It is also common to see two different ROC curves characterized by the area under the ROC curve, denoted by A_z. The highest A_z value is used to determine which test is best, because a higher A_z value means that the ROC curve is closer to the ideal operating point in the upper left corner of the ROC curve.

SUMMARY

- Scientific notation allows very large and very small numbers to be more conveniently represented.
- Learning to perform sequential calculations with a pocket calculator can save significant time in performing calculations in the clinic or laboratory.
- Many applications in nuclear medicine technology use ratio relationships.
- Dilution problems are examples of the application of ratio relationships: $C_1V_1 = C_2V_2$.
- The inverse square law proportionality:

$$1 \propto \frac{k}{d^2}$$

results in the intensity of radiation exposure I decreasing to one fourth when the distance is doubled.

- Units of radioactivity are the becquerel (Bq = 1 dps) or the curie (3.7×10^{10} dps).
- Conversion between mCi and MBq is accomplished by multiplying by 37 MBq/mCi.
- Exponents are described in the general form $base^{exponent} = number$.
- The general form of the radioactive decay equation is $A = A_0 e^{-\lambda t}$, or it may be expressed as $A = A_0 e^{-0.693 \times (t/t_{1/2})}$
- The decay constant λ and $t_{1/2}$ are inversely proportional to each other:

$$\lambda = \frac{0.693}{t_{1/2}}$$

- Decay factors (DF) are calculated from the exponential portion of the general decay equation $DF = e^{-0.693 \times (t/t_{1/2})}$ and are used to compute tables of DF values.
- The effective half-life t_E is calculated from the biological half-life t_B and the physical half-life t_P by the equation

$$\frac{1}{t_E} = \frac{1}{t_P} + \frac{1}{t_B}$$

- The intensity I of a radiation beam of high-energy photons is attenuated by the relationship $I = I_0 e^{-\mu x}$.
- A half-value layer (HVL) is the thickness of a particular material to absorb one half of the intensity of a beam of radiation. Each additional half-value layer reduces the beam again by one half.
- Standard deviation is a measure of the precision of data and is given by the symbol σ, defined as $\sigma = \left[\Sigma (x - \bar{x})^2 / (n-1) \right]^{1/2}$.
- The randomness of radioactive decay follows Poisson statistics, and the standard deviation is calculated by

$$\sigma_C = \sqrt{C}$$

- The *coefficient of variation (CV)* is defined as

$$CV = \left(\frac{\sigma}{\bar{x}} \right) \times 100$$

- The standard deviation for counting applications in the presence of background radiation is calculated by

$$\sigma_N = \sqrt{(C+B)}$$

- The chi-square test evaluates the reliability of consistent operation of counting equipment by evaluating variability in measurements.

- Sensitivity is the true positive fraction, the fraction or percentage of ill patients who have a positive test.
- Specificity is the true negative fraction, the fraction or percentage of well people who have a negative test.
- Accuracy is the fraction or percentage of patients being correctly diagnosed as ill or well.

REVIEW QUESTIONS

1. The radiation intensity from a point source of ^{99m}Tc is 9 mR/hr at 3 m from the source. If the distance is changed to 9 m, what is the new radiation intensity?
   a. 0.5 mR/hr
   b. 1.0 mR/hr
   c. 2.0 mR/hr
   d. 3.0 mR/hr

2. A technologist is sitting near a bone mineral densitometer, which is a point source of x-rays. If the x-ray beam intensity at 1 m from the x-ray beam is 0.20 mR/hr, what distance from the x-ray beam should the technologist move to decrease total weekly exposure to the occupational limit of 2 mR for a 40-hour workweek?
   a. 0.5 m
   b. 1.5 m
   c. 2.0 m
   d. 2.5 m

3. 10 mCi is equal to how many becquerels?
   a. 370 Bq
   b. 370 kBq
   c. 370 MBq
   d. 370 GBq

4. 20 mCi is equal to how many becquerels?
   a. 0.74 GBq
   b. 0.37 GBq
   c. 0.54 GBq
   d. 0.20 GBq

5. The dose equivalent for occupational, whole-body exposure is commonly limited to 50 mSv. How many rem is this?
   a. 5000 rem
   b. 500 rem
   c. 50 rem
   d. 5 rem

6. A source of ^{131}I ($t_{1/2}$ = 8.05 days) is delivered to the nuclear medicine department calibrated for 100 mCi at 8 AM on Monday. If this radioactivity is injected into a patient at noon on the following Tuesday, what radioactivity will the patient receive?
   a. 80 mCi
   b. 85 mCi
   c. 90 mCi
   d. 95 mCi

7. A patient was injected with ^{131}I on Monday at 10 AM. On Tuesday at 10 AM the thyroid probe was placed over the thyroid and 100,000 ct were produced. On Thursday at 10 AM the probe showed 25,000 ct. What is the effective half-life in this patient's thyroid?
   a. 12 hours
   b. 24 hours
   c. 48 hours
   d. 72 hours

8. A ^{99}Mo/^{99m}Tc generator is eluted Monday at 7 AM, producing 1.8 Ci of ^{99m}Tc in the eluate vial, in 20 ml saline. What volume of eluate should be withdrawn from the eluate vial into a syringe in order to inject a patient with 20 mCi of ^{99m}Tc at 3 PM (given the $t_{1/2}$ of ^{9m}Tc is 6.02 hours)?
   a. 0.56 ml
   b. 0.66 ml
   c. 0.76 ml
   d. 0.86 ml

9. If the HVL for some radionuclide in lead is 0.30 mm, what thickness of lead shielding is necessary to reduce the radiation exposure from 8 mR/hr to 1 mR/hr?
   a. 0.30 mm
   b. 0.45 mm
   c. 0.60 mm
   d. 0.90 mm

10. The linear attenuation coefficient in lead for ^{99m}Tc gamma rays (140 keV) is 23 cm^{-1}. What percentage of these gamma rays will be absorbed by a lead apron that contains 0.60 mm of lead?
    a. 75%
    b. 50%
    c. 25%
    d. 12.5%

11. A new gamma camera/computer system that uses a new method of calculating cardiac ejection fraction (EF) is installed in a nuclear medicine department. The department decides to calculate EF for the next 25 patients on both the old gamma camera and the new gamma camera before discontinuing the use of the old camera. In the future, if it is desired to convert the new EF value to that which would have been obtained on the old gamma camera (e.g., to assess if the patient's EF had changed), the mathematical analysis to be used is called
    a. Independent *t*-test
    b. Linear regression
    c. Standard error
    d. Chi-square

12. What is the standard deviation of 40,000 ct?
    a. 4000 ct
    b. 2000 ct
    c. 400 ct
    d. 200 ct

13. What is the coefficient of variation of 40,000 ct?
   a. 2%
   b. 1%
   c. 0.5%
   d. 0.25%

14. How many counts should be acquired into each pixel of a nuclear medicine flood image if we wish to be 95% confident that the true count in each pixel is within 1% of the measured counts in each pixel?
   a. 100,000 ct
   b. 40,000 ct
   c. 10,000 ct
   d. 4000 ct

15. A patient's thyroid is counted with the thyroid probe and produces 8000 ct. Then the patient is removed and the background is found to be 2000 ct. The (net counts) ± (standard deviation in the net counts) in this patient is
   a. 10,000 ± 100 ct
   b. 10,000 ± 77 ct
   c. 6000 ± 77 ct
   d. 6000 ± 100 ct

16. The gamma camera seems to be producing erratic results. A ^{57}Co flood source is counted 10 times, producing the following count values (1000, 975, 1032, 1096, 982, 997, 1012, 1090, 994, 977). What is the χ^2 value for these counts?
   a. 19.3
   b. 18.3
   c. 17.3
   d. 16.3

17. Which expression describes the operation of the gamma camera in question 16?
   a. Operating properly
   b. Showing too much variation
   c. Showing too little variation
   d. Not enough information to answer the question

18. One group of 20 patients is given a drug that is thought to have an effect on kidney function, and another group of 20 patients is given a placebo (i.e., sugar pill, which is known not to have an effect on kidney function). The nuclear medicine gamma camera is used to calculate the glomerular filtration rate (GFR) in these two groups of patients. What would be the proper statistical test to use to test the hypothesis that no difference in GFR exists between these two groups of patients?
   a. Chi-square test
   b. Paired *t*-test
   c. Independent *t*-test
   d. Linear regression analysis

19. A nuclear medicine test produces a positive test result in only 80 of the 100 patients known to be ill. Similarly, the test produces a negative test result in only 190 of the 200 patients known to be not ill. Which is correct?
   a. Sensitivity = 80%, specificity = 95%, accuracy = 90%, prevalence = 33%
   b. Sensitivity = 90%, specificity = 95%, accuracy = 90%, prevalence = 33%
   c. Sensitivity = 90%, specificity = 80%, accuracy = 90%, prevalence = 33%
   d. Sensitivity = 90%, specificity = 80%, accuracy = 70%, prevalence = 33%

20. One radiologist is known to be a lax reader compared with another radiologist who is known to be a strict reader. How would one expect their sensitivity and specificity to compare?
   a. The lax reader would have lower sensitivity and higher specificity.
   b. The lax reader would have higher sensitivity and lower specificity.
   c. The readers would be expected to have the same sensitivity and specificity.
   d. There is not enough information to answer the question.

21. A ^{99}Mo/^{99m}Tc generator is calibrated for 1.00 Ci of ^{99}Mo at 7 AM Monday. The generator is eluted daily Monday through Friday at 8 AM, but the workload is especially heavy on Friday so the generator is eluted again at 3 PM to obtain more ^{99m}Tc. Assuming 100% elution efficiency, how many mCi of ^{99m}Tc will be eluted at 3 PM Friday?
   a. 930 mCi
   b. 710 mCi
   c. 160 mCi
   d. 80 mCi

22. A radioactive source of ^{137}Cs ($t_{1/2}$ = 30 years) was calibrated on 10/23/2000 to contain 10 μCi. This is used as a daily accuracy check source in the dose calibrator. Presuming the dose calibrator is working properly, what activity should the dose calibrator show on 4/23/2006?
   a. 9.6 μCi
   b. 8.8 μCi
   c. 5.4 μCi
   d. 2.2 μCi

23. A source of ^{18}F ($t_{1/2}$ approximately 2 hours) is noted to contain 3 mCi at noon. What was the radioactivity at 8 AM that same day?
   a. 24 mCi
   b. 18 mCi
   c. 12 mCi
   d. 6 mCi

24. The biological half-life of ^{131}I in some particular patient is 30 days. The physical half-life is 193 hours. If the patient's thyroid is counted with the thyroid probe detector, what effective half-life will be observed?
    a. 26 days
    b. 6.3 days
    c. 5.1 days
    d. 1.2 days

25. A radioactive source decays from 20 mCi to 2.5 mCi in 18 hours. What is the physical half-life?
    a. 8 hours
    b. 7 hours
    c. 6 hours
    d. 5 hours

26. A sample shows a count rate of 36,000 cpm during a 3-minute counting period. Express this as the count rate ± standard deviation.
    a. 36,000 ± 220 cpm
    b. 36,000 ± 110 cpm
    c. 12,000 ± 55 cpm
    d. 12,000 ± 28 cpm

27. A long-lived radioactive source is counted for 1 minute and yields 10,000 ct. If this source is counted immediately again, there is a 95% probability that the result will be in the range:
    a. 9950 to 10,050 ct
    b. 9900 to 10,100 ct
    c. 9800 to 10,200 ct
    d. 9700 to 10,300 ct

28. A 5-ml sample of a standard diluted 1:10,000 produces 27,200 ct in the well counter. A 5-ml sample of patient plasma, counted for the same time as the diluted standard sample, produces 99,100 ct. What is the plasma volume?
    a. 10.8 L
    b. 2.74 L
    c. 1.73 L
    d. 0.91 L

29. Readers are encouraged to use Microsoft Excel to solve this problem. What is the mean of the following five numbers: 6.40, 7.20, 3.50, 9.20, 5.10?
    a. 9.01
    b. 6.28
    c. 5.97
    d. 4.83

30. Readers are encouraged to use Microsoft Excel to solve this problem. What is the standard deviation of the data in question 29?
    a. 4.02
    b. 3.26
    c. 2.15
    d. 1.92

31. Readers are encouraged to use Microsoft Excel to solve this problem. What is the coefficient of variation CV of the data in question 29?
    a. 34%
    b. 31%
    c. 28%
    d. 12%

32. Readers are encouraged to use Microsoft Excel to solve this problem. In a nuclear medicine technology training program, the students wonder if their final exam grade in their training program is related to their subsequent board score on the NMTCB exam. The five students attained the following pairs of scores (exam score, board score) = (72, 60), (84, 74), (88, 71), (68, 60), (91, 79). What is the linear correlation coefficient r between exam score and board score?
    a. 0.99
    b. 0.95
    c. 0.86
    d. 0.75

33. Using Table 1-7, what is the P value for the linear correlation coefficient r in question 31?
    a. $P = 0.001$
    b. $0.01 < P < 0.05$
    c. $0.05 < P < 0.1$
    d. $P > 0.10$

34. Using Table 1-7, does a linear correlation coefficient $r = 0.95$ for $n = 5$ data points indicate a statistically significant linear relationship between the x and y variables?
    a. Yes
    b. No
    c. Not enough information to answer the question

35. Readers are encouraged to use Microsoft Excel to solve this problem. What is the slope and intercept in the regression equation for problem 31?
    (board score) = intercept + (slope) × (exam score)
    a. intercept = 7.15, slope = 0.502
    b. intercept = 6.15, slope = 0.602
    c. intercept = 5.15, slope = 0.702
    d. intercept = 4.15, slope = 0.802

36. Using the regression equation in question 31, if the training program exam score was 84, what does the regression equation predict for the board score?
    a. 92
    b. 82
    c. 72
    d. 62

37. A thyroid uptake dose of 10 μCi is equal to how much radioactivity in SI units?
    a. 37 kBq
    b. 370 kBq
    c. 3.7 MBq
    d. 37 MBq

38. What is the proper number of significant figures for the quotient $(6.1 \times 10^{-2})/(0.1232)$?
  a. 0.49513
  b. 0.4951
  c. 0.495
  d. 0.50

39. What is the proper number of decimal places for the sum $(0.3) + (3.5264)$?
  a. 3.8264
  b. 3.826
  c. 3.83
  d. 3.8

40. It is known that 75% of a radionuclide decays away in 12 hours. If we start with 10 mCi, how much will be left after 6 hours?
  a. 7.5 mCi
  b. 5 mCi
  c. 2.5 mCi
  d. 1.25 mCi

41. A patient is prescribed to be treated with 150 mCi of ^{131}I ($t_{1/2} = 8.05$ days) on Monday at 8 AM. The clinic receives the unit dose in capsule form calibrated for Monday 8 AM. However the patient does not actually arrive for treatment until the following day, Tuesday at 4 PM. How much activity is available in the capsule on Tuesday at 4 PM? *Please use Table 1-4 to obtain your answer.*
  a. Between 141-150 mCi
  b. Between 131-140 mCi
  c. Between 121-130 mCi
  d. Between 57-62 mCi

42. A 52-pound (lb) pediatric patient is scheduled for a ^{99m}Tc renal study. The adult prescribed dose is 6 mCi, but for a 52-lb child, this hospital uses a dose factor of 35% for this size child. The dose factor is the percentage that the child dose should be, of the full adult prescribed dose. What dose amount should be administered to the child?
  a. 4.8 mCi
  b. 3.8 mCi
  c. 2.1 mCi
  d. 1.2 mCi

43. A radiologist orders an ^{111}In cerebrospinal fluid shunt study. The dose vial comes with a label indicating: activity 1.5 mCi, volume 1 ml. The ordering physician specifies an injection of 0.5 mCi in a 0.5-ml volume. The technologist will first need to withdraw 0.33 ml (which will contain the prescribed 0.5 mCi) from the dose vial, and then dilute it with saline to have the prescribed volume of 0.5 ml. What will be the final concentration in the dose to be injected?
  a. 3 mCi/ml
  b. 1.5 mCi/ml
  c. 1 mCi/ml
  d. 0.5 mCi/ml

44. A patient was treated with 150 mCi of ^{131}I. Measurements were made with a Geiger counter shortly after injection of the dose at a 1-m distance from the patient and showed an initial exposure rate of 19 mR/hr. State law allows a patient to be discharged when the radioactivity in the patient has decreased to less than 30 mCi. Over subsequent days, measurements are made with the Geiger counter of the radiation exposure at 1 m from the patient, showing decreasing mR/hr readings. The patient can be released from the hospital when the exposure rate from the patient has decreased to less than what mR/hr reading on the Geiger counter?
  a. 0.5 mR/hr
  b. 1.9 mR/hr
  c. 3.8 mR/hr
  d. 30 mR/hr

45. Dose calibrator accuracy is assessed over the years by measuring the activity of a long-lived radionuclide, such as a ^{57}Co source ($t_{1/2} = 270$ days). The ^{57}Co source was calibrated August 8, 2007, at 1.228 mCi. What must be the mCi reading of the dose calibrator on March 8, 2009, in order to indicate ±5% dose calibrator accuracy?
  a. Between 0.231-0.264 mCi
  b. Between 0.265-0.292 mCi
  c. Between 0.315-0.346 mCi
  d. Between 0.357-0.389 mCi

46. A ^{99m}Tc source is calibrated for 20 mCi at 8 AM. How much activity is left at 10:30 AM? *Please use Table 1-3 to select your answer.*
  a. 17.8 mCi
  b. 16.0 mCi
  c. 15.0 mCi
  d. 14.2 mCi

47. To insure an adequate first pass blood flow study with ^{99m}Tc, the injected bolus should have a small volume, necessitating the need for a concentration of >20 mCi/ml. What is the concentration available for patient injection if the ^{99m}Tc source is a vial containing 660 mCi in 25 ml of generator eluate?
  a. 26.4 mCi/ml
  b. 63.3 mCi/ml
  c. 20.9 mCi/ml
  d. 1.8 mCi/ml

48. The radiation dose to particular patient from an abdominal CT scan is 35 mGy as shown on the CT control console as the CT Dose Index (CTDI). The patient asks you how much is the radiation dose CTDI expressed in units of rads?
  a. 35 rad
  b. 350 rad
  c. 0.35 rad
  d. 3.5 rad

49. The integral uniformity for a gamma camera flood image is defined as ([hottest pixel counts] − [coldest pixel counts])/([hottest pixel counts] + [coldest pixel counts]) expressed as a percentage. A 40-Mct flood image is acquired and a region of interest (ROI) is drawn on the image showing that the hottest pixel contains 10,124 ct and the coldest pixel contains 9885 ct. What is the integral uniformity?
a. 0.54%
b. 1.19%
c. 2.38%
d. 4.76%

50. The radiation absorbed dose to the kidneys from a particular nuclear medicine scan is listed in the product literature from the radiopharmaceutical company as 1.7×10^{-3} mGy/MBq. What is the radiation absorbed dose expressed in units of rad/mCi?
a. 6.3×10^{-3} rad/mCi
b. 5.2×10^{-2} rad/mCi
c. 4.1×10^{-4} rad/mCi
d. 3.0×10^{-1} rad/mCi

REFERENCES

1. Bevington PR: *Data reduction and error analysis for the physical sciences*, ed 3, New York, 2003, McGraw-Hill.
2. Bushberg JT, Seibert JA, Leidholdt EM Jr, et al: *The essential physics of medical imaging*, ed 2, Philadelphia, 2002, Lippincott Williams & Wilkins.
3. Colton T: *Statistics in medicine*, Philadelphia, 1975, Lippincott Williams & Wilkins.

Physics of Nuclear Medicine

Paul E. Christian

OUTLINE

OBJECTIVES

After completing this chapter, the reader will be able to:
- Describe the properties of electromagnetic radiation.
- Describe the structure of the atom and its components and their properties.
- Explain the structure of the chart of the nuclides and define the line of stability.
- State the relationship of mass and energy in Einstein's equation.
- Write the correct form of radionuclide notation.
- List the nuclear families and state their characteristics.
- Name and describe the primary forms of radioactive decay.
- Diagram the schematics of the various radioactive decay processes.
- Define decay constant.
- Use the general form of the radioactive decay equation to calculate precalibration and postcalibration quantities of radioactivity.
- List the radioactive units and define curie and becquerel.
- Write the equations for average half-life and effective half-life and calculate effective and biological half-lives.
- Describe the interactions of charged particles with matter.
- Discuss the processes of excitation and ionization.
- Explain annihilation and the resultant products.
- Describe the photoelectric effect and explain the process.
- Describe Compton scattering and explain the resultant products of this process.
- Describe pair production and explain the resultant products of this process.
- Discuss the production of characteristic x-rays.
- Describe the process of the production of Auger electrons.
- Write the general form of the attenuation equation for gamma photons.
- Calculate the reduction of gamma radiation using the general attenuation equation.
- State the relationship between the linear attenuation coefficient and the half-value layer.

KEY TERMS

alpha decay
annihilation
Bateman equations
becquerel
beta decay

chart of the nuclides
Compton scattering
curie
decay constant
decay factor

effective half-life
electromagnetic radiation
electron capture
gamma decay
half-life

half-value layer (HVL)
isobar
isomer
isotone

isotope
linear attenuation coefficient
nuclear stability
pair production

photoelectric effect
positron decay
radioactive decay
transmutation

Physics is the study both of matter and energy and of the properties, forces, and interactions that influence the behavior of matter. Nuclear medicine applies the principles of physics to all aspects of radioactive decay, to the interaction between radiation and matter, and to the detection and measurement of quantities of radiation and radiation protection. Radiation is the motion of energy through space. A basic understanding of these principles is critical to the use of radioactive materials and radiation-detecting instrumentation.

ELECTROMAGNETIC RADIATION

Heat waves, radio waves, infrared light, visible light, ultraviolet light, and x-rays and gamma rays are all forms of **electromagnetic radiation** (Figure 2-1). They differ only in frequency and wavelength. Longer-wavelength, lower-frequency waves (heat and radio) have less energy than the shorter-wavelength, higher-frequency waves (visible light, x-rays, and gamma rays). The wave properties of light were first shown by

Christian Huygens in 1678 in his experiments with the separation of light into the color spectrum. The particulate characteristics of light were not appreciated until the experiments and research of Einstein, Planck, and Milliken in the early 1900s. Although electromagnetic energy has no mass, at very high frequencies it behaves more as a particle does, whereas at lower frequencies it behaves more as a wave does. The best way to think of electromagnetic radiation is as a wave packet called a *photon*. Photons are chargeless bundles of energy that travel in a vacuum at the velocity of light, c, which is 3×10^{10} cm/sec or 186,000 miles/sec.

The wavelength of electromagnetic radiation is symbolized by the Greek letter *lambda*, λ. Note that the Greek lambda used to refer to electromagnetic radiation should not be mistaken for the radioactive decay constant, which is discussed later in this chapter. Electromagnetic waves, as their name indicates, consist of fluctuating fields of electric and magnetic energy. Figure 2-2 shows the pattern of the wave cycle. Since light travels at a constant velocity, the oscillating

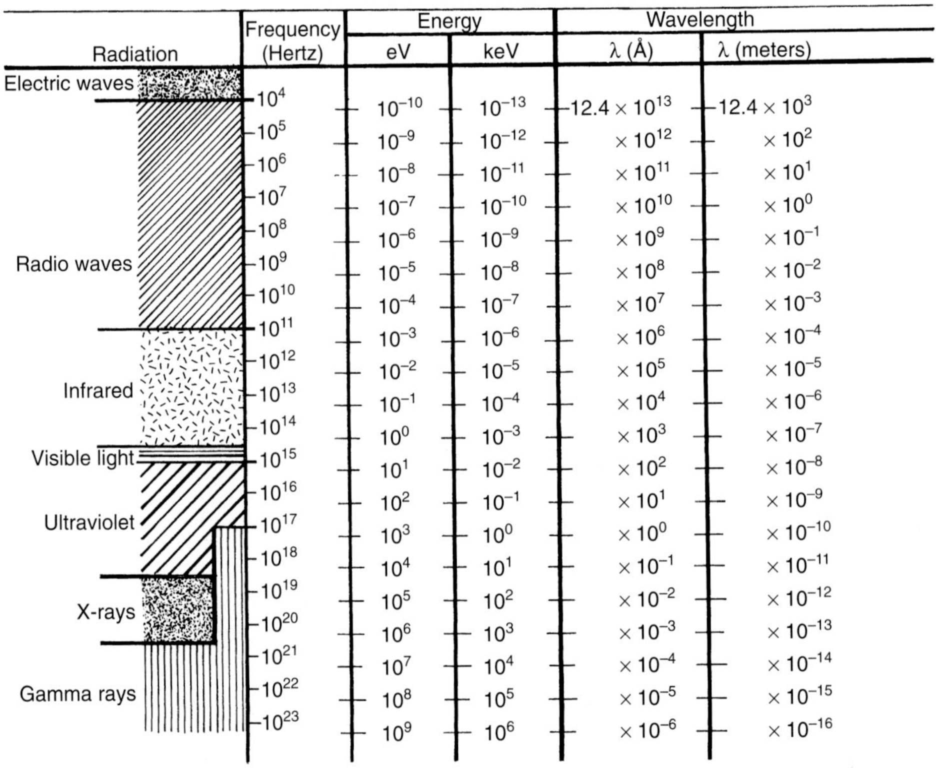

Radiation	Frequency (Hertz)	Energy		Wavelength	
		eV	keV	λ (Å)	λ (meters)
Electric waves	10^4	10^{-10}	10^{-13}	12.4×10^{13}	12.4×10^3
	10^5	10^{-9}	10^{-12}	$\times 10^{12}$	$\times 10^2$
	10^6	10^{-8}	10^{-11}	$\times 10^{11}$	$\times 10^1$
	10^7	10^{-7}	10^{-10}	$\times 10^{10}$	$\times 10^0$
	10^8	10^{-6}	10^{-9}	$\times 10^9$	$\times 10^{-1}$
Radio waves	10^9	10^{-5}	10^{-8}	$\times 10^8$	$\times 10^{-2}$
	10^{10}	10^{-4}	10^{-7}	$\times 10^7$	$\times 10^{-3}$
	10^{11}	10^{-3}	10^{-6}	$\times 10^6$	$\times 10^{-4}$
	10^{12}	10^{-2}	10^{-5}	$\times 10^5$	$\times 10^{-5}$
Infrared	10^{13}	10^{-1}	10^{-4}	$\times 10^4$	$\times 10^{-6}$
	10^{14}	10^0	10^{-3}	$\times 10^3$	$\times 10^{-7}$
Visible light	10^{15}	10^1	10^{-2}	$\times 10^2$	$\times 10^{-8}$
	10^{16}	10^2	10^{-1}	$\times 10^1$	$\times 10^{-9}$
Ultraviolet	10^{17}	10^3	10^0	$\times 10^0$	$\times 10^{-10}$
	10^{18}	10^4	10^1	$\times 10^{-1}$	$\times 10^{-11}$
	10^{19}	10^5	10^2	$\times 10^{-2}$	$\times 10^{-12}$
X-rays	10^{20}	10^6	10^3	$\times 10^{-3}$	$\times 10^{-13}$
	10^{21}	10^7	10^4	$\times 10^{-4}$	$\times 10^{-14}$
Gamma rays	10^{22}	10^8	10^5	$\times 10^{-5}$	$\times 10^{-15}$
	10^{23}	10^9	10^6	$\times 10^{-6}$	$\times 10^{-16}$

FIGURE 2-1 Electromagnetic spectrum.

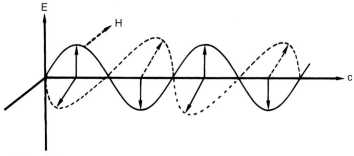

FIGURE 2-2 Component energy fields of electromagnetic wave. C, x axis = velocity; E, y axis = electric field *(solid line)*; H, z axis = magnetic field *(dotted line)*.

electromagnetic field wavelength and frequency are related by the equation:

$$c = \lambda v$$

where λ is the wavelength, v is the frequency, and c is the velocity of light. The time for one wave period, or cycle, is measured in cycles per second, called *hertz*. Planck described the relationship of the electromagnetic wave frequency to the energy as:

$$E = hv$$

where v represents the frequency of the electromagnetic wave and h is Planck's constant, 6.625×10^{-27} erg-sec/cycles. This equation can be manipulated to relate to energy and wavelength as:

$$E = \frac{12.4}{\lambda}$$

This equation expresses the energy in electron volts (eV) to the wavelength measured in angstroms (10^{-8} cm). The relationship indicates that photons with very short wavelengths have high energy and vice versa.

ATOMS AND MOLECULES

Matter is anything that occupies space and has mass. Ancient Greek philosophers theorized that all matter was composed of small indivisible pieces, which they called *atoms*. An atom is the smallest quantity of an element (e.g., hydrogen, carbon, oxygen) that retains all the chemical properties of that element. Atoms cannot be broken into smaller particles without losing their chemical properties. They are classified by their characteristics of weight, number of subparticles, and chemical properties. Two or more atoms may combine to form a molecule. A molecule is the smallest particle of a chemical compound that retains all the chemical characteristics of that compound. Molecules can have as few as two or as many as hundreds of atoms; therefore tens of thousands of different chemical compounds can be created by changing the number of atoms or the configuration of atoms within the molecule.

The atom is made up of two basic parts, the nucleus and the orbital electrons. A simple representation of an

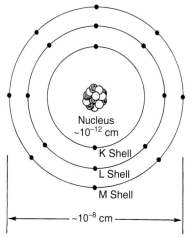

FIGURE 2-3 Bohr's atomic model with central nucleus surrounded by extranuclear region.

atom is a structure similar to a miniature solar system (Figure 2-3). This elementary model of an atom divides the atom into two portions: nuclear (in the center) and extranuclear (the surrounding area). Three principal types of subatomic particles compose an atom—protons, neutrons, and electrons. The nucleus is composed of two types of these particles—protons and neutrons; hence protons and neutrons are called *nucleons*. The nucleus is a cluster of these particles and gives the atom most of its mass.

The extranuclear region of the atom is the area outside the nucleus and is mostly empty space with electrons that orbit the nucleus like planets revolving around the sun. This region of the atom, specifically the outermost electrons, is responsible for all chemical interactions with other atoms and is the area in which most of the interactions of radiation and matter occur.

In 1960 the International Unions of Pure and Applied Physics and Chemistry set the standard substance physical scale to the carbon-12 (^{12}C) atom, whose mass is defined to be exactly 12.00000 atomic mass units (amu). All other atomic and particle weights are measured with reference to the ^{12}C atom.

Basic discussions of the composition of atoms are limited to the fundamental particles: electrons that orbit

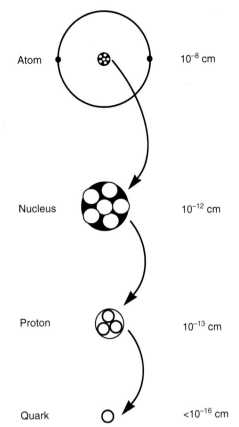

FIGURE 2-4 Size of the components within an atom.

the nucleus and the particles in the nucleus (protons and neutrons). Particle physics describes several families that hold many dozens of subatomic particles. For example, protons and neutrons are in the family called *hadrons;* electrons and neutrinos are in a family of "light"-mass particles called *leptons;* and photons are in a group called *bosons.*

In 1964 Murray Gell-Mann and George Zweig proposed that the hundreds of particles known at that time might be composed of combinations of simpler fundamental particles that they called *quarks* (Figure 2-4). Experiments since that time have shown that there are actually six quarks that compose subatomic particles.

Fortunately for the purposes of this book, a description of the composition of the atom and the processes of radioactive decay using the most common particles can be used.

Electrons

Electrons are the smallest of the subatomic particles and are found in the extranuclear region of the atom. Electrons are also called *negatrons* and are given the symbol e or e^-. They have one negative unit of charge (1.6×10^{-19} coulombs) and a small mass of 9.1×10^{-28} g, or 0.000549 amu, and travel at about one tenth the velocity of light. Since electrons carry a negative charge, they are deflected by electric or magnetic fields. Their mass allows

them to have kinetic energy that is proportional to the square of their velocity. Electrons are held in their orbits around the nucleus by binding energy, which in conjunction with their motion and centrifugal force keeps them from being attracted into the positively charged nucleus. An electrically neutral atom has an equal number of protons and electrons.

Protons

Protons are found within the nucleus of an atom and are symbolized by the letter p or p^+. They have one positive unit of charge, which is equal but opposite to the charge of the electron. The protons within the nucleus provide its positive charge. The proton has a mass of 1.67×10^{-24} g, or 1.00759 amu, which is 1835 times that of an electron. The total number of protons in an atom is the atomic number, symbolized by the letter Z, and is unique for each element: for example, one proton is hydrogen, two protons is helium, three protons is lithium.

Neutrons

A neutral particle within the nucleus of the atom had been theorized by Rutherford in 1920, but neutrons were not experimentally found until 1932 by Chadwick. Neutrons are slightly heavier than protons, have no electric charge, and have a mass of 1.00898 amu. For simplification, the mass of a neutron and a proton are considered to be the same—1 amu. Neutrons are symbolized by the letter n.

For this discussion a neutron can be considered a combination of a proton and an electron. Neutrons are unstable particles and break down into the simpler, more stable particles of a proton, an electron (beta-minus particle), and a neutrino. This instability of the neutron is the source of one type of radioactive decay. The decay process and the resultant particles are discussed later.

ATOMIC STRUCTURE

The model of the atom described by Niels Bohr in 1913 is one of the most easily understood representations. This miniature solar system has mostly empty space with the electrons in orbit around a small central nucleus. Three subatomic particles are used in this model. The electrons occupy specific orbits, or shells, around the centrally located nucleus. The electron shells are labeled K, L, M, N, O, P, and Q (see Figure 2-3), beginning with the innermost K shell. Specific amounts of energy hold each electron in its orbit. The innermost electrons are more tightly bound to the nucleus, and therefore more energy is required to remove them. Outer electrons are more loosely bound and only require smaller amounts of energy in order for them to be removed. Electrons can be removed from their orbits only by overcoming the *binding energy* for that shell. Binding energies are greatest for the innermost electrons, and the binding energy of specific electron shells is greater in heavier elements.

The electrons do not actually revolve around the nucleus in circular orbits in one plane; they move around the nucleus in a spherical pattern. Collectively, the electrons swarming about the nucleus to form an electron cloud. Individually the electrons change their distance from the nucleus and can even occasionally pass right through the nucleus.

Remember that the chemical properties of the atom are determined by the outermost electrons. The number of electrons that can occupy each orbit is limited. The formula $2n^2$ defines the number of electrons that can be contained in the major shells, where n is the shell number. For example, the K shell can contain only two electrons, the second shell can contain no more than eight, the third shell may contain 18, the fourth shell may contain 32, and so on. Each major shell is composed of several subshells.

The nucleus of an atom has an approximate diameter of 10^{-12} cm (see Figure 2-3) and is composed of a cluster of protons and neutrons. Most of the matter in the atom is located here; therefore the density of the nucleus is extremely high. Particles in the nucleus—protons and neutrons—are known as *nucleons*. The simplest atom, hydrogen, consists of one proton, no neutrons, and one orbital electron. The second element, helium, has a nucleus consisting of two protons, two neutrons, and two orbital electrons. More complex atoms have an increased number of protons and neutrons. In approximately the first 20 elements, the ratio of neutrons to protons is 1:1; however, elements with atomic numbers greater than 20 generally have more neutrons than protons in order to maintain **nuclear stability**. Very large atoms have a neutron-to-proton ratio of 1.6:1 (Figure 2-5).

As with electrons in the extranuclear orbit structure of the atom, the protons and neutrons in the nucleus are bound there with a specific amount of binding energy.

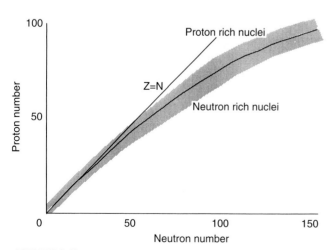

FIGURE 2-5 Neutron-proton ratio with line of nuclear stability.

Stability of the nucleus is determined by the total binding energy of nucleons in addition to the number and configuration of the proton-neutron arrangement. Protons and neutrons tend to pair up, creating a more stable nucleus, depending on the neutron-to-proton ratio. Nucleons move about within the nucleus and occupy certain energy states. Some nuclei hold additional energy in a nearly stable, or metastable, state. The nucleus can emit this extra energy in a manner called an *isomeric transition*, with the emission of electromagnetic radiation (gamma ray).

MASS-ENERGY RELATIONSHIP

In Einstein's equation $E = mc^2$, c represents the velocity of light measured in centimeters per second, m is mass measured in grams, and E is energy measured in ergs. According to this equation, matter can be converted into energy, and conversely, energy can create matter. This equation applies to a mass that is not moving and is therefore termed the *rest mass* of a particle of matter. When matter is converted to energy, the type of energy produced is of a form that is not imparted to or held by matter, such as heat or binding energy. Rather, it is pure energy, electromagnetic radiation.

The rest mass of an electron, 9.1×10^{-28} g, can be found by this equation to be equivalent to 0.511 MeV. Similarly, the rest mass of a proton can be found to be 931 MeV, and the rest mass of a neutron 939 MeV. This relationship is further defined in the discussions of radioactive decay and the interaction of radiation and matter.

Mass Defect

The relationship between mass and energy can be observed in the strong nuclear forces that exist in the nucleus. The sum of the masses of the nucleons in a ^{12}C atom is defined and measured as 12.00000 amu. However, the mass of a proton is 1.00759 amu; the mass of a neutron is 1.00898 amu; and the mass of an electron is 0.00054 amu. There are six protons, six neutrons, and six electrons in this atom, given the total mass of the individual particles as

$$6 \times 1.00759 = 6.04554$$
$$6 \times 1.00898 = 6.05388$$
$$\underline{6 \times 0.00054 = 0.00340}$$
$$12.10266 \text{ amu}$$

Since the carbon atom weighs 12.00000 amu, a difference of 0.10266 amu has been converted into binding energy of the particles in the nucleus. The difference in mass of the constituent particles and the total mass is called the *mass defect*. This amount of mass converts to 95.62779 MeV of nuclear binding energy. Particles can be removed from the atom only by expending a force greater than the binding energy.

Nuclear Stability

The number of protons and neutrons that form all possible configurations of the nucleus are graphed in Figure 2-5. Any configuration of protons and neutrons forming an atom is called a *nuclide*. Of the approximately 3100 nuclides, most are unstable and spontaneously release energy or subatomic particles in an attempt to reach a more stable state. This nuclear instability is the basis for the process called **radioactive decay.** Approximately 270 of the nuclides are in a stable form, comprising only 83 elements. The remainder of the approximately 3100 nuclides are radioactive and are referred to as *radionuclides.*

The cause of nuclear instability stems from the energy configuration of protons and neutrons in the nucleus. Although the structure of the nucleus might be thought of as being like a cluster of grapes, each nucleon has a certain energy state. For one specific radionuclide there is a specific release of particles and a specific amount of energy released by its unstable atoms in this decay process. For example, ^{131}I always decays by emitting beta-minus (β^-) particles and gamma rays of specific energies. From radioactive decay, each radionuclide has its own "fingerprint" of characteristic radiation(s).

In Figure 2-5 the approximately 270 stable nuclides follow along the center of the line of stability with radionuclide forms located on either side of this line. Radionuclides above the line of stability represent a region with a relative abundance of protons, termed *proton-rich* (or *neutron-poor*) *nuclei.* Radionuclides in this region achieve nuclear stability primarily by undergoing the decay processes of positron emission or **electron capture.** Radionuclides below the line of stability in the *neutron-rich* (or *proton-poor*) area undergo a radioactive decay process called **beta decay** in which a neutron becomes a proton followed by the release of a beta particle from the nucleus.

Some radionuclides are in a metastable form. These radionuclides carry a slight amount of excess nuclear energy, which can be emitted as electromagnetic radiation to allow the atom to reach a more stable form.

The plotting of nuclides by their number of protons (vertical axis) and neutron number (horizontal axis) is the basis for the **chart of the nuclides** (Figure 2-6). This chart contains all possible nuclides, both stable and unstable radioactive forms. The chart is useful in identifying daughter decay products from a particular radionuclide or series of decays. Each nuclide is represented in a small square containing information such as the

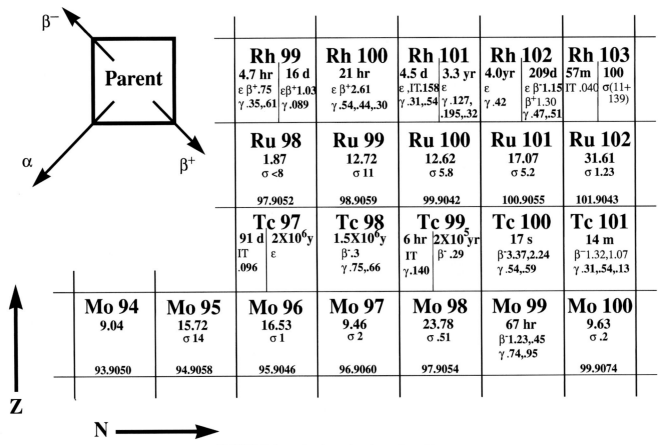

FIGURE 2-6 Section from the chart of nuclides.

half-life, decay mechanism, radiation type, and amount of energy being emitted.

NUCLEAR NOTATION AND NUCLEAR FAMILIES

There is a standard notation in the physical sciences for representing elements with a one- or two-letter chemical name symbol; it is taken primarily from the Greek names of the elements. The generalized symbol form commonly used in nuclear medicine appears as:

$$^{A}_{Z}X$$

where X is the chemical symbol, Z is the element's atomic number (number of protons), and A represents the atomic mass number of the atom (protons plus neutrons). Although the number of neutrons can be indicated as a trailing subscript number, it is usually not written because it can be calculated by subtracting Z from A. As an example, carbon with 6 protons and 8 neutrons would be written as C. Because an atom with 6 protons will always be a carbon atom, writing a 6 and C is a duplication of information; therefore by convention, it may be written as $^{14}_{6}C$ or simply as ^{14}C.

Although early scientists learned much about determining atomic weights and organizing the elements into the periodic chart, they did not immediately understand that there could be different atomic forms of the same element. The same element will always have a specific number of protons, as listed by the atomic number Z, and will have the same chemical properties; however, the number of neutrons can differ. The term *nuclide* refers to any configuration of the atom. The Greek terms *iso*, meaning *same,* and *topos*, meaning *place,* indicate that the atoms have the same position on the periodic table of elements. The term **isotope,** though sometimes erroneously used interchangeably with *nuclide,* actually defines a specific element with different forms of that element, each containing different numbers of neutrons. ^{97}Tc, ^{98}Tc, ^{99}Tc, ^{100}Tc, and ^{101}Tc are all isotopes of element 43 (see Figure 2-6) and follow a horizontal line on the chart of the nuclides. Since the periodic chart of the elements is far too small to contain all the different isotopes of each element, the chart of the nuclides is commonly used to list the 3100 isotopes of all the elements. It is relatively simple to identify the isotopes since the chart is laid out in a pattern following the line of stability listed by the number of protons and neutrons (see Figure 2-5). Isotopes for each element are found as a horizontal line, since the number of neutrons is plotted horizontally.

Additional families of nuclei are **isotones, isobars,** and **isomers.** Isotones are atoms of different elements that have the same number of neutrons but varying numbers of protons. The following are isotones: $^{98}_{42}Mo$, $^{99}_{43}Tc$, $^{100}_{44}Ru$, and, all having 56 neutrons and forming a vertical line on the chart of the nuclides (see Figure 2-6). The isotones are found in vertical columns on the chart, as the number of protons is represented on a vertical axis. Isobars are found on a 45-degree angle running from the lower right to upper left. Isobars are nuclides that have equal weights or the same mass number (protons plus neutrons). Examples of isobars are ^{99}Rh, ^{99}Ru, ^{99}Tc, and ^{99}Mo; they are found on a 45-degree angle in Figure 2-6.

Isomers are atoms that have identical physical attributes as far as the number of protons, neutrons, and electrons; however, they contain a different amount of nuclear energy. Isomeric forms of an atom are identified by putting an m after the mass number A. The m means the atom is currently in a metastable form and will emit gamma radiation from the nucleus to achieve the more stable energy configuration. The most commonly used radionuclide in nuclear medicine is an isomer—^{99m}Tc. Technetium-99 (^{99}Tc) is a more stable form with a half-life of 2.13×10^5 years. Other isomers that have been used in nuclear medicine are ^{113m}In and ^{87m}Sr. On the chart of the nuclides, isomers are designated by a vertical line within the square for a specific radionuclide.

Another format for diagramming nuclide information is presented with a hexagonal box for each nuclide, as in Figure 2-7 (the trilinear chart), where vertically adjacent neighbors are isobars. Oblique neighbors from upper left to lower right represent isotones, and obliquely adjacent neighbors from lower left to upper right represent isotopes. Isomers are identified with a vertical line through the hexagon. Within each hexagon is a box that identifies the element symbol, atomic number, and mass number. As an example of the information contained in this chart, ^{99}Mo and ^{99}Tc should be carefully examined. In Figure 2-7 molybdenum-99 has a physical half-life of 2.76 days and emits both beta and gamma radiation during radioactive decay. The maximum energy in MeV is listed as 1.230 for beta decay (β^-), and gamma-ray emissions are identified. Vertical downward arrows show that 92% of the time, molybdenum decays to the isomeric form of ^{99m}Tc and 8% of the time directly to ^{99}Tc. The left side of the hexagon representing technetium shows that isomeric transition (discussed later) will occur 100% of the time that ^{99m}Tc decays. Also indicated in the left side is the gamma energy of 0.140 MeV (or 140 keV). Technetium-99, as represented on the right half of the box, is also radioactive, with a half-life of 2.13×10^5 years. Decay is by beta radiation to its daughter product ruthenium-99, which is a stable element. Note that the ^{99m}Tc decays first to ^{99}Tc before it decays to stable ruthenium.

DECAY PROCESSES

Alpha Decay

Alpha particles (helium nuclei consisting of two protons and two neutrons) are radioactive decay products from radionuclides having large, unstable mass and

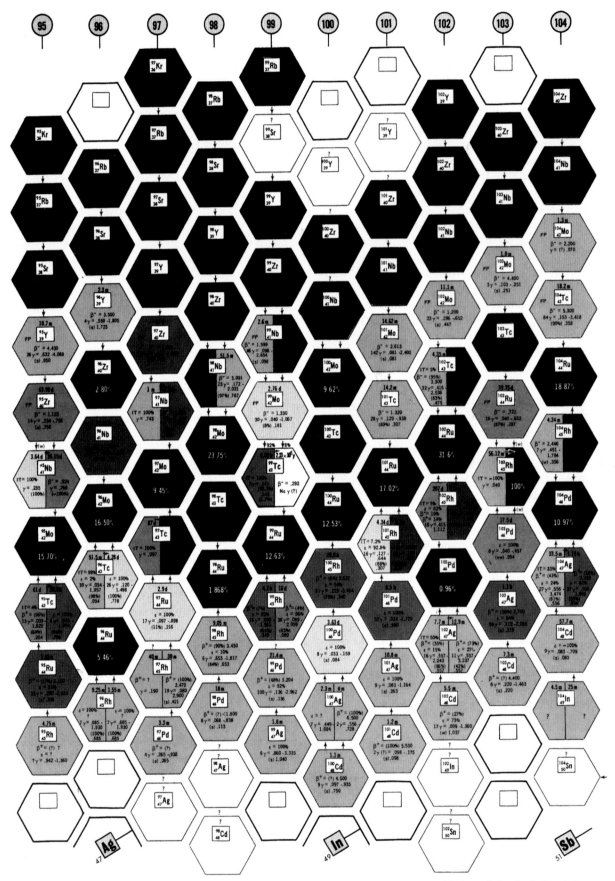

FIGURE 2-7 Trilinear chart of nuclides. Stable forms *(black background)*, instability *(dark- to light-shaded areas)*.

subsequent **alpha decay.** Using standard nuclear notation, the parent element M with atomic number Z and mass number A decays by alpha (α) emission as:

$$^A_ZM = {}^{A-4}_{Z-2}N + \alpha + energy$$

to the daughter product symbolized by N. Because alpha particles have a +2 charge and a large mass of 4 amu, they are very damaging to biological systems and therefore have no role in diagnostic nuclear medicine.

Beta Decay

The concept of a neutron being composed of a proton and electron is important in certain types of radioactive decay. A nucleus that is neutron rich becomes stable through the conversion of one of a neutron to a proton by the reaction:

$$n = p + \beta^- + \bar{v} + energy$$

As a result, a proton and an electron (β^-) have been created from the neutron. The mass number of the new nuclei is the same as that of the parent nuclei, because the masses of a neutron and proton are virtually the same; however, a different element is created. The formation of a different element by a radioactive decay process is called **transmutation,** or *isobaric radioactive decay.* The β^- particle that has been created in the nucleus through this decay process is ejected. In this decay process an antineutrino ($\bar{v}$) is created and carries away part of the energy of this reaction. The laws of conservation of momentum and energy are accounted for by this particle. Neutrinos (v) and antineutrinos have no electrical charge and a mass of almost zero. They travel at the velocity of light and are almost undetectable. The excess energy from the neutron is shared between the beta particle and antineutrino. This sharing of kinetic energy is not equal. Sometimes the electron receives more of the energy, and the neutrino receives less, or vice versa. As a result, the energy of the beta particle varies in a continuous energy spectrum with some maximum energy (E_{max}) that was available from the nucleus (Figure 2-8). This nuclear decay process is termed beta-minus (β^-) or simply beta decay. The parent element M with atomic number Z and mass number A decays by beta emission as:

$$^A_ZM = {}^A_{Z+1}N + \beta^- + \bar{v} + energy$$

The energy released by this process is shared as kinetic (motion) energy by the beta particle and the antineutrino. An example of a beta-emitting radionuclide used in nuclear medicine is ^{131}I, which decays as follows:

$$^{131}_{53}I = {}^{131}_{54}Xe + \beta^- + \bar{v} + energy$$

As shown in Figure 2-8 the average energy of a beta particle is about one third of the maximum energy, E_{max}.

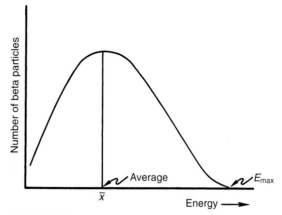

FIGURE 2-8 Generalized beta particle energy spectrum.

Positron (β^+) Decay and Electron Capture

A nucleus that is proton rich (neutron poor) can reduce its proton surplus by two possible decay processes:

$$p = n + \beta^+ + v + energy \text{ (positron decay)}$$

or

$$p + e^- = n + v + energy \text{ (electron capture)}$$

The first process is **positron decay,** and the second is electron capture.

Positron decay or emission results when a proton is converted to a neutron, a positron (β^+), a neutrino, and energy. In nuclear notation the general form of positron decay is written as:

$$\beta^+ + e^- = (0.511\,MeV) + (0.511\,MeV)$$

An example of positron decay is:

$$^{18}_9F = {}^{18}_8O + \beta^+ + v$$

An emitted positron loses kinetic energy through collisions with surrounding matter, because it is then moving slowly enough to be attracted to an electron. The positron and negatron spiral in toward each other, forming a temporary "positronium" atom for a brief instant before the two particles undergo **annihilation.** In the annihilation interaction the mass of each particle (positron and negatron) is converted into pure electromagnetic energy. Using Einstein's equation *(E = mc²),* the rest mass of each particle is converted into a 0.511-MeV photon; thus two 0.511-MeV photons are created. These two 0.511-MeV photons travel in opposite directions to conserve momentum (Figure 2-9). The 0.511-MeV photons are not gamma rays as they did not originate in a nucleus; they are correctly referred to as annihilation photons.

Electron capture occurs when an orbital electron travels in the proximity of the nucleus and is captured and combined with a proton to form a neutron. Remember from the cloud model of the atom that electrons spend a very small amount of their time in the proximity of the nucleus. Electron capture is generalized as:

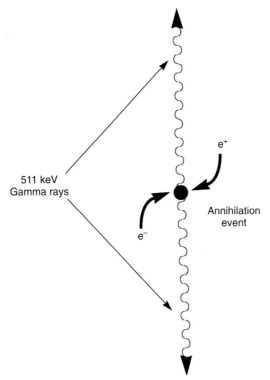

FIGURE 2-9 Annihilation of a positron and a negatron. The resultant pair of 0.511-MeV gamma rays travel 180 degrees apart.

$$^A_ZM + e^- = {}_{z-1}^A N + \nu + energy$$

An example is the decay of ^{125}I:

$$^{125}_{53}I + e^- = {}^{125}_{52}Te + \nu$$

Electrons involved in electron capture are usually those from the K or L shell. The probability for capture from another energy level is very low. A result of electron capture is the ionization of the atom with subsequent relocation of an outer-shell electron to fill the vacancy created by the capture event.

Proton-rich nuclei can reach stability through either positron emission or electron capture. These are always competing processes; however, the configuration of the nuclei and a high energy content of some nuclei increase the probability of positron emission. If the energy content is less, electron capture occurs. Some atoms can undergo either process with a certain probability.

A commonly used radionuclide in nuclear medicine, ^{67}Ga, undergoes electron capture. In addition to the changes that take place within the nucleus, characteristic x-rays are emitted because of energy changes that result from the electrons cascading down to fill vacant positions.

Gamma Decay

Gamma-ray emission represents a mechanism for an excited nucleus to release energy. The release of energy as a gamma (γ) ray may be part of another decay process,

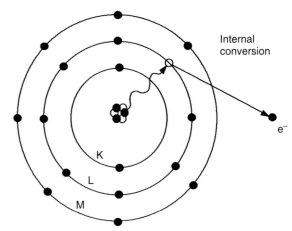

FIGURE 2-10 Internal conversion of L-shell electron. Energy transfer from nucleus ejecting orbital electron is alternative to gamma-ray emission. Internal conversion electron will have kinetic energy equal to gamma-ray energy minus binding energy.

such as alpha or β^-. In addition, it is the process for releasing energy from a metastable nucleus.

Gamma-ray emission usually occurs when there is more than 100 keV of excess energy in the excited nucleus. It should be remembered that gamma rays and x-rays have the same characteristics but are named based on their origin, gamma rays being emitted from the nucleus and x-rays from the electron shells. The ideal radionuclides for nuclear medicine are those that emit only gamma rays without emitting particulate radiation. These radionuclides thereby provide gamma rays for imaging without increasing patient radiation exposure. With particulate radioactive decay, the nucleus is most often left with additional energy, which is released promptly in the form of electromagnetic radiation.

When a metastable nucleus is present, a significant amount of time passes between any previous radioactive decay (such as from ^{99}Mo to ^{99m}Tc) and further release of energy. The release from the metastable state is termed an *isomeric transition*. In this transition the nucleus goes from a higher energy level to a lower energy level through emission of electromagnetic radiation (usually greater than 100 keV); this is sometimes termed **gamma decay**. The equation for an isomeric transition may be written as follows:

$$^A_ZM = {}^A_ZM + \gamma$$

An example of an isomeric transition is:

$$^{99m}_{43}Tc = {}^{99}_{43}Tc + \gamma$$

An alternative process to gamma-ray emission in metastable nuclei is termed *internal conversion*, which is the transfer of energy from the nucleus to an orbital electron, which is then ejected from the atom (Figure 2-10). Internal conversion reactions usually involve electrons from the K shell but occasionally involve electrons from the L or M shell. In this process the ejected electron is called a *conversion electron*. This leaves an ionized atom, which follows the normal process of reshuffling its electrons, resulting in the release of characteristic x-rays or Auger electrons.

Metastable nuclei are the purest sources of gamma rays for nuclear medicine imaging. The isomeric forms for these medically important radionuclides require that they be generator-produced within the nuclear medicine laboratory. Technetium-99m has become the most important radionuclide in nuclear medicine imaging.

SCHEMATICS OF RADIOACTIVE DECAY

The various decay processes of radionuclides can be represented diagrammatically to illustrate the relationship of individual processes that take place in radioactive disintegration. These diagrams show the relationship of the parent radionuclide to the daughter nuclide.

The diagrammatic representation of a decay scheme is based on representing the atomic number on the horizontal axis and the energy of the nucleus on the vertical axis (Figure 2-11, *top*). The parent nucleus, being larger, contains more energy and is represented as a horizontal line at the top of the diagram. Through the process of

radioactive decay the resulting daughter nucleus has less energy and is positioned lower on the diagram. Arrows are used to illustrate the emission of radiation. These arrows show the transition of the nucleus by alpha decay as a decrease in atomic number (Z), shifting to the left, indicating that the atomic number is decreased by 2 in the decay process. In β^- decay there is an increase in Z by 1, with a corresponding shift to the right. With positron decay and electron capture there is a decrease in Z by 1. Gamma emission is shown as a vertical down arrow, indicating the release of electromagnetic radiation and resulting only in a decrease in nuclear energy without a change in atomic number. The energy levels of the parent and daughter nuclei are represented as horizontal lines. The parent radionuclide, $_Z^A M$, is shown in general form as the decay process for β^- emission (Figure 2-12) to the daughter product $_{Z+1}^A M$. Two different diagonal arrows in this diagram represent two different energies of beta particle decay. In one case the longer diagonal line represents the emission of a beta particle going directly to the daughter nucleus without any additional energy release. This beta particle energy equals the difference between the parent and daughter energy levels. The shorter arrow represents release of a beta particle of lesser energy to an intermediate state with the prompt release of a gamma ray (vertical down arrow) to the daughter product. One individual atom of the parent radionuclide can release its energy in this beta decay by following either path; therefore one of two beta particles with different energies can be seen in this transition, and only those beta particles from the lower energy transition are accompanied by a gamma ray.

Figure 2-13 shows a simplified decay scheme for ^{131}I. The actual decay process for ^{131}I has several different

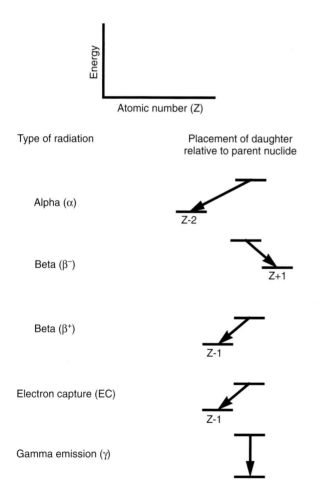

FIGURE 2-11 Axes *(top)* show directions of increasing energy and atomic number in decay schemes. Directional placement of each daughter nucleus is relative to parent in decay schemes.

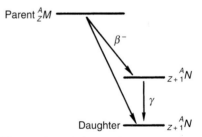

FIGURE 2-12 Hypothetical decay scheme representing beta particle emission.

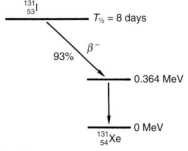

FIGURE 2-13 Generalized decay scheme for ^{131}I.

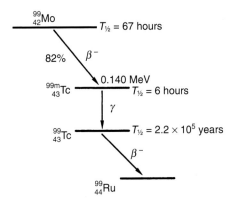

FIGURE 2-14 Generalized decay scheme for ^{99}Mo.

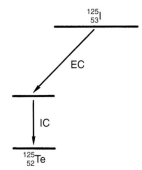

FIGURE 2-15 Generalized decay scheme for ^{125}I.

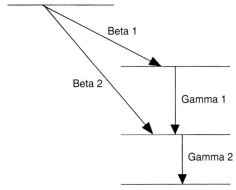

FIGURE 2-16 Decay by beta 1 is followed by emission of gamma 1 and gamma 2. Emission of higher-energy beta 2 is followed only by single gamma emission, gamma 2. Some radionuclides yield several gamma rays for single disintegration.

TABLE 2-1	Gallium-67 Photon Emissions	
Photons	Abundance Percentage	Mean Energy (keV)
Gamma 2	38	93.3
Gamma 3	21	184.6
Gamma 5	16	300.2
Gamma 6	4	393.5

beta energies, though only one is prominent (93%). With this beta particle there is a gamma transition releasing 0.364 MeV. Figure 2-14 shows the decay scheme for ^{99}Mo followed by the transitions of ^{99m}Tc and ^{99}Tc to ^{99}Ru. Approximately 82% of the transition from ^{99}Mo to ^{99m}Tc is by one particular beta energy. The radionuclide is then in the metastable form of ^{99m}Tc, which has a half-life of 6 hours. The isomeric transition of ^{99m}Tc is represented as a vertical line downward of a 0.140-MeV gamma ray to the daughter product ^{99}Tc. Technetium-99 has a long half-life (2.2×10^5 years) and decays by beta decay to yield stable ^{99}Ru.

Figure 2-15 shows the decay process for ^{125}I, which is used in research. The electron capture process is followed by an internal conversion process. The resulting daughter of tellurium, with the electron vacancy left by internal conversion, subsequently emits K-characteristic x-rays.

The radioactive decay schemes shown in Figures 2-11, 2-13, 2-14, and 2-15 have been simplified. Some radionuclides can emit several different gamma-ray energies, as illustrated in Table 2-1 for ^{67}Ga. Gallium-67 decays by electron capture to ^{67}Zn; the zinc nucleus then emits several energies of gamma photons. As indicated in Table 2-1 there is a gamma-ray abundance percentage for each ^{67}Ga atom that decays. For every 100 atoms, approximately 38% emit gamma rays at 93.3 keV, and so on. Decay schemes of this nature are helpful in identifying the most abundant peaks for selecting imaging windows. Two, three, or four peaks can be selected for

imaging on some instruments. In certain decay schemes, more than one gamma ray is emitted for each atom that decays. Figure 2-16 shows a radionuclide that yields more than one gamma ray for each atom that disintegrates. Decay by beta 1 leaves the daughter nucleus with energy that will be released by gamma 1 and gamma 2. Decay of beta 2 is followed only by gamma 2.

Mathematics of Decay

Individual atoms undergo spontaneous transformations to release energy and form daughter nuclei. There is no way of predicting when that transformation will occur for any one specific atom. However, when a large number of atoms are present, a certain probability of radioactive decay is obtained and a mathematical average rate of decay can be determined. A sample that contains N radioactive atoms has on average a certain number of atoms decaying per unit time represented as $\Delta N/\Delta t$. This can be described mathematically as:

$$\frac{\Delta N}{\Delta t} = -\lambda N$$

where λ is the decay constant of the radionuclide. In this equation the minus sign indicates that the rate of change $\Delta N/\Delta t$ is negative, and thus the number of atoms decreases with time. The decay constant λ therefore represents a probability or average percent of the atoms present that will decay in a certain time period. The units of λ are 1/time or time^{-1}. A value such as 0.10 hour^{-1} means that

TABLE 2-2	Decay Factors for ^{99m}Tc	
Hours	Decay Factor	Precalibration Factor
0	1.000	1.000
0.5	0.944	1.059
1	0.891	1.122
2	0.794	1.259
3	0.707	1.414
4	0.630	1.587
5	0.561	1.782
6	0.500	2.000
7	0.445	2.247
8	0.397	2.518
9	0.354	2.824
10	0.315	3.174
11	0.281	3.558
12	0.250	4.000

in each hour 10% of the atoms undergo radioactive decay. Through calculus the above equation is manipulated to derive the number of atoms remaining at any specific time*:

$$N_t = N_0 e^{-\lambda t}$$

where N_t is the number of atoms that remain at any time t, and N_0 is the number of radioactive atoms at the original time zero.

The factor $e^{-\lambda t}$ represents the fraction of radioactive atoms that remain after time t and is called the **decay factor**. The e represents Euler's number, the base of natural logarithms (2.718); it has been raised to the power $-\lambda t$. The decay factor ($e^{-\lambda t}$) is an exponentially decreasing function with time and can be determined using a calculator (see Chapter 1). The decay factors for various time intervals can be calculated; decay factors for ^{99m}Tc are given in Table 2-2.

The number of radioactive atoms (N) is, by the preceding definition ($\Delta N/\Delta t = -\lambda N$), proportional to the radioactivity (A). This equation can therefore be written to apply to radioactivity. It is called the *general decay equation*:

$$A_t = A_0 e^{-\lambda t}$$

---

*Derivation of the general decay equation $\dfrac{\Delta N}{\Delta t} = -\lambda N$

$$\frac{dN}{dt} = -\lambda N$$

$$\frac{dN}{N} = -\lambda dt$$

$$\int \frac{1}{N} dN = -\int \lambda dt$$

$$\frac{N_t}{N_0} = e^{-\lambda t}$$

$$N_t = N_0 e^{-\lambda t}$$

It is frequently difficult to work with the decay factor λ; it is much more practical to use another parameter $t_{1/2}$, known as half-life value. The decay constant λ and $t_{1/2}$ are related by the equation:

$$\lambda = \frac{0.693}{t_{1/2}}$$

where 0.693 is the value of the natural logarithm of 2. This relationship can be derived from the general decay equation by inserting values for the initial activity (A_0) and the activity at the time (t) when the activity (A_t) is at 50% of the activity at time zero. The decay equation may be represented by substituting the relationship of half-life for the decay constant and can be written as:

$$A_t = A_0 e^{-0.693t/t_{1/2}}$$

where the decay factor (DF) equals the exponential portion of this equation:

$$DF = e^{-0.693t/t_{1/2}}$$

The fraction of elapsed time relative to the half-life can be generated and used for determining the decay factor for any radionuclide, sometimes called the *universal decay table*. The calculation of decay factors is reviewed in Chapter 1. Since the decay factor represents an exponential function, it can be plotted either linearly or semilogarithmically (Figure 2-17). When reviewing this graphic representation, note that the number of atoms remaining is 0.50 at one half-life, and observe that the semilogarithmic plot (Figure 2-17, B) is represented as a straight line where the slope is determined by the decay constant.

RADIOACTIVITY UNITS

Radioactivity is quantitatively measured as the number of atoms that disintegrate per unit time. Two different units can be used to describe a quantity of radioactivity, the **curie** (Ci) and the becquerel (Bq). The curie was named in honor of Marie Curie, an early pioneer in the study of radioactivity and the becquerel in honor of Henri Becquerel who discovered radioactivity. One curie is defined as the amount of any radioactive material that decays at a rate of 3.7×10^{10} disintegrations per second (dps). This basic unit can be multiplied by standard mathematical scientific notation to yield larger and smaller multiples of the curie:

kilocurie (kCi) = $10^3 \times$ Ci = 3.7×10^{13} dps
curie (Ci) = $10^0 \times$ Ci = 3.7×10^{10} dps
millicurie (mCi) = $10^{-3} \times$ Ci = 3.7×10^7 dps
microcurie (μCi) = $10^{-6} \times$ Ci = 3.7×10^4 dps
nanocurie (nCi) = $10^{-9} \times$ Ci = 3.7×10^1 dps
picocurie (pCi) = $10^{-12} \times$ Ci = 3.7×10^{-2} dps

The Système International (SI) defines the other unit of radioactivity, the Bq. In 1894, Henri Becquerel

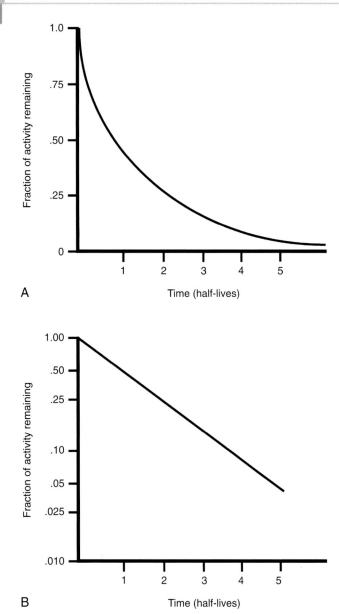

FIGURE 2-17 Fraction of radioactivity remaining (decay constant) as function of time is shown for a linear plot **(A)** and a semilogarithmic graph **(B)**. Slope of semilogarithmic straight line is determined by decay constant.

became the first person to identify radioactivity. One becquerel is the amount of radioactivity contained in a sample that decays at a rate of 1 dps. Because this unit is very small, nuclear medicine terminology uses multiples of the becquerel such as kilobecquerels (kBq) and megabecquerels (MBq).

Because most radioactivity in nuclear medicine is administered in doses of millicuries, or megabecquerels, it is important to be able to rapidly convert between these two units of measure. Multiply the number of millicuries by 37 MBq/mCi to convert to the number of megabecquerels. For example, 20 mCi × 37 MBq/mCi = 740 MBq. Conversely, convert the number of megabecquerels to millicuries by dividing by

37 MBq/mCi, for example, 111 MBq/(37 MBq/mCi) = 3 mCi.

The quantities of radioactivity administered to most patients are on the order of several millicuries (several hundred MBq). The total radioactivity contained in a ^{99}Mo-^{99m}Tc radionuclide generator is on the order of many Ci (many tens of thousands of MBq). The quantity of radioactivity contained in patient specimens or assayed in a scintillation well counter is on the order of nanocuries to microcuries (kilobecquerels).

Decay Calculations

Decay factors (DF) other than those in decay tables (see Table 2-2) for ^{99m}Tc can be found by multiplying those that correspond to the decay interval. For example, a 14-hour DF equals the 12-hour DF (0.250) times the 2-hour DF (0.794), or 0.198; this result could also be obtained by multiplying the 7-hour DF (0.445) by itself to get 0.198, or any other combination could be used.

Sometimes it is necessary to dispense or use a radiopharmaceutical before the calibration time. Precalibration DFs may be calculated from the inverse (1/DF) of the decay factor for the time interval. As an example, the precalibration decay factor for 2 hours equals 1/DF or 1/0.794 = 1.26.

Example 1:
A vial contains 10 mCi of ^{99m}Tc; how much radioactivity remains after 2 hours?

$$\text{DF for 2 hours} = 0.794$$
$$10\,\text{mCi} \times 0.794 = 7.94\,\text{mCi}$$

How much radioactivity was present 5 hours before for 10 mCi?

$$\text{Precalibration DF for 5 hours} = 1.782$$
$$10\,\text{mCi} \times 1.782 = 17.82\,\text{mCi}$$

How much of the 10 mCi remains after 36 hours?
DF for 12 hours is 0.250, which is applied three times:

$$10\,\text{mCi} \times 0.250 \times 0.250 \times 0.250 = 0.156\,\text{mCi}$$

Example 2:
Using the general decay equation, calculate the activity of 5 mCi/ml of ^{201}Tl after 48 hr ($t_{1/2}$ = 73 hours).

$$A_t = A_0 e^{-0.693t/t_{1/2}2}$$
$$A_t = 5\,\text{mCi/ml} \times e^{-0.693t/t_{1/2}}$$
$$A_t = 5\,\text{mCi/ml} \times e^{-0.693 \times (48hr)/(73hr)}$$
$$A_t = 5\,\text{mCi/ml} \times e^{-0.456}$$
$$A_t = 5\,\text{mCi/ml} \times 0.630$$
$$A_t = 3.17\,\text{mCi/ml}$$

Average Half-Life and Effective Half-Life

Average half-life describes the average lifetime of an atom in a sample of radioactivity. Mathematically, the average half-life can be calculated as

$$t_{ave} = 1.44 \times t_{1/2}$$

Although this term represents the average interval for which a group of atoms exists, it has no clinical use in patient dose calculations. The **decay constant** of a radionuclide represents the physical radioactive decay. It does not indicate the rate of biological turnover. Because rates are additive, the biological decay constant can be added to the physical decay constant to give the *effective* decay constant:

$$\lambda_{eff} = \lambda_b + \lambda_p$$

Since $\lambda = 0.693/t_{1/2}$, dividing both sides of the equation by 0.693 can represent this equation in terms of the half-life:

$$\frac{1}{t_{eff}} = \frac{1}{t_b} + \frac{1}{t_p}$$

where t_{eff} is the **effective half-life** (Figure 2-18), t_b is the biological half-life, and t_p is the physical half-life. This equation may be reorganized into the following form:

$$t_{eff} = (t_b \times t_p)/(t_b + t_p)$$

An example of effective half-life might be the determination of the disappearance of ^{99m}Tc-macroaggregated albumin (MAA) from the lungs. Assume that the biological half-life is 3 hours.

$$\frac{1}{t_{eff}} = \frac{1}{(3\,hr)} + \frac{1}{(6\,hr)}$$

The effective half-life (t_{eff}) in the lung is thus 2 hours.

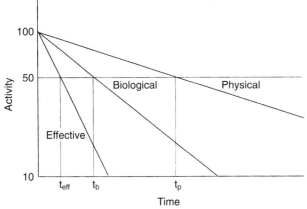

FIGURE 2-18 Semilogarithmic plot of physical (t_p) and biological (t_b) half-life components of shorter effective half-life, t_{eff}.

Parent-Daughter Radionuclide Relationships

As a radionuclide decays to form another nuclide, transmutation takes place when there is a change from one element to another. Some radioactive decay relationships are critical to the success of nuclear medicine, as these decay processes make possible radionuclide generator systems that produce radioactive elements as daughter products from the decay of a longer-lived parent radionuclide.

Parent-daughter sequential radioactive decay occurs when a radioactive parent radionuclide decays to a daughter product that is also radioactive and decays further. The process of sequential decay and its equations govern the use of radioactive generators, such as ^{99}Mo $\rightarrow$ ^{99m}Tc or ^{82}Sr $\rightarrow$ ^{82}Rb. The mathematical equation that governs sequential decay is the **Bateman equation**:

$$A_2 = A_1 \frac{\lambda_2}{\lambda_2 - \lambda_1}\left(e^{-\lambda_1 t} - e^{-\lambda_2 t}\right) + A_2(0)e^{-\lambda_2 t}$$

where A_1 is the quantity of radioactivity of the parent at time zero, A_2 is the daughter activity at any time t, and λ_1 and λ_2 are the decay constants for the parent and daughter respectively, and $A_2(0)$ is any initial daughter activity at time zero (0). With this equation the amount of radioactivity of daughter radionuclide may be computed.

In the case when the parent half-life is longer than the daughter half-life (called transient equilibrium) the time to maximum build up (t_{max}) of the daughter radionuclide may be calculated by the equation:

$$t_{max} = [1.44\, t_1 t_2/(t_1 - t_2)]\ln(t_1/t_2)$$

This equation is derived from the Bateman equation in the situation that we assume that there was initially no daughter radioactivity. In this equation t_1 is the half-life of the parent and t_2 is the daughter half-life. Thus the maximum amount of daughter radioactivity can be calculated as t_{max}. As an exercise the reader may calculate the time to the maximum build up of ^{99m}Tc from a ^{99}Mo generator assuming that the half-life of ^{99m}Tc is 6 hours and the half-life of ^{99}Mo is 66 hours (see Figure 6-5).

The reader is referred to Chapter 6 and the section entitled Generator Systems. The discussion in this section further describes the equations that govern radionuclide generators, including the parent-daughter relationships that create secular and transient equilibrium systems.

INTERACTIONS

Interactions of Charged Particles with Matter

Electrically charged particles (alpha particles, electrons, and positrons) have a high probability of interacting with the matter through which they move. Their mass and electrical charges interact with the mass of the nucleus and electrical charges of atoms. In addition, the kinetic energy of these particles and the properties of the surrounding matter determine how the particles will interact and how far these particles will travel. The density of matter, its atomic number, and its mass number influence the type and probability of these interactions.

Excitation and Ionization

Excitation is a process of absorbing small amounts of energy temporarily in the outer electron structure of an atom. Energy from a passing charged particle or from an interaction with electromagnetic radiation causes a short-lived or metastable excitation of an outer electron to a slightly higher energy level. The outer electron is not removed from the atom, and therefore no ionization occurs. Typically, excitation is very short-lived, and the atom spontaneously gives up the extra energy in the form of electromagnetic radiation.

Ionization of an atom results from the collision of radiation with the electron structure of an atom. Ionization occurs only when the radiation has sufficient energy to completely remove an electron from its orbit. The energy must therefore be larger than the binding energy of the particular orbital electron. For example, if the binding energy of an electron were 54 keV and the incident energy were 78 keV, the electron would be ejected from the atom with 24 keV (i.e., 78 keV − 54 keV) of kinetic energy. Ionization occurs in all forms of matter—solids, liquids, and gases.

Alpha Particles

An alpha (α) particle is equivalent to the nucleus of a helium atom ($^4_2$He). Alpha particles are produced by radioactive decay in very large, unstable atoms. Their high mass and double-positive electrical charge give them a high ionizing potential and a short path length in solids, liquids, or gases. They typically have energies between 3 and 8 MeV. Because it takes only about 34 eV to create one ion pair, the high energy of alpha particles along with their high mass and positive charge can create several hundred thousand ion pairs in only a fraction of a millimeter; this can be devastating to biological systems. Radionuclides that emit alpha particles have no use in nuclear medicine.

Beta Particles

The interaction of negatively charged beta particles in the proximity of the nucleus of an atom results in them being attracted to the positively charged nucleus. As the beta particle is deflected and slowed in its path, there is a release of energy as x-rays, called *bremsstrahlung radiation*. These x-rays are released in a continuous spectrum because of the variations in kinetic energy and path geometry of the beta particle. Bremsstrahlung interactions increase in probability with materials that have a high Z number.

A beta particle emitting radionuclides, such as ^{32}P, should not be shielded by a high-Z material such as lead. It is more appropriate to use a shielding material of low Z, such as plastic, because bremsstrahlung interactions are then less likely to occur. Bremsstrahlung interaction is the method used to produce x-rays in computed tomography (CT) scanners.

Annihilation

Positively and negatively charged electrons (positrons and negatrons) are antiparticles of each other. When positrons are produced in a decay process and are ejected from an atom, they have enough kinetic energy to travel a maximum of a few millimeters. The positron and an orbital electron from an atom are attracted to each other because of their opposite charges, spiral in toward each other, and interact in a process called *annihilation*. The path distance required for a positron to find an electron for this interaction depends on the positron energy and number of electrons in the immediate area of the atom from which the positron was originally emitted. In the annihilation process the mass of the two particles is converted into energy according to Einstein's equation $E = mc^2$. The rest masses of the positron and negatron are identical (0.511 MeV), giving a total energy of 1.022 MeV. The mass of each particle is converted into a 0.511-MeV photon (see Figure 2-9). The two photons travel in opposite directions, 180 ± 0.25 degrees from each other, to conform to the law of the conservation of momentum.

$$\beta^+ + e^- = 0.511\,\text{MeV} + 0.511\,\text{MeV}$$

The simultaneous detection of these two annihilation photons is the foundation for positron emission tomography (PET) imaging.

PHOTONS

Electromagnetic radiation in the narrow range referred to as visible light can be reflected or absorbed with little effect on matter. However, at the energies referred to as x-rays and gamma rays, the wavelength of the electromagnetic radiation becomes smaller than the size of the atom and the radiation penetrates through matter. Electromagnetic radiation, or photons, is far more penetrating in matter than are particulate types of radiation. There is no specific range for these photons, and their interaction with matter is based only on a probability of interaction. In matter, photons may undergo scattering, may have no interaction with matter, or, because they are simply energy, may be completely absorbed

TABLE 2-3	Interactions between Electromagnetic Radiation and Matter		
Interaction	**Interaction Site**	**Energy Range**	**Secondary Effects**
Photoelectric	Inner electron shells	Several keV to 0.5 MeV	Photoelectrons, characteristic x-rays
Compton	Outer electron shells	Several keV to several MeV	Compton electron, scattered photon
Pair production	Nuclear field	<1.02 MeV	Positron, electron, annihilation photons

and disappear. Although photons are more penetrating than particulate radiation, they demonstrate absorption, which diminishes exponentially with the distance traveled. For photons with energies associated with x-rays and gamma rays, three types of interactions occur: photoelectric, Compton, and pair production (Table 2-3).

Photoelectric Effect

The **photoelectric effect** is an interaction that takes place between an incident photon and an inner orbital electron. For the photoelectric effect to occur, the energy of the incident photon must be greater than the binding energy of the orbital electron. In the photoelectric effect the photon energy is totally absorbed, with some of its energy used to break the bond of the electron in its shell and the remaining energy given to the electron in the form of motion or kinetic energy (Figure 2-19). Therefore a generalized relationship for this interaction can be written as:

Photon energy = Electron binding energy + electron kinetic energy

The photoelectric effect usually occurs with electrons found in the K or L shell. Since an electron has been removed from the atom, there is no longer an electrically neutral balance between the number of protons and electrons; therefore the atom has been ionized with an inner shell vacancy created. In this interaction an ion pair has been formed—the positively charged atom and the negatively charged photoelectron—that leaves the atom.

The electron vacancy can be filled (1) by another orbital electron dropping in to fill a vacancy with the subsequent emission of a characteristic x-ray, or (2) by an Auger electron (discussed later). The ejected photoelectron is no different from any other free electron in matter and is involved in other interactions, depending on its kinetic energy. The disappearance of the incident photon is important clinically because the energy has been absorbed completely by the patient.

The probability of a photoelectric interaction occurring depends on the energy of the incident gamma ray and the atomic number of the material. Obviously, the photoelectric effect cannot occur unless the photon energy is above the binding energy. As a photon's energy increases, the probability for photoelectric interactions decreases (Figure 2-20). The probability of a photoelectric interaction increases dramatically with the atomic

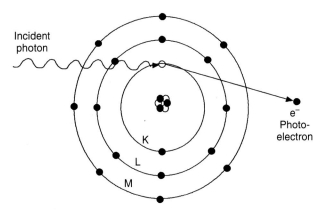

FIGURE 2-19 In photoelectric effect, incident photon is totally absorbed and transfers all its energy to resultant photoelectron.

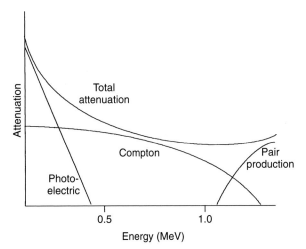

FIGURE 2-20 Interactions by photoelectric, Compton, and pair production combine to form attenuation coefficient. Probability of attenuation by photoelectric effect is dominant at low energy but decreases rapidly with increasing photon energy. Interactions through Compton scattering decrease more slowly, and pair production becomes dominant above 1.02 MeV.

number, that is, photoelectric interactions are unlikely to occur in low-Z materials such as water and tissue but are likely to occur in high-Z materials such as the iodine in a sodium iodide crystal or in lead. The photoelectric effect is therefore the primary type of interaction for detecting gamma rays with nuclear medicine instruments. All the gamma-ray energy is given to the crystal material in a thallium-activated sodium iodide crystal. The photoelectric effect is therefore one of the

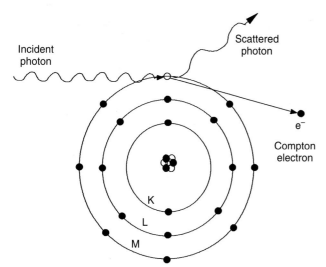

FIGURE 2-21 Compton scattering occurs in outer-shell electrons, with scattered photons having lower energy and a longer wavelength. Ejection of Compton electron produces an ionized atom.

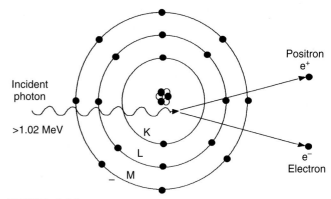

FIGURE 2-22 In pair production, photons with energy greater than 1.02 MeV may interact with strong forces near nucleus. Positron-electron pair is created with kinetic energy equal to excess above 1.02 MeV. Positron will undergo annihilation with electron.

most important interactions for nuclear medicine applications.

Compton Scattering

As its name implies, **Compton scattering** is an incomplete absorption of gamma rays or a scattering of gamma radiation. The Compton effect involves an inelastic interaction of photons with outer orbital electrons. As in the photoelectric effect, an electron is ejected from the atom; however, not all of the incident gamma-ray energy is absorbed, and a scattered photon of lower energy and longer wavelength is emitted. Figure 2-21 illustrates the incident photon at a high energy with short wavelength and a scattered photon with lower energy and longer wavelength. The energy and wavelength of the scattered photon are always lower than those of the incident photon, and the scattered photon's energy also depends on the atomic number of the scattering material, the incident photon's energy, and the angle of scatter. The energy of the scattered photon is related to the angle of deflection. The minimum energy loss of the scattered photon will be at a shallow scatter angle and can be calculated using the relationship:

$$E_{min} = \frac{E_0}{(1 + 2E_0/0.511)}$$

where E_0 is the incident photon energy (in MeV). As an example, for a 0.140-MeV gamma ray, $E_{min} = 0.090$ MeV; for a 0.364-MeV gamma ray, $E_{min} = 0.150$ MeV.

The maximum energy E_{max}, or *backscatter energy*, will be at a scatter angle of 180 degrees and can be calculated from:

$$E_{max} = \frac{E_0^2}{(E_0 + 0.2555)}$$

This maximum scatter energy for a 0.140-MeV photon is 0.049 MeV and for a 0.364-MeV photon is 0.214 MeV. The maximum scatter energy identifies the sharp increase in scatter on the gamma-ray spectrum, called the *Compton edge*.

The likelihood of Compton scattering increases with atomic number; therefore there is more Compton scattering in materials with high atomic numbers. Compton interactions are less likely to occur with higher-energy photons (see Figure 2-20).

Pair Production

Pair production is an interaction produced when a photon with energy greater than 1.02 MeV passes near the high electric field of the nucleus. The strong electrical force brings about the energy-mass conversion. When the photon comes near the nucleus, it disappears totally and two particles of matter are created, an electron and a positron, each possessing the mass equivalence of 0.511 MeV. For this interaction to occur, the initial photon must possess 1.02 MeV or more of energy. Any additional energy of the incident photon is converted into kinetic energy, which is given to the positron and negatron, thus conserving energy and momentum. The photon originally had zero charge, and the offsetting positive and negative charges of the negatron and positron ensure that the net charge remains zero.

The fates of the negatron and the positron are the same as if those particles were created by radioactive decay processes. The negatron interacts with surrounding atoms, possibly causing ionization and excitation. The positron loses some of its energy through interactions and ultimately undergoes annihilation with an orbital electron from an atom, producing a photon pair with 0.511 MeV each. Figure 2-22 illustrates the pair production process.

Figure 2-20 shows the dominance of pair production interactions for photons with very high energy. Note that

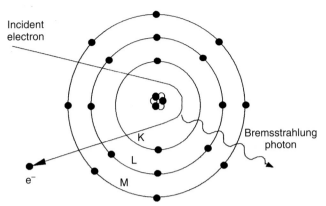

FIGURE 2-23 Deceleration of a charged particle passing near nucleus results in release of energy in the form of bremsstrahlung x-rays.

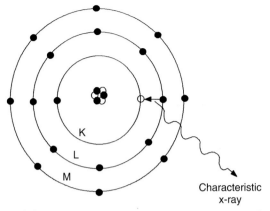

FIGURE 2-24 Characteristic x-rays are produced when an electron fills a lower shell vacancy. Energy of an x-ray represents an energy difference between two electron shells.

there can be no pair production interactions below 1.02 MeV.

EXTRANUCLEAR ENERGY RELEASE

Three distinct processes can occur in the electron structure of the atom to release energy. These result in the creation of bremsstrahlung radiation, characteristic x-rays, or Auger electrons.

Bremsstrahlung Radiation

Bremsstrahlung is a German word that simply means *braking radiation*. Bremsstrahlung is the process that results in the rapid deceleration of a charged particle as it comes under the intense positively charged electric field of the nucleus. The particle, whether it is an electron or a positron, has a very small mass in comparison with the nucleus. The rapidly moving particle is attracted toward or repulsed from the nucleus and, as it is rapidly decelerated, changes its direction. This deflection and deceleration, results in a significant loss of energy, which is emitted in the form of electromagnetic radiation in the x-ray region (Figure 2-23). In this type of interaction the conservation of energy and momentum must be maintained; therefore the energy of the initial charged particle is equal to the sum of the energy of the particle after deflection and the emitted bremsstrahlung x-ray.

The production of bremsstrahlung x-rays is greater for atoms with high Z values and can increase the total amount of radiation being produced and be more hazardous if thin lead shields are used. With thicker lead, the resulting bremsstrahlung emissions are attenuated within the shield. The production of bremsstrahlung radiation is not as significant in materials with low atomic numbers, such as plastic; therefore it is better to shield pure beta-emitting radionuclides such as ^{32}P with plastic shielding instead of thin lead. Bremsstrahlung interactions are the mechanism used to produce radiation in an x-ray tube.

Characteristic X-Rays

The production of characteristic x-rays occurs in atoms that have electron vacancies in their inner shells. As electrons drop down to fill these inner shells from outer orbits, there is a release of electromagnetic energy in the x-ray region (Figure 2-24). The energy of characteristic x-rays is determined by the energy shell difference; electrons filling the K shell are more energetic than those that fill an L shell because of the proximity to the nucleus and the higher binding energy.

Auger Electrons

Characteristic x-rays are produced as part of the process of reducing excess energy when electrons fill vacancies in inner shells. An alternative to characteristic x-rays is the Auger (pronounced *oh-zhay*) effect. In this interaction the surplus energy is given to another orbital electron, which is ejected (Figure 2-25). The ejected electron is called an *Auger electron,* and the atom is now left with two vacancies occurring in the electron structure. These vacancies are then filled by electrons from outer orbits, followed by the emission of characteristic x-rays or secondary Auger electrons. The production of Auger electrons results in increased radiation exposure when these processes take place within the body tissue.

ATTENUATION AND TRANSMISSION OF PHOTONS

As discussed previously, gamma photons interact with matter through photoelectric, Compton, and pair production processes. These interactions combine to form a value called the **linear attenuation coefficient,** μ is the sum of the photoelectric coefficient (τ), the Compton coefficient (σ) and the pair production coefficient (κ), or $m = \tau + \sigma + \kappa$. The linear attenuation coefficient μ is the probability of attenuation per distance traveled through

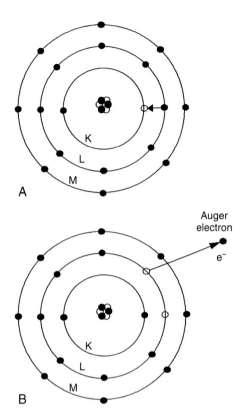

A

Auger
electron

B

FIGURE 2-25 Alternative process to production of characteristic x-rays is emission of Auger electron. As electron fills lower energy shell **(A)**, energy is transferred to release orbital electron. Atom **(B)** is left with two vacancies, which will be filled by outer orbital electrons with subsequent characteristic x-rays or additional Auger electron production.

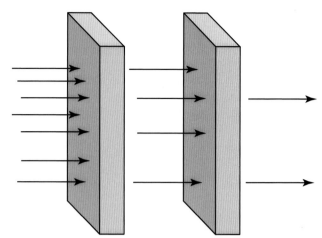

FIGURE 2-26 A beam of electromagnetic radiation passing through one half-value layer of absorber will lose half of the beam intensity. More absorbing material or additional half-value thickness absorbs more of the radiation. Complete blockage of a beam of radiation will require many half value layers until the intensity from the source is near background radiation levels.

an absorber; therefore μ has the unit of 1/distance (cm^{-1}). The general attenuation equation is:

$$I = I_0 e^{-\mu x}$$

where the initial intensity of radiation I_0 is reduced by the exponential function of the linear attenuation coefficient μ and distance traveled x, to obtain the value of the reduced intensity of the radiation field I.

The linear attenuation coefficient μ is related to the **half-value layer (HVL)** of the material by:

$$\mu = \frac{0.693}{HVL}$$

The HVL is the thickness of absorber necessary to diminish the intensity of the radiation to half its initial strength (Figure 2-26).

The general attenuation equation can be rewritten to incorporate the relationship to HVL as:

$$I = I_0 e^{-0.693x/HVL}$$

An example using these equations is the shielding of a source of ^{131}I with lead. The HVL for 364-keV gamma rays is 0.3 cm. The value of μ is then calculated to be 2.31 cm^{-1} (i.e., 0.693/0.3). Assuming 0.9 cm of lead

and an exposure rate of 5 mR/hr, the following can be calculated using the general attenuation equation:

$$I = 5(mR)/(hr)e^{-2.31 \times 0.9}$$
$$I = 5(mR)/(hr)e^{-2.079}$$
$$I = 5(mR)/(hr) \times 0.125$$
$$I = 0.625(mR)/(hr)$$

Since the thickness of the lead is equivalent to 3 HVLs, an alternative method to more simply solve this problem is to divide the intensity of the radiation field by 2, three times, or:

$$(5mR/hr/2/2/2) = 0.625 \, mR/hr$$

The measure of attenuation can also be calculated using another parameter, the mass attenuation coefficient, μ_{mass}, which depends on the material's density. The units of this coefficient are cm^2/g. The relationship between these two attenuation coefficients is represented as:

$$\mu_{mass} = \frac{\mu_{linear}}{density}$$

Using these attenuation relationships results in the following expression:

$$cm^2/g = \frac{cm^{-1}}{(g/cm^3)}$$

The mass attenuation coefficient can be broken down into its components for the processes of photoelectric, Compton, and pair production interactions.

Higher energy electromagnetic radiation requires a greater thickness of attenuating material than lower energy radiation. For example the HVL for ^{99m}Tc at 140 keV is only 0.03 mm of lead, whereas ^{18}F radiation at 511 keV requires 4.1 mm of lead for 1 HVL. Higher atomic number absorber material is more effective at stopping electromagnetic radiation. In addition, the density of the material also strongly influences the absorption of radiation. For example lead has an atomic number of 82 but has a density of only 11.3 g/ml, whereas tungsten (atomic number 74) has a much higher density at 19.3 g/ml. Therefore, because of the density differences, tungsten is a much better shielding material than lead for high energy radiation, such as at 511 keV for PET applications.

Another practical application of attenuation differences is to separate the measurement of vastly different energies of radioactive gamma ray emissions. For example when ^{99m}Tc is eluted from ^{99}Mo there is the potential for a slight amount of ^{99}Mo to break off from the system and contaminate the ^{99m}Tc. If the eluted ^{99m}Tc is placed into a lead shield of sufficient thickness then the shield effectively absorbs nearly all of the 140-keV gamma rays from the ^{99m}Tc but the 700- to 800-keV gamma radiation coming from any ^{99}Mo can be measured to determine the level of contamination. There will be a more detailed discussion of this technique in the chapter on radiochemistry.

SUMMARY

- Nuclear instability, the energy configuration of nucleons, is the cause of radioactive decay.
- The notation used in denoting various nuclides is $^A_Z X$, where X is the chemical symbol, Z is the element's atomic number (number of protons), and A represents the atomic mass number of the element (protons plus neutrons).
- Radioactive decay mechanisms important to nuclear medicine and PET are alpha decay, beta-minus decay, positron decay and electron capture, and gamma decay.
- Alpha particles (two protons and two neutrons) are emitted only by very large radionuclei, and alpha-emitting radionuclides are not used for imaging or internal therapy.
- Beta particles are high-speed electrons; they are associated with high local radiation exposure and

are therefore used for therapeutic radiopharmaceuticals. Their decay may also be followed by gamma emissions.
- Positron decay and electron capture are competing mechanisms for proton-rich radionuclides to lose energy.
- Isomeric decay is the loss of energy from the nucleus without a change in the number of nucleons (protons and neutrons), with the energy leaving as electromagnetic radiation.
- The general radioactive decay equation is $A_t = A_0 e^{-\lambda t}$ or $A_t = A_0 e^{-0.693t/t_{1/2}}$.
- The units of radioactivity are curies (3.7×10^{10} dps) or becquerels (1 dps).
- To convert mCi to MBq, multiply mCi by 37 MBq/mCi.
- Decay factors (DF) are calculated from the exponential portion of the general decay equation $DF = e^{-0.693t/t_{1/2}}$ and are used to compute tables of DF values.
- The effective half-life (t_{eff}) describes both the physical decay and the biological turnover of a radionuclide and is calculated from the equation:

$$\frac{1}{t_{eff}} = \frac{1}{t_b} + \frac{1}{t_p}$$

where t_b is the biological half-life and t_p is the physical half-life.
- The interaction of radiation and matter results primarily in the ionization of atoms.
- The interaction of gamma or x-ray photons and matter takes place by photoelectric, Compton, or pair production interactions.
- Annihilation reactions are between positrons and electrons (antiparticles of one another). The rest mass of each particle is converted into electromagnetic radiation through Einstein's equation $E = mc^2$. Two annihilation photons are produced, each with an energy of 511 keV, traveling 180 ± 0.25 degrees from each other.
- The attenuation of high-energy photons follows the general attenuation equation $I = I_0 e^{-0.693X/HVL}$.
- A material's half-value layer (HVL) is different for various energies with higher energy requiring thicker absorber.

Instrumentation

Mark Madsen

OBJECTIVES

After completing this chapter, the reader will be able to:
- Describe the construction and operating principles of gas-filled detectors, including ionization chambers, Geiger-Mueller detectors, and dose calibrators.
- Discuss efficiencies of detector systems relative to geometric efficiency, intrinsic efficiency and energy, temporal resolution, and dead time.
- Describe quality control procedures required for survey instruments.
- List the quality control procedures required for the dose calibrator and how each procedure is performed and results interpreted.
- Discuss quality control requirements for nonimaging scintillation detectors.

- Explain the basic operation of scintillation detectors and photomultiplier tubes.
- Describe the mechanisms to generate an energy spectrum with a scintillation detector.
- Discuss differences between liquid scintillation counting systems and scintillation crystal systems.
- Diagram the design of an Anger scintillation camera system and explain the function of each component.
- Diagram and discuss the properties of various camera collimators.
- Discuss spatial resolution and sensitivity of the scintillation camera.
- Diagram and describe the function of position logic circuitry for the scintillation camera.

- Describe the operation of a pulse height analyzer for energy discrimination.
- Explain images formation of the scintillation camera.
- List and discuss quality control procedures required for the scintillation camera system.
- Define NEMA standards and their application to nuclear medicine.

KEY TERMS

collimator
cutie pie
dead time
detector efficiency
dose calibrator
dynode
4π geometry
full-width-at-half-maximum (FWHM)
full-width-at-tenth-maximum (FWTM)

Geiger-Mueller detector
intrinsic resolution
ionization detector
line spread function
modulation transfer function (MTF)
multichannel analyzer (MCA)
National Institute of Standards and Technology (NIST)
photomultiplier tube (PMT)
point spread function
positron emission tomography (PET)

proportional counter
pulse height analyzer (PHA)
quench gas
scintillation camera
scintillation detector
single photon emission computed tomography (SPECT)
temporal resolution
well counter

RADIATION DETECTORS

Radioactive materials emit a variety of energetic particles that provide useful diagnostic information when those emissions are detected and analyzed. A wide variety of detection instrumentation has been developed and is in use in nuclear medicine and **positron emission tomography (PET)** imaging clinics. The applications for these instruments include the assaying radioactivity, surveying and monitoring for radioactive contamination, detecting radiotracers with probes, and imaging virtually every tissue and organ system in the body with a wide variety of studies. This chapter will discuss the instrumentation used for those applications along with the quality control procedures that are used to ensure that it is in proper working condition. All of the detectors described in this section are electronic. This is hardly surprising because only electronic devices have the speed and sensitivity to process the signals that are derived in the detection process. Where appropriate, this chapter will describe the basic electronic components that are integral to the detection process.

Ultimately, all detectors convert the energy deposited in the detection material into an electronic signal or pulse. The generic term for a device that transforms energy from one form to another is a transducer. For example, a microphone is a transducer that changes sound energy into an electric signal, whereas a speaker transduces electrical signals into sound. For radiation detectors, a number of materials such as air or cadmium telluride change absorbed radiation energy into electronic signals. Other examples include scintillators, which change the absorbed radiation into visible light and then require another transducer to change the scintillation light into an electronic signal.

Radiation deposits energy into detectors (and other materials) by imparting energy to electrons. In the case of beta decay, the energetic charged particles, either electrons or positrons, lose energy as they interact with the electrons in the materials they pass through, causing ionization of the atoms or excitation of outer shell electrons to higher energy levels. Gamma rays interact by either photoelectric absorption or Compton scatter to impart energy to electrons, which in turn lose that energy in material in the same way as beta particles.

Photoelectric absorption is usually the dominant interaction at low energy and is the most desirable interaction because it results in a signal that represents the full energy of the gamma ray. With photoelectric absorption, the incoming gamma ray is completely absorbed and all of its energy is transferred to an inner shell electron that is ejected from the atom. Photoelectric absorption is dominant in materials with a high atomic number and density. The likelihood that a gamma ray will be involved in a photoelectric absorption falls very rapidly with gamma ray energy.

Compton scattering plays an important role in gas ionization detectors, but provides a signal that is not useful to most imaging systems. With Compton scatter, an incoming gamma ray imparts a portion of its energy to a loosely bound electron, and the resulting lower energy scattered photon goes off in a different direction. The amount of energy lost in the interaction depends on the angle between the primary and scattered photons. Compton scatter causes a loss of contrast in imaging systems and can be partially removed by energy discrimination.

Before the specifics of radiation detectors are described, it is useful to consider the properties of detectors and how they influence the performance. These properties include efficiency, energy resolution, temporal (timing) resolution, and spatial resolution.

Detector Efficiency

Detector efficiency has a simple definition. It is the ratio of the number of detected events to the number of source emissions. Detector efficiency is often separated into two components: geometric and intrinsic efficiency. In order to register an event, an emitted gamma ray must hit the detector and it must also deposit some energy through a physical interaction.

Geometric Efficiency

Geometric efficiency is defined as the fraction of emitted photons (gamma or x-rays) that hit the detector and it depends on the detector configuration and its distance from the source. Mathematically it is defined by:

Equation 3-1

$$g_p = (\text{area of the detector}) \times \cos(\phi) 4\pi r$$

The term g_p is the geometric efficiency for a point source; r is the distance from the source to the detector (Figure 3-1, A). The $\cos(\phi)$ factor accounts for the apparent reduction in the area of the detector if it is not pointed directly at the source. When the detector is optimally positioned, $\phi = 0$ and $\cos(\phi) = 1$. Geometric efficiency is improved when the detector area is large and the source is close to the detector. The best configuration exists when the detector completely surrounds the source. That is approximated by the well design used in dose calibrators and well counters, and is achieved in liquid scintillation counters where the source is actually dissolved in the detector material.

Equation 3-1 is not convenient when the source is close to the detector. In that case, an alternate formulation is often used:

Equation 3-2

$$g_p = 0.5 \times [1 - \cos(\theta)]$$

Here, θ is the angle between the source and the edge of the detector (Figure 3-1, B). For example, if the source is sitting right on the detector, then $\theta = 90°$ and $g_p = 0.5$. This result makes sense since half of the emitted gamma rays will travel toward the detector and half will go in the other direction, away from the detector. If a source sitting inside a well counter makes an angle of 150 degrees with the detector edge, then $g_p = 0.5 \times [1 - \cos(150°)] = 0.93$. The solid angle geometry of a detector that completely surrounds a radioactive source is referred to as **4π geometry**. In this case the geometry efficiency would be 1.00.

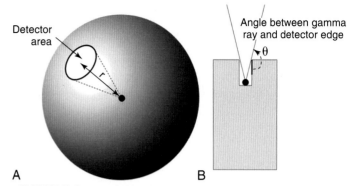

FIGURE 3-1 Geometric Efficiency. A, The geometric efficiency for a point source is the ratio of the detector area to the surface area of a sphere as given by Equation 3-1. **B,** Equation 3-2 is appropriate when the source is very close to or partially surrounded by the detector.

Intrinsic Efficiency

The fraction of gamma rays that are detected when they hit the detector is called the intrinsic efficiency (ε). Intrinsic efficiency is determined from:

Equation 3-3

$$\varepsilon = 1 - e^{-\mu t}$$

It depends on the thickness (t) and attenuation coefficient (μ) of the detecting material. To achieve an intrinsic efficiency near 1 requires that the product μt is large. The attenuation coefficient depends on the detector atomic number and density as well as the energy of the gamma rays. At low gamma ray energies, the attenuation coefficient for many detector materials is quite high and relatively thin detectors can be used, whereas the efficient detection of high energy photons such as annihilation radiation (511 keV) requires thick detectors.

The total attenuation coefficient includes both Compton scattering and photoelectric absorption interactions. Because interactions where all the gamma ray energy is deposited in the detector are often the only ones considered, the intrinsic efficiency may be calculated using only the photoelectric attenuation factor. This is referred to as the photopeak efficiency.

Scintillators are often used as detectors because they have high densities and high atomic numbers. Conversely, detectors based on gases, where the density of atoms in low, typically have very low intrinsic efficiency.

Energy Resolution

Detectors that produce an electronic signal for each individual interaction and whose amplitude reflects the amount of energy absorbed are said to have energy resolution. Energy resolution is advantageous for selective gamma ray detection and discrimination against Compton scattered radiation. Energy resolution is degraded by the amount of variation that occurs in the pulse height amplitude when an event is processed. In an

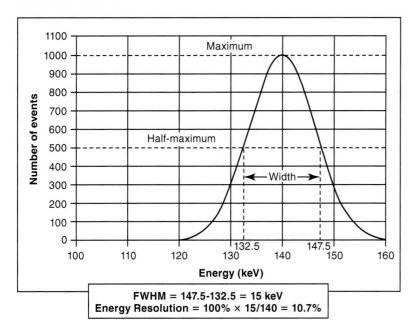

FIGURE 3-2 **Energy Resolution.** Energy resolution is specified by the ratio of the FWHM to the gamma ray energy. Small values of energy resolution imply good performance.

ideal detector, all pulses resulting from the complete absorption of a specific gamma ray (e.g., 140-keV gamma ray from ^{99m}Tc), would be the exact same size. A histogram plot of the number of events as a function of apparent energy as indicated by the pulse height would show all the events at the same spot on the *x*-axis. This plot is referred to as an energy spectrum. Real detectors have random distortions that result in different pulse amplitudes, even when the exact same energy is absorbed, and generate a spectrum that is spread out along the *x*-axis. The energy resolution of a detector is determined from the amount of spread that is manifested in the energy spectrum and is quantified from the following formula:

Equation 3-4

$$\text{Energy Resolution} = 100\% \times \text{FWHM (keV)}/E\gamma \text{ (keV)}$$

The **full-width-at-half-maximum (FWHM)** represents how wide the energy peak is at mid level (Figure 3-2). The energy resolution for a perfect detector would be 0% whereas those with high values have poor energy resolution. In general, scintillation detectors have moderate energy resolution; semiconductors are capable of very good energy resolution; and many ionization detectors such as the Geiger-Mueller (GM) detector and dose calibrator have no energy resolution.

Temporal Resolution and Dead Time

The conversion of gamma ray energy into an electronic pulse and the processing of the pulse requires a finite amount of time that is often referred to as **dead time.** If events happen too rapidly, they cannot be properly analyzed and information is lost. Detection systems can be classified as paralyzable or nonparalyzable depending on how they process an event. In nonparalyzable systems,

interactions that occur when the system is processing a previous event are ignored and they do not affect the ongoing processing of the first pulse. Electronic components like amplifiers, pulse height analyzers and counters generally act like nonparalyzable systems. With paralyzable systems, the system needs an uninterrupted time interval to finish processing any single event. If the event rate is too high, the detector will never be able to complete an event and it will shut down. The classic example of a paralyzable system is the GM detector, which needs an uninterrupted 100-microsecond (μsec) interval to recharge before it is ready for another event. Figure 3-3 shows a plot of the count rate response of paralyzable and nonparalyzable systems.

All event counting systems have count rate limitations. Sodium iodide well counters, for example, cannot accurately assay more than 1 μCi of activity. Although most gamma camera and single photon emission computed tomography (SPECT) studies are count limited, studies that monitor the first pass of high activity bolus injections operate in the range where count losses are evident. Many PET studies, especially in the three-dimensional mode, require corrections for count rate losses.

One other aspect of **temporal resolution** is pulse timing. For some applications, precise time determination of when an event has occurred provides important information. Coincidence detection of the annihilation photon pair is the basis of PET imaging where events are counted only if they are detected by opposed detectors within a very short time window (approximately 5 nanoseconds [nsec]). Coincidence detection requires fast electronics and is facilitated by detectors that are also fast in registering an interaction. Time of flight PET, which determines approximate source location from the differential timing between opposed detectors, requires event processing time in the range of 0.5 nsec.

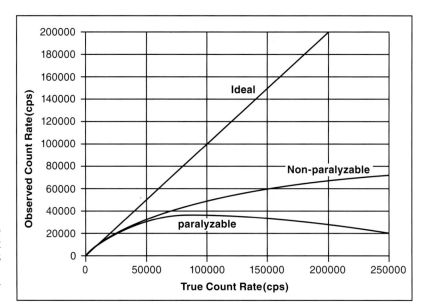

FIGURE 3-3 Count Rate Losses. Ideal detectors have a linear relationship between real and observed count rates. Most detectors lose increasingly more counts as the event rate increases. At very high count rates, paralyzable systems shut down, whereas nonparalyzable systems reach a constant maximum count rate.

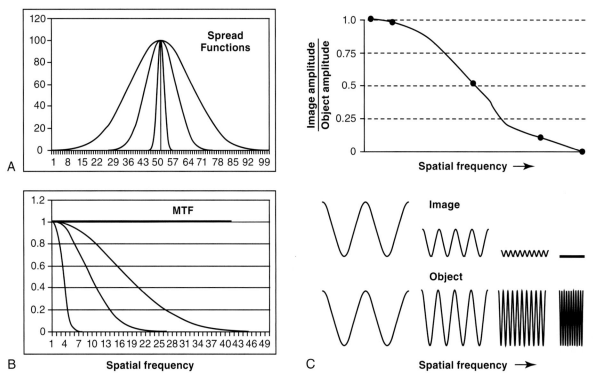

FIGURE 3-4 Modulation Transfer Function and Spread Functions. A, The finite spatial resolution if imaging systems causes points and lines to blur and the spread functions show the degree of blurring. **B,** The MTF has an inverse relationship with its associated spread function. A high-resolution (very compact) spread function has a very broad MTF. **C,** The MTF expresses how well an imaging system reproduces the contrast of a sinusoidal pattern as frequency increases. As seen in the lower right part of this figure, low frequency patterns are imaged with little or no losses in the resulting image, whereas high frequency patterns (corresponding to image detail) are substantially reduced.

Spatial Resolution

Spatial resolution refers to the amount of blurring that is produced by an imaging system. All imaging systems cause some blurring, and nuclear medicine imaging systems have the poorest spatial resolution of all the medical diagnostic modalities. Two ways to characterize system resolution are the **point spread function** and **line spread function.** These are obtained by imaging a point or line source of radioactivity and plotting the count profile through the image as shown in Figure 3-4, *A.* A source is considered to be a point if its dimensions are substantially less than the expected spatial resolution. Similarly, the width of a line source has the same constraints, whereas its length technically ought to span the field of view. For example, if the expected spatial resolution is 10 mm, the width of the line source or any dimension of the point source should be no larger than 2.5 mm.

The entire spread function conveys information about how the system blurs images. In the absence of scattered radiation, the point and line spread functions are well described by a Gaussian function and can be characterized by a single value related to the standard deviation of the Gaussian. By convention, the full-width-at-half-maximum (FWHM) of the spread function expressed in millimeters is used to represent the spatial resolution. As noted, this is a good characterization if the spread functions are Gaussian, but is incomplete if scattered radiation is present.

An alternate but equivalent way of representing spatial resolution is with the **modulation transfer function (MTF)**. The modulation transfer function is a plot of how well information is passed through the imaging system in terms of spatial frequency. Let's explore what that means. It turns out that any information that can be recorded (like an image) can be generated mathematically by adding together individual component images where the variation is only sinusoidal. A single sinusoidal component needs three parameters to describe it: the amplitude, the starting point (called the phase), and the spatial frequency. To make a complicated image, a large number of sinusoidal components varying in the x and y directions are needed. In general, the broad shapes in an image are defined by low spatial frequencies, and the detail (e.g., sharp edges) requires very high frequency spatial frequencies. Because of limited spatial resolution, imaging systems do not handle these components equally. Low spatial frequencies are recorded accurately (i.e., little or no change in amplitude), whereas high spatial frequencies are attenuated (the amplitude is decreased).

The MTF shows the spatial frequency efficiency behavior of an imaging system. As shown in Figure 3-4, C, it is a plot of the ratio of the image and the input sinusoidal amplitude as a function of spatial frequency. A perfect imaging system would have a MTF that was a line at 1.0 at all frequencies.

How are the spread functions related to the MTF? The MTF is generated from the Fourier transform of the point or line spread function. The Fourier transform is a mathematical operation that represents a function in terms of its frequency components. Transform pairs like the MTF and the spread function have an inverse relation; when one is compact, the other is broad. Figure 3-4, A-B, shows a comparison of a family of spread functions and the corresponding MTFs.

Since spread functions and MTFs contain the same information, why should we bother with them? There are several advantages to expressing resolution in terms of the frequency components. One advantage concerns image noise, the statistical fluctuations that are a fundamental part of the emission and detection of gamma rays. In the frequency domain it is easier to determine which portions of the image are most compromised by image noise and therefore how to optimize smoothing filters. The other advantage concerns resolution recovery. The blurring effect of spatial resolution is mathematically expressed by a complex operation called convolution. Compensating for the blurring, deconvolution, is even more complex. However, in the spatial frequency domain, blurring is expressed as a multiplication by the MTF. Resolution recovery can be therefore be accomplished by dividing the frequency components of the blurred image by the MTF.

GAS-FILLED DETECTORS

When gamma rays are directed toward any material, they will interact by either photoelectric absorption or Compton scattering. In both cases, energy is transferred from the gamma ray to an electron in the material. This creates a free, energetic electron. This electron will dissipate its energy by causing additional ionization and excitation of the atoms in the material. For each ionization, two charged entities are generated: the free electron (negative ion) and the remaining positively charged molecule (positive ion). In a gas, the resultant ions can easily be collected by charged electrodes referred to as the anode and cathode. The positively charged anode collects the negative ions while the negatively charged cathode collects the positive ions. The amount of charge collected by these terminals reflects the intensity of the radiation. Although the ability to collect charge makes gas ionization attractive as a means for detecting radiation, the low density atomic number of most gases make them inefficient absorbers of gamma rays.

The number of ions that are generated when a gamma ray interacts is generally too small to register individual events. The average energy to create an ionization in air is about 34 eV. If a 140 keV gamma ray is totally absorbed (a very rare event), then the number of ions that would be generated from this absorption is 140,000/34 = 4117. Less than 10% of these ions actually make it to the electrodes to be collected, so the signal is quite small. To overcome that limitation, a large number of events are summed together so that an electrical current is measured instead of individual events. Even though this current is very small, highly precise electrometers are capable of making the measurement.

A simple diagram of an ionization chamber is shown in Figure 3-5, A. A positively charged anode (usually a wire) and an outer shell cathode are connected in a circuit. When there are no ions created in the gas, no

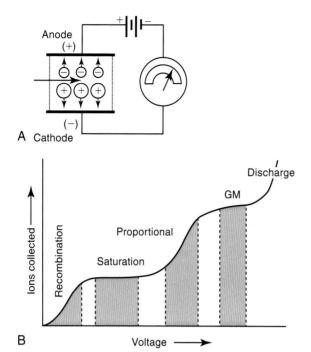

FIGURE 3-5 Gas Ionization Chambers. A, A simplified circuit of a gas ionization detector. Ions created by the radiation in the chamber are collected and generate a current. **B,** A plot of the number of collected ions for a fixed amount of radiation as a function of chamber voltage. Useful devices operate in the ionization region (saturation), proportional, and Geiger-Mueller regions.

current flows between the anode and cathode. If the gas volume between the anode and cathode is irradiated, ions form and a current will flow. The magnitude of the current depends on voltage difference between the anode and cathode, and the intensity of the radiation.

If the chamber is irradiated with a constant intensity, the number of ions that are collected depends on the anode voltage. Obviously, when there is no voltage on the anode, no ions will be collected. As the voltage on the anode is increased, a characteristic ionization curve is seen as shown in Figure 3-5, *B*. The shape of the curve is determined by the physical interactions of the ions as they travel to the anode and cathode. Five distinct regions are observed: recombination, saturation, proportional, Geiger-Mueller, and spontaneous discharge.

No radiation detection devices are operated in the recombination region. In order for ions to be collected, the negative ions (electrons) must get to the anode while the positive ions must get to the cathode. When the voltage attracting the charged ions is low, it is likely that some of the negative and positive ions will recombine and neutralize each other before they reach the terminals. As the voltage is increased, more of the ions are collected as the recombining fraction declines leading to the linear shape of curve in this region.

As the anode voltage is increased, eventually all of the ions that are formed by the radiation and can be collected reach the terminals, and further increases in voltage in a restricted range will not affect the number of ions collected and the curve flattens. This plateau is called the saturation region. In this region, several ionization chamber devices are operated, such as the ionization survey meter (**cutie pie**), personnel dosimeters, and the dose calibrator. Radiation detectors that work in the saturation region cannot detect individual events because the signal is just too weak. Most of these devices either integrate the collected charge (dosimeters) or measure the current from a large number of events (cutie pie and dose calibrator). These types of devices have no dead time and no energy resolution.

If the voltage is increased past the saturation region, the number of ions suddenly begins to increase again. This occurs because the negative ions (electrons) that are created by the radiation are accelerated toward the anode with sufficient energy to create new ionizations. The electrons from these new ionizations create even more ions. This amplification of ionization is called the Townsend avalanche effect and it is large enough that individual ionization events can be counted and the energy of the interaction can be estimated. The ultimate number of ions collected depends on two factors: (1) the anode voltage, and (2) the initial number of ions that were formed, which is directly related to the particle energy. Because the number of ions collected is directly proportional to the initial number of ions formed by the radiation, this portion of the curve is called the proportional region. Detectors that operate in this region are called **proportional counters.** Proportional counters are not found in most nuclear medicine clinics, but are often used in radiation protection labs to identify alpha- and beta-emitting radionuclides based on their energy spectra.

As the voltage on the electrodes is increased in the proportional region, the number of ions collected increases dramatically as the avalanche effect becomes more intense. Eventually, another plateau is reached, the **Geiger-Mueller (GM)** region. At this point, the amplification factor is so high that there is total discharge of the chamber for each ionizing event. The chamber sensitivity to any ions forming is very high in the GM region, but energy information is lost. Because there is a total discharge, the output signal size is the same whether there was a single initial ionization or a large amount of ionization. Ion chambers that operate in this region are called Geiger-Mueller or GM counters. GM detectors are good for surveying low-level radiation areas to identify small amounts of radioactive contamination, but are not good for high radiation areas. This is because they have a substantial recovery time (dead time) before they are capable of recording new events. If the radiation level is too intense, they cannot recover and are effectively

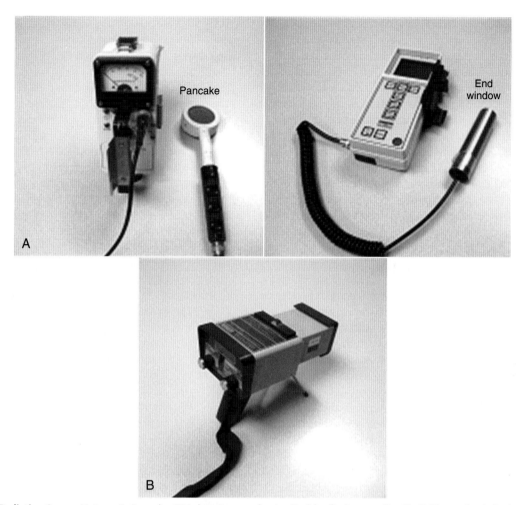

FIGURE 3-6 Radiation Survey Meters. A, Pancake GM detectors are best suited for finding small spills. **B,** The cutie pie ionization meter can be used to measure the exposure rate, even in high radiation areas.

turned off (paralyzed). Instead of air, argon, or neon at low pressure (0.8 atmosphere) is used as the sensitive element. A small amount of a **quench gas,** either chlorine or bromine, has been added to the detector chamber to stop the discharge so that the GM counter can recover for a new event. As the positive ions slam into the cathode, electrons are liberated that continue the discharge. The quench gas preferentially carries the positive charge and dissipates the extra energy at the cathode by dissociating without creating new ionizations.

If the voltage of a gas ionization chamber is raised beyond the GM region, spontaneous discharges will occur in the chamber, which not only make it useless but will eventually ruin the device.

Survey Meters

Gas detectors are ideal as survey meters because they are small and portable. Although their intrinsic efficiency for stopping gamma rays is low (<1%), they have sufficient sensitivity for detecting radioactive contamination and radiation levels that are above background. Because survey meters detect radiation through ionization it is natural to use units of exposure measured in mR or mR per hour, or the Système International counterpart, air kerma measured in mGy or mGy per hour. As the units imply, these devices can be operated in a rate mode or an integrating mode where the total exposure of a time interval is monitored. The two devices primarily used as survey meters are GM and ionization detectors (cutie pie) (Figure 3-6, *B*).

Geiger-Mueller Detector

The **Geiger-Mueller detector** operates in the Geiger-Mueller region of the ionization curve. As noted earlier, the GM detector yields a pulse when any ionization occurs in the detector gas, and an audio mode is often provided where each event produces a "click." The GM detector is more sensitive to low energy gamma rays than those above 200 keV, but it has no energy resolution. The recovery time for the anode to recharge after an event is about 100 μsec. Additional events that occur during this time interval (also called the dead time) prolong the recovery and can even stop the detector from operating when the exposure rate is too high. As a result GM detectors are confined to use in areas where the exposure level are below 1000 mR/hr. GM counters may have a variety of detachable detectors. The most common configurations are the end-window and pancake detectors shown in Figure 3-6, *A*.

Ionization Detector (Cutie Pie)

The cutie pie detector is an ionization chamber that works in the saturation region of the ionization curve. Unlike the GM detector, which measures individual ionization events, the cutie pie is a current measuring device and has no dead time because it measures the continuously produced current to assess exposure. It is not the best instrument for very low level radiation, but because it has no dead time, it is the appropriate device to use for the high levels of radiation you might find around a thyroid ablation dose or a new ^{99}Mo-^{99m}Tc generator. The cutie pie has an air chamber that is not sealed. As a result, changes in atmospheric pressure and room temperature will affect the reading.

Survey Meter Quality Control

Survey meters are battery driven and the first test that should be performed with each use is to verify that the batteries have sufficient charge by checking the battery level indicator. Every day the constancy of the survey meter must be checked by making an exposure reading by placing the sensitive element of the detector in contact with a long lived check source. Many survey meters have a low activity ^{137}Cs check source attached to the body of the meter for this purpose. Also attached to the meter is a calibration summary, which includes the expected measured exposure rate from the check source. The daily measurement should be within 10% of the recorded value.

The Nuclear Regulatory Commission (NRC) has specification recommendations for survey meter calibration, which are located in 10 CFR 35.61. These regulations require annual calibrations for all scales up to 10 mSv (1000 mR) per hour with two separate calibrations done at each scale setting. The annual calibration is usually performed with a high activity (3.1 GBq) ^{137}Cs source to achieve the scale readings required in 10 CFR 35.61. Dose rates for the different scales are adjusted by changing the source to detector distance. The vast

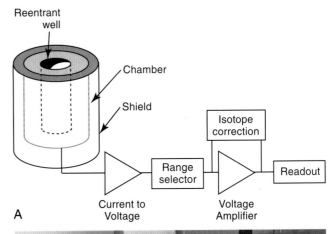

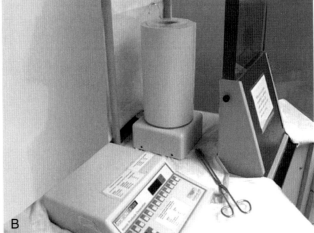

FIGURE 3-7 A, Dose calibrator diagram with chamber, shield, range selector, isotope correction, and readout. The dose calibrator has a reentrant well design and uses argon gas under high pressure. Accurate activity measurements are obtained when the selected isotope button matches the source being assayed. **B,** Photograph of a dose calibrator chamber (cylinder), electronics behind lead shield.

majority of nuclear medicine clinics send their survey meters to an outside facility for calibration.

Dose Calibrator

The NRC requires in 10 CFR 35.60 that any radioactivity administered to a patient or research subject must be assayed in a dose calibrator. If a clinic receives unit doses from a commercial radiopharmacy, they may rely on that calibration. However, if the sample is manipulated in any way or if the clinic prepares its own radiopharmaceuticals, then a dose calibrator is required. The **dose calibrator** is shown schematically in Figure 3-7, *A*. There is a thin-walled aluminum chamber configured as a reentrant well that contains argon at high pressure. Surrounding the chamber is a cylindrical shield (Figure 3-7, *B*) that both reduces the exposure to the operator from the radioactivity inside the well and increases the sensitivity of the system by scattering gamma rays back into the chamber.

The well configuration of the dose calibrator is large enough to accommodate vials or syringes and forms nearly 4π geometry around the source. The ions that are formed continuously when a radioactive sample is placed in the well generate a current that is measured with an electrometer. The amount of current depends on the activity of the sample and the types of radioactive emissions. The electronics of the dose calibrator converts the current into a voltage and modifies it with a calibration factor that is unique for each radionuclide. The calibration factors for all the commonly used radionuclides are determined by the manufacturer and are applied when the operator pushes the appropriate isotope button. The chamber power supply, electrometer, calibration factors, and readout are housed in a separate electronics module.

Potentially, all the radioactive emissions can contribute to the measured radioactivity. This can cause an underestimation of the radioactivity when a radionuclide emits low energy betas or gamma rays that are absorbed before they reach the chamber. For example, radionuclides that decay by electron capture, such as ^{123}I or ^{111}In emit low energy characteristic x-rays. When measured in a plastic syringe, there is little attenuation of the characteristic x-rays, but substantial attenuation of the x-rays occurs with a glass container. Correction factors for glass can be as large as 25% and are usually indicated by the manufacturer.

The dose calibrator should be conveniently located within the radiopharmacy or hot lab, but should be in an area where the radiation background is constant throughout the day. Dose calibrators have the capability of resetting the zero level by sampling the background under operator control. Obtaining the correct activity reading requires that the operator has selected the appropriate button for the radionuclide being assayed. The biggest source of error with dose calibrator measurements occurs when the activated radionuclide button does not match the source being assayed. Dose calibrators that are used for assaying PET radionuclides or large quantities of other high energy gamma emitters are often mounted below the counter top. This allows for thicker shielding and easier access.

Dose Calibrator Quality Control

There are well established quality control tests for monitoring the performance of dose calibrators and 10 CFR 35.60b requires that they be performed in accordance with nationally recognized standards or the manufacturer's instructions. Table 3-1 lists the tests along with the recommended frequency. These tests are generally required as part of the radioactive material license and are therefore regulated by either the NRC or an agreement state. Failure to do these tests as described in the license results in citable events.

TABLE 3-1	Dose Calibrator Quality Control Procedures	
Test	**Source**	**Frequency**
Constancy	^{57}Co, ^{133}Ba, ^{137}Cs, ^{68}Ge	Daily before clinical use
Linearity	^{99m}Tc	Installation and quarterly
Accuracy	NIST standard (^{57}Co, ^{133}Ba, ^{137}Cs, ^{68}Ge)	Annually
Geometry	^{99m}Tc	Installation

Constancy Test. The constancy test is done each day before clinical use to verify that the dose calibrator measurements are reliable. There are two portions to this test. First, the reading for the long-lived radioactive source standards should be made with the appropriate settings for each source. Most often the standards are ^{57}Co, ^{133}Ba, and ^{137}Cs, although in PET-only labs a ^{68}Ga source may also be used. The daily measurements from these sources are plotted as points either on graph paper or with a computer program that includes an acceptable range of ±5% and also accounts for the decay of the source. Measurements falling outside the range of acceptance should trigger a repair action. The second part of the constancy test is done with ^{137}Cs placed in the calibrator and measurements are recorded for all the commonly used radionuclide settings. Changes in the recorded values indicate a problem that requires repair.

Linearity Test. The linearity test checks that the calibrator is able to assay the correct activity over the entire range of radioactivity used in your laboratory. This test is done using a vial or syringe of ^{99m}Tc whose activity is at least as large as the maximum activity normally assayed. There are two methods that are commonly used to evaluate linearity. One uses attenuation shields to change the apparent activity of the source and the other follows the decay of a test source.

The decay method does not require any additional apparatus, but activity of a ^{99m}Tc source has to be measured 3 times a day for up to 4 days. The ^{99m}Tc source containing the appropriate activity is measured at selected times, typically 8:00 AM, 12:00 PM, and 4:00 PM. The exact time is not crucial but has to be accurately known. This is continued until the source is assayed at less than 10 μCi. For a 100 mCi source that will take about 84 hours. The assayed values are plotted as a function of the measurement times on a semilogarithmic graph and compared with the expected activity values using a 6-hour half-life.

The alternate linearity method requires the purchase of a set of cylindrical attenuation shields that cover the source and change its apparent activity. The attenuation factors associated with each shield must first be determined using a dose calibrator that has been demonstrated to be linear. The test begins as above with assaying of a source of ^{99m}Tc that represents the maximum activity used in the clinic. Activity measurements are recorded along with the shield identifier as the attenuation shields are place over source. The expected activity for each shield is calculated by dividing the source activity by the shield attenuation factor. The plot of measured activity versus expected activity should yield a straight line with a slope of 1.

With either method, deviations of the measured activity greater than 5% from the expected value requires action to determine the cause and may trigger a service call.

Accuracy Test. The accuracy of the dose calibrator must be validated annually using calibrated radioactive sources traceable to the **National Institute of Standards and Technology (NIST)**. At least two sources with different principal photon energies such as ^{57}Co or ^{137}Cs should be used. The sources are assayed and the date, time, and measured activity are recorded. The source activity is determined from the calibrated activity corrected for the decay occurring between the calibration and measurement dates. Deviations greater than 5% from the expected amount require action.

Geometry Test. The geometry test monitors how the activity measurement changes with sample volume or configuration. This test should be done using a syringe of the size that is normally used for injections and also with glass vials if your clinic uses generators and radiopharmaceutical kits. The procedure for syringes and glass vials is similar. A 1- to 2-mCi sample of ^{99m}Tc in a small volume (~0.5 ml) is placed in the vessel and the activity is measured and recorded. A fixed volume (0.5 ml for the syringe, 2 ml for the vial) of nonradioactive water or saline is added to the vessel and the new measurement is recorded. This process is repeated until the volume of the syringe or vial is 67% full. The measurements with added volume are compared to initial assay. If any samples lie outside of ±5%, a correction table or graph to convert from measured activity to the actual activity must be available close to the dose calibrator. The geometry test is performed at installation and must be repeated if the dose calibrator is relocated or serviced.

SEMICONDUCTOR DETECTORS

Although gas **ionization detectors** directly convert absorbed gamma ray energy into electric charge, they have several disadvantages. The average amount of energy required to form an ion pair is high (34 eV) and gas detectors have very low intrinsic efficiency for stopping gamma rays (<1%) because of the low density of gas. Like ionization detectors, semiconductor (or solid state) detectors also convert absorbed gamma ray energy directly into electric charge, but are significantly better than gas detectors. Semiconductors not only have much higher intrinsic efficiency than gases, but the average amount of energy required to form charge pairs (in this

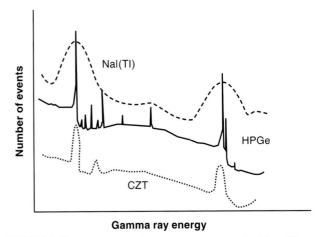

FIGURE 3-8 Comparison of energy spectra acquired by different detecting systems. The middle curve *(solid)* is from a HPGe and has superb energy resolution and can resolve many individual peaks. The upper curve *(broken line)* is from a NaI(Tl) detector with energy resolution that is substantially worse. CZT *(lower curve, dotted)* has significantly better energy resolution than NaI(Tl) although not as good as HPGe.

case mobile electrons and empty electron energy states called holes) is less than 2 eV. As a result, the signal from the absorption of a gamma ray is large enough that individual events can be processed with very good energy resolution. The more commonly used scintillation detectors discussed in the next section have only moderate energy resolution because of losses that occur in the collection of the scintillation light and in the conversion of the scintillation light into an electronic signal. With semiconductors the direct conversion of the absorbed energy into charge pairs eliminates the need for any additional stages with the associated signal losses. The improvement in energy resolution that is available from semiconductor detectors is illustrated in Figure 3-8.

A variety of semiconductor materials have been used as gamma ray detectors, although most of them have not been suitable for the gamma ray energies used in clinical nuclear medicine. It is possible to get exquisite energy resolution (~1% to 2%) with high purity germanium detectors (HPGe), but those detectors require liquid nitrogen cooling and because of the low atomic number of germanium are less efficient than the commonly used sodium iodide detectors discussed in the Scintillation Detectors section. HPGe detectors are used in research laboratories or radiation safety facilities where it is necessary to accurately identify individual radionuclide contaminants. For nuclear medicine applications, cadmium telluride (CdTe) or cadmium zinc telluride (CZT) are the semiconductor detectors of choice. These semiconductors have an effective atomic number of 50 with a density of 5.8 g/cm^3, yielding a much higher intrinsic efficiency than an equally thick NaI(Tl) crystal. It should be noted that sodium iodide crystals can be produced at any desired thickness, the effective thickness of CZT is limited to approximately 5 mm.

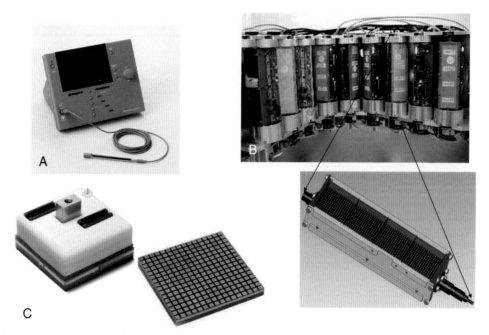

FIGURE 3-9 Examples of Solid State Semiconductor Detectors. A, Small surgical probe. **B,** Multiple imaging detectors for SPECT cardiac imaging. **C,** A small array of solid state imaging detectors.

A number of commercial devices used in nuclear medicine clinics are based on semiconductor detectors using CZT. These include hand held **probes** for lymphatic mapping, compact gamma cameras for scintimammography, and several cardiac SPECT systems. As shown in Figure 3-9, *A*, semiconductor probes can be made very compact and are well adapted for operating room procedures. CZT can be manufactured as a pixelated array of detectors where the **intrinsic resolution** is determined by the size of the individual detectors (Figure 3-9, *B-C*). Other advantages of pixelated detectors are discussed in the section on gamma cameras. The main problem associated with CZT pixelated arrays is the fabrication cost, which currently is significantly higher than that of sodium iodide specially for large area detectors.

SCINTILLATION DETECTORS

Scintillators emit low energy (visible) light photons when they absorb high energy x-rays or gamma rays. Scintillators are used in a wide variety of radiological imaging devices but are the primary detectors used in most nuclear medicine clinical procedures. Most scintillators used in the detection of gamma rays are inorganic crystals, although there are organic scintillators, which are generally used in the detection of low energy beta emitters.

Scintillations arise from energy transferred to electrons when a gamma ray interacts with the detector. Those energetic electrons have sufficient energy to excite a large number of electrons in the scintillator to a higher energy state. This means that the electrons will jump from lower energy states (called the valence band) to allowable high energy states (called the conduction band) that are separated by an energy gap of a few electron volts. The excited electrons will quickly fall back to the conduction band and will emit the energy associated with the band gap. Although a variety of mechanisms exist for dissipating this energy, one way is through the emission of photons whose energy is determined by the band gap, which for many materials is in the range of visible light. The fraction of energy emitted as photons can be enhanced by adding small amounts (parts per million) of an activator material such as thallium (Tl).

There are a wide variety of scintillators in use within nuclear medicine, and each of them has different properties that affect their performance. The key properties of some commonly used scintillators in nuclear medicine and PET are summarized in Table 3-2. The intrinsic efficiency is primarily determined by the density and effective atomic number of the detecting material. Although high density and atomic number are desirable for all gamma ray detectors, they are especially important for detecting the high energy annihilation photons. Energy resolution depends on the intensity of the scintillation and how well the light can be collected. Because the detector is often coupled to the glass window of a photomultiplier tube, the transmission of the scintillation to the photocathode is enhanced if the index of refraction of the detector is close to that of glass (1.5). None of the detectors are ideal in this regard and an optical coupling grease is used to minimize reflection between the surfaces.

TABLE 3-2	Properties of Commonly Used Scintillators				
Scintillator	Sodium Iodide NaI(Tl)	Cesium Iodide CsI(Tl)	Bismuth Germanate BGO	Lutetium Oxyorthosilicate LSO	Gadolinium Oxyorthosilicate GSO
Atomic number	51	54	74	66	59
Density (g/cm^3)	3.67	4.51	7.13	7.4	6.71
Index of refraction	1.85	1.8	2.15	1.82	1.85
Wavelength (nm)	410	565	480	420	430
Relative light output	100	45 (130)	15	75	41
Decay time (nsec)	230	1000	300	40	60

Scintillators require an additional stage to convert the scintillation into an electronic signal. The fraction of the light energy that results in an electronic signal is called the conversion or quantum efficiency. The conversion efficiency of the photomultiplier tube and avalanche photodiode (discussed later) depend on the wavelength of the scintillation. For example, photomultiplier tubes perform better with shorter wavelength light from sodium iodide (NaI[Tl]), whereas the infrared light emitted by cesium iodide (CsI[Tl]) is better suited for detection by avalanche photodiodes instead of photomultiplier tubes (PMTs). The resolving or dead time of a scintillation detector is determined by how long the scintillation light persists. This is important for precise timing in coincidence detection as well as for handling high counting rates.

Most detectors used for nuclear medicine studies rely on thallium activated sodium iodide, NaI(Tl). NaI(Tl) has a relatively high light output, and the output of other scintillators is often reported using NaI(Tl) as the standard. With an effective atomic number of 50 and a density of 3.67 g/cm^3, it has a relatively high intrinsic efficiency for gamma rays below 200 keV. Sodium iodide is manufactured in a wide variety of shapes and sizes, ranging from pixelated detectors as small as 2 to 3 mm to gamma camera detectors with dimensions of 55 × 40 cm. The disadvantages of NaI(Tl) include a sensitivity to cracking from mechanical stress and temperature changes as well as the need for hermetic sealing. NaI(Tl) is hygroscopic (absorbs water from the air) and turns yellow if exposed to any moisture, causing both a degradation of energy resolution and image artifacts.

Detector Electronics

Those devices that process individual gamma ray detection events produce electronic signals often referred to as pulses. The electronic pulses reflect the energy deposited in the detector by their size or pulse height. A number of electronic components are required to produce and analyze the event pulses. These include the detector material, a photon transducer (for scintillators), a preamplifier for powering the signal to the downstream components, an amplifier for shaping and increasing the pulse size, a pulse height analyzer for selecting specific energy ranges and scalars or rate meters for counting the number of selected events. These components are shown schematically in Figure 3-10.

Scintillators convert absorbed gamma ray energy into visible light and required an additional component to convert the scintillation into an electronic pulse. For more than 50 years, the **photomultiplier tube (PMT)** has been used in this application (Figure 3-11, *A*). Although PMTs are bulky vacuum tubes that have a conversion efficiency on the order of 25% to 30%, they have a very high gain and that has kept them competitive. The scintillation light photoelectrically ejects electrons from the front surface of the PMT, which is coated with a film of cesium antimony (the photocathode). These electrons are accelerated through a series of 8 to 11 electrodes called **dynodes** that are at successively higher voltage levels. The voltage level of the dynodes is controlled by a very stable high voltage supply that is typically set in the range of 800 to 1200 V. At each dynode, the impact of each incoming electron knocks out 4 to 5 additional electrons. The electronic signal increases geometrically so that the overall gain is on the order of several million. The resulting signal at the output of the PMT retains its dependence on the initial deposition of gamma ray energy. It is imperative that the high voltage power supplied to PMTs be stable, therefore it is usual practice to never turn off the power. Temperature changes in the clinic may cause drifting of the high voltage and electronics and the PMT gain will become unstable.

Although the PMT continues to be used as the photon transducer in scintillation detectors, other devices are posed to replace them. The solid state avalanche photodiodes (APD) is already being used in one commercial gamma camera (Figure 3-11, *B*). APDs are much more compact than PMTs, have a much higher conversion efficiency (60% to 90%), especially for infrared photons, and are insensitive to magnetic fields. However, the signal gain is substantially less than that of a PMT (200 vs. 1,000,000), and for gamma cameras using NaI(Tl), PMTs perform better, even with their shortcomings. Recently, solid state silicon photomultipliers (SPM) with

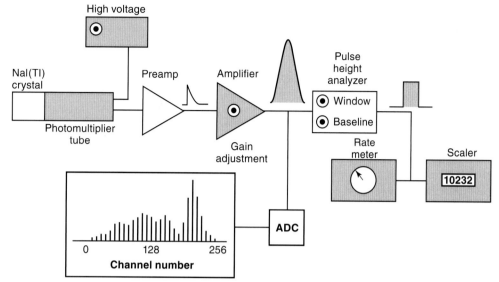

FIGURE 3-10 Scintillation Detector Electronics. The scintillation light from the detected event is converted into an electronic signal by the PMT. The PMT signal is shaped and amplified before the PHA judges whether the signal falls in the selected energy window. The pulse generated by window events is counted by a scaler or rate meter. *ADC,* Analog-to-digital converter.

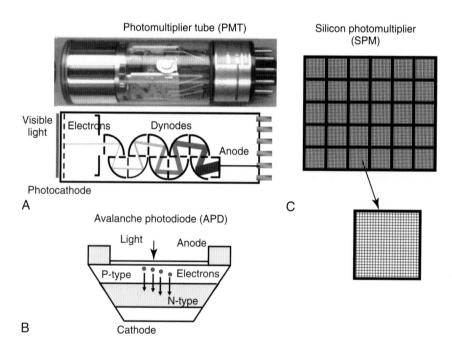

FIGURE 3-11 Photon Transducers. A, Photomultiplier tubes have been used for more than 5 decades to change visible light into an electronic signal. **B,** Avalanche photodiodes are solid state devices that have been used in several detecting systems in place of PMTs, but are limited by their relatively low amplification. **C,** Silicon photomultipliers combine the detection efficiency of the APD with the high gain amplification of the PMT.

high gains based on APD technology have been developed and are being incorporated into several research scintillation detectors. The sensitive element of the SPM has an array of very small photodiodes that operate like a GM tube (Figure 3-11, *C*). Any light detected by one of these subelements generates a high gain signal that indicates it has been hit. At low light levels like those associated with scintillation, a linear relationship exists between the light intensity and the number of subelements that fire. SPMs are being rapidly developed and it is likely that they will find their way into clinical devices in the near future.

The electronic pulses generated from the PMT or other photon converters generally do not have enough power to make it to the other components of the detecting systems. The role of the preamplifiers (preamps) is to boost the signal power and it functions in much the same way as a preamp in audio systems. Preamps are sometimes referred to as impedance matchers since they effectively reduce the high output impedance of devices like the PMT to match the effective impedance of the transmission cables.

The electronic signal generated by the PMT from the scintillation event rises very fast and then decays exponentially giving a long tail. The amplitude of this pulse carries the energy information, but it is not easy to analyze because of both its shape and low voltage level. The main amplifier changes the shape of the pulse so that it is more symmetrical and easier to determine its amplitude (pulse height). It also permits scaling the pulse to a convenient voltage range for pulse height analyzer.

Once the PMT high voltage level and the amplifier gain are set, the only thing that changes the size of the electronic pulse is the energy absorbed in the detector. As a result, the pulse height is an indicator of gamma ray energy. The **pulse height analyzer (PHA)** receives the output of the amplifier and determines if it falls within a selected energy range on the basis of the pulse height. The electronics within the PHA checks the height of the pulse against lower and upper voltage levels. If the pulse height is within the defined range, the PHA puts out a standard sized pulse that will be transmitted to a scaler or rate meter; otherwise no signal is generated. The PHA consists of three components: a lower level discriminator, an upper level discriminator, and an anticoincidence circuit that determines when the lower discriminator is triggered but not the upper energy discriminator, signaling that a pulse is received between the two windows.

The PHA is usually adjusted to collect photopeak events and a 15% to 20% energy window is set symmetrically over the photopeak. For ^{99m}Tc, a 15% energy window has a width of 21 keV and would range from 129.5 to 150.5 keV. A 20% energy window for ^{131}I at 364 keV has a width of 72.8 keV and ranges from 327.6 to 400.4 keV. In the early days of nuclear medicine, energy windows would be set manually by maximizing the count rate as the window was moved along the spectrum by increasing the baseline setting. In all modern counting systems, the energy windows are automatically set on the photopeak using software that finds the appropriate peaks in the spectra generated by a device called a **multichannel analyzer (MCA)**.

The MCA uses an analog to digital converter to change the electronic pulse into a number whose magnitude is determine by the pulse height. This number is linked to a memory location (channel) that is incremented each time it is accessed. Since the channels correspond to pulse height they also correspond to gamma ray energy. The MCA displays the contents of the channels and refreshes the display with each new event, giving a real-time display of the energy spectrum from the detector. Nearly all modern counting and imaging systems incorporate MCAs.

Spectroscopy with Sodium Iodide Detectors

A graph of the number of events from a detector as a function of pulse height is called an energy spectrum because of the direct relationship between the energy deposited in the detector and the associated pulse height (see Figure 3-8). Gamma ray spectra have several distinct features that are associated with different interactions that occur either in the detector or in the immediate vicinity of the detector. These features include the photopeak, Compton edge, Compton plateau, lead fluorescence peak, backscatter peak, escape peaks, and coincidence sum peak.

Photopeak. The total absorption of the gamma ray by photoelectric absorption or combined Compton scatter and photoelectric absorption results in pulses of the same average height leading to a distinctive feature on the energy spectrum called the photopeak (Figure 3-12, *A*). For most gamma ray energies used in nuclear medicine, total absorption is the most likely interaction, so the photopeak is usually the most prominent feature. Even

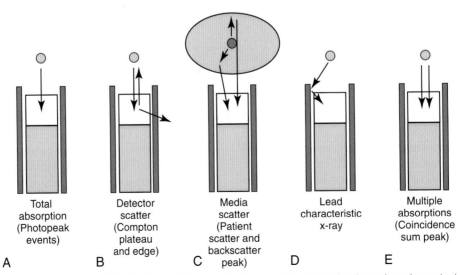

Total absorption (Photopeak events)

Detector scatter (Compton plateau and edge)

Media scatter (Patient scatter and backscatter peak)

Lead characteristic x-ray

Multiple absorptions (Coincidence sum peak)

A   B   C   D   E

FIGURE 3-12 Gamma Ray Interactions Resulting in Spectral Features. A, Photoelectric interaction (complete absorption). **B,** Compton interaction. **C,** Scatter from patient or backscatter. **D,** Lead characteristic x-ray production. **E,** Coincidence summed peak detection.

though all the gamma rays from any transition have the same energy, the photopeak is broadened because of the finite energy resolution of NaI(Tl).

Compton Plateau and Edge. Some gamma rays will have Compton scattering interactions in the detector and the scattered photon will leave without further absorption (Figure 3-12, *B*). In that case, a portion of the gamma ray energy will be given to the scattered electron resulting in an event. The amount of energy deposited in the detector depends on the scattering angle leading to a broad relatively flat feature on the spectrum called the Compton plateau. The range of the Compton plateau extends from 0 (small angle scatter where little energy is transferred to the detector) to the maximum electron energy transfer that occurs when the gamma ray is scattered at 180 degrees, directly opposite its initial direction (backscatter). The sharp drop-off associated with detector backscatter is another distinct feature called the Compton edge. For low-energy gamma rays like ^{99m}Tc, the Compton edge is at a relatively low energy and is often obscured by other features. It is more apparent on the energy spectra from ^{131}I and ^{18}F.

Media Scatter and the Backscatter Peak. Gamma rays from a radioactive source immersed in water or in a patient will have Compton scatter interactions (Figure 3-12, *C*). The scattered photons from these interactions often reach the detector where they are absorbed, imposing a scatter feature on the spectrum. The energy of these scatter photons ranges from the maximum gamma ray energy (small angle scatter where little energy is lost by the gamma ray) to backscatter, where the energy of the scattered photon is lowest. The backscattered photons are preferentially detected because they follow the same path as the primary gamma rays creating another distinctive peak on the energy spectrum. Scattered radiation within the source distribution (e.g., patient) are not useful since they will have originated outside the collimated field of view. By accepting only photopeak events the amount of scattered radiation is substantially reduced but is still present because of the less than perfect energy resolution of the detector.

Lead Fluorescent Peak. Most gamma ray detectors are surrounded by lead shielding to reduce the background count rate (Figure 3-12, *D*). When gamma rays are photoelectrically absorbed in the shielding, lead characteristic x-rays are emitted and absorbed in the detector creating a peak in the energy range of 80 to 88 keV.

Coincidence Sum Peak. The processing time for a detected event with NaI(Tl) is approximately 1 μsec. If more than one gamma ray absorption occurs within that time interval, the intensity of the scintillation is increased and the resulting pulse height is falsely associated with a single event of increased gamma ray energy (Figure 3-12, *E*). When this occurs frequently, it shows up as a distinctive peak. Coincidence sum peaks are generally only observed on most detectors when the event rates are very high, but they are common in well counters even

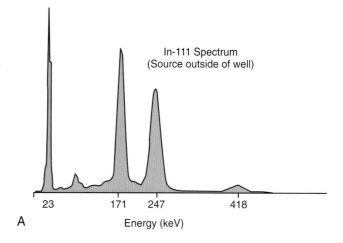

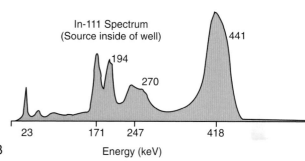

FIGURE 3-13 Comparison of ^{111}In Spectra. A, Source outside of the well or from a gamma camera demonstrates separate photopeaks. **B,** Source located in the well. Coincidence sum peaks from the simultaneous absorption of the two ^{111}In gamma rays along with the characteristic Cd x-ray becomes very likely in this geometry and cause a significant alteration of the spectrum.

when the event rate is low with radionuclides that emit multiple photons in a cascade. An example of an ^{111}In spectrum illustrating this is shown in Figure 3-13. Figure 3-13, *A*, shows the ^{111}In spectrum when the source is located outside the well. When the source is put inside the well, one obtains the spectrum shown in Figure 3-13, *B*, which shows coincidence peaks resulting from the simultaneous absorption of both 171- and 247-keV gamma rays as well as the absorption of the 23-keV characteristic x-ray.

Escape Peaks. When a gamma ray is photoelectrically absorbed, the initial energy transferred to the photoelectron is smaller than the gamma ray energy by about 28 keV, which is the binding energy of an iodine K shell electron. However, the iodine atom very quickly emits characteristic radiation as the inner shell vacancy is filled. Most often the characteristic radiation is also absorbed in the detector and it combines with the photoelectron to yield a signal corresponding to the full gamma ray energy. With low energy gamma rays (<100 keV) that are absorbed very close to the surface of the detector, the characteristic radiation may leave the surface without being absorbed creating a false peak that is 28 keV lower than the actual photopeak. This false peak is called the iodine escape peak and it is most apparent in the spectrum from ^{133}Xe. Other escape peaks associated with annihilation radiation can occur for very high energy gamma rays (>1.02 MeV) that have pair production interactions.

SCINTILLATION COUNTING SYSTEMS

Thyroid probes and well counters are remnants of the earliest era of nuclear medicine, but are still actively used. Well counters and thyroid probes use NaI(Tl) as the detector material with the standard electronic components discussed above. All of the devices produced in the last 10 years are computer controlled so that the operator does not have direct access to high voltage or amplifier adjustments.

Thyroid probes are used for iodine uptake studies, which may be performed with either ^{123}I or ^{131}I (Figure 3-14, *A*). The detectors are cylindrical with a diameter of 5 cm and to accommodate the high energy gamma rays from ^{131}I, they are often 5 cm thick. The detectors and the integrally mounted PMT are placed inside a housing that acts as a shield and the detector is recessed

by 5 to 10 cm to provide coarse collimation. The thyroid probe apparatus includes a mechanical support and a distance gauge for positioning the probe at a fixed distance from the patient's throat.

Well counters are used to count a variety of radionuclides; they are 7.5 cm in diameter and may be 5 to 7.5 cm thick. A hole large enough to accommodate a test tube is drilled into the detector so that the source can be located inside this well, creating nearly 4π geometry. Because of the high efficiency associated with well counters, very low activity samples below the nanocurie level can be accurately assayed and they are frequently employed for counting test samples and contamination survey wipes. The high efficiency limits the maximum amount of activity that can accurately assayed to about 1 μCi unless dead corrections are made. Well counters can be manually operated (Figure 3-14, *B*) or automated systems (Figure 3-14, *C*) where multiple samples can be counted and recorded sequentially under program control.

The quality control for well counters and thyroid probes is similar. Routine calibration is required to make

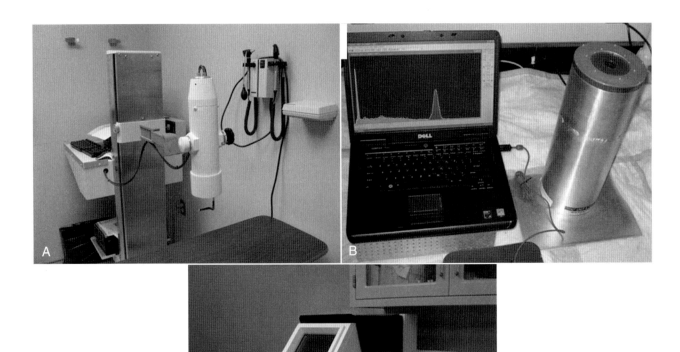

FIGURE 3-14 Nuclear Medicine NaI(Tl) Counting Systems. A, Thyroid probe with flat field collimator. **B,** Manual single sample well counter. **C,** Automated multisample well counter.

sure the photopeak settings for the radionuclides being assayed are correct. The calibration protocol is usually vendor specific and requires the counting of each specific radionuclide that is used with the detector on a quarterly basis. The stability of the system is checked with a constancy test using ^{137}Cs to verify that the gain settings or high voltage have not drifted. A chi-square evaluation is required at least quarterly and is done by collecting 10 measurements from the ^{137}Cs standard and verifying that result falls within the 0.1 to 0.9 probability range (see Chapter 1 for details). Energy resolution is also evaluated quarterly with a ^{137}Cs source or other monoenergetic source and may be reported as verification of the calibration procedure.

Coincidence Detection

Coincidence detection can be used for a variety of different scientific applications, but in nuclear medicine, it is primarily used for the detection of annihilation radiation from positron emitting radionuclides. Opposed detectors register events independently, but a valid count is only recorded if both detectors record an event within a specified time interval. Coincidence detection provides spatial resolution that primarily depends on the detector face size and better spatial resolution can be obtained by using smaller detectors. For conventional PET imaging systems, the coincidence time window is about 5 to 12 nsec. PET systems with fast detectors like lutetium oxyorthosilicate (LSO) and the optimized electronics may reduce the time window down to 0.6 nsec. This is fast enough to provide time-of-flight localization with an accuracy of about 9 cm. When this information is incorporated into the reconstruction algorithm, there is a substantial improvement in the noise level leading to better image quality, especially in large patients.

Liquid Scintillation Detectors

Low-energy beta emission from radionuclides such as ^{3}H and ^{14}C cannot penetrate the aluminum cans that protect NaI(Tl) detectors from moisture. These radionuclides are often used as research tracers for investigating macromolecules and require a different detection approach using liquid scintillators. For liquid scintillation counting the radioactive samples are dissolved in a solution that also contains organic liquid scintillators referred to as a scintillation cocktail. The radiotracer is in direct contact with the scintillating materials, and the beta energy that is emitted generates scintillations in the cocktail. The mixture often includes a secondary liquid scintillator, which absorbs the light from the primary scintillator and reemits it at a lower wavelength that is more suitable for the photomultipliers positioned on either side of the sample, inside a lighttight enclosure. The signals from the photomultiplier tubes are processed in a manner similar to that described for the conventional detectors.

A number of things can cause the scintillation light to be absorbed in the liquid scintillation cocktail before it can be detected. This absorption is referred to as quenching. The amount of quenching is affected by optical and chemical properties of the counting sample and a variety of techniques exist for quench compensation.

The only nuclear medicine procedure that requires liquid scintillation counters is the ^{14}C-14 urea breath test patients with ulcers. The bacteria *Helicobacter pylori* is the causative agent in many ulcers and produces the enzyme urease which is not present in normal human tissue. Patients with suspected *H. pylori* infection are administered ^{14}C-labeled urea. If urease is present, the urea ^{14}C is hydrolyzed into ammonia and $^{14}CO_2$, which is ultimately exhaled through the lungs. The exhaled breath of the patient is captured and dissolved into liquid scintillation samples for subsequent counting. The presence of $^{14}CO_2$ in the exhaled breath confirms active *H. pylori* infection.

GAMMA CAMERAS

The vast majority of all clinical nuclear medicine studies are based on the imaging of the internal distribution of one or more radiopharmaceuticals with a gamma camera. The term gamma camera refers to a device that can image the distribution of a gamma emitting radionuclide. A gamma camera requires a gamma ray detector, a **collimator** to act as the imaging forming aperture, pulse height analysis for selecting specific gamma ray energies and a computer for recording and displaying acquired events. Although many approaches to gamma ray imaging have evolved, they all incorporate these features. Gamma cameras that use scintillators as the detector are referred to as **scintillation cameras.** Scintillation cameras that have one large detector and obtain the event locations from averaging PMT signals are called Anger cameras after the inventor of that approach. A diagram of a clinical scintillation camera is shown in Figure 3-15. Gamma cameras that do not use a scintillation crystal and PMT currently use CZT as the detector are called solid state or semiconductor cameras.

Anger Scintillation Camera

In the late 1950s, Hal O. Anger developed the scintillation camera. Although his initial device had a very small field of view, it used only pinhole collimation and had to remain vertically oriented, but it had all of the design components of the modern gamma camera. This included one large NaI(Tl) detector that was covered by an array of PMTs, which was used to determine the position and energy of the detected events. Anger determined where events occurred by averaging the modified signals from all the photomultiplier tube where the weighting factors were determined by the physical location of each individual photomultiplier tube. This approach has become

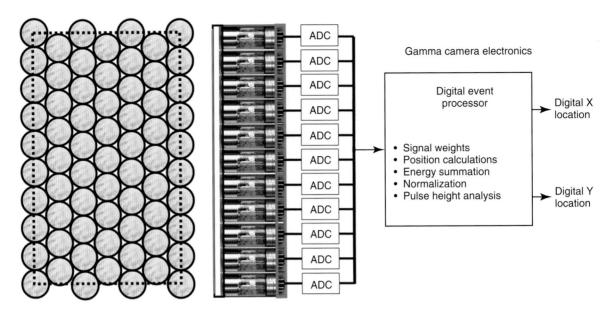

FIGURE 3-15 Schematic of a Scintillation Camera. An array of PMTs covers the large thin NaI(Tl) detector. Signals from many PMTs are digitized and summed with position weighting to determine the event location. Unweighted signals are summed to determine the energy of the detected event, and if the energy falls in the selected window, the event is registered. *ADC*, Analog-to-digital converter.

known as Anger logic and a variation of that logic circuit is still in use in most scintillation camera systems.

Modern Scintillation Cameras

Scintillation cameras based on the Anger design all use a large, thin NaI(Tl) crystal as the detector. General purpose gamma cameras often use a rectangular detector with approximate dimensions of 400 × 500 mm with a thickness of 9.6 mm. In order to determine the position and absorbed energy of a gamma ray interaction on the detector, an array of PMTs that spans the detector size is used. The PMT array consists of a close packed array of PMTs that are usually 50 to 75 mm (2 to 3 inches) across. PMTs with circular, hexagonal, and square shapes have all been used by different manufacturers. Circular or hexagonal tubes are packed in a hexagonal array as shown in Figure 3-15, while square tubes are packed rectilinearly. Between the detector and the PMT array, there may be a light pipe. The light pipe is a piece of transparent material such as optical quality glass, quartz, or optical quality plastic that allows the scintillation light to spread as it exits the crystal. In early implementations, the light pipe was very thick, but it has become progressively thinner and has even been eliminated in some commercial gamma cameras.

When the scintillation camera was first introduced, there were essentially no digital electronic systems, so all the signal processing had to be done with discrete analog components. For example, the PMT weighting factors were set determined by resistors or capacitors. In modern gamma cameras, digital signal processing is used for that

purpose. The PMTs still generate an analog signal whose amplitude is determined by the amount of light they collect. The output from each PMT is converted to a number by a high precision analog-to-digital converter (ADC). From that point, the processing of the information is handled algorithmically (Figure 3-15).

The scintillation light from the NaI(Tl) generates electronic signals in the PMTs closest to the detection event. The digitized signals from each PMT in the vicinity are added together to determine the energy associated with the event. If the magnitude of the combined signal falls within selected energy window, the event is valid. At the same time, the PMT signals are modified by weighting factors that depend on the location of each tube within the PMT array. Separate weighting factors are used to determine the x and y event locations. When the PMT signals modified by their position weighting factors are added together, the location of the event is determined with spatial resolution accuracy of about 3.5 mm, which is much smaller than the size of a PMT. This approach has a problem, however. Because the PMT signals depend on the amount of light collected, the apparent x and y values are also influenced by the total light collected, and the size of an image changes with gamma ray energy. To avoid that, the position signals are divided (normalized) by the energy signal, which as you recall, represents the total light signal. This normalization keeps the image size of a distribution constant regardless of the energy of the gamma ray. It also helps maintain good spatial resolution since it eliminates the blurring that would occur from the apparent fluctuation in pulse height that occurs because of the finite energy resolution of the scintillation camera.

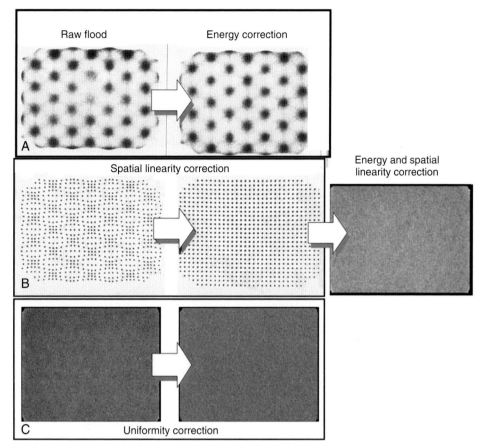

Raw flood   Energy correction

A

Spatial linearity correction

Energy and spatial
linearity correction

B

C   Uniformity correction

FIGURE 3-16 **Scintillation Camera Corrections.** **A,** Energy correction compensates for regional spectral shifts. **B,** Spatial linearity correction uses a lookup table from a calibration study to reposition events on the fly. **C,** A reference uniformity flood image is used to correct for any residual nonuniformities left after spatial linearity correction.

SCINTILLATION CAMERA CORRECTIONS

Scintillation camera manufacturers each have their individual patented devices and processes for correction techniques. This text will describe these correction techniques in general terms as an introduction to the processes for energy, linearity, and flood uniformity correction.

Energy Correction

Because the response of a PMT to the light generated from an absorbed gamma ray is not ideal, the method for localizing gamma ray interactions on the detector requires corrections to ensure accuracy of event position and to generate a usable image. The first correction that is applied is energy correction. The energy signal representing the total collected light from an interaction varies across the detector because the PMT coverage is not uniform. This results in energy spectrum shifts depending on whether the interaction occurs directly under a PMT or between them. With digital electronics, a matrix of energy windows is set with a finely adjusted PHA window for each pixel to keep the local photopeak centered. This not only improves the overall energy

resolution of the system, but ensures that each portion of the detector is only accepting photoelectric events and that scatter events are rejected. Energy correction is necessary for good camera performance, but far from sufficient because it does little to improve the main cause of poor uniformity, which is mispositioning of events (Figure 3-16, *A*).

Spatial Linearity Correction

The accuracy of the positioning of detected events is referred to as spatial linearity, and scintillation cameras that only rely on Anger logic or other centroid methods have poor spatial linearity. This is primarily the result of the less than ideal PMT response. Ideally, the signal from the PMT would change uniformly as a source is moved toward the PMT. In reality, the signal is relatively flat when the source is directly under the PMT and this behavior is accentuated for thin light pipes. Although thin light pipes result in a stronger signal that improves spatial resolution, they create more location distortion. This mispositioning of events not only creates a pincushion affect, it makes the field uniformity very poor (Figure 3-16, *B*). Fortunately, the distortion is very reproducible and can be mediated by having a table of position-based correction factors. The correction factors are obtained by imaging a precise rectangular array of holes exposed with a point source of ^{99m}Tc. The difference between the image and actual location of the holes provides the correction factors that are stored in a lookup table. When a valid event is detected, its calculated position points to the appropriate correction factors, which are applied with essentially no time loss. As can be seen in Figure 3-16, *B*, the application of spatial linearity correction has a profound effect on image uniformity.

Uniformity Correction

The image uniformity with combined energy and spatial linearity correction is probably sufficient for most conventional gamma camera planar imaging, but corrections for residual nonuniformities are required for **single photon emission computed tomography (SPECT)** imaging. Most commonly, a high count reference flood image is acquired (30 to 200 million counts) to form a correction map. Areas of the image with increased count density have factors that selectively ignore or skim counts. Using uniformity correction is the last step after energy and spatial linearity correction. Uniformity correction provides an image with uniformity of approximately ±3% with little loss in count sensitivity (Figure 3-16, *C*).

Photomultiplier Stabilization

Photomultiplier tubes are fairly unstable devices. Their gains are influenced by temperature, humidity, and magnetic fields; also, performance changes as they age. In order for energy and spatial linearity corrections to remain valid, they have to be a compensatory system to maintain the PMTs at their calibration levels. All gamma cameras have PMT stabilization of some kind. One common approach is to have one or more stable light-emitting diodes (LEDs) within the camera head that illuminates the PMT with a constant light intensity. PMT stability is maintained by varying the local high voltage levels to keep the response to this source constant. Another approach bases the PMT tuning on the relative count rate between two energy windows offset to the high energy side of the photopeak.

IMAGE ACQUISITION

Gamma cameras generate images by accumulating valid events (those that fall in the selected energy window). There are two basic approaches to acquiring gamma camera image data: list and frame mode. With list mode, the *x* and *y* locations along with a time stamp and potentially other information such as a gate signal are stored sequentially in a list of the events as they occurred. It is a straightforward process to generate an image from list mode data with a great deal of flexibility regarding

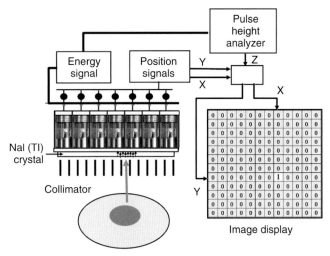

FIGURE 3-17 Scintillation Camera Image Formation. A valid event points to a location in a computer array corresponding to the event position on the detector. The location is incremented.

matrix size and frame time. Few gamma camera systems provide list mode capabilities at present.

By far the most common way of acquiring gamma camera events is in matrix or frame mode, which is illustrated in Figure 3-17. An image matrix is set up in computer memory for the designated acquisition. When a valid event is detected, the matrix location corresponding to the event *x* and *y* positions is incremented (i.e., one additional count is added to the contents). This continues until the acquisition reaches its predetermined stopping limit of either total accumulated counts or acquisition time.

Scintillation cameras can acquire images in different ways depending on the clinical application. These are generally classified as static, dynamic, gated, whole body, or SPECT studies. Static images or spot views are used to acquire images of the fixed distributions of the radiopharmaceuticals within the patient. Often a series of static images are acquired from several projection orientations. Dynamic studies record how the radiopharmaceutical distribution changes with time. Sequential image frames are acquired with the total number of frames and the imaging time per frame set by the operator. Dynamic studies can also be acquired with multiple phases where the frame time and number of frames in each dynamic phase can be set independently. The image matrix size used in dynamic studies is typically a 64 × 64 or 128 × 128 matrix; because the data density is somewhat low, fine image detail is not captured. Scintillation cameras can also accommodate cardiac and other physiological gating to capture the motion in organs like the heart that have repetitive motion. In gated blood pool imaging, images (usually a 64 × 64 matrix with 1.2 to 1.4 zoom) are acquired in multiple time bins that span the R-R interval of the electrocardiographic (ECG) signal obtained from the patient. Usually, the R-R interval is divided into 24 bins or frames where each time frame is

Parallel hole collimator

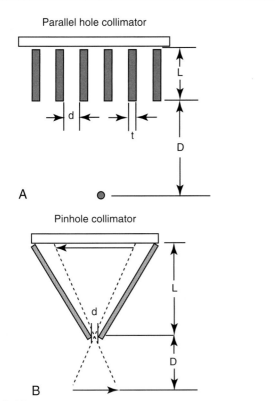

FIGURE 3-18 Collimator Parameters. A, Parallel hole collimator. B, Pinhole collimator.

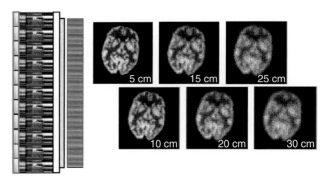

FIGURE 3-19 Parallel hole collimator resolution degrades the test image as the distance to between the collimator and the object increases.

20 to 50 msec depending on the patient's heart rate. A separate image is acquired for each time bin over several hundred heartbeats until an appropriate the image count density is reached.

Whole body imaging is used primarily for bone scans or tumor imaging studies. For these studies, the patient is translated on the bed in front of one gamma camera or more often two opposed gamma cameras. Some camera systems acquire separate spot images where the bed translates the whole field of view at the completion of each spot image, whereas others acquire the images continually as the patient moves uniformly between the detectors. For SPECT imaging, gamma cameras are mounted on a gantry that can rotate about the patient. SPECT acquisition and processing is discussed in detail in Chapter 9.

COLLIMATION

The collimator is the image-forming aperture of the gamma camera. Gamma rays are emitted in all directions from radioactive sources and cannot be focused like visible light. Collimators provide the means for projecting the gamma rays onto the detector by selective absorption. Only those gamma rays that travel on a trajectory that takes them directly through the collimator holes will hit the detector. This approach produces images but at the price of count sensitivity, since only less than 0.1%

of the gamma rays make it through the collimator. Collimators are made from high atomic number, high density materials such as lead and tungsten; even gold and uranium have been used for some research applications. Most collimators used in clinical imaging are multiholed with lead walls (septa) in a parallel geometry. The apertures of pinhole collimators are usually made from tungsten in order to prevent mechanical damage.

Collimator Resolution

The collimator contribution to spatial resolution depends on the configuration of the holes and is referred to as geometric resolution. For a parallel hole collimator, the geometric resolution can be estimated from a simple formula:

Equation 3-5
$$R_{coll} = d(D+L)/L$$

Referring to Figure 3-18, A, d is the hole size, L is the length of the hole and D is the distance from the source to the collimator. Anything that makes R_{coll} smaller improves spatial resolution. Decreasing the hole size and increasing the hole length both yield better spatial resolution. The standard distance for calculating collimator resolution is 100 mm from the front of the collimator, based on the recognition that internally distributed sources will often be that far away. Since collimator hole lengths are usually less than 40 mm, the sum D + L is dominated by D and the main effect of varying L is manifested in the denominator. Figure 3-19 illustrates how collimator spatial resolution degrades as the source to collimator distance increases.

Collimator Sensitivity

The count sensitivity of a parallel hole collimator is a bit more complicated but is also largely determined by the hole size and length:

Equation 3-6
$$S_{coll} = K(d/L)^2 \times d^2/(d+t)^2$$

The constant K depends on the geometry of the holes, which could be circular, hexagonal, triangular, or even square; d and L are the hole size and length described previously, and t is the septal thickness. The term $d^2/(d + t)^2$ accounts for the fraction of area available and is close to 1 for low energy collimators. For example, a high-resolution collimator may have a hole size of 1.2 mm and a septal thickness of 0.15 mm, leading to an area fraction of 0.8. The primary factor affecting the collimator sensitivity is $(d/L)^2$. To improve sensitivity, d/L should be large, which favors large hole size and short hole length to maximize sensitivity. Spatial resolution also depends on the d/L ratio but in the opposite way. Thus sensitivity is proportional to R_{coll}^2, and collimators represent a compromise between the competing factors of resolution and sensitivity. Since the optimal collimation can depend on the imaging situation, a variety of collimators of with different spatial resolutions are available. Collimators for imaging low energies (<160 keV) are typically classified as general purpose, high-resolution, or ultra–high-resolution collimators, although there is no standardization for these categories, and one vendor's general purpose collimator may be similar to another vendor's high-resolution collimator. For many clinical applications with ^{99m}Tc radiotracers, high-resolution collimators are most commonly used. General purpose collimators may be used for first pass cardiac and dynamic imaging, and ultra–high-resolution collimators may be used for bone spot imaging.

Imaging with parallel hole collimators demands a trade-off of resolution versus better sensitivity or inversely better resolution with poorer sensitivity. Other parallel hole collimators for imaging ^{67}Ga and ^{111}In are referred to as medium-energy collimators (<280 keV), and collimators for imaging ^{131}I (364 keV) are called high-energy collimators.

Pinhole Collimators

Clinically, pinhole collimators are most often used to image the thyroid gland or wrist or ankle joint, or is used for special pediatric applications. Although the pinhole sensitivity is low compared to a parallel hole collimator, it is capable of much better spatial resolution. Pinhole collimation can potentially make more efficient use of the detector area by magnifying the distribution being imaged. The magnification factor is L/D, where L is the distance from the detector to the pinhole and D is the distance from the pinhole to the source, as shown in Figure 3-18, B. Magnification also directly improves the effective intrinsic resolution (R_{int}) of the detector from its nominal value of R_{int} to $R_{int}D/L$. The geometric spatial resolution of a pinhole collimator is $d(L + D)/L$, where L and D are defined as before and d is the diameter of the pinhole. Since D is usually small compared to L, the geometric resolution is limited by the size of the pinhole, typically 4 to 7 mm. For very small distributions like those in research imaging of mice and rats, special pinhole collimators can provide submillimeter spatial resolution that exceeds the very best PET systems. Unfortunately pinhole imaging is not well suited for large distributions because of the strong decrease in sensitivity for sources that are not directly in-line with the pinhole and because of the varying magnification and field size for sources located at different distances from the pinhole.

Fabrication

Multihole low-energy collimators are either cast from molds or constructed from lead foils. All medium-energy and high-energy collimators are manufactured by casting molten lead alloy around a pattern of pins to form the holes in the collimator. Also, many low energy collimators are formed by the casting method. Foil collimators are constructed from corrugated foil sheets that when placed precisely together form holes from the pattern of the corrugation. The parameters that determine spatial resolution are the collimator thickness (i.e., hole length) and the hole size and shape. Longer and smaller holes produce better spatial resolution. These parameters also affect the count sensitivity but in an inverse way: shorter and larger holes produce better count sensitivity. The thickness of the hole walls (septa) also affects count sensitivity. The septal thickness is a trade-off between cross talk (septal penetration) between the holes and the count sensitivity. For low-energy gamma rays (<160 keV), the septal walls are less than 0.2 mm thick, whereas for a collimator designed for ^{131}I, the septal walls are 2 mm thick. As a result, high-energy collimators have poorer spatial resolution and sensitivity than their low-energy counterparts and are considerably heavier. It should be realized that collimators are relatively fragile devices that can easily be damaged by collisions with tables or other hard objects.

Most collimators used for conventional imaging are multihole parallel collimators as shown in Figure 3-20, A. These collimators produce a direct projection of the internal distribution of gamma emitting radionuclides onto the detector without any magnification. Several nonparallel hole collimators are available for either image minification or magnification. Small field of view gamma cameras may use diverging collimators (Figure 3-20, C) whose holes converge toward the detector to image large organs such as the lungs, which would not otherwise fit within the frame. Diverging collimators are generally avoided because they have the lowest sensitivity of any collimator design for a given spatial resolution. With converging collimators (Figure 3-20, D), the holes converge toward the patient, producing magnification and an improvement in count sensitivity compared with parallel hole collimation but at the cost of the usable field of view. Converging collimators are most often used for pediatric imaging studies. Fan beam collimators

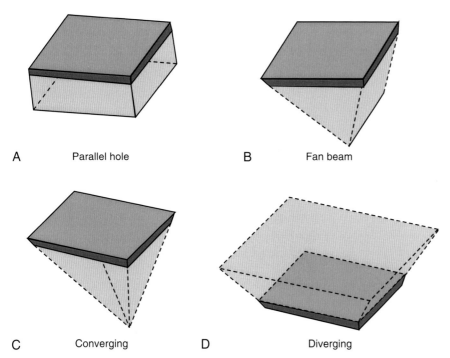

A   Parallel hole   B   Fan beam

C   Converging   D   Diverging

FIGURE 3-20 Collimator Geometries. A, Parallel hole. All the holes are aligned for parallel sampling with no magnification. **B,** Fan beam. In one direction, the holes converge to a focal point, in the other direction they are parallel yielding a focal line. **C,** Converging collimator. All the holes converge toward the patient, yielding a single focal point. **D,** Diverging collimator. The inverse of a converging collimator with the holes converging toward the detector.

(Figure 3-20, *B*) converge on only one axis to slightly improve both sensitivity and maintain resolution.

Gamma Camera Performance Specifications

The National Electrical Manufacturers Association (NEMA) provides standard testing methods for a wide variety of commercial products, including gamma cameras, SPECT, and PET systems. NEMA proscribes how a number of tests are to be performed that are used by the manufacturer to specify the operating performance of the imaging systems. NEMA does not specify what the results of the tests will be but specifies only the testing methods. These tests evaluate intrinsic spatial resolution and linearity, energy resolution, flood field uniformity, system spatial resolution, system sensitivity, count rate performance and multiwindow spatial registration. Box 3-1 gives typical values for each of these parameters for commercially available gamma camera systems.

The National Electrical Manufacturers Association introduced integral and differential uniformity parameters for quantifying uniformity. Both are based on having the flood image in a 64 × 64 matrix and applying the standard nine-point smoothing filter that is available on all computer systems. Integral uniformity is defined as 100% × (max − min)/(max + min), where *max* represents the maximum pixel value and *min* represents the minimum pixel value in either the useful field of view (UFOV) or the central field of view (CFOV). NEMA defines the UFOV as the field of view identified by the

---

BOX 3-1 | **Scintillation Camera Performance Specifications***

Field uniformity (integral uniformity): 3%-4%
Intrinsic spatial resolution (FWHM): 3.5-4.5 mm
System spatial resolution (FWHM): 8-12 mm
Energy resolution: 9%-10%
Multiwindow spatial registration: <2 mm

Temporal Resolution
Dead time: 1-2 μsec
Maximum count rate: 200,000-400,000 counts/second
20% loss rate: 80,000-120,000 counts/second

*These are typical values; some systems may have performance values outside these ranges.

---

manufacturer, whereas the CFOV is 75% of the UFOV. The integral uniformity is not affected by the location of the *max* and *min* values, which may be close to or distant from each other. The differential uniformity calculates the uniformity ratio over every possible 5 × 5 pixel region in either the UFOV or CFOV and reports the maximum value. A gamma camera could have a high integral uniformity (e.g., >5%), but could still be usable if the differential uniformity was below 5%. For most gamma cameras, the integral uniformity is specified at 3% to 4%, and the differential uniformity adds little useful information.

All spatial resolution values are expressed as the FWHM of a line spread function and is measured in mm. Intrinsic spatial resolution is the resolution of the detector without collimation and that falls in the range of 3.0 to 4.5 mm for ^{99m}Tc for most gamma cameras. System spatial resolution, also referred to as extrinsic spatial resolution, includes the blurring effects of the collimator at a source-to-collimator distance of 10 cm. The **full-width-at-tenth-maximum (FWTM)** is also reported. This parameter is sensitive to source scatter within the object (patient) being imaged. When no scatter is present, the FWTM is about two times the FWHM and is about three times the FWHM when there is scatter.

The spatial linearity parameter expresses the magnitude of the error in correctly positioning an event. With spatial linearity correction, this positioning error is less than 0.5 mm. Energy resolution is usually evaluated for ^{99m}Tc and has the same definition given earlier in the chapter. For ^{99m}Tc, the energy resolution for a NaI(Tl) scintillation camera is 9% to 10% and may be a factor of two less (5%) for gamma cameras with CZT detectors. Multiple energy window spatial registration testing monitors the correspondence between images acquired at different energies. The specification is 2 mm, which is well within the blur associated with the system spatial resolution, and displacements of that magnitude are not an issue.

Count rate performance can be represented by a graph that compares the observed count rate with the expected true count rate, but is most often directly specified by either the system dead time, the count rate where a 20% loss in counts occurs, or the maximum obtainable count rate. Conventional gamma cameras have a system dead time of 1 to 2 μsec and can achieve maximum counting rates of 200,000 to 400,000 counts per second. The 20% loss rate is the range of 50,000 to 100,000 counts per second. For most conventional planar and SPECT imaging, high count rates are not an issue and the count rate performance is more than adequate. Additional electronic processing can be added to gamma cameras to increase their count rate capability by an order of magnitude for high count rate applications such as coincidence imaging.

Pixelated Gamma Camera

Although Anger-type cameras are the most prevalent clinical devices, the design is not optimal for all imaging situations. Anger cameras have a "dead zone" along the perimeter of the detector. In large field of view cameras, that is not much of an issue, but as the area of the detector decreases, that dead zone becomes an increasingly large fraction of the total area. One way of avoiding that problem is to use pixelated detectors. A pixelated detector is an array of small individual detectors, each of which is independently capable of registering an event. As a result, pixelated cameras are said to have a live edge. Intrinsic spatial resolution in these cameras is determined by face size of the detectors, typically 2.5 to 3 mm across. The detectors may be semiconductors or

scintillators. With scintillators, as noted previously, some type of light transducer is required to convert the scintillation resulting from absorbed energy into an electronic signal. PMTs are generally too large to resolve the individual detectors and other devices such as position sensitive PMTs or APDs. Position sensitive PMTs (PSPMT) share the same design as PMTs but are able to localize the portion of the photocathode that the scintillation light impinges on. The Dilon Technologies (Newport News, Va.) breast imaging camera uses pixelated NaI(Tl) detectors with PSPMTs. Digirad (Poway, Calif.) cameras use pixelated CsI(Tl) detectors which emit infrared light that is well matched to APDs. In both cases, the location of the event is determined directly by the detector that involved in the interaction.

Semiconductor detectors are manufactured in pixelated arrays and several gamma cameras based on CZT are commercially available. This includes a scintimammography camera produced by Gamma Medica (Northridge, Calif.), the Spectrum Dynamics (Danville, Calif.) DSPECT cardiac SPECT system, and the General Electric (Waukesha, Wis.) Discovery 530c cardiac SPECT system. In addition to having a live edge, these cameras have energy resolution in the 4% to 6% range, which is nearly a factor of two better than scintillation cameras. The biggest challenge associated with CZT gamma cameras is obtaining pixelated arrays with uniform detectors. The price of these devices can be expected to drop and become more competitive as the manufacturing process improves.

GAMMA CAMERA QUALITY CONTROL

Nuclear medicine imaging studies are performed to diagnose a wide variety of pathologies. An imaging system that is not operating within specifications can compromise the quality of the images and adversely affect the patient by failing to diagnose a serious condition or by generating an artifact that may be interpreted as a positive finding. To insure that gamma cameras are working properly, it is important to have a quality assurance program that includes routine calibrations and testing procedures. These programs are necessary for responsible patient care and are required by accreditation agencies. It should be recognized however, that vigilance is necessary by both technologists and the physicians reading the gamma camera images. Although quality control tests uncover many problems with gamma camera performance, malfunctions can occur that are not manifested in the test images. The routine inspection of clinical images must be a part of a viable quality assurance program.

Accreditation

In recent years, the quality of imaging services has been a concern of health insurance companies and government agencies that provide healthcare funding. This concern has resulted in a trend toward clinic accreditation based on widely accepted standards. Most hospitals are accredited by The Joint Commission, which requires a formal quality assurance program that is reviewed by qualified expert for all imaging modalities including nuclear medicine. Clinics that are not covered by The Joint Commission may be accredited through the American College of Radiology (ACR) or the Intersocietal Commission for the Accreditation of Nuclear Medicine Laboratories (ICANL). These organizations have well-defined criteria that include detailed recommendations for acceptance testing and comprehensive annual tests as well as routine gamma camera quality control.

Quality Control Phantoms

A wide variety of phantoms have been described and are commercially available for gamma camera quality control. The most commonly used phantoms are described in this section (Figure 3-21).

Flood Field Phantom

For daily evaluation of extrinsic gamma camera field uniformity, one can either use a ^{57}Co flood field source (Figure 3-21, A) or a fillable flood phantom (Figure 3-21, B). Cobalt-57 flood sources are available in rectangular or round configurations and can be ordered with 5 to 20 mCi of activity. The fillable flood phantoms are also available in rectangular or round geometries. These phantoms are filled with water and allow the user to mix the desired radionuclide (most often ^{99m}Tc) in the selected amount (usually 5 to 10 mCi). The filling of these phantoms requires care to avoid bubbles, bulging of the phantom from too much water, and nonuniform mixing of the radionuclide. Because of these concerns, many clinics elect to use the ^{57}Co phantoms. Figure 3-22, A, shows a flood image with good uniformity across the entire field of the image.

Quadrant Bar Phantom

The weekly evaluation of gamma camera spatial resolution is often performed with a quadrant bar phantom.

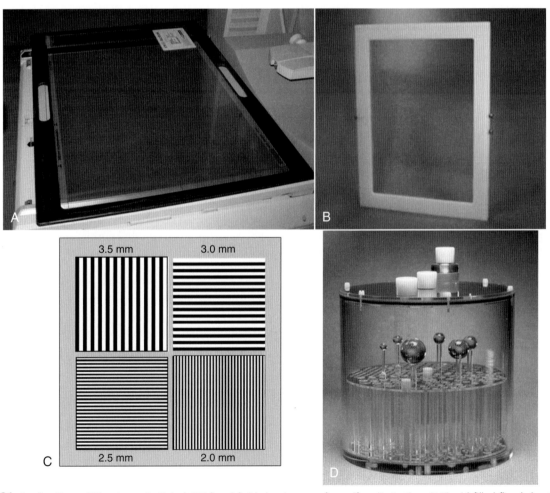

FIGURE 3-21 Quality Control Phantoms. A, Cobalt-57 flood field sheet source for uniformity testing. **B,** Liquid filled flood sheet source for ^{99m}Tc or other radionuclide uniformity testing. **C,** Quadrant bar phantom for spatial resolution evaluation. **D,** SPECT phantom for evaluating extrinsic spatial resolution.

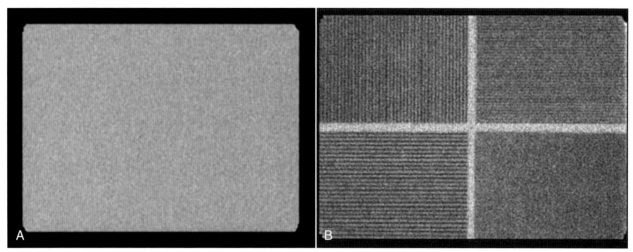

FIGURE 3-22 Routine Quality Control Images. A, Flood field image for evaluating uniformity. B, Transmission image of the quadrant bar phantom for evaluating intrinsic spatial resolution.

This consists of four sets of lead bars arranged orthogonally (Figure 3-21, C). Within each quadrant, the bars are all the same width and are separated by a distance equal to the bar width. To monitor intrinsic spatial resolution the bars widths range from 2 to 3.5 mm. Rectangular bar phantoms intended to monitor extrinsic resolution have bar widths that range from 3.2 to 6.4 mm. Figure 3-22, B, shows an image from a four-quadrant phantom image that demonstrates appropriate resolution of the camera.

SPECT Phantom

An alternate method of evaluating extrinsic gamma camera resolution is to image the rod pattern of a SPECT phantom. An example of a commonly used SPECT phantom is shown in Figure 3-21, D. Approximately 5 to 10 mCi of ^{99m}Tc or other radionuclide is uniformly mixed in the phantom. Images are acquired with the bottom of the phantom positioned directly on the collimator. SPECT quality control will be addressed in much more detail in Chapter 9.

Line Source

Line sources are used to quantitatively evaluate extrinsic spatial resolution. The sources are filled with ^{99m}Tc or other radionuclide and imaged using the selected collimator with the line source usually positioned 10 cm from the collimator surface. The line sources should be carefully filled so that the activity is uniformly distributed with no bubbles or other discontinuities. Line sources can be purchased or fabricated using capillary tubes or pipettes.

Spatial Linearity Phantom

Some manufacturers perform spatial linearity calibration after the gamma camera is installed. Most often, a lead

sheet sandwiched between aluminum plates with a precise rectangular array of holes is used. The linearity phantom is placed on the uncollimated gamma camera detector and is illuminated by a point source of ^{99m}Tc located several meters from the phantom. The phantom and the procedure are generally under the control of service personnel.

Acceptance Testing

After a gamma camera has been initially installed, it is a good practice to have the manufacturer's imaging specifications verified by an independent expert with experience testing gamma camera instrumentations. Tests should be performed for each of the parameters listed in Box 3-1 and the results compared to the expected results published by the manufacturer. Only when the all the specifications are met should the camera be accepted by the clinic. It is important to include acceptance testing during the purchase negotiations and to define the obligations of the manufacturer to meet the specifications before final payment is made. It is also important to require the manufacturer to provide any customized phantoms, apparatus or software needed to perform the acceptance tests. It is a good idea to contact the individual who will perform the evaluation before selection of the gamma camera and to involve that person in the early stages of the process.

Routine Gamma Camera Quality Control

There are several routine quality control tests that should be performed to make sure the gamma camera is suitable for patient use. These tests are usually performed by a technologist. The gamma camera should have the energy windows set for the radionuclides that will be used in the clinic on each day. Energy window settings are fairly automatic and often require calibration with just ^{99m}Tc.

It is usually recommended that the collimator be removed while the detector is exposed to a point source of activity that will yield a count rate in the range of 10,000 to 40,000 counts per second. The correct setting of the energy window can be verified by viewing the energy spectrum display that is available on all gamma camera systems.

Uniformity

There are a number of things that can cause nonuniformities in gamma camera images, including inappropriate photopeak setting, radioactivity contamination, malfunctioning electronic components, collimator or crystal damage, and crystal hydration. Uniformity should be evaluated daily before any clinical use of the camera. It can be evaluated intrinsically, usually with a ^{99m}Tc point source, or extrinsically, most often with a ^{57}Co flood source. Flood field images should have a high enough count density that statistical fluctuations do not obscure nonuniformities. Unlike acceptance testing where the goal is to accurately measure the integral uniformity of gamma camera, the daily test determines if the uniformity is within acceptable limits. The number of counts required to accurately determine the integral uniformity for a large field of view gamma camera is approximately 30 million, but only 5 to 10 million counts are required to see if the integral uniformity rises above an action limit that is usually set at 5%.

Intrinsic Uniformity

To measure intrinsic uniformity, the collimator is removed and a point source of ^{99m}Tc is positioned centrally either above or below the detector. The source-to-detector distance should be large enough that there is no significant change in count rate across the detector unless there is software to compensate for that problem. The NEMA recommendation of a source distance exceeding 5 times the largest detector dimension is more extreme than is necessary, and locating the source 2 meters away will be sufficient for even the largest clinical gamma camera. The activity of the ^{99m}Tc should be adjusted so that the gamma camera count rate is between 10,000 and 40,000 counts per second. It is reasonable to acquire the image in a 256 × 256 array for a total of 5 to 10 million counts. The flood field image should be reviewed and any structured pattern should be noted and addressed. If any artifact is present that will compromise clinical imaging, the gamma camera should not be used. Most vendors provide software for calculating the NEMA intrinsic uniformity. This value should be recorded and results that exceed 5% need to be investigated.

One other parameter that can easily be checked along with uniformity is the count sensitivity of the system.

This requires that the location of the source and detector remain constant from day to day. If the total number of acquired counts are divided by the source activity and the acquisition time, the resulting counts per seconds per μCi or per MBq should remain constant to within ±5%.

Extrinsic Uniformity

Many clinics prefer evaluating uniformity with the collimators on. Extrinsic uniformity monitors both the detector and the collimation and is therefore a more complete test of the imaging system. Although fillable liquid flood sources are available that can be loaded with 5 to 10 mCi of ^{99m}Tc, they require thorough mixing and may result in additional radiation exposure to the technologists. Most clinics prefer to use solid ^{57}Co flood sources, which can be purchased with activities of 5 to 15 mCi. Cobalt-57 has a half life of 272 days and the useful life of the flood source is about 3 years. The test requires the positioning of the ^{57}Co flood source so that it fills the field of views. Some clinics place the flood source directly on the collimator, whereas others locate it about 10 to 15 cm above the collimator. Usually a 15% or 20% energy window is centered on the 122 keV photopeak and a 10 million count flood is acquired in a 256 × 256 array. The flood image should be inspected for any structured nonuniformities and the integral uniformity should be calculated if the routine is provided by the vendor. The system sensitivity can be monitored by dividing the flood counts by the source activity and acquisition time.

Spatial Resolution

Gamma camera spatial resolution should be monitored on at least a weekly basis. In most clinics either a quadrant bar phantom or a SPECT phantom is used (Figure 3-23). The quadrant bar phantom can be used to measure spatial resolution either intrinsically or extrinsically with some caveats, whereas the SPECT phantom can only be used for extrinsic measurements.

Intrinsic Spatial Resolution

To monitor intrinsic spatial resolution, the collimator is removed and the quadrant bar phantom is placed on the detector. This needs to be done very carefully since any mechanical trauma can damage the crystal leading to a very expensive repair. It is prudent to protect the detector by using a thin piece of foam, cardboard, or other pad between the phantom and the crystal. A ^{99m}Tc point source should be centered over the phantom at a distance of about 1.5 m with enough activity to yield a count rate of 10,000 to 40,000 counts per second. A 3 to 5 million count image should be acquired with a pixel size of less than 1 mm. This will usually require a 512 × 512 matrix

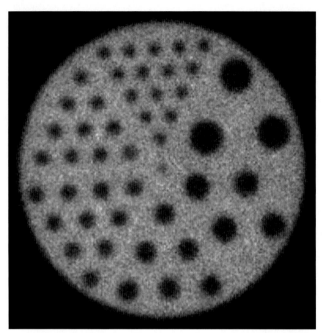

FIGURE 3-23 Extrinsic spatial resolution image of the rod sector of the SPECT phantom.

with some additional magnification. The acquired image should be reviewed to verify that smallest resolvable bar pattern is visible at the same contrast as previous measurements. It is good practice to acquire the phantom in different orientations to insure that resolution is uniformly good along the x and y directions.

Extrinsic Spatial Resolution

Extrinsic spatial resolution can be monitored with a quadrant bar phantom interposed between the collimator and a flood source. One million count images are acquired in a 256×256 matrix with some magnification (e.g., 1.5). This provides sufficient sampling since the collimator degrades the spatial resolution. This approach can be used to evaluate extrinsic spatial resolution as long as the collimator holes are smaller than any of the bar widths. Low energy collimators have 1- to 1.5-mm holes and can be used with the intrinsic quadrant bar phantoms. When the holes of the collimator are larger than the thickness of any of the bars, interference occurs, creating a false image called a Moiré pattern. Figure 3-24 shows the Moiré pattern created from the imaging of a quadrant bar phantom with a medium energy collimator. Quadrant bar phantoms with thicker bars are available for evaluating system resolution on the medium- and high-energy collimators.

Another way of monitoring spatial resolution is accomplished by imaging a SPECT phantom. As illustrated in Figure 3-23, a water filled SPECT phantom with 2 to 5 mCi of ^{99m}Tc added is placed with its bottom (the rod section) on the collimator. A static view is acquired in a 256×256 matrix for 3 to 5 million counts.

The image should be inspected to insure that the expected rod sectors are perceivable.

System Tuning

On some gamma cameras, routine calibration of the PMT stability system is required. Often this can be done weekly, but the manufacturer's recommendations should be followed. This test most often requires that the collimator is removed and the detector is exposed with a ^{99m}Tc point source. As counts are acquired, the individual PMTs are individually adjusted to maintain the target performance for energy and linearity correction.

Monthly Calibrations

Most gamma cameras require periodic uniformity correction that is typically performed each month. The system tuning described above is performed and then a very high count flood image is acquired that is used to determine regional correction factors. Each manufacturer has its own procedure for performing this calibration. In addition to uniformity correction, some gamma cameras also have energy and linearity correction procedures that are done on a routine basis. Because these tests are more complicated and require specialized phantoms, energy and linearity correction is most often performed by service personnel.

Annual Gamma Camera Quality Control Tests

The daily and weekly quality control tests make sure the major components of the gamma camera imaging system are working within acceptable limits. It is useful to perform more extensive and accurate testing annually. The results from annual tests can be compared with acceptance values in order to document any performance degradation. The following tests are recommended for annual evaluation: high count intrinsic uniformity, high count extrinsic uniformity with all commonly used collimators, system spatial resolution, system count sensitivity, and display system.

The annual intrinsic and extrinsic field uniformity tests are performed in the same way as the daily routine tests except that the total acquired counts should be at least 30 million. This increased count density reduces the image noise so that the integral uniformity result depends primarily on real nonuniformities. It is also a good idea to include a flood field image with the peak purposely set low (e.g., 120 to 140 keV) to look for early signs of crystal hydration. The annual spatial resolution test can be performed with the quadrant bar phantom or SPECT phantom, but some clinics prefer to measure the system resolution using a line source to obtain a quantitative result. Two images of the prepared line source located 10 cm from the collimator should be acquired, one with

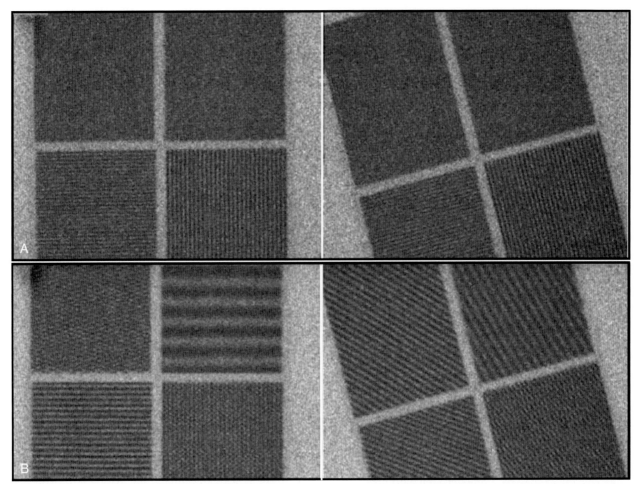

FIGURE 3-24 **Moiré Pattern with Quadrant Bar Phantom. A,** Quadrant bar phantom imaged in two orientations with a low energy high resolution (LEHR) collimator accurately showing the real bar pattern. No Moiré effect is observed since the collimator hole size is small compared to the phantom bar widths. **B,** Quadrant bar phantom imaged with a medium-energy collimator. All the apparent bar patterns are artifacts resulting from Moiré interference patterns. In the left image, bars are larger than those actually in the phantom, and in the right image, the bars are both the wrong size and are oriented at angle inconsistent with the actual bars.

the source oriented along the gamma camera x-axis and the other with the source oriented along the gamma camera y-axis. The image should have at least 100,000 counts and a pixel size less than 2 mm. This can be accomplished with a 256×256 matrix with some magnification. The system FWHM in the x and y directions is determined from the count profile obtained from the line images.

The system count sensitivity should be checked on the most commonly used collimator. It is determined from the total counts acquired from a known activity for a fixed length of time. A source can be prepared by drawing approximately 1 mCi of ^{99m}Tc (accurately measured in a dose calibrator) into a 5-ml syringe with a total volume of 3 to 4 ml. The source should be located at a fixed and reproducible distance approximately 10 cm from the collimator. An image of the source is acquired for 1 minute and the system sensitivity (counts/minute/µCi) is determined by dividing the image counts by the source activity expressed in µCi.

Displays

The displays that are used by the physicians to view the nuclear medicine studies should be evaluated to make sure that it is has no patterned artifacts and has maintained its resolution and luminance. Standard display test patterns are widely available and can be downloaded at no cost.

Several other annual tests are sometimes recommended. A brief description of these is included for completeness, however, it should be recognized that these parameters are generally very stable in a gamma camera and are not likely to fail without manifesting a change in uniformity, spatial resolution, or count sensitivity, which would be evident in the other tests.

Energy Resolution

The energy resolution for a gamma camera can be inferred from the multichannel analyzer display. The energy window should be set to match the specified energy resolution at 140 keV (~9% to 10%) and a spectrum acquired. If the energy window intersects the photopeak at the 50% level, then the energy resolution is within specification.

Multiwindow Spatial Registration

Although there is a well defined NEMA procedure for measuring multiwindow spatial registration (MWSR), it requires multiple sources or image acquisitions. An alternate method that is easier to perform requires the imaging of a quadrant bar phantom with two different energies. A source should be prepared consisting of ^{111}In or ^{67}Ga. A million-count bar image should be acquired with the energy window set to the first gamma ray energy. The energy window should be change to the second gamma ray energy and a second million-count image should be acquired. These two images should be added together. If no distortion is observed, the MWSR is adequate, but if the image looks like a double exposure, the camera settings that affect image registration need attention.

Count Rate Capability

The temporal resolution of a gamma camera can be checked in several different ways and any one of them is sufficient for the annual evaluation. The maximum count rate is determined by moving a 1-mCi point source of ^{99m}Tc progressively closer to an uncollimated detector while observing the gamma camera count rate. The peak count rate is recorded and it should be within ±5% of previous measurements.

A more elaborate test shows how the observed count rate becomes nonlinear at higher activities. A 5-mCi ^{99m}Tc source in an open lead pig is positioned about 1.5 m away from the detector. A stack of identical copper plates is used to shield the source. The count rate and plate thickness are recorded each time a plate is removed. From these recordings, a true versus observed count rate plot can be generated. The count rate associated with 20% count losses can be easily interpolated from the graph. The camera dead time can be directly determined using the two-source method. Two approximately equal sources are prepared that will each result in about 20% count rate losses (about 80,000 to 120,000 counts per second for most gamma cameras). Source 1 is counted first and the count rate is recorded. Without moving source 1, source 2 is added and the count rate is again recorded. Finally, source 1 is removed and the count rate for source 2 is determined. Dead time is determined from the following equation:

Equation 3-7

$$\text{Dead time} = \frac{2R_{1\&2}}{(R_1 + R_2)^2} \times \ln\left(\frac{R_1 + R_2}{R_{1\&2}}\right)$$

R_1 and R_2 are the count rates for the individual sources and $R_1\&_2$ is the count rate for the combined sources.

IMAGE QUALITY

In this final section of the chapter, the basic principles of image quality will be discussed. The information contained in a gamma camera image is limited by a number of factors that include the distribution of the radiopharmaceutical within the patient, the statistical fluctuations or image noise, method of image sampling, and the overall spatial resolution. These factors contribute to a property called the signal-to-noise (SNR) ratio. The SNR is strongly correlated with detection. Areas of an image with a high signal-to-noise ratio contain information that is easily conveyed to an observer, whereas the information is obscured in those areas with a low SNR.

Sampling

Gamma camera images are digitally sampled into an array of elements referred to as pixels. The number of pixels and the pixel size are determined by the image matrix and any acquisition magnification that is applied. The optimal sampling for an image depends on the system spatial resolution since that sets the limit for the smallest object that can be displayed. For example, if the system resolution is 10 mm, an object that is 1 mm across can be imaged, but it will be blurred so that its apparent size in the image will be 10 mm. The proper sampling of the image requires a pixel size that is approximately 2.5 times smaller than the system resolution. For the example given above, this would require a pixel size of less than 4 mm. If no acquisition magnification is used, that would require a 256 × 256 matrix for a large field of view camera. If the pixel size is too coarse, the spatial resolution is degraded as illustrated in Figure 3-25. That situation should always be avoided because the information lost from undersampling cannot be recovered.

What about oversampling? A modest amount of oversampling often produces a more pleasing image even though there is no additional information contained. Oversampling by more than a factor of two is counterproductive. The larger arrays require more storage, and image manipulations use more computer resources. Although there are no permanent losses associated with having too fine a pixel since pixels can always be added together to obtain a smaller matrix, image quality in the highly oversampled image can suffer from having an insufficient number counts in each pixel. With the spatial resolution available in gamma cameras for clinical imaging, there is little need to ever exceed a 256 × 256 matrix or have pixels smaller than 2 mm even at the highest count densities. For dynamic studies or other procedures where the number of counts is limited, 128 × 128 or even 64 × 64 matrices may be adequate.

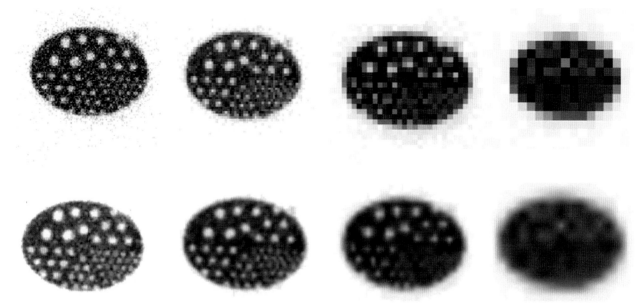

FIGURE 3-25 Gamma Camera Image Sampling. A SPECT phantom was imaged with sampling that varied from 32 × 32 (19.6-mm pixels) *(right)* up to 256 × 256 (2.4-mm pixels) *(left)*. **A,** Images are displayed in same matrix as they were acquired. **B,** The images were all interpolated to a display matrix of 256 × 256.

Object and Target Size

For the purposes of this discussion, object refers to some real entity that is being imaged that has a well defined size and shape. The image of the object is a target that may catch the attention of someone observing the image. At the same contrast, large targets are much more obvious or detectable than small objects as can be appreciated from Figure 3-26. There is a size correspondence between the target and the object until the object size approaches the spatial resolution of the imaging system. Regardless of how small the object gets, the target will be blurred to the same size. The blurring affects the contrast of the target and is often referred to as the partial volume effect. This is illustrated in Figure 3-26.

Contrast

Contrast is a ratio that represents difference between an area of interest and its surroundings. In Figure 3-26, the targets along each row have the same contrast, whereas contrast decreases along the columns. Contrast is a very important consideration in imaging since it is strongly associated with the capability of detecting image information. Because the distribution of radiopharmaceuticals depends on organ function and physiology, nuclear medicine and PET images can provide diagnostic information that is superior to computed tomography (CT) or magnetic resonance imaging (MRI), despite their superior image quality in terms of spatial resolution and image noise.

The contrast in an image depends on the subject contrast and the properties of the imaging system. Subject contrast refers to the contrast within the patient which is determined by the distribution of the radiopharmaceutical. Nuclear medicine procedures are designed to optimize subject contrast in a number ways. For many procedures (e.g., bone scans), images are not acquired until background activity has had a chance to clear from the blood. In others, the patient fasts or is well-hydrated to improve the uptake or clearance of the radiopharmaceutical. Different radiopharmaceuticals may have more specific uptake and it is the goal of achieving better subject contrast that drives development of new tracers.

Image contrast refers to the contrast that exists in the gamma camera image. Image contrast is often very different from subject contrast because the gamma camera compresses the three dimensional patient distribution into a two-dimensional representation. Underlying and overlying activity often combine to substantially reduce the contrast available in an image. As noted earlier, the blurring effect of the imaging system spatial resolution also serves to reduce contrast. This implies that the technologist can affect image contrast through selecting a certain collimator, keeping the patient immobile, and carefully positioning the gamma camera close to the patient. The selection of the radiopharmaceutical can also have a significant effect on image contrast. For example, metaiodobenzylguanidine (MIBG) labeled with ^{123}I yields images with better contrast than when it is labeled with ^{131}I because better spatial resolution and decreased scatter is associated with [123]I. Image quality is also enhanced in that case because more MIBG ^{123}I can be administered leading to images with a higher count density and reduced noise.

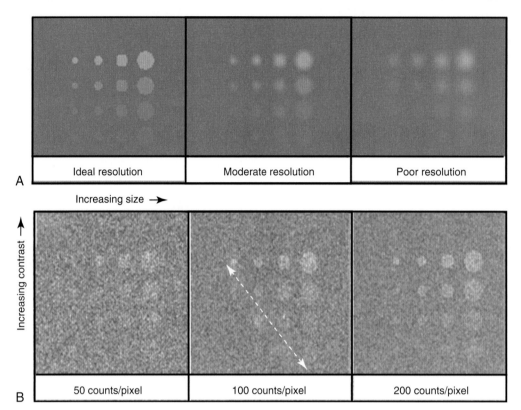

FIGURE 3-26 **Detection Test Pattern.** Across the rows, the target contrast is constant while the size of the targets increases. Down the columns, the target size is constant while the contrast decreases. **A,** Images without noise showing the effect of spatial resolution on contrast and size. **B,** Noisy images at three count densities. Targets of similar signal-to-noise ration occur along the diagonal direction indicated by the arrow.

Noise

Noise in an image refers to statistical fluctuations. As with any type of detection, gamma camera images have statistical fluctuations that depend on the number of acquired events. If no processing has been done to an image (e.g., smoothing or image arithmetic operations) the expected standard deviation for a count sample is equal to the square root of the number of counts. Noise obscures details in images when the standard deviation associated with an area becomes close to the count density. Since count density increases linearly with the number of events whereas the standard deviation increases with the square root of the number of events, noise is a problem associated with low counts. The effect of count density on noise is illustrated in Figure 3-26. As the count density increases, the number of targets that can be reliably seen increases. It is always desirable, though not always possible, to acquire images with a high count density. Actions that would increase count density such as administering more activity or imaging longer are constrained by radiation dose concerns or patient comfort.

Signal-to-Noise Ratio

The effects of noise and contrast can be combined together along with target size information to yield the SNR. Suppose an observer looking at an image sees a potential abnormal area (a target) because of a contrast difference. The number of counts in that target area above the surrounding background is the signal. The signal therefore depends on the size of the target and its contrast with the background. The observer will compare the target area with similar sized areas in the background to gauge the amount of variance in the image. This is the noise and if the signal is large compared to the noise, the observer will flag the target area as abnormal. For gamma cameras, a simple formula can be used to estimate the expected SNR (represented by k) in terms of target size and contrast and count density:

Equation 3-8

$$k = dCn^{1/2}$$

Here d represents the size across the target in the image, C is the contrast between the target and the background, and n is the count density in counts/cm^2. This formula can be arranged to estimate what count density is required to detect an abnormality.

Equation 3-9

$$n = k^2/(C^2 d^2)$$

Typically, this expression is used to define the limits of detection in terms of target size and contrast. For this formula to be useful, a threshold value for k has to be used. What is the minimal acceptable value for the SNR? For most imaging situations, it has to be between 3 and 4. If an observer has a SNR threshold of 2 for example, he will make a false positive call 5% of the time or for every 1 out of 20 noisy areas he views. Since images often have hundreds or more areas that are scanned, false positives would occur on virtually every image with a $k = 2$ threshold. With $k > 3$, the chance of a false positive drops below 0.3%, which makes the chance of a routine false positives remote.

It is instructive to use Equation 3-9 to estimate the minimal required count density for some imaging examples. For simplicity, we will assume that $k = 3.2$ is an adequate threshold SNR and that we will be looking for a target whose size matches the system spatial resolution ($d = 1$ cm). The minimum count density needed to reliably detect a 1-cm abnormality with a contrast of 0.1 is $(3.2)^2/(0.1 \times 1)^2 = 1000$ counts/cm^2. That count density is well within the range of most nuclear medicine studies that use ^{99m}Tc. In some imaging situations like dynamic studies, the count density is more than a factor of 10 smaller. At that count density the largest target of the same contrast ($C = 0.1$) that could be detected is 3.2 cm and that is why we can use coarser matrices for those studies.

What if the contrast were reduced to 0.01 for the 1-cm target? Then the required count density would increase to 100,000 counts/cm^2, which is far beyond practicality for any radionuclide imaging, and the detection of such low contrast 1-cm targets is impossible. How many counts would be required to detect a 5-mm target with a contrast of 0.1? That is problematic since the spatial resolution for most clinical gamma camera imaging will be more than 5 mm, d would never be that small. However, if the gamma camera could achieve that resolution, then 4,000 counts/cm^2 would be required.

In summary, the contrast, count density and spatial resolution that are available with clinical gamma camera imaging sets limits on what is detectable and that governs how the acquisition parameters are determined for the studies that are performed. Good imaging techniques that optimize spatial resolution can have a significant affect the quality of the image information and the detectability of disease.

SUMMARY

- Detectors in nuclear medicine are designed for gamma rays with energies that range from 30 keV to 1 MeV.
- Detection efficiency depends on fraction of emitted gamma rays that hit the detector (geometric efficiency) and the fraction of those that hit and are absorbed in the detector (intrinsic efficiency).
- Intrinsic efficiency depends on the gamma ray energy, the atomic number, and density of the detector and the detector thickness.
- Energy resolution allows a detector to selectively count gamma rays of different energies and to reject Compton scattered radiation.
- Spatial resolution is a measure of image blurring and is quantified by the FWHM of a point or line spread function.
- Detector event dead time results in lost events at high count rates.
- Gas ionization chambers have very low intrinsic efficiency and generally have no energy resolution, but they are useful as survey meters and for measuring radioactivity as dose calibrators.
- GM detectors have large dead times and are best suited for surveying low level contamination. Cutie pie detectors do not have dead time and are best suited for surveying high level radiation areas.
- Survey meters require annual calibration.
- The dose calibrator is a regulated device that requires routine quality control tests for constancy, linearity, accuracy, and geometric effects.
- Semiconductor detectors have very good energy resolution. Cadmium zinc telluride (CZT) is a semiconductor that is already being used in nuclear medicine imaging systems.
- Scintillation detectors provide the best intrinsic efficiency for most nuclear medicine and PET applications. Scintillation detectors convert gamma ray energy to visible light and require an additional stage (photomultiplier tube or avalanche photodiode) to convert the light to an electronic signal.
- Thallium activated sodium iodide, NaI(Tl), is the most commonly used detector in nuclear medicine applications.
- Scintillation counters require a preamplifier to power the event signal to an amplifier that amplifies and shapes the signal for the pulse height analyzer. The pulse height analyzer selects signals that fall within a selected energy range.
- Multichannel analyzers that provide an energy spectrum of detected events are part of most gamma ray detecting systems including gamma cameras.
- Most scintillation gamma cameras follow the design of Hal Anger and use a large NaI(Tl) crystal with an array of photomultiplier tubes to determine the position and energy of a detected event.
- Energy, spatial linearity and uniformity corrections along with PMT stabilization are required for gamma camera imaging.
- All gamma cameras require collimation to form an image from detected gamma rays. Parallel hole collimators are most often used in conventional and SPECT imaging.
- Collimators have very low count sensitivity, and the spatial resolution degrades as the source to collimator distance increases.

- Gamma camera images are acquired as digital computer images with a matrix size of 128×128 or 256×256.
- Routine quality control of gamma cameras includes daily intrinsic or extrinsic uniformity images and weekly resolution images.
- Acceptance testing should evaluate the manufacturer's specification and should include tests for energy resolution, count rate performance, and multiwindow spatial registration.
- Image quality depends on the signal-to-noise ratio that incorporates information about the size, contrast, and count density of imaged areas.

Computer Science

Paul E. Christian, Mark D. Wallenmeyer

OUTLINE

OBJECTIVES

After completing this chapter, the reader will be able to:
- Describe the representation of data in decimal, binary, octal, and hexadecimal format.
- Explain the function of the CPU.
- Describe the operation and use of input/output devices.
- Explain the principles of data storage.
- Describe the operation of disk drives.
- Discuss the use, advantages, and limitations of data storage media.
- Explain the operation of ADCs and the camera/computer interface.
- List environmental factors for computers.
- Diagram and explain digital storage of images.

- Discuss the advantages and disadvantages of different image size matrices.
- Explain the acquisition of gated cardiac data.
- Describe image processing operations.
- Calculate a nine-point smooth for a 3×3 matrix.
- Perform image region-of-interest placement and curve generation.
- Explain the principles of normalization and calculate normalized background-corrected counts.
- Diagram computer network configurations.
- Discuss uses for nonimaging computers.
- Define the Internet, and discuss nuclear medicine applications.

KEY TERMS

binary
bit
Bluetooth
byte
CD-ROM
central processing unit (CPU)
Digital Imaging and
  Communications in Medicine
  (DICOM)

DVD-ROM
Multi-gated cardiac acquisition
image matrix
list mode acquisition
network
normalization
operating system
picture archiving and
  communications system (PACS)

pixel
region of interest (ROI)
Universal Serial Bus (USB)
word

Computer: an electronic machine that stores instructions and information to perform rapid and complex calculations or to store, manipulate, and retrieve information.

By this definition the computer is distinguished from the calculator, a device used to make simple computations. In addition the computer is capable of not only storing information (numbers, data, images, or text) but also following a set of instructions to make complex calculations and manipulate the information in some specific order. This can be as simple as adding two numbers or as complicated as calculating the values in single photon emission computed tomography (SPECT) and positron emission tomography (PET) three-dimensional (3D) image volumes using advanced reconstruction algorithms. Not only are calculations performed, but also information can be evaluated, such as calculating logical evaluations and sorting information in a database.

Computers have become an integral part of the nuclear medicine department, with applications not only to imaging but also to less demanding but repetitive tasks such as billing, scheduling, patient reports, nuclear pharmacy records, and administrative and general office applications.

This chapter concentrates primarily on the application of computers to acquire, store, and process images. Image processing is discussed in general, and specific applications are presented in the clinical chapters, which appear later.

BASIC COMPUTER COMPONENTS

Central Processing Unit

The nucleus of the computer is called the **central processing unit (CPU)** (Figure 4-1). Its three primary functions are to regulate the system operation and perform computations, to interact with memory to execute programs and store data, and to coordinate the control of input and output devices. The CPU as the central management area for program execution has two primary components: the control unit (CU) and the arithmetic logic unit (ALU).

Transistors execute instructions and other operations. Their switching from one state to another is controlled by a high-speed clock that "ticks" at rates now greater than 3 billion times per second (3 gigahertz). With each clock cycle the control unit coordinates the steps necessary to complete each instruction. Each instruction activates other areas within the CPU to perform operations, activates the ALU, and directs communication with memory and other devices. The ALU performs all arithmetic and executes all logic operations.

Memory

Because the CPU acts as the brain of the computer, it retains information by storing it in memory. Memory can be thought of as a group of mailboxes; each memory element has a specific address to store a single byte or word until it is needed. Memory consists of two basic types: read-only memory (ROM) and random-access memory (RAM). The contents of ROM are permanent and remain in memory even when the machine is turned off. RAM is sometimes referred to as "read-and-write memory" and can be changed. When programs are loaded into the computer from an external storage device or when data are input into the computer, they reside in RAM. When the computer is turned off, information stored in RAM is lost.

ROM chips reside within the CPU and are used to store the instructions that "boot" the computer and read the first set of instructions from disk. They can also contain information that tests various internal components of the system, identifies and checks the amount of available memory, and identifies external devices.

When a computer is turned on, the electrical signal follows a permanently programmed path to the CPU and ROM chips that start the boot program. Additional ROM chips contain the basic input/output system (BIOS). The BIOS chips check the disk drive to locate the **operating system,** such as DOS, Windows, UNIX or Linux. The BIOS instructions then load and start the operating system program found on the disk drive. The BIOS also communicates with other areas, such as the memory, keyboard, monitor, and disks.

RAM chips provide the computer with its tremendous flexibility in performing a wide variety of functions. Outside of being developed to perform computations, the computer is the only tool ever made that was not devised to perform a specific function. RAM therefore provides the computer capability to contain programs, data, documents, graphics, and spreadsheets, all stored as zeroes and ones. Certain types of RAM chips also contain programs that store flood uniformity and energy correction matrices inside the scintillation camera.

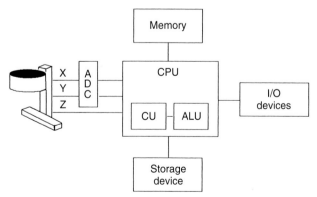

FIGURE 4-1 Nuclear medicine computer with the camera interfaced via an analog-to-digital converter *(ADC)* to digitize *X* and *Y* signals. The central processing unit *(CPU)* controls the communication of information to the memory, input/output devices, and storage devices. *ALU,* Arithmetic logic unit; *CU,* control unit; *I/O,* input/output.

The speed at which information can be stored and retrieved from memory greatly affects the speed of the CPU. Faster RAM chips are more expensive, and the fastest memory might not always be used in the CPU. Slow memory might require the processor to sit idle for several clock cycles while it waits for requested data to be passed to it. A solution to this problem is the addition of fast external RAM *cache memory.* Cache memory is typically built in as part of the main circuitry of the CPU. The cache memory fetches data from RAM and delivers it to the CPU. The first time data are retrieved might take several clock cycles, during which the CPU is idle. The cache also stores a copy of the data retrieved in its high-speed memory chips. As soon as the cache detects that the CPU is idle, it fetches data, or instructions, from memory addresses adjacent to the address for the data the software requested originally. The next time the software asks for data to be sent to the CPU, the cache checks to see if the data have already been stored in its high-speed memory and then delivers the requested data immediately.

For slightly more than the last decade, nuclear medicine computers have used the capability to bypass the CPU during image acquisition. This is accomplished using direct memory access (DMA), which uses both hardware and software to allow data to be passed directly into memory. DMA therefore does not require the interruption of another program running in the CPU to store counts or images as they are acquired. In early nuclear medicine computers the scintillation events from the camera were acquired faster than the information could be processed and stored in the computer. DMA takes the CPU out of the loop for data acquisition, allowing counts to be stored in image arrays at very high count rates. DMA also allows computers to acquire one image while processing another simultaneously.

The internal architecture of ordinary computers relies on several clock cycles to execute each instruction. In an automobile manufacturing plant this would be like completely building each car before starting the next. An innovative variation in computer design is the reduced–instruction set computer (RISC). RISC architecture essentially implements an assembly-line approach to completing tasks within the CPU. A combination of hardware and software efficiently reorganizes the list of tasks into more efficient instructions. The instructions are then carried out in an assembly-line fashion, or pipeline processing. Pipeline processing permits loading of the next instruction while preceding orders are being carried out. The efficiency of the assembly line and faster execution of simple instructions produces a tremendous gain in speed. There has been a tremendous growth of RISC technology in the last several years because of their overwhelming speed in performing image processing and handling graphics. A long list of operations on each data element and a large number of data elements, such as an image or series of images, are efficiently handled by RISC

systems. Repeated computations such as those involved in SPECT slice reconstruction can be performed quickly on RISCs. At this time some RISC technology is now a part of current high-performance Intel chips, and machines can perform many millions of operations per second. RISC architecture has significantly impacted personal computers during recent years by vastly improving performance.

Input/Output Devices

Input/output (I/O) technology is the practical application of computer science. I/O devices allow the user to enter or execute instructions, provide access to data, and then finally obtain the results of the program with a meaningful output of results. Since computers understand or communicate only in zeros and ones, I/O devices also provide the means by which humans communicate with the computer.

Mouse. In 1968 Douglas Engelbart created a pointing device for computer users to interact with information on the screen. Because of its small size and tail-like cable, the device was nicknamed a *mouse.* Although the mouse never can replace a keyboard, it allows rapid interaction with screen information for pointing to and selecting information from a menu or direct interaction with graphics, such as drawing a **region of interest** (**ROI**). The mouse has become very popular in recent years because it enables the user to point to various graphic displays or windows and to quickly point to and select items from a displayed list.

A mechanical mouse contains a ball that protrudes from a hole in the bottom of the housing. As the housing is moved, the ball rotates and turns two rollers mounted at a 90-degree angle from each other. These rollers turn potentiometers that measure the amount of vertical and horizontal movement.

An optical mouse has no moving parts. A light from a tiny built-in lamp illuminates the grid surface, and a lens focuses the image of the lines onto a photodetector. As the mouse is moved, the photocathode converts the spatial information of the mouse movement into cursor movements that are translated to the screen. A mouse, whether mechanical or optical, usually has two or three buttons to activate the functions of the screen cursor. The mouse is used to position the cursor, and the buttons are used to activate functions.

The mouse is now available in many different formats. Many new computers now come with the traditional mouse which has a wire attached to it, which has a round connection on it. Other mouse configurations include Universal Serial Bus (USB), wireless, and Bluetooth technologies.

Trackball. A trackball is another pointing device that works very much like a mechanical mouse; in fact, it could be thought of as a mouse turned upside down. Instead of the ball rolling along a surface, the user rolls the ball within the housing to turn the rollers that measure the indicated movement in two directions. This type of device is good to use when space is limited and moving a traditional mouse could be inconvenient. The trackball is stationary and does not move like the mouse does.

Keyboards. The traditional input device is known as the keyboard. The keyboard serves many different function, and can be customized depending on the computer. A traditional keyboard will contain all the letters of the alphabet, along with numbers from 0 to 9. Many of the keyboards that are now available include a 10-key input pad. This is a numeric keypad similar to the layout of a touch-tone phone. This allows for rapid input of numerical values, which may be valuable when inputing such things as wipe test values. Many keyboards available now have specifically designed function keys as well. Keys can be assigned to perform specific tasks such as opening a program on your computer or opening a web browser.

Modem. A modem can be used to connect computers over a standard telephone line or high-speed line. The word *modem* comes from two terms: *mo*dulate and *dem*odulate. The modem produces a continuous frequency, or carrier wave, to transmit information. Once two modems are connected and the carrier signal is established between the two units, the wave of the carrier is either amplitude, frequency, or phase modulated to carry binary (a binary digit, a 0 or 1) information. Data packets—a group of bits—are transmitted, and the two modems communicate check signals to ensure that data are received accurately. The speed of data transmission over telephone lines is measured in thousands of bits per second, or kbps; on high speed data lines, speed is measured in millions of bits per second, or mbps.

Moving large data and image files is best achieved using higher-speed connections such as ISDN, DSL, T1, T3, or higher-speed connections between facilities such as fiber optic connections.

Drives and Data Storage

Hard Drive. The most common form of data storage is the magnetic hard disk drive. Magnetic disk drives, have storage capacities ranging from a few hundred kilobytes (10^3 bytes) to many gigabytes (10^9 bytes). A computers primary hard disk drive is a hard disk made of an aluminum platter coated on both sides with a thin layer of ferromagnetic material. Microscopically small areas can be magnetized to store a zero or one to encode binary data. The disk is organized into concentric circles called *tracks* and pie-shaped areas called *sectors* (Figure 4-2).

These divisions organize the disk so that data can be recorded in a logical manner and accessed quickly. Before disks can be used, they are formatted to create the magnetic tracks and sectors. A hard disk (Figure 4-3, *A*) spins at a speed as high as 15,000 revolutions per

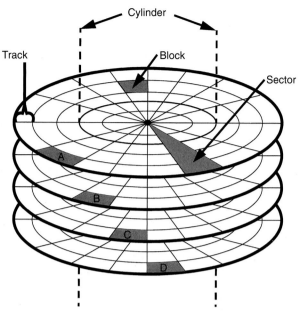

FIGURE 4-2 Disks are laid out in concentric rings called tracks and pie-shaped sectors that identify locations for storing data. A specific sector on a specific track identifies one block of data, which can be 256, 512, or 1024 bytes. Multiplatter disks may also have vertical cylinders of data on a track. Disks can quickly write data by not having to move the read/write heads from a track by writing to multiple platters in sequence denoted as *A, B, C, D*.

minute. A pair of small electromagnets called *read/write heads* (Figure 4-3, *B*) located on an access arm are positioned close to the disk. The read/write heads can be quickly positioned by a stepper motor over the various tracks. As the disk rotates, the read/write heads bring each sector on a particular track past the heads. Binary data can therefore be written to or read from the disk at very high speed. Access time or seek time to a particular track or sector can be a small fraction of a second on hard disks, sometimes a few thousandths.

The distance between the disk surface and the read/write heads is about 10 microinches; therefore hard disk systems usually are sealed to protect them from dust particles, fingerprints, and other foreign material. The heads literally fly over the surface of the disk on a thin cushion of air. Contact between the disk and the read/write heads is called a "head crash," at this high speed it can damage either the heads or the disk surface.

Large–storage capacity disks may have multiple platters (see Figure 4-3), and each platter can be formatted into several hundred tracks. The capacity of a disk drive may be several hundred gigabytes. Most nuclear medicine computers performing SPECT or PET imaging need a hard disk that can hold at over one hundred gigabytes to allow room for the operating system and sufficient space for storing many patient data sets. Data are laid onto the disk in blocks of information. A block usually consists of 256 bytes; however, some disk systems have larger blocks—512 or 1024 bytes.

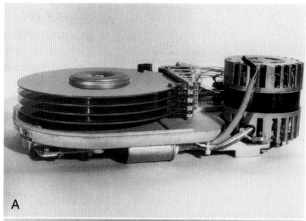

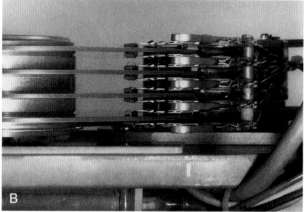

FIGURE 4-3 A, The disk drive shown here has four platters with read/write heads on both sides of each platter. An actuator arm positions the heads in and out while the disk rotates at high speed, allowing data to be written and retrieved very quickly. **B,** Each platter has a set of read/write heads on each side in extremely close proximity to the disk.

The location of files (information) on the disk is identified by a directory or file allocation table, usually found at the beginning of the disk. The file allocation table stores information about the disk's structure, the track and sector location, and the length of each file. Each time a file is to be read or written, the operating system orders the hard disk controller to move the read/write heads to the disk file allocation table. The operating system reads the table to determine the location of an existing file or to find available space in which to write a new file. Some nuclear medicine computers require that a single file of images be written onto a continuous sequence of blocks on the disk. The fastest way to write data onto a multiplatter disk is to write on several platters, one after another onto the same track so that time is not lost in mechanically moving the actuator arm to change tracks. Figure 4-3 shows the use of several blocks and platters creating a vertical cylinder of disk space for rapid access. Some imaging techniques, such as gated SPECT and 3D PET studies, require significant amounts (dozens of megabytes) of disk space. Most new systems break up a file into clusters of data strewn onto various regions on the disk. When the operator deletes a file, the computer simply erases the file location from the directory, though the information remains on disk until it is overwritten. Some systems allow recovery of deleted files by reestablishing the information in the directory.

Optical disks. Optical disk drives provide one media to write large amounts of data on a very small area of disk. The first types of optical disks were nonerasable and are called "Write Once Read Many" (WORM) drives. WORM drives use an intense laser beam focused onto the polished surface of the disk to essentially burn the surface to encode a bit. WORM drives are best suited for storing large quantities of data that will be kept for a long time. The platters in these optical drives can be changed once the disk is filled.

Magneto-optical drives provide an erasable medium for optical encoding of data. The disk is coated with an aluminum substrate protected by a sheet of plastic. An intense laser beam rapidly heats a tiny spot on the disk so that the crystals in the alloy can be aligned by the magnetic field of a write head. Bits are stored by magnetically aligning the crystals so that a reflected laser beam encodes binary data. A low-intensity laser beam is used to read the data. Magneto-optical disks are about 5 inches in diameter and contain tens of thousands of tracks for writing data. Magneto-optical disks can store about 1 gigabyte of data and are valuable for archiving images. Magneto-optical disks on nuclear medicine and PET computers are often replaced by CDs or DVDs, which are a quick and relatively inexpensive write-only archive media that can store several gigabytes of data.

CD-ROM. The CD-ROM (compact disc read-only memory) was originally designed by Sony and Philips in the early 1980's to contain music for playback, to improve the quality of sound that the user would hear. Since then, the CD-ROM has undergone many changes. Now, the CD (as it is commonly known as), is capable of storing not only music, but many different file formats, including data, images, and video. The typical CD can hold around 700 megabytes of information, which correlates to approximately 300,000 text pages. The original CD-ROM was a "read-only memory" disc. This meant that once data was written to it, the data could not be altered or deleted. The CD-RW is a compact disc that can be rewritten as needed. It functions much like the old floppy disks, but holds much more information. The CD-RW can typically be rewritten approximately 1000 times before the material in the CD becomes unwritable. The shelf life of a CD-ROM is 10 to 15 years. This should be taken into consideration when deciding what type of optical back up device to use.

DVD-ROM. The DVD-ROM (digital versatile disc/digital video disc read-only memory) is another variation of an optical disc that has the ability to hold approximately six times as much data as the CD-ROM. The DVD was introduced in 1993, designed to be a way to replace the video cassette. The storage capacity of a typical single sided

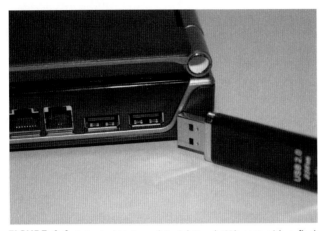

FIGURE 4-4 A typical Universal Serial Bus (USB) port with a flash (thumb) drive. USB ports serve a variety of purposes to connect different types of devices, such as keyboard, mouse, flash drives, external hard drives, and external CD/DVD drives.

DVD is 4.7 gigabytes, where a double-sided disc will hold 8.5 gigabytes of information on one disc. Like the CD-ROM, the DVD-ROM has evolved into a recordable disc as well. The DVD-R/RW, DVD+R/RW, and DVD-RAM (random access memory) discs are available to read/write information to. Like the CD-ROM, the DVD can be rewritten approximately 1000 times. The average shelf life is comparable to the CD-ROM.

USB

Universal Serial Bus is a port for connecting different peripherals to the computer. Information that is sent through the USB port is bidirectional. This makes it a very useful tool for external devices, such as portable hard drives, floppy disc drives, keyboards, and mice. It is the most common type of port on computers that are available today (Figure 4-4). The USB flash drive, or thumb drive, is a small device that can hold much more information than a typical 3.5-inch floppy disc. Storage capacities of these new storage devices are greater than 8 gigabytes.

Bluetooth

Bluetooth technology is a short-range radio frequency technology that will allow the connection of two different electronic devices, such as a cell phone and ear piece, or laptop computer and mouse. Bluetooth technology is now available in the whole electronics industry and is making its way into the automotive industry because of its wireless technology. Bluetooth technology was first introduced in 1998. The purpose of the first Bluetooth technology was to replace wired technology used to transfer voice and data.

Data Representation

The most fundamental building block of all computers is the transistor; essentially the transistor is a switch that can be placed only in the on or off positions. Information stored by this switch is therefore **binary** and can be used to represent 0 or 1. Also, the binary state can be used to signify a logical condition of true or false. All numbers and all logical conditions within the computer are represented in the binary form. The binary configuration, 0 or 1, is called a *binary digit* or **bit**.

The customary decimal counting system of values 0 through 9 is not sufficient to represent all the numbers; therefore additional columns are used to represent powers of 10 (10, 100, 1000, etc.). Similarly in binary counting, columns are represented by powers of 2 (2^0, 2^1, 2^2, etc.; or 1, 2, 4, 8, etc.).

The binary counting method is used for number representation in the computer, though other systems can also be used by the computer within the system. Counting systems containing 8 bits (octal) or 16 bits (hexadecimal) can also be used. The equivalent values to usual decimal counting follow:

Binary	Decimal										
	1024	512	256	128	64	32	16	8	4	2	0 or 1
Power	2^{10}	2^9	2^8	2^7	2^6	2^5	2^4	2^3	2^2	2^1	2^0
0	0	0	0	0	0	0	0	0	0	0	0
1	0	0	0	0	0	0	0	0	0	0	1
2	0	0	0	0	0	0	0	0	0	1	0
3	0	0	0	0	0	0	0	0	0	1	1
4	0	0	0	0	0	0	0	0	1	0	0
5	0	0	0	0	0	0	0	0	1	0	1
10	0	0	0	0	0	0	0	1	0	1	0
15	0	0	0	0	0	0	0	1	1	1	1
16	0	0	0	0	0	0	1	0	0	0	0
60	0	0	0	0	0	1	1	1	1	0	0
128	0	0	0	1	0	0	0	0	0	0	0
200	0	0	0	1	1	0	0	1	0	0	0
350	0	0	1	0	1	0	1	1	1	1	0

The decimal number 21 is represented as the sum of decimal numbers—16 + 4 + 1:

$$1 \times 2^4 = 16$$
$$0 \times 2^3 = 0$$
$$1 \times 2^2 = 4$$
$$0 \times 2^1 = 0$$
$$1 \times 2^0 = \underline{1}$$
$$21$$

or all powers of 2 or in binary, resulting in 0 000 000 000 010 101. Note that 16 numbers are present in these examples, all zeros or ones. Most computers process numbers in groups of 16, 32, or 64 bits.

In hexadecimal counting (base 16) the usual decimal numbers 0 through 9 are supplemented with letters to obtain the full representation of numbers until the next column is needed. Sometimes computer users see numbers or need to enter certain codes that are in either octal or hexadecimal characterization.

Decimal	Octal	Hexadecimal
0	0	0
1	1	1
2	2	2
3	3	3
4	4	4
5	5	5
6	6	6
7	7	7
8	10	8
9	11	9
10	12	A
11	13	B
12	14	C
13	15	D
14	16	E
15	17	F
16	20	10
17	21	11
18	22	12
19	23	13
20	24	14

As mentioned, a bit represents a limited amount of information. A series of bits is needed to encode larger numbers. Eight bits form a **byte.** The maximum number that can be stored in a byte is 2^8, or 256 entries. Since the first number is 0, numbers from 0 to 255 can be stored in a single byte. Two bytes can be put together to form a **word;** a word is therefore 16 bits in length and is capable of storing a number as large as 2^{16}, or 65,536. Words are frequently used to represent the number of counts in a single image picture element, called a **pixel.** The range of counts that could be stored in a single word is 0 to 65,535. The most basic storage element of infor-

mation on a magnetic tape or disk is to store the data in groups of bytes, called a *block*. For example, a disk sector might store a block of 256, 512, or 1024 bytes. Information, whether numbers, text, or executable programs, is called a *file*. The size of a file can be listed as the number of bytes needed to store the information.

Memory requirements are usually indicated as thousands of bytes (kilobytes), millions of bytes (megabytes), or billions of bytes (gigabytes). When discussing the size of memory or the size of a file on disk, the prefix *kilo* does not refer to the usual definition of 1000: it refers to 1024. Therefore 4 kilobytes of memory is 4×1024, or 4096 bytes.

To effectively communicate with the computer, humans need to exchange information not as zeros and ones or other numeric representation but as standard written alphanumeric symbols. A set of numbers to represent alphanumeric characters has been established as the American Standard Code for Information Interchange (ASCII). Using this standard code, a byte can represent a letter of the alphabet, a number, a punctuation character, or a keyboard control character. Text files for word processing can be stored with one byte of information for each character of the document. In addition, ASCII code allows concise communication between the computer operator via the keyboard, computer, and display monitor, allowing the direct translation from alphanumeric characters into binary information. Text files, programs, and data all appear as binary information inside the computer. The confusion of data or text files for programs creates havoc within the computer and can halt operation of the system.

IMAGE ACQUISITION

Camera Interface

Capturing images from the scintillation camera first requires the conversion of analog *x, y,* and *z* pulses into digital information. As previously mentioned, digitization is accomplished by the ADCs to provide a quantitative location of the scintillation event. The digital location information locates the appropriate pixel into which the gamma event can be recorded. If the output is from an analog scintillation camera, separate from the computer, then the energy pulse has already been processed by a pulse height analyzer and determined to be within the selected energy range. If the particular system is a digital camera/computer, the digitized *z* pulse is compared with the selected window settings for pulse height analysis. If the *z* pulse has been determined to be within the appropriate window, the scintillation event is recorded in the pixel identified by the *x* and *y* locations, adding 1 to the current pixel value (Figure 4-5). Scintillation events are stored in the proper pixel locations until the acquisition time has elapsed or until the selected number of counts or count density has been reached.

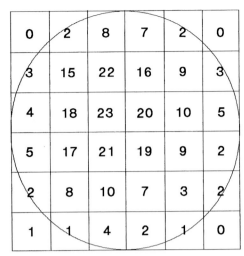

FIGURE 4-5 Scintillation detector (*circle*) gamma events are input to an array of pixels in the computer. Counts are accumulated by each pixel to store a representation of the image. Arrays of 64 × 64, 128 × 128, and 256 × 256 are most commonly used to store digital images.

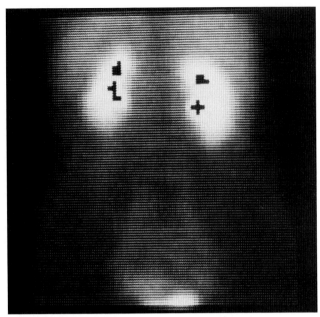

FIGURE 4-6 Each pixel can store only a limited number of counts; pixel overflow results when the number of counts exceeds the maximum value a pixel can hold. This kidney scan shows pixel overflow in the area of the renal pelvis.

Matrix Size

At present, image matrices are represented as a square matrix with the camera field of view inscribed within the square. The camera field-of-view shape therefore inscribes a circle, hexagon, square, or rectangle within the matrix (see Figure 4-5), depending on camera shape. The image density for each pixel is determined by the number of gamma-ray counts stored within a pixel. For image display the highest pixel count is assigned the brightest intensity on the display, with other pixel counts assigned to appropriate intermediate intensities. Before acquisition the image pixel data depth can be selected as an acquisition parameter. A pixel able to contain only 1 byte (8 bits) of information allows the storage of 256 different numbers, 0 to 255. If the counts per pixel reach the maximum of 255, pixel rollover may occur when the 256th count is reached, and the pixel value goes back to 0 (Figure 4-6). Pixel rollover is prevented on some systems with the maximum of 255 being retained; however, counts greater than 255 are not recorded, and quantitative information is lost. Acquiring data with a pixel depth in word mode (16 bits) lessens the likelihood of reaching the maximum count of 65,535. A consequence of storing higher-density images is that they take twice as much memory and disk space for storage.

Most computer systems allow the selection of 64 × 64, 128 × 128, 256 × 256, or 512 × 512 matrices. Static image acquisition usually contains sufficient counts to produce a high–spatial resolution image. If a large–field-of-view camera (400 mm) has a full-width-at-half-maximum (FWHM) resolution of 4 mm, high-resolution images should be stored in a matrix size of at least 100 pixels (400 mm/4 mm). A camera can visualize about two bars per the FWHM when there are sufficiently high

counts. The selected **image matrix** should be multiplied by this value (i.e., 2) to get a 200-pixel matrix. Static images acquired in a 256 × 256 matrix therefore are visually indistinguishable from analog images; that is, no evidence of the image matrix is seen. Figure 4-7, *A* to *C*, shows a bone scan image displayed as 256 × 256, 128 × 128, and 64 × 64 images, respectively. The image resolution deteriorates as the selected acquisition matrix size gets smaller. In Figure 4-7, *D*, the 64 × 64 data have been used to interpolate intermediate pixels to create a 256 × 256 display image. Note that the interpolated image appears as a smoothed version of the 64 × 64 data without recovering the resolution available with 256 × 256 acquired data.

Dynamic images do not usually contain enough counts to warrant the use of high-resolution matrices; dynamic studies are performed to record physiological information. The time per image is therefore critical to ensure that meaningful physiological information is not missed by acquiring images too slowly. Blood flow studies of organs such as the kidneys and brain should be acquired at 1 frame/sec. The series of images should be continued for a long enough period to obtain valuable information and to not miss the injection bolus. Image resolution for these studies typically uses a 64 × 64 or 128 × 128 matrix. More rapid physiological phenomena, such as first-pass cardiac studies, require acquisition framing rates of 25 frames/sec in a 64 × 64 matrix.

Slower functional processes that take place over a period of many minutes, such as kidney function, need frame rates of 20 to 30 seconds with an image resolution of 64 × 64 or 128 × 128 pixels. Hepatobiliary images

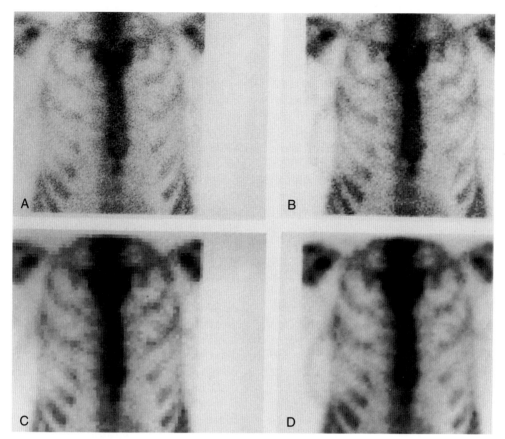

FIGURE 4-7 Digitized bone scan is shown in high-resolution 256 × 256 matrix **(A)**, a 128 × 128 matrix **(B)**, and a 64 × 64 matrix **(C)**. Both the 256 × 256 and 128 × 128 matrices are adequate for high-resolution imaging; the 64 × 64 matrix begins to lose detail because the pixel size is much larger than the resolution of the camera. Interpolation of the 64 × 64 image data into a 256 × 256 **(D)** matrix fails to recover image resolution, though the image might be more aesthetically pleasing.

require acquisition at 1 to 3 min/frame, and the high-count density allows image matrices of 128 × 128 or 256 × 256 to be recorded. Again, the data storage requirements must be considered. A word mode study of 60 1-minute images in a 256 × 256 matrix requires 7,864,320 bytes (60 frames × 256 × 256 × 2 bytes per word).

Gated blood pool studies and SPECT image files are similar in size and storage format to dynamic studies. SPECT image files from a single detector camera can be acquired as 60 images of 64 × 64 pixels, or 245,760 words. Significant file space might be required when using multidetector SPECT cameras and acquiring 120 images in a high-resolution matrix of 128 × 128 pixels using 3,932,160 bytes.

On some computer systems, dynamic, gated, or SPECT image files must be stored on sequential data blocks on the disk. When many image files have been acquired and deleted, there might not be enough sequential blocks of available storage, and data acquisition will not be allowed until appropriate space is available. In this case the disk must be "squeezed" to move data so that there are no free data blocks between files. Most newer systems do not require contiguous blocks, and

information from one file can be distributed into several groups of blocks spread over the disk. The file allocation table on the disk keeps track of the location of the various parts of the file and is totally transparent to the user. Disks that can distribute information in this way cannot be squeezed.

The acquisition of whole-body images into a digital form requires a very high-resolution matrix. The minimum matrix length should be at least a 512-pixel array; however, high-resolution cameras should use a 1024-2048 image matrix. Information acquired into an image matrix size smaller than these arrays has an image resolution far below those acquired by spot film imaging.

Many types of imaging are applied to small organs, such as the thyroid and the heart, compared to the size of the detector. In acquiring computer images of these organs it is sometimes helpful to use hardware magnification, or zoom, to improve the resolution of the acquired image matrix in addition to presenting a larger image for viewing. When the hardware zoom mode is turned on, the x and y signals from the gamma camera are amplified by the zoom factor to fill the image matrix from the center point of the camera, and the outside perimeter of the image is lost. Although zooming increases resolution, there is a decrease in the number of counts per pixel, resulting in a noisier image.

Magnification of areas on digitized images can also be performed. Most commonly, magnification is used to improve the visual display, though there is no increase in resolution. Software zoom is commonly applied to increase the size of the heart on SPECT myocardial perfusion imaging, because although the patient's whole chest fills the field of view, the only area of interest is the myocardium. Software zoom of areas on a digitized bone scan also can be useful in better appreciation of small detail, such as the vertebrae or hip joints.

Pixel Size Calibration

As you were able to see in the previous section, the smaller the pixel size, the better the resolution. A 256×256 matrix has a smaller pixel size than does a 64×64 matrix. This can be seen by imaging two point sources at a given distance and measuring the number of pixels between the sources with the camera software. For example, if you put two point sources 10 cm apart and image them on the face of the collimator, then use the camera software to measure the number of pixels between them, you get 40 pixels. You then divide the number of pixels by the distance to get pixels per centimeter as shown below:

$$40 \, \text{pixels}/10 \, \text{cm} = 4 \, \text{pixels/cm or } 2.5 \, \text{mm/pixel}$$

Frame versus List Mode

Data acquisition of the gated radionuclide ventriculogram (RVG) requires synchronization of dynamic data acquisition with the cardiac cycle. More commonly known as **multiple gated acquisition (MUGA)**, or **equilibrium radionuclide angiography (ERNA)**, the RR interval of the ECG is divided equally into a series of frames or images (frame mode). From 16 to 32 images are used to acquire the data through the length of time for one cardiac cycle. An additional input to the computer to receive the R wave signal from an ECG is required. Data are acquired each time an R wave occurs. The time for each image frame is selected by dividing 60 seconds by the heart rate times the number of images in the sequence. For a 24-frame study with a heart rate of 60, each frame represents only 42 msec of data acquisition. With the detection of an R wave, acquisition begins with image data rapidly filling each frame in the sequence. If a new R wave is detected before the last frame is reached, acquisition into the first frame of the sequence begins again. Data from several hundred cardiac cycles are required to obtain a statistically accurate image. Images acquired in a 64×64 matrix with a hardware magnification are typically acquired for approximately 5 million counts. Usually this is accomplished in less than 10 minutes per view.

This technique acquires all data as R waves are detected. In patients with arrhythmias the quality of the data is compromised by premature ventricular contractions (PVCs) and the compensatory beats that follow PVCs. One technique to filter out bad beats is *dual buffering,* which allows information from a single cardiac cycle to be held in temporary image memory buffers. Before this information is added to the final set of data, the length of the cardiac cycle is determined to see if the RR interval is within a selected percentage of the patient's normal cardiac cycle. Heart rates outside the window indicate that the buffer should be cleared, and no data from this cardiac cycle are saved. While the first beat is evaluated, images from the following beat are placed into the second buffer for RR interval evaluation. Data acquisition therefore alternates back and forth between the two buffers, evaluating RR intervals and placing only good cardiac intervals into the saved file of images.

Another mechanism for capturing gated cardiac data is **list mode acquisition.** In list mode, the arrival of a z pulse indicates that a gamma ray of proper energy has been detected. A timing mark is then stored along with the x and y locations of the scintillation event. In addition, when R waves are detected from the physiological trigger, a physiological marker is placed in the list of data. List mode acquisition requires a significant amount of disk space (several megabytes) to store a single study. The advantage of this technique is that after data have been acquired as a list of gamma-ray events, the data can be evaluated, the desired RR interval can be selected from the acquired data, and images can be constructed only from those of desired heart rate. If the reformatted data are found unacceptable, a new RR interval can be selected and a new series of images can be formatted.

Data obtained from a gated cardiac study are most commonly evaluated by generating a time-activity curve of counts in the left ventricle. If the RR interval has been selected inappropriately, with too many R waves arriving early, image data do not fill the last images of the dynamic sequence equally; therefore counts in the last few frames can be artificially low, and the volume curve can tail off at the end. Also, if too many beats have been obtained from inadequately acquired data, the cardiac ejection fraction value may be wrong.

In recent years, gated SPECT myocardial perfusion studies have proven helpful in evaluating myocardial perfusion, but this technique also displays the slice image as an ECG-gated cinematic study. Thus not only is perfusion evaluated by the radiopharmaceutical concentration but diminished perfusion also is correlated with corresponding decreased myocardial wall motion and thinning associated with myocardial infarction.

Some time of flight PET systems (discussed in Chapter 10) also use list mode acquisition to record the arrival of events recorded by the ring of detectors that make up a PET scanner. The list mode events must then be sorted in order to organize the event list information into a format that can be then used to reconstruct image slices.

IMAGE DISPLAY AND PROCESSING

Display Terminals

The most common type of communication device is the keyboard and monitor. The typewriter-like keyboard allows alphabetic and numeric characters to be entered into the computer. In addition, the keyboard of a computer has additional keys not found on a typewriter, such as control (CTRL), alternate (ALT), escape (ESC), and arrow keys to move the cursor. Most keyboards also have a series of 10 or 12 function keys that can be defined by different programs to perform special functions.

The display monitor comprises the other half of the video display terminal. Nuclear medicine systems use a high-quality flat-panel monitors. High-resolution monitors create an array of about 1280 pixels across and 1024 pixels down or higher resolutions.

Flat-panel color monitors have a matrix of red, green, and blue pixel elements. Each pixel is a thin film transistor. An electrical signal is sent to activate each pixel and the strength of each signal is measured in steps up to 256 levels (one byte) to create a variable intensity scale for each color. With three colors (red, green, and blue), each with a variable intensity level, a color palette of 16.8 million colors ($256 \times 256 \times 256$) can be displayed.

Gamma-ray scintillation events that occur at specific detector locations are stored as digital images by accumulating gamma-ray counts. As discussed previously, each pixel is stored as a byte or word, and an image is represented as an array or matrix of pixels. Once the information is stored, the image is displayed on a high-resolution monitor. Each pixel on the image is assigned a grayscale value based on the number of counts. Images are typically displayed with the brightest pixel assigned to the maximum display intensity. Display screens and software usually allow images to be displayed as either black on white or white on black. Although the human eye can differentiate fewer than 100 shades of gray, most computer systems generate an 8-bit image, assigning display intensities from 0 to 255. The maximum pixel count is therefore assigned a display intensity of 255, and all other pixels are assigned scaled values from 255 down to 0. Some display systems may be assigned only 64 shades of gray, which is sufficient for viewing. Display artifacts can arise when too few shades of gray are assigned to the display. For example, an image displaying only 16 shades of gray shows the discrete count thresholds that will generate isocount lines where changes in count rate across the image jump from one count threshold to another.

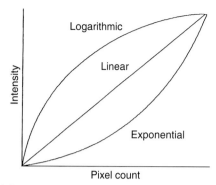

FIGURE 4-8 Grayscale intensity can be assigned as a linear relationship relative to the pixel count. An exponential relationship suppresses low counts, providing background subtraction. A logarithmic relationship enhances low-count intensities.

The relationship between the number of counts and display intensity is usually linear (Figure 4-8), which provides a uniform shading between all count levels. Most computers also allow a logarithmic and an exponential relationship between pixel count and intensity. An exponential relationship suppresses the number of gray scales assigned to low-count values while expanding the number of shades of gray assigned to higher pixel counts (see Figure 4-8). This in effect reduces the low-count pixels, removing background. Conversely, the logarithmic relationship assigns more gray levels to low-count pixels and compresses the number of shades of gray assigned to high pixel values, enhancing differences in low-count densities.

Background subtraction is another enhancement technique to allow better appreciation of slight differences in count. Background enhancement selects a count threshold that is set to the lowest intensity and reassigns intensities between the threshold and the maximum pixel count.

The use of color is another technique to provide image enhancement. Typically a selected color table is used to enhance the differences between pixel count densities and to provide some visual background erase. The red, green, and blue guns of the CRT can be assigned intensity values from 0 to 255 and can be mixed to generate more than 16 million colors. A color table that has only 10 different colors with discrete steps has the same effect of creating isocontour colors in the image as black-and-white images with limited shades of gray. The most effective color tables are those that have gradual and continuous shades of color. For example, the colors of the rainbow—from violet through red, representing low- to high-count values, respectively—provide some aesthetically pleasing images. Another commonly used color table, the "hot iron" table, assigns gray scales from black to dark red through orange and white for the hottest pixel values. The result is an enhancement similar to an exponential scale to suppress low-count densities.

Image Algebra

The simplest image processing operations are those representing the mathematical operations of add, subtract, multiply, and divide. Nuclear medicine computers allow images to be manipulated with these simple functions. For example, a dynamic flow study originally acquired at 1 frame/sec can be reformatted through the addition of three images into one to create a dynamic set with each image representing 3 seconds. Image addition is usually performed to improve the count density of images or to compress a sequence of dynamic images into a smaller number of frames, which can be used more easily to identify time-activity changes within the images. Subtraction is commonly applied to an image matrix in one of two ways: (1) subtraction of a numeric value from all pixels and (2) subtraction of one image from another. Subtraction of a number from the pixel count from each pixel of an image is used to perform background subtraction as an alternative to grayscale enhancement; this technique might be applied to an image where body background is to be eliminated from the image. Subtraction of one frame from another has many clinical uses, such as creation of a cardiac stroke volume image by subtracting the end-systolic image from the end-diastolic image, which leaves only the counts representing areas of myocardial contraction. Another example of frame subtraction is parathyroid imaging, where a technetium image of the thyroid is subtracted from a thallium image of the thyroid and parathyroids. The resultant image is a picture of only parathyroid tissue.

Reframing

Many times, a procedure may be performed using certain parameters that need to be adjusted after the acquisition has taken place. Reframing can adjust the images and compile them to form a better image for interpretation. The most common acquisition that reframing needs to be done with is the flow study. Frames from the flow study can be added together to enhance the image quality and provide a better image. If a flow study is acquired at 1 second per frame for 60 seconds, the study could be reframed many different ways. Adding 2 frames to each other would produce 30 frames at 2 seconds per frame. Or, adding 3 frames together would produce 20 frames at 3 seconds per frame. Acquiring a study in this manner provides much more flexibility when processing the information.

Interpolation

Interpolation is the process of changing the matrix size after the image has been acquired. The matrix can be changed from a larger size to a smaller size, or from a smaller size to a larger size. When an image is interpolated, there is no loss of data. The data is will be redistributed from one pixel to the adjacent pixels. Because of the shifting of counts from one pixel to the next, smoothing (linear) should be applied to the image to ensure an even distribution of counts.

Cinematic Display

A dynamic sequence of images may be displayed as a continuous-loop movie known as a *cinematic display.* The images to be displayed are formatted into an area of memory known as a *buffer* so that information can be retrieved quickly. Some systems may have insufficient memory, and a display buffer is created on disk. Dynamic studies, gated blood pool images, and SPECT images can all be displayed in a cinematic mode. The rate at which images are displayed can be changed; for example, the beating heart from a gated blood pool study can be displayed in real time in a closed loop to provide an image of the beating heart. Longer dynamic studies, such as 30-minute kidney studies, can be displayed to compress the set of images into a few seconds. The observer therefore has a better appreciation of physiological changes that occur over a long time.

Three-Dimensional Display

Although commercial SPECT systems have been available for more than 25 years, techniques to view the vast amount of data contained in a series of slice images have remained limited. Surface display and volume rendering are two techniques for 3D viewing. Surface displays are created by selecting a count threshold for generating a 3D isocount surface. The problem, therefore, becomes to correctly set this threshold to include only clinically useful information; the proper threshold setting is critical for proper clinical interpretation of the 3D object. Because this display shows only a solid outer surface of the organ, information inside the organ is not seen; therefore the most suitable organs for surface displays are thin organs with cold abnormalities, such as the heart and the brain cortex. A very smooth set of slice images creates a smoother surface than the reconstructed slices for directed viewing. Volume rendering is a display technique that provides a translucent appearance to a 3D volume (Figure 4-9). Stacks of reconstructed transverse slices (an image volume) are reprojected into planar images from multiple directions around the object volume like the original planar images (Figure 4-10, *A*). In this reprojection process the maximum pixel count along each projection line is selected as the maximum activity that would be seen for an individual pixel. This projection of the highest concentration of radioactivity provides the image a translucent appearance and also produces an image with very little noise. This technique is excellent for identifying hot abnormalities in SPECT image data and can be applied to a variety of studies, such as finding hot lesions on bone SPECT and identifying hepatic hemangiomas on labeled red-cell studies (Figure 4-10, *B*). The volume-rendered projections are viewed cinematically to produce a dramatic and aesthetically pleasing display. Complex 3D volumes such as a whole-body PET study may be quickly evaluated using volume rendering and displaying the images to see an image of the patient's rotation in space. The human eye easily tracks moving objects, such as an abnormal hot tumor on the display, and the observer's brain will quickly identify the 3D relationship of all objects and organs that are seen.

Image Smoothing

Image smoothing is performed to reduce noise from the random effects of radionuclide counting. The simplest technique is to average the counts of a given pixel with that of its eight surrounding neighbors and replace the center pixel count with the new value.

The most common type of simple image smoothing is the nine-point smooth, which is a filtering technique used to modify a specific pixel value according to the values of its neighbors. The nine-point smooth uses a 3×3 matrix centered over each pixel in the image. The filter weighting values 4, 2, and 1 multiply the center and adjacent pixel values to allow the original value and closest pixels to have more influence on the result of filtering (Figure 4-11). The new computed value after filtering is placed into the pixel location of a new filtered image. Nine-point smoothing blends each pixel value with those of its neighbors, creating a smoother, more aesthetic image (see Figure 4-11). However, this smoothing results in a slight loss of resolution, and detail is slightly blurred. Filters can be based not only on a 3×3 matrix but also on a 5×5, 7×7, or larger filter matrix. In addition, filters with negative values around the edges can enhance or sharpen the edges of organs. These filters are sometimes used in applications for automatic edge detection programs.

Filtering of dynamic image sets can use a temporal filter, which performs weighted averaging of an image

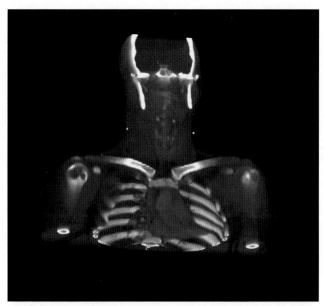

FIGURE 4-9 Three-dimensional surface rendering of CT data creates a volume projection with cut planes on the base to generate a cross-sectional axial slice and a coronal plane cut through the anterior ribs just behind the sternum.

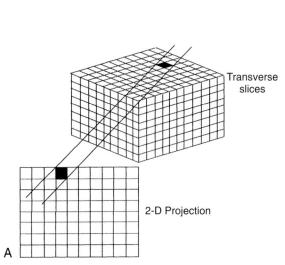

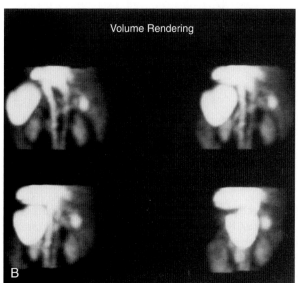

FIGURE 4-10 A, Volume rendering displays are generated from a stack of transverse slices by reprojecting the data into two-dimensional (2D) projections for cinematic viewing. The highest-count pixel along the path for reprojection is placed into the 2D image. **B,** Volume-rendered translucent display of a hepatic hemangioma study shows the exact anatomical location of a hot lesion in the liver as seen from four different angles.

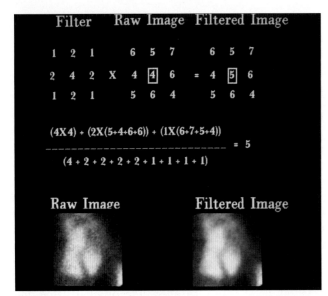

FIGURE 4-11 A nine-point smooth filter with values of 4, 2, and 1 is applied to the center pixel value (4) of a 3 × 3 pixel area of the raw image. Multiplying the raw image center point by 4, the side values by 2, and the corner pixel values by 1 and then dividing by the filter sum produces a new value (5), which is placed into the filtered image. Raw and nine-point smoothed gated cardiac images are shown at bottom.

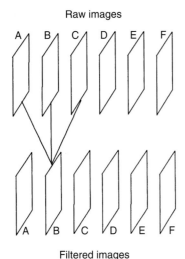

FIGURE 4-12 Dynamic series of images can be temporally smoothed by adding the previous and following images. Image *B* in the filtered image set is composed of an average of *A*, *B*, and *C* from the raw images.

with those that occur just before and after a dynamic image sequence. For example, Figure 4-12 shows an example of filtering frame *B* by multiplying the original frame *B* by a weighting value of 2 and adding 1 times the preceding frame *A* and 1 times the following image, frame *C*. Temporal filtering is applied most frequently to gated cardiac images with the filter applied in a closed loop. Temporal filtering removes noise without a loss of spatial resolution, as occurs with the nine-point smooth.

REGION OF INTEREST

Image Quantitation

Digital nuclear medicine images are many times acquired to derive quantitative information. Counts in a particular area can be extracted from the image by defining an ROI on the displayed image using a mouse, joystick, trackball, or light pen. ROIs can be defined as a rectangle or ellipse or manually drawn as an irregular shape. The ROI program usually allows an option to display or print the counts within the region, the number of pixels in the region, and the average count per pixel. Most computer systems allow 16 to 32 regions to be drawn on a single image. When defining ROIs, the area defined should be physiologically meaningful. For example, when drawing an ROI over the kidney, should the area include the whole kidney and renal pelvis, cortex, and collecting system, or simply the cortex? Different information can be extracted from the images, depending on how the ROI has been defined. Some clinical programs perform automated ROI definition. These programs can use a specific count threshold, maximum slope, isocount level, second derivative, or other criteria to identify the edge of an organ. A combination of techniques such as isocount level mixed with the profile maximum slope (second derivative) can be used in automatically defining the region of the left ventricle on a gated blood pool study.

Some nuclear medicine computer systems allow ROIs to be manipulated just as images can be manipulated. It might be desirable to add or subtract regions. For example, a region defining the renal pelvis could be subtracted from a region defining the whole kidney, thereby leaving the area of the renal cortex. ROIs can be saved with the patient's study to allow reprocessing the information at a later time with the originally defined regions.

Curves

Quantitative information from a single image is derived by setting an ROI and obtaining the ROI counts. The ROI counts in sequential images from a dynamic study can be used to plot the radioactivity-versus-time change or time-activity curve. Physiological information from dynamic studies might be appreciated more easily by generating time-activity curves. Curve displays are widely applied to a variety of clinical applications. Curves provide useful information in evaluating the accumulation and washout of radiopharmaceutical from the kidney, changes in left-ventricular volume on gated studies (Figure 4-13), and changes in radionuclide distribution on gastrointestinal studies. Curves should be displayed to best demonstrate diagnostic information. When multiple curves are displayed on the same graph, such as the individual kidneys in a renal study, it is important that the curves be properly distinguished from

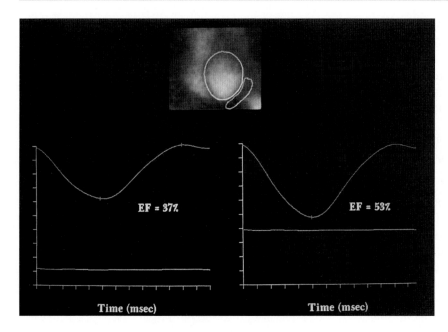

FIGURE 4-13 Regions of interest of the left ventricle and background can be drawn, and time-activity curves can be generated. Curves on the left demonstrate the left-ventricular curve (*upper*) and background curve (*lower*). The background curve contains less activity and is smaller. Curves on the right show a higher background curve (*lower*) after area normalization. With normalization of the background counts, the ejection fraction is correctly computed at 53%.

one another and correctly labeled as to their region (e.g., left kidney, right kidney). Curve display software many times allows the user to select the options for the format of the display: a continuous line versus dots at each data point, the intensity or color of the curves, and display of axis labels. Curve information should also be scaled properly; that is, the extent of the data range along both the *x*- and *y*-axes changes the appreciation of changes in radioactivity. The appropriate scale of each axis should allow the observer to view most accurately changes of clinical significance in the study. For example, a renal scan with a *y*-axis that is very short would display only a small change in radioactivity in a normal renal study.

The manipulation of curves is also valuable in data interpretation. Simple algebraic functions are useful for applications such as adding curves from two separate regions, performing subtraction of a background curve from an organ curve, or multiplying one curve to match the scaling of another curve.

Because of statistical limitations in counts, it is sometimes helpful to smooth curve data. Commonly a 1-2-1–weighted smooth is done for each curve point with its preceding and following neighbors. Another technique to reduce noise in curve data is to fit the curve points to a mathematical formula that allows additional quantitative information to be derived. Most commonly, a straight-line linear fit or an exponential function is fitted to the data. The fitted curve can then allow quantitative numbers to be measured, such as the slope of a linear function or the half-time of an exponential curve.

Normalization

Normalization is a concept in nuclear medicine that implies that a measurement has been brought to a

standard. For instance, two images with different maximum counts may have their intensities normalized if the image with the lowest maximum count is multiplied so that the maximum count matches the maximum count in the second image. The two images, therefore, would be displayed with the same maximum intensity. Normalization is most commonly applied to two ROIs or curves. For example, the counts in ROI-1 are normalized to a second, larger ROI-2 by multiplying ROI-1 counts by the ratio of the number of pixels in ROI-2 divided by the number of ROI-1 pixels. Region normalization is performed most commonly to subtract the background counts of one region from the counts of a different size region.

As an example, consider the subtraction of background in calculating the left-ventricular ejection fraction (EF) from a gated blood pool study (see Figure 4-13). Assume that the counts in an end-diastolic (ED) ROI are 89,485 and 56,375 in the end-systolic (ES) ROI. The left-ventricular ejection fraction can be calculated using the equation:

$$EF = (ED - ES)/ED \times 100$$

In this example, ignoring background, the EF would be:

$$(89,485 - 56,375)/89,485 \times 100 = 37\%$$

This value is erroneously low because body background has not been subtracted. Assume that the ED ROI contains 89,485 counts with an area of 586 pixels, that the ES counts are 56,375 in 416 pixels, and that a background region contains 9134 counts in 89 pixels. To subtract the proper amount of background activity from the ED ROI, the area covered by the ROIs must be of the same size, thus the process of region count normalization. Since the background region is smaller than the left-ventricle region, the background region counts are multiplied by a ratio of the region sizes (number of left-ventricle pixels per number of background pixels).

$$\text{Normalized background counts} = \frac{\text{Background} \times \text{Number of heart pixels}}{\text{Number of background pixels}}$$

The background region contains 9134 counts in 89 pixels, and the ED heart region contains 586 pixels; the normalized ED background becomes 9134 × (586/89), or 60,140 counts. This can be subtracted from the ED count of 89,485, giving a background-subtracted ED count of 29,345. The same normalization calculation can be made for the ES region, which contains 56,375 counts in 416 pixels; the normalized background is 9134 × (416/89), or 42,693 counts. Subtracting this normalized background from the ES left-ventricle counts gives a net of 13,682 counts. With these normalized background-subtracted values, a background-corrected EF is calculated as:

$$(29,345 - 13,682)/29,345 \times 100 = 53\%$$

With proper subtraction of background, the EF value has now been significantly changed.

These same principles of normalization can be applied to curve mathematics. Multiplying the background curve by the ratio of the organ region size divided by a smaller background region size properly increases the background curve for subtraction, significantly changing the EF value. Note that the background curve on the lower right of Figure 4-13 is increased after correct scaling by normalization and that the EF values have changed.

CLINICAL APPLICATIONS

Most hospitals use clinical applications programs provided by a computer manufacturer. Before commercial sale of this software, the company must provide evidence to the U.S. Food and Drug Administration (FDA) of clinical utility along with a description of the program. The accuracy of derived values can vary slightly from one computer system to the next. For example, if one patient-gated blood pool study were processed on several different brands of computers, some variation in the left-ventricular EF value would be found. These variations come from how automated or manual edge detection techniques are implemented, background placement is selected, and so on. It is assumed that there is not enough variation to change the diagnosis of the patient. Validation of program results is important along with establishing normal values of quantitative results.

Clinical applications programs designed specifically for use in the hospital can be written using a programming language such as C or by using a *macro protocol*. A macro is a chain of simple computer operations that are combined to form a practical and meaningful method of evaluating image data. For example, a simple macro can be written to perform image normalization and subtraction of two images, adding frames in a dynamic study or image displays. More involved macros, such as for a renal study, perform a long sequence of operations, such as adding frames of a flow study, displaying the summed image, setting ROIs, generating curves, subtracting normalized background, displaying curves, and performing calculations. Clinical programs or macro protocols should be carefully planned and written to ensure accuracy of the results. Errors or bugs should be identified and removed to ensure that accurate and clinically useful information is being obtained. Any calculated values should be tested on several sets of data to validate the results.

Networks

Networking of computers in nuclear medicine not only has become common but also is an important enhancement to the nuclear medicine clinic. The connection of two or more computers from the same manufacturer is often simple, and the transfer of images and programs can be performed with ease. However, initial complications may occur when networking systems come from different manufacturers; hardware differences, communications problems, and different image file formats are common challenges. Standard networking protocols such as Ethernet allow reliable communication between systems. Files are usually pushed from one system to another by communications software, which takes only a few seconds to transfer an image file. Additional programs might be required to convert image files properly from one manufacturer's format to that of another.

Several different configurations can be used to create a **network**. Figure 4-14 shows two possible arrangements of networks: a central host computer and a bus network. Host networking connects several computers to a larger central host computer for storing and processing all data. The host computer usually has more than one processing terminal for image manipulation and display. Large-capacity disks, optical disks, and tape are available for image storage and archiving. A bus network connects several computers along a single communications line. Each computer has a unique name, and the destination computer is specified when transferring files.

Hospital and Radiology Information Systems

The hospital information system (HIS) is a database used by the hospital to store medical records. The HIS can be made up of many different components into one system. Other information systems specific to different sections

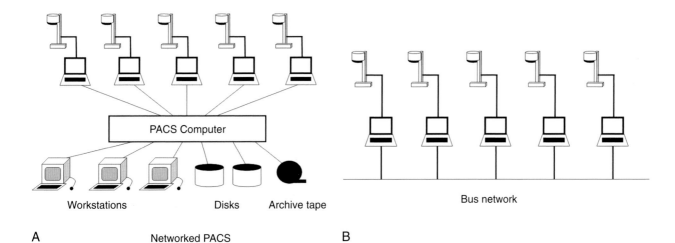

FIGURE 4-14 Nuclear medicine networks can have a variety of configurations. **A,** Acquisition computers send images to a central host computer, which acts as a server for workstations and peripheral devices. **B,** A bus network, such as Ethernet, allows a line for communication between imaging computers.

of the hospital can be integrated into the HIS so that all patient records can be viewed at one location, such as the patient bedside, nurses station, or the physician's office. The HIS can contain many different systems, such as the patient's medical record, electronic health records, laboratory results, radiology information systems, and picture archiving and communications system (PACS). These systems are designed to allow the end user (the health care profession) to do their job with as much ease, effectiveness, and efficiency as possible.

The radiology information system (RIS) should not be confused with the HIS. The RIS is designed specifically for the radiology department to manage the registration, scheduling, patient tracking, and patient workflow that needs to be managed in the radiology department. The RIS is typically integrated with the PACS (discussed in the next few sections) to allow the images from a patient to be displayed along with the information that is stored in the RIS.

Both the HIS and RIS are very network dependent. A hospital or clinic must have the high-speed computer infrastructure for these systems to be efficient.

Digital Imaging and Communications in Medicine

Digital Imaging and Communications in Medicine (DICOM) is a standard that was set forth by a group of manufacturing companies, service organizations, consulting companies, biomedical professional organizations, trade associations, and other government agencies to improve the compatibility and efficiency of moving information between imaging systems and information systems in the health care environment.

In 1985, the American College of Radiology (ACR) and the National Electrical Manufacturers Association (NEMA) introduced the first standard of DICOM, which was called ACR/NEMA 300. This standard has gone through many improvements and versions. Today, DICOM has become the overall standard for medical imaging vendors and hospital organizations for transferring data and images between vendor computer formats.

DICOM data is set up in data sets. DICOM files may include information that cannot be removed from the data set. For example, if an image is acquired, certain information is attached to that image in the data set so that it will never be lost. This is called the data element. Such information is the patient's name, medical record number, accession number, date, and technologist. Without this DICOM standard, hospitals and clinics would need a different computer for each imaging system in their department. DICOM allows the radiology/nuclear medicine department to purchase the best possible systems for their needs without worrying about who the manufacturer is.

Picture Archiving and Communications System

In most departments all nuclear medicine images are acquired digitally and are transferred from one system to another. Physicians view and interpret images directly from the computer screen, thus eliminating the need for film. Such a system is called a **picture archiving and communications system (PACS)**. The filmless nuclear medicine department should have hardware and procedures in place to allow archiving of image data, a backup copy of these data, and enough storage capacity to keep many patient studies available for immediate retrieval. Image data should be kept for several years, consistent with the practice of maintaining a film library for a specified period.

There are obvious advantages to moving images from various cameras to other computers for viewing. Images from one vendor camera may be transferred to another vendor's camera, but the internal file layout or format will likely be different. This transfer of images is easier if both cameras speak the same "file" language.

The Internet

The Internet, or the "information superhighway," can be most simply described as a network of networks. Hundreds of thousands of networks are connected together to form the Internet. The Internet was born from a U.S. Department of Defense project to connect various military research sites. During the 1970s and 1980s this network expanded to include military, government, educational, and commercial computer centers. Computers send information in an envelope called an *Internet protocol (IP)* packet of data to a specific "address." Although no one owns the Internet, there are organizations that promote the global exchange of information and provide technical direction, management, and security.

The organization of computers on the Internet is controlled by an addressing system. A postal mailing address for a residence or business has information from the largest geographic area to a specific city, street, and number. Internet addresses have a set of names and numbers associated with both the computer and the computer network. In order to connect devices on a network, the use of IP addresses are employed. Even if the devices are not connected to the internet, the use of IP addresses is the standard used. Every computer or device that is connected together has a unique IP address. An IP address consists of four sets of numbers called octets. These numbers in machine code are binary numbers, yet when displayed to the end user, the following dotted-decimal format represents a number that is easier for the user to remember. Each number is called an octet, and can be from 0 to 255. Examine the following:

- 192.168.123.132 (displayed to the user)
- 11000000.10101000.01111011.10000100 (binary code)

As previously described, 8-bit numbers have a range of 0 to 255, so four of these numbers compose the IP addresses for up to 4,228,250,625 computer devices connected worldwide. Data files to be transferred on the Internet are broken up into small, manageably sized data packets that may actually be routed in different directions on the Internet but arrive and are reorganized into their original format at their destination. The transmission and reorganization of a file is transparent to the computer user and is part of the beauty of the software that uses the IP.

Computers within large institutions may be directly connected to the Internet, or their network may be connected to the Internet. Access to the Internet may also be provided using either standard telephone lines or special high-speed data lines that connect to another computer that resides on the Internet. Home service is most commonly obtained through a commercial network provider for which customers pay a monthly fee. Often, nuclear medicine computers may not be connected to the Internet because of the concern over security issues, or they may be protected behind a computer firewall to prevent outside access. Any computer directly connected to the Internet should have appropriate security of user accounts and protection of data. Computer network system administrators may prevent unauthorized access to sensitive patient data and protect programs.

The Internet provides computer users with the ability to exchange and obtain information. Electronic mail (e-mail) uses a standard format of data called *simple mail transfer protocol (SMTP)* to allow various types of computers and software to send and receive mail. As previously mentioned, e-mail must be addressed not only to a specific mail server computer on a certain Internet domain, but also to a specific individual account.

The transfer of information files between systems can be done using file transfer protocol (FTP). This protocol uses a standard transfer method of data between Internet sites. Users may use FTP to enter computers where they have permission to look at a listing of files in different directories and *get* or *put* files. To use FTP, the user must have a fairly specific idea of the computer to be accessed and the file directory to be reviewed to obtain the desired information.

The most rapidly expanding part of the Internet is the World Wide Web (WWW). The WWW is based on *hypertext* documents. Hypertext documents have "links" to other documents on the same computer or information at another location, which could be in another city or even country. Hypertext documents differ from other types of connectivity on the Internet in that they provide not only text but also image files, video files, and sound files, which are transferred at the click of a mouse button. A hypertext document is written in a special format language called *hypertext markup language (HTML)*. Special formatting codes within these documents instruct the local computer to display a certain size font and text, where to position an image file on the page, and so on. Links to other documents appear as colored text or small icons, which are activated by clicking on them with the mouse button. This may access a video, image, or sound file or may simply connect to another document.

Access to the WWW is obtained using "browser" software that interprets hypertext documents. A browser such as Internet Explorer is usually included with the operating system or can be downloaded onto a computer for free. Browser software also contains access to search engines (Google, Bing, Yahoo, etc), which allow the user to type in words that describe any topic of interest, and then a list of sites using hypertext links is presented on the screen. The user may then move around or "surf" through documents at various sites to locate information.

The WWW provides tremendous opportunities for locating or exchanging information between Web sites. For example, a nuclear medicine department could create a Web server with documents relevant to its research, continuing education programs, or teaching files, all of which can be available online to anyone with access to the Internet. At this time, many large teaching hospitals have Web sites with a variety of information.

SUMMARY

- Computers are built into many nuclear medicine instruments and image devices.
- Instructions and information are stored in binary format so that the CPU can execute programs and read and write data.
- Image data are stored in either byte or word mode depending on the data depth necessary to store the information without pixel rollover.
- The gamma camera signals for the location and energy of scintillation events. Analog signals are converted into digital form by ADCs.
- Computer memory in the CPU is allocated to store images in a computer matrix at a prescribed data density (byte or word mode).
- Scintillation camera acquisitions may be static planar, whole body, dynamic, gated, SPECT, or gated SPECT.
- The matrix size is selected to optimize the spatial resolution based on the type of acquisition being performed.
- A matrix size of 256×256 is used for most planar studies; in the case of low-count studies a 128×128 matrix may be used.
- Dynamic studies may be 64×64 or 128×128 for rapid imaging sequences where the count density and spatial resolution are low; slow dynamic acquisitions will have higher resolution and the image matrix size should be 128×128 or 256×256.
- SPECT acquisitions are commonly 64×64 with a zoom factor for cardiac studies. High-count or high-resolution studies are usually performed with 128×128 matrices.
- Pixel size may be calculated by:
  pixel size (mm/pixel) = camera dimension (mm)/ (zoom factor × matrix size)
- Normalization must be used when performing ROI quantitative measurements in order to account for differences in the ROI size between organ and background regions.
- Images are converted from Cartesian coordinate matrices into frequency space so that filtering can be applied to reduce noise and improve organ visualization.
- Imaging studies need to be stored for future reference because most studies are not filmed and digital viewing is used for interpretation by the physicians. Long-term storage should be on a medium that has sufficient durability, and online storage should have a data backup mechanism.
- PACS systems allow long-term data storage and distribution of images throughout the health care enterprise.
- DICOM image format allows imaging modalities to communicate to transfer and view studies conveniently.
- The environment for computers and data storage media should be kept clean, and the environment should have controlled temperature, humidity, electric fields, power quality, and static electricity.

SUGGESTED READING

Lee K: *Computers in nuclear medicine: a practical approach*, ed 2, New York, 2005, Society of Nuclear Medicine.

Laboratory Science

Kristen M. Waterstram-Rich

OBJECTIVES

After completing this chapter, the reader will be able to:
- Use laboratory glassware appropriately, including beakers, flasks, graduated cylinders, pipets, and burets.
- Use an analytical balance to perform mass measurements accurately.
- Use and calibrate a centrifuge to separate solids from liquids.
- Use a pH meter.
- Describe the electronic structure of atoms.
- Explain the structure of the periodic table of elements and discuss characteristics of various groups.
- Explain ionic and covalent bonds.
- Use the laws of constant composition and multiple proportions.

- Describe the gram atomic weights, gram molecular weights, and the mole.
- Describe molarity, molality, and normality.
- Explain the characteristics and production of colloids.
- Demonstrate and use chemical reaction equations.
- Describe oxidation-reduction reactions and electrolytic reactions.
- Define acids, bases, and neutralizing reactions.
- Define and measure pH.
- Explain the mechanisms of buffering solutions.
- Describe the simple nomenclature of organic compounds.

KEY TERMS

anion
atom
atomic mass
atomic number
Avogadro's number
cation
centrifuge
chelate
colloid
compound

covalent bond
electron
empirical formula
ion
isotope
ligand
mole
molecular formula
molecule
neutron

noble gas
periodic table
pipet
proton
solute
solution
solvent
volumetric flask

Throughout history, humans have combined chemicals to create new substances or products. Some of these creations that were initiated by chemical reaction were unintentional, even accidental—some were planned. Having the ability to predict how chemicals will react and how to manipulate chemical reactions to obtain a desired outcome is essential to producing or compounding the radiopharmaceuticals used in nuclear medicine. Furthermore, the rationale for producing particular radiopharmaceuticals or for incorporating the use of pharmaceuticals into a particular procedure is based on the expansion of these fundamental chemistry principles to areas of organic and biochemistry.

Radiochemistry and radiopharmacy will be addressed in Chapter 6; however, this chapter provides basic information on chemical reactions. The concepts of atomic structure, chemical equations, moles, acids, bases, and buffers will be addressed. Knowledge of chemical reactions can be applied to all aspects of life, and a nuclear medicine technologist is expected to apply this knowledge to the specialty of nuclear medicine.

GLASSWARE AND INSTRUMENTATION

Glassware

The fundamental part of any scientific laboratory is the equipment, the most basic of which is the glassware. Figure 5-1 shows those items most commonly used in routine laboratory manipulations.

Beakers, Flasks, and Graduated Cylinders. The most frequently used glassware is the beaker. Beakers range in capacity from a few milliliters to several liters and are used in the preparation of **solutions** and as weighing vessels when a high degree of accuracy is not required.

Erlenmeyer flasks are also used in these procedures and, because of their conic shape and small mouth, offer the advantage that solutions can be prepared by swirling the contents of the flask with little risk of spilling. This feature also makes the Erlenmeyer flask an ideal vessel for the substance in titrations. Neither the beaker nor

the flask provides the accuracy (±5% to 10%) required for precise volume measurement.

Volume measurements requiring an accuracy of ±1% to 2% can be achieved by the use of the appropriate graduated cylinder (see Figure 5-1). However, many laboratory procedures require the preparation of solutions accurate in concentration to ±0.001%. This precision can be attained by use of a **volumetric flask**. Flasks marked *TC* are calibrated "to contain" a specific volume, depending on the size of the flask, and allow volume measurement within the accuracy limits noted above.

Pipets and Burets. In the normal course of laboratory work, many occasions arise where a precise volume of a solution or **solvent** is required and an appropriate-sized volumetric flask is not available. In such cases a small (<5 ml) or nonintegral volume is usually required, and a **pipet** or buret must be used.

Pipets (see Figure 5-1) are transfer vessels used to measure and deliver a precise volume of solution or pure liquid. They are generally of two types: those that must be filled and drained manually and automatic pipets that measure and deliver a fixed volume when activated.

The ordinary pipets, which require manipulation, are of two styles: one is calibrated to deliver a fixed volume, whereas the other is graduated and may be used to deliver any increment of volume up to the full capacity of the pipet. Both styles are available in sizes ranging from micro-volumes (a fraction of a milliliter) to a capacity of several hundred milliliters.

Care must be exercised in the use of pipets, because some are calibrated to deliver the stated volume by normal drainage (some solution remains in the tip of the pipet) and others are calibrated to deliver the entire volume drawn into the pipet, which requires "blowing out" the last traces of the solution. The blow-out pipets are identified by one or two bands placed near the top.

Automatic pipets are especially important to the radioimmunoassay laboratory, where knowing the accurate volumes of radioactive solutions is required.

Procedures such as titrations, in which an accurately measured but unknown volume of solution must be

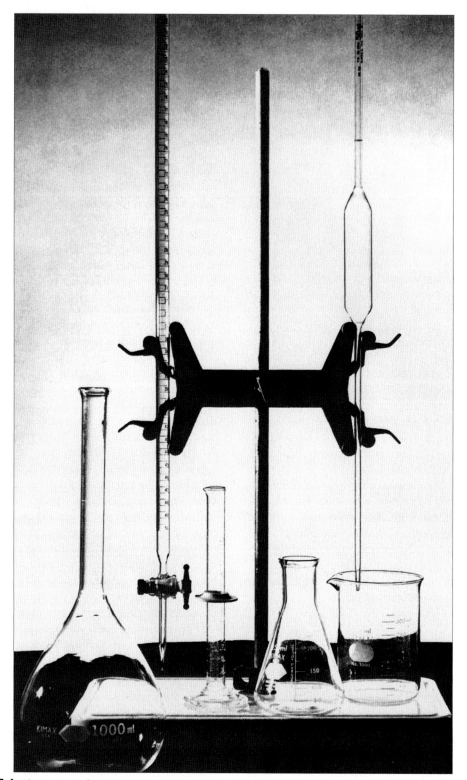

FIGURE 5-1 Glassware. *Left to right,* Volumetric flask, buret, graduated cylinder, Erlenmeyer flask, pipet, and beaker.

determined, are conveniently performed by use of a buret. The buret, which is graduated, allows a direct reading of the volume used in reaching the end point, that is, the point at which the added titrant has reacted with the entire quantity of substance present in the sample.

Instrumentation

Just as certain types of glassware are important to the laboratory, so also are several instruments. All nuclear pharmacy or radioassay laboratories must be equipped with a minimum of three instruments: an analytical balance, a **centrifuge,** and a pH meter.

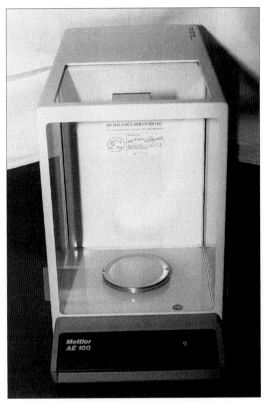

FIGURE 5-2 Analytical balance.

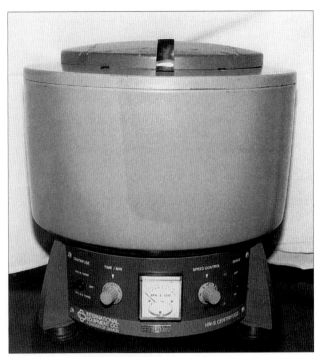

FIGURE 5-3 Centrifuge.

The Analytical Balance. The analytical balance (Figure 5-2) is vital to any laboratory in which mass measurements of solids are routinely required, usually in small quantities (<1 g). The balance shown in Figure 5-2 allows mass measurements accurate to ±0.1 mg.

The balance is designed so that as the units on the weight dials are changed, the instrument automatically adds or removes weights from a knife-edge counterbalance inside the instrument. Newer, currently available analytical balances are automatic taring and provide a direct digital readout of weight. If handled with care, the balance will give dependable results with a minimum of service.

The Centrifuge. Quite often it is necessary to separate solids from liquids, such as separating red blood cells from the plasma. When such separations are necessary, a centrifuge is used (Figure 5-3).

The centrifuge is composed of a balanced motor and shaft on which cups or holders are mounted. A container holding the mixture to be separated is placed in one cup, and a counterbalance container (having the same weight as the sample container) is placed in the cup opposite the sample.

The centrifuge exerts a strong centrifugal force on the sample by spinning the material at relatively high speeds (500 to 1500 revolutions per minute [rpm]). In the case of blood, the heavier red blood cells settle to the bottom of the container, leaving the lighter plasma on top. The plasma can then be drawn off, thus effecting a separation of the two components.

The pH Meter. The measurement of pH is generally accomplished by two methods, one of which provides reasonably accurate values, and the other provides more precise values. The less sensitive method makes use of a paper containing a universal indicator. The universal indicator is a mixture of organic dyes, which themselves are acids and bases, and it changes color on being converted from one form to the other, that is, acid to base or base to acid. These color changes occur at specific pH values.

Accurate pH values, which are usually necessary in radioimmunoassay analysis or the preparation of radiopharmaceuticals, are determined by use of a pH meter (Figure 5-4).

A pH meter has two electrodes. (Note that the one in Figure 5-4 contains both electrodes in a single probe.) One electrode of known potential (a calomel electrode) serves as a reference and involves the following electrode reaction:

$$2Hg + 2Cl^- \rightleftharpoons Hg_2Cl_2 + 2e^-$$

This reaction has a constant potential of −0.27 V. The second electrode (a glass electrode) consists of a meter wire dipped into a solution of known pH, and this solution is separated by a thin glass membrane from the solution whose pH is to be determined. The potential across the glass membrane, and thus the half-cell voltage of this electrode, is a function of the pH of the solution outside the membrane. A third component of a pH meter is a voltmeter or potentiometer capable of measuring voltages accurate to at least ±0.01 V. The voltmeter

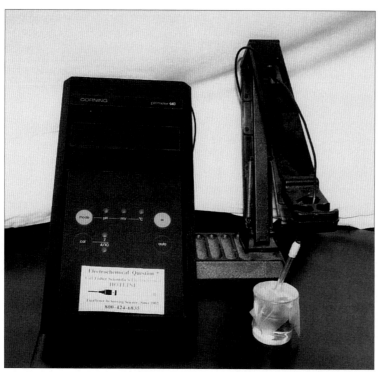

FIGURE 5-4 pH meter.

or potentiometer is designed, based on the potential difference of the two electrodes, to give a reading in pH units.

ELEMENTS AND COMPOUNDS

In introducing the study of chemistry as it applies to nuclear medicine and nuclear pharmacy, it is desirable to define the word *chemistry*. Chemistry can best be defined as the study of matter and the changes that matter undergoes.

All matter exists in one of three physical states—solid, liquid, or gas. Each substance differs in physical and chemical properties from all other substances.

Physical properties are the attributes characteristic of a substance, such as odor, color, hardness, luster, density, and structure. These properties depend on the conditions imposed on the substance and may be affected by a change in temperature, pressure, or radiation. However, a substance, be it an element or a **compound,** that has undergone a change in physical properties because of a change in conditions will exhibit the initial properties when that substance is returned to the original condition. For example, sulfur, which is a yellow solid at room temperature, becomes a liquid when heated to 113° C and returns to the yellow solid when allowed to cool. Physical changes are readily reversible.

In contrast to a change in physical properties, chemical change results in a complex and deep-seated change. Chemical change always results in the formation of one or more "new" substances, each of which has chemical and physical properties unique to itself. Most chemical changes are reversible only with great difficulty, and many—for example, the burning of wood or paper—are irreversible.

Electronic Structure

Because each element has unique chemical and physical properties, it is logical to ask why this is so. To answer this question, the very nature of the elements, that is, their constitution and behavior, must be examined.

Experimental evidence has shown that all elements are made up of minute particles called **atoms.** An atom is the smallest unit of an element that can exist and still maintain the properties of the element. All atoms of a given element are identical in chemical properties, and the atoms of each element differ in properties from the atoms of all other elements. To understand why this is so requires knowledge of the structure of atoms and the components necessary to their formation.

Structurally, all atoms can be described as a sphere composed of two parts. One part is a small, compact nucleus located at the center of the sphere; the second part, a region of space surrounding the nucleus, is populated by small particles called **electrons (e−).**

The nucleus is primarily composed of two types of particles—**protons (p+)** and **neutrons (n0).** Protons are small particles, each of which has a charge of +1, whereas neutrons, also small particles, have no charge and are therefore neutral. Since like charges repel, other particles within the nucleus overcome these repulsive forces and act as the "nuclear glue" that holds the protons together in the nucleus.

The mass of an atom is, for all practical purposes, contained in the nucleus and equal to the sum of the masses of the protons and neutrons. Each proton and neutron has arbitrarily been given a value of 1 atomic mass unit (amu), which has been found by experiment to be equal to 1.67×10^{-24} g. By definition, the number of protons in the nucleus of an atom is the same as the **atomic number** of the element. Since the mass of the neutron is known to be essentially the same as that of the proton, all the mass of the atom is attributed to the protons and neutrons, and the sum of the two is equal to the **atomic mass** of the atom, which is expressed in amu. Thus the atomic mass minus the atomic number equals the number of neutrons present in the nucleus.

The net charge of an atom of an element is zero; that is, it is neutral. Therefore, since protons have a positive charge (+1), there must be one negative charge present for each proton in the nucleus. These negatively charged particles are called *electrons,* each of which has a net charge of −1. For most purposes, the mass of the electron is considered to be zero, because when compared to the mass of the proton and neutron, its mass is negligible (5.5×10^{-4} amu). The number of electrons present in an atom, which is equal to the number of protons, also signifies that the number of electrons is equal to the atomic number.

As previously noted, electrons are found in the space surrounding the nucleus; however, they are not found at fixed points but are circulating about the nucleus and occupy specific regions with respect to the nucleus and with respect to other electrons (Figure 5-5). The relative distance of an electron from the nucleus, and the shape and the orientation of the region it occupies with respect to other regions, has been determined by a combination of spectroscopic evidence and a mathematic treatment known as *quantum mechanics.* However, the results of these treatments are useful in that they allow a description of each electron of an atom in terms of its general position, its relative energy, and the shape of the region that it will occupy. Each electron can be described by a set of four quantum numbers (note that lowercase letters refer to single particles, whereas capital letters refer to systems):

1. The principal quantum number is designated by the letter *n,* which can have a positive integral value, with the exception of 0, that is, 1, 2, 3, and so on. This quantum number indicates the relative distance from the nucleus at which the electron is found, and also its relative energy. These are major energy levels and are often called *shells.*

2. The secondary quantum number is designated by ℓ. The values of ℓ have a range of positive, integral numbers from 0 to n − 1; that is, if n = 3, then ℓ = 0, 1, and 2. This quantum number describes the geometric shape of the subenergy level in which the electron is found. These subenergy levels are found within a major energy level and are usually referred to as *orbitals.*

3. The magnetic quantum number is designated by *m.* The numerical value of m can vary from negative ℓ to positive ℓ; that is, if ℓ = 1, m = −1, 0, +1. This quantum number defines the orientation of the orbital in space; that is, because an s orbital is spherically symmetric (Figure 5-6), it has no discernible orientation. However, orientations of the three p orbitals are mutually perpendicular along the x-, y-, and z-axes (Figure 5-7).

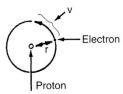

FIGURE 5-5 Bohr's model of hydrogen atom. *v,* Velocity of electron; *r,* average radius of orbit of electron about nucleus.

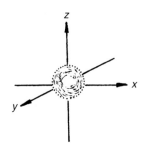

FIGURE 5-6 Atomic s orbitals.

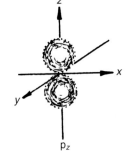

FIGURE 5-7 Atomic p orbitals.

TABLE 5-1	**Relationship of Quantum Numbers**													
Shell (n)	1	2		3										
Subshell (ℓ)	0	0	1	0	1		2							
m value	0	0	−1	0	+1	0	−1	0	+1	−2	−1	0	+1	+2
s value	±½	±½	±½	±½	±½	±½	±½	±½	±½	±½	±½	±½	±½	±½
Number of electrons*	↑↓	↑↓	↑↓	↑↓	↑↓	↑↓	↑↓	↑↓	↑↓	↑↓	↑↓	↑↓	↑↓	↑↓

*↑ denotes e⁻ with +½ spin; ↓ denotes e⁻ with −½ spin.

4. The spin quantum number is designated s. This quantum number can have only one of two numeric values ($+\frac{1}{2}$ or $-\frac{1}{2}$) because only two electrons may occupy the same orbital (the Pauli exclusion principle) and must have opposite spins. Electrons, which are negatively charged, are mutually repulsive. Evidence has shown, however, that electrons are not simply charged particles moving in space but are also spinning about an axis while undergoing translational motion. The spin of the electron gives rise to a magnetic field, and the fields arising (as north and south poles of a magnet are attracting) consequently reduce the degree of repulsion from like charges. This permits two electrons that have common n, ℓ, and m quantum numbers to occupy the same orbital.

The quantum numbers used to identify an electron do not describe the energy of the electron quantitatively. However, the larger the n and ℓ values for the electron, the further the electron will be from the nucleus, and consequently these electrons will have a greater energy than those electrons of lower n and ℓ values. Also, the number of orbitals of equivalent energy contained within a major energy level is given by $m = -1$ to $+1$. For example, the second major energy level, $n = 2$, contains two types of subenergy levels. When $\ell = 0$, $m = 0$, indicating that only one orbital of this type is present, which is termed an *s orbital*. However, when $\ell = 1$ and $m = -1$, 0, and +1, indicating that there are three orbitals of this type, each of equivalent energy, they are called *p orbitals*. Thus the second energy level is composed of a total of four subenergy levels or orbitals. For higher values of n, in addition to s and p orbitals, there are also d and f orbitals.

It follows that no two electrons can have the same set of quantum numbers; this is known as the *Pauli exclusion principle* (Table 5-1).

An examination of Table 5-1 indicates that the total number of electrons that a given shell (n) can accommodate is equal to $2n^2$.

At this point it is necessary to describe the order in which the major and subenergy levels will be filled by electrons. An electron will always enter the lowest energy level available, and obviously the greater the attraction between an electron and the nucleus, the lower the

energy of the electron will be. Thus the first electron will enter the 1s orbital of the first energy level, and the second electron, differing in quantum number from the first electron only in the sign of the spin quantum number, will also enter the 1s orbital; these electrons will be paired. Recall that a given shell can accommodate $2n^2$ electrons. In this case $n = 1$ and $2n^2 = 2$, so the first energy level is filled.

The next electron must now enter the second energy level, $n = 2$, and will occupy the 2s orbital; the same will be true for the next electron. The 2s orbital now containing two electrons, whose spins are paired, is filled, and the next electron must enter one of the three 2p orbitals. One might expect the next electron to enter the same p orbital to give paired electrons; however, spectroscopic evidence indicates that this electron enters one of the two remaining empty p orbitals and has the same spin number as the first p electron. This behavior is summarized by Hund's rule, which states that for an atom where orbitals of equal energies are being filled, the electrons will remain unpaired until each orbital is half filled, that is, one electron in each of the orbitals.

To facilitate the assignment of electrons to the lowest energy orbital available, the following sequence is helpful:

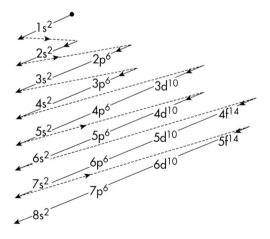

The arrows and broken lines indicate the proper order of filling. The symbols and their significance are as follows:

Example:
Given the term $4p^3$, indicate the n, ℓ, m, and s values.

1. $n = 4$, the fourth energy level.
2. Since p electrons are involved, $\ell = 1$.
3. With ℓ being 1, $m = -1, 0, +1$ (the three p orbitals), each of which can accommodate two electrons for a total of 6.
4. The superscript 3 denotes the presence of three electrons in the p orbitals. Following Hund's rule, each orbital (p_x, p_y, p_z) will contain one electron, all of which will have parallel spins ($s = +\frac{1}{2}$).

Had the electrons cited in the example been the electrons of highest energy in a neutral atom, the element to which they belong would be known. These being the highest-energy electrons would indicate that all orbitals of lower energy had been filled. Thus counting the number of electrons (using the diagram) and recalling that the number of electrons is equal to the atomic number of the element reveals that the element corresponding to the atom has an atomic mass of 33. The **periodic table** (Figure 5-8) shows element number 33 to be arsenic (As).

Periodic Table of the Elements

Early in the nineteenth century, chemists noted a relationship between atomic weight and properties of the elements. Although many of the elements had not yet been discovered, chemists were able to recognize those elements having similar properties and group them into families. Around 1870 several chemists segregated the known elements into groups (families) and showed that properties were a function of atomic number rather than atomic weight and that the properties of a given element, both physical and chemical, were similar to those elements having an atomic number differing by 8, 18, 32, and so on. For example, lithium (Li; atomic number 3), sodium (Na; atomic number 11), potassium (K; atomic number 19), and rubidium (Rb; atomic number 37) exhibited similar physical properties in being shiny, ductile, malleable, and good conductors of electrical current. Chemically, these elements are similar in that they form compounds with other elements in the same proportions. Thus *one* atom of Li or Na reacts with *one* atom of fluorine (F), forming lithium fluoride (LiF) or sodium fluoride (NaF), but *two* atoms of Li or Na react with *one* atom of oxygen to form lithium oxide (Li_2O) or sodium oxide (Na_2O). Other families such as fluorine, chlorine, bromine, iodine, and astatine, or oxygen, sulfur, selenium, tellurium, and polonium are groups of elements exhibiting similar chemical and physical properties.

The periodic table contains the elements known at this time (see Figure 5-8). Elements of similar properties are grouped together in columns (placed vertically) to form a family having the same electron configuration in the outermost shell. For example, Li, Na, and so on, each contain *one* electron in the outer shell, whereas F, Cl, and so on, each contain *seven* electrons in the outer shell. However, the elements in a row (placed horizontally) differ from one another in chemical and most physical properties. From a consideration of the electron configuration of the elements, it is apparent that the elements in a given row differ in electron configuration from all other elements contained in that row. Thus sodium, having one electron in the 3s atomic orbital, differs from the element of the next higher atomic number, magnesium (Mg), which has two electrons in the 3s atomic orbital, and so on.

The information contained in the periodic table is not restricted to electron configuration of the outer shell, but also indicates the complete structure of the electrons and the relative atomic mass of each element. Each element is identified by its chemical symbol, as shown in Figure 5-9. The number above the chemical symbol is the atomic number (Z number) of the element and the number below the symbol is the average atomic mass (A number) of the element. For example, the element fluorine (Figure 5-9) has an atomic number, or Z number, of 9, which indicates the number of protons and electrons present in the atom. The number 18.9984 shown below the symbol indicates the average atomic mass, or A number, of the element. Recalling that the atomic mass number minus the atomic number gives the number of neutrons present in the nucleus and that the masses of the neutron and proton are essentially identical, the atomic mass of an element is expected to be an integer. Obviously, the value for fluorine or any other element is not integral and indicates that all atoms of an element are not identical. The nonintegral atomic mass arises from the fact that all atoms of a given element do not contain the same number of neutrons. If some atoms contain a greater or lesser number of neutrons in the nucleus than other atoms, the average atomic mass of a collection of such atoms will not be integral. Atoms that differ only in the number of neutrons present in the nucleus are called isotopes.

Stable Electron Configurations: The Noble Gases

Chemists of the nineteenth century also noted that certain elements were unreactive and would not combine with other elements to give compounds. It is now known that these elements are members of the eighth group shown in the periodic table and constitute a family of elements. These elements all exist in the gaseous state under normal conditions and, because they are inert, are commonly referred to as the **noble gases**. In the periodic table (see Figure 5-8), each of the noble gases contains eight electrons in the outer shell, thereby indicating that for these elements the s and p orbitals within the outer shell are completely filled.

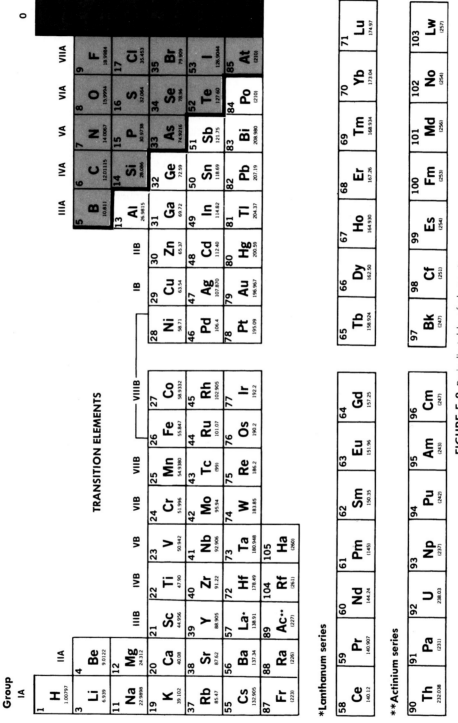

FIGURE 5-8 Periodic table of elements.

Elements other than the noble gases combine with other elements and do so in such a way that the resulting electron configuration of the elements undergoing reaction is changed to an electron configuration of the noble gases. *This gives a stable electron configuration to each element, one that all elements strive to attain.* For this to be true, the reacting elements must either donate to, accept from, or share electrons with another element. For example, sodium, which has an electron configuration of $1s^22s^22p^63s^1$, differs in electron configuration from the noble gas neon (Ne) (in which the second energy level is completely filled, $1s^22s^22p^6$) by one electron; that is, sodium contains one more electron, $3s^1$. Therefore, for sodium to attain an electron configuration identical with neon, it must donate (transfer) the 3s electron to another element.

Assume that sodium is undergoing a reaction with fluorine $1s^22s^22p^5$, and note that the electron configuration of fluorine differs from that of the noble gas neon by one electron. However, fluorine needs to acquire one electron to attain noble gas configuration, whereas sodium had only to donate one electron to achieve the same electron structure. An equation for the reaction of one atom of sodium with one atom of fluorine may now be written (Figure 5-10).

It can be seen that the electron structures of sodium (1+), fluorine (1−), and neon (neutral) are identical; that is, each has an electron structure of $1s^22s^22p^6$. Note at this point that only electrons were involved in this reaction and that the sodium atom transferring an electron to the fluorine atom acquires a net charge of 1+, and the fluorine atom accepting the electron from sodium acquires a net charge of 1− (compare the number of protons in the nucleus to the total number of electrons present for sodium and fluorine in the products).

Although the foregoing is a rather simple example, an understanding of the chemistry of most elements can be explained in the same manner. *Most elements undergo reaction by donating, accepting, or sharing electrons so as to attain the electron configuration of a noble gas.* The transition metals are an exception to the rule.

Ionic Compounds

The reaction of sodium with fluorine, as discussed in the previous section, involves a complete transfer of electrons and results in the formation of charged particles called **ions.** In those reactions involving a complete transfer of electrons, the ion resulting from the element donating electrons is called a **cation** (in this case a sodium ion, Na^{1+}), and the element accepting electrons is called an **anion** (fluoride ion, F^{1-}). The elements occupying the left part of the periodic table are known as metals and tend to undergo chemical reaction by donating electrons. Conversely, the nonmetals, which occupy the right part of the periodic table, tend to undergo chemical reaction by accepting electrons. Each metallic element differs from the other metals in its ability to donate electrons, and the nonmetallic elements differ from one another in their ability to accept electrons. The ability of an element to accept electrons is known as its *electronegativity,* with the element having the greatest ability to accept electrons (fluorine) arbitrarily being assigned a value of 4. This is the Pauling scale; others exist and are in common use. The ability of all other elements to accept electrons is compared numerically to fluorine. These values are shown in Table 5-2.

Thus in the foregoing reaction between sodium and fluorine, the fluorine atom (electronegativity 4.0) readily acquires an electron from sodium (electronegativity 0.9), resulting in ions, both of which are isoelectronic with neon. Elements that tend to react by transfer of electrons must differ in electronegativity by approximately 2.5 electronegativity units.

At this point it must be noted that the sodium and fluorine ions produced in this reaction, though they have electron configurations identical with that of neon, differ from the noble gas in that sodium still contains 11 protons in its nucleus and fluorine retains its 9 protons. The sodium ion produced now possesses one more proton in its nucleus than it has electrons in the energy levels surrounding it; therefore sodium in this state must have a net charge of 1+. Similarly, fluorine, now containing one additional electron, must have a net charge of 1−. Since opposite charges attract each other, it should

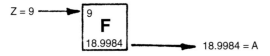

FIGURE 5-9 Periodic chart representation of fluorine (F).

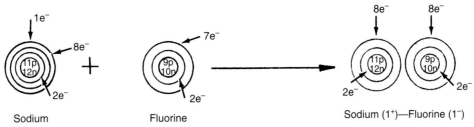

Sodium   Fluorine   Sodium (1⁺)—Fluorine (1⁻)

FIGURE 5-10 Reaction of sodium atom and fluorine atom to produce ionic compound.

TABLE 5-2	Electronegativity Values of Selected Elements					
H 2.1						
Li 1.0	Be 1.5	B 2	C 2.5	N 3.0	O 3.5	F 4.0
Na 0.9	Mg 1.2	Al 1.5	Si 1.8	P 2.1	S 2.5	Cl 3.0
K 0.8	Ca 1.0	Sc 1.3	Ge 1.8	As 2.0	Se 2.4	Br 2.8
Rb 0.8	Sr 1.0	Y 1.2	Sn 1.8	Sb 1.9	Te 2.1	I 2.5

not be surprising that the resulting ions approach each other and are held together by these electrostatic attractions to form an ionic compound. *All elements that undergo reactions to form ions result in the formation of ionic compounds.*

Covalent Compounds

Elements whose electronegativities differ by less than 2.5 also undergo reaction to attain electron configurations identical with one of the noble gases. However, in this case neither element is sufficiently electronegative to completely acquire the electrons of the second element, the result being that they react in a manner so as to share the electrons in their valence shell (valence electrons are those in the outermost shell). For example, in the reaction of carbon (C) (electronegativity 2.5) with chlorine (Cl) (electronegativity 3.0), the compound formed *has no charge.* If circles (o) and exes (x) are used to indicate the electrons involved in the reaction, and given that the electrons of lower energy (in shells closer to the nucleus) are still present, the reaction can be represented as follows:

$$\text{o}\overset{\text{o}}{\underset{\text{o}}{\text{C}}}\text{o} + 4\,{}^{x}_{x}\overset{xx}{\underset{xx}{\text{Cl}}}{}^{x}_{x} \rightarrow {}^{x}_{x}\overset{xx\;\;ox\;\;xx}{\underset{xx\;\;xo\;\;xx}{\text{Cl}{}^{x}_{o}\text{C}{}^{o}_{x}\text{Cl}}}{}^{x}_{x}$$

Although the chlorine and the carbon atoms have not reacted by electron transfer, each of the atoms has attained the electron configuration of a noble gas by sharing its valence electrons. Unlike sodium fluoride (NaF), the compound carbon tetrachloride (CCl_4) formed in this reaction is a **molecule** in which the four chlorine atoms and the carbon atom are bound to one another and function as one unit. The product CCl_4 is called a *molecule.* The bond in this case, rather than being ionic as that of NaF, *is covalent. All compounds that are formed by the sharing of electrons rather than the transfer of electrons are said to have* **covalent bonds.**

Even though these bonds are described as being covalent, it is apparent that the electronegativities of the two elements (see Table 5-2) are not the same; therefore the electrons used in forming the bonds between the carbon atom and the four chlorine atoms cannot be shared equally. This leads to the conclusion that the electron pair in each of these bonds is more strongly attracted to chlorine than to carbon. Covalent bonds formed from two different elements of unequal electronegativity must be *polar covalent,* meaning that the electrons forming the bond are more strongly attracted to one atom than to the other.

Those elements of essentially the same electronegativity react to form bonds that are completely covalent; that is, the electrons of the bond are shared equally between the two atoms. For example, oxygen (O), which composes 20% of the earth's atmosphere, exists as the molecule O_2. It is apparent that the electronegativity of each oxygen atom in the molecule is the same; therefore the electrons that bond these atoms cannot be attracted more strongly by one atom than by the other. This results in an equal sharing of electrons, *and the bond is completely covalent.* Other examples of nonpolar covalent bonds are nitrogen (N_2, which is 80% of the earth's atmosphere), hydrogen (H_2), and the halogens (F_2, Cl_2, Br_2, I_2). As will be discussed later, the carbon-hydrogen bond in organic molecules is essentially nonpolar covalent because both carbon and hydrogen have electronegativity values of approximately 2.5.

Coordinate Covalent Bonds

Those compounds containing coordinate covalent bonds are similar to those compounds containing covalent bonds in that the bonding electrons are shared by two atoms. However, the electrons used in forming these bonds are donated by *one atom only.* As an example, consider the reaction in which a molecule of sulfuric acid is formed from the following elements:

$$2\text{H}_{\square} + \text{o}\overset{\text{oo}}{\underset{\text{oo}}{\text{S}}}\text{o} + 4\,{}^{x}\overset{xx}{\underset{xx}{\text{O}}}{}^{x} \rightarrow \text{H}{}^{x}_{\square}\overset{xx\;\;oo\;\;xx}{\underset{xx\;\;oo\;\;xx}{\text{O}{}^{x}_{o}\text{S}{}^{o}_{x}\text{O}}}{}^{x}_{\square}\text{H}$$

or

$$\text{H}-\text{O}-\overset{\displaystyle \text{O} \atop \uparrow}{\underset{\downarrow \atop \displaystyle \text{O}}{\text{S}}}-\text{O}-\text{H}$$

The symbol "—" represents a covalent bond, and ↑ represents a coordinate covalent bond in which the arrow points toward the atom that did not contribute any electrons to bond formation.

Considering each bond in the sulfuric acid molecule and the electrons used in forming each bond, it is apparent that the hydrogen-oxygen bonds and two of the sulfur-oxygen bonds are polar covalent, whereas the remaining two sulfur-oxygen bonds are coordinate covalent bonds, in that the electrons used in forming these bonds are contributed by the sulfur atom only.

Complex Ions and Chelates

The formation of coordinate covalent bonds need not occur by reaction of neutral elements, as shown in the previous section. In many reactions a coordinate covalent bond is formed by the interaction of a neutral molecule with an ion. In reactions of this type the driving force, or reason for reaction, is that an atom contained within the neutral molecule has not attained the electron configuration of a noble gas. In previous discussions the metals were assumed to react by transfer of their electrons to form ionic compounds. However, elements such as aluminum (Al) have been found to form compounds in which the bonds are largely polar covalent. This being true, it is apparent that the aluminum atom needs three electrons to attain the noble gas configuration of argon (Ar). Consequently, aluminum chloride ($AlCl_3$), in a nonpolar solvent, reacts with anhydrous chloride gas (Cl_2) according to the following equation:

The electrons used in forming the fourth chlorine-aluminum bond are donated by the chloride ion, resulting in the formation of a coordinate covalent bond. The ions that provide the bonding electrons are called **ligands.**

A second example of coordinate covalent bond formation is one in which a positive ion undergoes reaction with a neutral molecule, as illustrated in the following reaction:

The products resulting from reactions of neutral molecules with either a cation or an anion are called *complex ions.*

Although elements such as aluminum and nitrogen can share one pair of electrons with simple ions to form complex ions, other elements, especially the transition elements, must accept two or more pairs of electrons to attain a noble gas electron configuration. These complexes are especially important in nuclear medicine and in many cases involve the formation of **chelates** in which the electron pairs (two or more pairs) are donated by functional groups present in the ligand molecule. The

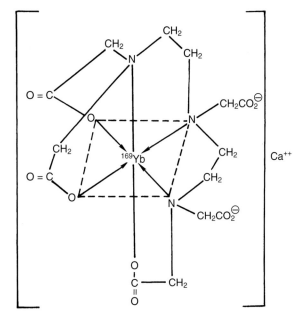

FIGURE 5-11 Ytterbium-pentetic acid (Yb-DTPA) complex. *Arrows,* Coordinate covalent bonds; *dotted line,* plane through these atoms.

term *chelate,* from the Greek word *ché-lé* (claw), is reserved for these ligands. The complex ytterbium-pentetic acid (Yb-DTPA) (Figure 5-11), used as a cisternographic imaging agent, is an excellent example of a chelate. In this case the electrons used in forming the coordinate covalent bonds are donated by the functional groups present in the pentetic acid molecule.

Although the structures of many complex ions of technetium are still under investigation, it is reasonable to assume that their structures are similar to those formed by ytterbium.

LAWS OF CONSTANT COMPOSITION AND MULTIPLE PROPORTION

The fact that elements generally react with other elements to attain a noble gas electron configuration leads to the conclusion that any two elements that undergo reaction must do so in a definite ratio of atoms, that is, one Na to one F and one C to four Cl. It then follows that the elements must also react to definite ratios by weight. This is stated by the *law of constant composition:* a compound, regardless of its origin or method of preparation, always contains the same elements in the same proportions by weight.

In some cases, depending on reaction conditions, an element will combine with another to give products that differ in the ratio of atoms of the two elements. For example, sodium usually reacts with oxygen to form sodium oxide (Na_2O), but under other conditions they react to form sodium peroxide (Na_2O_2). However, in each case the ratio of sodium to oxygen is definite. This is stated by the *law of multiple proportions:* When two elements combine to form two or more different compounds, the ratio of the mass of one element that combines with a fixed mass of a second element is a simple ratio of whole numbers, for example, 2:1 or 3:2.

Sample Problems

Example 1:

When subjected to quantitative elemental analysis, two samples of a compound containing only carbon and oxygen give the following data:

	Weight of Sample	Weight of C Found	Weight of O Found
Sample 1:	0.7335 g	0.2002 g	0.5333 g
Sample 2:	0.6162 g	0.1682 g	0.4480 g

Do these data uphold the law of constant composition? If the law is upheld, the percentage of carbon and oxygen must be the same in each sample. To determine this, the ratio of the weight of each element to the total weight of the sample must be equal to the ratio of the percent of the element to 100%.

Sample 1:

$$\text{Percent carbon} = \frac{0.2002}{0.7335} = \frac{\%C}{100\%} \%C = 27.29$$

$$\text{Percent oxygen} = \frac{0.5333}{0.7335} = \frac{\%O}{100\%} \%O = 72.71$$

Sample 2:

$$\text{Percent carbon} = \frac{0.1682}{0.6162} = \frac{x\%C}{100\%} \%C = 27.29$$

$$\text{Percent oxygen} = \frac{0.4480}{0.6162} = \frac{x\%O}{100\%} \%O = 72.71$$

The percentage of carbon and oxygen being the same for both samples indicates that they are of identical composition and thus support the law of constant composition.

Example 2:

A third sample, obtained from a different source, was also found to contain only carbon and oxygen and gave the following data upon analysis:

	Weight of Sample	Weight of C Found	Weight of O Found
Sample 3:	0.3599 g	0.1543 g	0.2056 g

Show that these data illustrate the law of multiple proportions. Follow the procedure used in example 1. Sample 3:

$$\text{Percent carbon} = \frac{0.1543}{0.3599} = \frac{\%C}{100\%} \%C = 42.87$$

$$\text{Percent oxygen} = \frac{0.2056}{0.3599} = \frac{\%O}{100\%} \%O = 57.13$$

Obviously this composition indicates that sample 3 was obtained from a compound different from that of samples 1 and 2. Although the samples differ in composition, the law of multiple proportions states that the ratios of the masses of the elements in each compound should be related as simple whole numbers. Thus:

For example 1: $\dfrac{\%O}{\%C} = \dfrac{72.71}{27.49} = 2.66$

For example 3: $\dfrac{\%O}{\%C} = \dfrac{57.13}{42.87} = 1.33$

Therefore the ratios of oxygen to carbon in sample 1 and sample 3 are related by the ratio of 2.66:1.33 or 2:1.

GRAM ATOMIC WEIGHTS, GRAM MOLECULAR WEIGHTS, AND THE MOLE CONCEPT

The chemistry discussed thus far has been based on the interactions of individual atoms. Although this description is a valid one, the isolation and use of single atoms in the laboratory is neither practical nor possible. The smallest sample that can be accurately measured in the laboratory will contain 10^{15} to 10^{17} atoms or molecules.

For a reaction to be accurately described by a chemical equation, it is necessary only that the number of atoms or molecules of the reactants be present in the *ratio* given by the coefficients for these substances. In the following reaction, the ratio of hydrogen (H_2) molecules to oxygen (O_2) molecules must be 2:1.

$$2H_2 + 1O_2 \rightarrow 2H_2O$$

The chemist, being unable to count the number of atoms or molecules necessary for a given reaction, must resort to an indirect method to achieve this ratio. The fact that each element possesses a unique atomic mass (see Figure 5-8) indicates that even though equal weights of hydrogen and oxygen could be measured, the number of molecules of hydrogen present in the sample would be 16 times that of the oxygen molecules; that is, one hydrogen molecule has a weight of 2 relative to a weight of 32 for one oxygen molecule. A convenient method that allows the measurement of the required quantities of the reactants by accurate weighing of each substance is based directly on their gram atomic weight (gaw) or gram molecular weight (gmw). By definition, these are the weights in grams that are numerically equal to the atomic weights (amu) or molecular weights (the sum of the atomic weights of all atoms present in the molecule) of the elements or compounds involved. From this definition, it is apparent that 1 gmw of any two substances will contain the same number of atoms or molecules. The number of atoms or molecules in 1 gaw or 1 gmw has been shown by experiment to be 6.02×10^{23}. This number is called **Avogadro's number,** and 1 gaw or 1 gmw of any substance is commonly referred to as 1 **mole.**

These concepts are illustrated in the following examples:

Example 1:
How many moles (gaw) of chromium (Cr) are contained in 28 g? From the periodic chart the atomic weight of chromium is found to be 52 amu; therefore the weight of Cr contained in 1 mole (gaw) is 52 g.

$$\frac{1\,mole}{52\,g} = \frac{x\,mole}{28\,g}$$
$$x = \frac{(28\,g)(1\,mole)}{52\,g}$$
$$x = \frac{28}{52}\,mole$$
$$x = 0.538\,mole$$

Example 2:
How many grams are contained in 0.59 moles (gram molecular weights) of sulfuric acid? Because sulfuric acid (H_2SO_4) is a molecule, its molecular weight must first be determined.

$$2H \times 1\,amu = 2\,amu$$
$$1S \times 32\,amu = 32\,amu$$
$$4O \times 16\,amu = 64\,amu$$

Molecular weight $= 98\,amu$

Therefore 1 mole (gmw) would contain 98 g of sulfuric acid, and:

$$\frac{98\,g}{1\,mole} = \frac{x\,g}{0.59\,mole}$$
$$x = \frac{(98\,g)(0.59\,mole)}{1\,mole}$$
$$x = (98\,g)(0.59)$$
$$x = 57.82\,g$$

Example 3:
How many molecules are contained in 0.50 mole of nitrogen (N_2)? One mole (gmw) of N_2 (28 g) would contain Avogadro's number of molecules (6.02×10^{23}). Therefore:

$$\frac{6.02 \times 10^{23}\,molecules}{1\,mole} = \frac{x\,molecules}{0.50\,mole}$$
$$x = \frac{(0.50\,mole)(6.02 \times 10^{23})\,molecules}{1\,mole}$$
$$x = (0.50)(6.02 \times 10^{23})\,molecules$$
$$x = 3.01 \times 102^{23}\,molecules$$

Example 4:
How many moles of water (H_2O) are present in a sample containing 5×10^{12} molecules? One mole of H_2O contains 6.02×10^{23} molecules. Therefore:

$$\frac{1\,mole}{6.02 \times 10^{23}\,molecules} = \frac{x\,mole}{5.0 \times 10^{12}\,molecules}$$
$$x = \frac{(1\,mole)(5.0 \times 10^{12})\,mole}{6.02 \times 10^{23}\,molecules}$$
$$x = \frac{(5.0 \times 10^{12})\,mole}{6.02 \times 10^{23}}$$
$$x = 0.83 \times 10^{-11}\,mole$$
$$x = 8.3 \times 10^{-12}\,mole$$

EMPIRICAL AND MOLECULAR FORMULAS

All substances now known were initially obtained from natural resources or chemical reactions, and in many cases their elemental composition and structures were unknown. The elements present in such compounds must be determined by *qualitative chemical analysis* and the relative amount of each element by *quantitative chemical analysis.* The information obtained in these analyses is useful in determining the **empirical formula** of a substance.

The ratio of the elements contained in a substance (the relative number of each kind of atom present) is indicated by the empirical formula. However, the empirical formula may not truly reflect the **molecular formula** of the substance, which may be a whole number multiple of the empirical formula. For instance, the organic substance oxalic acid, which is a constituent of some plants, has an empirical formula of CHO_2 but a molecular formula of $C_2H_2O_4$.

Example:
A compound, on analysis, was found to have the following composition by weight:

$$Carbon\,(C) = 50.7\%$$
$$Hydrogen\,(H) = 4.25\%$$
$$Oxygen\,(O) = 45.1\%$$

What is the empirical formula of the compound?
Because percentage is based on 100, it may be assumed that a 100-g sample of the compound would contain:

50.7 g C
4.25 g H
45.1 g O

Because a definite atomic weight (and gram atomic weight) is a unique property of each element, the relative abundance of each element is obtained by the following:

$$\text{Carbon:} \frac{50.7\,g}{12\,g} = \frac{x\,gaw}{1\,gaw}$$

$$x = \frac{50.7\,g}{12\,g}(1\,gaw)$$

$$x = 4.23\,gaw$$

$$\text{Hydrogen:} \frac{4.25\,g}{1\,g} = \frac{x\,gaw}{1\,gaw}$$

$$x = \frac{(4.25\,g)(1\,gaw)}{1\,g}$$

$$x = 4.25\,gaw$$

$$\text{Oxygen:} \frac{45.1\,g}{16\,g} = \frac{x\,gaw}{1\,gaw}$$

$$x = \frac{(45.1\,g)(1\,gaw)}{16\,g}$$

$$x = \frac{45.1}{16}\,gaw$$

$$x = 2.82\,gaw$$

However, each element must be present in an integral value of its atomic weight, or gram atomic weight. To obtain integral values for each element, the above values of the gram atomic weight must be divided by the smallest value obtained. Thus:

$$\text{Oxygen:} \frac{2.82\,gaw}{2.82\,gaw} = 1$$

$$\text{Carbon:} \frac{4.23\,gaw}{2.82\,gaw} = 1.5$$

$$\text{Hydrogen:} \frac{4.25\,gaw}{2.82\,gaw} = 1.5$$

These values indicate that the empirical formula of the compound is $C_{1.5}H_{1.5}O_1$. Obviously, these values are not integral, and the actual number of atoms present in the molecule must be a multiple of these. Multiplying the value for each element by two results in an empirical formula of $C_3H_3O_2$, indicating an integral or whole number value for each element.

Further analysis of this substance indicates its molecular weight to be 142. What is the molecular formula of the compound?

The molecular weight of the compound is derived from the following empirical formula:

Carbon	(3)(12) =	36
Hydrogen	(3)(1) =	3
Oxygen	(2)(16) =	32
Empirical weight		= 71

Inasmuch as the molecular formula must be a multiple of the empirical formula, that is, $142/71 = 2$, the molecular formula is $C_6H_6O_4$.

Empirical or molecular formulas may be characteristic of several different compounds and provide no information pertinent to the structure of the molecule.

SOLUTIONS AND COLLOIDS

Much of the chemistry encountered in nuclear medicine involves solutions. A solution is a homogeneous mixture of two substances: the **solute** can be a gas, liquid, or solid, and the solvent is generally a liquid. One must choose a solvent that will dissolve the solute and yet not undergo chemical reaction with the solute.

In working with solutions one must know the concentration of the solute in a given volume of solution and therefore must be familiar with the methods and units used in defining concentrations.

Molarity

Molarity expresses the number of moles of solute contained in 1 L of solution.

$$\text{Molarity (M)} = \frac{\text{Number of moles of solute}}{\text{Number of liters of solution}}$$

Sample Problems

Example 1:

What is the molarity of a solution prepared by dissolving 16 g of barium chloride ($BaCl_2$) in sufficient water to give a total volume of 450 ml?

Step 1: How many moles of $BaCl_2$ are in the 16-g sample?

$$1\,mole\,(BaCl_2) = 137.5\,g + 2(35.5\,g)$$
$$1\,mole\,(BaCl_2) = 208.5\,g$$
$$\frac{1\,mole}{208.5\,g} = \frac{x\,mole}{16.0\,g}$$
$$x = \frac{(16.0\,g)(1\,mole)}{208.5\,g}$$
$$x = \frac{16.0\,mole}{208.5}$$
$$x = 0.077\,mole$$

Step 2:

$$\text{molarity (M)} = \frac{mole}{liter}$$
$$M = \frac{0.077\,mole}{0.450\,L}$$
$$M = \frac{0.171\,mole}{L\,(molar)}$$

Example 2:

How would 20 L of 6.0 M sodium hydroxide (NaOH) solution be prepared from solid NaOH?

Step 1: How many grams of NaOH are in 6.0 moles?

$$1 \text{ mole (NaOH)} = 23\,g + 16\,g + 1\,g$$
$$1 \text{ mole (NaOH)} = 40\,g$$
$$\frac{x\,g}{6.0\,\text{moles}} = \frac{40\,g}{1\,\text{mole}}$$
$$x = \frac{(40\,g)(6.0\,\text{moles})}{1\,\text{mole}}$$
$$x = (40)(60)\,g$$
$$x = 240\,g \text{ in } 6.0 \text{ mole of NaOH}$$

Step 2: One liter of 6.0 molar (M) solution requires 240 g of NaOH. Therefore for 20 L of 6.0 M solution, 20×240 g $= 4800$ g of NaOH dissolved in sufficient water to give a total volume of 20 L.

Example 3:
How could the solution prepared in Example 2 be used to obtain 1.0 L of 0.50 M NaOH solution?

Step 1: The 6.0 M NaOH must be diluted with additional water. What volume of the 6.0 M solution contains 0.50 moles of NaOH?

$$\frac{1.0\,L}{6.0\,\text{mole (NaOH)}} = \frac{x\,L}{0.50\,\text{mole (NaOH)}}$$
$$x = \frac{(1.0\,L)(0.50\,M)}{(6.0\,M)}$$
$$x = \frac{0.50\,L}{6.0}$$
$$x = 0.083\,L$$

Step 2: If 0.083 L of 6.0 M NaOH contains 0.50 moles of NaOH, then to obtain a 0.50 M solution, one must add enough water to bring the volume to exactly 1.0 L.

Molality

A molal solution is defined as the number of moles of solute contained in 1 kilogram (kg) of solvent.

$$\text{Molarity (m)} = \frac{\text{Number of moles of solute}}{\text{Number of kilograms of solvent}}$$

Whereas 1 L of a *molar* solution is prepared by the addition of sufficient solvent to the solute to give a total volume of 1 L, a *molal* solution is prepared when the solute is dissolved in 1 kg (in the case of water, 1 L) of solvent. The total volume of a 1 molal solution will generally be greater than that of a 1 molar solution.

Sample Problem

Example:
Calculate the molality of a solute prepared by dissolving 20.4 g of sodium chloride (NaCl) in 192 g of H_2O.

Step 1: How many grams are contained in 1 mole of NaCl?

$$1 \text{ mole (NaCl)} = 23\,g + 35.5\,g$$
$$1 \text{ mole (NaCl)} = 58.5\,g$$

Step 2: How many moles are contained in 20.4 g of NaCl?

$$\frac{1\,\text{mole}}{58.5\,g} = \frac{x\,\text{mole}}{20.4\,g}$$
$$x = \frac{(20.4)(1\,\text{mole})}{58.5\,g}$$
$$x = \frac{(20.4)}{58.5\,g}\,\text{mole}$$
$$x = 0.349\,\text{mole}$$

Step 3: From the definition of molality,

$$m = \frac{.0349\,\text{mole}}{0.192\,kg}$$
$$m = 1.82\,\text{molal solution}$$

Note that most solutions are usually expressed in terms of molarity rather than molality.

Normality

A third method of expressing concentration, and one that is generally more useful than that of molarity or molality, is normality (N). Normality is defined as the number of equivalents (Eq) of solute per liter of solution. The number of equivalents present in a solution, rather than being defined as the number of moles of solute per liter, is defined as the number of moles of reactant species contained in 1 mole of the solute. For example, as previously discussed, in the reaction $H^+ + {}^-OH \rightarrow H_2O$ the reactants must arise from two different substances, one of which provides H^+ and another that provides ^-OH (conventionally OH^-, also ionically OH^-). Those compounds that give H^+ ions are called *acids*, which will be discussed later. Two of the most common acids are hydrochloric acid (HCl) and sulfuric acid (H_2SO_4). Both of these acids may be considered to be completely ionized in aqueous solution to give the H^+ ion and the corresponding anions. It should be apparent that ionization of 1 mole of HCl will give rise to 1 mole of H^+ ion, whereas the ionization of 1 mole of H_2SO_4 will give rise to 2 moles of H^+ ion. Thus in comparing HCl with H_2SO_4, 0.5 mole of H_2SO_4 will provide the same number of H^+ ions that would be provided by 1 mole of HCl. Therefore the weight of H_2SO_4 that will provide 1 Eq of H^+ ion (1 mole) is half its molecular weight: 98 g/2 = 49 g, whereas the weight of HCl required to produce 1 Eq (1 mole) of H^+ is equal to its molecular weight (36.5 g). Similarly, the substances that provide OH^- ion (called *bases*) will have equivalent weights dictated by the number of moles of OH^- that will be provided by 1 mole of the base. Thus:

$$\text{Normality (N)} = \frac{\text{Number of equivalents}}{\text{Number of liters of solvent}}$$

and

$$Normality\ (N) = \frac{(Moles\ of\ solute)("Moles"\ of\ reactant\ provided)}{1L\ of\ solution}$$

$$= \frac{Equivalents}{Liter} = \frac{Eq}{L}$$

A second type of reaction that uses *normal* solutions is that in which an oxidation-reduction is involved. This type is yet to be discussed, and suffice it to say at this point that the equivalent weight of a reagent in an oxidation-reduction reaction is determined by the number of electrons that it accepts or donates.

How are equivalent weights calculated? The equivalent weight, in grams, of an acid is calculated when the gram molecular weight of the acid is divided by the number of potential hydrogen ions contained in the molecule. For a base the gram molecular weight is divided by the number of hydroxide ions.

Sample Problems

Example 1:
What is the equivalent weight of HCl?

$$Equivalent\ weight = \frac{gmw}{Number\ of\ H^+\ ions}$$

$$Equivalent\ weight = \frac{36.5\ g}{1} = 36.5\ g$$

Example 2:
What is the equivalent weight of H_2SO_4?

$$Equivalent\ weight = \frac{gmw}{Number\ of\ H^+\ ions}$$

$$Equivalent\ weight = \frac{98\ g}{2}$$

$$Equivalent\ weight = 49\ g$$

Example 3:
What is the equivalent weight of 1 mole of calcium hydroxide, $Ca(OH)_2$?

$$Equivalent\ weight = \frac{gmw}{Number\ of\ H^-\ ions}$$

$$Equivalent\ weight = \frac{74\ g}{2}$$

$$Equivalent\ weight = 37\ g$$

The normality of a solution must be a whole number multiple of a corresponding molar solution.

Example 4:
What is the normality of a 90 ml sample of a solution that contains 10 g of NaOH?

Step 1:

$$1\ equivalent\ weight\ of\ NaOH = \frac{1\ gms\ of\ NaOH}{1\ OH^-\ ion}$$

$$1\ equivalent\ weight = \frac{40\ g}{1} = 40\ g\ of\ NaOH$$

Step 2: The number of equivalents of NaOH in solution:

$$\frac{1\ Eq}{40\ g} = \frac{x\ Eq}{10\ g}$$

$$x = \frac{(1\ Eq)(10\ g)}{40\ g}$$

$$x = \frac{10}{40}\ Eq = 0.25\ Eq\ of\ NaOH$$

Step 3: Normality equals equivalents/liter. Therefore:

$$N = \frac{Eq}{L} = \frac{0.25}{0.09}$$

$$N = 2.78\ normal$$

NOTE: Because normality equals molarity for NaOH, this solution is both 2.78 N and 2.78 M.

Example 5:
What are the normality and molarity of 100 ml of an aqueous solution containing 50.0 g of phosphoric acid (H_3PO_4)?

Step 1: How many grams of H_3PO_4 are contained in 1 gew (gram equivalent weight)?

$$1\ gew = \frac{1\ gmw}{Number\ of\ H^+\ ions}$$

$$1\ gew = \frac{98.0\ g}{3} = 32.7\ g\ of\ H_3PO_4$$

Step 2: What is the number of equivalents in 50 g of H_3PO_4?

$$\frac{1\ Eq}{32.7\ g} = \frac{x\ Eq}{50.0\ g}$$

$$x = \frac{(1\ Eq)(50.0\ g)}{32.7\ g}$$

$$x = \frac{50.0\ g}{32.7\ g} = 1.53\ Eq\ of\ H_3PO_4$$

Step 3: By definition,

$$N = \frac{1.53\ Eq}{0.100\ L}$$

$$N = 1.53\ normal$$

Step 4: Because H_3PO_4 is triprotic (3 H^+ ions), the molarity of this solution will be

$$m = \frac{N}{3} = \frac{15.3}{3}$$

$$m = 5.10\ molar\ H_3PO_4$$

Colloids

A second type of mixture, one that is important in nuclear medicine, is the **colloid**. Unlike true solutions, colloids consist of minute particles suspended in a dispersing medium. Colloid particles vary in shape and range in size from 10^{-9} to 10^{-7} m in diameter. Although several important types of colloids exist, the present discussion is restricted to the colloid in which a solid is dispersed in a liquid—a *sol*.

Although one might expect the particles to settle out on standing, the dispersed colloid particles remain suspended in the dispersing medium indefinitely. This behavior is attributed to a constant bombardment of the dispersed particles by the molecules of the dispersing medium; thus the colloid particles are in constant motion. This phenomenon is called *Brownian movement* and may be observed with the proper type of microscope.

Unlike true solutions, colloids exhibit an optical effect characterized by the scattering of light when a narrow beam is passed through them. The scattering of light is attributable to the deflection of light by the colloid particles and is called the *Tyndall effect*.

A third property characteristic of colloids is an electrical charge effect in which charged particles such as ions are bound or adsorbed on the surface of the colloid particle. An important example, probably involving this effect, is the ^{99m}Tc-labeled sulfur colloid used for liver imaging.

TABLE 5-3	Common Ions, Their Symbols, and Charge	
Ion	**Chemical Symbol**	**Charge**
Hydroxide	OH^-	1–
Nitrate	NO_3^-	1–
Nitrite	NO_2^-	1–
Phosphate	PO_4^{3-}	3–
Carbonate	CO_3^{2-}	2–
Bicarbonate	HCO_3^-	1–
Sulfite	SO_3^{-2}	2–
Sulfate	SO_4^{-2}	2–
Bisulfate	HSO_4^-	1–
Ammonium	NH_4^-	1+
Stannous or tin (II)	Sn	2+
Stannic or tin (IV)	Sn	4+
Ferrous or iron (II)	Fe^{2+} (FeO)	2+
Ferric or iron (III)	Fe^{3+} (Fe_2O_3)	3+
Cuprous or copper (I)	Cu^+ (Cu_2O)	1+
Cupric or copper (II)	Cu^{2+} (CuO)	2+
Permanganate	MnO_4^-	1–
Manganese (IV)	Mn^{4+} (MnO_2)	4+
Manganese (II)	Mn^{2+} (MnO)	2+
Pertechnetate	TcO_4^-	1–
Technetium (IV)	Tc^{4+} (TcO_2)	4+
Chromate	CrO_4^{2-}	2–
Chromium (III)	Cr^{3+}	3+
Mercurous	Hg^+	1+
Mercuric	Hg^{2+}	2+
Cyanide	CN^-	1–
Thiocyanate	SCN^-	1–

CHEMICAL REACTIONS AND EQUATIONS

The ability to predict chemical reactions and correctly write and understand the chemical equations describing the reactions is of utmost theoretical and practical importance. The basis for one type of chemical reaction—the combination reaction, in which two elements react to produce one substance—and the chemical equations describing this reaction are discussed earlier in this chapter. In addition to combination reactions, the following types of chemical reactions must also be considered:

1. Metathesis or double decomposition
2. Oxidation-reduction
   a. Replacement
   b. Electrochemical

Because all reactions are described by a chemical equation, it is necessary to learn the terms and symbols used in writing equations. The symbols indicating the physical state of substances involved in a reaction are as follows:

1. A gas is indicated by (g) and may alternatively be indicated by the symbol (↑), for example, O_2 (g) or O_2 (↑).

2. A liquid is designated by (l), for example, H_2O (l).
3. A solid is indicated by (s) or, if there is a product precipitating from solution, by the symbol (↓), for example, $BaSO_4$ (↓).
4. The symbol → separates the reactants from the products of the reaction.

A correct chemical equation also requires that the equation be balanced; that is, the number of atoms of each element appearing as reactants must be found in equal number in the products. The steps needed to complete and balance an equation are as follows:

1. Determine the correct formulas for those compounds obtained as products from a knowledge of the valence or oxidation numbers of the elements of the charge on ions involved in the reaction. The valence or oxidation number of monatomic ions is equal to the net charge of the cation or anion. The charge of many complex ions is not readily discernible and should be memorized. Once determined, the formula of a compound cannot be changed in subsequent balancing operations (Table 5-3).
2. Balance those ions of elements other than hydrogen, oxygen, and polyatomic ions.

3. *Then* balance the hydrogen and oxygen atoms.
4. The correct coefficients for reactants and products must be the smallest whole number possible, for example:

$$2H_2 + O_2 \rightarrow 2H_2O$$

not

$$4H_2 + 2O_2 \rightarrow 4H_2O$$

5. Finally, the sum of the charges of the reactants must equal the sum of the charges of products.

The balanced equation specifies the ratio or quantity of reactants required and the ratio or quantity of products produced. This is called the *stoichiometry* (element-equality) of the reaction. The following example illustrates these steps and the stoichiometry of a reaction:

Example:
Complete and balance the following equation:

$$Fe(OH)_3 + H_2SO_4 \rightarrow$$

Step 1: From Table 5-3, the hydroxide ion has a charge of 1−. Therefore the iron present in $Fe(OH)_3$ must have a charge of 3+. Similarly, for H_2SO_4 each hydrogen has a charge of 1+, and so the sulfate anion must have a charge of 2−. Products formed in this reaction must involve an interchange of cations and anions by the two reactants. Therefore ferric ion combines with sulfate ion, and hydrogen ion combines with hydroxide ion. *All products formed must be neutral, that is, have no charge.* Iron having a 3+ charge and sulfate having a 2− charge dictates that the correct formula for this product must be $Fe_2(SO_4)_3$. The remaining product is H_2O, and the equation showing both reactants and products is as follows:

$$Fe(OH)_3 + H_2SO_4 \rightarrow Fe_2(SO_4)_3 + H_2O \text{ (unbalanced)}$$

Step 2: Because each reactant and product contains hydrogen, oxygen, or both, those compounds containing iron may be used in stating the balancing procedure.

Reactant: 1 Fe^{3+}
Product: 2 Fe^{3+}

Therefore:

$$2Fe(OH)_3 + H_2SO_4 \rightarrow Fe_2(SO_4)_3 + H_2O \text{ (unbalanced)}$$

It is now convenient to balance the polyatomic sulfate ion.

Reactant: 1 SO^-
Product: 3 SO^-

Therefore:

$$2Fe(OH)_3 + 3H_2SO_4 \rightarrow Fe_2(SO_4)_3 + H_2O \text{ (unbalanced)}$$

Step 3: Complete the balancing of elements, considering hydrogen and oxygen.

Reactants: 12 H^+
Product: 2 H^+

Thus

$$2Fe(OH)_3 + 3H_2SO_4 \rightarrow Fe_2(SO_4)_3 + 6H_2O \text{ (balanced)}$$

Check the oxygen, other than those contained in sulfate ions.

Reactant: 6 O^{2-}
Product: 6 O^{2-}

Step 4: The coefficients of reactants and products cannot be reduced to smaller whole numbers; therefore they are correct as written in step 3.
Step 5: Because all compounds, reactants, and products are electrically neutral, the sum of the charges of the reactants equals that of the products, and the equation, complete and balanced, is that shown in step 3.

The stoichiometry of the balanced equation states that two molecules or moles of $Fe(OH)_3$ react with three molecules or moles of H_2SO_4 to yield one molecule or mole of $Fe_2(SO_4)_3$ and six molecules or moles of H_2O.

All balanced equations give the information shown in this example. The value of the chemical equation lies in the fact that it is the basis for calculating the amount of product produced from a given quantity of reactants and, conversely, allows calculation of the quantities of reactants required to produce a desired quantity of products.

Metathesis Reactions

The term *metathesis* means mutual exchange and is often referred to as *double decomposition*. When two compounds undergo metathesis, both compounds are decomposed and two new compounds are formed. The positive ions of each compound react with the negative ions of the other compound, as shown in the following equation:

$$A^+B^- + C^+D^- \rightarrow A^+D^- + C^+B^-$$

These reactions generally involve ionic compounds as reactants and nearly always give ionic products, one of which is usually a solid.

Examples:
Predict the products obtained in the following reactions and balance the equations:

1. $CdSO_4 + KOH \rightarrow$
2. $Pb(NO_3)_2 + H_2S \rightarrow$

(See Table 5-3 for ionic charges.)
Double decomposition would give:

1. $CdSO_4 + KOH \rightarrow Cd(OH)_2\downarrow + K_2SO_4 \text{ (unbalanced)}$
2. $Pb(NO_3)_2 + H_2S \rightarrow PbS\downarrow + HNO_3 \text{ (unbalanced)}$

Balance equation 1.
Reactant: 1 Cd^{2+}
Product: 1 Cd^{2+}; therefore the reactant KOH must be multiplied by 2 to balance K^+ ions.

$$CdSO_4 + 2KOH \rightarrow Cd(OH)_2\downarrow + K_2SO_4$$

Inspection of this equation shows that both SO^- and OH^- ions occur in equal numbers in both the reactants and the products, and the equation as shown is balanced.

Balance equation 2.
Reactant: 1 Pb^{2+}
Product: 1 Pb^{2+}; therefore Pb^{2+} ions are balanced.

Thus

Reactant: 1 S^{2-}
Product: 1 S^{2-}; therefore S^{2-} ions are balanced.

Thus

Reactant: 2NO_3^{1-}
Product: 1NO_3^{1-}; therefore the product HNO_3 must be multiplied by 2 to balance NO_3^{1-} ions.

$$Pb(NO_3)_2 + H_2S \rightarrow PbS\downarrow + 2HNO_3$$

Inspection shows that the H^+ ions occur in equal numbers in both the reactants and products, and the equation is balanced.

Oxidation-Reduction Reactions

Oxidation-reduction reactions, commonly called *redox reactions*, are those reactions in which certain atoms gain or lose electrons and thus undergo a change of oxidation number. The oxidation number of a monatomic ion is its charge. For example, the oxidation number of F^- ion is −1 (or it can be expressed 1−). If the oxidation number changes during a reaction ($2F^- \rightarrow F_2 + 2e^-$), an oxidation or reduction has occurred (F^-, oxidation number −1, has undergone oxidation to give neutral F_2). The process of oxidation always involves the loss of electrons, and consequently the oxidation number of the element involved changes in a positive direction. For example, the ion Fe^{2+} readily undergoes oxidation by loss of an electron to give Fe^{3+}. For each reactant undergoing oxidation there must be a second reactant that undergoes reduction. The reactant undergoing reduction must gain one or more electrons, and thus its oxidation number changes in a negative direction. For example, if the reaction in which Fe^{2+} was oxidized to Fe^{3+} is reversed so that $Fe^{3+} + 1e^- \rightarrow Fe^{2+}$, a reduction has occurred. Changes in oxidation number generally occur within the limits of ±5 as indicated here:

$$
\begin{array}{c}
\text{Oxidation} \\
\longrightarrow \\
-5\ -4\ -3\ -2\ -1\ 0\ +1\ +2\ +3\ +4\ +5 \\
\longleftarrow \\
\text{Reduction}
\end{array}
$$

Confusing though it may seem, an oxidizing agent is a reactant that, by acquiring electrons from a second reactant, causes an increase in oxidation number of the second reactant. Conversely, a reducing agent is the reactant that donates electrons and brings about a reduction of the oxidation number of the other reactant (the oxidizing agent). This change is illustrated in the equation:

Oxidation number = 0		Oxidation number = 0
Ca	+	S →
Reducing agent		**Oxidizing agent**
Oxidation number = +2 (or ⁺⁺)		Oxidation number = −2 (or ⁼)
Ca^{++}	+	S^-
Oxidized		**Reduced**

In all redox reactions the total number of electrons lost by the reducing agent must equal the total number of electrons gained by the oxidizing agent.

The oxidation states of substances involved in redox reactions are undergoing change, and many equations cannot be balanced by simple inspection. However, the total ionic charge of the reactants must equal that of the products, and the number of atoms of each element in the reactants must equal the number of atoms of the same elements in the products. In balancing redox equations, several rules must be observed.

1. The oxidation state of all elements is zero; that is, the number of electrons and protons are equal, and the charge is zero.
2. The oxidation state of a monatomic ion is equal to the charge of that ion. Some elements maintain the same oxidation number in the majority of compounds in which they are found, as shown in Table 5-4.
3. The sum of all oxidation numbers of the atoms of a compound must equal zero.

Those elements generally exhibiting only one oxidation state are shown in Table 5-4.

For example, chlorine in the compound $HClO_3$ (chloric acid) has an oxidation number of +5. In determining the oxidation number of chlorine from the formula, one must make use of Table 5-4, which states that oxygen always has an oxidation number of −2 and that hydrogen, in most compounds, has an oxidation number of +1. Because there are three oxygens in the

TABLE 5-4	Elements Generally Exhibiting One Oxidation State	
Element	Common Oxidation Number	Rare Oxidation Number
Hydrogen	+1 (H^+)	−1 (H^-)
Alkali metals (Na, K, and so on)	+1 (Na^+)	
Alkaline earth metals (Mg, Ca, and so on)	+2 (Mg^{2+})	
Oxygen	−2 (O^{2-})	−1 (O^-), +2 (O^{2+})
Fluorine	−1 (F^-)	
Chlorine, bromine, and iodine	−1 (Cl^-)	Cl: +1, +3, +5, +7 Br: +1, +3, +5 I: +1, +5, +7

$HClO_3$ molecule, the sum of the oxidation numbers for oxygen is required to be 3(−2), or −6, and hydrogen has an oxidation number of +1. Because rule 3 states that the sum of all oxidation numbers for each compound must equal zero, and the sum of the oxidation numbers of hydrogen and oxygen (+1 + [−6]) equals −5, the oxidation number of chlorine must be +5. Note that the oxidation number of the atoms involved in a compound is determined by their electronegativity and the electronegativity of the elements to which they are bonded.

Now that the rules for balancing redox equations have been established, consider the use of these rules in the following examples. The most convenient method of balancing charge is to use half-reactions. Half-reactions involve only the ions undergoing a change in oxidation number during reaction.

Example 1:
Balance the following equation:

$$HNO_3 + H_2S \rightarrow NO + S + H_2O \text{ (unbalanced)}$$

Determine the oxidation state of each atom on both sides of the equation to find which atoms have undergone a change of oxidation number. Consider each compound separately.

$$\overset{+1 \quad +5 \quad 3(-2)}{H \quad N \quad O_3} + \overset{2(+1) \quad -2}{H_2 \quad S} \rightarrow$$
$$\overset{+2 \quad -2}{N \quad O} + \overset{0}{S} + \overset{2(+1) \quad -2}{H_2 \quad O} \text{ (unbalanced)}$$

In arriving at these oxidation numbers, the use of the foregoing rules and Table 5-4 reveals that hydrogen always has the oxidation numbers of +1 and oxygen −2. The sum of the oxidation numbers of hydrogen atoms in HNO_3 is +1, and, because there are three oxygen atoms in this substance, the sum for oxygen atoms is 3(−2) = −6. Rule 3 states that the sum of the oxidation numbers for the HNO_3 molecule must be zero; therefore

nitrogen must have an oxidation number of +5; that is, the equation (hydrogen +1, plus oxygen −6 = −5) requires that the oxidation number of nitrogen be +5.

$$H(+1) \text{ } N(+5) \text{ } O_3 (-6) \text{ or } (+1) + (+5) + (-6) = 0$$

The equation states that the product containing nitrogen is NO, and following the procedure just described reveals that nitrogen in the product has an oxidation number of +2.

$$\overset{+2 \quad -2}{N \quad O} \text{ or } (+2) + (-2) = 0$$

Therefore the half-reaction in which nitrogen is involved is as follows:

$$N^{5+} + 3e^- \rightarrow N^{2+}$$

Similarly, it is found that sulfur occurs as a reactant in H_2S and has an oxidation number of −2.

$$\overset{2(+1) \quad -2}{H_2 \quad S} \text{ or } (+2) + (-2) = 0$$

Sulfur occurs in the product in the elemental form, and by rule 1 it must have an oxidation number of zero. The half-reaction involving sulfur is:

$$S^{2-} - 2e^- \rightarrow S^0$$

Inspection of the equation shows that the oxidation numbers of hydrogen and oxygen remain the same in both the reactants and products; that is, they do not change. Consider the half-reactions and recall that the number of electrons acquired by the oxidizing agent must equal the number of electrons donated by the reducing agent; it may readily be noted that the half-reaction involving nitrogen must be multiplied by 2 and the half-reaction involving sulfur be multiplied by 3. The six electrons donated by sulfur must equal the six electrons accepted by nitrogen.

$$2(N^{5+} + 3e^- \rightarrow N^{2+})$$
$$3(S^{2-} - 2e^- \rightarrow S^0)$$

Applying the coefficients of the half-reactions, the full equation in which nitrogen and sulfur are balanced must be written as:

$$2HNO_3 + 3H_2S \rightarrow 2NO + 3S + H_2O \text{ (unbalanced)}$$

The atoms of the remaining elements must now be balanced, and balancing must be done by inspection.

Nitrogens are balanced.
Sulfurs are balanced.
Reactant: 8 Hs
Product: 2 Hs

Multiplying H_2O (the product) by 4 balances Hs and gives the equation:

$$2HNO_3 + 3H_2S \rightarrow 2NO + 3S + 4H_2O$$

Inspection shows that the oxygens are also balanced and that the equation has been balanced by a simple inspection process. Consider a second example of a redox reaction.

Example 2:

$$K_2Cr_2O_7 + HCl \rightarrow KCl + CrCl_3 + H_2O + Cl_2 \text{ (unbalanced)}$$

Following the process outlined in the preceding example reveals that the elements undergoing oxidation and reduction are as follows:

$$2(Cr^{6+} + 3e^- \rightarrow Cr^{2+}) \text{ reduction (oxidizing agent)}$$
$$3(Cl^- - 2e^- \rightarrow Cl) \text{ oxidation (reducing agent)}$$

Note that not all the Cl^- ion in the reaction undergoes oxidation, as some is used in forming the products KCl and $CrCl_3$, in which the oxidation number of -1 is retained.

Multiplying, to balance changes in oxidation number, gives:

$$K_2Cr_2O_7 + 6HCl \rightarrow KCl + 2CrCl_3 + H_2O + 3Cl_2 \text{ (unbalanced)}$$

Balancing the remaining elements gives

$$K_2Cr_2O_7 + 14HCl \rightarrow 2KCl + 2CrCl_3 + 7H_2O + 3Cl_2 \text{ (balanced)}$$

Electrolytic Reactions

A special type of oxidation-reduction is that involving an electric current supplied by an external source and using an electrolytic cell (Figure 5-12).

The anode is highly electron deficient and may be thought of as being positive in charge, whereas the cathode is rich in electrons and therefore has a large negative charge. This being the case, positive ions (cations) in solution or in the liquid state migrate to the cathode and are reduced by a transfer of electrons from the cathode to the cation. Conversely, the anions, being negatively charged, migrate to the anode and in transferring electrons to the anode undergo oxidation. These processes are summarized as follows:

Cathode: $A^+ + 1e^- \rightarrow A^0$ (reduction)
Anode: $B^- - 1e^- \rightarrow B^0$ (oxidation)

Electrolysis is used primarily in the industrial production of certain elements such as elemental sodium and chlorine. A second important process involving electrolysis is that of electroplating, in which elemental chromium, nickel, or silver is deposited or plated on the surface of other metals as a protective or decorative coating.

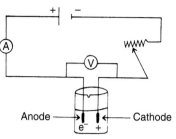

FIGURE 5-12 Oxidation-reduction involving use of electric current. *A*, Amperage; *V*, voltage.

ACIDS AND BASES

Understanding the chemistry and theory of acids and bases is vital to the practice of nuclear medicine because the acidity of the body fluids must remain essentially constant. All compounds and, more importantly, solutions of the compounds are acidic, basic, or neutral. The properties of acids and bases are as follows:

Acids	Bases
1. Taste sour	1. Taste bitter
2. Cause certain organic dyes, called *indicators*, to change color; for example, blue litmus paper in the presence of an acid changes to red	2. Cause certain organic dyes, called *indicators*, to change color; for example, red litmus paper in the presence of a base changes to blue
3. Release CO_2 from carbonate salts	3. Feel slick (slimy)
4. Include these common materials: vinegar, citrus juices, soda (seltzer and all carbonated beverages)	4. Include these common materials: aqueous ammonia solution, soap, and lye (NaOH)

Concepts of Acids and Bases

Acids and bases have been defined in the historic evolution of chemistry by the Arrhenius (1884), Brönsted-Lowry (1923), and Lewis (1923) concepts. Each of these concepts remains useful in the current understanding of acid-base chemistry.

Arrhenius defined an acid as a substance that yields hydrogen ion (H^+) or hydronium ion (H_3^+O) when dissolved in water, and bases as those substances that yield hydroxide ions (OH^-) when dissolved in water.

The Brönsted-Lowry concept provides a more general definition of acids and bases. It defines an acid as a substance that can provide (or donate) a proton (H^+) to a second substance, which by definition is a base. For example, acetic acid can donate a proton directly to a base such as ammonia.

$$\underset{\text{Acid}}{CH_3COOH} + \underset{\text{Base}}{NH_3} \rightarrow \underset{\substack{\text{Acetate} \\ \text{ion}}}{CH_3COO^-} + \underset{\substack{\text{Ammonium} \\ \text{ion}}}{NH_4^+}$$

Brönsted-Lowry acids and bases are not restricted to aqueous solutions, as are Arrhenius acids and bases;

therefore this concept is valid for any solvent system. Thus the following reaction can occur:

$$H_2SO_4 + NaCl \rightarrow H_2Cl + NaSO_4$$
Acid   Base   Acid   Base

Sulfuric acid is used as both a reactant and a solvent.

Lewis, in 1923, proposed a still more general definition of acids and bases. The Lewis concept defines an acid as any compound that can *accept* an *electron pair,* and a base as any compound that can *donate* an *electron pair.* Acid-base reactions of this type often involve the formation of a coordinate covalent bond and are illustrated by the reaction of boron trifluoride with ammonia as follows:

Acid Base

Boron trifluoride, which has an empty orbital, can accept the two nonbonding electrons of the nitrogen in ammonia (recall that the second energy level can accommodate eight electrons).

Neutralization Reactions

Most reactions that have been discussed previously in this chapter cannot be classified as neutralization reactions. The process of neutralization involves the reaction of acids with bases as defined by the Arrhenius concept, H^+ or H_3^+O and OH^-. The products of neutralization are invariably a salt and water. If equal quantities, as defined by normality of an acid and base, are mixed, the resulting solution is neither acidic nor basic. The discipline of medicine makes use of acids and bases not only in clinical diagnostic procedures but also as agents in treating certain injuries and disorders. Antacids, containing aluminum and magnesium hydroxides, are commonly used to neutralize excess stomach acid (HCl). Sodium bicarbonate (a base) finds use as a neutralizing agent in the treatment of acid burns, and picric acid is often used to accelerate the rate of mitosis.

A general equation describing the neutralization process may be written as follows:

$$HA + BOH \rightarrow AB + H_2O$$
Acid + Base $\rightarrow$ A salt + Water

The driving force for all neutralization reactions is the formation of the stable water molecule, and equations for these reactions can be balanced by simple inspection.

$$H_2SO_4 + NaOH \rightarrow Na_2SO_4 + H_2O \text{ (unbalanced)}$$

Inspection gives the following:

1. SO_4^{2-} ions are balanced
2. *Reactant:* 1 Na^+
   Product: 2 Na^+

3. Multiplying the reactant NaOH by 2 gives:

$$H_2SO_4 + 2NaOH \rightarrow Na_2SO_4 + H_2O \text{ (unbalanced)}$$

4. Multiplying the product H_2O by 2 to balance hydrogen gives:

$$H_2SO_4 + 2NaOH \rightarrow Na_2SO_4 + 2H_2O$$

Inspection shows that the oxygen atoms are balanced; therefore the equation is balanced.

Calculations

Laboratory procedures using neutralization reactions are quite common and are generally used to determine unknown quantities of acids or bases present in biological or chemical samples. A useful relationship for calculation of the quantity of an acid or base in a given sample is:

$$V_1N_1 = V_2N_2$$

where

V_1 = Volume of the standard solution (prepared in the laboratory)
N_1 = Normality of the standard solution
V_2 = Volume of the unknown solution
N_2 = Normality of the unknown solution

The usefulness of this equation becomes readily apparent when applied it to the evaluation of results of neutralization reactions obtained by titrimetric procedures. Because the normality of the standardized solution of acid or base (equivalents per liter or equivalents per milliliter) is known, one can titrate a known volume or weight of a sample containing an unknown quantity of acid or base and, by the use of the volume-normality relationship given above, ascertain the quantity of acid or base present in the sample.

Titrations are performed by taking an aliquot (V_2, a precisely measured volume) of the solution containing an unknown quantity (N_2 in the foregoing equation) of acid or base and placing it in a titration vessel, usually an Erlenmeyer flask. A standard solution of acid or base whose concentration is precisely known is then carefully delivered into the titration flask by use of a buret. The point at which neutralization occurs (i.e., the end point) is detected by use of an organic indicator that changes color when neutralization occurs. The volume, V_1, of standard acid or base required to exactly neutralize the substance in the "unknown" is read from the buret. At this point the values of V_1, N_1, and V_2 are known, and by use of the relationship $V_1N_1 = V_2N_2$, the number of equivalents (N_2) of the substance contained in the unknown can be calculated. The following examples illustrate the usefulness of titrimetric procedures as analytical tools.

Example 1:
What is the normality of a hydrochloric acid solution, 25 ml of which requires 37 ml of 0.30 N NaOH solution for neutralization?

$$V_1(NaOH) = 37\,ml$$
$$N_1(NaOH) = 0.30\,N$$
$$V_2(HCl) = 25\,ml$$
$$N_2(HCl) = ?$$

Using $V_1N_1 = V_2N_2$, solve for N_2.

$$(37\,ml)(0.30\,N) = (25\,ml)(N_2)$$
$$N_2 = \frac{(37\,ml)(0.30\,N)}{25\,ml}$$
$$N_2 = \frac{11.1}{25}\,N$$
$$N_2 = 0.44\,N$$

Example 2:
Given 30.0 ml of 0.25 M phosphoric acid (H_3PO_4) solution, what volume of 0.25 M calcium hydroxide [$Ca(OH)_2$] solution would be required for neutralization?

Step 1: Because the equation is valid only when concentrations are expressed as normalities, the normality of both the H_3PO_4 and $Ca(OH)_2$ solutions must first be found. H_3PO_4 is a triprotic acid (3 H^+ ions); therefore:

$$Normality = 3\,(Molarity)$$

or

$$N = 3\,(0.25\,M)$$
$$N = 0.75 \text{ for } H_3PO_4$$

$Ca(OH)_2$ is a dibasic (2 OH^- ions) base; therefore:

$$Normality = 2\,(Molarity)$$

or

$$N = 2\,(0.25\,M)$$
$$N = 0.50 \text{ for } Ca(OH)_2$$

Step 2: Using $V_1N_1 = V_2N_2$

$$V_1(H_3PO_4) = 30.0\,ml$$
$$N_1(H_3PO_4) = 0.75\,N$$
$$V_2(Ca[OH]_2) = ?$$
$$N_2(Ca[OH]_2) = 0.50\,N$$
$$(30.0\,ml)(0.75\,N) = (V_2)(0.50\,N)$$
$$V_2 = \frac{(30\,ml)(0.75\,N)}{0.50\,N}$$
$$V_2 = \frac{22.5}{0.50}\,ml$$
$$V_2 = 45.0\,ml \text{ of } Ca(OH)_2$$

Strong versus Weak Acids and Bases

The foregoing discussion of acids and bases implies that all acids and bases dissociate completely in aqueous medium giving either a H_3O^+ ion or a OH^- ion. In reality, only *strong acids* such as HCl, HBr, HI, H_2SO_4, and HNO_3 may be considered to be completely ionized in aqueous solutions; thus

$$H_2SO_4 + 2H_2O \rightarrow 2H_3O^+ + SO_4^{2-}$$

The common bases NaOH and KOH are *strong bases* and dissociate completely when dissolved in water; thus:

$$NaOH + H_2O \rightarrow Na^+ + OH^- + H_2O$$

Many acids are defined as being weak in that they do not completely dissociate in water because the conjugate base of the acid is of nearly the same base strength as water. Some of the common weak acids are acetic acid, carbonic acid, phenol, water, and boric acid. For example, less than 0.5% of the acetic acid molecules in a 1 M solution undergo reaction with water to produce H_3O^+ ion; the remaining 99.5% of the molecules remain undissociated. Equations for such reactions are written as follows:

$$CH_3COOH + H_2O \rightleftharpoons CH_3COO^- + H_3O^+$$

The double arrow separating reactants and products indicates that a dynamic equilibrium is established in which the rate of the reverse reaction, thus:

$$H_3O^+ + CH_3COO^- \rightarrow CH_3COOH + H_2O$$

is equal to the rate of the forward reaction:

$$CH_3COOH + H_2O \rightarrow CH_3COO^- + H_3O^-$$

Thus at equilibrium the concentration of each species in the solution remains constant. The disproportionate length of the arrows in the equation simply indicates that the acetic acid remains largely undissociated.

A similar situation exists for aqueous solutions of *weak bases*, for example, NH_3, Na_2CO_3, and H_2O. Thus a 0.1M solution of NH_3 in water undergoes reaction to the extent of 0.5%.

$$NH_3 + H_2O \rightleftharpoons NH_4^+ + OH^-$$

EQUILIBRIUMS AND EQUILIBRIUM CONSTANT

The extent of dissociation of weak acids and bases and the resulting equilibriums have been studied exhaustively. These studies have resulted in a mathematic statement that allows calculation of the degree of dissociation. The mathematic expression describing the general equilibrium reaction:

$$HY + H_2O \rightleftharpoons Y^- + H_3O^+$$

is expressed as follows:

$$K_{HY} = \frac{[Y^-][H_3O^+]}{[HY][H_2O]}$$

NOTE: The brackets indicate concentration of the species in moles per liter.

The equation states that the mathematic product of the concentrations of the reaction products divided by the mathematic product of the concentrations of the reactants is a constant (this is valid only at a given temperature). For example, the equilibrium expression for:

$$NH_3 + H_2O \rightleftharpoons NH_4^+ + OH^-$$

is expressed as follows:

$$K_{NH_3} = \frac{[NH_4^+][OH^-]}{[NH_3][H_2O]}$$

Inasmuch as water is present in large excess in most solutions, its concentration remains essentially constant; therefore the term for the concentration of water is incorporated with the equilibrium constant, and the mathematic expression is normally:

$$K_{NH_3} = \frac{[NH_4^3][OH^-]}{[NH_3]}$$

Experiments have shown that K_{NH3} is equal to 1.8 × 10^{-5} m at 25° C. In general, the larger the numeric value of K, the stronger the acid or base, depending on whether H_3O^+ or OH^- ion is one of the products.

A most important equilibrium reaction is that involving pure water, because reactions involving acids and bases are normally conducted in aqueous medium. Even though water is neutral, it was classified as both a weak acid and a weak base in the preceding section.

Experiments have shown that water undergoes autoionization, in which one molecule of water functions as an acid and a second molecule functions as a base, giving the following equation:

$$H_2O + H_2O \rightarrow H_3O^+ + OH^-$$

Even though autoionization is occurring, water is neutral, because the concentration of H_3O^+ ion is exactly equal to the concentration of OH^- ion. The equilibrium expression for water is:

$$K = \frac{[OH^-][H_3O^+]}{[H_2O]}$$

or

$$K_W = [H_2O]K = [OH^-][H_3O^+]$$

The concentration of water being constant gives:

$$K_W = [OH^-][H_3O^+]$$

K_W has been determined experimentally to be 1 × 10^{-14} M^2. For pure water:

$$[H_3O^+] = [OH^-] + \sqrt{1 \times 10^{-14}} = 1 \times 10^{17} M$$

THE pH CONCEPT

An aqueous solution, no matter whether acidic, basic, or neutral, must have a concentration of H_3O^+ and OH^- ions, the product of which must equal 1 × 10^{-14}.

$$K_W = [H_3O^+][OH^-] = 1 \times 10^{-14} M^2$$

Any solution in which $[H_3O^+]$ is equal to $[OH^-]$ must be neutral, and any solution in which $[OH^-]$ and $[H_3O^+]$ are unequal must be either basic or acidic. However, at all times $[H_3O^+] \times [OH^-]$ equals 1 × 10^{-14} M^2. As with the solutions discussed previously in this chapter, the concentration of H_3O^+ is expressed as moles/liter. This has been further simplified and is commonly expressed in terms of pH (from the French term *puissance d'hydrogene,* meaning "power of hydrogen") as a number between 0 and 14.

The pH of a solution is defined as being equal to the negative log of the $[H_3O^+]$, thus:

$$pH = -\log[H_3O^+]$$

and a neutral solution having a concentration of H_3O^+ equal to 10^{-7} has a pH of 7.

$$pH = -\log[H_3O^+] = -\log 10^{-7} = 7$$

For those solutions in which $[H_3O^+]$ is larger than 10^{-7}, the solution will contain a concentration of H_3O^+ ions greater than that of OH^- ions, and will therefore be acidic. Whenever the $[H_3O^+]$ is greater than $[OH^-]$, the pH will be less than 7, and for those solutions in which the $[H_3O^+]$ is less than $[OH^-]$, the pH will be greater than 7 and the solution will be basic.

Values of pH		
1, 2, 3, 4, 5, 6	7	8, 9, 10, 11, 12, 13, 14
Acidic	*Neutral*	*Basic*

In an analogous manner, the pOH of a solution is the negative log of $[OH^-]$; therefore, knowing that pH is equal to $-\log[H_3O^+]$ and that K_W is equal to 1 × 10^{-14}, it follows that pOH must equal 14 − pH. For example, if a solution is found to have a $[H_3O^+]$ of 1 × 10^{-3} M, the pH of the solution will be $-\log(1 \times 10^{-3})$, or 3, and the pOH therefore must be 14 − 3, or 11.

Example 1:
What is the pH of a solution that has a $[H_3O^+]$ of 2.3 × 10^{-5} M? Use the relationship $pH = -\log[H_3O^+]$, and proceed as follows:

$$pH=-\log(2.3\rightarrow10^{-5})$$
$$pH=-\log(2.3+\log10^{-5})$$
$$pH=-(0.36+[-5]\log10)$$
$$pH=-(0.36-5)$$
$$pH=-(4.64)$$
$$pH=4.64 \text{ (The solution is acidic.)}$$

Example 2:
A solution is found to have a concentration of OH^- equaling 3.0×10^{-8} M. What is its pH?

a. Using $pOH = -\log[OH^-]$, find pOH.

$$pOH=-\log(3.0\rightarrow10^{-8})$$
$$pOH=-(\log3.0+[-8]\log10)$$
$$pOH=-(0.477+[-8])$$
$$pOH=-(-7.523)$$
$$pOH=7.52$$

b. Using $pH + pOH = 14$, find pH.

$$pH+7.52=14$$
$$pH=14-7.52$$
$$pH=6.48 \text{ (The solution is acidic.)}$$

Example 3:
Find the $[H_3O^+]$ of a solution that has a pH of 9.8 using $pH = -\log[H_3O^+]$.

$$9.8=-\log[H_3O^+]$$
$$\log[H_3O^+]=-10+0.2$$

Using antilogs, find the $[H_3O^+]$.

$$[H_3O^+]=(\text{antilog }0.2)(\text{antilog}-10)$$
$$[H_3O^+]=1.58\rightarrow10^{-10} \text{ M}$$

Example 4:
Given the following information for a solution of acetic acid:

$$K_a=1.8\rightarrow10^{-5}$$
$$[HOAc]=0.5\,M \text{ (HOAc is acetic acid.)}$$

Find the pH of the solution.

a. The equilibrium reaction is:

$$HOAc \rightleftharpoons H^+ = OAc^-$$
$$0.5\,M\times M+x\,M$$

We know that:

$$K_a=\frac{[H^+][OAc^-]}{[HOAc]}$$

Assuming that x M of HOAc dissociates, the concentrations at equilibrium are:

$$[HOAC]=0.5-x$$
$$[H^+]=x$$
$$[OAc]=x$$

Thus:

$$1.8\times10^{-5}=\frac{x^2}{5\times10^{-1}-x}=\frac{x^2}{5\times10^{-1}}$$

Because HOAc is a weak acid, it is largely undissociated, and x, compared to 5.0×10^{-1}, is very small and may be eliminated from the denominator without seriously affecting the value calculated for x.

$$x^2=(1.8\times10^{-5})(5\times10^{-1})$$
$$x^2=9\times10^{-6}$$
$$x=3\times10^{-3}\,M=[H^+][OAc^-]$$

b. Using $pH = -\log[H_3O^+]$, proceed as follows:

$$pH=-\log(3\times10^{-3})$$
$$pH=-(\log3+[-3]\log10)$$
$$pH=-(-2.52)$$
$$pH=2.52 \text{ (The solution is acidic.)}$$

BUFFER SOLUTIONS

All biological systems are dependent on fluids that are maintained within very narrow limits of pH. For example, human blood must be maintained within a pH range of 7.3 to 7.5 and therefore requires a means by which these pH limits can be maintained. The mechanism by which this is achieved is referred to as *buffering* and involves a solution that contains a mixture of substances, some that are acidic and others that are basic. Again, with blood as an example, the substances involved in the buffering effect are carbonates, bicarbonates, carbonic acid, the phosphates (PO_4^{3-}, HPO_4^{2-}, and $H_2PO_4^-$, and certain proteins that function by maintaining the pH of blood in the range of 7.3 to 7.5.

A relatively simple buffer system is one consisting of a mixture of acetic acid and its conjugate base acetate ion. To understand how this system can function to maintain a pH within a small range, recall that acetic acid, which is a weak acid, is described by an equilibrium expression. Examine what occurs when a "foreign" acid or base is introduced into the acetic acid–acetate ion buffer system.

This equation shows that undissociated acetic acid is present and is available to react with any base entering the system. For example, if a small quantity of sodium hydroxide is added to the system (HOAc + NaOH → NaOAc + H₂O), the concentration of acetic acid will decrease while the concentration of acetate ion will increase. Conversely, when an acid such as HCl is added to the system (NaOAc + HCl → HOAc + NaCl), the concentration of acetic acid increases while the concentration of acetate ion is decreased. The concentration of the buffer system components will undergo change, but the expression governing the equilibrium will still be valid.

Although buffer solutions will not maintain a fairly constant pH if large quantities of acids or bases are added to them, it is remarkable how much they can accommodate without an appreciable change in pH. This is illustrated in the following example:

Example:
Consider 1 L of the acetate buffer that is 0.1 M in acetic acid and 0.1 M in sodium acetate.

$$HOAc \rightleftharpoons H^+ + OAc^- \quad K_a - 1.6 \times 10^{-5}$$

0.1 M   x M + x M

$$NaOAc \rightarrow Na^+ + OAc^- \text{ (100\% ionized)}$$

0.1 M   0.1 M   0.1 M

a. Calculate the pH of the following buffer solution:

$$K_a = \frac{[H^+][OAc^-]}{[HOAc]} = \frac{[H^+](1 \times 10^{-1} + x)}{(1 \times 10^{-1} + x)} = 1.8 \times 10^{-5}$$

Because the acetic acid contributes a negligible amount of the total quantity of OAc^-, the $[OAc^- + x]$ may be assumed to be 0.1 M. Similarly, the $[HOAc^- x]$ may be assumed to be 0.1 M; therefore

$$1.8 \times 10^{-5} = \frac{[H^+](1 \times 10^{-1})}{(1 \times 10^{-1})}$$

and

$$[H^+] = 1.8 \times 10^{-5} \text{ M}$$

The pH of the solution will be, to a first approximation, as follows:

$$pH = -\log[H^+] = -\log(1.8 \times 10^{-5})$$
$$pH = -(\log 1.8 + [-5]\log 10)$$
$$pH = -(0.26 - 5)$$
$$pH = 4.74$$

b. Calculate the pH of the solution after addition of 0.1 mole of HCl, assuming that the increase in total volume of the buffer solution will be negligible.

$$HCl + NaOH \rightarrow NaCl + HOAc$$

0.01M   0.01M   0.01M   0.01M

The reaction states that for each equivalent of HCl added, 1 equivalent of OAc^- will be consumed, thus forming an equivalent of HOAc. The concentrations now become

$$HOAc \rightleftharpoons H^+ + OAc^-$$

(0.01M + 0.01M)   x M + (0.1 − 0.01M)

Following the same rationale as used in part a, calculate the $[H^+]$.

$$K_a = \frac{[H^+][OAc^-]}{[HOAc]}$$
$$\frac{[H^+][0.09]}{[0.11]} = 1.8 \times 10^{-5}$$
$$[H^+] = \frac{(1.1 \times 10^{-1})(1.8 \times 10^{-5})}{(9 \times 10^{-2})}$$
$$[H^+] = 0.22 \times 10^{-4} = 2.2 \times 10^{-5} \text{ M}$$

Thus:

$$pH = -\log[H^+] = -\log(2.2 \times 10^{-5})$$
$$pH = -(\log 2.2 + [-5]\log 10)$$
$$pH = -(0.34 - 5)$$
$$pH = 4.66$$

Comparing the pH of the original buffer solution (4.74) with the pH of the solution after addition of 0.01 mole of HCl (4.66) it is seen that the pH has changed by only 0.08. As a problem to solve, what change in pH would be expected if 0.01 mole of NaOH had been added to the original solution? Similarly, the buffer systems involved in maintaining a narrow pH range for blood involve simple acid-base reactions such as those just described.

ORGANIC COMPOUNDS

The chemistry discussed in this chapter has involved, with the exception of acetic acid, substances referred to as being *inorganic*. Inorganic substances comprise all those elements and compounds derived from elements other than carbon, the number of which can be counted in the thousands. Organic chemistry is best defined as the chemistry of carbon, and organic compounds recorded in the literature are numbered in the millions. Carbon differs from all other elements in its unique ability to form strong covalent bonds to other carbon atoms, thus resulting in myriads of compounds, ranging from those of low molecular weight to highly complex molecules containing thousands of carbon atoms. A thorough discussion of organic chemistry is beyond the scope of this chapter; however, the importance of organic chemistry as applied to nuclear medicine specifically and to all living systems generally requires some foundation in this subject.

Historically, organic chemistry as a discipline is relatively young because philosophical and theological thought held that organic substances, being found primarily in living systems, required a vital force for their creation and that humans would never accomplish the creation or synthesis of these substances. In 1828 the German chemist Friedrich Wöhler, while working with the inorganic substance ammonium cyanate ($NH_4^+ CNO^-$), found that when it was heated the substance was converted to the nonionic organic substance urea

$$(H_2N-\overset{\displaystyle O}{\overset{\|}{C}}-NH_2),$$

which is a metabolic product excreted in urine. This discovery gave rise to great controversy in the scientific community, and serious investigation in organic chemistry did not occur until the mid-1800s.

Types of Organic Compounds and Nomenclature

Organic compounds are divided into families or homologous series in which all members of a given family exhibit essentially the same type of chemical reactivity. Each family of simple organic compounds is characterized by a *functional group*, the most reactive site of the molecule, which determines the chemical reactions that all members of the family will undergo. The main families of organic compounds and their characteristic functional groups are given in Table 5-5.

TABLE 5-5	Families of Organic Compounds and Their Functional Groups			
Family	**Structure**	**IUPAC Name**	**Suffix**	**Functional Group**
Alkanes		Methane	–ane	(None)
Alkenes		Ethene	–ene	
Alkynes	H—C≡C—H	Ethyne	–yne	—C≡C—
Arenes (aromatic compounds)		Benzene	–ene	
Alcohols		Ethanol	–ol	—O—H
Phenols		Phenol	–ol	—O—H
Ethers		Diethylether	–ether	—O—
Halides		Bromomethane	The substituents *chloro-, fluoro-,* etc., are prefixed to parent alkane	—X(F, Cl, Br, I)
Aldehydes		Ethanal	–al	

Continued

TABLE 5-5   Families of Organic Compounds and Their Functional Groups—cont'd

Family	Structure	IUPAC Name	Suffix	Functional Group
Ketones	$H_3C-CO-CH_3$	2-Propanone	–one	$-CO-$
Carboxylic acids	CH_3-COOH	Ethanoic acid	–oic	$-CO-OH$
Esters	$CH_3-CO-O-CH_2-CH_3$	Ethyl ethanoate	–oate	$-CO-O-C-$
Amides	$CH_3-CO-NH_2$	Ethanamide	–amide	$-CO-N\backslash$
Amines	CH_3-NH_2	Methamine	–amine	$-C-N\backslash$
Thiols	CH_3-CH_2-SH	Ethanethiol	–thiol	$-C-S-$

IUPAC, International Union of Pure and Applied Chemistry.

As previously noted, each compound possesses a name unique to itself; this is also the case with organic compounds. Although many organic compounds, especially those isolated as naturally occurring products in the early years of organic chemistry, are still referred to by the names (common or trivial) given them by their discoverers, the multitude of organic compounds now known requires a systematic method of naming them. Currently, the generally accepted rules for naming organic compounds are those set down by the International Union of Pure and Applied Chemistry (IUPAC). Using alkanes as an example, the IUPAC rules are as follows.

Those molecules in which all the carbon atoms are bonded to form a continuous chain are called *normal alkanes* (Table 5-6). All other alkanes are named as though they had been derived from the hydrocarbon with the longest continuous chain; this being the parent compound (see Rule 1).

$$CH_3-CH-CH-CH-CH_3$$

with substituents CH_3, CH_3, CH_2, and CH_3.

EXAMPLE:

Rule 1: The longest chain consists of six carbon atoms; therefore the parent hydrocarbon is *hexane.* However, unlike hexane the above molecule has three branches in which CH_3 groups have been substituted for hydrogens of the parent compound. The CH_3 groups belong to a family of alkyl groups, which are derived from the alkanes by removal of one hydrogen atom. These are named by replacement of the "-ane" ending of the alkane by "-yl" (Table 5-7).

Rule 2: The carbon atoms of the parent structure are numbered from the end that will give the *lowest numbers* to those carbons to which the alkyl groups are attached.

$$CH_3-CH-CH-CH-CH_2-CH_3$$

with OH and branches CH_3, numbered 1 2 3 4 5 6.

Number as previously shown and *not* as follows.

TABLE 5-6	Normal Alkanes (C_nH_{2n+2})		
Number of Carbons	**Name**	**Expanded Formula**	**Condensed Formula**
1	Methane	$H-C-H$ (with H above and below C)	CH_4
2	Ethane	$H-C-C-H$ (with H above and below each C)	CH_3-CH_3
3	Propane	$H-C-C-C-H$ (with H above and below each C)	$CH_3-CH_2-CH_3$
4	Butane	$H-C-C-C-C-H$ (with H above and below each C)	$CH_3-(CH_2)_2-CH_3$
5	Pentane	$H-C-C-C-C-C-H$ (with H above and below each C)	$CH_3-(CH_2)_3-CH_3$
6	Hexane	$H-C-C-C-C-C-C-H$ (with H above and below each C)	$CH_3-(CH_2)_4-CH_3$

Starting with pentane, the alkanes are named systematically with a numeric prefix indicating the number of carbon atoms: pent-, hex-, hept-, oct-, non-, dec-, undec-, dodec-, tridec-, tetradec-, pentadec-, hexadec, heptadec-, octadec-, nonadec-, eicos- (20), heneicos- (21), docos-, tricos-, tetracos-, and so on.

TABLE 5-7	Alkyl Groups Derived from the Alkanes by Removal of One Hydrogen	
	Common Alkyl Groups	**Derived From**
Methyl	CH_3-	Methane
Ethyl	CH_3-CH_2-	Ethane
Propyl	$CH_3-CH_2-CH_2-$	Propane
Isopropyl	$CH_3-CH-CH_3$	Propane
Butyl	$CH_3-CH_2-CH_2-CH_2-$	Butane
sec-Butyl	$CH_3-CH-CH_2-CH_3-$	Butane
Isobutyl	$HC-CH_2-$ (with CH_3 above and CH_3 below HC)	Butane
tert-Butyl	CH_3-C- (with CH_3 above and CH_3 below C)	Butane

Rule 3: The groups attached to the parent structure are given both a name and a number to indicate their point of attachment. If the same group occurs as a substituent in the molecule more than once, the prefixes di-, tri-, tetra-, and so on, are used to specify the number of times this group appears. If more than one type of group is attached to the parent compound, these groups are named in alphabetical order. Therefore the correct name for the compound just shown is "2,3,4-trimethylhexane."

A comma (with no space) is used between numbers and a hyphen between the number and the name of the substituent.

Note in Table 5-7 that the isobutyl and *tert*-butyl groups are not shown to be derived from one of the normal alkanes. The names given these groups arise from an older nomenclature in which both of the alkanes containing four carbon atoms were called *butanes*. This pair of structural isomers consists of the normal butane and a second compound having the structure that is called *isobutane*. Inspection of the structure

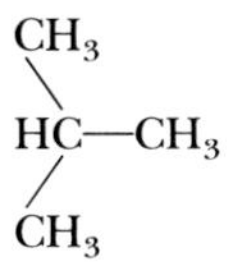

$$
\begin{array}{c}
CH_3 \\
| \\
HC-CH_3 \\
| \\
CH_3
\end{array}
$$

of isobutane shows that two alkyl groups can be derived, depending on the hydrogen that is removed. The prefixes secondary and tertiary are used to indicate the carbon through which the alkyl substituent is attached. If the carbon of the alkyl group, at the point of attachment, is bonded to only one other carbon, the alkyl group is designated as primary; if bonded to two other carbons, the alkyl group is secondary; and it is tertiary if bonded to three other carbons, for example, the *sec*-butyl and *tert*-butyl groups.

The IUPAC rules for naming all organic compounds generally follow these rules with the following modifications: (1) the ending (suffix) of the name is dictated by the main functional group present in the compounds, (2) the longest continuous chain (parent compound) must contain the main functional group, and (3) the chain is numbered so that the main functional group receives the lowest possible number.

EXAMPLE:

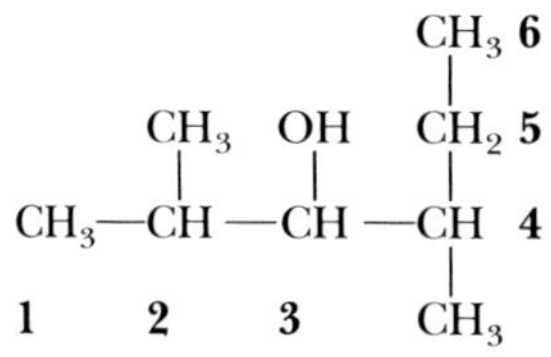

$$
\begin{array}{c}
\qquad\qquad CH_3\ \mathbf{6} \\
\qquad\qquad | \\
CH_3\ \ OH\ \ CH_2\ \mathbf{5} \\
|\qquad |\qquad | \\
CH_3-CH-CH-CH\ \ \mathbf{4} \quad \text{2,4-Dimethyl-3-hexanol} \\
\mathbf{1}\quad\ \mathbf{2}\quad\ \mathbf{3}\quad CH_3
\end{array}
$$

Alkanes. Also called *saturated hydrocarbons*, these compounds are a major source of energy but are of little importance in nuclear medicine. Perhaps their greatest use in nuclear medicine would be as solvents; however, as a point of interest the saturated hydrocarbon cyclopropane:

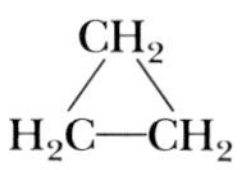

$$
\begin{array}{c}
CH_2 \\
/\quad\ \backslash \\
H_2C-CH_2
\end{array}
$$

(with the prefix "cyclo-" indicating a ring or cyclic system) is used as a general anesthetic.
Alkenes. This family of hydrocarbons, which contains a carbon-carbon double bond (C=C) is a potentially useful group of substances in labeling procedures. Although several substances are currently under investi-

gation, their usefulness as imaging agents has yet to be proved. Potential agents may arise through addition of radioactive reagents to the carbon-carbon double bond.

$$
R-HC{=}CH-R' + HI \rightarrow R-\overset{\displaystyle H}{\underset{\displaystyle H}{C}}-\overset{\displaystyle H}{\underset{\displaystyle I}{C}}-R'
$$

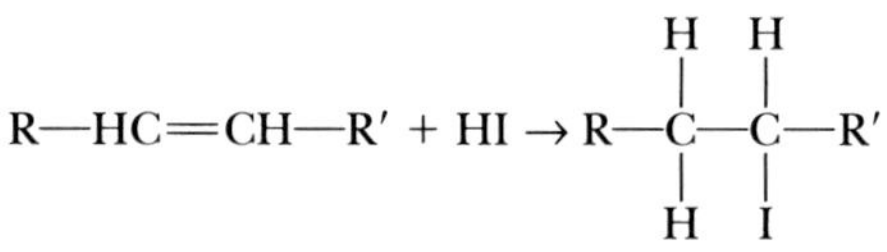

The alkynes, having chemical properties similar to the alkenes, are also of interest as potential sources of radiopharmaceuticals.
Arenes and Aromatic Compounds. This family of compounds contains at least one aromatic ring, which is characterized by benzene, the simplest of the aromatic compounds.

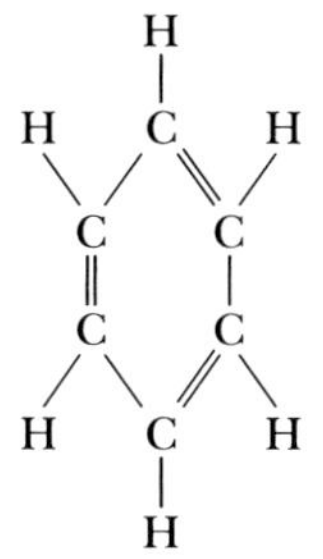

The chemistry of these compounds differs greatly from that of the alkenes and alkynes in that rather than addition reactions, they undergo substitution reactions in which one or more hydrogens are replaced by another atom or group. For example, the iodination of benzene is:

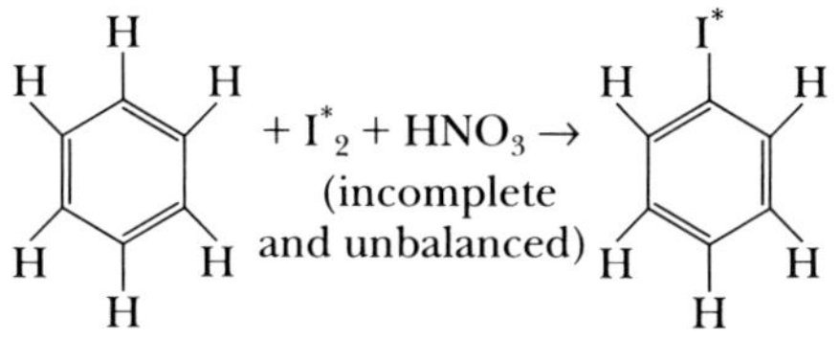

$$+ I^*_2 + HNO_3 \rightarrow \text{(incomplete and unbalanced)}$$

This reaction is found to be especially useful in the preparation of *ortho*-iodohippuric acid, which has found use as a renal function agent.

Among other aromatic substances containing a radioactive halogen are the estrogens, which have been approved for experimental imaging procedures in humans.

An especially important radiolabeled, aromatic compound used for determination of thyroid function is T_3.

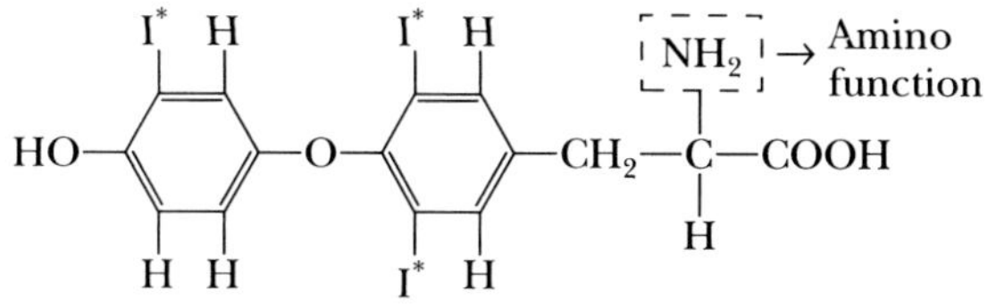

3,5,3'–Triiodothyronine (T₃)

Alcohols and Phenols. Alcohols and phenols contain the functional group —OH. Inspection of the structures of rose bengal and T₃ shows that each contains a phenolic hydroxyl (—OH) function as a part of the molecule. Likewise, brominated estrone, mentioned in the preceding section, also contains this functional group.

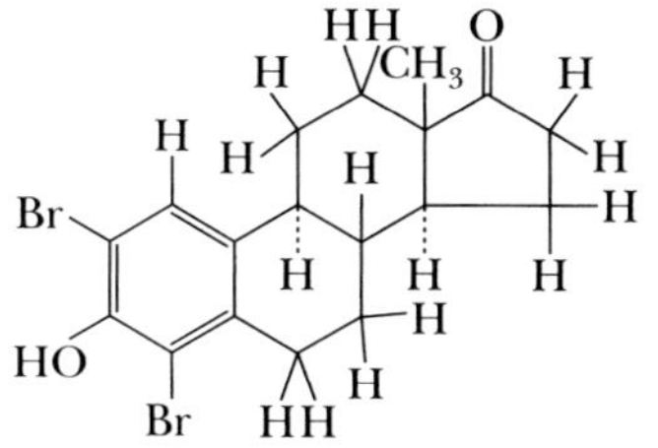

2,4–Dibromoestrone

Molecules containing this structural feature are highly important in preparation of radiopharmaceuticals.

Ethers. The ether linkage, R—O—R, also occurs in rose bengal and T₃, and its importance as a structural feature, as with the phenolic —OH function, lies in its ability to facilitate substitution reactions in which radioactive halogens are introduced into the aromatic ring.

Halides. Radiopharmaceuticals that contain halogens, especially those containing radioactive bromine or iodine, again for example, rose bengal, T₃, and brominated estrogen, are of utmost importance and have great effectiveness in the practice of nuclear medicine, solely because of the presence of the radioactive halogen in these molecules. However, the functional molecules are of equal importance in that they determine the organ or site in which the total radioactive substance is localized.

Aldehydes and Ketones. The carbonyl function

is common to both aldehydes and ketones. The presence of this functional group is not especially important to the labeling of organic molecules, but, as previously noted, its presence is vital in determining the biodistribution of the radioactive substance.

Carboxylic Acids. Several compounds containing the carboxyl function have been noted in previous sections. In addition, pentetic acid (DTPA) forms a complex with ^{169}Yb to give ^{169}Yb-pentetic acid (^{169}Yb-DTPA), a cisternographic imaging agent.

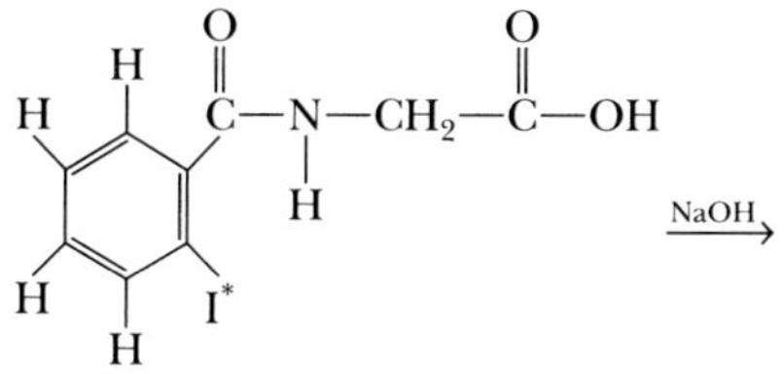

o-Iodohippuric acid

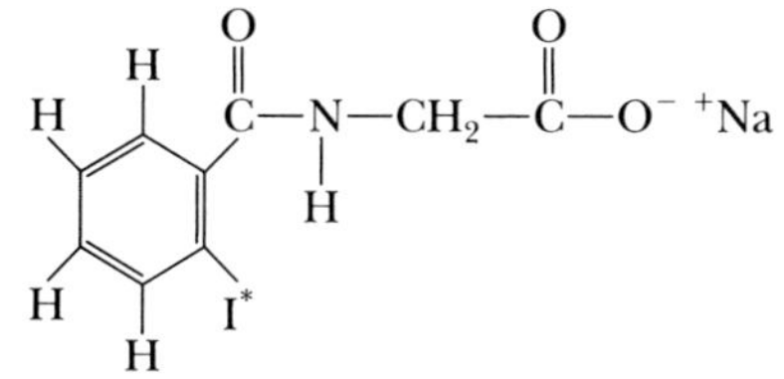

Hippuran

The sodium salt of o-iodohippuric acid, hippuran, in filtering through the glomeruli of the kidneys, provides an effective means of evaluating kidney function, especially important to patients who have received a kidney transplant.

Esters, functioning as derivatives of carboxylic acids, are formed by means of an acid-catalyzed condensation reaction between a carboxylic acid and an alcohol. These substances have not as yet been found to be useful as precursors to radiopharmaceuticals.

Amides. Hippuran (previous section), in addition to the carboxylate group, also contains an amide function. Components of all biological tissues have amide functions, which usually are referred to as *peptide linkages*. The protein human serum albumin (HSA), whose structure is not completely known, when labeled with ^{99m}Tc, is used as a blood pool imaging agent.

Amines and Thiols. Amines and thiols are the nitrogen and sulfur analogs of the alcohols. Substances in which the amino groups (—NH₂) are an important structural component are the proteins and amino acids from which they are derived.

Of the compounds useful in nuclear medicine, one of the most important is pentetic acid (DTPA; see the previous section on carboxylic acids).

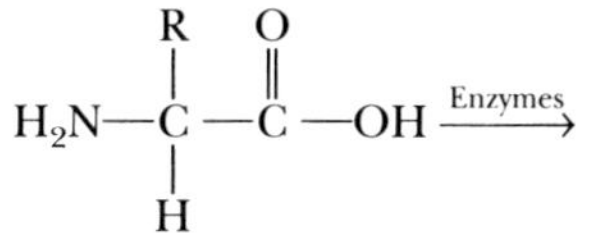

Amino acid

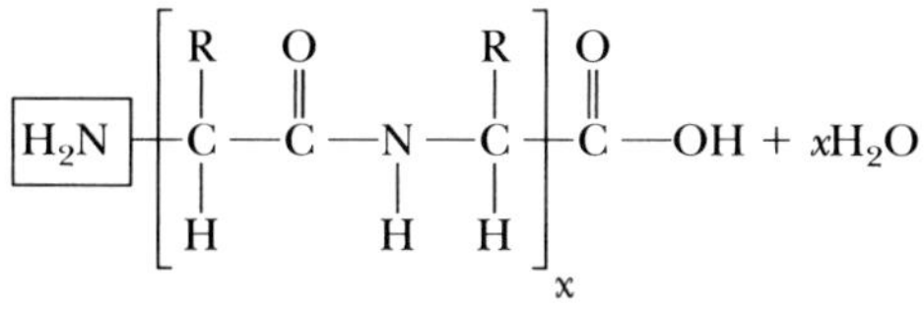

Protein

SUMMARY

- A thorough understanding of each of the radiopharmaceutical compounds requires knowledge of not only their structure and biological fate but also the chemical processes by which they are prepared. A discussion of the procedures used in preparing these substances is contained in Chapter 6.

- Volume measurements requiring an accuracy of ±1% to ±2% can be achieved by the use of the appropriate graduated cylinder.

- Solutions accurate in concentration to ±0.001% can be attained using a volumetric flask.

- Pipets are transfer vessels used to measure and deliver a precise volume of solution or liquid. Two types are (1) those that must be filled and drained manually, and (2) automatic pipets, which measure and deliver a fixed volume when activated.

- Care must be exercised in the use of pipets because some are calibrated to deliver the stated volume by normal drainage (some solution remains in the tip of the pipet), and others are calibrated to deliver the entire volume drawn into the pipet, which requires "blowing-out" the last traces of solution.

- Procedures such as titrations are performed by use of a buret.

- The centrifuge is used to separate solids from liquids, such as red blood cells from plasma.

- Law of constant composition: a compound, regardless of its origin or method of preparation, always contains the same elements in the same proportions by weight.

- Empirical or molecular formulas may be characteristic of several different compounds and provide no information pertinent to the structure of the molecule.

- A solution is a homogeneous mixture of two substances—the solute and the solvent.

- Colloids consist of minute particles that are suspended in dispersing medium.

- Oxidation-reduction reactions, commonly called *redox reactions,* are those reactions in which certain atoms gain or lose electrons and thus undergo a change of oxidation number.

- A technologist should understand the chemistry and theory of acids and bases because the acidity of the body fluids must remain essentially constant.

- Neutralization reactions are quite common and are generally used in determining unknown quantities of acids or bases present in biological or chemical samples.

SUGGESTED READINGS

Chang R: *Chemistry*, ed 7, New York, 2002, McGraw-Hill.
Harris DC: *Quantitative chemical analysis*, ed 6, New York, 2003, WH Freeman.
Wade LG Jr: *Organic chemistry*, ed 5, New York, 2003, Prentice Hall.

Radiochemistry and Radiopharmacology

Sally W. Schwarz, Reiko Oyama, Carolyn J. Anderson

OBJECTIVES

After completing this chapter, the reader will be able to:

- Discuss nuclear stability and its relationship to radioactive decay.
- Describe the basic mechanisms for radionuclide production in a reactor.
- Describe the fundamentals of particle accelerator operation and the production of radionuclides using particle accelerators.
- Describe generator kinetics in the production of radionuclides, and detail the difference between transient and secular equilibrium.
- Diagram wet column and dry column molybdenum-technetium generators, and explain the elution process.
- Describe the chemical properties of the pertechnetate ion.
- Explain the technetium labeling processes used by reduction methods.

- Discuss the chemical and labeling processes of gallium and indium radiopharmaceuticals.
- Describe the pharmacokinetics of thallium as a myocardial perfusion imaging agent.
- Explain iodination techniques.
- List and describe the properties of PET radiopharmaceuticals and advantages of using these compounds.
- Describe the differences between quality control relative to radionuclide purity, radiochemical purity, and chemical impurities.
- Describe how particle sizes are measured.
- Discuss the difference between sterile compounds and compounds containing pyrogens, and tests for ensuring these properties.

PRODUCTION OF RADIONUCLIDES

Nuclear Stability

Approximately 275 different nuclei have shown no evidence of radioactive decay and hence are considered stable with respect to this type of transformation. Figure 6-1 shows the relationship of the number of neutrons to the number of protons in the known stable nuclei. In the light elements, stability is achieved when the numbers of neutrons and protons are approximately equal. As the elements become heavier, the ratio of neutrons to protons (n/p ratio) for nuclear stability increases from 1 to about 1.5. If a nucleus has an n/p ratio too high for stability (neutron rich), it will undergo radioactive decay in a manner such that the n/p ratio decreases to approach the line of stability. The consequence is the production of a negative beta particle (β^-) as shown by the following example:

$$n \rightarrow p + e^- + \bar{v} \, (\beta^- \text{ decay})$$

The decay energy is the energy difference between parent and daughter nuclide. The $\bar{v}$ (antineutrino) carries away the energy difference between the β^- particle and the decay energy.

If the n/p ratio is too low for stability, radioactive decay occurs in a manner that will reduce the number of protons and increase the number of neutrons by the net conversion of a proton to a neutron. This is accomplished through either positron emission (β^+) or absorption by the nucleus of an orbital electron (electron capture [EC]). Examples are shown in the following reactions:

$$p \rightarrow n + e^+ + v \, (\beta^+ \text{ decay})$$
$$p + e^- \rightarrow n + v \, (\text{electron capture})$$

The v (neutrino) carries away the energy difference between the β^+ particle and the decay energy.

Beta decay often leaves the daughter nucleus in an excited state. This excitation energy is removed either by gamma-ray emission or by a process called internal conversion. Generally, emission of a gamma ray occurs immediately after the beta decay (within 10^{-12} seconds), but in some cases the nucleus may remain in the higher energy state for a measurable length of time. When this

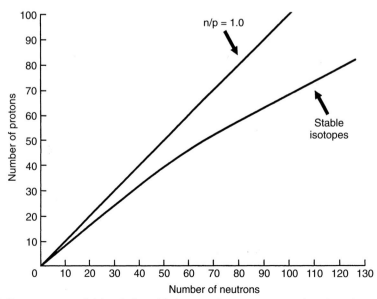

FIGURE 6-1 Neutron-proton (n/p) ratio in stable isotopes becomes greater than 1 as the mass increases.

occurs, the excited nucleus is said to be in a **metastable** state, indicated by the letter *m*. An example is ^{99m}Tc, which decays with a half-life of 6 hours to ^{99}Tc. The transition of a radionuclide from an upper energy state to a lower energy state by the emission of gamma rays is referred to as an **isomeric transition.**

If a nucleus is capable of emitting a gamma ray, there is also a probability that the photon may eject an electron from an extranuclear shell. This process is an alternative to isomeric transition and is known as **internal conversion.** As an upper-level electron undergoes a transition to occupy the lower energy electron site, an x-ray is emitted, characteristic of the electron shell that is being filled. In a process similar to internal conversion, these x-rays may cause the ejection of an additional outer shell electron known as an **Auger electron.** The process continues until all inner shell vacancies have been filled by "cascading" electrons from outer shells, with corresponding emissions of x-rays or Auger electrons.

Positron decay leaves the daughter nuclide two electron mass units lower than the parent, requiring at least 1.022 MeV (2×0.511 MeV/electron) of transition energy. Once released from the nucleus, the β^+ reacts with an electron, resulting in the release of two 0.511-MeV photons, which are called **annihilation radiation,** emitted in opposite directions. Some positron-emitting radionuclides decay to excited states of the daughter nuclide. These excited daughter nuclides can further decay by isomeric transitions, as discussed earlier.

Alpha decay occurs primarily for nuclei heavier than lead. In alpha decay the proton number is reduced by 2 and the mass by 4 units. It is represented by the following equation:

$$^A_Z X \left(\begin{matrix} A-4 \\ Z-2 \end{matrix} \right) Y + {}^4He$$

The probability of alpha decay is greater for nuclei with an even number of neutrons or protons than for nuclei with an odd number. Radionuclides that decay by alpha emission are not useful in nuclear medicine imaging, but may have future therapeutic applications.

Radionuclides used to label **radiopharmaceuticals (RaPhs)** for nuclear medicine imaging should decay by either gamma or positron (β^+) emission. Gamma radiation emitted from RaPhs readily penetrates tissues and escapes from the body, allowing external detection by gamma cameras. Positron-emitting radionuclides produce two 0.511-MeV gamma photons emitted in opposite directions from the positron-electron annihilation. The angle of nearly 180 degrees of the emitted 0.511-MeV photons is exploited in positron emission tomography (PET) to allow electronic collimation of the radiation and determination of the three-dimensional location of the decay event.

Reactor-Produced Radionuclides

The two major principles of a nuclear reactor are that neutrons induce fission in uranium and that the number of neutrons released by this fission is greater than one. Thus:

$$^{235}U + n \rightarrow \text{fission products} + 2.5\,(n)$$

For each neutron consumed, an average of 2.5 new neutrons are released with an energy of 1.5 eV. These new neutrons can be used to fission other ^{235}U nuclei, leading to the release of more neutrons, self-propagating the reaction. These nuclear chain reactions are controlled by the use of moderators and neutron absorbers (materials used to reduce neutron energy [thermalize] to 0.025 eV) in a reactor so that an equilibrium state is reached. Radionuclides can be produced in a nuclear reactor by two methods: (1) irradiation of material within the neutron flux (neutrons $\times$ cm^{-2} $\times$ sec^{-1}) or (2) separation and collection of the fission products.

Thermal Neutron Reactions. The neutrons around the core of a nuclear reactor are low-energy (thermal) neutrons that typically induce the following types of nuclear reactions:

Equation 6-1

$$^A_Z X + n \rightarrow {}^{A+1}_Z X + \gamma$$

Equation 6-2

$$^A_Z X + n \rightarrow {}^A_{Z-1} Y + p$$

In a reaction of the first type, the target atom X, with atomic number Z and atomic mass A, absorbs a neutron, and energy is emitted in the form of gamma rays. This is written as an (n, γ) reaction. The following are examples:

$$^{98}Mo\,(n, \gamma)\,^{99}Mo$$
$$^{112}Sn\,(n, \gamma)\,^{113}Sn$$

In the second type of reaction, a proton is emitted after absorption of a neutron by the target atom. Since this changes the atomic number of the nucleus, an isotope of a different element (Y) is formed. Examples of this type of nuclear reaction (n, p) are as follows:

$$^{14}N\,(n, p)\,^{14}C$$
$$^3He\,(n, p)\,^3H$$

The (n, γ) reaction forms a radioisotope from a stable isotope of the same element, precluding production of high specific activity material. The **specific activity** is defined as the activity of a radioactive isotope per gram of that same element. In an (n, p) reaction the product nuclide is an isotope of a different element, enabling the production of high specific activity, **carrier-free** (no stable isotope of the same element) radioisotopes.

The previously described reactions will produce neutron-rich products, decaying primarily by β^- emission. Radionuclides that decay by β^- emission are not generally used in imaging. However, products of (n, γ) reactions include parent isotopes used in nuclear generators. In a radionuclide generator the daughter radionuclide is the isotope of interest and is usually separated from the parent isotope by column chromatography. Examples of the parent-daughter system of radionuclide generators are as follows:

$$^{98}\text{Mo}(n, \gamma)^{99}\text{Mo} \xrightarrow{t_{1/2} = 67 \text{ hours}} {}^{99m}\text{Tc}(t_{1/2} = 6 \text{ hours})$$
$$^{112}\text{Sn}(n, \gamma)^{113}\text{Sn} \xrightarrow{t_{1/2} = 115 \text{ days}} {}^{113m}\text{In}(t_{1/2} = 1.7 \text{ hours})$$

Fission Product Separation. The fission process itself results in the formation of lighter radionuclides of unequal mass, some of which are used in nuclear medicine (^{99}Mo, ^{131}I, ^{133}Xe) (Figure 6-2). The neutron interacts with the ^{235}U nucleus to form unstable ^{236}U, which then undergoes fission. An example of a fission reaction occurring in a nuclear reactor is as follows:

$$n + {}^{235}_{92}\text{U} \rightarrow {}^{236}_{92}\text{U} \rightarrow {}^{89}_{36}\text{Kr} + {}^{144}_{56}\text{Ba} + 3n$$

Similar to products of (n, γ) reactions, fission products tend to decay by β^- emission, and only a limited number have found use in nuclear medicine. However, unlike radionuclides formed from (n, γ) reactions, fission products can be produced carrier free. For example, fission-produced ^{99}Mo is formed from uranium, whereas thermal neutron–produced ^{99}Mo is made from bombarding a ^{98}Mo target. Unfortunately a major problem associated with fission-produced radionuclides is the difficulty in chemically separating the product of interest from the others formed to obtain a radiochemically pure preparation.

Accelerator-Produced Radionuclides

Accelerators are devices that increase the energy of charged particles to enable a nuclear reaction on impact with a target. The invention of the **cyclotron** in 1930 was a successful attempt to overcome the difficulties associated with the length of high-energy linear accelerators. The basic principles of the cyclotron are shown in Figure 6-3. In the simplest cyclotron design the particles are accelerated in spiral paths inside two semicircular, flat,

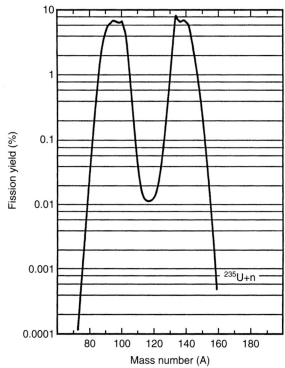

FIGURE 6-2 Relative yields of fission products of various mass formed after uranium fission.

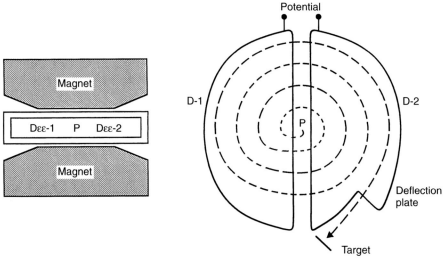

FIGURE 6-3 Schematic diagram of the operation of a positive ion cyclotron.

evacuated metallic cylinders called *dees*. The dees are placed between the two poles of a magnet so that the magnetic field operates on the ion beam, constraining it to a circular path. At the gap between the dees the ions experience acceleration due to the imposition of an electrical potential difference. The beam particles originate from the ion source at the center of the cyclotron, acquiring energy for each passage across the gap. Eventually the high-energy particle beam reaches the periphery of the dees, where it is deflected onto an external target. Fixed-frequency cyclotrons can accelerate positively charged ions up to about 50 MeV for protons. Techniques have now been developed to use cyclotrons at much higher energies. Linear accelerators can accelerate particles up to energies of several hundred MeV.

The majority of cyclotrons built before 1980 accelerated positively charged particles such as protons ($_1^1H^+$) or deuterons ($_1^2H^+$), ^3H particles, and α particles. The first negative-ion cyclotron designed specifically for PET was built by Computer Technology and Imaging, Inc. (CTI; Knoxville, Tenn.).

Medical cyclotrons currently being marketed accelerate negative ions, either hydrogen or deuterium ions. The negative ion design allows for a simple deflection system, in which the beam is extracted by interaction with a very thin carbon foil. The carbon foil strips electrons from H^-, resulting in the formation of positively charged proton, which changes direction without a final magnetic deflection due to the change in charge on the particle. The proton beam then bombards the target in a manner similar to that in a positively charged particle cyclotron. It is also possible to extract the beam at two points with the negative ion machines, allowing production of two radioisotopes simultaneously. Siemens CTI currently markets a proton-only machine. GE Medical Systems (Uppsala, Sweden) (Figure 6-4), Ebco (Vancouver, Canada), and IBA (Louvain, Belgium) market machines that have both proton and deuteron capability.

The cost of radionuclide production depends on the method employed. In a reactor there are many positions for thermal neutron irradiation of samples, allowing several isotopes to be produced simultaneously. This allows the cost of operation to be divided among several reactor-produced radionuclides. The overall price of fission products produced in a nuclear reactor is largely associated with the extensive separation process.

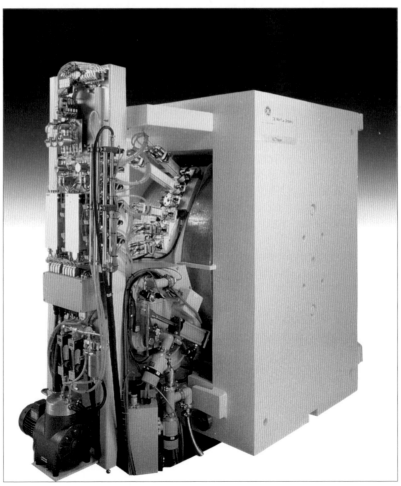

FIGURE 6-4 GE PETtrace negative ion cyclotron.

Generator	Parent $t_{1/2}$	Daughter $t_{1/2}$	Daughter E_γ (%)
^{99}Mo-^{99m}Tc	2.78 day	6 hr	140 keV (90)
^{81}Rb-^{81m}Kr	4.7 hr	13 sec	190 keV (65)
^{113}Sn-^{113m}In	115 day	1.7 hr	393 keV (64)
^{68}Ge-^{68}Ga	280 day	68 min	511 keV (176)
^{62}Zn-^{62}Cu	9.3 hr	9.8 min	511 keV (196)
^{82}Sr-^{82}Rb	25 day	1.3 min	511 keV (192)

TABLE 6-1 Decay Properties for Parent and Daughter Radionuclides of Several Generators

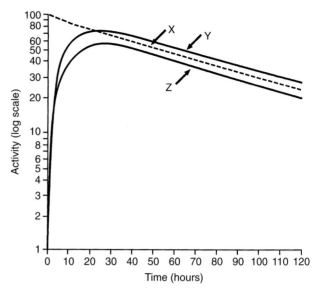

FIGURE 6-5 Growth and decay of daughter radionuclide in a transient equilibrium situation. At equilibrium, daughter activity (Y) actually exceeds parent activity (X). Point Z is the daughter activity present in a ^{99}Mo-^{99m}Tc generator. Daughter (^{99m}Tc) activity is less than that of parent (^{99}Mo), as only 86% of the ^{99}Mo present decays to ^{99m}Tc.

Alternatively, the cost of accelerator-produced isotopes is quite high. Because the machine is most frequently used to produce a single radionuclide, the entire cost of operating the accelerator must be charged for each production.

Generator Systems

Certain parent-daughter systems involve a long-lived parent radionuclide that decays to a short-lived daughter. Since the parent and daughter nuclides are not isotopes of the same element, chemical separation is possible. The long-lived parent produces a continuous supply of the relatively short-lived daughter radionuclide and is therefore called a **generator**. The generator systems used in nuclear medicine are listed in Table 6-1.

The two types of parent-daughter relationships are transient and secular equilibrium. In a **transient equilibrium** system the half-life of the parent is a factor 10 to 100 times greater than that of the daughter, whereas in a **secular equilibrium** the half-life of the parent is 100 to 1000 times greater than that of the daughter. The ^{99}Mo-^{99m}Tc generator, where ^{99}Mo has a 67-hour half-life and ^{99m}Tc has a 6-hour half-life, is an example of transient equilibrium (Figure 6-5). The generator system ^{113}Sn($t_{1/2}$ = 115 days)-^{113m}In($t_{1/2}$ = 1.7 hours), shown in Figure 6-6, is an example of secular equilibrium. The time required to reach equilibrium dictates how frequently each generator can be eluted and depends on the half-lives of the parent and daughter.

Equations Governing Generator Systems. Assuming there is initially no daughter activity present in a generator, the daughter activity at any given time can be calculated from the following general equation:

Equation 6-3

$$A_2 = \frac{\lambda_2}{\lambda_2 - \lambda_1} \times A_1^0 \left(e^{-\lambda_1 t} - e^{-\lambda_2 t} \right)$$

where A_1^0 is the parent activity at time zero, A_2 is the daughter activity at time t, and λ_1 and λ_2 are the decay constants for the parent and daughter, respectively. This general equation can be simplified for the special cases

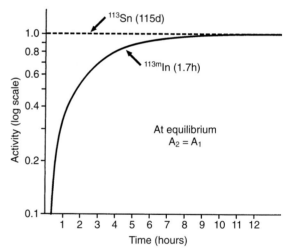

FIGURE 6-6 Growth and decay in ^{113}Sn-^{113m}In generator as an example of secular equilibrium.

of transient and secular equilibrium. In both cases a state of radioactive equilibrium is reached after a certain time in which the decay rates of the parent and daughter are equal.

In the case of transient equilibrium, as the time t becomes sufficiently large, $e^{-\lambda_2 t}$ is negligible compared with $e^{-\lambda_1 t}$, and the equation can be simplified as follows:

Equation 6-4

$$A_2 = \frac{\lambda_2}{\lambda_2 - \lambda_1} \times A_1^0 \left(e^{-\lambda_1 t} \right)$$

Because $A_1 = A_1^0 e^{-\lambda_1 t}$ where A_1 is the parent activity at time t, this equation can be rewritten as:

Equation 6-5

$$A_2 = \frac{\lambda_2}{\lambda_2 - \lambda_1} \times A_1$$

Assuming the parent only decays to the daughter, at equilibrium the daughter activity will be greater than the parent activity by the factor $\lambda_2/(\lambda_2 - \lambda_1)$. At equilibrium, both activities then appear to decay with the half-life of the parent. In the specific case of the ^{99}Mo/^{99m}Tc generator, there is only 86% decay of the ^{99}Mo to ^{99m}Tc. This makes the factor (0.86) $\lambda_2/(\lambda_2 - \lambda_1)$, which simplifies to (0.86 × 1.1). Therefore the actual ^{99m}Tc activity present at transient equilibrium is 0.946 times the ^{99}Mo activity.

In the case of secular equilibrium, the parent activity does not decrease significantly during many daughter half-lives. The decay constant of the parent (λ_1) is much smaller than that of the daughter (λ_2), and the following approximation can be made:

Equation 6-6

$$\lambda_2 - \lambda_1 \cong \lambda_2$$

This approximation can be used to further simplify equation 5 to yield the following expression:

Equation 6-7

$$A_2 = A_1$$

Therefore at equilibrium the daughter activity is equal to the parent activity, as shown in Figure 6-5.

^{99}Mo-^{99m}Tc Generator. The ^{99}Mo-^{99m}Tc generator is commonly used in nuclear medicine because of the ideal half-life (6 hours) and optimum energy (140 keV, 90% abundance) of ^{99m}Tc. A large number of RaPhs are made with ^{99m}Tc, and they are discussed later in the chapter. Molybdenum-99 ($t_{1/2}$ = 67 hours) forms the anionic species molybdate (MoO$_4^{2-}$) and paramolybdate (Mo$_7$O$_{24}^{6-}$) in an acidic medium. These anions are loaded on the generator column containing positively charged alumina (Al$_2$O$_3$) that has previously been washed with saline (pH 5). The generator is eluted with normal saline (0.9% NaCl), and ^{99m}Tc is produced as **pertechnetate** (^{99m}TcO$_4^-$).

The two types of ^{99}Mo-^{99m}Tc generators used in nuclear medicine are the wet column and dry column generators (Figure 6-7). The wet column generator contains a reservoir of normal saline that is connected to the alumina column. After elution of this generator, saline remains on the column, leading to the formation of water radiolysis products, which are reducing agents. This causes reduction of the ^{99m}Tc and decreased ^{99m}Tc pertechnetate (^{99m}TcO$_4^-$) yields, since the reduced ^{99m}Tc species do not elute from the column. This problem has been addressed by purging the saline reservoir with oxygen gas. Previous attempts to add oxidizing agents to the column to decrease the formation of reduced ^{99m}Tc species resulted in ^{99m}Tc RaPh formulation problems.

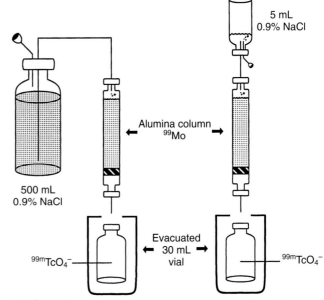

FIGURE 6-7 Schematic diagram of a wet column ^{99}Mo-^{99m}Tc generator (left) that has a 0.9% NaCl reservoir. A dry column ^{99}Mo-^{99m}Tc generator (right).

The dry column generator system was developed to alleviate poor elution yields of ^{99m}TcO$_4^-$ by removing saline from the column after elution. This decreases the amount of radiolysis products formed. The dry column generator employs a 5- to 20-ml saline charge, which is applied to an exterior port of the generator. An evacuated vial draws saline through the generator to remove ^{99m}Tc-pertechnetate, followed by air to dry the column. Leaving air on the column promotes oxidation of any reduced ^{99m}Tc species back to the +7 valence state of ^{99m}Tc pertechnetate, which can then be eluted from the generator. The ^{99m}Tc-pertechnetate can be dispensed as it is eluted from the generator as a RaPh for thyroid and Meckel diverticulum imaging. Aliquots of the bulk ^{99m}Tc-pertechnetate solution can also be added to manufacturers' kits to produce a number of ^{99m}Tc-labeled RaPhs, such as bone methylene diphosphonate (MDP), kidney (pentetic acid [DTPA], glucoheptonate [GHP], mercaptoacetyltriglycine [MAG3]), lung macroaggregated albumin (MAA) and cardiac agents methoxyisobutyl isonitrile (MIBI) tetrofosmin.

^{82}Sr-^{82}Rb Generator. Rubidium-82, a positron-emitting radionuclide, is used primarily as a myocardial perfusion agent for PET imaging. The rubidium cation (Rb$^+$) is an analogue of potassium (K$^+$) and therefore gives a similar biodistribution. Strontium-82 ($t_{1/2}$ = 25 days) is accelerator produced by bombardment of a molybdenum target with 700- to 800-MeV protons. Strontium-85 is also produced as a radionuclidic impurity. The allowable limit for ^{82}Sr is 0.02 mCi/mCi ^{82}Rb, and for ^{85}Sr is 0.2 mCi/mCi ^{82}Rb. The generators regularly meet this requirement after a first elution of the generator to waste.

The ^{82}Sr is loaded onto a stannic oxide column, and ^{82}Rb ($t_{1/2}$ = 76 seconds) is eluted with normal saline (0.9% NaCl). The 76-second half-life of ^{82}Rb allows repeat imaging studies after 10 half-lives of the ^{82}Rb, approximately 14 minutes, but poses difficulties in dose preparation for patient administration. Also the limited chemistry of this alkali metal ion severely restricts potential applications for this radionuclide in nuclear medicine. In an effort to overcome the short half-life, a calibrated continuous infusion system has been developed, allowing elution of the generator directly into an intravenous catheter. The ^{82}Rb generator is approved by the U.S. Food and Drug Administration (FDA) and produced by Bracco Diagnostics, Inc. (Princeton, N.J.) for myocardial perfusion imaging.

^{81}Rb-^{81m}Kr Generator. Krypton-81m, a gamma ray–emitting nuclide with a photon energy of 190 keV (65% abundance), was used as a lung-imaging agent. Rubidium-81 ($t_{1/2}$ = 4.7 hours), cyclotron produced by the reaction ^{79}Br(α, 2n) ^{81}Rb or ^{82}Kr(p, n) ^{81}Rb, is loaded onto a generator column containing a strong cation-exchange resin (Bio-Rad AG MP-50). The noble gas ^{81m}Kr ($t_{1/2}$ = 13 seconds) is eluted by passing humidified oxygen over the generator column. The ^{81m}Kr and O_2 are delivered to the patient via a non-rebreathing face mask. The major disadvantages of the ^{81}Rb-^{81m}Kr generator are the high cost and the 12-hour expiration time of the generator due to the 4.5-hour half-life of the parent isotope. This limits the use of the generator to the day of delivery only. The generator was an FDA-approved RaPh used for lung ventilation imaging, but is no longer available in the United States.

^{68}Ge-^{68}Ga Generator. Gallium-68 ($t_{1/2}$ = 68 minutes) emits a 2.92-MeV positron in 89% abundance, making it very useful in PET imaging. The ^{68}Ge-^{68}Ga generator[14] is not FDA-approved, but the number of ^{68}Ga RaPhs that are being investigated, both in animal models and clinically, is increasing. Clinically investigated ^{68}Ga RaPhs include ^{68}Ga–macroaggregated albumin (MAA), ^{68}Ga-citrate, ^{68}Ga–ethylenediaminetetraacetic acid (EDTA), ^{68}Ga-DOTA-Tyr^3-octreotide (^{68}Ga-DOTATOC), and ^{68}Ga-DOTA-Tyr^3-octreotate (^{68}Ga-DOTA-TATE).[48] Due to recent improvements in ^{68}Ge-^{68}Ga generator technology, there has been renewed interest in the development of ^{68}Ga RaPhs. Until recently, the ^{68}Ge-^{68}Ga generator that was commercially available consisted of ^{68}Ge loaded onto a tin dioxide column and ^{68}Ga was eluted using 1 M HCl.[29] Disadvantages of this generator included the large elution volume (3 ml) and the high acid concentration, which required extensive buffering before use. Additionally, the presence of trace metals made complexation of ^{68}Ga challenging. More recently, a generator was developed and is produced by Cyclotron Co. (Obninsk, Russia) and is marketed and distributed by Eckert and Ziegler Eurotope GmbH (Berlin, Germany). The current product is not validated for human use. In this generator, the ^{68}Ge is loaded onto a TiO$_2$ column and the ^{68}Ga is eluted with 5 ml of 0.1 N HCl (Figure 6-8). Most of the activity (80% to 90%) is eluted in the second 1-ml fraction. The use of dilute HCl and the smaller volume of ^{68}Ga eluate makes this generator much more practical for RaPh development. In addition, specific activities up to 1 GBq/nmol ^{68}Ga-labeled DOTATOC were accomplished.[5]

^{62}Zn-^{62}Cu Generator. Copper-62, a positron-emitting radionuclide (98% abundance) with a 9.7-minute half-life, is an attractive radionuclide for PET imaging. Copper-62 labeled pyruvaldehyde bis (N^4-methylthiosemicarbazone) (^{62}Cu-PTSM) has been used in clinical investigations for heart and brain blood flow measurement.[19] The parent isotope, ^{62}Zn, is cyclotron

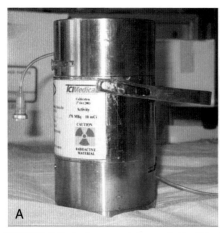 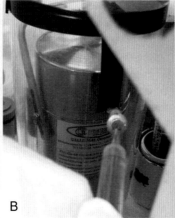 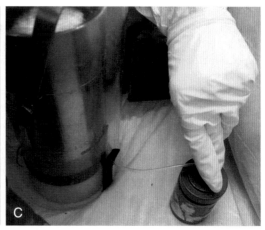

FIGURE 6-8 A, Commercially available ^{68}Ge-^{68}Ga generator (TCI Medical, Albuquerque, N.M.) showing inlet and outlet tubing. **B,** Eluant injected into inlet tubing. **C,** Effluent (^{68}Ga) collected in shielded vial.

produced via the ^{63}Cu(p, 2n) ^{62}Zn reaction. Facilities for the production of ^{62}Zn exist at a number of commercial facilities as well as at several clinical PET centers. The major disadvantage is the short half-life of the parent isotope, ^{62}Zn (9.3 hours), which requires generator replacement at 1- or 2-day intervals. Two different ^{62}Zn-^{62}Cu generator systems have been developed.[18,19] In one design, ^{62}Zn is loaded onto a column containing Dowex 1 × 8 anion exchange resin, which retains Zn^{2+} and allows Cu^{2+} to be eluted using 0.2 N HCl/1.8 N NaCl or 2 N HCl.[40] The other system employs a column containing a strong cation exchange resin adsorbent (CG-120, Amberlite), and ^{62}Cu is eluted in 0.2 M glycine.[23] The eluant in the latter generator is suitable for direct intravenous injection.

Clinical use of a ^{62}Cu-tracer requires a convenient method for routine, repetitive, high-yield RaPh synthesis using the eluate of a ^{62}Zn-^{62}Cu generator. While previous work with ^{62}Cu-PTSM relied on a fairly simple remote system for RaPh synthesis,[32] ^{62}Cu RaPh preparation has been further simplified by integration of reagent mixing operations into the 20 × 30 × 40–cm housing of a modular generator unit, available from Proportional Technologies, Inc. (Houston, Tex.).[23,46] This modular generator can directly deliver the ^{62}Cu-PTSM in a sterile, pyrogen-free solution suitable for intravenous injection. The RaPh synthesis time is the 40-second period required for generator elution. Such a modular ^{62}Zn-^{62}Cu generator system, nationally or regionally distributed from commercial medium-energy cyclotron facilities, may effectively support PET imaging centers as a source of short-lived RaPh for evaluation of tissue perfusion.

TECHNETIUM RADIOPHARMACEUTICALS

Technetium-99m was discovered in 1937 by Perrier and Segre in a sample of naturally occurring ^{98}Mo that had been irradiated by neutrons and deuterons. It was introduced into nuclear medicine in 1957 with the development of the ^{99}Mo-^{99m}Tc generator at the Brookhaven National Laboratory. The first clinical use of technetium, in 1961 at the University of Chicago, heralded a new era

for nuclear medicine. The widespread use of ^{99m}Tc as the radionuclide of choice for a variety of nuclear medicine imaging procedures has been based mainly on its physical properties. These properties include a $t_{1/2}$ of 6 hours; a 140-keV photon (88% abundance) which provides good tissue penetration and imaging characteristics for use in single photon emission computed tomography (SPECT). Additionally there is no beta emission which reduces radiation absorbed dose, and Tc-99m is available from the ^{99}Mo-^{99m}Tc generator, although as of this writing (2010), reactor shut-downs in Europe and Canada have lead to shortages of ^{99}Mo for this generator system, and consequently has limited the number of gamma scintigraphy and SPECT procedures using ^{99m}Tc.

Oxidized Technetium Complexes

Technetium is obtained from a generator in normal saline (0.9% NaCl) as the pertechnetate ion, ^{99m}TcO$_4^-$. In this form Tc is in the +7 valence state as pertechnetate and has all seven of the outer electrons involved in covalent bonding. This is the most stable of all valence states of technetium in aqueous solution. The single negative charge of pertechnetate and the geometry of the compound—oxygens in the four corners of a tetrahedron—give it a charge and size similar to the iodide ion (Figure 6-9). As a result the biodistribution of ^{99m}TcO$_4^-$ is similar to the iodide anion (I$^-$), with uptake in the thyroid, salivary glands, gastric mucosa, and choroid plexus. It concentrates in the thyroid through an anion transport mechanism, but it is not organified like iodide. This allows imaging of the thyroid. Since ^{99m}TcO$_4^-$ is secreted by the gastric mucosa, it may be used to locate Meckel diverticulum since most symptomatic patients contain ectopic gastric mucosa, which should appear on the image at the same time that stomach activity appears. Pertechnetate is excreted primarily via the gastrointestinal tract and the kidneys.

Since ^{99m}TcO$_4^-$ crosses the placental barrier, the fetal radiation dose must be considered when determining the suitability of a study employing pertechnetate for a pregnant woman.

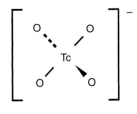

Tetrahedral
V = 4 × 10^{-23} cm^3

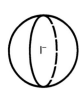

Spherical
V = 4.22 × 10^{-23} cm^3

FIGURE 6-9 Spatial comparison of TcO$_4^-$ and I$^-$ ions.

Oral administration of potassium perchlorate, Lugol solution (a solution of 5% iodine and 10% potassium iodide), or a saturated solution of potassium iodide (SSKI) before administration of $^{99m}TcO_4^-$ influences the distribution of the RaPh. Perchlorate is approximately the same size as pertechnetate and competitively inhibits the uptake of $^{99m}TcO_4^-$ into the thyroid and salivary glands, choroid plexus, and gastric mucosa. Stable iodine-127 is also taken up by these tissues and blocks the uptake of $^{99m}TcO_4^-$. Historically, pertechnetate was used for brain imaging, but localization in the choroid plexus caused a false positive brain image. This uptake can be blocked using either a stable iodine or potassium perchlorate preparation, but superior ^{99m}Tc brain imaging agents have been developed to replace $^{99m}TcO_4^-$.

Other than pertechnetate, the only RaPh containing technetium possibly in a +7 valence state is technetium-sulfur colloid. Technetium-99m sulfur colloid (^{99m}Tc-SC) was first introduced in 1966 for hepatic imaging. This agent is prepared from commercially available kits that contain sodium thiosulfate, phosphoric or hydrochloric acid, gelatin, and a buffer. Sodium thiosulfate and gelatin are added to an acidified solution of ^{99m}Tc-pertechnetate. The mixture is heated in a boiling water bath for 5 minutes. Following heating, the vial is vented and a buffer is added. ^{99m}Tc-SC exists as ^{99m}Tc-heptasulfide co-precipitated with colloidal sulfur particles, which are generated from acid decomposition of the sodium thiosulfate. The final suspension is maintained at a pH of 5.5 to 6.0 to avoid conversion of the heptasulfide back to pertechnetate. See Figure 6-10 for the schematic production of ^{99m}Tc-SC. The particle size is <1 μm. Gelatin is used as a stabilizer to prevent aggregation of the colloidal particles, which would result in lung uptake when injected.

After intravenous (IV) injection, ^{99m}Tc-SC is rapidly cleared from the blood. The mechanism of action is phagocytosis, cells of the reticuloendothelial system (RES) engulf the colloidal particles. In normal subjects approximately 85% of the ^{99m}Tc-SC is localized in the liver, 10% in the spleen, and the remainder in the bone marrow. It is used for liver and spleen imaging.

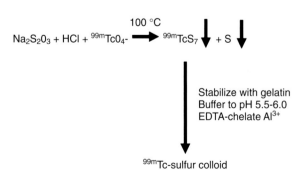

FIGURE 6-10 Schematic production of ^{99m}Tc-sulfur colloid kit formulation.

Additionally gastric emptying studies can be performed by adding ^{99m}Tc-SC to egg whites or whole eggs then cooking the eggs. After oral administration, the gastric emptying can be imaged.

Filtering of the ^{99m}Tc-SC suspension with a 0.22-μm filter removes the larger colloidal particles. The ^{99m}Tc-SC particles ≤100 nm, can be used for bone marrow imaging and lymphoscintigraphy because the smaller particles (mini ^{99m}Tc-SC) are more efficiently phagocytized by the RES cells in lymph nodes and marrow. Lymphoscintigraphy is a method using a radioactive tracer to check the lymph system for disease, and can be used to find the sentinel lymph node, the first node to receive lymph from a tumor. Lymphoscintigraphy can be performed using mini ^{99m}Tc-SC, ^{99m}Tc-antimony trisulfide colloid, and ^{99m}Tc–human serum albumin nanocolloids. The last two RaPhs are commercially available as kit formulations in Europe and Australia.

More recently, an agent marketed by Neoprobe (Dublin, Ohio) for sentinel lymph node mapping is under investigation. Technetium-99m diethylenetriamine pentaacetic acid (DTPA)–mannosyl-dextran (Lymphoseek), is composed of a dextran backbone to which multiple units of mannose and DTPA are synthetically attached (Figure 6-11). This agent accumulates in lymphatic tissues by binding to a mannose-binding protein receptor that resides on the surface of macrophage cells.[45] Patients with breast cancer who would have sentinel node biopsy participated in a clinical study to image their axial lymph nodes with either Lymphoseek or mini ^{99m}Tc-SC. In this initial study, the molecular targeted agent Lymphoseek showed more rapid and superior injection site clearance, suggesting that this agent would be more selective for positive versus negative lymph nodes.

Reduced Technetium Complexes

To alter the biodistribution of technetium it is necessary to attach it to carriers. First the technetium must be chemically reduced from the +7 valence state to a lower oxidation state, where it is a more reactive species capable of combining with a large number of compounds. This can be accomplished using a number of reducing agents, such as stannous chloride, iron ascorbic acid, or electrolytic methods. Stannous chloride is the reducing agent used most frequently in kit formulations for ^{99m}Tc RaPh.

Blood Pool Imaging Agents. Labeling of red blood cells (RBCs) with ^{99m}Tc provides an intravascular tracer useful for a variety of imaging procedures, including radionuclide ventriculography (RVG) and hemangioma and gastrointestinal bleeding studies. RBCs can be labeled with ^{99m}Tc using either in vivo or in vitro methods.

A common method for in vivo labeling of RBCs involves injection of stannous chloride ($SnCl_2$), usually in the form of a pyrophosphate kit reconstituted with 0.9% NaCl, into the patient to "tin" the cells. A time of

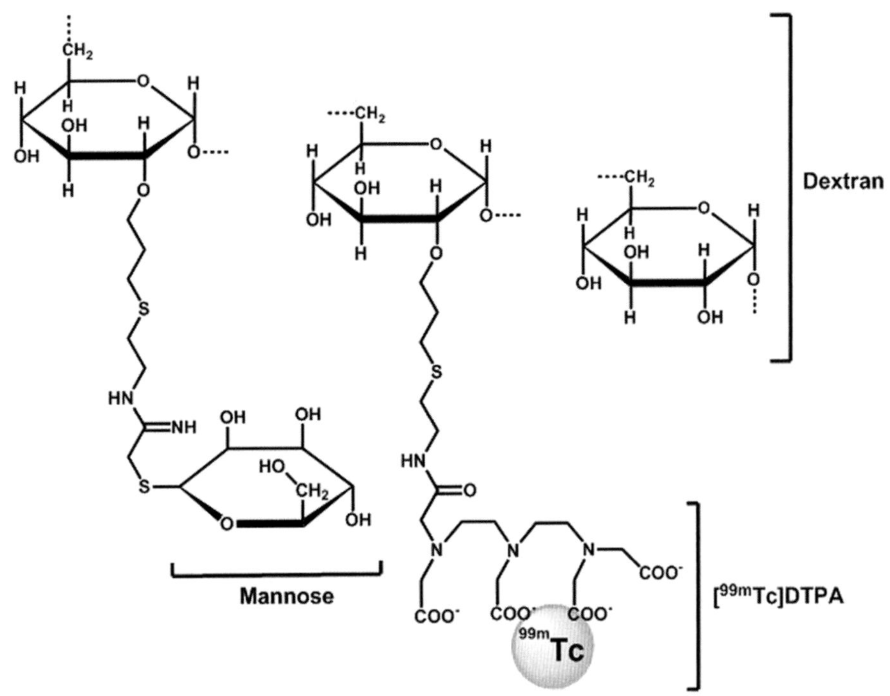

FIGURE 6-11 Lymphoseek. Attachment of mannose and ^{99m}Tc-DTPA to dextran backbone.

15 to 30 minutes is required, which allows the stannous chloride to be diluted in the total blood volume, before the ^{99m}Tc-pertechnetate injection. The stannous chloride reduces the ^{99m}Tc and allows the ^{99m}Tc to bind to the RBCs. Despite the speed and ease of in vivo RBC labeling, the low labeling efficiency of 80% results in sufficient free ^{99m}TcO$_4^-$ to complicate interpretation of images in studies such as gastrointestinal bleeding. A modified in vivo RBC labeling method has been developed that improves labeling efficiency. The patient's blood is tinned as in the first method; then a sample of the patient's blood is withdrawn into an anticoagulated syringe containing ^{99m}TcO$_4^-$. After incubation of the syringe at room temperature for 10 to 15 minutes, the contents are reinjected into the patient. This allows ^{99m}Tc labeling of a smaller volume of blood, which results in higher labeling efficiency.

An in vitro method for labeling RBCs with ^{99m}Tc is the use of a commercially available kit, Ultratag (Covidien; Mansfield, Mass.). An aliquot of the patient's blood, anticoagulated with heparin or acid-citrate-dextrose (ACD), is removed and added to the reaction vial containing stannous chloride. The stannous chloride diffuses across the RBC membrane. Sodium hypochlorite (Syringe I) is then added to the vial to reduce any extracellular stannous chloride. Syringe II, which contains citric acid, sodium citrate and dextrose, is added to complex the remaining Sn^{2+}, which remains in the extracellular space, and enhance the oxidation of Sn^{2+}. Next,

^{99m}Tc-pertechnetate is added to the kit formulation; it diffuses across the RBC membrane and is reduced and bound intracellularly. Approximately 80% of the ^{99m}Tc binds to the beta chain of globin portion of hemoglobin, and 20% to the heme. The final radiochemical purity of this preparation is greater than 90%.

Human serum albumin (HSA) labeled with ^{99m}Tc is another intravascular tracer that has been used. Commercially available kits contain the albumin and the stannous chloride reducing agent. Addition of ^{99m}TcO$_4^-$ results in the formation of ^{99m}Tc-HSA, which can be used as a blood pool imaging agent.

Skeletal Imaging Agents. In 1972 phosphate derivatives were labeled with technetium for skeletal imaging. Before this, skeletal imaging was performed using radioisotopes of strontium (^{85}Sr and ^{87m}Sr) or fluorine (^{18}F). These isotopes had either unfavorable decay characteristics, which resulted in high radiation absorbed doses, or undesirably short half-lives. The first technetium phosphate evaluated was an inorganic phosphate, ^{99m}Tc-polyphosphate.

There are two basic types of phosphate derivatives: inorganic phosphates that have phosphorus-oxygen bonds (P–O–P) and organic phosphates that have phosphorus-carbon bonds (P–C–P) (Figure 6-12). The inorganic phosphates are composed of differing lengths of the basic POP unit ([–P–O–P–]$_n$). When there is only one POP, the phosphate is pyrophosphate; when there is more than one POP unit, it is a polyphosphate. The

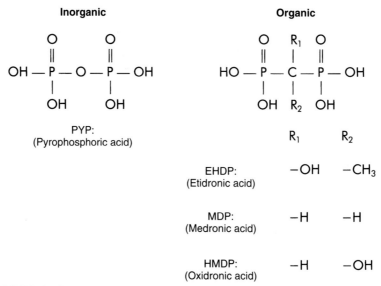

FIGURE 6-12 Inorganic and organic phosphate agents used for skeletal imaging.

polyphosphates undergo hydrolysis in vivo by alkaline phosphatases, which degrade them to the basic P–O–P unit, pyrophosphate. Since the P–C–P bonds of the organic phosphates are more resistant to the phosphatase hydrolysis, these compounds are more stable in vivo. This results in more rapid blood clearance and greater skeletal uptake than with the inorganic phosphates.

Technetium labeling of a phosphate is accomplished by reaction of the phosphate with stannous chloride to form a stannous phosphate chelate, followed by addition of ^{99m}Tc pertechnetate, which is reduced and complexed with the phosphate. The most commonly used ^{99m}Tc bone agents are ^{99m}Tc–hydroxymethylene diphosphonate (HMDP) and ^{99m}Tc–methylene diphosphonate (MDP). The mechanism of uptake is adsorption on the mineral phase, the hydroxyapatite, of the bone.

Lung Imaging Agents. Macroaggregated albumin (MAA) is formed by heat denaturation of the protein in an aqueous solution. Particles formed have diameters of 10 to 90 µm, with the majority between 10 and 40 µm. All commercially available MAA products use stannous chloride as the reducing agent. Since the smallest vessels in the lung vasculature range from 7 to 10 µm in diameter, labeled macroaggregates greater than 10 µm are readily trapped, allowing for lung visualization through the mechanism of capillary blockade.

Renal Imaging Agents. Technetium-99m pentetate (DTPA) and ^{99m}Tc-glucoheptonate (GHP) are two chelates used for renal imaging studies (Figure 6-13). These low molecular weight, water-soluble compounds are rapidly eliminated from the body. Technetium-99m DTPA is excreted exclusively by glomerular filtration. Technetium-99m GHP is cleared through glomerular filtration in addition to tubular secretion, with some retention of activity in the renal cortex. These tracers can also be used for brain imaging. Technetium-99m-2,3-

dimercaptosuccinic acid (DMSA) is another chelating agent that has been labeled with ^{99m}Tc and used for renal imaging. The cortical retention of this agent appears to be superior to other currently available agents, with 50% of the injected activity retained in the renal cortex 1 hour after administration. The commercial kit preparation is supplied by Amersham, (Piscataway, N.J.) is light sensitive, and should be stored between 2° and 8° C. After preparation the ^{99m}Tc-DMSA has a shelf life of 4 hours and should be stored in the refrigerator.

The technetium renal agent, ^{99m}Tc-mertiatide (mercaptoacetyltriglycine [MAG3]) (see Figure 6-13), supplied by Covidien (Mansfield, Mass.), was synthesized as a replacement for ^{131}I-hippuran which is no longer available. The ^{99m}Tc-mertiatide has rapid blood clearance and renal excretion via tubular secretion and glomerular filtration, similar to ^{131}I-hippuran.[44] The preferential nuclear properties of ^{99m}Tc make ^{99m}Tc-mertiatide superior to ^{131}I-hippuran as a renal agent. The kit method of preparing ^{99m}Tc-mertiatide requires boiling for 10 minutes. The quality-control method for the kit formulation employs Sep-Pak chromatography, which is discussed later under quality control.

Cardiac Imaging Agents. One of the goals of nuclear medicine has been to develop a ^{99m}Tc complex that has a biodistribution similar to ^{201}Tl. Several technetium agents have been developed for use in myocardial imaging. One of these cardiac agents is ^{99m}Tc-methoxyisobutyl isonitrile (MIBI), also known as ^{99m}Tc-sestamibi (Cardiolite, Miraluma; see Figure 6-14). The kit method of production is a 10-minute boiled preparation involving a ligand exchange labeling reaction. This results in the formation of a ^{99m}Tc-hexakis-isonitrile complex with ^{99m}Tc in an oxidation state of +1. The mechanism of myocardial localization is not known, though it has been determined that it does not occur via

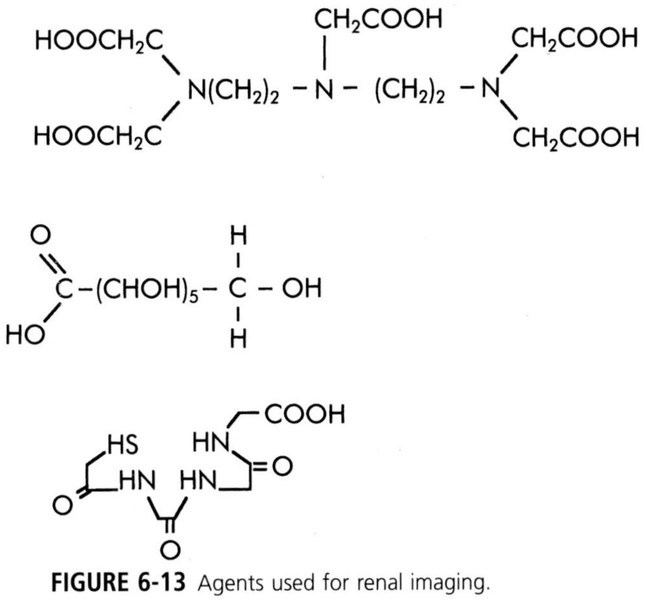

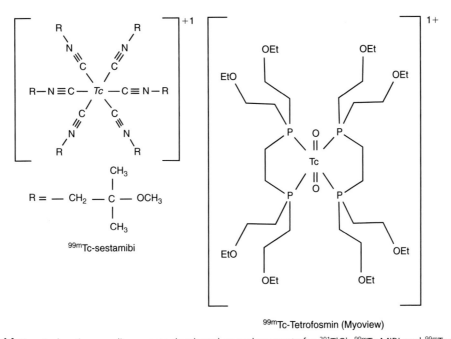

FIGURE 6-13 Agents used for renal imaging.

FIGURE 6-14 Two technetium cardiac agents developed as replacements for ^{201}TlCl, ^{99m}Tc-MIBI and ^{99m}Tc-tetrofosmin.

the Na$^+$/K$^+$ pump, which is the mechanism of uptake for ^{201}Tl.[41] ^{99m}Tc-sestamibi has approximately 65% cardiac extraction efficiency; minimal or no redistribution occurs. The amount of liver uptake that occurs has presented some problems in reading the resulting cardiac images.[10,13] The mechanism of localization for ^{99m}Tc-sestamibi in various types of breast tissue (benign, inflammatory, malignant, fibrous) has not been established.

Another cardiac agent is ^{99m}Tc-tetrofosmin (Myoview), a cationic ^{99m}Tc-complex of an ether-substituted phosphine ligand (see Figure 6-14). The kit formulation of ^{99m}Tc-tetrofosmin involves an exchange reaction during the 15-minute, room-temperature incubation. The non-reconstituted kit should be stored in the refrigerator, protected from light. Uptake into the myocardium reaches a maximum of 1.3% of the injected dose (ID) at 5 minutes postinjection, falling to 1% ID by 2 hours. The mechanism of uptake into the myocardium has not been established. Imaging may be initiated 15 minutes postinjection.

See the section on thallium chloride for a discussion of cardiac pharmacological stress agents.

Hepatobiliary Imaging Agents. A group of *N*-substituted iminodiacetic acid ligands that contain hydrophilic groups for ^{99m}Tc complexation and possess the necessary hepatocellular specificity have been developed. The first of this group of RaPh was ^{99m}Tc-lidofenin (HIDA).[28] A variety of ^{99m}Tc-iminodiacetic acid analogues that have different groups substituted on the aromatic ring have also been developed (Figure 6-15). Both disofenin and mebrofenin offer improved hepatocellular specificity, more rapid blood clearance, and reduced renal clearance. These agents provide information regarding hepatocyte function, outline the biliary tract, and provide evidence of bile flow or obstruction. The mechanism of uptake for the hepatobiliary imaging agents is a membrane bound anion transport system. After transport, the hepatobiliary agent is bound to glutathione S-transferase and transported to the biliary caniculus where it is excreted into the bile.[35] The same membrane bound system transports and excretes bilirubin. The uptake and clearance are therefore affected by increasing levels of bilirubin. Technetium-99m disofenin (Hepatolite) and ^{99m}Tc-mebrofenin (Choletec) show display competitive uptake of the RaPh even in cases of significantly elevated bilirubin levels.

Hepatobiliary excretion of a compound has been found to be related to several physicochemical characteristics: (1) a molecular weight of 300 to 1000; (2) the presence of a strong anionic polar group ionized at plasma pH; (3) the presence of a nonpolar group to decrease renal excretion; (4) lipophilic character; and (5) binding to plasma proteins, which can promote transfer into the hepatocyte.[24] The original work done on ^{99m}Tc-HIDA determined the structural configuration to exist as a dimer (Figure 6-16).[27] The ^{99m}Tc atom serves as a bridge between two ligand molecules. Dimerization is one of the major factors determining the hepatobiliary route of excretion for this RaPh.

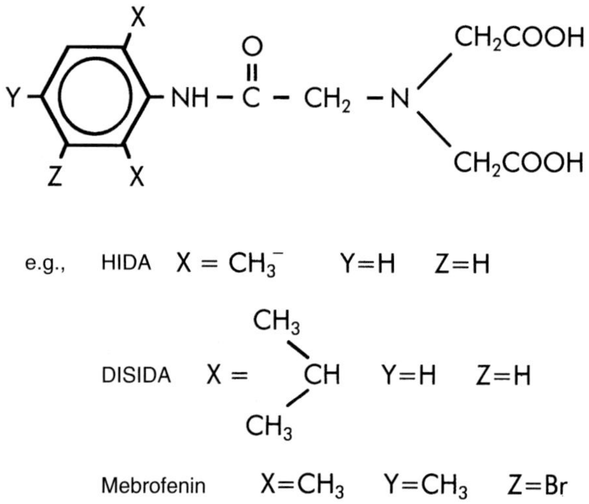

Brain Imaging Agents. With the advent of single photon emission computed tomography (SPECT) came renewed interest in brain imaging. One of the lipophilic brain agents marketed by Amersham is ^{99m}Tc-hexamethyl propylamineoxime (HMPAO), also known as exametazime. The lipophilicity of the ^{99m}Tc-exametazime (Ceretec) allows it to be rapidly extracted into the brain (about 6% ID at 1 minute after injection). It then immediately hydrolyzes to a more polar metabolite that does not diffuse out of the brain. Evidence has been presented to indicate that the retention of ^{99m}Tc-exametazime is accomplished by an intracellular reaction with glutathione.[34] The main problem with the original commercial kit formulation is instability; it must be used within 30 minutes of preparation, and quality control must be done before injection. A modification of the kit formulation of HMPAO is the immediate addition of methylene blue to the kit preparation after the addition of ^{99m}TcO$_4^-$ to stabilize the ^{99m}Tc-exametazime. After preparation of ^{99m}Tc-exametazime, the kit can be used for 4 hours. Since the final injection is a dark blue color and therefore cannot be checked for the presence of particulate matter, it must be injected through a 0.45-μm filter, which is provided by the manufacturer.

Additionally, white blood cells (WBCs) have been labeled with technetium using ^{99m}Tc-exametazime. The original kit formulation, not the stabilized kit formulation, must be used for ^{99m}Tc-WBC labeling. Radiolabeling is accomplished in the presence of plasma, in vitro. Unlike the labeling of WBCs using ^{111}In-oxine, transferrin does not adversely affect the ^{99m}Tc-labeling process. Although diagnostic equivalent images can be obtained with ^{99m}Tc-labeled WBCs, the 6-hour half-life of technetium can make imaging 24 hours after injection difficult,

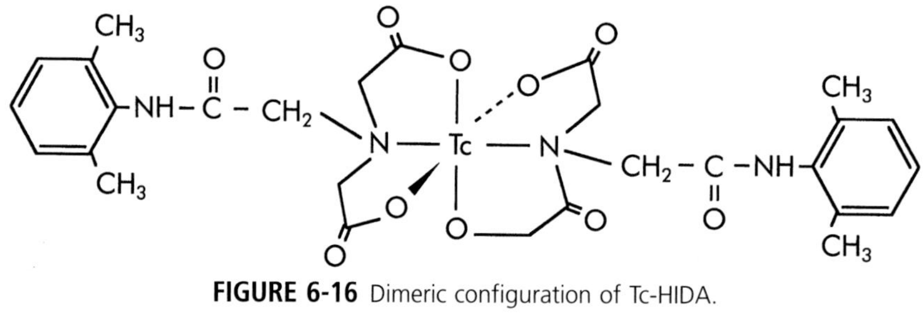

FIGURE 6-15 ^{99m}Tc-hepatobiliary analogues developed with different groups substituted on the aromatic ring of the iminodiacetic acid structure.

FIGURE 6-16 Dimeric configuration of Tc-HIDA.

when abscess-to-background ratios are typically maximized.

A second commercial ^{99m}Tc brain agent is ^{99m}Tc-L,L-ethylcysteinate dimer (ECD). Technetium-99m ECD (Neurolite), produced by Bristol Meyers Squibb (BMS; Princeton, N.J.), has approximately 5% of the injected dose extracted into the brain within 2 minutes postinjection. This lipophilic agent shows more rapid brain clearance and a higher brain/soft tissue ratio than ^{99m}Tc-HMPAO.[27] This RaPh is not degraded by hydrolysis, but is enzymatically metabolized to a nonpolar species which is retained in the brain. The commercial kit formulation is stable for 6 hours allowing increased utilization.

Peptide Imaging Agents. ^{99m}Tc-labeled Deprotide peptide (NeoTect) is a new type of technetium imaging agent that identifies somatostatin receptor–bearing pulmonary masses in patients presenting with CT or chest x-ray pulmonary lesions, highly suspect for malignancy. The kit contains sodium glucoheptonate and stannous chloride. The glucoheptonate is rapidly labeled with the ^{99m}Tc pertechnetate. The ^{99m}Tc-glucoheptonate then exchange labels the peptide during the 10 minute incubation in a boiling water bath or heat block.

Complexes for Labeling of Targeting Molecules Using ^{99m}Tc(I)-Carbonyl Precursors. The recent development of a ^{99m}Tc precursor complex by Alberto at the University of Zurich has opened up the design of a new class of ^{99m}Tc-labeled RaPhs for targeting molecular processes. $[^{99m}Tc(OH_2)_3(CO)_3]^+$ is a highly versatile synthon that is soluble in aqueous solution and highly stable when exposed to air. Half of the coordination sphere is shielded, whereas the other half is available to exchange by incoming chelators. The preparation of $[^{99m}Tc(OH_2)_3(CO)_3]^+$ starts from $^{99m}TcO_4^-$ followed by a six-electron reduction using BH_4^- as the one-step reducing agent. The reaction is carried out in the presence of one atmosphere of CO under heating at 95° C for 30 minutes.

A kit to prepare $[^{99m}Tc(OH_2)_3(CO)_3]^+$ was formulated by Covidien under the trade name Isolink. The kit contains boranocarbonate $H_3BCO_2^{2-}$ (BC), which serves both as the reducing agent and the source of CO. BC can be lyophilized for the kit formation, and is stable in neutral to alkaline pH in aqueous solution. $[^{99m}Tc(OH_2)_3(CO)_3]^+$ is synthesized in quantitative yield by adding generator eluate to the vial with subsequent heating to 98° C for 20 minutes. $[^{99m}Tc(OH_2)_3(CO)_3]^+$ is stable for hours if kept under N_2, but is slowly reoxidized when exposed to air.

The versatile $[^{99m}Tc(OH_2)_3(CO)_3]^+$ can be stabilized by monodentate, bidentate, or tridentate ligands that contain nitrogen, oxygen or, sulfur-containing coordinating groups. Histidine is a versatile tridentate chelator if not coupled to a biomolecule by the amine or the carboxylic group through peptide formation. Through alkylation at the α-NH_2 group, histidine has been introduced in the peptide neurotensin, providing an efficient tridentate, histidine-based ligand.[4] $[^{99m}Tc(OH_2)_3(CO)_3]^+$ can be used to label an endless array of ligand-biomolecule conjugates, and the use of this precursor in kit formation will undoubtedly result in clinically used RaPh in the future. For further detail and information on this subject, please see the thorough review by Alberto.[1]

Manufacturers' Package Inserts

A package insert or prescribing information is a document provided along with a prescription medication to provide additional information about that drug. In the United States, the FDA determines the requirements for patient package inserts. Package inserts follow a standard format and include the same types of information. For RaPhs or kits used for the preparation of RaPhs the sections include the following:

1. Description: provides the amount of each ingredient that is contained in the preparation, the route of administration, and the pH of the final product
2. Physical characteristics: includes the half-life and the principal radiation emission data
3. External radiation: lists such things as the specific gamma ray constants and half-value layer in lead
4. Clinical pharmacology: explains how the RaPh is distributed in the body, metabolized, and eliminated, and describes the mechanism of localization and pharmacokinetics
5. Clinical trials: describes the uptake and distribution in various patient groups with differing pathologies
6. Indications and use: describes the uses (indications) for which the RaPh has been FDA-approved
7. Contraindications: lists situations in which the RaPh should not be used—for RaPh it usually states none known
8. Warnings: covers serious side effects that could occur
9. Precautions: addresses how to prepare and use the RaPh; this includes safe handling of the radioactive material, use of the material during pregnancy, use with nursing mothers, and use in pediatrics
10. Adverse reactions: lists all side effects observed in all studies of the RaPh
11. Dosage and administration: gives recommended dosage(s)
12. Radiation dosimetry: lists the radiation doses to organs and tissues of an average patient (70 kg) per the maximum dosage listed for each approved indication
13. Instructions for preparation of the kit: (if appropriate) states the general preparation scheme

14. Radiochemical purity: states the method to determine the purity of the RaPh
15. How supplied: lists the physical characteristics of the RaPh or kit formulation and how it should be stored

GALLIUM AND INDIUM RADIOPHARMACEUTICALS

The four radionuclides of indium and gallium that have been used in nuclear medicine applications are ^{67}Ga, ^{68}Ga, ^{111}In, and ^{113m}In. As discussed previously, ^{68}Ga and ^{113m}In are generator produced. Cyclotron production of ^{67}Ga ($t_{1/2}$ = 78 hours) and ^{111}In ($t_{1/2}$ = 67 hours) can be accomplished by several different nuclear reactions:

$$^{67}Zn(p, n)\ ^{67}Ga$$
$$^{68}Zn(p, 2n)\ ^{67}Ga$$
$$^{111}Cd(p, n)\ ^{111}In$$
$$^{109}Ag(\alpha, 2n)\ ^{111}In$$

Analysis of the decay schemes for ^{67}Ga and ^{111}In indicates the following gamma photon energies and abundances: ^{67}Ga, 93 keV (40%), 184 keV (24%), 296 keV (22%), and 388 keV (7%); ^{111}In, 173 keV (89%) and 247 keV (94%). The physical half-lives and decay characteristics of ^{67}Ga and ^{111}In make them well-suited for nuclear medicine. The gamma energies of ^{111}In are in the optimum range of detectability for the commercially available gamma cameras, and the abundance of gamma emissions provides 183 photons for every 100 disintegrations. Although the gamma energies of ^{67}Ga are in a range suitable for detection, their abundances are low. Therefore more than twice as much ^{67}Ga as ^{111}In would have to be injected to obtain a comparable image.

In aqueous solution, gallium and indium exist only as Ga^{3+} and In^{3+}, making RaPh production simpler than with ^{99m}Tc, because a reduction does not have to be performed. The solution chemistry of both indium and gallium is similar to that of iron, with In^{3+} and Ga^{3+} forming very strong complexes with the plasma protein transferrin. To see the desired biodistribution using an indium or gallium RaPh, a complex must be formed that is stronger than that of the metal with transferrin.

The solubility of indium hydroxides varies with the pH. At values higher than 4.5, indium hydroxide becomes very insoluble. In aqueous solution the free hydrated Ga (III) ion is stable only under acidic conditions. Hydrolysis occurs as the pH is raised, leading to the formation of insoluble gallium hydroxide. Unlike indium hydroxide, gallium hydroxide is amphoteric, dissolving in alkaline as well as acidic solutions. Thus, as pH is raised to ~3, $Ga(OH)_3$ precipitates but then redissolves as $Ga(OH)_4^-$ at pH greater than 7.4.[20]

The most widely used ^{67}Ga RaPh is ^{67}Ga-citrate, an agent used for imaging tumors and sites of inflammation.

On injection of the ^{67}Ga-citrate, more than 90% of the gallium becomes bound to plasma proteins, particularly transferrin, resulting in slow clearance from the plasma. However, when transferrin is saturated with stable gallium or iron prior to injection of radioactivity, the plasma and urinary clearance are improved. Under these conditions the gallium distribution shifts from soft tissue to bone, though uptake by tumors does not seem to be affected. Alternatively, increasing ^{67}Ga protein transferrin binding causes an increase in soft tissue activity and decreased tumor activity. The mechanisms of ^{67}Ga localization in tumors and sites of inflammation are not completely understood, but the uptake into intracellular components by one or more mechanisms, possibly involving binding of ^{67}Ga-transferrin binding to transferring receptors, is strongly indicated.

Because of the great stability of indium and gallium with transferrin, only very strong chelates can be used in vivo to direct the localization of the radionuclides to other sites. Strong chelators such as EDTA or DTPA can be easily labeled with Ga(III) or In(III) using citrate or acetate as a transfer ligand. ^{111}In-DTPA has been used for renal and brain imaging and is currently used for cisternography.

Platelets and WBCs can be labeled with ^{111}In to provide agents for imaging inflammatory processes and thrombi. A weak complex is formed between the ^{111}In and 8-hydroxyquinoline (oxine). Because the ^{111}In-oxine complex is weak, the radiometal rapidly exchanges with transferrin in the plasma. In the absence of plasma, the complex diffuses across the cell membrane and the metal binds to intracellular sites. Isolation of the desired blood component from plasma permits easy labeling of either platelets or WBCs. This is routinely accomplished using centrifugation or sedimentation.

Procedures to label WBCs and platelets with ^{111}In-oxine vary, but the overall process can be summarized as follows:

1. Draw the patient's blood into an anticoagulated syringe and sediment the WBCs or platelets by centrifugation. Remove and save the leukocyte-poor (LPP) or platelet-poor plasma (PPP).
2. Wash the cells with 0.9% NaCl (saline) to remove plasma transferrin. Remove the saline wash and resuspend the cells in saline.
3. Add ^{111}In-oxine to the cell suspension and incubate 15 minutes at room temperature.
4. Add a portion of the LPP or PPP to the ^{111}In-labeled WBCs or ^{111}In-labeled platelet preparation. Centrifuge the cells.
5. Resuspend the labeled cells in the remaining LPP or PPP for reinjection.

Overall labeling efficiencies (percentage of ^{111}In bound to cells) for WBCs is 70% to 90% and for platelets is 50% to 70%. Care must be taken to avoid damaging the cells during the labeling procedure.

Indium-111 has also been conjugated to octreotide as an agent for the scintigraphic localization of primary and metastatic somatostatin receptor–positive neuroendocrine tumors.[2] Somatostatin is a naturally occurring 14-amino-acid peptide responsible for hormonal regulation of a number of organ systems. However, octreotide (Sandostatin), an eight-amino-acid analogue of somatostatin, has a much longer biological half-life and even greater regulatory properties than the native peptide.[2] For these reasons it is a much better peptide for labeling than somatostatin. A labeled form of octreotide is commercially available as the DTPA-chelated compound ^{111}In-DTPA-octreotide (^{111}In-pentetreotide, OctreoScan). The most commonly diagnosed tumors have been carcinoids and gastrinomas, with a lower success rate noted for insulinomas and neuroblastomas. In the kit formulation, ^{111}In is complexed using sodium citrate, added to the pentetreotide, and incubated for 30 minutes at room temperature. Quality control must be performed before patient administration using C_{18} Sep-Pak chromatography.

Monoclonal antibodies (MAbs) have been labeled with ^{111}In using bifunctional chelates. The chelating agent is first conjugated to the antibody, and then ^{111}In binds to the conjugated MAb via the chelating agent. The MAb B72.3 (satumomab) is an intact MAb that is directed to a high molecular weight, tumor-associated glycoprotein. The expression of this glycoprotein has been demonstrated in a variety of adenocarcinomas. This MAb was conjugated using a derivatized DTPA ligand, then radiolabeled with ^{111}In. The kit formulation contained 1 mg of satumomab pendetide (OncoScint). Indium-111 acetate was prepared by addition of ^{111}In chloride to a vial of sodium acetate buffer. The ^{111}In-acetate was then transferred to the MAb reaction vial. The vial is incubated for 30 minutes at room temperature and filtered through a low protein-binding 0.22-μm filter. The preparation should be stored at room temperature and used within 8 hours of preparation. The indication for OncoScint was the determination of the extent and location of extrahepatic malignant disease in cases of colorectal or ovarian carcinoma, but the kit is no longer available.

THALLIUM CHLORIDE

Thallium-201 is a monovalent cationic metal used in cardiac imaging. It is ultimately obtained from a ^{201}Pb-^{201}Tl generator. ^{201}Pb is produced by bombarding natural thallium metal with protons, according to the following nuclear reaction:

$$^{203}\text{Tl}(p, 3n)\,^{201}\text{Pb} \xrightarrow[\text{(EC)}]{t_{1/2}=9.4\,\text{h}}\, ^{201}\text{Tl}$$

The ^{201}Pb is then complexed, and undesirable target material is removed by ion exchange chromatography. The purified lead radioisotopes are affixed to another

column. ^{201}Pb decays by electron capture with a $t_{1/2}$ of 9.4 hours to give ^{201}Tl. A second purification by column chromatography is required to remove the ^{203}Pb radiocontaminant, which is present at the end of purification at a level less than 0.5% per mCi ^{201}Tl at calibration. The ^{201}Tl is isolated carrier-free, has a $t_{1/2}$ of 74 hours, and decays by electron capture with gamma emissions between 140 and 170 keV.

Thallium clears rapidly from the blood, with maximum concentration in the heart approximately 10 to 30 minutes after injection in the resting state and 5 minutes after stress induced either by exercise or pharmacological intervention at the time of administration. Uptake of ^{201}Tl into the myocardium occurs intracellularly in proportion to blood flow. Additionally, adequate tissue oxygenation is required to support ^{201}Tl uptake in myocardial cells, because oxygen supports the Na-K-ATPase concentrating mechanism. Similarities between ^{201}Tl$^+$ and K$^+$ include monovalent charges, comparable ionic radii, and involvement in the membrane Na-K-ATPase pump.

A number of pharmaceuticals are available for use with ^{201}Tl or ^{99m}Tc in cardiac imaging to simulate exercise stress testing in patients who cannot exercise adequately. The newest agent is regadenoson (Lexiscan). It is an adenosine agonist, has a low affinity for the A_{2A} receptor, and produces coronary vasodilation and increase in coronary blood flow (CBF). The dose administered is 0.4 mg/5 ml IV push over 10 seconds, followed by the injection of 5 ml of 0.5% NaCl. The RaPh is usually injected 10 to 20 seconds post regadenoscan. The drug can be reversed using aminophylline 100 mg injected IV over 60 seconds. The side effects noted are systemic vasodilation, including dizziness, headache, and flushing, and GI effects, such as nausea and vomiting.

Adenosine (Adenocard) is another coronary vasodilator for use in perfusion imaging. It is an endogenous nucleoside, produced by enzymatic dephosphorylation of ATP, which causes direct coronary vasodilation. It activates adenosine-A2 receptors in coronary arterial wall and leads to an increase in the adenosine cyclase and cyclic adenosine monophosphate (cAMP) levels, decreases transmembrane calcium uptake which results in vasodilation. The initial dose of 0.14 mg/kg/min (total dose of 0.84 mg/kg) is infused over 6 minutes. It has a very short biological half-life, less than 10 seconds, which allows rapid reversal of the pharmacological effect without injection of another drug. The most common adverse effects are facial flushing and shortness of breath.

Dipyridamole (Persantine) is the original coronary vasodilator. It indirectly raises endogenous adenosine blood levels by blocking cell membrane transport and reuptake of endogenous adenosine therefore causing vasodilation. The dose employed is 0.142 mg/kg/min (0.570 mg/kg total) and is infused over 4 minutes. The most frequent adverse reaction reported was chest pain/angina pectoris. Parenteral aminophylline (50 to 250 mg) can be administered by intravenous injection of 50 to

100 mg over 30 to 60 seconds. If symptoms persist the dose may be increased to a total of 250 mg. This drug should be available during dipyridamole stress testing for relieving adverse reactions such as bronchospasm or chest pain.

IODINATED RADIOPHARMACEUTICALS

Sodium iodide, either ^{123}I- or ^{131}I-labeled, is used for thyroid imaging, uptake measurements, and therapy (in the case of ^{131}I) as a capsule or a solution for oral administration. Iodine-123 ($t_{1/2}$ of 13.2 hours) decays by electron capture with emission of a 159-keV gamma (83%), whereas iodine-131 ($t_{1/2}$ of 8 days) decays by β^- emission with subsequent gamma emission of 364 keV (82%). Iodine-131 has also been used to label monoclonal antibodies for in vivo tumor imaging and therapy. Human serum albumin labeled with ^{125}I ($t_{1/2}$ of 60 days; decays by electron capture with a 35-keV gamma emission) is used to measure plasma volume, and ^{125}I-labeled antibodies are used for radioimmunoassay.

The most commonly used cyclotron produced radiohalogen is ^{123}I. It has gradually replaced the reactor produced ^{131}I as the isotope of choice for diagnostic RaPh labeling. Due to the lower gamma energy of 159 keV, ^{123}I delivers a much lower radiation dose to the patient and is ideally suited for use in a gamma camera.

To label proteins, particularly antibodies, with iodine, the use of mild iodination methods that do not denature the protein is important. Iodination of proteins involves the formation of positively charged iodine species that react with various groups within the protein. Under general conditions used for iodination, the tyrosine residues in the protein are iodinated to the greatest extent, giving monoiodotyrosine and diodotyrosine. The method of iodination chosen depends on the application. Retention of biological activity of the protein is probably the most important consideration in the choice of the labeling technique.

Cyclotron production of ^{123}I can be accomplished by several methods. Enriched ^{124}Te can be bombarded with protons, resulting in the ^{124}Te(p, 2n) ^{123}I reaction. The most likely contaminant of this reaction is ^{124}I, which emits a high-energy photon that can affect image resolution. Alternatively, this can be produced by the ^{127}I(p, 5n) ^{123}I, where the main contaminant is ^{125}I. This contaminant does not pose a problem in imaging but will deliver a higher radiation dose to the patient because of the half-life of 65 days.

As the field of PET has grown, interest in ^{124}I as PET radionuclide has increased. The half-life of 4.2 days is long enough for localization with monoclonal antibodies and the 23% positron decay allows imaging with PET. Receptor specific ligands have been synthesized with ^{123}I for SPECT imaging and now with ^{124}I for PET imaging. The most common reactions for the production of ^{124}I are proton or deuteron irradiation of enriched tellurium:

^{124}Te(p, n) ^{124}I or ^{124}Te(d, 2n) ^{124}I depending on the cyclotron and particle availability.[36]

PET RADIOPHARMACEUTICALS

The most frequently used positron-emitting radionuclides for PET imaging are ^{15}O ($t_{1/2}$ = 2 minutes), ^{13}N ($t_{1/2}$ = 10 minutes), ^{11}C ($t_{1/2}$ = 20 minutes), and ^{18}F ($t_{1/2}$ = 110 minutes). Their decay characteristics are listed in Table 6-2. Unlike the larger radionuclides used in conventional nuclear medicine, most PET radionuclides are identical to those found in naturally occurring biomolecules, and therefore the biochemical and physiological processes in the body can be studied directly. Although fluorine is not usually native, labeling with ^{18}F only minimally changes the structure of a biomolecule, because its size is similar to the hydrogen it replaces. The short half-lives of these isotopes require production and RaPh synthesis close to where the PET imaging takes place. This often requires an on-site cyclotron; however, for ^{18}F-labeled RaPh, centralized radiopharmacies that supply regional hospitals and PET centers are becoming more common.

TABLE 6-2	Decay Properties of Several Short-Lived Positron-Emitting Radionuclides Used in Nuclear Medicine		
Nuclide	$t_{1/2}$ (min)	E_β^+ max (MeV)	**Preferred Method of Production**
^{15}O	2	1.72	^{14}N (d, n) ^{15}O
^{13}N	10	1.19	^{16}O (p, α) ^{13}N
^{11}C	20	0.96	^{14}N (p, α) ^{11}C
^{18}F	110	0.64	^{18}O (p, n) ^{18}F

Oxygen-15

Oxygen-15 is cyclotron produced using either the ^{14}N(d, n) ^{15}O or the ^{15}N(p, n) ^{15}O nuclear reaction. With a half-life of 2.04 minutes, PET RaPh labeled with ^{15}O are limited to a few simple molecules such as ^{15}O-labeled water, ^{15}O-labeled oxygen gas, ^{15}O-labeled carbon dioxide, and ^{15}O-labeled carbon monoxide. The short half-life and the low radiation absorbed dose from ^{15}O-labeled RaPh allow amounts of activity up to 100 mCi to be administered in imaging procedures, which can be repeated at 8- to 10-minute intervals.

Oxygen-15 labeled oxygen gas can be used directly to study oxygen metabolism, or the ^{15}O-labeled oxygen can be converted to ^{15}O-labeled CO, CO_2, or H_2O. Labeled carbon oxides are produced by passing ^{15}O-labeled oxygen through an activated carbon furnace. The furnace temperature determines whether ^{15}O-labeled carbon monoxide or ^{15}O-labeled carbon dioxide is produced. High specific activity ^{15}O-labeled carbon dioxide can be produced that allows ^{15}O-labeled carbon dioxide to be safely administered to patients by inhalation. ^{15}O-labeled carbon monoxide binds to hemoglobin found in the RBC, allowing the study of RBC volume.

Oxygen-15 labeled water can be produced by passing ^{15}O-labeled oxygen gas and hydrogen gas over a palladium catalyst using a commercial synthesis module made by CTI. This allows ^{15}O-labeled water to be produced at the scanner site. A second method for ^{15}O-labeled water production is a carbonic acid–mediated exchange reaction.[47] Oxygen-15–labeled carbon dioxide is bubbled through saline. Both methods provide ^{15}O-labeled water in a form suitable for immediate IV injection. The most common use for ^{15}O-labeled water is as a tracer for cerebral and myocardial perfusion.

A diagnostic test exists for evaluating symptomatic carotid artery occlusion utilizing ^{15}O-labeled water and ^{15}O-labeled oxygen gas. By measuring the oxygen extraction fraction in the brain, the risk of subsequent stroke can be determined. A study is currently being conducted to determine whether this test can be used to identify stroke patients who may benefit from carotid artery bypass surgery.[21]

Nitrogen-13

Currently ^{13}N is cyclotron produced by the ^{16}O(p, α) ^{13}N nuclear reaction. This nuclear reaction is performed in-target using a 5-mM solution of ethanol in water to yield ^{13}N in the form of ammonia.[6] Ethanol is used as a scavenger to reduce the amount of ^{13}N-nitrates formed.[8] The ^{13}N-ammonia is delivered from the target through an anion exchange resin, then through a Millipore 0.22-μm filter, used for end-product sterilization. This tracer is partially extracted, but the extraction fraction decreases at high perfusion rates. The trapping mechanism for ^{13}N-ammonia involves incorporation of ^{13}N into glutamine due to the enzymatic action of glutamine synthetase. It is primarily used as a myocardial perfusion imaging agent. It can be used for rest-stress imaging in place of SPECT, or in the case of an equivocal SPECT scan, but requires a 60-minute interval between injections to allow for ^{13}N to decay.

Carbon-11

Carbon-11 is generally produced by the ^{10}B(d, n) ^{11}C or ^{14}N(p, α) ^{11}C nuclear reactions. Carbon-11 labeled carbon monoxide (^{11}CO), carbon dioxide (^{11}CO$_2$), cyanide (^{11}CN$^-$), methyl iodide (^{11}CH$_3$I), and methyl triflate (^{11}CH$_3$Tr) are the most commonly used synthetic precursors. The number of different ^{11}C-labeled compounds that have been synthesized as RaPhs for PET studies is extensive. This chapter briefly discusses a few of the more clinically useful ones.

One compound routinely prepared is ^{11}C-acetate, a tracer used in the study of myocardial metabolism. Commercial modules for synthesis of ^{11}C-acetate are available

from CTI, Bioscan, and GE. Carbon-11 carbon dioxide is bubbled through the grignard, methylmagnesium bromide, and the intermediate formed is hydrolyzed with acid, distilled, and then sterile-filtered.[39]

Carbon-11 labeled acetate is converted to acetyl coenzyme A by the enzyme acetyl CoA synthetase after myocardial uptake. Acetyl coenzyme A enters the tricarboxylic acid cycle (TCA or Krebs cycle) and is predominately metabolized to the end product ^{11}CO$_2$. Because the TCA cycle is closely linked to oxidative phosphorylation, ^{11}C-acetate metabolism can provide an index of oxidative metabolism. Carbon-11 labeled acetate is currently being utilized to evaluate prostate carcinoma.[38] In addition, it is being investigated to evaluate hepatocellular carcinoma.[25] It is hypothesized that tumor cells preferentially incorporate C-11 acetate metabolites into the membrane lipids in tumor cells, because cell growth and proliferation inevitably necessitate membrane constitutes.[50]

Carbon-11 labeled glucose is also used to study metabolism. Early methods to prepare ^{11}C-glucose were lengthy compared to the 20-minute half-life of ^{11}C; however, modifications have corrected this. The glucose analogue 2-deoxy-D-glucose labeled with ^{11}C in the C-1 position has been synthesized rapidly from the ^{11}C cyanide precursor. This analogue of glucose has similar characteristics except that it fails to undergo intracellular enzymatic glycolysis beyond initial phosphorylation. It is metabolically trapped in brain and myocardial cells and has been used for measurement of cerebral and myocardial glucose metabolism.[11]

Carbon-11 labeled methyl iodide can be made using two methods. One method is a liquid-phase process that involves the reduction of ^{11}C-carbon dioxide to ^{11}C-methanol using lithium aluminum hydride, then addition of hydriodic acid to form ^{11}C-methyl iodide. Siemens CTI produces a commercial liquid-phase ^{11}C-methyl iodide module. However, this technique is more cumbersome and often results in low radiochemical yields and specific activity.

The second method of ^{11}C-methyl iodide production involves a gas-phase process, and a commercial module is available from GE. Using this system, ^{11}C-carbon dioxide is first reduced to ^{11}C-methane by heating in the presence of hydrogen gas over a nickel catalyst at 360° C. The ^{11}C-methane intermediate is converted by recirculation, through an iodination column at 690° C, to ^{11}C-methyl iodide, which is then trapped on a porous polymer support. This precursor can then be released as a gas for RaPh labeling applications. The gas-phase process yields high specific activity and requires about 12 minutes. Turnaround time between successive batches of ^{11}C-methyl iodide is about 30 minutes.

A new ^{11}C-labeled RaPh, 2-[4′-(C-11-methylamino) phenyl]-6-hydroxybenzothiazole (Pittsburgh Compound B, or ^{11}C-PIB), has been developed to evaluate people who are at risk of developing Alzheimer's disease.[31] A

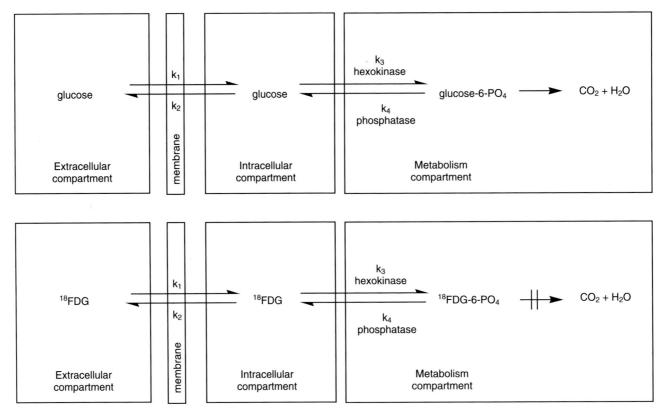

FIGURE 6-17 Fluorodeoxyglucose (FDG) undergoes metabolism similar to glucose, by hexokinase, but is metabolically trapped, because phosphorylization cannot proceed.

neutral analogue of thioflavine T (arylbenzothiazole) has high affinity for beta amyloid (Aβ) and neurofibrillary tangles (NFB), which are characteristic markers in the brains of patients with Alzheimer's disease. After preparing the precursor, ^{11}C-methyl iodide, as described previously, it is added to the normethyl PIB precursor, heated at 90° C for 5 minutes. The protecting group is removed using hydrochloric acid to form ^{11}C-PIB.

Fluorine-18

Fluorine-18 fluoride is produced either by the [18]O(p, n) ^{18}F or the [20]Ne(d, a) ^{18}F nuclear reaction. The proton irradiation of enriched ^{18}O-labeled water is the preferred method for producing [18]F.

Fluorine-18 fluoride is produced using a particle accelerator typically in a cyclotron with an energy of 11 MeV to 20 MeV with a beam current ranging from 20 to 60 microamperes. Though ^{18}F can be produced at energies below 4 MeV using high beam currents, the technical difficulties of designing successful targets to handle the high beam currents have limited the use of lower energies.

The target body is constructed of metals such as silver, copper, titanium, nickel, or stainless steel. The target has small cavities for the target water, which are 0.1- to 3-ml in volume and covered by thin metal foils. The production of ^{18}F for most ^{18}O-labeled water targets is excellent,

with yields of greater than 1.0 to 10 Ci at end of a 2-hour bombardment (EOB). Since ^{18}F has a relatively short half-life (109.8 minutes), rapid automated chemistry systems are required to process it into a usable RaPh.

The most frequently used ^{18}F-labeled RaPh is 2-deoxy-2-[^{18}F]fluoro-D-glucose (FDG). Some of the FDA-approved indications for FDG are lung, breast, cervical, colorectal, head and neck, thyroid, melanoma, lymphoma, and esophageal cancers; refractory seizures; and myocardial viability.

The mechanism of ^{18}F-FDG trapping follows the glucose biochemical pathway. Fluorine-18 FDG is transported into the cell and metabolized by phosphorylation with hexokinase to ^{18}F-FDG-6 phosphate. However, unlike glucose, ^{18}F-FDG-6-phosphate is then trapped in the cell because of the stereochemical and structural demands of the enzyme responsible for further catabolism (Figure 6-17).

The most commonly used method for production of ^{18}F-FDG involves the method developed by Hamacher and associates.[20] The method utilizes a nucleophilic displacement reaction with mannose triflate. Nucleophilic fluorination reactions are inhibited by water, so it is essential that the aqueous solution of ^{18}F-fluoride be completely dried before starting the reaction of the triflate with [18]F. Initially the ^{18}F is mixed with a counterion by elution of the anion exchange cartridge using

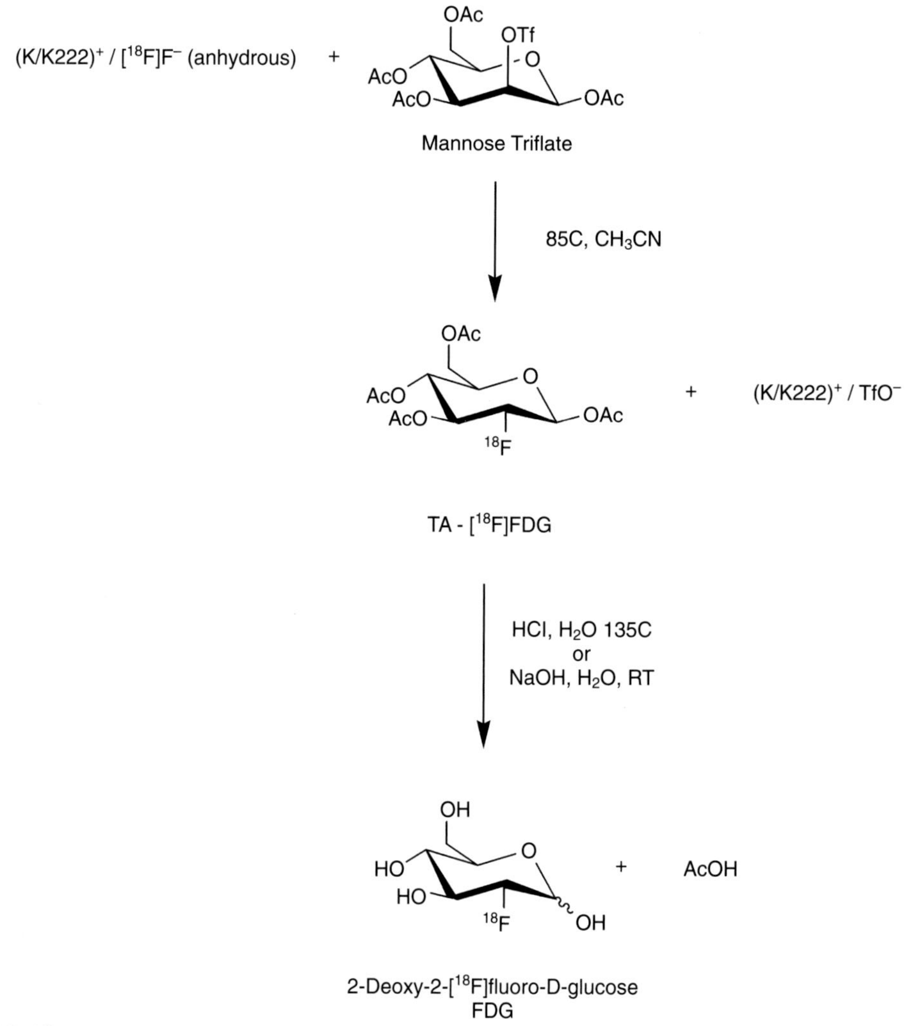

FIGURE 6-18 Fluorodeoxyglucose (FDG) synthetic scheme using Kryptofix chemistry with acid or base hydrolysis.

potassium carbonate, traces of water are removed by distillation, and then acetonitrile is added to resolubilize the dried complex of ^{18}F-fluoride.[31] Fluorine-18 fluoride (in acetonitrile) is added to the mannose triflate precursor and displaces the triflate. Acid hydrolysis of the acetylated intermediate, tetra acetyl-^{18}F-glucose (TA-^{18}F-FDG), gives ^{18}F-FDG (Figure 6-18). The Hamacher synthesis uses Kryptofix as a phase transfer catalyst to increase the reactivity of the ^{18}F-anion.[20]

FDG synthesis modules available on the market employ similar chemistry methods to prepare the ^{18}F-FDG. GE Healthcare TRACERlab MX$_{FDG}$ module (Figure 6-19) uses a nucleophilic reaction with Kryptofix and base hydrolysis[23] and CTI Explora FDG synthesizer also uses a nucleophilic reaction with Kryptofix but has acid hydrolysis.

Another GE FDG synthesizer which can be used for FDG production is the TRACERlab FX$_{FN}$. This is a module that produces tracers via the nucleophilic substitution method. The resulting tetra acetyl-^{18}F-glucose is trapped on a standard reverse-phase extraction cartridge,

and the acetyl groups are removed using acid or base hydrolysis.[17]

The use of a neon gas target containing 1% F$_2$ provides labeled fluorine gas, ^{18}F^{19}F. The production of ^{18}F involving F$_2$ gas using this nuclear reaction is inherently carrier added, and there are practical limits on the specific activity that can be obtained. Using ^{18}O gas via the ^{18}O(p, n) ^{18}F produces ^{18}F$_2$ using a no carrier added reaction, allowing higher specific activities for production of ^{18}F-FDOPA.[42] The positron-emitting fluorinated L-dopa analogue 6-^{18}F-fluoro-L-3,4-dihydroxyphenylalanine, ^{18}F-FDOPA (Figure 6-20), has been used as an imaging agent for brain dopamine neurons. The chemical structure of fluorodopa differs from L-dopa only at the 6 position of the catechol moiety where a fluorine atom replaces a hydrogen atom. Fluorodopa F-18 Injection was added to the *United States Pharmacopoeia* (USP) in 1991. Because dopamine cannot cross the blood-brain barrier, its precursor, ^{18}F-FDOPA, the analogue of L-dopa that crosses the blood-brain barrier, is administered. Once ^{18}F-FDOPA crosses into the brain, it is

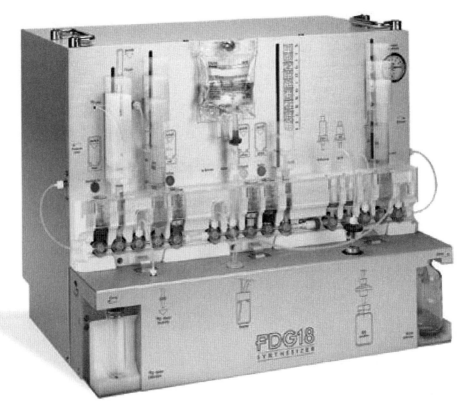

FIGURE 6-19 General Electric Medical Systems TRACERlab MX$_{FDG}$ synthesis module for the automated production of fluorodeoxyglucose (FDG).

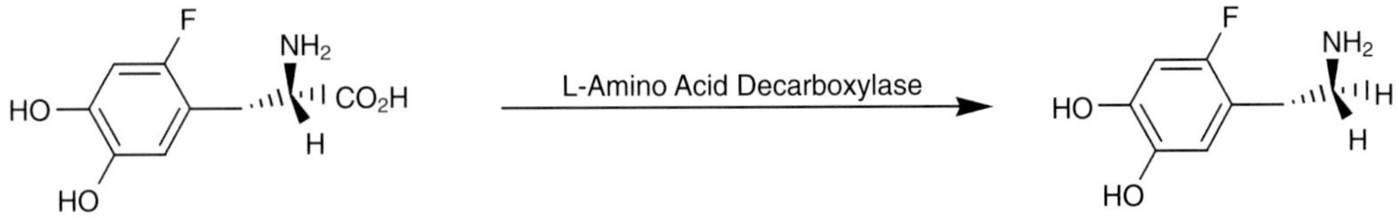

6-FDOPA   6-Fluorodopamine

FIGURE 6-20 FDOPA decarboxylation to FDA.

converted to 6-^{18}F-fluorodopamine (^{18}F-FDA) by decarboxylation (see Figure 6-20), is actively stored in sympathetic synaptic vesicles in the brain, and can be released by sympathetic nerve stimulation. Fluorine-18 FDOPA has been used to study parkinsonism and other neurological disorders. It is also being used to investigate endocrine disorders.[26]

The TRACERlab FX$_{DOPA}$, manufactured by GE, produces FDOPA using the one-pot synthesis of deVries.[12] The method uses a fluorodestannylation reaction followed by acidic removal of the protecting groups.

FLT (3′-deoxy-3′-fluorothymidine) is a pyrimidine nucleoside taken up by cells. It is phosphorylated by thymidine kinase 1 (TK1) and proceeds to be synthetically incorporated into DNA. F-18 FLT is the radiolabeled form of thymidine, which, after phosphorylation, leads to intracellular trapping within the cell similar to the mechanism of FDG. The retention of FLT within

the cell, therefore, provides a measure of cellular TK1 activity, an enzyme which is closely related to cellular proliferation, which is upregulated in the *S* phase of the cell cycle. It has been utilized in several oncological applications as a probe to measure cell proliferation.

The synthesis of ^{18}F-FLT is a nucleophilic displacement reaction, similar to FDG, but requires purification using preparative high-pressure liquid chromatography (HPLC). The major problem with this synthesis has been the low yield of the reaction. Solutions have focused on using differing starting materials. In 2000, Machulla and colleagues[28] developed a nucleophilic synthesis starting with an internally protected dimethoxytriphenylmethyl anhydrothymidine (DMTThy) precursor, which increased the FLT yield to ~14%. Adding an additional protective group to the amine at the 3 position of the pyridine ring increased the FLT yield to ~40%.[37] This modified synthesis has been performed using the GE TRACERlab MX$_{FDG}$ synthesis module.

THERAPEUTIC RADIOPHARMACEUTICALS

Sodium ^{32}P-phosphate is an FDA-approved RaPh indicated for treatment of polycythemia vera, chronic myelocytic leukemia, and chronic lymphocytic leukemia, and for palliation of metastatic bone pain. It is prepared as a solution for IV administration. Chromic ^{32}P-phosphate is a suspension of ^{32}P used for intracavity installation for treatment of peritoneal or pleural effusions caused by metastatic disease. Phosphorus-32 decays by β^- emission with a $t_{1/2}$ of 14.3 days. The major toxicity noted is significant marrow suppression in approximately one third of patients receiving this RaPh. The duration of response is 1.5 to 11 months.

Strontium-89 chloride (Metastron) has been approved by the FDA for relief of bone pain in cases of painful skeletal metastases. The compound behaves biologically as calcium does and localizes in hydroxyapatite crystal by ion exchange. Strontium uptake occurs preferentially at sites of active osteogenesis. This allows primary bone tumors and areas of metastatic involvement to accumulate significantly higher concentrations of strontium than surrounding normal bone. Strontium-89 decays by β^- emission with a $t_{1/2}$ of 50.6 days. This RaPh causes bone marrow suppression. Typically, platelets will be depressed by about 30% compared to preadministration levels. The Medi-Physics package insert indicates that Metastron should be used with caution in patients with platelet counts below 60,000 and white cell counts below 2,400.

In 1997, ^{153}Sm-EDTMP (Quadramet) was approved by the FDA for relief of bone pain for similar indications as ^{89}Sr-chloride. Samarium-153 decays only by β^- emission and has a $t_{1/2}$ of 46.3 hours. Samarium-153 is complexed with a bone-seeking ligand, EDTMP, which localizes in bone metastases by chemisorption. The duration of response is 1 to 12 months. The main toxicity of this radiotherapeutic is mild transient bone marrow suppression.

In February 2002 the first radiolabeled MAb received FDA approval for radioimmunotherapy. Yttrium-90 labeled MX-DTPA-anti-CD20 antibody (^{90}Y-ibritumomab tiuxetan [Zevalin]) is used to treat patients with non-Hodgkin lymphoma (NHL).[51] Yttrium-90 has a half-life of 64.2 hours, a mean beta energy of 0.936 MeV, and a tissue penetration of 2.5 mm. The unlabeled MAb, rituximab, targets the CD20 antigen present on the surface of normal and malignant B-lymphocytes, and also has FDA approval for treating patients with NHL. The Zevalin therapeutic regimen is administered in two steps. Initially a single infusion of rituximab (250 mg/m^2), is followed by ^{111}In-labeled Zevalin at a fixed dose of 5.0 mCi (1.6 mg total antibody dose). After 7 to 9 days a second infusion of rituximab (250 mg/m^2) is followed by ^{90}Y-labeled Zevalin (0.4 mCi/kg, maximum 32 mCi). If the platelet count is in the range of 100,000 to 149,000 cells/mm^3, the dosage must be reduced to 0.3 mCi/kg). Both labeled antibodies should be administered over 10 minutes.[51] For a review on the phases I to III clinical trials of Zevalin, see Witzig.[47]

In June, 2003, ^{131}I-labeled anti-CD20 monoclonal antibody (^{131}I-tositumomab, BEXXAR) was approved by the FDA for radioimmunotherapy of NHL. Tositumomab is a murine IgG$_{2a}$ directed against the CD20 antigen, similar to rituximab. The therapeutic regimen BEXXAR,[3] includes the use of both tositumomab and ^{131}I-tositumomab. The ^{131}I is covalently linked to the antibody via the tyrosine amino acids. Clinical studies evaluated the efficacy of the BEXXAR therapeutic regimen in 130 patients with rituximab-naïve follicular NHL. The overall response rates ranged from 49% to 64% and the median durations of response ranged from 13 to 16 months. Initially tositumomab 450 mg is injected intravenously over 60 minutes, which is followed by the dosimetric IV infusion of 5.0 mCi ^{131}I labeled tositumomab (35 mg) over 20 minutes.

Whole body biodistribution and dosimetry calculation are performed. The calculation for each patient is performed to determine the amount of ^{131}I-tositumomab (in mCi) to deliver 75 cGy total body dose (TBD), or in patients with platelets $\geq$100,000 and <150,000 platelets/mm^3, 65 cGy TBD.[3]

Two products have been developed to treat certain patients with unresectable hepatocellular carcinoma. TheraSpheres are tiny glass beads (20 to 30 µm), and SIR-Spheres are resin spheres (20 to 40 µm). Both products are microspheres, labeled with ^{90}Y, which decays 100% by β^- emission. These products are therapeutic devices which are injected directly into the liver via catheter. The microspheres are trapped in tumors at the precapillary alveolar level. Beta radiation is delivered internally to tumor at site of active growth. Patients can be released after infusion of the microspheres, since the ^{90}Y decays only by β^- emission. After administration, the bremsstrahlung radiation produced from the β^- interaction in the body, can be imaged and used to determine qualitative distribution in the liver.

REGULATORY ISSUES: RADIOPHARMACEUTICAL QUALITY ASSURANCE

Radiopharmaceutical compounding and quality control (QC) are regulated by USP Chapters <797> and <823>. Chapter <797>, *Pharmaceutical Compounding—Sterile Preparations*, includes requirements for traditional RaPhs. Risk levels are assigned according to potential for microbial contamination during compounding. Immediate-use provision is intended only for those situations where there is a need for emergency or immediate patient administration of compounded sterile preparations (CSPs). Immediate-use CSPs are exempt from low risk RaPh requirements if the RaPh can be prepared, dispensed, and administered within 1 hour of preparation. An example of an immediate-use RaPh would be ^{99m}Tc-MAA, prepared on-call by a nuclear medicine technologist (acting under the authority of an authorized user physician), and administered for an emergency lung scan. Low risk RaPh would be compounded from sterile components in an International Organization of Standardization (ISO) Class 5 (an enclosure that allows 100 particles of 0.5 μm and larger per cubic foot of air) primary engineering control (PEC) with not more than two entries into the original sterile vial, and the beyond-use dating for the RaPh is ≤12 hours. The ISO Class 5 PEC must be located in an ISO Class 8 (an enclosure that allows 100,000 particles of 0.5 μm and larger per cubic foot of air) area or a segregated compounding area. The segregated area must be demarcated by a line on the floor, or be a separate room. The room can have no unsealed windows, no connection to outdoors, and no high traffic flow areas. There can be no sink next to the ISO Class 5 PEC. Personnel must be appropriately gowned and gloved in the work area. An example of low risk compounding would be the preparation of ^{99m}Tc kit formulation. The ^{99m}Tc generator must be eluted according to manufacturer's directions in a demarcated, ISO Class 8 or cleaner environment.

Medium and high risk RaPhs involve more complex manipulations, and may involve use of non-sterile components. The requirements for the preparation of these RaPhs are outlined in separate sections of USP Chapter <797>. High risk PET RaPh compounding is addressed in USP Chapter <823>, and is described later in this section. Chapter <797> specifically states that Chapter <823> supercedes Chapter <797> for PET compounding, but upon release of PET RaPh as a final drug product, for any further manipulations such as dispensing, the contents of Chapter <797> apply. For all RaPhs, the USP monographs, if available, are the minimum standards that must be achieved to produce these compounds.

Chapter <797> outlines training requirements for nuclear medicine personnel to compound low risk RaPhs. Training can be achieved using audiovisual instruction sources, produced by expert personnel, as well as written publications. Personnel must pass a written exam after training, and initially complete media-fill testing, using aseptic manipulations, to demonstrate compounding skills. This testing must be repeated at least annually.

Preparation of traditional RaPhs requires written procedures for appropriate gowning and gloving, including procedures for hand washing. Gowning requirements include dedicated shoes or shoe covers, head cover, masks and eye protection, gowns with fitted sleeves, and sterile gloves disinfected with sterile 70% isopropanol (IPA). These procedures must be documented through observational audits and gloved fingertip sampling using microbiological contact plates. Garb exposed in patient care areas may not reenter the compounding area.

Additionally the ISO Class 5 PEC must be cleaned using appropriate disinfectants (such as sterile 70% IPA, alternated on a defined schedule with a disinfectant effective against spore-forming microorganisms) at the beginning of each shift, and checked on a regular basis using contact and air settling plates.

Radiopharmaceuticals for positron emission tomography (PET) are currently prepared according to USP Chapter <823>, *Rapharmaceuticals for Positron Emission Tomography—Compounding*. This Chapter requires that written specifications must be in place for all components used in any PET drug compounding. Written acceptance criteria for the identity, purity, and quality must be established for each PET drug. Production procedures must be in writing in the form of standard operating procedures including a written batch record for each PET drug production. PET RaPh final product containers must be assembled in a Class 100 environment (laminar flow hood [LFH] or isolator) before moving the final vial assembly to the chemistry production module. Quality control requirements are defined in Chapter <823>. These are described in the following section on RaPh quality control requirements for PET drugs.

On December 10, 2009, FDA published final rule for the manufacture of PET drug—21 CFR Part 212 (Part 212) "Current Good Manufacturing (CGMP) for PET drugs."[15] This rule becomes effective on December 12, 2011. Part 212 establishes CGMP for PET production, separate from regular drug CGMP rule (Parts 210 and 211). CGMP for PET are the minimum standards that each manufacturer must follow to ensure the PET drug meet requirements of the act regarding safety, has the identity and strength defined, and meets the quality and purity characteristics that it is supposed to have over its shelf-life.

Part 212 requires that producers of all PET drugs submit either a New Drug Application (NDA) or an Abbreviated New Drug Application (ANDA) for each of their PET drugs, regardless whether they are produced for commercial distribution, before December 12, 2011. An ANDA ("generic" version) may be submitted to FDA for fludeoxyglucose F 18 injection, sodium fluoride F 18 injection and ammonia N 13, since NDAs have been accepted by the FDA for these 3 PET drugs which provide the reference listed drug (RLD) needed for submission of an ANDA.

Part 212 provides that CGMP may be met for investigational and research PET drugs for human use, produced under an Investigational New Drug (IND) application (21 CFR Part 312.1-312.7), or under the approval of a Radioactive Drug Research Committee (RDRC) (21 CFR 361.1), by producing those PET drugs in accordance with Part 212, *or* in accordance with the USP General Chapter <823>. As a guide to making the choice between Chapter <823> and Part 212 for production of investigational PET drugs covered under an IND for Phase 0-2, Chapter <823> is an acceptable choice, but as the IND moves into Phase 3, or if there is the intent to commercialize the PET drug, Part 212 rule should be followed.

RADIOPHARMACEUTICAL QUALITY CONTROL

Radionuclidic Purity

Radionuclidic purity is defined as the proportion of the total radioactivity present as the stated radionuclide. As such, measurement of radionuclidic purity requires determination of the identity and amounts of all radionuclides that are present. Radionuclidic impurities can have significant effects on the overall radiation dose to the patient and the quality of the images obtained. The identities and amounts of radionuclidic impurities found in a RaPh depend on the method of radionuclide production used. As an example, ^{99m}Tc obtained from a generator prepared using neutron bombardment–produced ^{99}Mo has different impurities than ^{99m}Tc obtained from a generator containing fission-produced ^{99}Mo. The requirements for radionuclidic purity as listed by the USP[42] for sodium ^{99m}Tc-pertechnetate solution are listed in Table 6-3.

An assay using a multichannel analyzer for detection and identification of all gamma-emitting radiocontaminants present in a sample is usually performed by the manufacturer. In the case of ^{99m}Tc, one expected radionuclidic impurity is parent ^{99}Mo. It is necessary for the user to assay routinely for ^{99}Mo breakthrough using a gamma-ionization dose calibrator and a lead vial holder thick enough to absorb the 140-keV gamma emission of ^{99m}Tc but thin enough to allow penetration of the 720- and 740-keV gamma emissions of ^{99}Mo (Figure 6-21). The Nuclear Regulatory Commission (NRC)–allowable

^{99}Mo contamination is less than 0.15 µCi/mCi of ^{99m}Tc. NRC regulations require that every elution from a ^{99}Mo-^{99m}Tc generator be tested for ^{99}Mo breakthrough and that the records be maintained for 3 years.

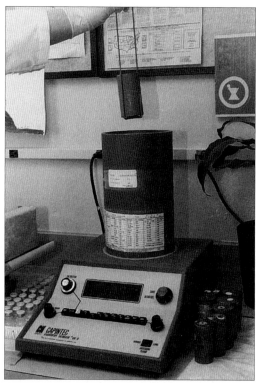

FIGURE 6-21 Molybdenum-99 assay chamber being placed in a dose calibrator.

Radiochemical Purity

Radiochemical purity is defined as the proportion of the stated radionuclide that is present in the stated chemical form. The radiation absorbed dose, the biological distribution, and thus the quality of the image are directly related to the radiochemical purity. Several chromatographic methods can be used to determine radiochemical purity, including gel-permeation chromatography, gas-liquid chromatography, and paper chromatography. The method applicable to routine in-house quality control of technetium RaPh is paper or instant thin-layer chromatography (ITLC).

Chromatography involves the separation of a chemical mixture into its components along a stationary phase (adsorbent) as a result of different velocities in the mobile phase (migrating solvent). Radiochromatography differs from regular chromatography only in that the presence of the component is determined by the location of its radioactivity rather than by some other physical or chemical property. The R_f of a compound is defined as the measure of its migration distance, where:

TABLE 6-3	NRC-Allowable Radionuclidic Impurities in ^{99m}Tc-Pertechnetate	
Neutron Bombardment: ^{98}Mo (n, γ) ^{99}Mo	**Fission-Separation ^{99}Mo**	
^{99}Mo < 0.15 µCi/mCi ^{99m}Tc	^{99}Mo < 0.15 µCi/mCi ^{99m}Tc	
All other gamma-emitting radionuclides	**Other gamma-emitting radionuclides**	
0.5 µCi/mCi ^{99m}Tc	^{131}I < 0.05 µCi/mCi ^{99m}Tc	
<2.5 µCi/administered dose	^{103}Ru 0.05 µCi/mCi ^{99m}Tc	
	^{89}Sr < 0.0006 µCi/mCi ^{99m}Tc	
	^{90}Sr < 0.00006 µCi/mCi ^{99m}Tc	
	Remaining β + γ < 0.1 µCi/mCi	
	α < 0.001 µCi/mCi ^{99m}Tc	

NRC, Nuclear Regulatory Commission.

$$R_f = \frac{\text{Distance of center of spot from origin}}{\text{Distance of solvent from origin}}$$

When the $R_f = 1$, the component migrates with the solvent front, but when the $R_f = 0$, the component remains at the point of application (origin).

The ideal separation of a component in a solvent system gives an R_f value greater than 0 but less than 1. A component that migrates at the solvent front ($R_f = 1$) or remains at the origin ($R_f = 0$) is not truly separated. However, for routine rapid quality control of technetium RaPh and the separation of known impurities, free pertechnetate ($^{99m}TcO_4^-$) and reduced hydrolyzed ^{99m}Tc from the labeled RaPh, R_f values of 1 and 0 are considered acceptable.

A typical thin-layer radiochromatogram of ^{99m}Tc-sulfur colloid with $^{99m}TcO_4^-$ contaminant is shown in Figure 6-22. The radioactivity associated with the peaks may be measured in several ways. The simplest method, which was used to obtain the data, involves the use of a radiochromatogram scanner (Figure 6-23). In this system the detector is moved across the paper chromatography strip, a ratemeter indicates the count rate, and the counts are graphically printed out by a strip chart recorder. A manual counting system can also be employed, in which the chromatogram is cut into strips, and each strip is counted using a well counter or an ionization dose calibrator.

The radiochemical purity of a RaPh preparation can be calculated using the following expression:

$$\text{Percentage of radiochemical purity}$$
$$= (\text{Counts in Area R}) \text{ divided by}$$
$$(\text{Counts in Area R} + \text{Counts in Area I}) \times 100$$

where R refers to the RaPh and I refers to the impurity

Routine rapid radiochromatography can be performed to evaluate the percentage of radiochemical purity of ^{99m}Tc RaPh. The most commonly employed procedure involves the use of instant thin-layer chromatography silica gel–impregnated (ITLC-SG) glass-fiber sheets as the solid support. These strips are developed in solvents such as saline, acetone, and methyl ethyl ketone (MEK). ^{99m}Tc RaPh can be divided into three groups based on their chromatographic behavior.

1. *Oxidized, particulate.* This group contains ^{99m}Tc-sulfur colloid. Because the technetium is present in the +7 oxidation state, it is not necessary to analyze for reduced hydrolyzed ^{99m}Tc in these preparations. The chromatographic system used involves a single solvent (saline, acetone, or MEK) to determine the amount of $^{99m}TcO_4^-$.

2. *Reduced, particulate.* This group includes the ^{99m}Tc-labeled lung perfusion imaging agent MAA. The rapid chromatographic procedures described for sulfur colloid can be used only to determine $^{99m}TcO_4^-$. It is not possible to separate reduced hydrolyzed ^{99m}Tc (which is colloidal at physiological pH) and the ^{99m}Tc-MAA using this rapid system. It is possible, however, to use an indirect method to detect reduced hydrolyzed ^{99m}Tc impurity levels. The RaPh is first filtered through a Millipore filter with a 1-μm pore diameter,

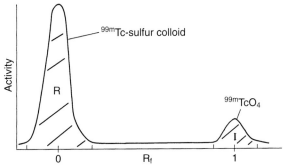

FIGURE 6-22 Radiochromatogram scan of ^{99m}Tc-sulfur colloid *(R)* indicating radiochemical purity. The only radiocontaminant present is $^{99m}TcO_4^-$ *(I)*.

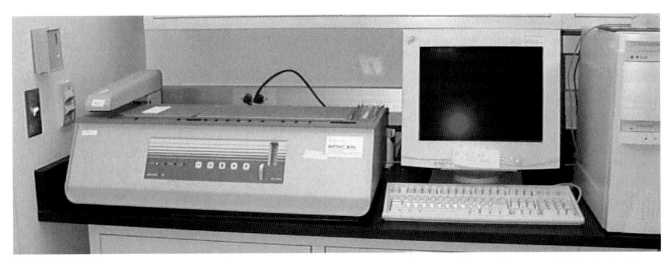

FIGURE 6-23 Radiochromatogram scanner used for radiochemical purity analysis and calculation of percent radiochemical purity.

TABLE 6-4	Chromatographic Systems Used for Quality Control of ^{99m}Tc Radiopharmaceuticals					
				R_f		
RaPh	**Solvent**	**Solid Support**	**Free ^{99m}TcO$_4^-$**	**Free ^{99m}TcO$_2$**	**^{99m}Tc-RaPh**	
Sulfur colloid	Acetone or saline	ITLC-SG	1.0	—	0	
Macroaggregated Albumin (MAA)	Acetone or saline	ITLC-SG	1.0	—	0	
Pyrophosphate (PYP)*						
Methylene Disphosphonate (MDP)*	Acetone	Whatman 31ET	1.0	0	0	
Hydroxymethylene diphosphonate (HDP)*	Saline	ITLC-SG	1.0	0	1.0	
Pentetate (DTPA)*						
Glucoheptonate (GHP)*						
2,3-dimercaptosuccinic acid (DMSA)	Saline	ITLC-SG	1.0	0	0	
Disofenin*	20% NaC1	ITLC-SA	1.0	0	0	
Mebrofenin*	H$_2$O	ITLC-SG	1.0	0	1.0	
Sestamibi	100% EtOH	Aluminum oxide TLC	0	0	1.0	

*Each of these Tc-99m RaPhs requires the use of both solvents and solid supports detailed in the table above in order to determine the radiochemical purity. For example Mebrofenin would require the use of 20% NaCl with ITLC-SA and and H$_2$O with ITLC-SG to determine the radiochemical purity.

which retains the ^{99m}Tc-MAA but allows the colloidal reduced hydrolyzed ^{99m}Tc to pass through. Once the macroparticles have been removed, rapid chromatography on the filtrate (using either saline, acetone, or MEK) enables the determination of free ^{99m}TcO$_4^-$ and reduced hydrolyzed ^{99m}Tc.

3. *Reduced, soluble.* This group contains the soluble, reduced ^{99m}Tc-RaPh, including DTPA, glucoheptonate, methylene diphosphonate, pyrophosphate, DMSA, and albumin. The chromatographic procedure for this group involves two solvents (saline and an organic solvent, such as acetone or MEK) to determine the percentages of ^{99m}TcO$_4^-$, reduced hydrolyzed ^{99m}Tc , and labelled RaPh.

The Rf values of the technetium RaPh and the relevant impurities are outlined in Table 6-4 for each of these groups. The steps in a typical chromatographic procedure for a reduced, soluble ^{99m}Tc-RaPh are as follows:

1. Place 1 ml of saline in a small glass vial; repeat this procedure using 1 ml organic solvent in another small glass vial.
2. Mark two 1 × 6-cm ITLC chromatography strips at 2 cm and 5 cm with a pencil.
3. Place a small spot of the RaPh in the center of each strip (near the mark located 2 cm from the bottom of the strip) using a tuberculin syringe.
4. Place one strip into each solvent before the spot has air-dried to prevent air oxidation of the RaPh. Allow the solvent front to move up each strip until it has reached the line at 5 cm.
5. Cut the strips in the middle between the pencil markings and count each portion of the strips for activity, or use a radiochromatogram scanner (see Figure 6-23) to measure the amount of activity along the intact strips.

6. In the dual solvent system, the percentage of free ^{99m}TcO$_4^-$ is calculated from the strip developed in the organic solvent, and the percentage of reduced hydrolyzed ^{99m}Tc is determined using the strip developed in saline. Subtraction of the percentages of these two impurities from 100% yields the overall radiochemical purity of the ^{99m}Tc RaPh.

Radiochemical testing using ITLC is easily performed in any nuclear medicine laboratory. Testing each lot of a RaPh kit on a weekly basis is a reasonable approach for routine radiochemical testing. Additional testing should be performed if there are questions concerning purity of a given preparation. Several of the newer technetium RaPh require more specific types of quality control methods.

In the preparation of the lipophilic ^{99m}Tc-exametazime, three radiochemical impurities can be present: a secondary ^{99m}Tc-amine complex, ^{99m}TcO$_4^-$, and reduced hydrolyzed ^{99m}Tc. A combination of three chromatographic systems is necessary for radiochemical purity determination: 0.9% NaCl (ITLC-SG); MEK (ITLC-SG); and acetonitrile-water, (Whatman Paper) 1:1. In the 0.9% NaCl (saline) solvent the ^{99m}TcO$_4^-$ migrates at the solvent front, whereas the ^{99m}Tc-exametazime, secondary ^{99m}Tc-amine complex, and reduced hydrolyzed ^{99m}Tc remain at the origin. In the MEK solvent, ^{99m}TcO$_4^-$ and ^{99m}Tc-exametazime migrate at the solvent front, whereas the secondary ^{99m}Tc-amine complex and the reduced hydrolyzed ^{99m}Tc remain at the origin. Use of the acetonitrile-water (1:1) solvent causes ^{99m}TcO$_4^-$, ^{99m}Tc-exametazime, and the secondary ^{99m}Tc-amine complex to migrate with the solvent front, whereas the reduced hydrolyzed ^{99m}Tc remains at the origin. The calculations used for determining the percentage of ^{99m}Tc-exametazime are shown in Figure 6-24.

The radiochemical purity of ^{99m}Tc-mertiatide is determined using Sep-Pak chromatography. The Sep-Pak is

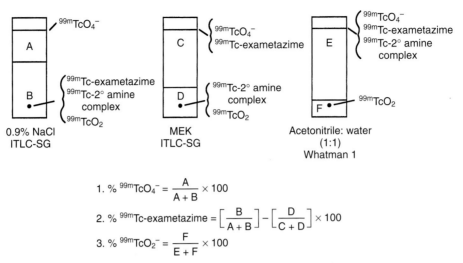

1. $\% \ ^{99m}TcO_4^- = \dfrac{A}{A + B} \times 100$

2. $\% \ ^{99m}Tc\text{-exametazime} = \left[\dfrac{B}{A + B}\right] - \left[\dfrac{D}{C + D}\right] \times 100$

3. $\% \ ^{99m}TcO_2^- = \dfrac{F}{E + F} \times 100$

FIGURE 6-24 Chromatographic system used for radiochemical purity determination for ^{99m}Tc-exametazime and calculation of percentage of radiochemical purity.

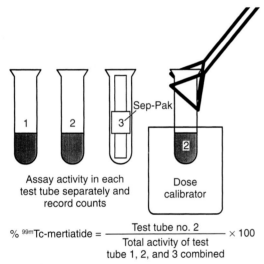

$\% \ ^{99m}Tc\text{-mertiatide} = \dfrac{\text{Test tube no. 2}}{\text{Total activity of test tube 1, 2, and 3 combined}} \times 100$

FIGURE 6-25 Calculation of percent radiochemical purity of ^{99m}Tc-mertiatide.

made of C_{18} hydrocarbon chains that retain nonpolar compounds. Initially the Sep-Pak is prepared by washing with 100% ethanol to remove nonpolar impurities, then with 0.001 N HCl to remove polar impurities followed by 5 ml of air to remove remaining solvent form the cartridge. A sample of the ^{99m}Tc-mertiatide is then placed on the Sep-Pak and eluted with a 0.001 N HCl solution, which elutes any polar impurities present in the preparation. This fraction is retained and labeled fraction 1. Then the Sep-Pak is eluted with an ethanol-saline (1:1) solution, which solubilizes and elutes the ^{99m}Tc-mertiatide. This fraction is labeled 2, and the Sep-Pak, containing reduced hydrolyzed impurities is labeled 3. Fractions 1, 2, and 3 are counted in the dose calibrator. Figure 6-25 shows the calculation for ^{99m}Tc-mertiatide purity determination.

A single solid support, aluminum oxide, and a single solvent, 100% ethanol, are used for quality control of ^{99m}Tc-sestamibi. The ^{99m}Tc-sestamibi migrates at the solvent front. Pertechnetate is thought to form a complex with the aluminum and remains at the origin. The reduced hydrolyzed ^{99m}Tc also remains at the origin.

Technetium-99m-tetrofosmin quality control requires the ITLC-SG as the solid support and a 35/65 (v/v) mixture of acetone and dichloromethane. After spotting the ITLC-SG, the solvent is allowed to migrate 18 cm. The strip is removed from the solvent and cut into three pieces one cut at 3 cm and one cut at 12 cm above the origin which is 3 cm above the bottom of the strip. The percent ^{99m}Tc-tetrofosmin will be equal to the activity of the center piece of the strip, divided by the total activity of the three pieces, multiplied by 100.

Completion of quality control, involving C_{18} Sep-Pak chromatography, is recommended before patient administration for ^{111}In-pentetreotide. The Sep-Pak is prepared for use by initially flushing with 10 ml of methanol, followed by 10 ml of water, followed by an additional 5 ml of water. A sample of ^{111}In-pentetreotide is placed on the Sep-Pak and eluted with 5 ml of water. The fraction is labeled fraction 1. The Sep-Pak is then eluted with 5 ml of methanol, which solubilizes ^{111}In-pentetreotide. This is labeled fraction 2, and the Sep-Pak is labeled fraction 3. Each fraction is assayed in the dose calibrator, and the percent purity of the ^{111}In-pentetreotide is determined (Figure 6-26).

Chemical Impurities

Chemical impurities are all the nonradioactive substances present in a RaPh preparation that either affect labeling or directly cause adverse biological effects. In microgram concentrations, aluminum can affect the formation of ^{99m}Tc-labeled RaPh. The NRC states the

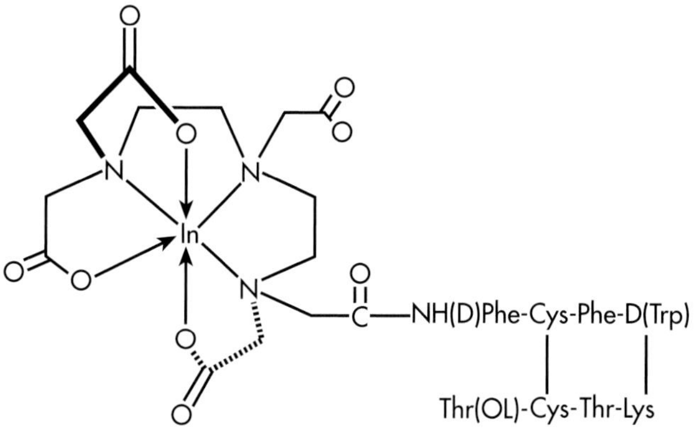

FIGURE 6-26 Spatial configuration of ^{111}In-pentetreotide (OctreoScan).

concentration of aluminum should <10 µg/ml. The presence of excess Al^{3+} can cause formation of colloidal ^{99m}Tc-Al particles, resulting in liver uptake, aggregation of sulfur colloid to larger particles with resultant capillary blockade and lung visualization, and ^{99m}Tc-RBC aggregation, which results in uptake of the damaged cells in lungs and spleen.

Aluminum can be detected using a spectrophotometric method. Aluminum solutions of known concentrations are reacted with aluminon reagent (the ammonium salt of aurin tricarboxylic acid), and the absorbance in the visible region of the spectrum is measured. A standard curve is then prepared by plotting the absorbance versus the aluminum concentration; this curve can be used to determine aluminum concentrations of unknown samples. A more convenient method for aluminum determination is the use of a commercially available indicator paper impregnated with aluminon reagent that turns pink when Al^{3+} is present in a spot of the eluant solution. A standard solution of Al^{3+} (10 µg/ml) is used as a color comparison.

Most of the commercially available technetium kits contain stannous ion as the reducing agent. In most cases more stannous ion is contained in each kit than is actually required to reduce and bind the technetium that is added; this excess of stannous ion has been found to cause some problems. For example, liver uptake has been noted on an otherwise normal bone scan, which may be attributable to the formation of ^{99m}Tc-tin colloids. Another problem that can occur with excess stannous ion is inadvertent RBC labeling. As mentioned previously, excess stannous ion injected into a patient receiving a reduced [99m]Tc RaPh remains in the circulation. This can cause RBC labeling on subsequent administration of ^{99m}Tc-pertechnetate for brain or thyroid imaging.

Microbiological Testing

Sterility Testing. The objective of sterility testing is to provide assurance that the sterilization process was conducted properly. The sterility test required by the

USP[42] involves inoculation of the product in both fluid thioglycolate and soybean-casein digest media. Fluid thioglycolate provides conditions primarily intended for growth of anaerobic bacteria; however, it will also detect aerobic bacteria. Soybean-casein digest medium is suitable for the culture of both fungi and aerobic bacteria. The official sterility test requires 14 days, but because of the short half-life of ^{99m}Tc, the USP[42] allows for the release of these RaPh before the completion of the tests. The cold kits used to prepare the [99m]Tc RaPh are tested for sterility and pyrogen content.

Pyrogen/Bacterial Endotoxin Test (BET). Pyrogens are any agents that cause a rise in temperature and are generally considered to be heat-stable by-products of the growth of bacteria, yeasts, and molds. The word *pyrogen* is often used to mean bacterial endotoxin. Prior to 1977, the USP required that all intravenously administered pharmaceuticals (including radiopharmaceuticals) be tested for the presence of pyrogens by monitoring of three healthy rabbits for 3 hours after IV injection of the test sample. The test was positive if any rabbit showed an increase of 0.6° C or more above the baseline temperature or if the sum of the three temperature increases exceeded 1.4° C.

In 1977 the FDA gave conditional approval for the use of the limulus amebocyte lysate (LAL) bacterial endotoxin testing (BET) as an alternative to the rabbit test for pyrogen testing, to use for final release for certain products. The LAL is isolated from the horseshoe crab *(Limulus)*. LAL reacts with gram-negative bacterial endotoxins in nanogram or greater concentrations to form an opaque gel. Gram-negative endotoxins are recognized as the most important source of pyrogen contamination. The BET test is both a rapid and a very sensitive in vitro method. The test requires 60 minutes to complete. The USP[42] now requires BET testing.

The Endosafe Portable Test System (PTS) is a software-driven spectrophotometer for measuring and documenting endotoxin, which is approved by the FDA. The system utilizes an assay in which the bacterial endotoxin initiates activation of enzymes in LAL, which finally cleaves a synthetic substrate. Cleavage results in the release of the chromophore, p-nitroaniline (PNA). PNA is a yellow color that is measured by the PTS spectrophotometer at 385 to 410 nm. The system uses a cartridge that contains four channels to which LAL reagent and the chromogenic substrate have been applied. Two channels contain an endotoxin spike and serve as positive product controls. The other two channels are for the test sample. PTS is particularly suited for PET drugs because the test requires approximately 20 minutes. Since the system requires <0.1 ml of diluted product (1:100 dilution can be validated), it allows reduced radiation exposure for the quality control (QC) operator.

Manufacturers are required to perform sterility and BET testing on all their products before release into the marketplace. The short half-life of ^{99m}Tc, however, prohibits testing of ^{99m}Tc-labeled RaPh for sterility prior to patient administration. It then becomes imperative that the user emphasize aseptic technique. The use of laminar airflow enclosures improves the environment for RaPh formulation, because these enclosures contain high-efficiency particulate air (HEPA) filters to remove particles of 0.3 μm and larger with an efficiency of 99.97%. Vertical laminar airflow hoods are preferred in a radiopharmacy, because horizontal flow presents a potentially serious contamination hazard to personnel by forcing radioactivity out into the room. If the laminar airflow cabinet is reinforced, it can support a leaded glass shield to provide radiation protection for the technologist during preparation of the RaPh.

Quality Control Requirements for PET Drugs. Currently PET drugs are being compounded according to the USP monograph requirements, if available, and USP Chapter <823>,[42] On December 10, 2009, the FDA finalized the PET CGMP rule for PET drugs which includes both production and quality control requirements. At the same time, Guidance "PET Drugs—Current Good Manufacturing Practice (CGMP)" was published which describes the FDA's current thinking on CGMP.[16] It provides practical examples of methods or procedures that PET drug production facilities can use to comply with the CGMP requirements. Quality control procedures for PET drugs are now outlined in the FDA Guidance document and are comparable to the current Chapter <823> requirements.

Part 212 requires pre-release quality control testing be performed for each batch of PET RaPh drug having a half-life of ≥20 minutes, or on a QC *sub-batch* for PET drug having a half-life <20 minutes. Examples of QC sub-batches would include ^{15}O-water and ^{13}N-ammonia, where the initial batch is used to perform QC tests, then subsequent batches prepared with the same initial reagents, can be released without QC testing.

Required QC tests at end of synthesis (EOS) include identity testing; pH; visual appearance; radiochemical and chemical testing, including specific activity testing or a mass limit test; residual solvent analysis; and BET (<175 endotoxin units [EU]/volume of the administered product [V]).

Each of these tests must include adequate standards testing as part of the analysis. Final products administered intravenously must be filtered through a 0.22-μm filter to ensure sterility, and the filter must be tested for integrity post-filtration and pre-release.

Sterility testing is required post-release for every batch of PET RaPh prepared for human use. An aliquot of the batch must be inoculated for sterility within 30 hours EOS (FDA Guidance).[16] Radionuclidic purity testing, commonly involving gamma analysis with a multichannel analyzer (MCA), must be performed on a regularly defined interval.

As an example the following tests should be performed pre-release for each batch of ^{18}F-FDG:[43]

1. Identity testing for ^{18}F-FDG involves decay analysis over a defined period of time. This test is performed using a dose calibrator. The half-life is determined mathematically using linear regression. The acceptable $t_{1/2}$ = 109.7 (with an allowable range of 105 to 115 minutes).

2. The pH must be between 4.5 and 7.5. An aliquot of each batch ^{18}F-FDG is tested either with pH paper or a pH meter.

3. The batch is checked visually (using adequate shielding) to ensure a clear colorless solution that is free of particulate matter.

4. The radiochemical purity and identity of ^{18}F-FDG can be determined by using an activated silica gel thin-layer chromatographic (TLC) plate developed in acetonitrile-water (95:5). A nonradioactive USP FDG standard should be spotted with the ^{18}F-FDG. This system allows separation of ^{18}F-FDG ($R_f \cong 0.4$); ^{18}F-fluoride ($R_f \cong 0$); and ^{18}F-FDG, nonhydrolyzed intermediate ($R_f \cong 0.6$). Acceptable radiochemical purity is ≥90%.

5. The chemical purity of each batch of ^{18}F-FDG must be checked pre-release. If the synthetic method of ^{18}F-FDG production involves the use of Kryptofix, which is a toxic substance, current USP[42] requires determination of the concentration of Kryptofix in the final product. The current USP-approved[42] method to test for the presence of Kryptofix, developed by Chaly and Dahl,[7] involves a TLC QC procedure using a silica gel TLC plate developed in a mixture of methanol–30% ammonium hydroxide (9:1). The developed plate is dried, and an iodine vapor chamber is used for visualization. A yellow spot ($R_f \cong 0.4$) indicates the presence of Kryptofix. The USP[42] test takes about 30 minutes to complete. Mock and colleagues[31] have also developed a color spot test for FDG that can determine the presence of Kryptofix to as low as 20 μg/ml in about 5 minutes. The test uses pretreated strips of plastic-backed silica gel TLC, saturated with iodoplatinate reagents that are overspotted with drops of ^{18}F-FDG and Kryptofix standard solutions. The test requires less than 10 minutes to perform but must be validated against the USP[42] method. The Kryptofix concentration must be ≤50 μg/ml. Residual solvent concentrations such as acetonitrile, ethanol, and ether must be tested if they are used in the synthesis before release of ^{18}F-FDG. Gas chromatographic methods have been developed for the measurement of residual solvents that allow precision and linearity over the range of concentration levels suggested by the FDA[9] and required by the USP.[42] The concentration of acetonitrile must be ≤0.04% w/v (0.4 mg/ml), ethanol 0.5% w/v (5 mg/ml), and ether 0.5% w/v (5 mg/ml).

6. Every batch must be tested for BET. The acceptable endotoxin limit is 175 EU/V. The V is usually defined as the batch volume of the FDG.

Post-release sterility testing must be performed for each batch of ^{18}F-FDG. The product should be inoculated in both fluid thioglycolate and soybean-casein digest media within 30 hours EOS (FDA Guidance).[16]

Certain QC tests may be performed as a periodic quality indicator test (PQIT).[16] One example of this type of test is the radionuclidic purity analysis. This test should be performed on a defined interval by γ-ray spectroscopy using a suitable gamma counting device. An MCA is often used to determine the presence of any gamma photon energy other than that characteristic of ^{18}F, including 511 keV, 1.02 MeV, or Compton scatter. The radionuclidic purity must be ≥99.5%.

SUMMARY

- A nucleus with an n/p ratio too high for stability results in the production of a negative beta particle.
- A nucleus with an n/p ratio too low for stability results in the production of a positron or absorption by the nucleus of an orbital electron (electron capture).
- Beta decay often leaves the daughter nucleus in an excited state. The excitation energy is removed either by gamma-ray emission or by internal conversion.
- Radionuclides that decay by alpha emission are not useful in nuclear medicine imaging, but may have future therapeutic applications.
- Radionuclides used to label RaPh for nuclear medicine imaging should decay by a process that results in photon emissions.
- The ^{99}Mo-^{99m}Tc generator is an example of transient equilibrium.
- The actual ^{99m}Tc activity present at transient equilibrium is 0.946 times the activity of ^{99}Mo.
- The ^{113}Sn-^{113m}In generator is an example of secular equilibrium.
- At equilibrium the daughter activity is equal to the parent activity.
- The time required to reach equilibrium dictates how frequently each generator can be eluted and depends on the half-lives of the parent and daughter.
- ^{99m}TcO$_4^-$ is Tc in the +7 valence state and concentrates primarily in the thyroid, salivary glands, gastric mucosa, and choroid plexus.
- Pretreatment of potassium perchlorate, Lugol solution, or a saturated solution of potassium iodide (SSKI) influences the distribution of technetium.
- To alter the biodistribution of technetium, it is necessary for it to be chemically reduced; this is accomplished by using reducing agents.
- Stannous chloride is the reducing agent used most frequently in kit formulations for ^{99m}Tc RaPh.
- Labeling of red blood cells (RBCs) with ^{99m}Tc provides an intravascular tracer useful for many nuclear medicine procedures. RBCs can be labeled either in vivo or in vitro.
- Peptide imaging agents can identify somatostatin receptors.
- On injection of ^{67}Ga-citrate, 90% of the gallium becomes bound to plasma proteins, particularly transferrin, resulting in a slow release from plasma.
- Pharmacological cardiac stress agents include dipyridamole, adenosine, and regadenoson.
- The most frequently used positron-emitting radionuclides for PET imaging include ^{15}O, ^{13}N, ^{11}C, and ^{18}F.
- The most frequently used ^{18}F-labeled RaPh is 2-deoxy-2-[^{18}F]fluoro-D-glucose (FDG).
- The mechanism of ^{18}FDG trapping follows the glucose biochemical pathway.
- The radiation absorbed dose, the biological distribution, and the quality of the image are directly related to the radiochemical purity.
- Quality assurance for RaPh includes sterility and pyrogen testing, and testing for radionuclidic purity, radiochemical purity, and chemical purity.

REFERENCES

1. Alberto R: New organometallic technetium complexes for radio pharmaceutical imaging, *Top Curr Chem* 252:1-44, 2005.
2. Bauer W, Briner U, Doepfner W, et al: SMS 201-995: a very potent and selective octapeptide analogue of somatostatin with prolonged action, *Life Sci* 31:1133, 1982.
3. BEXXAR, Research Triangle Park, NC, March 2005, GlaxoSmithKline, (package insert).
4. Blauenstein P, Garayoa EG, Ruegg D, et al: Improving the tumor uptake of ^{99m}Tc-labeled neuropeptides using stabilized peptide analogues, *Cancer Biother Radiopharm* 19:181, 2004.
5. Breeman WAP, deJong M, deBlois E, et al: Radiolabelling DOTA-peptides with ^{68}Ga, *Eur J Nucl Med Mol Imaging* 32:478-485, 2005.
6. Brodack JW, Kaiser SL, Welch MJ: Laboratory robotics for the remote synthesis of generator-based positron-emitting radiopharmaceuticals, *Lab Robot Autom* 1:285, 1989.
7. Chaly T, Dahl JR: Thin layer chromatographic detection of Kryptofix 2.2.2. in the routine synthesis of [^{18}F]-2-fluoro-deoxyglucose, *Nucl Med Biol* 16:385, 1989.
8. Channing MA, Dunn BB, Kiesewetter DO, et al: The quality of [^{13}N]ammonia produced by using ethanol as a scavenger, *J Labelled Comp Radiopharm* 35:334, 1994.
9. Channing MA, Huang BX, Eckelman WC: Analysis of residual solvents in 2-[^{18}F]FDG by GC, *Nucl Med Biol* 28:469, 2001.
10. Coleman RE, Maturi M, Nunn AD, et al: Imaging of myocardial perfusion with Tc-99m SQ 3Q217: dog and human studies, *J Nucl Med* 27:893, 1986.
11. Dence CS, Herrero P, Schwarz SW, et al: Imaging myocardium enzymatic pathways with carbon-11 radiotracers, *Methods Enzymol* 385:286-316, 2004.
12. deVries EFJ, Luurtsema G, Brussermann M, et al: Fully automated synthesis module for the high yield one-pot preparation of 6-[^{18}F]fluoro-L-DOPA, *Appl Radiat Isot* 51:389, 1999.
13. Dudczak R, Leitha T, Kletter K, et al: Comparison of Tc-99m-methoxyisobutyl-isonitrile (MIBI) for myocardial imaging in man, *J Nucl Med* 29:794, 1988.
14. Ehrhardt GJ, Welch MJ: A new germanium-68/gallium-68 generator, *J Nucl Med* 19:925, 1978.
xx Federal Register / Vol. 74, /December 10, 2009, p. 65409
xxx Federal Register / Vol. 74, /December 10, 2009, p. 65538

15. Füchtner F, Steinbach J, Mading P, et al: Basic hydrolysis of 2-[18F]fluoro-1,3,4,6-tetra-O-acetyl-C-glucose in the preparation of 2-[18F]fluoro-2-deoxy-D-glucose, *Appl Radiat Isot* 47:61, 1966.

16. Fujibayashi Y, Matsumoto K, Yonekura Y, et al: A new zinc-62/copper-62 generator as a copper-62 source for PET radiopharmaceuticals, *J Nucl Med* 30:1938, 1989.

17. Green MA, Mathias CJ, Welch MJ, et al: Copper-62-labeled pyruvaldehyde bis (N4-methylthiosemicarbazonato) copper (II): synthesis and evaluation as a positron emission tomography tracer for cerebral and myocardial perfusion, *J Nucl Med* 31:1989, 1990.

18. Green MA, Welch MJ: Gallium radiopharmaceuticals chemistry, *Nucl Med Biol* 16:435, 1989.

19. Grubb RL Jr, Powers WJ, Derdeyn CP, et al: The carotid occlusion surgery study, *Neurosurg Focus* 14:1-9, 2003.

20. Hamacher K, Coenen HH, Stocklin G: Efficient stereospecific synthesis of NCA 2-[18F]fluoro-2-deoxy-D-glucose using aminopolyether supported nucleophilic substitution, *J Nucl Med* 27:235, 1986.

21. Haynes NG, Lacy JL, Nayak N, et al: Performance of a 62Zn/62Cu generator in clinical trials of PET perfusion agent 62Cu-PTSM, *J Nucl Med* 41:309, 2000.

22. Hirom PC: The physiochemical factors required for the biliary excretion of organic cations and anions, *Biochem Soc Trans* 2:327-329, 1974.

23. Ho CL, Yu CH, Yeung DWC: 11C-acetate PET imaging in hepatocellular carcinoma and other live masses, *J Nucl Med* 44:213-221, 2003.

24. Jager PL, Chirakal R, Marriott CJ, et al: 6-L-18F-Fluorodihidroxyphenylalanine PET in neuroendocrine tumors: basic aspects and emerging clinical applications, *J Nucl Med* 49:573-586, 2008.

25. Leveille J, Demonceau G, DeRoo M, et al: Characterization of technetium-99m-L,L-ECD for brain perfusion imaging. Part 2. Biodistribution and brain imaging in humans, *J Nucl Med* 30:1902, 1989.

26. Loberg MD, Fields AT: Chemical structure of technetium-99m-labeled N-(2,6-dimethylphenyl-carbamoylmethyl)-iminodiacetic acid (99mTc-HIDA), *Int J Appl Radiat Isot* 29:167, 1978.

27. Loc'h C, Maziere B, Comar D: A new generator for ionic gallium-68, *J Nucl Med* 21:171, 1980.

28. Machulla HJ, Blocher A, Kunztsch M, et al: Simplified labeling approach for synthesizing 3′-deoxy-3′[18F]fluorothymidine ([18F]FLT), *J Radioanal Nucl Chem* 243:843-846, 2000.

29. Mathis CA, Wang Y, Holt DP, et al: Synthesis and evaluation of 11C-labeled 6-substituted 2-arylbenzothiazoles as amyloid imaging agents, *J Med Chem* 46:2740-2754, 2003.

30. Mathias CJ, Margenau WH, Brodack JW, et al: A remote system for the synthesis of copper-62-labeled Cu(PTSM), *Int J Rad Appl Instrum A* 42:317-320, 1991.

31. Mock BH, Winkle W, Vavrek MT: A color spot test for the detection of Kryptofix 2.2.2 in [18F]FDG preparations, *Nucl Med Biol* 24:193, 1997.

32. Neirinckx RD, Burke JF, Harrison RG, et al: The retention mechanism of technetium-99m-HMPAO: intracellular reaction with glutathione, *J Cereb Blood Flow Metab* 8:54, 1988.

33. Nunn AD, Loberg MD: Hepatobiliary agents. In Spencer RP, editor: *Radiopharmaceuticals: structure-activity relationships*, New York, 1981, Grune & Stratton, pp 539-548.

34. Nye JA, Avila-Rodriguez MA, Nickles RJ: A new binary compound for the production of 124I via the 124Te(n,p) 124I reaction, *Appl Radiat Isot* 65:407-412, 2007.

35. Oh SJ, Mosdzianowski C, Chi DY, et al: Fully automated synthesis system of 3′-deoxy-3′-[18F]fluorothymidine, *Nucl Med Biol* 31:803-809, 2004.

36. Oyama N, Miller TR, Dehdashti F, et al: 11C-acetate PET imaging of prostate cancer—detection of recurrent disease at PSA relapse, *J Nucl Med* 44:549-555, 2003.

37. Pike VW, Eakins MN, Allan RM, et al: Preparation of [1-11C] acetate: an agent for the study of myocardial metabolism by positron emission tomography, *Int J Appl Radiat Isot* 33:505, 1982.

38. Robinson GD, Zielinski FW, Lee AW: Zn-62/Cu-62 generator: a convenient source of copper-62 radiopharmaceuticals, *Int J Appl Radiat Isot* 31:111, 1980.

39. Sands H, Delano ML, Gallagher BM: Uptake of hexakis (t-butylisonitrile) technetium (I) and hexakis (isopropylisonitrile) technetium (I) by neonatal rat myocytes and human erythrocytes, *J Nucl Med* 27:404, 1986.

40. Shen B, Ehrlichmann W, Uebele M, et al: Automated synthesis of n.c.a. [18F]FDOPA via nucleophilic aromatic substitution with [18F]fluoride, *Appl Radiat Isotop* 67:1650-1653, 2009.

41. Taylor A Jr, Eshima D, Fritzberg AR, et al: Comparison of iodine-131 OIH and technetium-99m MAG3 renal imaging in volunteers, *J Nucl Med* 27:795, 1986.

42. USP, 29-NF 24, Rockville, Md, 2005, United States Pharmacopeial Convention, Inc.

43. Walhaus TR, Lacy J, Whang J, et al: Human biodistribution and dosimetry of the PET perfusion agent 62Cu-PTSM from a compact modular 62Zn/62Cu generator, *J Nucl Med* 39:1958, 1998.

44. Wallace AM, Hoh CK, Vera DR, et al: Lymphoseek: a molecular radiopharmaceutical for sentinel node detection, *Ann Surg Oncol* 10(5):531-538, 2003.

45. Welch MJ, Kilbourn MR: A remote system for the routine production of oxygen-15 radiopharmaceuticals, *J Labelled Comp Radiopharm* 12:1193-1200, 1985.

46. Win Z, Al-Nahhas A, Rubello D, et al: Somatostatin receptor PET imaging with Gallium-68 labeled peptides, *Q J Nucl Med Mol Imaging* 51:244-250, 2007.

47. Witzig TE: Radioimmunotherapy for patients with relapsed B-cell non-Hodgkin's lymphoma, *Cancer Chemother Pharmacol* 48(suppl 1):S91, 2001.

48. Yoshimoto M, Waki A, Yonekura Y, et al: Characterization of acetate metabolism in tumor cells in relation to cell proliferation—acetate metabolism in tumor cells, *Nucl Med Biol* 28:117-122, 2001.

49. Zevalin, San Diego, Calif, January, 2002, IDEC Pharmaceuticals, Cambridge, Mass., August, 2005, Biogen Idec.

SUGGESTED READING

Fowler JS, Wolf AP: The synthesis of carbon-11, fluorine-18 and nitrogen-13 labeled radiotracers for biomedical applications. In *Nuclear science series: nuclear medicine*, Washington, DC, 1982, Technical Information Center, U.S. Department of Energy.

Kilbourn MR: Fluorine-18 labeling of radiopharmaceuticals. In *Nuclear science series, nuclear medicine*, Washington, DC, 1990, National Academy Press.

Kowalsky RJ, Falen SW: *Radiopharmaceuticals in nuclear pharmacy and nuclear medicine*, Washington, DC, 2004, American Pharmacists Association.

Krenning EP, Bakker WH, Kooij PPM, et al: Somatostatin receptor scintigraphy with indium-111-DTPA-D-phe1-octreotide in man: metabolism, dosimetry and comparison with iodine-123-tyr-octreotide. *J Nucl Med* 33:652, 1992.

Rydberg J, Liljenzin JO, Choppin G: *Radiochemistry and nuclear chemistry*, ed 3, Oxford, England, 2001, Butterworth-Heinemann.

Saha GB: *Fundamentals of nuclear pharmacy*, New York, 2004, Springer-Verlag.

Steigman J, Eckelman WC: Chemistry of technetium in medicine. In *Nuclear science series, nuclear medicine*, Washington, DC, 1992, National Academy Press.

Swanson DP, Chilton HM, Thrall JH: *Pharmaceuticals in medical imaging*, New York, 1990, Macmillan.

Verbruggen AM: Radiopharmaceuticals: state of the art, *Eur J Nucl Med* 17:346, 1990.

Welch MJ, Kilbourn MR: Positron emitters for imaging. In Freeman L, editor: *Freeman and Johnson's clinical radionuclide imaging*, vol 1, ed 3, Orlando, Fla, 1984, Grune & Stratton.

Radiation Safety in Nuclear Medicine

Peter A. Jenkins, Karen S. Langley

OBJECTIVES

After completing this chapter, the reader will be able to:
- List and define units of radiation, absorbed dose, and dose equivalent.
- Discuss sources of radiation exposure to the general population.
- List the regulatory limits for radiation exposure.
- Define ALARA and detail a comprehensive ALARA program for nuclear medicine.
- Discuss patient radiation exposure and describe exposure to critical organs (with examples).
- Explain the appropriate use of ionization chamber detectors.
- Use Geiger counters and scintillation detectors for laboratory surveys and decontamination procedures.

- Describe the appropriate clinical use of the dose calibrator to be in compliance with federal and state regulations.
- Discuss the use of personnel monitoring devices.
- List the criteria for posting warning signs for exposure to radiation.
- Discuss the receipt, disposition, and disposal of radioactive materials and radioactivity.
- Discuss the methods of testing for and controlling radioactive contamination.
- Define the criteria that constitute a misadministration.
- Discuss the necessary precautions when using therapeutic radionuclides.
- Describe the effects of ionizing radiation.

KEY TERMS

absorbed dose
acute radiation sickness syndrome (ARS)
airborne radioactivity area
as low as reasonably achievable (ALARA)
byproduct material
central nervous system (CNS) syndrome
Department of Transportation (DOT)
deterministic effects
disintegrations per minute (dpm)

dose equivalent
effective dose equivalent
efficiency
exposure
gastrointestinal (GI) syndrome
hemopoietic syndrome
high radiation area
International Council on Radiation Protection (ICRP)
medical event
minimum detectable activity (MDA)
National Council on Radiation Protection (NCRP)

Nuclear Regulatory Commission (NRC)
quality management program (QMP)
radiation area
radiation safety committee (RSC)
radiation safety officer (RSO)
restricted area
stochastic effects
very high radiation area
written directive

Definitions and Acronyms

Absorbed dose is the energy deposited in a given mass. The traditional unit of absorbed dose is the rad and for the SI unit it is the Gy. Note that the rad is derived from the unit of energy (erg) and the unit of mass (g) 1 rad = 100 erg/g. Similarly, the Gy is derived from the SI unit for energy (Joule) and the SI unit for mass (kg) 1 Gy = 1 J/kg.

Acute radiation sickness syndrome (ARS) typically refers to systemic dysfunctions that occur as a result of exposure to acute, high-dose radiation. The most often referred to ARS (and the threshold for symptoms) include:

Transient Phase	0 to 100 rad
Hemopoietic	100 to 800 rad
Gastrointestinal	800 to 3000 rad
Central Nervous System	>3000 rad
Lethal Dose$_{50/60}$	400 to 600 rad (with no medical intervention)

Airborne radioactivity area is a room, enclosure, or area in which airborne radioactive materials, composed wholly or partly of licensed material, exist in concentrations (1) in excess of the derived air concentrations (DACs) specified in Appendix B, of 10 CFR 20.1001–20.2401,* or (2) to such a degree that an individual present in the area without respiratory protective equipment could exceed, during the hours an individual is present in a week, an intake of 0.6% of the annual limit on intake (ALI) or 12 DAC-hours (10 CFR 20).*

As low as reasonably achievable (ALARA) means making every reasonable effort to maintain exposures to radiation as far below the dose limits in this part as is practical and consistent with the purpose for which the licensed activity is undertaken, taking into account the state of technology, the economics of improvements in relation to state of technology, the economics of improvements in relation to benefits to the public health and safety, and other societal and socioeconomic considerations, and in relation to utilization of nuclear energy and licensed materials in the public interest.*

Byproduct material is radioactive material (except special nuclear material) yielded in or made radioactive by exposure to the radiation incident to the process of producing or using special nuclear material.*

Central nervous system (CNS) syndrome follows a wholebody dose over 3000 rad (30 Gy). CNS disorder affects the entire CNS. Immediate signs and symptoms will include convulsions, ataxia, tremor, and lethargy. Because onset of manifest illness is very rapid, symptoms of other ARS may be observed only for individuals not receiving lethal dose.

Counts per minute (cpm) is a unit of undefined radiation quantification. It is not corrected for radiation type or detector efficiency and is typically used for general survey meters (e.g., GM detector).

Department of Transportation (DOT) governs the use of the nation's transportation systems. Included in these regulations are rules defining radioactive materials and prescribing authorized modes for their transport.

Deterministic effects, or nonstochastic effects, are effects that are understood to occur when dose reaches a given threshold or amount. The severity of effect varies with the dose. Examples are skin erythema and cataract formation.

Disintegrations per minute (dpm) is a unit of radiation quantification that accounts for detector efficiency: dpm = cpm/ efficiency.

Dose equivalent (H_T) means the product of the absorbed dose in tissue, quality factor, and all other necessary modifying factors at the location of interest. The units of dose equivalent are the rem and sievert (Sv).*

Effective dose equivalent (H_E) is the sum of the products of the dose equivalent to the organ or tissue (H_T) and the weighting factors (W_T) applicable to each of the body organs or tissues that are irradiated ($H_E = \Sigma W_T H_T$).*

Efficiency for a detector is dependant on the detector properties and on the details of the counting geometry. Typically, efficiency refers to the *absolute* efficiency of the detector system. Efficiency is calculated by: E = number of pulses recorded/number of radiation quanta emitted by source.†

Exposure is specifically defined as the amount of charge liberated in air from interactions with x-rays or gamma radiation, 0 to 3 MeV. The unit of exposure is the roentgen (R). 1 R = 2.58 × 10^{-4} C/kg.

---

*U.S. Nuclear Regulatory Commission: *Title 10, Code of Federal Regulations,* Part 20, Standards for protection against radiation, Washington, DC, 2005, U.S. Nuclear Regulatory Commission.
†U.S. Nuclear Regulatory Commission: Consolidated guidance about materials licenses. In *NUREG-1556, vol 9, Program-specific guidance about medical use licenses,* Washington, DC, 2005, U.S. Nuclear Regulatory Commission.

Continued

Definitions and Acronyms—cont'd

Gastrointestinal (GI) syndrome follows about 800 to 1000 rad (8 to 10 Gy) whole-body irradiation. It includes the hemopoietic symptoms and adds severe nausea, vomiting, and diarrhea very soon after exposure due to the destruction of the intestinal epithelium and the complete destruction of the bone marrow. Vomiting, reduced lymphocyte count, and reduced CNS function occur within 1 to 2 hours of irradiation. Onset of manifest illness will occur 1 to 3 days postirradiation. Mortality is very high and requires aggressive, hospitalized therapy that may last several months.

Hemopoietic syndrome is a systemic illness caused by high dose, acute exposure to ionizing radiation and is exhibited in the blood-forming and respiratory (mucosal) tissues. It appears after a whole-body dose of about 200 rad (2 Gy). Vomiting may occur (5% to 50% of population) 3 to 6 hours postirradiation and will usually subside in less than 24 hours. Manifest illness, which will include moderate to severe leukopenia, occurs from 2 days to 2 weeks postirradiation. Mortality is minimal (200 rad) to low (200 to 600 rad) with aggressive therapy. Hospitalization may range from 45 to 90+ days, depending on dose and other confounding factors.

High radiation area is an area, accessible to individuals, in which radiation levels from radiation sources external to the body could result in an individual receiving a dose equivalent in excess of 0.1 rem (1 mSv) in 1 hour at 30 cm from the radiation source or 30 cm from any surface that the radiation penetrates.*

International Council on Radiation Protection (ICRP) is an advisory body made of representatives from all over the world that issues recommendations and guidance in the areas of radiation protection.

Medical event is defined by the NRC as the administration of byproduct material or radiation from byproduct material that results in any of the following (10 CFR 35.3045)‡:

1. A dose that differs from the prescribed dose or dose that would have resulted from the prescribed dosage by more than 0.05 Sv (5 rem) effective dose equivalent, 0.5 Sv (50 rem) to an organ or tissue, or 0.5 Sv (50 rem) shallow dose equivalent to the skin; and
   a. The total dose delivered differs from the prescribed dose by 20% or more
   b. The total dosage delivered differs from the prescribed dosage by 20% or more or falls outside the prescribed dosage range, or
   c. The fractionated dose delivered differs from the prescribed dose, for a single fraction, by 50% or more
2. A dose that exceeds 0.05 Sv (5 rem) effective dose equivalent, 0.5 Sv (50 rem) to an organ or tissue, or 0.5 Sv (50 rem) shallow dose equivalent to the skin from any of the following:
   a. An administration of a wrong radioactive drug containing byproduct material
   b. An administration of a radioactive drug containing byproduct material by the wrong route of administration
   c. An administration of a dose or dosage to the wrong individual or human research subject
   d. An administration of a dose or dosage delivered by the wrong mode of treatment, or
   e. A leaking sealed source
3. A dose to the skin or an organ or tissue other than the treatment site that exceeds by 0.5 Sv (50 rem) to an organ or tissue and

50% or more of the dose expected from the administration defined in the written directive (excluding, for permanent implants, seeds that were implanted in the correct site but migrated outside the treatment site).

Minimum detectable activity (MDA) is an a priori value used to demonstrate the capability of a detection system. MDA is defined for a discrete number of events in a given time period; however, it is often estimated for survey rate meters. MDA is largely dependant on detection efficiency.

National Council on Radiation Protection (NCRP) is a nonprofit corporation chartered by Congress in 1964 to provide information and recommendations concerning radiation protections to members of the public.

Nuclear Regulatory Commission (NRC) is a federal governing body that has the primary mission of protecting public health and safety and the environment from the effects of radiation from nuclear reactors, materials, and waste facilities. The NRC also regulates nuclear materials and facilities to promote the common defense and security.

Quality management program (QMP) is a program that establishes a set of policies and procedures that ensure proper administration of radiopharmaceuticals to patients. The revision of 10 CFR 35 did not include a reference to QMP but does require procedures for administration that require a written directive. Essentially, the only change from the old QMP program (old 10 CFR 35.32) to the new 10 CFR 35.40‡ is the dropping of the annual program review requirement. However, this annual review is still included as a recommendation.

Radiation area is an area, accessible to individuals, in which radiation levels could result in an individual receiving a dose equivalent in excess of 0.005 rem (0.05 mSv) in 1 hour at 30 cm from the radiation source or from any surface that the radiation penetrates.*

Radiation safety committee (RSC) may be required, based on the type of radioactive material license and the scope and conditions of the license. The purpose of the RSC is to set policy for the entire institution and is responsible for the use of all radioactive materials under specific license conditions. The RSC is made up of individual representatives from specifics areas of radioactive materials use, including management.

Radiation safety officer (RSO) is an individual responsible for the day-to-day operation of an institution's radiation safety program. RSOs must meet minimum training and experience requirements in order to oversee the radiation safety program and comply with the regulatory minimum qualifications.

Restricted area means an area whose access is limited by the licensee for the purpose of protecting individuals against undue risks from exposure to radiation and radioactive materials. Restricted areas do not include areas used as residential quarters, but separate rooms in a residential building may be set apart as restricted areas.*

Stochastic effects are effects that are considered random in nature. For instance, cancer is a stochastic effect of radiation exposure. Typically, stochastic effects are listed as occurrence rates (i.e., 1 in 10,000) or percent increase (i.e., 10% increase lifetime fatal cancer risk). Stochastic effects may be observed in some cells, tissues, organs, or persons, but not others.

‡U.S. Nuclear Regulatory Commission: *Title 10, Code of Federal Regulations*, Part 35, Human uses of byproduct material, Washington, DC, 2005, U.S. Nuclear Regulatory Commission.

Definitions and Acronyms—cont'd

Very high radiation area is an area, accessible to individuals, in which radiation levels from radiation sources external to the body could result in an individual receiving an absorbed dose in excess of 500 rad (5 Gy) in 1 hour at 1 m from a radiation source or 1 m from any surface that the radiation penetrates. NOTE: At very high doses received at high dose rates, units of absorbed dose (e.g., rad and gray)

are appropriate, rather than units of dose equivalent (e.g., rem and sievert).*

Written directive is an authorized user's written order for the administration of byproduct material or radiation from byproduct material to a specific patient or human research subject.‡

RADIATION SAFETY PROGRAM

The radiation safety program is a vital part of any nuclear medicine department that affects all aspects of the department, patients, and employees. Without a comprehensive, viable radiation safety program, nuclear medicine could not be practiced. The program is one of the first things that must be developed when establishing a new department, and without a radiation safety plan, a license to possess radioactive materials cannot be obtained. If the radiation safety program fails, an institution could lose its privilege to use radioactive materials.

The radiation safety program for a nuclear medicine department should be designed to ensure that all radiation regulations are met and to provide efficient procedures for all radiation safety aspects of the nuclear medicine program. In recent years, the **Nuclear Regulatory Commission (NRC)** has adopted a risk-informed, performance-based approach to regulations. In the past, many programs simply adopted procedures considered "best practices." While the NRC does not currently require the adoption of specific procedures, it is advisable to review the procedures presented by the NRC and guidance organizations and use aspects of these recommendations that best fit a specific program. The radiation safety program should provide sufficient detail and guidance to avoid regulatory deficiencies but still allow small variances to allow for a more efficient practice of nuclear medicine.

The safety program should be designed to:

- Ensure safety and control of radioactive materials.
- Control radiation **exposure** in controlled and non-controlled areas.
- Provide adequate general protection.
- Provide exposure monitoring (external and internal).
- Provide adequate radiation safety instrumentation.
- Require and enforce proper training and practices.
- Ensure management involvement.

Procedures and policies should be written in such a manner that they are sufficiently clear to obtain proper performance. The goal is to develop a risk-informed, performance-based program. The radiation safety program is greater than a series of procedures; it must involve everyone likely to be exposed from activities within the department and must include patients and family members, housekeeping staff members, receptionists, maintenance and security personnel, as well as technologists, nurses, and doctors. The program does not need to be a large, complex set of rules and procedures that only a few at an institution can understand, nor does it need to be so simple and vague that no one understands what is expected or needs to be done to meet the requirements.

Things to consider when developing program include:

- Scope of the program
- Auxiliary support (health/medical physics)
- License conditions
- State regulations (may be more strict than NRC regulations)
- Institutional requirements

Personnel Responsible for the Radiation Safety Program

Each employee that uses radioactive material will have a role in the radiation safety program of the institution. The role of each individual will vary from facility to facility and be largely based on the scope and complexity of the radiation safety program. However, the role of the nuclear medicine technologist (NMT) is integral to all aspects of radiation safety. Often, it is the chief NMT who develops, maintains, and enforces the radiation safety program, but all technologists in the department should be involved and understand every aspect of the program. Each technologist must always ensure they follow the program's specific requirements through proper handling techniques, instrument surveys, calibrations, patient name and dose verifications, contamination control, spill response, and effective record-keeping of these processes.

Typically, the radioactive materials license, based on local, state, and federal radiation regulations, will be the primary document that will determine the specific minimum personnel and procedures that will be required for each program. After the license, each institution may have specific policies or procedures that must be followed. These policies and procedures may originate with the institutional administration or the institution may have a **radiation safety committee (RSC)**. It is vital that these are not overlooked. Often they are in place because the scope of radioactive materials use is greater than a single program or department within the institution. The following sections further explain the roles of institutional administration and/or RSC in the use of radioactive materials.

An institution may have an in-house radiation safety group, headed by a **radiation safety officer (RSO)**, who will be involved to lesser or greater extent in the development and maintenance of the radiation safety program. Large institutions, with varied uses of radioactive material for diagnosis, therapy, and research, may have a separate individual who is the RSO whose major responsibility is this program. In smaller institutions, the RSO could be a single physician or a qualified NMT directly running the program. Additionally, an institution may have in-house expertise in the form of health or medical physicists. These individuals are specially trained in radiation physics and its effect and interaction with all living things and are typically very knowledgeable in radiation regulations. The radiation safety group or medical physics group may be able to provide additional support and expertise to meet radiation regulations. They may also offer specialized services that will help meet regulatory requirements for which procedures will need to be developed (e.g., sealed-source leak tests, detector calibrations).

Training within the Radiation Safety Program

The training program in support of the radiation safety program should include every individual who may be involved with the activities of the nuclear medicine department. The primary purpose of any training should be to educate. The training that an individual or group of individuals receives should specifically address their role in the radiation safety program. The radiation safety program may succeed or fail depending on the understanding of those involved in it. Individuals should receive instruction on departmental and institutional policies and procedures as well as the basic principles of radiation protection.

Radiation safety training should be developed specifically for each group of individuals involved with the department adapted to the specific audience. The training may range in detail and length depending on the individuals, or groups of individuals, being trained. Separate training modules should be developed for each target audience and include the information that is most important for that group. Housekeeping staff members may need instruction on when it is appropriate to remove trash from the department, while security personnel may need instruction on **restricted areas** and access privileges to the department. These personnel may also require instruction on sign recognition and meaning, job limitations in restricted areas, restricted area access, inventory security, and basic radiation protections concepts (e.g., time, distance, and shielding).

The training program should address specifically who needs training, what training they will receive, when they will receive the training, and how often refresher training will be required (if at all). The program should also outline what methods of training are acceptable and how understanding of the training will be shown. For some, understanding may be shown by issuing a short quiz, though this is not always required. And, of course, the training program should address the issue of records: what training was given, when it was given, and who attended.

The NRC recommends the following training topics for users of **byproduct material** and ancillary personnel[10]:

Users of byproduct material:

- Basic radiation biology (e.g., interaction of ionizing radiation with cells and tissues)
- Basic radiation protection to include concepts of time, distance, and shielding
- Concept of maintaining exposure **as low as reasonably achievable (ALARA)** (10 CFR 20.1101)[14]
- Risk estimates, including comparison with other health risks
- Posting requirements (10 CFR 20.1902)[14]
- Proper use of personnel dosimetry (when applicable)
- Access control procedures (10 CFR 20.1601, 10 CFR 20.1802)[14]
- Proper use of radiation shielding, if used
- Patient release procedures (10 CFR 35.75)[16]
- Instruction in procedures for notification of the RSO and AU, when responding to patient emergencies or death, to ensure that radiation protection issues are identified and addressed in a timely manner. The intent of these procedures should in no way interfere with or be in lieu of appropriate patient care (10 CFR 19.12, 10 CFR 35.310, 10 CFR 35.410, 10 CFR 35.610)[12,16]
- Occupational dose limits and their significance (10 CFR 20.1201)[14]
- Dose limits to the embryo/fetus, including instruction on declaration of pregnancy (10 CFR 20.1208)[14]
- Workers' right to be informed of occupational radiation exposure (10 CFR 19.13)[12]
- Each individual's obligation to report unsafe conditions to the RSO (10 CFR 19.12)[12]
- Applicable regulations, license conditions, information notices, bulletins, and so on. (10 CFR 19.12)[12]

- Where copies of the applicable regulations, the NRC license, and its application are posted or made available for examination (10 CFR 19.11)[12]
- Proper record-keeping required by NRC regulations (10 CFR 19.12)[12]
- Appropriate surveys to be conducted (10 CFR 20.1501)[14]
- Proper calibration of required survey instruments (10 CFR 20.1501)[14]
- Emergency procedures
- Decontamination and release of facilities and equipment (10 CFR 20.1406, 10 CFR 30.36)[14,15]
- Dose to individual members of the public (10 CFR 20.1301)[14]
- Licensee's operating procedures (e.g., survey requirements, instrument calibration, waste management, sealed-source leak testing) (10 CFR 35.27)[16]

Ancillary personnel:

- Storage, transfer, or use of radiation and/or radioactive material (10 CFR 19.12)[12]
- Potential biological effects associated with exposure to radiation and/or radioactive material, precautions or procedures to minimize exposure, and the purposes and functions of protective devices (e.g., basic radiation protection concepts of time, distance, shielding) (10 CFR 19.12)[12]
- The applicable provisions of NRC regulations and licenses for the protection of personnel from exposure to radiation and/or radioactive material (e.g., posting and labeling of radioactive material) (10 CFR 19.12)[12]
- Responsibility to report promptly to the licensee any condition that may lead to or cause a violation of NRC regulations and licenses or unnecessary exposure to radiation and/or radioactive material (e.g., notification of the RSO regarding radiation protection issues) (10 CFR 19.12)[12]
- Appropriate response to warnings made in the event of any unusual occurrence or malfunction that may involve exposure to radiation and/or radioactive material (10 CFR 19.12)[12]
- Workers may request radiation exposure reports, as per 10 CFR 19.13 (10 CFR 19.12).[12]

Training and Experience Regulations

Training and experience requirements are addressed in 10 CFR 35, starting in section 50 and extend through 999, in association with the types of procedures. Important aspects of the training requirements are the qualifications in the specific type of procedure to be performed as well as the requirement to have knowledge and experience that is directly related to the radiation safety of the procedure performed. Proper credentials include academic training, formal certifications by professional boards recognized by the NRC, and actual experience in the field. The requirements become more prescriptive as the amount of radiation or risk increases. For example, ^{131}I-uptake studies and therapy are addressed separately from other, more general nuclear medicine uptake and imaging procedures and are spelled out with training additional to that required for more routine diagnostic imaging (10 CFR 35.394).[16]

Training is also important when moving from one institution to another. Personnel may have a common background and understanding of the nuclear medicine field, but different locations may have different license conditions or approaches to meeting license conditions for radiation safety. Workers must be made aware of those differences[12]; therefore supplemental training must be given to meet this requirement when new personnel arrive.

Radiation-Monitoring Equipment

The selection of the proper radiation detector is very important when showing compliance with radiation regulations. The use of the wrong detector for a given survey can give false readings and lead to potential problems. When selecting the appropriate instrument, it is vital to consider the type of radiation and the detector **efficiency** for the given detector. For instance, a typical Geiger-Mueller (GM) meter may be fine to detect high energy photons of ^{131}I (depending on desired detection limit), but is typically too insensitive for detecting very small quantities of ^{99m}Tc contamination when an NaI(Tl) detector would be better. When selecting the instruments, consider the type of survey that will be performed, the desired detection limit, the type and energy of the radiation, and the detector efficiency of the detection system. The NRC has given the guidelines in Table 7-1 to use for detector selection.

Radiation detection equipment must be calibrated annually. Calibration typically requires the service of an outside business (often the manufacturer), unless the institution is large enough to have in-house calibration facilities. It is also good practice to perform "daily checks" on the detector systems each day of use to ensure proper function. Daily checks typically involve measuring a known source of activity and ensuring proper response of the meter. A few of the most commonly encountered detection systems for radiation safety purposes in a nuclear medicine department include GM instruments, ionization chamber instruments, scintillation instruments, and well counters.

Geiger-Mueller Instruments. A portable survey meter using a GM tube (Figure 7-1) is most commonly used for area surveys for contamination. The GM tube (see Chapter 3) provides high gas amplification, resulting in an ability to detect individual ionizing events. The GM meter is operated to display the rate at which the individual events are detected, usually using a rate meter,

TABLE 7-1	Typical Survey Instruments			
Detectors	**Radiation**	**Energy Range**		**Efficiency**
Portable Instruments Used for Contamination and Ambient Radiation Surveys				
Exposure rate meters Count rate meters	Gamma, x-ray	mR-R		N/A
Geiger-Mueller	Alpha	All energies (dependent on window thickness)		Moderate
	Beta	All energies (dependent on window thickness)		Moderate
	Gamma	All energies		<1%
NaI scintillator	Gamma	All energies (dependent on crystal thickness)		Moderate
Plastic scintillator	Beta	C-14 or higher (dependent on window thickness)		Moderate
Stationary Instruments Used to Measure Wipe, Bioassay, and Effluent Samples				
Liquid scintillation counter	Alpha	All energies		High
	Beta	All energies		High
	Gamma			Moderate
Gamma counter (NaI)	Gamma	All energies		High
Gas proportional	Alpha	All energies		High
	Beta	All energies		Moderate
	Gamma	All energies		<1%

From U.S. Nuclear Regulatory Commission: Consolidated guidance about materials licenses. In *NUREG-1556, vol 11, Program-specific guidance about licenses of broad scope*, Washington, DC, 1999, U.S. Nuclear Regulatory Commission.

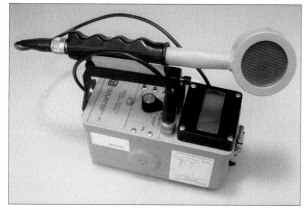

FIGURE 7-1 A Geiger-Muller tube used as a portable survey meter to survey for contamination.

which is calibrated in counts per minute (cpm). This simplicity of design results in an instrument that is inexpensive and reliable.

A typical GM probe consists of a gas-filled tube with a metal housing. Usually, one section of the housing is replaced with a thin window, such as mica, which is covered with a removable cap, often plastic. With the cap removed, all except the lowest energy beta particles (e.g., ^{3}H) are able to penetrate the thin window and are readily detected. With the cap in place, only higher-energy beta particles and x-rays and gamma rays penetrate. Another commonly encountered GM detector is the compensated GM detector. A compensated GM is usually constructed with a GM tube surrounded by a tissue-equivalent plastic. This compensating shield "flattens" out the energy response of the GM tube and allows for a wider range of use.

A GM meter is not the best instrument for measuring exposure rates, though it is often used in nuclear medicine labs because it is inexpensive. Geiger-Mueller meters are often energy-dependent and also have a large dead time, resulting in significant loss at high count rates. However, it is possible, though not ideal, to calibrate a GM meter in mR/hr with a calibration source of energy comparable to the energy of radiations that will be monitored, though a compensated GM is better suited for exposure-rate readings. The unit must be calibrated at least annually and in accordance with license requirements. The meter reading of a check source is measured and a label with this reading is attached to the meter. Each time the meter is used, the current count rate is compared to the value established at calibration to ensure proper function.

The use of detectors is in some respects based on the detector efficiency. Geiger-Mueller meters have very low efficiency for photons of the energy encountered in nuclear medicine but are often used, however, because of the low cost and ease of use. However, before using the GM meter to perform exposure-rate surveys, a thorough analysis of limitations and acceptable uses should be performed. Similarly, before a GM meter is used for contamination surveys, a thorough analysis of the efficiency for the particular radionuclide should also be done.

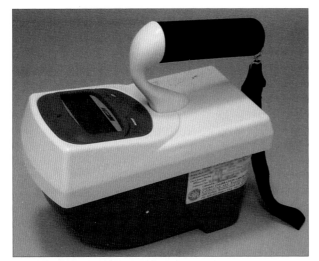

FIGURE 7-2 An ionization chamber is used to measure high exposure rates and is used for large sources of radioactivity and measures in mR/hr.

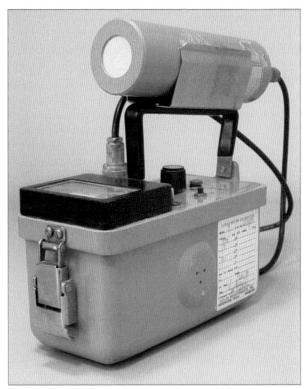

FIGURE 7-3 Thin-crystal end-window NaI(Tl) detectors are used to survey for low-energy materials, sources, and contamination. They are typically more efficient for detection of ^{99m}Tc and ^{125}I contamination than a Geiger-Mueller detector.

Ionization Chamber Instruments. Survey instruments operated in the ionization region of the gas amplification curve are designed to measure radiation exposure or exposure rate. These instruments operate in the current mode rather than pulse mode, and so require the detection of a large number of events. Ion chambers are unable to detect very small amounts of activity such as those associated with contamination. Adequate sensitivity for low exposure levels is obtained by using a rather large air-filled chamber. Ionization survey meters (Figure 7-2) may be used to measure high exposure rates accurately and should be used when surveying a large source of radioactivity, such as a generator or a patient treated with a therapeutic amount of radioactive iodine.

A portable ionization chamber may have a removable cap. This allows detection of the presence of higher-energy beta particles, such as those from ^{32}P or ^{89}Sr. The concept of exposure is defined only for x-rays and gamma rays, however, so a measurement of beta-particle intensity is not possible.

Scintillation Instruments. Scintillation detectors (Figures 7-3 and 7-4) using a sodium iodide (NaI) crystal are used not only as portable devices but also as fixed devices, such as well counters. In portable devices, a probe consisting of a crystal and photomultiplier tube (PMT) is connected to electronics similar to that found with a GM tube. The high sensitivity of the scintillation detector makes it particularly useful for detecting very low levels of activity. For quantitative measurements, however, it is necessary to calibrate the detector with the radionuclide of interest and also to use the same geometry. A system such as this may be used, for example, in checking the thyroid of personnel who have cared for ^{131}I-therapy patients. As a survey instrument, thin-window NaI(Tl) detectors are often the detector of choice for gamma-emitting radionuclides in the

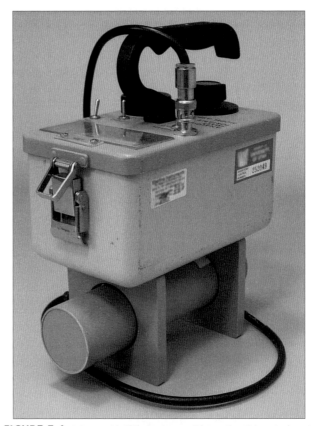

FIGURE 7-4 A larger NaI(Tl) detector without the thin window is more efficient at detecting higher-energy gamma emissions such as those from ^{131}I or ^{137}Cs than the thinner crystal with thin end window.

diagnostic energy region. Closed-window (no window, only aluminum crystal housing) detectors are often the choice for high-energy, gamma-emitting radionuclides (e.g., ^{137}Cs, ^{60}Co).

Well Counter. A sodium iodide well counter is used for determination of radioactivity, usually in **disintegrations per minute (dpm)**, from wipe tests and leak tests. As described in Chapter 3, the well counter may be used to accurately measure very small amounts of radioactivity. Routine quality control of the well counter should also include daily calibration with a standard, usually ^{137}Cs. The gain or high voltage at which proper calibration occurs should be recorded. A 1-minute count at a fixed window width should also be recorded. This allows monitoring for any drift in the system. A check of the full-width-at-half-maximum (FWHM) of the ^{137}Cs photopeak should be obtained monthly. Spread in the photopeak may be indicative, among other possibilities, of degradation of the crystal. (See Chapter 3 for additional discussion of testing.)

Detection Efficiency

Detection efficiency, or sensitivity, is a vital concept to understand in order to comply with radiation regulations. For instance, sealed-source leak-test surveys must be able to detect at least 185 Bq (5 nCi) of activity. If the incorrect detector is used to perform the test and the sensitivity is greater than what is required, the negative survey results may lead to the assumption that the source is not leaking, when in fact it may be.

The efficiency, or sensitivity, of a detector is dependant on many factors. The type of detector (e.g., GM, NaI scintillation, plastic scintillation, proportional), the detector size and shape (larger areas and volumes are more sensitive), the distance from the detector to the radioactive material (geometry), the type of radiation being measured (alpha, beta, and gamma radiation), the energy of the measured radiation, and other aspects of a detector all determine its efficiency.

Often times, when detector sensitivity is discussed, it refers to the absolute efficiency of the detector. Absolute efficiency is simply defined as the number of counts observed by the detector divided by the number of quanta emitted from the radioactive source[6]:

$$E = \frac{\text{number of pulses recorded}}{\text{number of radiation quanta emitted}}$$

Efficiency can be presented in any units that are convenient to the specific application. Common efficiency units are cpm/dpm.

Once the efficiency for a detector (and geometry) is known, it can be determined whether or not a detector is capable of detecting radioactivity at the level given in the regulation. **Minimum detectable activity (MDA)** is an a priori value used to demonstrate the capability of

a detection system, and it is calculated with the following formula:

$$\text{MDA} = \frac{2.71 + 4.66\sqrt{\text{bkg}}}{E \times t}$$

where

bkg = the observed background
E = the detector efficiency (in cpm/dpm)
t = the count time (in seconds)
MDA has units of activity (Bq, pCi, etc.)

Minimum detectable activity is defined for a discrete number of events in a given time period; however, it is often estimated for survey rate meters. One approximation of MDA for survey meters is

$$\text{MDA}\left(\frac{\text{dpm}}{100\ \text{cm}^2}\right) = \frac{2.71 + 4.65\sqrt{(R_b)(2T)}}{(2T)(E)\left(\frac{A}{100}\right)}$$

where

R_b = background count rate (in cpm)
T = counting instrument time constant (in minutes)
E = detector efficiency (in cpm/dpm)
A = probe area in cm^2

Example:
Leak-test surveys were performed on a sealed source. The detection system must be able to detect at least 185 Bq. The well-counting system available has a detection efficiency of 0.02 cpm/dpm (2%) for the radionuclide of concern. Assuming the wipe is counted for 30 seconds, and a 1-minute background count yielded 50 counts (this example will use bkg = 25, because 50 counts in 1 minute is 25 counts in 0.5 minutes), is the system adequate to meet regulatory requirements?

$$\text{MDA} = \frac{2.71 + 4.65\sqrt{25}}{0.02 \times 30\ \text{s}} = 43.3\ \text{dps}$$

Because the MDA is less than the required detection limit, this detection system is adequate for the purpose of counting leak tests for the given radionuclide.

Care must be taken to ensure that the detection system is capable of meeting MDA for all radionuclides in inventory. Note that the only factor in the MDA that can be easily manipulated is the count time. By increasing the count time, the MDA is lowered. For example, if the efficiency was 0.002 and the background was 200, what would be the MDA for a 30-second count?

$$\text{MDA} = \frac{2.71 + 4.65\sqrt{100}}{0.002 \times 30\text{s}} = 820\ \text{dps}$$

In this situation, the detection system would be inadequate to count the wipes from the test. However, if the amount of time to count the samples can be determined, the MDA of the regulations can still be met and the cost of new equipment can be avoided. Solving the MDA equation for time results in:

$$t = \frac{2.71 + 4.65\sqrt{bkg}}{E \times MDA}$$

This equation shows that MDA of 185 Bq (with a detection efficiency of 0.002 cpm/dpm and a background of 100 cpm) can be met if the sample is counted for 133 seconds. It is good practice to count longer than is necessary to meet MDA because the MDA is not actually the amount of activity that is detectable (see *Committee to Assess Health Risks from Exposure to Low Levels of Ionizing Radiation* under Suggested Reading for a complete MDA discussion).

Annual Dose Limits

The purpose for survey instrumentation and exposure monitoring is to ensure that exposures to the occupational worker, patient, public, and the environment are within the required limits and ALARA. The annual dose limits are found in 10 CFR 20.1201 and are summarized in Box 7-1. These limits represent the combined dose from both external as well as internal exposures.

BOX 7-1 | Dose Limits per 10 CFR 20

Public
100 mrem (0.100 mSv) effective dose equivalent
500 mrem (0.500) effective dose equivalent for a preapproved exposure related to a medical procedure. Note that this must be preapproved and justified.

Occupational
1. An annual limit, which is the more limiting of
   a. The total effective dose equivalent being equal to 5 rems (0.05 Sv); or
   b. The sum of the deep dose equivalent and the committed dose equivalent to any individual organ or tissue other than the lens of the eye being equal to 50 rems (0.5 Sv).
2. The annual limits to the lens of the eye, to the skin of the whole body, and to the skin of the extremities, which are
   a. A lens dose equivalent of 15 rems (0.15 Sv), and
   b. A shallow dose equivalent of 50 rem (0.5 Sv) to the skin of the whole body or to the skin of any extremity.
   Minors are limited to 10% of the occupational limit.

Pregnant Occupational
50 mrem per month, 500 mrem over gestation period.

From U.S. Nuclear Regulatory Commission: *Title 10, Code of federal regulations*, Part 19, Notices, instructions and reports to workers—inspection and investigations, Washington, DC, 2005, U.S. Nuclear Regulatory Commission.

Exposure Monitoring

Personnel who are working in areas where there is a reasonable likelihood of receiving a measurable exposure to radiation should be issued personnel dosimeters. The conditions of the radioactive materials regulations require that dosimeters be issued to personnel who could receive in excess of 10% of the occupational limit[16] (i.e., 500 mrem/yr). Many workers are unlikely to receive such a radiation exposure but should be monitored to demonstrate compliance with institutional ALARA goals, to provide useful information to employees regarding their working environment, and to provide data for the RSO to assess any changes in the working environment.

As the primary means of exposure monitoring, workers are often issued a whole-body dosimeter that is worn on the body between the neck and the waist. Whole-body badges are usually exchanged monthly, bimonthly, or quarterly, though more or less frequent cycles are possible. In addition to the whole-body badge, monitors for the hands are issued to workers handling radioactive materials. Ring badges containing a thermoluminescence dosimeter (TLD) chip are often used for this. The ring badge is worn with the sensitive material facing toward the palm of the hand, on the hand that is likely to receive the highest exposure. Furthermore, the ring badge is worn under protective gloves to prevent accidental contamination of the ring that does not reflect exposure to the skin and hand.

Photographic film, TLDs, and optically stimulated laser (OSL) dosimeters are the most common options for personnel dosimeters. These materials satisfy the requirement for permanent exposure record when used in conjunction with vendor-supplied reporting. Each one of these, when used as whole-body dosimeter, has a series of filters that attenuate the radiation and assist in determining the energy and quantity of the radiation accumulated, and from this the exposure is translated to dose. When TLDs are used as ring badges, they do not usually have these filters, and other assumptions have to be made to estimate the dose. The film badge darkens with the energy deposited and is then developed and the density assessed. The TLD and OSL badge stores the energy in matrices in the TLD materials, which release the energy by application of heat or laser light when processed. The amount of energy is then related back to the amount of radiation. They are all sensitive to high temperatures as well as radiation. Therefore it is important to leave them in a controlled low background area when not in use. Do not leave them in such places as the dashboard of a vehicle.

Pocket ionization chambers (Figure 7-5) and digital pocket dosimeters are detectors that are more active than the passive dosimeters listed previously. They can be read while being used to see what exposure is accumulating. This is handy in a radiation field where an individual

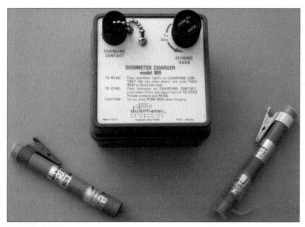

FIGURE 7-5 Pocket ionization chambers, seen as pencil-sized cylinders, are portable ion chambers. The pocket dosimeters are charged and reset to zero exposure setting while on the charger (seen in the center). Dosimeter may be read by looking through the lens in the end of the dosimeter to see the accumulated amount on the scale at any time.

TABLE 7-2	NRC ALARA Investigation Levels	
Part of Body	Investigational Level I (mrem/yr)	Investigational Level II (mrem/yr)
Whole body; head; trunk including male gonads; arms above the elbow; or legs above the knee	500 (5 mSv)	1500 (15 mSv)
Hands; elbows; arms below the elbow; feet; knee; leg below the knee; or skin	5000 (50 mSv)	15,000 (150 mSv)
Lens of the eye	1500 (15 mSv)	4500 (45 mSv)

ALARA, As low as reasonably achievable; *NRC*, Nuclear Regulatory Commission.
From U.S. Nuclear Regulatory Commission: Consolidated guidance about materials licenses. In *NUREG-1556, vol 9, rev 1, Program-specific guidance about medical use licenses,* Washington, DC, 2005, U.S. Nuclear Regulatory Commission.

needs to monitor the total exposure. The pocket ionization detector is a simple electrometer and can be damaged if dropped or discharged by static electricity. The digital pocket dosimeters look like pagers and can be read while they are worn. They are not, however, considered a permanent record and are better used as a supplement to managing occupational dose in higher radiation environments.

The reports that provide the results of personnel monitoring should be reviewed and initialled when received by the RSO. Any unusual exposure or exposure exceeding the applicable ALARA limit (Table 7-2) should be promptly investigated. If the exposure exceeds ALARA Level I, it is necessary to evaluate the cause. If the exposure exceeds ALARA Level II, the employee must be notified in writing and an explanation must be generated and corrective action proposed. A summary report of personnel monitoring, giving any Level I or II exposures, should be included in the quarterly RSC meeting. Depending on the size of the institution, either the original or a duplicate report should be posted for personnel to review and initial. Records of personnel monitoring must be maintained as permanent records.

For the pregnant worker, other conditions may exist. As soon as a worker learns she is pregnant, she should notify her supervisor and the RSO. The pregnant employee should read the information on the risks of radiation in pregnancy as contained in U.S. Nuclear Regulatory Commission (NRC) Regulatory Guide 8.13, *Instruction Concerning Prenatal Radiation Exposure, Rev. 3, 1999.* As a "declared pregnant worker," she will be asked to sign a statement that she is pregnant and has been informed of the risks. The exposure limits are 500 mrem to the fetus during gestation. This is monitored by a separate badge, which should be worn at the abdomen. To provide quicker feedback on exposure, this badge may be exchanged more frequently than the whole-body badge. Mutually agreed-on work restrictions may be in effect for a pregnant employee. Unless the worker's exposure will exceed 50 mrem/mo in a particular job, these restrictions should not affect the worker's choice of job assignments, particularly those that may result in financial gain (e.g., on call). The employer must, however, provide the pregnant employee with opportunities for work in situations that are likely to result in lower exposures. The worker may also choose not to declare pregnancy, in which case none of these conditions are in effect.

In addition to the monitoring that provides a permanent record, pocket dosimeters are useful in situations where there is the possibility for high exposure in a relatively short period. For example, the pregnant technologist working on call should be able to obtain immediate exposure information, allowing for a change in working conditions if necessary. These monitors, however, do not provide the permanent record required by regulatory agencies.

In addition to external exposure monitoring, internal monitoring of radionuclides, from inhalation or ingestions, must also be considered. If the dose from internally deposited radionuclides is likely to contribute more than 10% of the annual dose limit, a regular internal monitoring program must be instituted. This typically requires knowledge of the airborne concentration, which may not be easily determined, as well as the labeling of the radionuclide in the body. Without a simple method to continuously monitor airborne concentrations and specific biokinetics, internal assessment has traditionally been addressed by demonstrating that there has been no uptake. This is determined by performing bioassays of those individuals handling large quantities of dispersible material at certain time intervals such that any significant amount of internally deposited radionuclide would be detected. Negative bioassay results at the given time intervals has been considered an acceptable method to demonstrate compliance with internal dose regulations without measuring airborne concentrations. In nuclear medicine the only practice routinely requiring bioassays is the handling of high-activity therapeutic amounts of ^{131}I sodium iodide.

Typical bioassay procedures state that personnel who handle therapeutic quantities of unsealed radioactive sodium iodide or who are in the room during patient administration of these amounts must have a thyroid bioassay between 6 and 72 hours following involvement. Personnel handling smaller therapeutic amounts of radioactivity, such as for hyperthyroid treatments or when handling encapsulated material, need less frequent bioassays. However, a consistent policy with a 6- to 72-hour time frame helps prevent forgotten bioassays. The bioassay is performed by taking a count of the level of the thyroid in a manner analogous to a thyroid uptake. Care should be taken to ensure that count times and geometry are sufficient to ensure that the MDA is less than the required trigger limit. If an amount of radioiodine greater than a specified trigger limit is detected, follow-up actions are required. The radioiodine procedures are reviewed to determine the cause. The employee is usually restricted from further iodine work until the activity has decreased to an acceptable level.

The contribution of the internal **dose equivalent** due to internal uptake must also be added to the individual's external dose. This may be done by contacting the whole-body badge supplier and requesting that the calculated dose be added to the individual's record. Negative findings do not require that any correction to the monitoring record be made.

Material Inventory and Accountability

Material accountability should be one of the main areas of focus for every radiation safety program. The loss of control of material may be grounds for license suspension, which would effectively shut down a nuclear medicine program. That being said, material inventory should become part of daily procedures and record-keeping. Simple, well-designed control measures will go a long way to ensure accountability is maintained. Policies and procedures should cover all aspects of material handling from the time of order to the time of disposal.

Ordering of materials should be done only by authorized users or their designee. It is often a good idea to control the number of individuals who are authorized to order radioactive materials to minimize incorrect orders or to avoid missed orders. Materials should be ordered only from properly authorized vendors. Procedures for ordering materials should be established that will address deliveries during normal business hours and after hours.

Records of ordering and receipt should include authorized user, radionuclide, physical/chemical form, activity, and supplier.

The **U.S. Department of Transportation (DOT)** determines the labeling and packaging requirements. The labeling for radioactive materials is distinctive and designed to give some important basic information. Unless the shipment is exempt, there will be a package label of a Radioactive White I, Yellow II, or Yellow III, which communicates the general level of exposure from the package. On the label is also marked the transportation index (TI) information, which is a unitless number that communicates the degree of control to be exercised when handling the package and is equal to the mrem/hr at 1 m (Figure 7-6 and Table 7-3).

Certain packages of radioactive material require special receipt procedures. For these packages (see 10 CFR 71[17] for a complete list of criteria), external radiation and surface contamination levels must be verified within 3 hours of receipt if delivered during normal working hours, or within the first 3 hours of the next work day if delivered after-hours. Packages should be inspected for leakage, damage, and correct radionuclide and quantity before accepting delivery.

Once material has been properly received, it must be inventoried. Typically, computer databases are used to help departments keep track of materials and quantities on hand. It is extremely important to keep good records of all materials to ensure that sources are not inadvertently lost (e.g., disposed, stolen, misplaced) or possession limits exceeded. Inventory records should include

TABLE 7-3	Transport Index	
Transport Index	Maximum Radiation Level at any Point on the External Surface	Label Category
0	Less than or equal to 0.005 mSv/hr (0.5 mrem/hr)	WHITE I
More than 0, but not more than 1	Greater than 0.005 mSv/hr (0.5 mrem/hr) but less than or equal to 0.5 mSv/hr (50 mrem/hr)	YELLOW II
More than 1, but not more than 10	Greater than 0.5 mSv/hr (50 mrem/hr) but less than or equal to 2 mSv/hr (200 mrem/hr)	YELLOW-III
More than 10	Greater than 2 mSv (200 mrem) but less than or equal to 10 mSv/hr (1000 mrem/hr)	YELLOW III (Must be shipped under exclusive use provisions; see 49 CFR 173.441(b))

From U.S. Department of Transportation: *Title 49, Code of Federal Regulations,* Parts 172.403, Pipeline and hazardous materials safety administration, Washington, DC, 2005, U.S. Department of Transportation

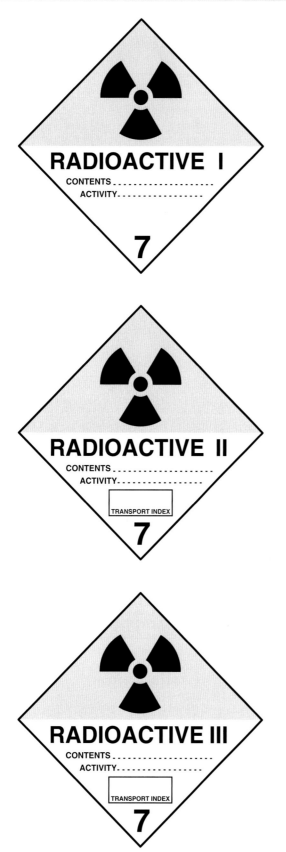

FIGURE 7-6 Transportation labels for radioactive materials: White I label, Yellow II label and Yellow III label. The number (I, II, or III) indicates the relative level of exposure from the radioactive package.

records of receipt, transfer, and disposal. Regular, periodic physical inventories should be conducted to account for all licensed material. Semiannual physical inventories of sealed sources are required. It is often good practice to perform these inventories on a more frequent basis, especially for programs that store or seldom use some sealed sources in inventory.

All sealed sources must be properly labeled and stored in a secure location. If the storage location conceals the source (e.g., in a cupboard or refrigerator), the outside of the storage place must also be clearly marked. Semiannual leak tests of the sealed sources must also be completed per 10 CFR 35.67. A leak test consists of wiping the surface of the source (except open-face sources) with a filter or other type paper. The wipe is then counted on an appropriate instrument, usually a well counter, to determine if any activity is leaking from the source. It is a good practice to do these leak tests at regular intervals along with physical inventory. If a source is found to be leaking, a report must be filed with the NRC within 5 days, as described in 10 CFR 35.3067.

Safe-Use Guidelines

Safe-use guidelines typically imply methods to reduce exposure and the spread of contamination. The most often discussed dose-reduction methods include time, distance, and shielding. Simply put, the less time a person is around a radiation source, the lower the exposure; the more distance between a person and a radiation source, the lower the exposure; and the more shielding between a person and a radiation source, the lower the exposure.

Time. Instinctively it is easy to understand that the more time spent around a radiation source, the larger the exposure will be, and the less time around the source, the lower the exposure. However, when determining the appropriate amount of time to spend around a patient who has been administered radioactive material, it is important to consider the effect on work performance, patient and visitor perception, and actual exposure rate from the patient. It may be appropriate to consider the use of shielding and distance in order to maximize the amount of time spent with a patient. Safe-use guidelines and the ALARA principle underline the need to minimize exposure, but it may not always be practical to simply reduce the amount of time spent around a radioactive source.

Distance. When dealing with point sources of radiation, the exposure is rate proportional to the inverse-square of the distance ($1/d^2$). For instance, assume the exposure rate at 1 m is X mR/hr. By changing the distance to 2 m, the exposure is cut to $\frac{1}{4}$: $X/2^2 = X/4$. Though typical patients who are administered with radioactive material do not resemble a point source, it is a good approximation for laboratory syringes.

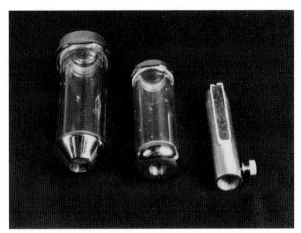

FIGURE 7-7 Syringe shields used for dose preparation and administration.

TABLE 7-4	Transmission Factors per Number HVL	
Number HVL	**Transmission Factor (= $\frac{1}{2}^N$)**
0	1
1	0.5
2	0.25
3	0.125
4	0.0625
5	0.03125
6	0.015625
7	0.0078125
8	0.00390625
9	0.001953125
10	0.000976563

Shielding. Shielding of the correct density, material, and thickness can be the most effective means to reduce radiation exposure in a nuclear medicine laboratory. For instance, the greatest exposure to the technologist occurs during the administration of radioactive materials. The simple practice of using syringe shields (Figure 7-7) and transport shields will greatly reduce exposure; however, not all shields are appropriate. For instance, many believe that lead aprons used in diagnostic x-ray procedures are an effective tool for reducing exposure from radiopharmaceuticals. Lead aprons often are constructed of many different materials; none of them are actually lead. These aprons are designed for protection at specific photon energies. The photon energies encountered in the nuclear medicine environment are many times larger than those in diagnostic x-ray. For this reason, lead aprons are not an effective shielding tool in nuclear medicine.

It is convenient to discuss shielding needs in numbers of half-value layers (HVLs). (Chapter 2 discussed the derivation of HVLs.) Recall that an HVL is the amount of material needed to reduce the radiation intensity by one half. It is a function of material composition, density, radiation type, and energy. Table 7-4 lists the transmission factor for different number of HVLs. Keep in mind that HVL is a function of energy, material, and density. Tables of HVLs as a function of energy, material, and density are commonly available.

Contamination Control. Radioactive contamination is radioactive material where it is not wanted. Contamination control is usually very simple to achieve through simple practices of good housekeeping and personal hygiene. Most technologists observe universal precautions that will prevent the majority of the spread of contamination onto their person. Proper protective equipment is the first line in controlling the spread of contamination. By frequently changing gloves, washing hands, using secondary containers, and working with materials only in designated areas, most contamination will be contained to the immediate work area. Most often when contamination is found on floors or other work surfaces, it is through carelessness when handling dispersible material. Contamination is typically not an issue in laboratories where individuals practice simple, commonsense principles to keep things clean.

Contamination control procedures should include procedures for marking radioactive work areas, proper laboratory attire, acceptable handling measures and practices, and adequate contamination surveys. Since radioactive material cannot be observed with any of the five human senses, each individual must practice good hygiene and keep work areas clean, and contamination surveys must be performed properly.

Radiation Area Surveys

Regular surveys should be performed to ensure that material handling procedures are adequate, radiation areas are properly posted, and radioactive contamination is not present. There are several surveys that are required to be performed. The most common surveys are exposure-rate surveys, contamination surveys, and sealed-source leak-test surveys. Each survey is required to be performed at a set interval. Surveys must be performed with the proper equipment to ensure that the radiation can be detected at the level given in the regulations.

Exposure-rate surveys are used to quantify the exposure rate in different areas. Surveys must be performed in unrestricted areas to ensure that members of the public are not exposed to dose rates that would contribute more than 100 mrem in 1 year or 2 mrem in 1 hour to any member of the public. Exposure-rate surveys must also ensure that exposure rates to employees do not exceed the limits of the designated areas (i.e., radiation area). Surveys should be performed with an instrument capable of detecting 0.1 mR/hr. Surveys should be performed often enough to ensure that changes in work conditions do not result in unexpected exposures. Daily, weekly, monthly, and quarterly survey periods should be considered for different areas.

Surveys for radioactive contamination must be conducted such that both fixed and removable

TABLE 7-5	Surface Contamination Limits		
Restricted			
Nuclide	**Contamination Level (dpm/100 cm²)**		
^{32}P, ^{58}Co, ^{59}Fe, ^{60}Co, ^{75}Se, ^{85}Sr, ^{90}Y, ^{111}In, ^{123}I, ^{125}I, ^{131}I, ^{153}Sm, ^{169}Yb, ^{177}Lu, ^{198}Au	2000		
^{51}Cr, ^{57}Co, ^{67}Ga, ^{99m}Tc, ^{197}Hg, ^{201}Tl	20,000		
Unrestricted			
Nuclide*	**Average†‡¶**	**Maximum†§¶**	**Removable†‖¶**
^{125}I, ^{126}I, ^{131}I, ^{133}I, ^{90}Sr	1000	3000	200
Beta-gamma emitters, except as noted above	5000	15,000	1000

*Where surface contamination by multiple nuclides exists, the limits established for each nuclide should apply
†As used in this table, dpm is the rate of emission by radioactive material, as determined by correcting the counts per minute (cpm) observed by an appropriate detector for background, efficiency, and geometric factors associated with the instrumentation.
‡Measurements of average contaminant should not be averaged over more than 1 m². For objects of less surface area, the average should be derived for each such object.
§The maximum contamination level applies to an area of not more than 100 cm².
‖The amount of removable radioactive material per 100 cm² of surface area should be determined by wiping that area with filter or soft absorbent paper, applying moderate pressure, and assessing the amount of radioactive material on the wipe with an appropriate instrument of known efficiency. When removable contamination on objects of less surface area is determined, the pertinent levels should be reduced proportionally and the entire surface should be wiped.
¶The average and maximum radiation levels associated with surface contamination resulting from beta-gamma emitters should not exceed 0.2 mrad/hr at 1 cm and 1.0 mrad/hr at 1 cm, respectively, measured through not more than 7 mg/cm² of total absorber.
From U.S. Nuclear Regulatory Commission: Consolidated guidance about materials licenses. In *NUREG-1556, vol 9, rev 1, Program-specific guidance about medical use licenses,* Washington, DC, 2005, U.S. Nuclear Regulatory Commission.

contamination may be identified. Special care must be taken when considering the appropriate instrument to use for performing such surveys. As discussed earlier in this chapter, detector efficiency for each detector and each radionuclide must be determined to ensure that regulatory limits can be met. For instance, a GM meter, operated in count-rate mode, used for fixed contamination surveys of ^{99m}Tc may be inadequate; however, the same detector may be usable in a counting system (i.e., discrete count times). Procedures should reflect the acceptable detection methods for each survey type. Table 7-1 lists some meter selection guidelines. Table 7-5 lists the NRC's recommended contamination levels for restricted and unrestricted areas. However, each lab may adopt the NRC's recommendation or establish lab-specific limits. If lab-specific limits are used, justification must be submitted to the NRC (or agreement state) for approval of limits before their use.

Posting and Labeling

Posting is an integral part of the effort to control unwanted exposures. The information in this section is taken directly from 10 CFR 20.1003 and 10 CFR 20.1902. Areas must be posted to correctly alert or inform personnel that may need to access the area.

a. *Posting of radiation areas.* The licensee shall post in each radiation area a conspicuous sign or signs bearing the radiation symbol and the words "CAUTION, RADIATION AREA." **Radiation area** means an area, accessible to individuals, in which radiation levels could result in an individual receiving a dose equivalent in excess of 0.005 rem (0.05 mSv) in 1 hour at 30 cm from the radiation source or from any surface that the radiation penetrates.

b. *Posting of high radiation areas.* The licensee shall post in each **high radiation area** a conspicuous sign or signs bearing the radiation symbol and the words "CAUTION, HIGH RADIATION AREA" or "DANGER, HIGH RADIATION AREA." High radiation area means an area, accessible to individuals, in which radiation levels from radiation sources external to the body could result in an individual receiving a dose equivalent in excess of 0.1 rem (1 mSv) in 1 hour at 30 cm from the radiation source or 30 cm from any surface that the radiation penetrates.

c. *Posting of very high radiation areas.* The licensee shall post in each **very high radiation area** a conspicuous sign or signs bearing the radiation symbol and words "GRAVE DANGER, VERY HIGH RADIATION AREA." Very high radiation area means an area, accessible to individuals, in which radiation levels from radiation sources external to the body could result in an individual receiving an **absorbed dose** in excess of 500 rad (5 Gy) in 1 hour at 1 m from a radiation source or 1 m from any surface that the radiation penetrates. Note that for very high doses received at high dose rates, units of absorbed dose (e.g., rad and Gy) are appropriate, rather than units of dose equivalent (e.g., rem and sievert).[14]

d. *Posting of airborne radioactivity areas.* The licensee shall post in each **airborne radioactivity area** a conspicuous sign or signs bearing the radiation symbol and the words "CAUTION, AIRBORNE RADIO-ACTIVITY AREA" or "DANGER, AIRBORNE RADIOACTIVITY AREA." Airborne radioactivity area means a room, enclosure, or area in which airborne radioactive materials, composed wholly or partly of licensed material, exist in concentrations (1) in excess of the derived air concentrations (DACs) specified in Appendix B, Sec. 20.1001 to 20.2401, or (2) to such a degree that an individual present in the area without respiratory protective equipment could exceed, during the hours an individual is present in a week, an intake of 0.6% of the annual limit on intake (ALI) or 12 DAC-hours.[14]

e. *Posting of areas or rooms in which licensed material is used or stored.* The licensee shall post, in each area or room in which there is used or stored an amount of licensed material exceeding 10 times the quantity of such material specified in Appendix C to part 20, a conspicuous sign or signs bearing the radiation symbol and the words "CAUTION, RADIOACTIVE MATERIAL(S)" or "DANGER, RADIOACTIVE MATERIAL(S)."

Sign	Intended Use
CAUTION RADIATION AREA	To signify areas in which radioactive material is used or stored in amounts exceeding quantities specified by state and federal regulatory agencies, typically when the quantities exceed 10 times the quantity specified in Appendix C of Part 20 of the NRC regulations.[17]
CAUTION HIGH RADIATION AREA	To signify areas accessible to personnel in which a major portion of the body of a person could receive more than 5 mrem in an hour.
CAUTION AIRBORNE RADIOACTIVITY AREA	To denote areas accessible to personnel in which a major portion of the body of a person could receive a dose in excess of 100 mrem in any 1 hour.
CAUTION RADIOACTIVE MATERIALS	To signify that the airborne activity level in the area may transiently exceed the restricted area limit or may exceed 0.6% of the Annual Limit of Intake (ALI) or 12 DAC hours.

Release of Patients Administered Radioactive Materials

The NRC allows the release of patients who have been administered radioactive material if the exposure from the release of the patient will not exceed 500 mrem to any individual member of the public or the individual's immediate family from the administration of the radioactive materials. There are three different methods that are acceptable to use for determining patient release eligibility: administered activity, measured dose rate, or patient-specific dose calculation. Each method is specifically outlined in the NRC's guidance document: NUREG 1556, Volume 9, Appendix U.[10] When releasing patients, it must first be determined whether the patient should be released based on medical concerns; this will be the decision of the patient's primary caregiver and the nuclear medicine physician. Additionally, the dose to the public and the patient's family must be considered on an individual basis. Table 7-6 lists the activities and the dose rates at which patients may be released.

Depending on the activity administered or the dose rate at 1 m from the patient, the patient may be required to receive written instructions. These instructions include information on minimizing doses to other individuals. If a patient is breast-feeding, additional instructions may be required that provide instructions on the discontinuation or interruption of breast-feeding and the consequences of failing to comply with the recommendation. Table 7-7 lists the activities for which written instructions are required, and Table 7-8 contains the activities for written instructions for patients who are breast-feeding.

Radioactive Waste

The objective of radioactive waste management is to prevent human contact with concentrations of material or radiation levels significantly above background level. Most of the waste material generated in nuclear medicine may be disposed of by holding the material in storage for extensive decay, diluting and dispersing the material to the atmosphere or sanitary sewer system, or returning the spent material to the manufacturer or supplier (10 CFR 20.2001).[14] Rarely, these techniques are inadequate, and materials are concentrated and shipped for land burial. Recommended techniques for safe disposal follow. As with all aspects of nuclear medicine, records of the disposal must be maintained by the department.

Return to Manufacturer or Supplier. Returning waste to the manufacturer or supplier is very useful for long-lived materials found in nuclear medicine. Departments using molybdenum generators may be able to return the old, partially decayed generator to the manufacturer. As part of the purchase of new long-lived sealed ^{57}Co flood source or dose calibrator constancy checks, the old

TABLE 7-6	Activities and Dose Rates for Authorizing Patient Release			
	Activity at or Below Which Patients May Be Released		Dose Rate at 1 m, at or Below Which Patients May Be Released*	
Radionuclide	(GBq)	(mCi)	(mSv/hr)	(mrem/hr)
^{111}Ag	19	520	0.08	8
^{198}Au	3.5	93	0.21	21
^{51}Cr	4.8	130	0.02	2
^{64}Cu	8.4	230	0.27	27
^{67}Cu	14	390	0.22	22
^{67}Ga	8.7	240	0.18	18
^{123}I	6	160	0.26	26
^{125}I	0.25	7	0.01	1
^{125}I implant	0.33	9	0.01	1
^{131}I	1.2	33	0.07	7
^{111}In	2.4	64	0.2	20
^{192}Ir implant	0.074	2	0.008	0.8
^{32}P†	—	—	—	—
^{103}Pd implant	1.5	40	0.03	3
^{186}Re	28	770	0.15	15
^{188}Re	29	790	0.2	20
^{47}Sc	11	310	0.17	17
^{75}Se	0.089	2	0.005	0.5
^{153}Sm	26	700	0.3	30
^{117m}Sn	1.1	29	0.04	4
^{89}Sr†	—	—	—	—
^{99m}Tc	28	760	0.58	58
^{201}Tl	16	430	0.19	19
^{90}Y†	—	—	—	—
^{169}Yb	0.37	10	0.02	2

*If the release is based on the dose rate at 1 m in this column, record of release must be maintained.

†Activity and dose rate limits are not applicable in this case because of the minimal exposures to members of the public resulting from activities normally administered for diagnostic or therapeutic purposes.

Adapted from U.S. Nuclear Regulatory Commission: Consolidated guidance about materials licenses. In *NUREG-1556, vol 9, rev 1, Program-specific guidance about medical use licenses,* Washington, DC, 2005, U.S. Nuclear Regulatory Commission.

source may be exchanged if it was purchased from the same manufacturer. Programs may exist where the contaminated materials used with long-lived materials, such as for ^{89}Sr therapy, may be returned. The specific requirements for such returns must be arranged in advance with the manufacturer or supplier, who will also usually supply the appropriate paperwork, copies of which are maintained by the department.

Dry Waste. Most of the dry waste generated in nuclear medicine consists of items contaminated with radionuclides with relatively short physical half-lives. Radioactive waste with half-lives of 120 days or less may be stored for extensive decay before disposing of the material per 10 CFR 35.92. State and federal regulatory authorities permit the disposal of short-lived radionuclides by decay-in-storage programs. The material is typically held in storage a minimum of 10 half-lives or decayed to a level such that it is not distinguishable from background, and then is carefully monitored with an appropriate survey instrument of good sensitivity. If the survey indicates that the material has decayed to a level not distinguishable from background levels (when measured in a low background area), it may then be transferred to the appropriate regular trash for disposal (e.g., needle containers to biohazard waste). Before disposing of the material, all radiation signs and symbols must be obliterated or defaced. This is most easily and safely accomplished as the item is placed in waste, so that it is not necessary to later go through a waste bag. The radionuclides for which decay is used are usually separated by half-lives to minimize the time shorter half-lived material must be stored and therefore the space required for decay in storage.

Long-lived materials, usually found only in research programs, may require the material to be shipped to a federally approved low-level radioactive material land burial site. Waste materials shipped for disposal must be properly packaged and labeled according to DOT requirements. A number of commercial companies act as brokers in the handling of radioactive waste material destined for either burial or incineration.

Liquid Waste. Small quantities of liquid waste that are either soluble or dispersible in water can be discharged in a designated sink to a sanitary sewer system provided the collective amounts disposed of by this method do not exceed concentrations and annual amounts specified in

TABLE 7-7	Activities and Dose Rates Above Which Instructions Should Be Given When Authorizing Patient Release			
Radionuclide	Activity Above Which Are Required		Dose Rate at 1 m Above Which Instructions Are Required*	
	(GBq)	(mCi)	(mSv/hr)	(mrem/hr)
^{111}Ag	3.8	100	0.02	2
^{198}Au	0.69	19	0.04	4
^{51}Cr	0.96	26	0.004	0.4
^{64}Cu	1.7	45	0.05	5
^{67}Cu	2.9	77	0.04	4
^{67}Ga†	1.7	47	0.04	4
^{123}I†	1.2	33	0.05	5
^{125}I	0.05	1	0.002	0.2
^{125}I implant	0.074	2	0.002	0.2
^{131}I	0.24	7	0.02	2
^{111}In†	0.47	13	0.04	4
^{192}Ir implant	0.011	0.3	0.002	0.2
^{32}P‡	—	—	—	—
^{103}Pd implant	0.3	8	0.007	0.7
^{186}Re	5.7	150	0.03	3
^{188}Re	5.8	160	0.04	4
^{47}Sc	2.3	62	0.03	3
^{75}Se	0.018	0.5	0.001	0.1
^{153}Sm	5.2	140	0.06	6
^{117m}Sn	0.21	6	0.009	0.9
^{89}Sr‡	—	—	—	—
^{99m}Tc	5.6	150	0.12	12
^{201}Tl†	3.1	85	0.04	4
^{90}Y‡	—	—	—	—
^{169}Yb	0.073	2	0.004	0.4

*The activity values were computed based on 1 mSv (0.1 rem) total effective dose equivalent.

†These radionuclides are not byproduct material and are not regulated by the Nuclear Regulatory Commission (NRC). Information is presented for the convenience of readers of this guide, who should be alert to differences that might exist between regulations of the NRC and state requirements for non-NRC regulated material.

‡Activity and dose rate limits are not applicable in this case because of the minimal exposures to members of the public resulting from activities normally administered for diagnostic or therapeutic purposes.

Adapted from U.S. Nuclear Regulatory Commission: Consolidated guidance about materials licenses. In *NUREG-1556, vol 9, rev 1, Program-specific guidance about medical use licenses*, Washington, DC, 2005, U.S. Nuclear Regulatory Commission.

10 CFR 20, Appendix B,[14] and there are no additional restrictions placed on this process by state or local municipalities. The maximum permitted concentrations specified by regulatory authorities are based on the total water discharge rates of the licensee (water discharge rate can generally be assumed to be equal to the water consumption rate; hence water bills provide a record of the licensee's water discharge rates) and the released radioactivity. To demonstrate compliance with the concentration limits, the released concentrations can be averaged over extended periods, such as a month. Records of the date of disposal and the type and amount of radioactivity must be maintained by the department.

Gaseous Waste. Certain gases, principally ^{133}Xe, are often disposed of after their use by discharging them to the atmosphere. This does not apply to unused xenon, which is held for decay. This method of waste disposal is discussed in the Control and Evaluation of Airborne Activity section. An important alternative method of disposing ^{133}Xe is to use activated charcoal to trap the gas after its use. The activated charcoal traps containing the ^{133}Xe are periodically placed in storage for an extended period to permit most of the radioactivity to decay before reuse of the filter. Several precautions are important with this method. Other gases, such as CO_2 and water vapor, compete with the xenon for trapping by the charcoal. Thus the traps can become saturated and ineffective in trapping ^{133}Xe and should be periodically replenished with fresh charcoal.

Section 2005 in Part 20 of Title 10 of the *Code of Federal Regulations* defines a category of waste that can be disposed of without regard to its radioactivity: ^{3}H and ^{14}C in liquid scintillation cocktails or animals that have a concentration less than 185 Bq/g (0.05 mCi/g). This category of waste can be found in many hospitals and universities involved with clinical and biomedical research. It has to be treated only as hazardous waste and can be incinerated as nonradioactive.

TABLE 7-8	Activities That Require Written Instructions and Records for Patients Who Are Breast-Feeding				
	Activity Above Which Instructions Are Required		Activity Above Which a Record Is Required		Examples of Recommended Duration of Interruption of Breast-Feeding*
	(MBq)	(mCi)	(MBq)	(mCi)	
^{131}I NaI	0.01	0.0004	0.07	0.002	Complete cessation (for this infant or child)
^{123}I NaI[†]	20	0.5	100	3	
^{123}I OIH[†]	100	4	700	20	
^{123}I MIBG[†]	70	2	400	10	24 hr for 370 MBq (10 mCi) 12 hr for 150 MBq (4 mCi)
^{125}I OIH	3	0.08	10	0.4	
^{131}I OIH	10	0.3	60	1.5	
^{99m}Tc DTPA	1000	30	6000	150	
^{99m}Tc MAA	50	1.3	200	6.5	12.6 hr for 150 MBq (4 mCi)
^{99m}Tc-pertechnetate	100	3	600	15	24 hr for 1100 MBq (30 mCi) 12 hr for 440 MBq (12 mCi)
^{99m}Tc DISIDA	1000	30	6000	150	
^{99m}Tc glucoheptonate	1000	30	6000	170	
^{99m}Tc MIBI	1000	30	6000	150	
^{99m}Tc MDP	1000	30	6000	150	
^{99m}Tc PYP	900	25	4000	120	
^{99m}Tc red blood cell in vivo labeling	400	10	2000	50	6 hr for 740 MBq (20 mCi)
^{99m}Tc red blood cell in vitro labelling	1000	30	6000	150	
^{99m}Tc sulphur colloid	300	7	1000	35	6 hr for 440 MBq (12 mCi)
^{99m}Tc DTPA aerosol	1000	30	6000	150	
^{99m}Tc MAG3	1000.0	30	6000	150	
^{99m}Tc white blood cells	100	4	600	15	24 hr for 1100 MBq (30 mCi) 12 hr for 440 MBq (12 mCi)
^{67}Ga citrate[†]	1	0.04	7	0.2	1 mo for 150 MBq (4 mCi) 2 wk for 50 MBq (1.3 mCi) 1 wk for 7 MBq (0.2 mCi)
^{51}Cr EDTA	60	1.6	300	8	
^{111}In white blood cells[†]	10	0.2	40	1	1 wk for 20 MBq (0.5 mCi)
^{201}Tl chloride[†]	40	1	200	5	2 wk for 110 MBq (3 mCi)

DISIDA, Di-isopropyliminodiacetic acid; *DTPA,* diethylenetriamine pentaacetic acid; *EDTA,* ethylenediaminetetraacetic acid; *MAA,* macroagregated albumin; *MAG3,* mercaptylacetyltriglycine; *MBIG,* metaiodobenzylguanidine; *MDP,* methyl diphosphonate; *MIBI,* 2-methoxy isobutyl isonitrile; *OIH,* ortho-iodohippurate; *PYP,* pyrophosphate.

*The duration of interruption of breast-feeding is selected to reduce the maximum dose to a newborn to less than 1 mSv (0.1 rem), although the regulatory limit is 5 mSv (0.5 rem). The actual doses that would be received by most infants would be far below 1 mSv (0.1 rem). Of course, the physician may use discretion in the recommendation, increasing or decreasing the duration of interruption.

[†]These radionuclides are not byproduct material. These are now regulated by the Nuclear Regulatory Commission (NRC) based on the Energy Policy Act of 2005 dated August 8, 2005. Information is presented for the convenience of readers of this guide, who should be alert to differences that might still exist between regulations of the NRC and state requirements for the new-NRC regulated material.

Adapted from U.S. Nuclear Regulatory Commission: Consolidated guidance about materials licenses. In *NUREG-1556, vol 9, Program-specific guidance about medical use licenses,* Washington, DC, 2005, U.S. Nuclear Regulatory Commission.

Radioactive Spill Emergency Procedures

With even the most careful attention to radiation safety procedures, it is possible for an accident to occur, usually a spill. The emergency procedures manual would ideally cover all types of potential emergencies, but this is often impractical. At the minimum, the emergency procedures should cover the most likely and the most hazardous type of emergencies. The specific procedures will vary from program to program but will often have many similar procedures. Because many types of emergencies (mostly spills) may include personnel contamination, procedures for handling personnel and area control and decontamination must be posted in any area where unsealed radioactive material is routinely handled. If there is a possibility that a spill could occur, resulting in an immediate room shutdown, the procedure should be posted in more than one location.

A procedure to handle a radioactive spill should include the following:

1. *Clear the area.* Have anyone else in the immediate area move to a more distant location and remain there until checked for contamination. If there is any chance of shoe contamination of these people, have them remove their shoes at a boundary quickly defined as the clean area. If there are non-contaminated personnel present, ask one of them to assist.
2. *Notify a supervisor or the RSO.* The posted form must clearly list current notification numbers.
3. *Contain the spill with absorbent paper.* If the radioactive material is high activity, attempt to shield the source, if this can be done quickly.
4. *Evaluate the severity.* Do this to determine the best way to decontaminate and whether assistance from the radiation safety office should be obtained.
5. *Decontaminate personnel.* Removing and bagging outer clothing, including shoes, will remove most contamination. Skin contamination is removed by gentle washing with tepid water and soap or a commercial decontaminating agent. Do not irritate or abrade the skin, which may cause absorption of the contaminant. Check the effectiveness with a low-range GM survey meter or sodium iodine detector, and continue until the radiation level is at or near background. Residual radioactivity on the hands may be removed by using powder-lined gloves taped at the wrist, causing the radioactivity to be released with sweat.
6. *Decontaminate the spill area.* Use personnel and radiation safety precautions appropriate for the radioactivity and type of radionuclide. For low-activity spills, immediately start using absorbent paper. Work from the outside to the center of the spill. If necessary, wash with small amounts of decontaminant, making sure that the liquid does not spread the contamination. Place all contaminated materials in a plastic bag, label it, and place it in radioactive waste. For high-activity spills with greater possibility for high exposure to personnel, it is reasonable to plan the decontamination procedure before starting, including an assessment of the exposure rate. Depending on the findings, it may be necessary to use more than one person or to allow some time for decay.
7. *Survey.* Use a low-range GM tube. Record the findings, noting the location and reading. When no additional contamination is removable, take wipe tests to confirm successful decontamination. Record these results.
8. *Write up a report.* Describe the accident and steps taken to clean up the spill.

An all too common spill may occur when injecting a patient who is being stressed on a treadmill. The radioactive material often lands on the treadmill and may also land on the patient. In this case, stop the treadmill, have the patient step off (if possible onto a towel or absorbent paper), and contain the radioactivity. Have the patient step out of his or her shoes to a clean area, and decontaminate the skin if necessary. Decontaminate the treadmill as much as possible. If any radioactivity remains, have patients wear booties until no radioactivity is detectable on the treadmill.

Special Consideration for Facilities that Store and Use ^{133}Xe or Other Volatile Materials. The nuclear pharmacy and rooms in which gaseous radioactive material is used should be maintained at a negative pressure with respect to the surrounding areas. Maintaining such an area at negative pressure means that the direction of airflow at the boundaries of the room is into the room. Thus airborne activities generated within the room are removed by the exhaust system that maintains the negative pressure, and the activity should not, to any appreciable extent, passively diffuse into the surrounding nonrestricted areas such as corridors or waiting areas. The exhaust system serving areas in which volatile radioactive materials are used or stored should serve only those areas (a dedicated system), should provide enough ventilation to sufficiently dilute radioactivity released within the room, and should exhaust the radioactivity at release points properly located away from the general population, for example, on the rooftop of the building and away from any air intakes. Measurements should be made to demonstrate that the airflow at the boundaries of such rooms is toward the room, and measurements should be periodically made thereafter, about every 6 months, to show that the situation is unchanged.

It is important to properly store radioactive gases and volatiles. Containers of ^{133}Xe are generally stored in a fume hood so that any inadvertent leakage of activity is routed away from the immediate work area. Optimum storage of ^{131}I sodium iodide solution intended for oral administration involves several considerations. Although the fraction of the vial activity that is gaseous is kept at a low value (about 0.0001 to 0.001) by maintaining it at a basic pH, the volatile fraction can be further reduced by keeping the stored vials refrigerated and in the dark. According to manufacturers of ^{131}I sodium iodide, the basic pH minimizes the labeled I_2 species, whereas reduced temperature assists in controlling the volatile HI component. Also, when preparing the radioactivity for patient administration, it is important to minimize agitation or handling of the vial and to avoid exposure of the contents to bright light.

It is generally recommended that information be posted in imaging rooms in which ^{133}Xe is used that specifies the period of time that the room should be evacuated by personnel following an accidental release of gas within the room. A common criterion used to calculate the evacuation time is to delay reentry until the average concentration of ^{133}Xe in the room has decreased to the occupational limits specified for restricted areas. (This criterion is very conservative, because the airborne activity to which radiation workers are exposed in restricted areas may be averaged over the 520 working hours of a calendar quarter to demonstrate compliance with the specified limit of airborne activity concentration.) Such a calculation employs the volume of room air into which the activity was released and the net ventilation rate of the room. In equation form, the time of evacuation can be expressed as follows:

$$T = (V/Q)\ln(A/CV)$$

where

T is the time of evacuation in minutes
A is the released activity of ^{133}Xe in mCi
V is the room air volume in ml (1 ft^3 = 28,300 ml)
Q is the net ventilation rate of the room in ml/min
C is the airborne activity concentration limit of ^{133}Xe in the air of a restricted area (3×10^{-5} µCi/ml)

Example:
Compute the evacuation time that should be posted in a ^{133}Xe imaging room if the greatest radioactivity used is 30 mCi, the dimensions of the room are 10 ft × 12 ft × 8 ft, and the net ventilation rate of the room is 250 ft^3/ min.

$$T = V/Q\ln 9(A/CV)$$

where

$V = 960$ ft^3 = 2.7×10^7 ml
$Q = 250$ ft^3/min = 7.1×10^6 ml/min
$C = 3 \times 10^{-5}$ µCi/ml
$A = 30$ mCi = 3×10^4 µCi

$$T = \frac{2.71 \times 10^7 \text{ ml}}{7.1 \times 10^6 \text{ ml/min}}$$
$$\frac{3 \times 10^4 \text{ µCi}}{(3 \times 10^{-5} \text{ µCi/ml})(2.7 \times 10^7 \text{ ml})}$$

$T = 3.8 \ln 37$ minutes
$T = 13.7$ minutes

Evaluation of the average concentrations of airborne activity in nonrestricted areas should also be performed and documented. The practice of maintaining rooms in which gaseous activities are used at a negative pressure with respect to the surrounding non-restricted areas helps to ensure that the airborne levels in those areas are at acceptably low values. However, it is prudent to periodically document the low levels by conducting airborne-activity surveys to measure the levels. Such surveys, usually conducted during representative use of the gaseous or volatile radionuclide, permit the evaluation of the peak or worst-case airborne concentration levels. If the measured peak levels are less than the nonrestricted

area concentration limit for a specific radionuclide, there is compliance. If the transient peak levels are significantly higher than the nonrestricted area limit, however, a calculation should be made over an extended time—from a month to a year—to demonstrate that the time-averaged concentration is less than the applicable limit.

A special case is the evaluation of the average concentration at the site where a ventilation system serving a gaseous activity use area, such as a ^{133}Xe imaging room, releases the air to the atmosphere. For the release site to be a nonrestricted area, the average airborne activity of the exhaust must be less than the nonrestricted area limit for the radionuclide under consideration. Calculation of the average concentration requires knowledge of the discharge rate of the exhaust and the activity released from the site in a given period. The following example illustrates such a calculation.

Example:
A room used for ^{133}Xe examinations has a continuously operating ventilation system with a measured discharge rate of 2000 ft^3/min, and it is assumed that all the administered activity for an average patient workload of 12 examinations per week is released from the ventilation exhaust. If the average administered activity is 10 mCi per patient, show that the average concentration at the release point, based on a representative week, is less than the NRC limit for ^{133}Xe in the air of a nonrestricted area, 3×10^{-7} mCi/ml (a useful conversion factor is 28,300 ml/ft^3). The total estimated release of activity per week is:

$$(12 \text{ patients/wk})(10 \text{ mCi/Patient}) = 120 \text{ mCi/wk} = 1.2 \times 10^5 \text{ µCi/wk}$$

The total volume of air released per week is:

$$(2000 \text{ ft}^3/\text{min})(10,080 \text{ min/wk})(28,300 \text{ ml/ft}^3) = 5.7 \times 10^{11} \text{ ml/wk}$$

The average concentration for the week is then:

$$c = \frac{1.2 \times 10^5 \text{ µCi/wk}}{5.7 \times 10^{11} \text{ ml/wk}} = 2.1 \times 10^{-7} \text{ µCi/ml}$$

The computed average in this example represents 70% of the NRC limit. Although such a situation satisfies the commission's regulation, it provides a small margin of safety and does not fulfill the ALARA goal of licensees voluntarily reducing environmental releases to 10% or less of the legal requirements. When results indicate that air concentrations are in excess of the desired level, several corrective actions can be taken. These actions include increasing the discharge rate, decreasing the released activity by using activated charcoal filters to trap most of the radioactive xenon, and considering the location of the exhaust (e.g., on a rooftop) as a restricted area. However, the last approach is often operationally burdensome—the boundary of the restricted area must be clearly established and posted—and access to the location must be restricted.

When charcoal filters are used to reduce the concentration released to the atmosphere, the user must be able to demonstrate that the filters are effective and are performing as assumed. Measurements to determine the trapping efficiency and whether a filter has become saturated should be periodically performed.

Emergency Room Support: Planning and Preparation

There is an ever increasing focus on medical facilities' ability and readiness to respond to large, mass casualty emergencies. Many of the scenarios for which facilities prepare for involve the contamination of patients with radioactive materials or radiation-induced injuries. In the context of medical response to large radiological events, facilities must not only be prepared to diagnose and treat radiation-induced injuries, but they must also be prepared to handle radiation detection and decontamination of patients. Neither the treatment of radiation-induced injuries nor the detection and decontamination of patients is a trivial task. However, as a facility plans for these types of events, it should consider all the resources available in order to increase its readiness and chances for success in any response to the event.

There are several principles to understand about emergency room procedures and handling patients who may have been involved in an accident that involves radiation exposure, radioactive materials, or both. The administration of first aid, resuscitation, and medical stabilization are priorities in addition to the immediate treatment of serious injuries. There are four basic types of radiation accident patients:

1. *External irradiation only.* These are patients who are not radioactive but have been exposed to radiation from some external source.
2. *Internal contamination only.* This often occurs in an industrial accident and external contamination may not be present.
3. *Embedded radioactive source.* These patients have typically been involved in an industrial accident with sources or fragments of a source of radioactive material inside the body.
4. *External contamination.* Patients may have been involved in a transportation or industrial accident or spill of radioactive materials.

In planning for and responding to these types of events, nuclear medicine technologists can play a unique role because of their training and experience. Specifically, the nuclear medicine technologist possesses knowledge and skills that are immediately useful to a facility as it prepares for and responds to radiological emergencies.

Each day nuclear medicine technologists handle radioactive material, measure radiation exposure, and engage in many other activities that would need to be repeated during a large, radiological event. Some areas that they may provide insight during the planning and response phases include:

- Contamination detection, quantification, and removal
- The use of portable survey meters
- Measuring radiation exposure and dose
- Speaking with patients and family members about radiation and its effects

Nuclear medicine technologists should not be overlooked by facility planners when preparing for radiological events. Not only are they already part of the staff and familiar with the institution, but they possess a unique set of skills and knowledge that will be invaluable in planning for and responding to radiological events.

The typical emergency room written plan should include the prevention of contamination to personnel, equipment, and the facility. The plan should include assessment for the presence of radioactive contamination and decontamination procedures. Reassessment for external contamination follows decontamination until criteria have been reached for allowable nonremovable contamination. After the external contamination procedures are completed, the assessment for internal contamination is performed with possible treatment for internal contamination and follow-up.

Program Audits

A review of the radiation safety program should be conducted quarterly to ensure that procedures are followed. The review, which is conducted by a medical physicist, or other appropriate personnel, should include a visual check of personnel safety practices and camera quality-control records. The department policy and procedures and related records must be reviewed annually by a medical physicist. The results should be presented to the RSC.

Patient Precautions

The radiation dose that the patient receives is considered acceptable in that the study provides needed medical information, which is a benefit. To ensure that the use of radioactivity is beneficial, procedures must be in place so that the correct patient receives the correct amount of radioactivity for an appropriate study. All studies must be properly requisitioned. When the patient arrives, his or her identity must be clearly ascertained. This may be done in a number of ways, such as by checking an inpatient wristband or asking for date of birth, which may be checked against the requisition. The radiopharmaceutical to be used must be checked, and the proper material must be selected. For example, if kits are prepared in the department, color coding may be used so that a bone agent is not confused with pertechnetate. Before administration, the radionuclide must be assayed, the radioactivity must be compared with the recommended amount, and the syringe must be properly labeled. Last, the correct route of administration must be used, and care must be taken to prevent administration of a useless radiation dose to the patient, such as by extravasation.

Additional precautions, using a **written directive**, must be taken for medical procedures that have a higher risk to the patient, for example, using any ^{131}I or ^{125}I procedures greater than 30 µCi, or any other unsealed-source therapy procedures such as ^{32}P or [89]Sr. For these procedures, a written directive must be completed by the authorized user (i.e., the nuclear medicine physician authorized for unsealed-source therapy procedures). The written directive must identify the patient, the procedure, radiopharmaceutical form, and route of administration. The directive must be signed and dated. Before administration, the patient must be identified in two ways. Before administration by the authorized user, the material must be assayed and documentation must be provided that the radioactivity is within 10% of the prescribed amount. There must also be documentation that the administration is in accordance with the written directive, for example, by having the physician who administers the material sign the dose slip. The written documentation must be kept on file. The description of how these additional precautions will be addressed and the mechanism for review should be contained in the institution's **quality management program (QMP)**. It is no longer a requirement of the materials license that a QMP be in place; however, it is still a good practice to maintain a QMP to ensure patient safety and regulatory compliance. At specified intervals (e.g., quarterly) the paperwork should be reviewed to further evaluate whether problems have occurred. The files of patients who fall into the previous categories should be reviewed for accuracy and completeness during inspections by federal or state regulators.

If an error is made in dosing a patient, the incident should be documented. It must then be determined if the event is one that should be reported to the appropriate regulatory agency. Incidents that must be reported are **medical events**. Medical event is defined by the NRC as the administration of byproduct material that results in any of the following (10 CFR 35.3045)[16]:

1. A dose that differs from the prescribed dose or dose that would have resulted from the prescribed dosage by more than 0.05 Sv (5 rem) **effective dose equivalent**, 0.5 Sv (50 rem) to an organ or tissue, or 0.5 Sv (50 rem) shallow dose equivalent to the skin, and one of the following conditions:
   a. The total dose delivered differs from the prescribed dose by 20% or more.
   b. The total dosage delivered differs from the prescribed dosage by 20% or more or falls outside the prescribed dosage range.
   c. The fractionated dose delivered differs from the prescribed dose, for a single fraction, by 50% or more.
2. A dose that exceeds 0.05 Sv (5 rem) effective dose equivalent, 0.5 Sv (50 rem) to an organ or tissue, or 0.5 Sv (50 rem) shallow dose equivalent to the skin from any of the following:
   a. An administration of a wrong radioactive drug containing byproduct material
   b. An administration of a radioactive drug containing byproduct material by the wrong route of administration
   c. An administration of a dose or dosage to the wrong individual or human research subject
   d. An administration of a dose or dosage delivered by the wrong mode of treatment
   e. A leaking sealed source
3. A dose to the skin or an organ or tissue other than the treatment site that exceeds by 0.5 Sv (50 rem) to an organ or tissue and 50% or more of the dose expected from the administration defined in the written directive (excluding, for permanent implants, seeds that were implanted in the correct site but migrated outside the treatment site).

In the case of a medical event, it is necessary to notify the appropriate regulatory agency within 24 hours of discovery. Additional notification must be made to the referring physician and the affected patient, unless it is medical opinion of the physician that informing the patient would be harmful. It is highly unlikely that a diagnostic study would meet the whole body or organ dose requirement of a medical event. Although generally not required, it is good practice to document any incorrect administration, investigate the cause, and determine possible methods to prevent reoccurrence.

Studies of women of childbearing age also require additional precautions. Before beginning the study, the last menstrual period (LMP) must be ascertained and documented, such as on the requisition. If a woman is pregnant or late in her menstrual cycle, the nuclear medicine physician and the referring physician must decide if the study should be performed. If the study is performed, documentation of the administered radioactivity and type of study should be recorded so that the probable dose to the fetus may be calculated. If the woman is breast-feeding, she should discontinue for a designated time following the study. The NRC in 10 CFR 35.3047 has added the requirement that if the resulting dose equivalent to an embryo/fetus is more than 5 rem and it is not approved in advance, it must be reported to the NRC or agreement state regulators within 1 calendar day with a written report to follow within 15 days. If there is a breast-feeding child and a dose of greater that 50 rem total effective dose is received or if the exposure resulted in unintended permanent functional damage to an organ or physiological system to the child as determined by a physician, then this must also be reported within 1 calendar day.

SOURCES OF RADIATION EXPOSURE

This chapter deals with the control of radiation. It is important to understand that there are many sources besides the activities of nuclear medicine that may cause radiation exposure and cannot be controlled. These help provide context to the risks from medical applications of radiation.

The primary source of exposure for much of the population is what is called *background radiation*. Humans have always been exposed to background levels caused by the following:

1. Terrestrial radiation from the presence of naturally occurring radioactivity in the soil, primarily caused by uranium and its by-products. The levels of radiation may vary significantly, depending on the location. For example, the Colorado plateau in the Rocky Mountains has higher levels of terrestrial radiation because of greater amounts of uranium.
2. Cosmic radiation that results from the interaction of particles from outer space with the atmosphere and high-energy photons from outer space. Cosmic radiation levels will be higher at a higher altitude because of less shielding from the atmosphere.
3. Internal radioactivity due to naturally occurring radioactivity deposited in the body. An example is ^{40}K, a naturally occurring isotope of potassium.

The average annual whole-body radiation dose equivalent in the United States is approximately 0.82 mSv (82 mrem)/yr, varying from about 0.65 mSv (65 mrem)/yr in the Atlantic and Gulf Coast regions to about 1.4 mSv (140 mrem)/yr in the Colorado plateau. Recent estimates of the annual radiation dose to the population have also included the contribution due to radon gas. The estimated whole-body dose equivalent due to radon is approximately 2 mSv (200 mrem)/yr, though the only tissue of concern is the lung.[4] Thus, the average total estimated whole-body dose equivalent is 3 mSv (300 mrem)/yr, of which 1 mSv (100 mrem)/yr is due to penetrating radiations (Figure 7-8).

The only other significant source of radiation to the general population in the United States is medical radiation exposure, presumably for beneficial reasons. As shown in Table 7-9, the average per capita radiation dose equivalent due to medical radiation is approximately 0.53 mSv (53 mrem)/yr.[8] This estimate includes

TABLE 7-9	Annual Effective Dose Equivalent in the U.S. Population	
Source	**Dose (mSv)**	**% of Total**
Natural Sources		
Radon	2.0	55
Other	1.0	27
Medical		
Diagnostic x-rays	0.39	11
Radiopharmaceuticals	0.14	4
Occupational	0.009	0.3
Consumer Products	0.05-0.13	2
Nuclear Industry		
Weapons testing research, etc.	0.0011	1
ROUNDED TOTALS	3.6	100

Compiled from National Council of Radiation Protection: *Ionizing radiation exposure of the population of the United States,* Report No. 93, Washington, DC, 1987, National Council of Radiation Protection.

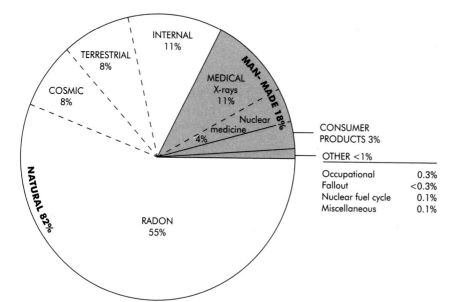

FIGURE 7-8 Percent contribution of various radiation sources to the total average effective dose equivalent in the U.S. population.

0.39 mSv (39 mrem)/yr due to diagnostic x-rays and 0.14 mSv (14 mrem)/yr resulting from the use of radiopharmaceuticals.

The remaining contributors to the average per capita radiation dose equivalent are consumer products, nuclear industry, weapons testing, and perhaps of most interest, occupational exposure.[2] Although the average whole-body dose equivalent for nuclear medicine personnel is estimated to be 3 mSv (300 mrem)/yr, the number of personnel is small (approximately 10,000) compared with the total population. Thus the dose averaged over the population results in about 0.001 mSv (0.1 mrem) of the occupational exposure contribution. The total annual effective dose equivalent due to both natural and man-made sources in the United States is estimated to be 3.6 mSv (360 mrem)/yr.[8]

RADIATION REGULATIONS

The NRC is responsible for the regulation of the civilian uses of byproduct, source and special nuclear material. The regulations are found in Title 10 of the *Code of Federal Regulations* as referenced throughout this chapter. The general requirements are found in 10 CFR 20, *Standards for Protection Against Radiation* and the sections that further relate to medical uses are found in 10 CFR 35, *Medical Use of Byproduct Material*. That being said, there is actually much more to the overall picture of the regulatory process than there is space to address here.

The regulations themselves have developed from a series of statutes and acts that are enforced by the NRC, the Environmental Protection Agency (EPA), the Food and Drug Administration (FDA), the Occupational Safety and Health Administration (OSHA), and the Department of Transportation (DOT). The regulations are needed to enable these agencies to administer and enforce these acts. The regulations go through a process of development that includes the recommendations of recognized advisory committees along with the detailed procedures requiring public notice and allowing a period for public comment. It is intended to ensure that the problem that the regulation is intended to address is examined along with the impacts on affected parties, financial and social costs, as well as benefits. Proposed rules are published in the *Federal Register,* describing the intended rule, and comments are solicited.

There are a number of advisory groups that provide guidance to the regulatory process in the area related to the safe handling of radiation. Two major advisory groups include the **National Council on Radiation Protection (NCRP)** and the **International Council on Radiation Protection (ICRP)**, which apply to practices related to the peaceful use of atomic energy. The NCRP was founded in 1964 as a nonprofit corporation chartered by the U.S. Congress and charged with the scientific development, evaluation, and application of basic radiation concepts, measurements, and units, as well as dissemination of information and recommendations on radiation in the public interest. The ICRP has close official relationships with a number of international organizations, which include the International Commission on Radiation Units and Measurements (ICRU), the World Health Organization (WHO), and the International Atomic Energy Agency (IAEA). These organizations have a close but separate relationship and provide guidance for the setting of radiation protection criteria, standards, and practices. Professional societies such as the Society of Nuclear Medicine, the Health Physics Society, the American College of Radiology, and the American Association of Physicists in Medicine, along with public comment, are also included in the regulatory process.

Throughout the development of the standards and regulations, there is an implied principle that the benefits outweigh the risk for the particular use. The regulatory process includes a review that indicates who is at risk, how many are at risk, and approximately how much risk should be present in order to generate a risk characterization. Also analyzed are the non-risk factors that impact economic, political, and social areas, as well as legal and physical constraints that can dictate or limit possible options. The individual states themselves have an important impact on the regulation of the use of radiation. There are currently areas where no federal agency has had express regulatory responsibility such as general x-ray producing machines and machine-generated radioactive material such as positron emission tomography (PET) isotopes. In these cases, the states have been able to regulate these areas if they deemed it necessary. There are laws passed by Congress whereby the NRC as well as the EPA can give some of their regulatory and enforcement authority to the states. When this takes place, the states are then known as *agreement states*. The majority of the states, more than 33, are agreement states. There is one authority, however, that cannot be given to the states and that is the regulation of nuclear reactors, which remains with the NRC.

Guidance documents have been written by the NRC to provide suggested procedures that are meant to ensure compliance with the regulation. Entities with relatively simple licensing needs can use these procedures fairly directly with a caution that they can be more restrictive than the actual license or the regulatory requirement. *The Regulatory Guide* series provides the licensees and applicants guidance on implementing specific parts of the NRC's regulations. The NUREGs are reports or brochures on regulatory decisions, results of research, results of incident investigations, and other technical and administrative information. NUREG 1556, *The Consolidated Guidance about Materials Licenses*, has several volumes and is used extensively by the NRC for medical licensees.

Regulations have been constructed around risk-versus-benefit considerations, as already mentioned, with an effort to keep the estimated risk within the levels accepted by society for other activities. Dose limits have changed over the years with a great deal of influence from the NCRP and ICRP. The recommendation is that radiation workers should face the same risk as the average worker in a safe industry or business, which is a 5×10^{-3} lifetime probability of suffering a job-related fatality. This concept was kept in mind when creating requirements to combine the external dose as well as the internal committed dose into the annual limit. This is relatively easy to do for short-lived radionuclides, but it can be very difficult and time-consuming for industries with long-lived radioactive material. (For additional reading on this area, see *Physics of Radiology* by A.B. Wolbarst.[18])

Based on the risk-benefit principle, doses are smaller for the public versus an occupational worker or a patient. For a pregnant worker, there is an additional consideration balancing the higher sensitivity of the fetus. A pregnant worker may further limit her exposure if necessary if she declares her pregnancy in writing and at that point is given monthly limits in addition to a limit for the gestation period. Patients do not have a dose limit, but there are precautions taken to minimize unnecessary radiation to a pregnant patient and training of the medical personnel to be conscious of minimizing the dose in general wherever possible.

Shipping and Receiving of Radioactive Material

When radioactive material is in commercial transport, it is the DOT, not the NRC, who dictates how a package is shipped, packaged, and labeled, and the amount of contamination allowed on the packaging (49 CFR 173.443)[9] when transported. The transportation of hazardous materials in the United States has been regulated for over 100 years. The original emphasis was on explosive material, and then other materials were added such as flammables, corrosives, and poisonous materials. These regulations have evolved in a much more complex regulatory environment but the basic concepts of containment in transit and communication of the hazards to involved personnel still apply.

The DOT regulations are found in 49 CFR, Parts 100 to 500. In order to make a shipment, the delivery person must have the required training commensurate with the type of materials being shipped according to 49 CFR 107. Once a radioactive material shipment is received into a facility, the NRC has regulatory authority for how it is handled and the requirements for receiving the radioactive material (10 CFR 20.1906).[14]

Notice to Employees

The Notice to Employees, NRC form 3, per 10 CFR 20.1911[14] (Figure 7-9)[13] or the agreement state's version,

is required to be posted in enough places where workers will be likely to see it on their way to work in areas where radioactive materials are used. It gives information as to workers' rights, the ability to report problems anonymously, and where to call to report problems or request an inspection. The notice also provides a description of where the copies of their radiation exposure, the license, operating procedures, and records are found. The form also includes the employee's responsibilities to know the regulations applicable to their work and obey them.

RADIATION DOSE

The concepts and definition of exposure, dose, dose equivalent, and effective dose equivalent are used daily in the practice of nuclear medicine. They are, however, often used incorrectly or misunderstood. The following is a brief overview of these concepts.

Radiation Exposure

Exposure is defined as the amount of charge (coulomb [C]) liberated in a volume (in units of mass, kg) of air from the interaction of x-rays or gamma rays of energy 0 to 3 MeV. Note that the unit of exposure is not defined for particles, nor is it defined for ionization in matter other than air. This is important to remember when extrapolating exposure-rate measurements to units of dose (discussed in the following sections). The unit of exposure is the roentgen (R). The roentgen is defined as $1\ R = 2.58 \times 10^{-4}\ C/kg$.

Absorbed Dose

Absorbed dose *(D)* is defined as the amount of energy *(E* in ergs or Joules) deposited in a unit mass *(m* in g or kg): $D = E/m$. Unlike exposure, the concept of absorbed dose applies to all types of materials and to all types of ionizing radiation. The unit of absorbed dose is the rad (rad) or gray (Gy). The rad has been replaced by the SI unit Gy but is still used in U.S. regulatory documents. Absorbed dose is defined as 1 rad = 100 erg/gm or 1 Gy = 1 J/kg; note that 100 rad = 1 Gy.

Note that exposure is the measure of the amount of ionizing radiation, while absorbed dose is a measure of the amount of energy absorbed in a given mass. Often, measurements are taken using a meter that will give results in units of exposure in order to show compliance with dose limits. However, this is usually considered a conservative estimate because it is often assumed that 1 R = 1 rad for x-rays and gamma rays. The amount of absorbed dose from a given exposure varies from tissue to tissue and individual to individual; however, typical conversion factors for R to rad are less than 1, so this is considered a conservative approach.

NRC FORM 3
(3-2005)
Part 1

UNITED STATES NUCLEAR REGULATORY COMMISSION
Washington, DC 20555-0001

NOTICE TO EMPLOYEES

STANDARDS FOR PROTECTION AGAINST RADIATION (PART 20); NOTICES, INSTRUCTIONS AND REPORTS TO WORKERS; INSPECTIONS (PART 19); EMPLOYEE PROTECTION

WHAT IS THE NUCLEAR REGULATORY COMMISSION?

The Nuclear Regulatory Commission is an independent Federal regulatory agency responsible for licensing and inspecting nuclear power plants and other commercial uses of radioactive materials.

WHAT DOES THE NRC DO?

The NRC's primary responsibility is to ensure that workers and the public are protected from unnecessary or excessive exposure to radiation and that nuclear facilities, including power plants, are constructed to high quality standards and operated in a safe and secure manner. The NRC does this by establishing requirements in Title 10 of the Code of Federal Regulations (10 CFR) and in licenses issued to nuclear users.

WHAT RESPONSIBILITY DOES MY EMPLOYER HAVE?

Any company that conducts activities licensed by the NRC must comply with the NRC's requirements. If a company violates NRC requirements, it can be fined or have its license modified, suspended or revoked.

Your employer must tell you which NRC radiation requirements apply to your work and must post NRC Notices of Violation involving radiological working conditions.

WHAT IS MY RESPONSIBILITY?

For your own protection and the protection of your co-workers, you should know how NRC requirements relate to your work and should obey them. If you observe violations of the requirements or have a safety concern, you should report them.

WHAT IF I CAUSE A VIOLATION?

If you engaged in deliberate misconduct that may cause a violation of the NRC requirements, or would have caused a violation if it had not been detected, or deliberately provided inaccurate or incomplete information to either the NRC or to your employer, you may be subject to enforcement action. If you report such a violation, the NRC will consider the circumstances surrounding your reporting in determining the appropriate enforcement action, if any.

HOW DO I REPORT VIOLATIONS AND SAFETY CONCERNS?

If you believe that violations of NRC rules or the terms of the license have occurred, or if you have a safety concern, you should report them immediately to your supervisor. You may report violations or safety concerns directly to the NRC. However, the NRC encourages you to raise your concerns with the licensee since it is the licensee who has the primary responsibility for, and is most able to ensure, safe operation of nuclear facilities. If you choose to report your concern directly to the NRC, you may report this to an NRC inspector or call or write to the NRC Regional Office serving your area. If you send your concern in writing, it will assist the NRC in protecting your identity if you clearly state in the beginning of your letter that you have a safety concern or that you are submitting an allegation. The NRC's toll-free SAFETY HOTLINE for reporting safety concerns is listed below. The addresses for the NRC Regional Offices and the toll-free telephone numbers are also listed below. You can also e-mail safety concerns to allegation@nrc.gov.

WHAT IF I WORK WITH RADIOACTIVE MATERIAL OR IN THE VICINITY OF A RADIOACTIVE SOURCE?

If you work with radioactive materials or near a radiation source, the amount of radiation exposure that you are permitted to receive may be limited by NRC regulations. The limits on exposure for workers at NRC licensed facilities whose duties involve exposure to radiation are contained in sections 20.1201, 20.1207, and 20.1208 of Title 10 of the Code of Federal Regulations (10 CFR 20) depending on the part of the regulations to which your employer is subject. While these are the maximum allowable limits, your employer should also keep your radiation exposure as far below those limits as is "reasonably achievable."

MAY I GET A RECORD OF MY RADIATION EXPOSURE?

Yes. Your employer is required to advise you of your dose annually if you are exposed to radiation for which monitoring was required by NRC. In addition, you may request a written report of your exposure when you leave your job.

HOW ARE VIOLATIONS OF NRC REQUIREMENTS IDENTIFIED?

NRC conducts regular inspections at licensed facilities to assure compliance with NRC requirements. In addition, your employer and site contractors may conduct their own inspections to assure compliance. All inspectors are protected by Federal law. Interference with them may result in criminal prosecution for a Federal offense.

MAY I TALK WITH AN NRC INSPECTOR?

Yes. NRC inspectors want to talk to you if you are worried about radiation safety or have other safety concerns about licensed activities, such as the quality of construction or operations at your facility. Your employer may not prevent you from talking with an inspector. The NRC will make all reasonable efforts to protect your identity where appropriate and possible.

MAY I REQUEST AN INSPECTION?

Yes. If you believe that your employer has not corrected violations involving radiological working conditions, you may request an inspection. Your request should be addressed to the nearest NRC Regional Office and must describe the alleged violation in detail. It must be signed by you or your representative.

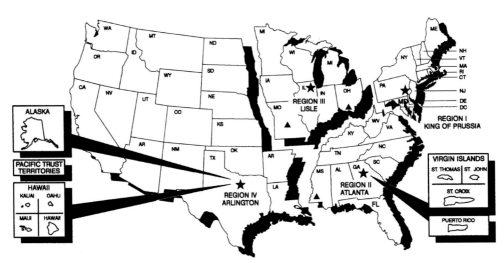

▲ - Callaway Plant Site in Missouri and Grand Gulf Plant Site in Mississippi are under the purview of Region IV. The Portsmouth Gaseous Diffusion Plant in Ohio is under the purview of Region II.

FIGURE 7-9 U.S. Nuclear Regulatory Commission radiation protection standards *Notice to Employees.*

NRC FORM 3
(2-2005)
Part 2

HOW DO I CONTACT THE NRC?

Talk to an NRC inspector on-site or call or write to the nearest NRC Regional Office in your geographical area (see map below). If you call the NRC's toll-free SAFETY HOTLINE during normal business hours, your call will automatically be directed to the NRC Regional Office for your geographical area. If you call after normal business hours, your call will be directed to the NRC's Headquarters Operations Center, which is manned 24 hours a day. You can also e-mail safety concerns to allegation@nrc.gov.

CAN I BE FIRED FOR RAISING A SAFETY CONCERN?

Federal law prohibits an employer from firing or otherwise discriminating against you for bringing safety concerns to the attention of your employer or the NRC. You may not be fired or discriminated against because you engage in certain protected activities, including but not limited to,

- ask the NRC to enforce its rules against your employer;

- refuse to engage in activities which violate NRC requirements;

- provide information or are about to provide information to the NRC or your employer about violations of requirements or safety concerns;

- are about to ask for, or testify, help, or take part in an NRC, Congressional, or any Federal or State proceeding.

WHAT FORMS OF DISCRIMINATION ARE PROHIBITED?

It is unlawful for an employer to fire you or discriminate against you with respect to pay, benefits, or working conditions because you help the NRC or raise a safety issue or otherwise engage in protected activities. Violations of Section 211 of the Energy Reorganization Act (ERA) of 1974 (42 U.S.C. 5851) include actions such as harassment, blacklisting, and intimidation by employers of (i) employees who bring safety concerns directly to their employers or to the NRC; (ii) employees who have refused to engage in an unlawful practice, provided that the employee has identified the illegality to the employer; (iii) employees who have testified or are about to testify before Congress or in any Federal or State proceeding regarding any provision (or proposed provision) of the ERA or the Atomic Energy Act (AEA) of 1954; (iv) employees who have commenced or caused to be commenced a proceeding for the administration or enforcement of any requirement imposed under the ERA or AEA or who have, or are about to, testify, assist, or participate in such a proceeding.

HOW DO I FILE A DISCRIMINATION COMPLAINT?

If you believe that you have been discriminated against for bringing violations or safety concerns to the NRC or your employer, you may file a complaint with the NRC, the U.S. Department of Labor (DOL), or appropriate state entities. If you desire a personal remedy, you must file a complaint with the DOL pursuant to Section 211 of the ERA or with appropriate state entities. Your complaint to the DOL must describe in detail the basis for your belief that the employer discriminated against you on the basis of your protected activity, and it must be filed in writing either in person or by mail within 180 days of the discriminatory occurrence. Additional information is available at the DOL web site at www.osha.gov. Filing an allegation, complaint, or request for action with the NRC does not extend the requirement to file a complaint with the DOL within 180 days. To do so, you may contact the Allegation Coordinator in the appropriate NRC Region, as listed below, who will provide you with the address and telephone number of the correct OSHA Regional office to receive your complaint. You may also check your local telephone directory under the U.S. Government listings for the address and telephone number of the appropriate OSHA Regional office.

WHAT CAN THE DEPARTMENT OF LABOR DO?

If your complaint involves a violation of Section 211 of the ERA by your employer, it is the DOL, NOT THE NRC, that provides the process for obtaining a personal remedy. The DOL will notify your employer that a complaint has been filed and will investigate your complaint.

If the DOL finds that your employer has unlawfully discriminated against you, it may order that you be reinstated, receive back pay, or be compensated for any injury suffered as a result of the discrimination and be paid attorney's fees and costs.

Relief will not be awarded to employees who engage in deliberate violations of the Energy Reorganization Act or the Atomic Energy Act.

WHAT WILL THE NRC DO?

The NRC will evaluate each allegation of harassment, intimidation, or discrimination to determine whether sufficient information exists to initiate an investigation. Following this evaluation, an investigator from the NRC's Office of Investigations may interview you and review available documentation. Based on the evaluation, and, if applicable, the interview, the NRC will assign a priority and a decision will be made whether to pursue the matter further through an investigation. The assigned priority is based on the specifics of the case. The NRC may not pursue an investigation of low priority cases to the point that a conclusion can be made whether the harassment, intimidation, or discrimination actually occurred. If you do not object, the NRC may refer lower priority cases to the involved licensee for a response and will request that the licensee independently review such issues. Even if NRC decides not to pursue an investigation, if you have filed a complaint with the DOL, the NRC will monitor the results of the DOL investigation.

If the NRC or the DOL finds that unlawful discrimination has occurred, the NRC may issue a Notice of Violation to your employer, impose a fine, or suspend, modify, or revoke your employer's NRC license.

UNITED STATES NUCLEAR REGULATORY COMMISSION REGIONAL OFFICE LOCATIONS

A representative of the Nuclear Regulatory Commission can be contacted by employees who wish to register complaints or concerns about radiological working conditions or other matters regarding compliance with Commission rules and regulations at the following addresses and telephone numbers.

REGIONAL OFFICES

REGION	ADDRESS	TELEPHONE
I	U.S. Nuclear Regulatory Commission, Region I 475 Allendale Road King of Prussia, PA 19406-1415	(800) 432-1156
II	U.S. Nuclear Regulatory Commission, Region II Atlanta Federal Center 61 Forsyth Street, S.W., Suite 23T85 Atlanta, GA 30303-3415	(800) 577-8510
III	U.S. Nuclear Regulatory Commission, Region III 2443 Warrenville Road, Suite 210 Lisle, IL 60532-4352	(800) 522-3025
IV	U.S. Nuclear Regulatory Commission, Region IV 611 Ryan Plaza Drive, Suite 400 Arlington, TX 76011-8064	(800) 952-9677

To report safety concerns or violations of NRC requirements by your employer, telephone:

NRC SAFETY HOTLINE

1-800-695-7403

To report incidents involving fraud, waste, or abuse by an NRC employee or NRC contractor, telephone:

OFFICE OF THE INSPECTOR GENERAL HOTLINE

1-800-233-3497

FIGURE 7-9, cont'd

TABLE 7-10	Comparison of Types of Radiation, Quality Factor, and Absorbed Dose	
Type of Radiation	**Quality Factor (Q)**	**Absorbed Dose Equal to a Unit Dose Equivalent***
X-ray, gamma, or beta radiation	1	1
Alpha particles, multiple-charged particles, fission fragments, and heavy particles of unknown charge	20	0.05
Neutrons of unknown energy	10	0.1
High-energy protons	10	0.1

*Absorbed dose in rad equal to 1 rem or the absorbed dose in gray equal to 1 Sv.
Adapted from U.S. Nuclear Regulatory Commission: Title 10, *Code of Federal Regulations*, Part 20, Standards for protection against radiation, Washington, DC, 2005, U.S. Nuclear Regulatory Commission.

TABLE 7-11	Comparison of Quality Factor (10 CFR 20) and Radiation Weighting (ICRP 60)	
Type of Radiation	**Q**	**W$_R$**
X-ray, gamma, or beta radiation	1	1
Alpha particles, multiple-charged particles, fission fragments, and heavy particles of unknown charge	20	20
High-energy protons	10	5
Neutrons: unknown energy	10	—
Thermal	2	5
0.01 MeV	2.5	10
0.1 MeV	7.5	10
0.5 MeV	11	20
>0.1 MeV to 2 MeV	5.5 to 3.5*	20
>2 MeV to 20 MeV	3.5*	5

*10 CFR 20.1004 lists neutron energies from 2.5×10^{-8} to 4×10^2 MeV. Approximations listed here for comparison.
Adapted from U.S. Nuclear Regulatory Commission: Title 10, *Code of Federal Regulations*, Part 20, Standards for protection against radiation, Washington, DC, 2005, U.S. Nuclear Regulatory Commission; International Commission on Radiological Protection: *Report 60: Recommendations of the International Commission on Radiological Protection 60*, vol 21, Nos. 1 and 2, New York, 1991, Pergamon.

Radiation-Weighted Dose

As noted in earlier chapters, various types of radiation interact with matter differently; even radiation of the same type but of differing energies will cause dissimilar effects. In a biological system, these varying effects can change the overall outcome on the system from absorbed dose. To account for this difference in effects by different radiation and energies, the concept of radiation-weighted dose was developed. It should be noted that weighted doses are used for radiological protection and regulatory purposes.

Radiation-weighted dose accounts for the absorbed dose as well as the type of radiation. In U.S. regulatory terms, this unit is referred to as *dose equivalent*. Dose equivalent *(H)* is defined as the quantity of the absorbed dose and a radiation-modifying value called the quality factor. The quality factor *(Q)* is an attempt to account for these varying effects for different radiation types. Table 7-10 lists the radiation quality factors as defined by the NRC. The unit of dose equivalent is the rem: H (rem) $= D$ (rad) $\times Q$. Dose equivalent can also be expressed in SI units. The SI unit for weighted dose is the sievert (Sv): 100 rem = 1 Sv. Care should be taken when converting from units of Sv to dose equivalence. Beginning in the mid-1970s, the International Commission on Radiation Protection (ICRP) introduced other radiation-weighted doses that are also expressed in Sv.

The ICRP defines equivalent dose similar to dose equivalent. Equivalent dose (also denoted as H) is calculated similarly as dose equivalent, but instead of multiplying by the quality factor, dose is multiplied by a radiation weighting factor. Table 7-11 lists some quality and radiation weighting factors. Other than the values of the weighting factors, there is little difference between dose equivalent and equivalent dose. Dose equivalent and equivalent dose are often given for a specific organ. When given for a specific organ, dose is expressed as H_T (T for tissue or organ) to differentiate between whole-body dose and organ dose.

Obviously, different organs in the body are more sensitive to the effects of radiation than others. In order to account for this fact, the ICRP developed the unit of **effective dose equivalent** (H_E or EDE). The EDE adds an additional modifying factor to the concept of absorbed dose that accounts for the relative radiosensitivity of different organs, the tissue weighting factor (w_T): $H_E = D \times w_T \times w_R$. For dose from multiple radiation types, H_E is the sum of all radiation types: $H_E = \Sigma D_R \times w_{T,R} \times w_R$.

Currently, EDE for U.S. regulatory purposes is based on values shown in Table 7-12 for the tissue-weighting factor. However, the ICRP has made more recent recommendations that are also listed in Table 7-13.[7] Caution must be used when evaluating EDE to ensure that proper radiation and tissue weighting factors are applied. As stated before, the U.S. regulations are based on older ICRP recommendations, but recent scientific publications are based on the more recent ICRP recommendations.

Because internally deposited radionuclides may deliver dose to tissues or organs of the body over a period of time, the concept of committed dose has been defined. Committed dose equivalent (CDE) is simply the committed dose equivalent to the organ or tissue over the irradiated time. For occupational use, time is assumed to be

TABLE 7-12	Comparison of Tissue Weighting Factors	
Tissue or Organ	W_T (ICRP 26 and NRC)	W_T (ICRP 60)
Gonads	0.25	0.2
Bone marrow (red)	0.12	0.12
Colon	—	0.12
Lung	0.12	0.12
Stomach	—	0.12
Bladder	—	0.05
Breast	0.15	0.05
Liver	—	0.05
Esophagus	—	0.05
Thyroid	0.03	0.05
Skin	—	0.01
Bone surface	0.03	0.01
Remainder	0.3	0.05

Adapted from Cember H: *Introduction to health physics*, ed 3, New York, 1996, McGraw-Hill.

TABLE 7-13	Risk Coefficients for Selected Organs
Tissue	Risk Coefficient (Probability of Biological Change per Sv)
Gonads	40×10^{-4} Sv^{-1} (40×10^{-6} rem^{-1})
Breast	25×10^{-4} Sv^{-1} (25×10^{-6} rem^{-1})
Red bone marrow	20×10^{-4} Sv^{-1} (20×10^{-6} rem^{-1})
Lung	20×10^{-4} Sv^{-1} (20×10^{-6} rem^{-1})
Thyroid	5×10^{-4} Sv^{-1} (5×10^{-6} rem^{-1})
Bone surfaces	5×10^{-4} Sv^{-1} (5×10^{-6} rem^{-1})
Remainder	50×10^{-4} Sv^{-1} (50×10^{-6} rem^{-1})
TOTAL	165×10^{-4} Sv^{-1} (165×10^{-6} rem^{-1})

Adapted from National Council of Radiation Protection: *Recommendations on limits for exposure to ionizing radiation*, Report No. 91, Washington, DC, 1987, National Council of Radiation Protection

50 years, and for nonoccupational used, it is assumed to be 70 years.

$$CDE = H_T(t) = \int_{t_0}^{t_0+t} \dot{H}_T dt$$

where

t is the time of irradiation (50 years for occupational exposure, 70 years for nonoccupational)
H_T is the dose equivalent rate at time *t* in tissue *T*

The concept of CDE can be expanded to estimate the dose from an internally deposited radionuclide to the entire body. This concept is called as the *committed effective dose equivalent* (CEDE). Similar to CDE, CEDE accounts for the dose over a period of time. Again, 50 years is assumed for occupational exposure, and 70 years is assumed for nonoccupational exposure. CEDE adds

the additional tissue weighting factor in order to estimate whole-body effective dose equivalent from the dose to an organ or tissue.

$$CDE = E(t) = \sum_T w_T CDE = \sum_T w_T H_T(t)$$

BIOLOGICAL EFFECTS OF IONIZING RADIATION

The radiation safety practices that have been described are intended to minimize the dose received (i.e., energy deposited) to the body due to ionizing radiation. This is necessary because biological effects due to radiation have been observed, either directly as in the case of high, single exposures, or in some percentage of a population, as in the case of somewhat lower exposures. A knowledge of these biological effects helps to assess the risks associated with exposure to radiation.

Acute Effects

A high, single radiation exposure to all or most of the body results in acute effects (i.e., those showing rapid onset, severe symptoms, and a short course). At a minimum whole-body dose of 2 Sv (200 rem), radiation sickness will be observed. Note that this results from a dose to the whole body delivered in a short time, a situation that would occur only because of a severe radiation accident. Within 1 or 2 hours of exposure, nausea, vomiting, and, at higher doses, diarrhea will be observed. Neurological symptoms such as headache, decreased blood pressure, and fatigue are also observed. This is called the *prodromal stage*. Except with the highest doses, a latent period follows, during which the victim shows no visible signs or symptoms of radiation injury.

The radiation syndrome (the signs and symptoms) exhibited, depends on the whole-body dose received. The dose levels given are approximate in that there is fortunately little human data. At doses of 100 Gy (10,000 rad) cerebrovascular damage results in death in a matter of hours. Although the exact cause of death is unknown, it appears that vascular damage results in rapid accumulation of cerebral fluid, resulting in disorientation, diarrhea, convulsions, coma, and death. At doses of 10 Gy (1000 rad) and higher, the damage that results in death is due to damage of the gastrointestinal system. Following a short latent period, the victim will exhibit severe diarrhea, dehydration, loss of weight, and exhaustion. Death occurs in approximately 3 to 10 days. Death of the immature cells of the epithelial lining of the intestine, which are normally sloughed off and replaced, results in inability to absorb necessary nutrients and maintain body fluid balance. At doses of approximately 0.2 to 0.8 Gy (200 to 800 rad), the dose is not high enough to seriously affect the gastrointestinal tract. It is high enough to kill mitotically active precursor blood cells. It will be the hematopoietic system, then, that will be affected. In humans, a rather long latent period lasts a few weeks. During this time, as mature blood cells die off naturally, the supply of immature cells is inadequate for replacement. At about 3 weeks, fatigue, petechial hemorrhages, ulceration of the mouth, and bleeding may occur. More seriously, infections and fever from white blood cell depression may occur. If other symptoms are not too severe, infection may be controlled by antibiotics.

One way of expressing the lethality of a dose is the LD_{50}. This means the dose that will result in a specified endpoint, in this case, death, to 50% of the population. For humans, the LD_{50} is thought to be about 3 to 3.5 Gy (300 to 350 rad) for healthy adults irradiated but with no medical intervention. With medical intervention, particularly prevention and treatment of infection, it may be possible to raise this by a factor of two.[4]

Cataract Induction

The lens of the eye differs from other organs in that dead and injured cells are not removed. Damage to the lens caused by a single dose of approximately 5 Sv (500 rem) will induce opacities that interfere with vision within a year. When the dose occurs over a protracted time, a total dose of 8 Sv (800 rem) or larger is required, and the cataract appears several years after the last exposure.[8] The 1980 Biological Effects of Ionizing Radiation report[1] concludes that cataract induction should not be a concern for the doses currently permitted radiation workers. For example, even if a worker received 0.05 Sv/yr to the eyes for a working lifetime of 40 years (both high estimates), the lifetime dose would be 2 Sv, which is still well below the threshold.

Fertility Effects

Doses of a few Sv to the human testes can lead to permanent sterility; smaller doses cause only a temporary reduction in the number of sperm cells. A single dose of 4 Sv (400 rem) to the ovaries is required to produce permanent sterility; at 0.5 Sv (50 rem), temporary amenorrhea can occur. Occupational exposure levels will not result in fertility effects.[5]

Late Effects

Radiation has also been shown to produce effects that may occur long after the dose is received because of damage to cells that is expressed much later. If this cell is a germ cell (oocyte or sperm), damage may result as a genetic mutation. Damage to all other cells of the body, somatic cells, may result in leukemia or cancer in the exposed individual. These are **stochastic effects,** meaning there is a probability of occurrence that has no threshold, increases with increasing doses to the individual, but

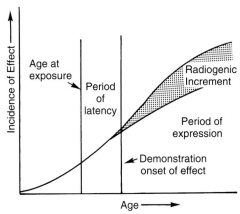

FIGURE 7-10 Graph illustrating the periods of latency and expression.

does not increase with severity as a function of the dose. For example, a dose of both 0.1 Sv (10 rem) and 1 Sv (100 rem) may cause leukemia to develop later in life, but in both cases the leukemia is the same in severity. The difference is that the probability of occurrence will be greater with the higher dose.

Knowledge of somatic late effects of radiation is based on studies of groups of people who were exposed to ionizing radiation. There have been a number of such groups, the largest of which are the survivors of the bombing of Hiroshima and Nagasaki, who have been carefully followed. Many other examples exist, often with irradiation to specific areas of the body, such as children irradiated for an enlarged thymus who developed subsequent thyroid cancer and women irradiated for pneumothorax who developed subsequent breast cancer. In all cases the dose received and the time to acquire the dose is estimated and the data plotted (Figure 7-10). Animal studies will expand the data. The data points in Figure 7-10 demonstrate the difficulty that arises in estimating the risk at low doses. Most of the data available are for high total doses and often high dose rates, defined as greater than 0.1 Gy/min. The doses of concern are at much lower doses and dose rates. It is necessary to attempt to interpret the data to develop a mathematical model that may be used to predict the response at low doses. Groups such as the National Academy of Sciences Committee on the Biological Effects of Ionizing Radiation (BEIR V) have done extensive reviews and analysis of the data. The two most common models, as shown in Figure 7-11, are the linear model (*curve 1*) and linear-quadratic model (*curve 2*). There is disagreement, however, about which model should be used for estimating risk. The most current recommendation is to use the linear model, but with the proviso that the risk at low-dose rates, as found in most diagnostic situations, is a factor of two or more lower than predicted by that model.

Two additional difficulties are present in estimating late effects. A natural incidence, often rather large, of cancers and leukemia is observed. Also, a latent period

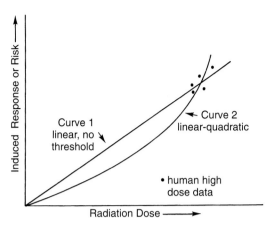

FIGURE 7-11 Dose response relationships.

TABLE 7-14	Risk Coefficients for Selected Organs			

Tissue or Site	Age of Exposure (yr)	Years at Risk*	Absolute Risk Coefficient†	
			Male	Female
Leukemia	0-9	5-26	1.7	1.1
	10-19	5-26	0.85	0.54
	20-34	5-26	1.1	0.67
	50+	5-26	1.6	0.99
Lungs	10-19	10-33	0.30	0.3
	20-34	10-33	0.56	0.56
	35-49	10-33	0.86	0.86
	50+	10-33	1.2	1.2
Breast	0-9	10-35	—	3.8
	10-19	10-35	—	7.6
	20-29	10-35	—	4.9
	30-39	10-35	—	4.9
	40-49	10-35	—	1.3
	50+	10-35	—	0.8
Thyroid	0-9	10-34	1.5	5.0
	10-19	10-34	1.5	5.0
	20-34	10-34	0.5	1.5
	35-49	10-34	0.5	1.5
	50+	10-34	0.5	1.5

*Number of excess cases of cancer per million persons per year per rem of organ dose (low-level, low-LET radiation) averaged over the specified period of expression.
†Following the radiation exposure.
From Rall JE, et al: *Report of the National Institutes of Health Working Group to Develop Epidemiological Tables,* NIH publication No. 85-2748, Washington, DC, 1985, U.S. Government Printing Office.

follows exposure before the effect is observed. Beyond the latent period, there will be an increase in the incidence of the cancer or leukemia, the radiogenic increment (Figure 7-10). This may increase at a constant rate with time or extend for a given number of years beyond exposure, depending on the cancer.

Organs and tissues differ greatly in their susceptibility to cancer induced by radiation. The organs most sensitive to radiation-induced carcinogenesis are the active bone marrow, thyroid, female breasts, and lungs.[3] Risk coefficients of radiation-induced malignancies are listed in Table 7-13. Because of the relatively high susceptibility of female breast and thyroid tissues, women have an overall greater somatic risk than men. Radiation-induced leukemia is better understood than other types of radiocarcinogenesis because of the natural rarity of the disease, the relative ease of its induction, and its short latent period. However, the combined risk of induced solid tumors (such as thyroid, lung, and female breast) exceeds that of leukemia. The fatal risk from all malignancies is likely to be on the order of 10^{-2}/Sv; that is, the probability of death due to a radiation-induced malignancy is approximately 1 chance in 100 per Sv of whole-body radiation dose. The ranges of fatal risk estimates are listed in Table 7-14. The risk factors shown in Table 7-14 were derived to apply to acute doses of about 10 rem or more and should not be used for doses comparable to natural background levels or even many occupational exposures. In fact, the 1980 BEIR report refuses to discuss the effects of exposures below 0.1 Sv (10 rem) and states, "Below these doses, the uncertainties of extrapolation of risk were believed by some members of the committee to be too great to justify the calculation." Accordingly, the use of the risk factors for lower doses will yield upper-limit estimates of the fatal cancer risk of radiation exposure. Incidentally, the malignancy will result in death roughly half the time. Thus, the risk of cancer induced by radiation is of the order of 2×10^{-2}/Sv.

The risks due to radiation may be compared with other occupational or overall risks. The American Cancer

Society[2] has reported that approximately 30% of adults in the 20- to 65-year age bracket will develop cancer at some time from all possible causes including cigarettes, food, drugs, air pollutants, and naturally occurring background level radiation. Thus, in any group of 10,000 workers not exposed to radiation on the job, about 3000 will develop cancer. If each of this entire group of 10,000 workers were to receive an occupational exposure of 10^{-2} (1 rem), the risk factor of 2×10^{-2}/Sv (2×10^{-4}/rem) would predict an additional two cases of cancer.

An interesting measure of risk is the life expectancy lost on the average because of radiation-induced cancer. It is estimated that the average loss of life expectancy due to radiation exposure is about 1 day/rem of whole-body dose equivalent. Table 7-15 lists comparative loss of life expectancy attributed to selected health risks.

Another useful comparison is the relative fatal risk of certain everyday endeavors. For example, an NCRP publication[11] states that a one-in-a-million risk of death has been attributed to each of the following:

400 miles by air
60 miles by car
¾ of a cigarette

TABLE 7-15	Estimated Loss of Life Expectancy from Selected Health Risks
Health Risk	**Estimated Days of Life Expectancy Lost, Average**
Smoking 20 cigarettes per day	2370
Overweight (by 20%)	985
All accidents	435
Auto accidents	200
Alcohol consumption (U.S. average)	130
Home accidents	95
Drowning	41
10 mSv (1 rem)/yr for 30 yr	30
Natural background radiation	8
All catastrophes (earthquakes, floods, etc.)	3.5
10 mSv (1 rem)/year occupational radiation dose equivalent	1

From U.S. Nuclear Regulatory Commission: Instruction concerning risk from occupational radiation exposure. In *Draft regulatory guide*, Washington, DC, 1980, U.S. Nuclear Regulatory Commission.

20 minutes of being a man of age 60
0.1 mSv (10 mrem) of whole-body radiation

In conclusion, the only somatic effect thought to occur at occupationally permitted levels is cancer induction. The probability of death due to radiation-induced cancer is conservatively believed to be less than $10^{-2}/Sv$ ($10^{-4}/rem$) when applied to the situation of a few Sv received over several years. This risk, approximately 1 chance in 100/Sv of whole-body dose, is low when compared to the risks of fatality associated with smoking, driving, or being overweight.

Genetic Effects

Radiation may also result in a genetic mutation. A mutation is an inherited change in a gene, a finite segment of DNA within a chromosome. Mutations are, generally speaking, dominant or recessive. Dominant genes are expressed in the first generation. Recessive genes are expressed only when matched with similar recessive genes, and so may not be expressed for a number of generations. The genetic mutations that occur are not unique. Rather, there may be an increase in the occurrence of mutations that occur naturally or spontaneously in the population.

Radiation genetic-risk estimates have been derived primarily from mouse data. Large-scale human genetic studies that have been carried out to date show no significant increase in genetic endpoints with increasing dose. In particular, ongoing studies of Japanese bomb survivors have shown no statistically significant increase in five different genetic endpoints. However, based on the mouse data, there is reason to believe that humans receive radiation-induced genetic effects in a somewhat similar fashion. The current estimate of radiation-induced genetic effects is that the risk of serious genetic disorders is 6 to 35 first-generation cases per 10^6 live births per 10 mSv.

The doubling dose is the dose of radiation that will double the spontaneous mutation rate in a biological system. Data from mouse studies and Japanese survivors have been used by groups such as BEIR V to estimate the doubling dose in humans. The current estimate as given in BEIR V is 1 Sv (100 rem).

Developmental Effects

At high doses of in utero exposure (single exposures greater than approximately 0.25 Sv), effects on the fetus have been observed. These effects include growth and developmental retardation, congenital abnormalities, and prenatal or neonatal death. Below this level, these effects are not observed or are at levels low enough to be indiscernible above the normal incidence of abnormalities, which is approximately 6% of live births. The effects are dose-related and are also related to the time in pregnancy. The three periods of concern are preimplantation, which extends to roughly 10 days after conception; organogenesis, which extends to 7 weeks after conception; and fetal development through birth.

During preimplantation, radiation damage results in either death of the fertilized egg or survival with no measurable effect. Outwardly, no effect would be noticed other than a failure to conceive.

Irradiation during organogenesis is the period of most concern. For this reason, it is often noted that radiation should be particularly limited during the first trimester. The implanted egg multiplies rapidly and differentiation occurs with development of organ systems. The effect of radiation is to produce congenital abnormalities. In early organogenesis, these may be skeletal effects, whereas in late organogenesis, neurological effects are noted. In addition, there may be some form of growth retardation due to loss of cells. Much of the information available, however, is based on studies of mice and rats, which develop at a rate that varies from humans in extent and timing. This makes it difficult to extrapolate to the expected human effect. These effects have not been observed at less than a 0.1 Sv (10 rem) dose delivered to the embryo.

After organogenesis, the fetus continues to grow and develop. Irradiation during this stage at higher doses may result in growth retardation or damage to organs. There is contradictory evidence that lower doses result in an increased incidence of leukemia.[4]

In nuclear medicine, the possibility for exposure to the embryo or fetus is very small. Of particular concern is that there not be an accidental exposure of the fetal thyroid due to administration of radioactive iodine. The fetal thyroid takes up iodine after the tenth week of pregnancy. Because pregnancy may be easily ascertained, any woman of childbearing age who receives radioactive sodium iodide should have pregnancy status confirmed.

SUMMARY

- A radiation safety program must be comprehensive and be integrated throughout all aspects of the nuclear medicine practice.
- Aspects of the program must include safety and control of radioactive materials and control of exposure; provide adequate radiation protection, external monitoring, and appropriate radiation safety instrumentation; require proper training and practices; and ensure management involvement.
- Radiation safety programs may involve federal, state, and local regulations and institutional policies.
- Radiation safety training should be appropriate for all personnel (e.g., physicians, technologists, ancillary personnel, housekeeping personnel, security personnel, engineers).
- Radiation-monitoring equipment should be appropriate for the scope of the nuclear medicine practice.
- Radiation-detection equipment must be calibrated annually.
- Daily checks and other periodic testing must be conducted according to a schedule defined by the radiation safety program.
- Radiation detection equipment usually involves GM detectors, ionization chambers, dose calibrators, and scintillation detectors.
- The detection efficiency must be determined and the MDA determined for certain detectors.
- Annual dose limits are set for both external and internal exposures.
- Exposure may be monitored with whole-body badges, finger badges, and digital or pocket dosimeters.
- Pregnant workers should declare their pregnancy to the RSO as soon as they learn of their pregnancy, to facilitate minimizing fetal dose.
- A fetal monitoring badge should be worn on the abdomen.
- The exposure limit to the fetus during gestation is limited to 500 mrem.
- Job restrictions may be agreed upon between the pregnant worker and employer.
- Bioassays may be required for workers who administer therapeutic doses.
- An inventory of radioactive materials must be kept to include receipt, use, and disposal of materials.
- Receipt procedures must be followed to inspect, check exposure rates and contamination, and record the receipt measurements.
- Semiannual inventories of sealed sources must be conducted and recorded.
- Sealed sources must be wipe tested for leakage and results must be recorded.
- Safe use of radioactive materials includes the appropriate application of time, distance, and shielding.
- ALARA principles must be applied in all aspects of practice.
- Contamination control practices are employed, including frequent changing of gloves, hand washing, and good housekeeping practices.
- Radiation surveys are conducted to quantify and record exposure rates in designated areas. Both removable and fixed contamination must be identified.
- Signs are posted in work areas that are appropriate for the materials and exposure levels encountered in that area.
- Patient release criteria are prescribed by the radionuclide, exposure rate, and exposure to the public or family members.
- Dry radioactive waste that has a half-life of 120 days or less may be decayed in storage for disposal. Materials may be disposed of typically following 10 half-lives and monitoring with appropriate instrumentation, which demonstrates that the material is not above background levels.
- Emergency procedures should be written and include the following: clear the area, notify supervisor or RSO, contain the spill, evaluate severity, decontaminate personnel, decontaminate spill area, survey, and write report.
- Written directives are used for greater than 30 µCi of ^{125}I or ^{131}I and for therapeutic radionuclides as a part of the QMP.
- Medical events are documented and reported according to federal, state, and local regulations.
- Radioactive materials are shipped in compliance with DOT regulations.
- The biological effects of ionizing radiation include acute effects, cataract induction, fertility effects, late effects, and genetic effects.

REFERENCES

1. Advisory Committee on the Biological Effects of Ionizing Radiations: *The effects on populations of exposure to low levels of ionizing radiation*, Washington, DC, 1980, Division of Medical Science, National Academy of Sciences, National Research Council.
2. American Cancer Society: *Cancer facts and figures: probability of developing invasive cancer over selected age intervals, by sex, US, 1999-2000*, New York, 2005, American Cancer Society.
3. Environmental Protection Agency: *Proposed federal radiation protection guidance for occupational exposure*, Washington, DC, 1981, U.S. Environmental Protection Agency Office of Radiation Programs.
4. Hall EJ: *Radiobiology for the radiologist*, ed 3, Philadelphia, 1978, JB Lippincott.

5. International Council of Radiation Protection: Report no. 41: nonstochastic effects of ionizing radiation, *Ann Intern Comm Radiol Protect* 1(3), 1977.

6. Knoll B: *Radiation detection and measurement*, ed 3, New York, 2000, Wiley.

7. National Council of Radiation Protection: *Recommendations on limits for exposure to ionizing radiation*, Report No. 91, Washington, DC 1987, The National Council on Radiation Protection.

8. Pochin EE: Why be quantitative about radiation risk estimates? Lauriston S. Taylor lecture no. 3, Washington, DC, 1978, National Council of Radiation Protection.

9. U.S. Department of Transportation: Research and Special Programs Administration, In *Part 173: Shippers general requirements for shipment and packaging*, Washington, DC, 2005, U.S. Department of Transportation.

10. U.S. Nuclear Regulatory Commission: Consolidated guidance about materials licenses. In *NUREG-1556, vol 9, Program-specific guidance about medical use licenses*, Washington, DC, 2005, U.S. Nuclear Regulatory Commission.

11. U.S. Nuclear Regulatory Commission: Consolidated guidance about materials licenses. In *NUREG-1556, vol 11, Program-specific guidance about licenses of broad scope*, Washington, DC, 1999, U.S. Nuclear Regulatory Commission.

12. U.S. Nuclear Regulatory Commission: *Title 10, Code of Federal Regulations*, Part 19, Notices, instructions and reports to workers—inspection and investigations, Washington, DC, 2005, U.S. Nuclear Regulatory Commission.

13. U.S. Nuclear Regulatory Commission: *Title 10, Code of Federal Regulations*, Part 19, Notices, instructions and reports to workers: inspection and investigations, Washington, DC, 2008, U.S. Nuclear Regulatory Commission.

14. U.S. Nuclear Regulatory Commission: *Title 10, Code of Federal Regulations*, Part 20, Standards for protection against radiation, Washington, DC, 2005, U.S. Nuclear Regulatory Commission.

15. U.S. Nuclear Regulatory Commission: *Title 10, Code of Federal Regulations*, Part 30, Rules of general applicability to domestic licensing of byproduct material, Washington, DC, 2005, U.S. Nuclear Regulatory Commission.

16. U.S. Nuclear Regulatory Commission: *Title 10, Code of Federal Regulations*, Part 35, Human uses of byproduct material, Washington, DC, 2005, U.S. Nuclear Regulatory Commission.

17. U.S. Nuclear Regulatory Commission: *Title 10, Code of Federal Regulations*, Part 71, Packaging and transportation of radioactive material, Washington, DC, 2005, U.S. Nuclear Regulatory Commission.

18. Wolbarst AB: *Physics of radiology*, ed 2, Madison, Wis., 2005, Medical Physical Publishing.

SUGGESTED READING

Committee to Assess Health Risks from Exposure to Low Levels of Ionizing Radiation, National Research Council: *Health risks from exposure to low levels of ionizing radiation: BEIR VII phase 2*, Washington, DC, 2006, National Academies Press.

National Council on Radiation Protection: *Radionuclide exposure of the embryo fetus*, Report No. 128, Washington, DC, 1998, National Council on Radiation Protection.

National Council on Radiation Protection, Meinhold C: *Limitation of exposure to ionizing radiation*, Report No. 116, Washington, DC, 1993, National Council on Radiation Protection.

Shapiro J: *Radiation protection: a guide for scientists, regulators, and physicians*, ed 4, Cambridge, Mass, 2002, Harvard Press.

Turner JE: *Atoms, radiation and radiation protection*, ed 2, New York, 1995, Wiley Interscience.

Patient Care and Quality Improvement

Kathy Thompson Hunt, Donna C. Mars, Denise A. Merlino

OBJECTIVES

After completing this chapter, the reader will be able to:

- Identify steps that must be taken before patient arrival for a nuclear medicine procedure.
- List ways to ensure positive outcomes with various types of patient encounters.
- Describe appropriate techniques for interacting with various age groups.
- Demonstrate the proper techniques for transferring patients.
- Identify commonly prescribed medications including their indicated use.
- Describe the dosage, contraindications, and side effects of medications used in conjunction with nuclear medicine procedures.
- Describe and demonstrate proper venipuncture technique including the administration of intravenous medications.
- Describe and demonstrate precautions for using and disposing of biohazardous waste including sharps.
- Describe and demonstrate the proper monitoring and care of intravenous lines
- Describe and demonstrate the standard precaution guidelines.
- Identify and discuss the three categories of intravascular radiopaque contrast media.
- Discuss the difference between high osmolar, low osmolar, and isomolar contrast media.

- Match clinical symptoms of adverse reactions to iodinated contrast media to the level of treatment required.
- Determine the information needed from the patient or the patient's medical record before administering any type of contrast media.
- Demonstrate proper aseptic and sterile techniques.
- Describe how to obtain accurate respiration rate, pulse rate, and blood pressure measurements.
- Describe actions to be taken in various medical emergencies.
- Describe the care and monitoring of ancillary equipment associated with the care of patients.
- Discuss quality improvement programs and their relationship to nuclear medicine services.
- Identify the various components to a comprehensive quality management program within medical imaging.
- Describe methods to provide quality improvement in customer service.
- Discuss techniques to obtain and analyze data relative to patient care, including problem solving.
- List the forces that drive quality within medical imaging.
- Identify the key terms and coding systems important to describe the procedures and services performed by nuclear medicine professionals.

KEY TERMS

Ambulatory Payment Classifications (APC)
anaphylactic reaction
anaphylactoid reaction
antecubital
blood urea nitrogen (BUN)
bradycardia
Centers for Medicare and Medicaid Services (CMS)
central venous line
chronic obstructive pulmonary disease (COPD)
compliance
contrast-induced nephropathy (CIN)
current procedural terminology (CPT)
decubitus
diastolic pressure
dyspnea
electronic medical record (EMR)
extravasation
Food and Drug Administration (FDA)
gadolinium-based contrast media (GBCM)
glomerular filtration rate (GFR)

Healthcare Common Procedure Coding Systems (HCPCS)
Health Insurance Portability and Accountability Act (HIPAA)
hepatitis B virus (HBV)
high osmolality contrast media (HOCM)
Hospital Outpatient Prospective Payment System (HOPPS)
human immunodeficiency virus (HIV)
hypertension
hypoglycemia
Independent Diagnostic Testing Facilities (IDTF)
infiltration
International Classification of Diseases (ICD)
intradermal
intrathecal
intravenous drip infusion pump
isomolar
low osmolality contrast media (LOCM)
Medicare Physician Fee Schedule (MPFS)
National Uniform Billing Committee (NUBC)

nephrogenic systemic fibrosis (NSF)
Occupational Safety and Health Administration (OSHA)
osmolality
osmotoxic
paramagnetic metals
peripherally inserted central catheter (PICC)
personal protective equipment (PPE)
power or pressure injector
quality assurance (QA)
quality control (QC)
quality improvement (QI)
quality management (QM)
radiology benefit management (RBM)
radiopaque contrast media (ROCM)
Society of Nuclear Medicine (SNM)
stoma
syncope
syringe infusion pump
systolic pressure
tachycardia
The Joint Commission
total quality management (TQM)
venipuncture

PATIENT CARE

It is the responsibility of the nuclear medicine technologist (NMT) to provide quality care to the patient during all procedures. The NMT is often the only person available to provide basic care to the patient while performing the nuclear medicine procedure. It is also the responsibility of the NMT to provide excellent customer-oriented, quality services and maintain confidentiality in accordance with the **Health Insurance Portability and Accountability Act of 1996 (HIPAA)**. This chapter discusses the various responsibilities associated with the first encounter with the patient, including patient assessment and care of the patient. This chapter also provides a framework for continuous performance improvement and compliance concepts in nuclear medicine.

PATIENT PREPARATION

The NMT is often the primary contact for the patient from scheduling to completion of the procedure. It is very important for the technologist to remember that establishing trust and cooperation begins within the first 30 seconds of meeting the patient.

There are multiple settings for nuclear medicine, such as outpatient diagnostic centers, physicians' offices, mobile units, and hospitals. Patient encounters are modified based on the setting, but basic quality service must be maintained, and efforts to continuously improve the process must be pursued.

The first step is usually to review the referring physician's order to correlate the procedure with the patient's history and to determine if there are any contraindications. The format used by physicians when ordering a procedure will also vary with the setting. A hospitalized patient will have orders written in the medical chart or entered electronically in the information system. Orders for an outpatient may be electronically transmitted, verbally ordered, or presented on arrival in written format. Restrictions may be placed on the method of ordering procedures, the format of the order, or required components based on institutional policy or legal requirements. Federal or state regulation may dictate and define what constitutes a medical order.

Some nuclear medicine procedures require specific, standardized patient preparation. Standardized protocols should be established with the scheduling source, for example, nursing units, physician offices, or clinics. A reminder by nuclear medicine personnel regarding patient preparation at the time of scheduling can help prevent delays in performing the procedure. The scheduling source should also be aware of any conflicting exams, such as barium radiographs, other nuclear medicine procedures, or interfering medications.

Basic information included on the request should be the patient's name, identification number, referring physician's name, and clinical indications for the procedure.

Hospitalized patients will have additional information, such as room number and mode of transportation.

Arrangements must be made for the availability of the radiopharmaceutical required for the procedure. Orders must be placed for radiopharmaceuticals not routinely stocked. When ordering radiopharmaceuticals, the timing from preparation to injection must be a consideration. Ample time must be allowed when ordering from a nuclear pharmacy so that arrival of the patient and the radiopharmaceutical dose are synchronized. A simplified flow chart of the process of scheduling a patient is presented in Figure 8-1. Several preparations must be made before the patient's arrival:

- Quality control measurements must be performed on all equipment—for example, daily quality control on the dose calibrator and gamma camera.

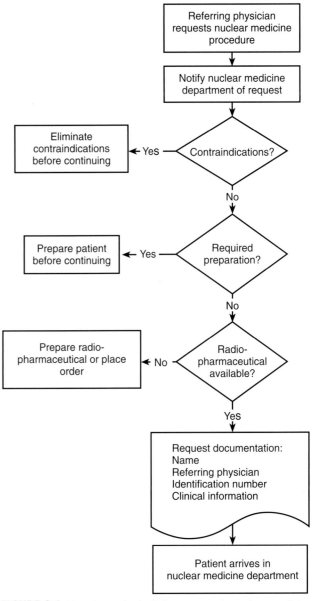

FIGURE 8-1 Flowchart of scheduling process in nuclear medicine department.

- Personnel must be trained in the technical aspects of procedures and in customer service.
- Necessary supplies must be assembled.
- Radiopharmaceutical doses must be checked in according to Nuclear Regulatory Commission (NRC) and state regulations.
- Interventional agents must be ordered, if applicable.
- Emergency equipment and supplies must be available.

PATIENT ENCOUNTER

It is very important that the first contact the patient experiences with the health care personnel is positive. The greeting the patient receives will set the tone for the entire procedure. The person greeting the patient, whether it is the transporter, technologist, or clerical personnel, must do so in a friendly, professional manner. It is important to remember that most patients have limited knowledge of nuclear medicine procedures and the term *nuclear* alone may initiate fears that have to be addressed before the patient's procedure. The patient must be clearly identified on arrival by using person-specific information. For outpatients, this process may include asking the person's name, birth date, or phone number. With hospitalized patients, matching the name and medical record number on an arm band to the order can serve as a means of identifying the patient. The Joint Commission requires two patient identifiers be used when identifying patients. The intent of the requirement is to ensure the correct patient is matched to the correct procedure. Electronic identification, such as bar coding technology, will comply with this requirement if it uses two or more person-specific indicators.

When the patient arrives in the nuclear medicine department, further investigation must be made to ensure that the correct procedure is scheduled and that there are no contraindications. Before beginning the procedure, the technologist must obtain a complete medical history including the verification of adherence to any patient preparation required before the procedure. The medical history will give the technologist information concerning any contraindications, such as previous procedures, medications or disease states that may interfere with the procedure. Interfering procedures, medications or disease states may call for special precautions or result in an alternative protocol being performed. For outpatients, a thorough medical history may not be available; therefore, it is the technologist's responsibility to obtain the history from the patient. Technologists usually have access to the medical records of hospitalized patients. These records may be available as a hard copy referred to as a medical chart or in an **electronic medical record (EMR)**.

Patients expect to receive an explanation of what is expected of them, how the procedure will be performed, any discomfort they may experience, the required length of time for the procedure, and how and when they will hear about the results. Effective communication at this point will help ensure cooperation throughout the procedure. It is important to use terminology appropriate to the patient's understanding. The American Medical Association (AMA) has determined that written material relating to the medical procedure must be geared to that of a fifth-grade reading level to ensure that the patient is able to comply with the necessary preparation and understand the upcoming procedure.

The technologist must determine the extent of the patient's physical ability. Patients who are physically challenged may have special care needs. Assistance must be provided for those patients who are unable to move on and off imaging tables. The geriatric patient may have a hearing loss, making it difficult to hear and follow instructions. Pediatric cases require special handling techniques, and the psychiatric patient may have special needs. Language interpreters fluent in the patient's native language or sign language need to be used to address language barriers.

The following sections present information and skills related to age specific care, body mechanics, medications and their administration, infection control, use of specialized equipment, and basic patient-care skills such as obtaining vital signs and responding to the patient during emergency procedures.

Establishing a quality or performance improvement process, which involves strategic planning, process management, customer satisfaction, analysis and management of data, and specific problem-solving tools and techniques for the individual technologist and nuclear medicine teams, is also discussed.

AGE-SPECIFIC CARE

During a career in nuclear medicine, a person will have the opportunity to work with diverse age groups. Although each patient should be treated as an individual, there will be situations where patients will be very similar to others in their age group. This is due to the different developmental stages each person passes through during a lifetime. How a technologist works with a small child may be very different from how the technologist works with an adult. Understanding the different developmental stages and learning how to identify normal behavior for the age group will help the technologist provide quality care.

Developmental Stages for Children/Adolescents

0 to 6 Months. Children during this developmental stage are self-oriented. Their feeling of security is based on their own needs being met. They see themselves as the center of the world and discover that if they cry a caregiver will come. A young infant needs to be touched and responds well to being held or wrapped in a tight blanket. Physically, an infant is able to make large muscle movements (arms and legs) and eventually is able to roll over. Loud noises will scare children of this age, and they have the tendency to cling to parents when in unfamiliar surroundings.

Technologists working with infants during this development stage should prepare the imaging room before the child's arrival. If possible, the parents should be allowed to stay with their child. Often, having the parents feed the infant before the exam may cause the infant to fall asleep, thus making the imaging easier. Since infants cannot say what is wrong, it is very important for the technologist to be observant and carefully watch and listen to the child for signs of a problem.

6 to 15 Months. Children in this age group are curious about everything. They want to explore their world, pick items up, and place everything in their mouth. Since they are able to sit up and are learning to crawl, children in this age group are very mobile. They do not like to be separated from their caregiver and are able to express their emotions clearly.

When working with this age group, restraining devices must be used since children are more mobile. They should be held or restrained at all times. Because children at this age are beginning to develop a memory, a scrub uniform or laboratory coat may cause children to become upset. Limiting the number of strangers entering the room and having a parent close by may help ease a child's anxiety. Remember, children in this age group want to put everything in their mouths. To prevent injuries, health-care supplies, such as gauze or needles, should be kept out of the child's reach.

15 to 24 Months. At this developmental stage, children become more independent. They are able to communicate more, play alone or with others, and are very active. Since they are more independent, they are unhappy with loss of control and, if any restraints are used, children in this age group will become very resistant.

Technologists should take the time to develop a rapport with the child. Allowing toddlers to hold their favorite toy or blanket will provide comfort and a sense of security. While understanding that a child may become frustrated with restraints, children this age must be watched or restrained at all times.

3 to 5 Years. Preschool children are very independent and can be separated from their caregiver. They do not like to be told what to do and can express their feelings verbally. Children in this age group understand cause-and-effect relations only in relation to their own needs, wants, and experiences. They are able to identify with adults and like to imitate or show off learned skills. Preschool-aged children can understand and follow simple game rules.

When working with children in this age group, the technologist should remember to maintain constant communication and reassurance. Comments made by the technologist will be taken literally, so it is important

to remain truthful. It is important that the technologist explain why the procedure is being performed and that it is not a punishment. Otherwise, this age group may demonstrate their frustration by a variety of behaviors such as throwing objects, having a temper tantrum, or holding their breath. The technologist should look for what is causing the distress and, depending on the circumstance, either ignore the behavior or physically move the child away from the situation to prevent injury. Establishing trust with a child may help calm their fears and ease frustration. Allowing children to safely hold medical equipment, talking with them throughout the procedure, and showing interest in their thoughts and feelings will help them adjust to unfamiliar surroundings. Children in this age group want to be "helpers." Praising children for their help and cooperation along with allowing them to have choices will help them feel a sense of independence.

6 to 12 Years. Children in this age group are highly verbal. They want to talk and ask a lot of questions. They are able to understand and follow directions, make decisions, and accept responsibility for their actions. They do not want to be treated "like a kid" but still want the caregiver present to help or show approval.

It is highly likely that children from this age group will be seen in a nuclear medicine department because injury or accidents are a major cause of health concerns in this population. Patients in this age group need to be reassured with clear and simple explanations about what is happening to them. Often, a child's fear of the unknown is greater than his fear of reality. It is important for the technologist to allow time before and after the procedure for questions and discussions. A child's cooperation can be gained by explaining what is expected and allowing him to manipulate the equipment, if appropriate.

13 to 17 Years. This is a significant time for adolescents in that it represents a transition from childhood into adulthood. Adolescents experience changes in cognitive development and are able to reason and solve problems. Self-image is important and they become more focused on body awareness and modesty. They show less dependence on family for affection and emotional support.

When working with adolescents, it is important to explain why a procedure is necessary. As much as possible, involve the patient in decision making and planning; for example, let the patient choose a time and the individuals present during the procedure. Special consideration for the patient's privacy is important especially during an examination. Adolescents may have difficulty accepting new authority figures and may resist complying with procedures. It is important to recognize the patient's fears and treat the patient as an individual.

The Adult Patient

Age 19 to 65 Years. This age group spans many years. Although individuals in this group are considered adults, there are different thought processes and concerns associated with each decade of years. Young adults (i.e., younger than 25 years) are trying to find their place in life. They are entering new roles and responsibilities at work and at home as they move from dependence to independence. As they get older, the threat of poor health adds additional stress and concerns. When working with adult patients, it is important to access what illness means to each individual. The care and information provided is based on an individual's level of maturity and their ability to problem solve and make decisions. It is important to take the time to explain why a procedure is being performed. Some adult patients may need just a few details whereas others may want a more extensive explanation. Always provide a nonjudgmental atmosphere when caring for adult patients. Identify the needs of the patient and provide for physiological needs such as changes in sight, hearing, and memory.

Ages 66 Years and Older. During this stage, aging adults have to adjust to physical changes that may affect them emotionally. These physical changes place this population at higher risk for many problems or diseases such as stroke, diabetes, high blood pressure, heart problems, and fractures. Because of this increased risk, members of this age group are likely to be taking one or more medications that may interfere with a nuclear medicine procedure.

It is important that the technologist treats older patients with compassion, patience, and respect. Older patients may need additional time to understand and react to what is being said and to express their thoughts. When speaking with an older patient, technologists should face the patient and make sure their eyes are on the same level as the patient's. This may require the technologist to sit in a chair to talk to a patient in a wheelchair. Since older patients may have difficulty hearing, always speak slowly and use short, simple, and direct sentences. Never assume that the patient heard and understood what was said. Since aging patients are more susceptible to falls, make sure the imaging area is safe and free of clutter. If a patient uses a walker, cane, or wheelchair, make sure it is placed within easy reach of the patient. Since an aging patient's skin is more susceptible to tears or bruises, special attention should be given to the patient before applying tape or using restraints when securing the patient on the imaging table. At all times, maintain aging patients' dignity and privacy.

BODY MECHANICS

The principles of proper body alignment, movement, and balance are referred to as body mechanics (Figure 8-2). Practicing the concepts of body mechanics is important in terms of the health and wellness of the technologist as well as the safety of the patient.

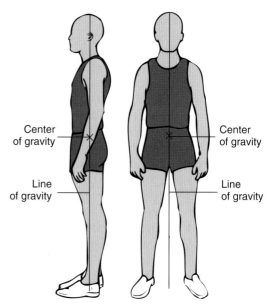

FIGURE 8-2 Correct body alignment.

Concepts of Body Mechanics

Base of support—Provide wide and stable base of support by standing with feet a shoulder width apart with one foot slightly advanced.

Center of gravity—Keep objects close to the body. The weight of an object is multiplied by a factor of 10 for every inch it is held away from the body.

Body alignment—When lifting objects off the floor, bend the knees and keep the back straight and avoid twisting the trunk.

Lifting Tips

- Avoid lifting heavy objects above shoulder or below waist level.
- Keep stomach muscles tight, using legs for lifting and abdominal muscles for support.
- Bend the knees when lifting from below the waist level.
- Avoid using back muscles to lift.

Pushing/Pulling Tips

- When moving heavy objects or equipment, push rather than pull while using leg and abdominal muscles.
- If pulling is necessary, do so by walking forward; in other words, do not walk backwards while pulling an object.

Carrying Tips

- Hold loads with arms and legs working together.
- Avoid bending the neck to the side when carrying a load on the shoulder.

- Vary carrying techniques and pause for rest when carrying for long distances.

Patient Transfers

The first step is to determine that the technologist has the correct patient by using two patient identifiers. The next step is to assess the patient's ability to move and explain to the patient his or her role in the transfer. Safety should be of primary concern when transferring patients by a wheelchair or stretcher. If needed, safety straps can be used with wheelchairs, stretchers, and imaging tables. Stretcher side rails should be in place during transport of the patient. The use of restraints requires a physician's order.

To transfer a patient from the bed to a wheelchair, start by lowering the bed to the level of the wheelchair seat and elevating the head of the bed. Position the wheelchair at a 45-degree angle to the bed with wheels locked, and raise foot supports out of the way. Position the patient on the edge of the bed by placing one arm under the patient's shoulders and the other arm under the knees to raise the patient to a sitting position. Allow time for the patient to adjust to the upright position. Take precautions to ensure patient safety by supporting the patient. Many patients suffer from orthostatic hypotension after long periods of rest and feel lightheaded or faint when changing to an upright position suddenly. After this adjustment period, most patients will be able to move to the wheelchair with only minimal assistance.

Orthopedic or neurologically impaired patients require more assistance. Always position the patient's strongest side toward the area to which he or she is being transferred. Stand facing the patient. Reaching under the patient's shoulders, place hands over the scapulae. The patient's hand may rest on the technologist's shoulders. While using proper body mechanics, lift upward. If the patient has an injured leg or foot, the technologist should place her feet on either side of the affected foot. A technologist can use their own knee to block the patient's knee and provide additional support. Pivot the patient toward his or her strong side and into the wheelchair.

To move a patient from the wheelchair to a locked imaging table, place the wheelchair at a 45-degree angle to the table with the patient's strongest side toward the table. Lock the wheels, raise foot supports, and help the patient stand, using the face-to-face assist. Have the patient place one hand on the footstool handle and one arm on the technologist's shoulder and step onto the footstool, with strong side first, pivoting with the patient's back to the table. Ease the patient to a sitting position. Place one arm around the patient and the other arm under the patient's knees. With a single motion, place the legs on the table while lowering the head and shoulders into the supine position.

If a patient is unable to stand, a stretcher should be used. Start with the patient in the supine position with knees flexed and feet flat. Position the stretcher parallel to the imaging table toward the patient's strongest side and lock the stretcher wheels and the imaging table. Place one arm under the patient's shoulders and the other arm under the pelvis. Instruct the patient to push with feet and elbows as the technologist assists in the transfer to the imaging table. The maneuver should be repeated until the patient is secure on the imaging table.

Use "draw sheet" lifts or a slide board when a patient is unable to assist in the transfer. Both techniques require the use of two or more people. A draw sheet is a sheet folded in half that is placed under the patient. To use a draw sheet, turn the patient on their side and place the folded draw sheet on the bed with the fold against the patient's back. Roll the top sheet until the sheet roll is against the patient's back. Turn the patient to the opposite side, moving over the rolled sheet. Straighten the sheet roll and return the patient to a supine position. Align the patient's head and torso in order to move the patient as one unit while supporting the patient's head. When transferring the patient, the sheet is rolled up close to each side of the patient to provide a handhold for lifting and pulling the patient onto the imaging table. A slide board can be used in conjunction with the draw sheet. Roll the patient onto his or her side and insert the board under the draw sheet, being sure to include the patient's head and torso. The slide board provides a hard surface to make the transfer easier. The use of antistatic spray will prevent the build-up of static electricity on the board. (Figures 8-3 and 8-4).

If a patient cannot be transferred by these techniques, a hydraulic lift may be necessary. It is important that the technologist is familiar with how to operate the equipment before using the device. Basic features of a hydraulic lift include support arms attached to a base, a manual pump for raising the support arms, a release knob used for lowering the support arms, and a spreader bar to which a transfer sling is attached. If a hydraulic lift is necessary, the patient should arrive in the nuclear medicine department in a wheelchair already sitting on the transfer sling. The transfer sling should be positioned equally around both sides of the body. Do not put anything (e.g., cushion, pad) between the patient and the sling since this may cause the patient to slide out of the sling. A hydraulic lift should never be used for transporting a patient from one location to another location.

To lift the patient from the wheelchair, move the hydraulic lift slowly toward the patient and position the spreader bar over the patient's chest (Figure 8-5). Attach the transfer sling to the hydraulic lift based on the manufacturer's recommendations. Using the manual pump, gently lift the patient above the wheelchair. Once the patient has cleared the wheelchair, the wheelchair can be

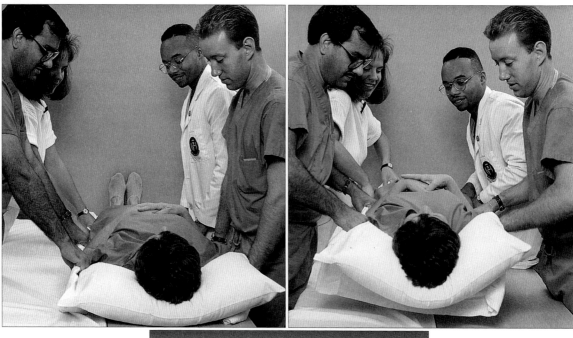

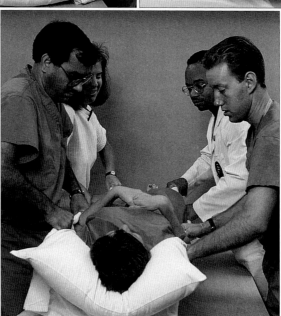

FIGURE 8-3 Patient transfer using a draw sheet.

removed and the lift can be positioned over the imaging table. The patient can now be carefully lowered to the imaging table by operating the release knob. This procedure can be reversed when returning the patient to the wheelchair.

MEDICATIONS AND THEIR ADMINISTRATION

Technologists are required to be competent in the administration of all medications, including radiopharmaceuticals, and nuclear medicine enhancing (interventional) medications, such as furosemide and cholecystokinin

(CCK). The **Food and Drug Administration (FDA)** has reclassified radiopharmaceuticals and contrast media as drugs, where they once were classified as biologicals. **The Joint Commission** also includes radiopharmaceuticals and contrast media in its definitions of drugs. It is the ultimate responsibility and duty of the technologist to be familiar with the routes of administration, pharmacology, and adverse effects of all medications used in nuclear medicine procedures. Most institutions require technologists to demonstrate competency in all medications that are administered in conjunction with a procedure. There are varying mechanisms to demonstrate competencies, including annual in-service workshops with a written

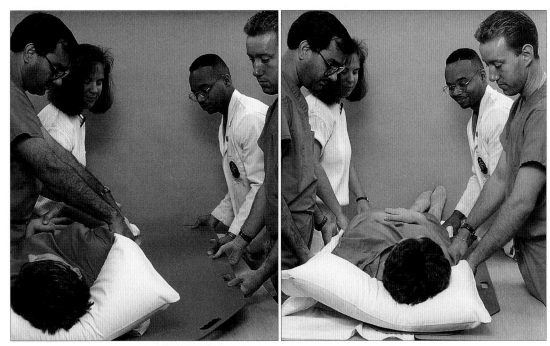

FIGURE 8-4 Patient transfer using a slide board.

exam and evaluation by a physician, nurse, or pharmacist. Department policies should include all potential medications to be administered for each procedure and highlight clinical information, such as the dose and route of administration, as well as potential adverse reactions and the steps to take if an adverse reaction occurs. Consult the *Scope of Practice for Nuclear Medicine Technologists* published by the Technologist Section of the **Society of Nuclear Medicine (SNM)**, the *Essentials and Guidelines for an Accredited Educational Program for the Nuclear Medicine Technologist* published by the Joint Review Committee on Educational Programs in Nuclear Medicine Technology, the *Components of Preparedness* and *Pharmaceuticals List* published by the Nuclear Medicine Technology Certification Board (NMTCB), or the *Content Specifications for the Examination in Nuclear Medicine Technology* published by the American Registry of Radiologic Technologists (ARRT) for additional information on each of the pharmaceuticals and radiopharmaceuticals that are within the scope of practice for an NMT to administer.

A written or verbal order that is properly documented must accompany each procedure. A viable written order for each nuclear medicine medication (such as including the addition of a pharmacological interventional drug) must be documented before administration. Verify the order by checking the patient's written or electronic records. The medication may be ordered by its generic or trade name. The generic name of a medication identifies its chemical family. Different pharmaceutical companies may manufacture the same generic substance under a different proprietary or trade name. A useful resource that lists medications alphabetically according to their generic classes, trade names, or indications is the *Physician's Desk Reference* (PDR) (Tables 8-1 and 8-2). All medications administered must be properly documented in the patient's medical record. Proper documentation includes the medication name, dose, route of administration, and the name and credentials of the person administering the medication. Appropriate documentation also serves as the basis for billing and compliance as discussed later in this chapter.

The Six Rights

The correct administration of pharmaceuticals includes the six rights system as follows:

1. Right dose
2. Right medication
3. Right patient
4. Right time
5. Right route
6. Right documentation

Several additional points must be remembered when administering medications:

- Know the indications and side effects of the medication before administration.
- Follow the established rules of the aseptic technique.
- Read the label three times: before and after withdrawal of the medication and before administration. The technologist is responsible for any medication

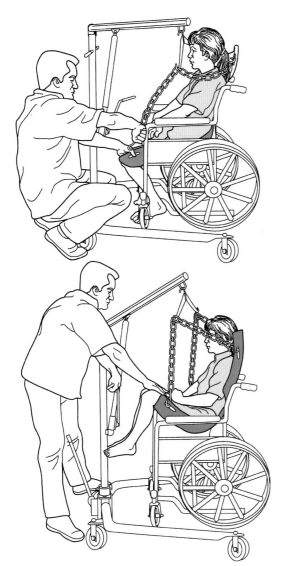

FIGURE 8-5 A hydraulic lift transfer.

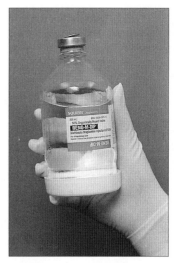

FIGURE 8-6 Check the name of medication, its strength, and the expiration date.

that he or she administers, regardless of who has prepared it.

• Check medication for proper concentration and expiration date (Figure 8-6).
• Check two patient identifiers before administration.
• Monitor the patient for side effects. Be familiar with any medication that may require an antidote and where the emergency cart is located.
• A medication error must be reported according to institutional policy. The referring physician must also be notified.

Routes of Medication Administration

Medications may be administered by topical, sublingual, oral, or parenteral routes.

Topical Route—Medication is applied to a limited area for a local effect. The medication is absorbed through the skin and into the bloodstream. Examples are solutions, creams, or transdermal patches applied directly to the skin.

Sublingual Route—Medication is placed beneath the tongue and is absorbed into the bloodstream. An example of a sublingual medication is nitroglycerin. Administration of nitroglycerin results in a dilation of the coronary arteries. This produces a systemic effect to counteract angina pectoris.

Oral Route—Oral medications are supplied in a variety of forms, such as tablets, capsules, granules, and liquids. Sodium iodine ^{123}I or ^{131}I is often administered by mouth, usually in capsule or liquid form, for thyroid uptakes, scans, and therapy. Oral medications are administered as follows:

• Wash hands.
• Read the label and prepare for administration.
• If a physician is administering the medication, show the physician the label before administration.
• If a physician requests the technologist to administer the medication, check the patient's two identifiers and read the label again before administering. Stay with the patient while the medication is swallowed, and offer water if permitted.

Parenteral Route—Medications injected directly into the body and are classified according to the depth of the injection (Figure 8-7).

• *Subcutaneous* (under the skin) medications are injected at a 45-degree angle using a ⅝-inch needle with a 23 to 25 gauge. The most common injection

TABLE 8-1	Overview of Clinical Pharmacology	
Class	**Why Used**	**Examples (Brand Names) Other Uses**
Antihistamines		
Allergies	Prevent allergic reactions	Diphenhydramine (Benadryl)
		Astemizole (Hismanal)
Antiinfectives		
Antibiotics	Treat/prevent	
	Bacterial infections	Aminoglycosides (IV) gentamicin, tobramycin—nephrotoxic
		Penicillins, cephalosporins amoxicillin (Amoxil), Unasyn, Timentin, cefazolin, cefuroxime, ceftriaxone (Rocephin)
		Quinolones ciprofloxacin (Cipro), ofloxacin (Floxin)
		Other miscellaneous clindamycin, erythromycin, metronidazole, trimethoprim/sulfamethoxazole (Bactrim), vancomycin, doxycycline fluconazole (Diflucan)
Antifungals	Treat/prevent	Amphotericin B—nephrotoxic
	Fungal infections	Cyclophosphamide, ifosfamide—nephrotoxic
Antineoplastics	Treat cancer	Doxorubicin, fluorouracil, methotrexate, cisplatin, carboplatin, vincristine, vinblastine
Autonomic		
Anticholinergics	Inhibit effects of parasympathetic nervous system activity	Atropine, preop for salivation; causes dry mouth, constipation
		Ipratropium (Atrovent)—inhaled for COPD
Adrenergics	Bronchodilation	Albuterol (Ventolin)—inhaled for asthma
	Increase HR, BP	See Cardiac drugs
Coagulation		
Anticoagulants	Treat/prevent blood clots: for DVT/PE, AMI, Afib	Heparin (IV)
		Warfarin (Coumadin)
Thrombolytics	Break up clots for AMI	TPA, streptokinase
Cardiovascular		
Cardiac drugs	Increase heart's contraction	Digoxin (Lanoxin)—also for Atrial fibrillation, dobutamine (Dobutrex)
		Dopamine
		Low dose increases urine output.
		High dose increases heart contractility
	Treat arrythmias	Lidocaine, bretylium
Antilipemic	Treat elevated cholesterol	Lovastatin (Mevacor)
		Cholestyramine (Questran)
Hypotensives	Reduce blood pressure	ACE-inhibitors—also CHF, diabetes, captopril (Capoten), enalapril (Vasotec)
		β-Blockers—also post MI, atenolol (Tenormin), metoprolol (Lopressor)
		Calcium channel blockers diltiazem (Cardizem), verapamil (Calan), Nifedipine (Adalat, Procardia)
		Central A_2 agonists clonidine, methyldopa (Aldomet)
		Peripheral A_1 antagonists prazosin (Minipress), terazosin (Hytrin)
Vasodilators	Angina, acute MI	Nitrates nitroglycerin, isosorbide dinitrate (Isordil)
CNS-Agents		
Analgesics and antipyretics	Pain and fever	Aspirin—also antiplatelet (stroke, MI, angina)
		Acetaminophen (Tylenol)
		NSAIDs—can be nephrotoxic esp with ACE inhibitor, ibuprofen (Motrin), indomethacin (Indocin)—also for gout
Analgesics	Pain	Opiates morphine, meperidine (Demerol)
	Reverse opiate-induced sedation and respiratory depression	Opiate antagonist naloxone (Narcan) (IV), phenytoin (Dilantin)
Anticonvulsants	Prevent seizures	Carbamazepine (Tegretol)
		Valproic acid (Depakene)
Psychotherapeutics	Depression	Amitriptyline (Elavil)
	Psychosis, agitation	Fluoxetine (Prozac)
		Haloperidol (Haldol)
Anxiolytics	Anxiety, insomnia	Benzodiazepines midazolam (Versed), lorazepam (Ativan)

Continued

TABLE 8-1	Overview of Clinical Pharmacology—cont'd		
Class	**Why Used**	**Examples (Brand Names) Other Uses**	
Water/Electrolytes			
Diuretics	Remove fluid	Loop—also in CHF, furosemide (Lasix)	
		Thiazide—also in hypertension, hydrochlorothiazide	
Gastrointestinals			
Miscellaneous	Prevent acid secretion	H₂ blockers ranitidine (Zantac), cimetidine (Tagamet)	
		Proton pump inhibitors Omeprazole (Prilosec)	
Prokinetics	Speed passage of food out of stomach	Metoclopramide (Reglan)	
		Cisapride (Propulsid)	
Antiemetics	Prevent/treat nausea/vomiting	Promethazine (Phenergan)	
		Ondansetron (Zofran)	
Hormonal			
Adrenals	Supplement, antiinflammatory	Prednisone administered orally	
		Methylprednisolone (IV)	
		Triamcinolone (Azmacort)—inhaled-asthma	
Antidiabetics	Replace insulin	Insulin (many kinds)	
	Stimulate insulin release	Sulfonylureals glipizide (Glucotrol), glyburide (DiaBeta, Micronase)	
	Increase glucose uptake	Metformin (Glucophage)	
		Contraindication: must not give within 2 days of radiological procedures, and then hold metformin until renal function returns	
Thyroid	Replace	Levothyroxine (Synthroid)	
	Suppress	Propylthiouracil	
Miscellaneous			
Asthma/COPD	Relax bronchial muscle	Theophylline (Theo-Dur), aminophylline	
Gout	Acute	colchicine, allopurinol	
	Chronic	Benztropine (Cogentin)	
Parkinson's disease	Restore dopamine/ACh balance	Carbidopa-levodopa (Sinemet)	

ACE, Angiotensin- converting enzyme ; *CHF,* congestive heart failure; *COPD,* chronic obstructive pulmonary disease; *MI,* myocardial infarction.
From McEvoy GK, editor: *American hospital formulary service—drug information,* Bethesda, Md, 1996, American Society of Health-System Pharmacists. Modified by Ted Morton, PharmD, Baptist Memorial Hospital, Memphis, Tenn.

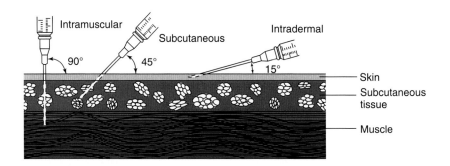

FIGURE 8-7 Comparison of the angles of needle insertion.

sites are the upper arm or outer aspect of the thigh. Injection volume is usually 2 ml or less. (Example: allergy injections.)

• *Intramuscular* (into the muscle) medications are injected into the deltoid muscle of the upper arm, the upper quadrant of the gluteus maximus muscle in the hip, or the vastus lateralis muscle of the lateral thigh at a 90-degree angle. The injection volume may be up to 5 ml, and the needle size can range from 22 to 25 gauge. (Example: vitamin B₁₂ injections.)

• *Intradermal* (between the layers of skin) medications are administered using a tuberculin syringe with a very small needle (26 or 27 gauge). (Example: tuberculin skin test and injections for lymphoscintigraphy.)

TABLE 8-2	Nonradioactive Pharmaceuticals Used in Nuclear Medicine		
Pharmaceutical Generic (Trade Name)	Indication	Dosage	Adverse Effects
Acetazolamide (Diamox)	Brain imaging	1 g in 10 ml sterile water, IV over 2 min	Tingling sensations in extremities and mouth, flushing, light-headedness, blurred vision, headache
Adenosine (Adenocard)	Cardiac imaging	140 µg/kg/min for 6 min, or 50 µg/kg/min increased to 75, 100, and 140 µg/kg/min each min to 7 min	Chest, throat, jaw, or arm pain; headache, flushing, dyspnea, ECG changes
Aminophylline	Cardiac imaging	50-250 mg IV	Nausea, vomiting, headaches
Captopril (Capoten)	Renal imaging	25-50 mg orally 1 hr before study	Orthostatic hypotension, rash, dizziness, chest pain, tachycardia, loss of taste
Cimetidine (Tagamet)	Meckel diverticulum imaging	Adult: 300 mg/kg Pediatric: 20 mg/kg in 20 ml saline, IV over 2 min with imaging 1 hr later	Diarrhea, headache, dizziness, confusion, bradycardia
Dipyridamole (Persantine)	Cardiac imaging	0.57 mg/kg IV over 4 min (0.142 mg/kg/min)	Chest pain, nausea, headache, dizziness, flushing, tachycardia, shortness of breath, hypotension
Dobutamine (Dobutrex)	Cardiac imaging	Incremental dose rate of 15 µg/kg/min up to 15 (child); up to 40 µg/kg/min every 3 min (adult)	Angina, tachyarrhythmia, headache, nausea, vomiting
Enalaprilat (Vasotec IV)	Renovascular hypertension evaluation	0.04 mg/kg in 10 ml saline, IV over 5 min	Orthostatic hypotension, dizziness, chest pain, headache, vomiting, diarrhea
Furosemide (Lasix)	Renal imaging	Adult: 20 to 40 mg Pediatric: 0.5 to 1 mg/kg, IV over 1 to 2 min	Nausea, vomiting, diarrhea, headache, dizziness, hypotension
Glucagon	Meckel diverticulum imaging	Adult: 0.5 mg (range 0.25-2 mg) Pediatric: 5 µg/kg, IVor IM	Nausea, vomiting
Morphine (Astramorph, Duramorph)	Hepatobiliary imaging	0.04 mg/kg, diluted in 10 ml saline, IV over 2 min; range 2-4.5 mg)	Respiratory depression, nausea, sedation, light-headedness, dizziness, sweating
Pentagastrin (Peptavlon)	Meckel diverticulum imaging	6 µg/kg (subcutaneously)	Abdominal discomfort, urge to defecate, nausea, flushing, headache, dizziness, tachycardia, drowsiness
Phenobarbital (Luminal)	Pediatric hepatobiliary imaging	5 mg/kg/day orally for 5 days	Respiratory depression, nausea, vomiting, dizziness, drowsiness, headache, paradoxical excitement in children
Naloxone hydrochloride (Narcan)	Hepatobiliary imaging	0.8 mg IV	Change in mood, increased sweating, nausea, nervousness, restlessness, trembling, vomiting
Regadenoson (Lexiscan)	Cardiac imaging	0.4 mg/5 ml IV rapid 10 sec injection followed by immediate 5 ml saline flush Inject radiopharmaceutical 10-20 sec later	Dyspnea, headache, flushing, chest discomfort, dizziness, angina pectoris, chest pain, nausea
Recombinant TSH/ rhTSH (Thyrogen)	Thyroid imaging	0.9 mg IM for 2 consecutive days	Nausea, headache, swelling and tenderness of thyroid
Sincalide (Kinevac)	Hepatobiliary imaging	0.02 µg/kg in 10 ml saline, IV over 5 min	Abdominal pain, urge to defecate, nausea, dizziness, flushing

ECG, Electrocardiogram; IM, intramuscular; IV, intravenous.
Modified from Park HM, Duncan K: Non-radioactive pharmaceuticals in nuclear medicine, J Nucl Med Technol, 22(4):240-249, 1994.

- *Intravenous* (IV) medications are administered using various types of equipment depending on the type of injection and the substance to be injected. Intravenous injections are the route most often used in nuclear medicine and will be discussed in more depth later.
- *Intrathecal* medications such as contrast media or radiopharmaceuticals are administered using a spinal needle to inject medications directly into the subarachnoid space of the spinal cord. The NMT's responsibility with this parenteral method is to assist the physician by preparing a sterile environment and to assist during administration of the medication. (Example: nuclear cisternogram injection)

Intravenous Equipment

Venipuncture may be accomplished with a butterfly needle set, a syringe and needle, or an IV catheter. A butterfly needle set or winged infusion set consist of a flexible tubing attached to a needle with two plastic "wings" on either side. The needle is held by grasping the wings between the thumb and index finger. Before the butterfly needle set is inserted into the vein, the tubing may be filled with saline or sterile water to avoid injecting air. The butterfly set can be used for multiple injections and is often used for bolus injections followed by a saline flush. It is very effective when medications are administered through small or shallow veins because the needle can be inserted at a shallow angle. The technologist may use a butterfly needle set when the injection site is difficult to obtain with a syringe and needle.

The use of syringes and needles is generally restricted to withdrawing blood samples or for single injections. Needles are supplied in various diameters and lengths, and the gauge of a needle indicates the diameter. As the gauge increases, the diameter of the bore decreases. The length of the needle is measured in inches and is determined by the depth needed for the injection. The needle length may vary from $\frac{1}{2}$ inch for intradermal use to $4\frac{1}{2}$ inches for intrathecal (spinal cord) injections (Figure 8-7).

Intravenous catheters frequently are used when repeated IV injections, infusions, or bolus injections are administered. An over-the-needle catheter is composed of a silicon catheter with a stylet/needle inside the catheter lumen. Administering medications through an intravenous catheter is discussed later in the chapter. The **Occupational Safety and Health Administration (OSHA)** requires the use of safety-engineered sharps devices to minimize potential health risk to employees. New devices have been developed, including needleless IV access systems and syringes with built-in safety features to retract or protect the needle (Figures 8-8 and 8-9). OSHA

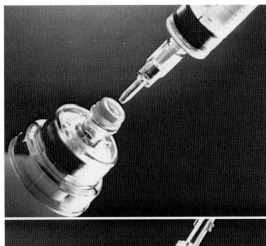

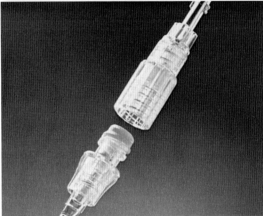

FIGURE 8-8 Example of needleless IV access system.

recognizes that these devices may not be available for every situation in a nuclear medicine department since radiation safety must also be a concern.

Preparation for Venipuncture

The **antecubital** or median cubital vein on the anterior surface of the elbow is usually used. Other sites that may be used include the median basilic veins, cephalic veins, veins of the anterior wrist, or veins of the posterior hand (Figure 8-10). Dilate the vein by applying the tourniquet 4 to 6 inches above the venipuncture site. Ask the patient to make and hold a tight fist. Put on gloves. Palpate the area, using the first or second finger to locate a vein. Appropriate veins for venipuncture will demonstrate a rebound sensation on palpation. Avoid superficial veins or veins that feel hard or knotty with palpation. Prepare the site by cleansing the area with 70% isopropyl alcohol or some of the newer patient preoperative skin preparations that include chlorhexidine gluconate with isopropyl alcohol. Cleanse the area by applying the agent to the center of the site and working outward from the center in a circular motion.

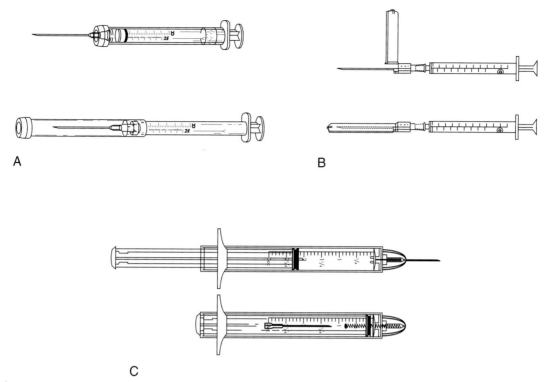

A

B

C

FIGURE 8-9 Examples of syringes with built-in safety features to retract or protect the needle. **A,** Self-sheathed protected position. Hypodermic syringe with "self-sheathing" safety feature. **B,** Protected position. Added feature attached to syringe needle. **C,** Retracted protected position. Hypodermic syringe with "retractable technology" safety feature.

Venipuncture Procedure

Venipuncture technique is the same whether using a butterfly needle set, needle and syringe, or IV catheter. Anchor the vein by stretching the vein firmly in the opposite direction of the course of the needle. To insert a needle, remove the needle cover and turn the bevel upward (except in the pediatric population). Pediatric injection techniques are discussed in detail in the Chapter 23. Hold needle and penetrate the skin just below the point where the vein is to be entered. With a syringe and needle, the needle is inserted at a 30-degree angle. An intravenous catheter may be inserted at a 20- to 30-degree angle. A butterfly needle set may be inserted at a shallow angle depending on the vein selected. Avoid touching the insertion site after cleansing it. Advance the needle quickly but cautiously, penetrating the vein with the needle point. As the vein is entered, usually there is a sensation of resistance followed by an ease of penetration and a flashback of blood into the tubing with the butterfly needle set, or into the needle hub when using a needle and syringe. While continuing to hold the skin taut, carefully advance the needle in a direct line with the vein to prevent puncture of the vein's posterior wall.

To confirm that the needle is in the vein, withdraw a small amount of blood into the needle and syringe before injecting the radiopharmaceutical. To confirm placement of needle using a butterfly set, inject sterile water or saline before injecting the radiopharmaceutical. Observe for signs of possible **infiltration** such as swelling or burning sensation in the area of injection. If signs are present, discontinue the injection immediately. If no signs are present, release the tourniquet and withdraw the needle. Apply pressure immediately with a dry gauze or cotton ball and maintain pressure for approximately 1 minute or until bleeding stops. Use paper tape to secure the butterfly needle, if used (Figure 8-11).

To insert an over-the-needle catheter, remove the needle cover and turn the bevel of the stylet/needle up. Anchor the vein and insert the needle at a 20- to 30-degree angle as previously described. Lower the needle until it is almost flush with the skin, and enter the vein. This is to prevent piercing of the posterior wall of the vein. Check for vein entry by observing a flashback of blood, and advance the needle $\frac{1}{4}$ inch farther into the vein to establish the catheter tip. Holding the stylet/needle hub with one hand, use the thumb and forefinger of the other hand to gently advance the catheter off the stylet/needle and into the vein. Do not reinsert the stylet/needle into the catheter. Release the tourniquet and relax the tension on the skin. To prevent excessive flashback of blood, use the index finger to apply pressure on the vein above catheter. A 2 × 2 inch sterile gauze pad may be placed under the catheter hub to prevent leakage of

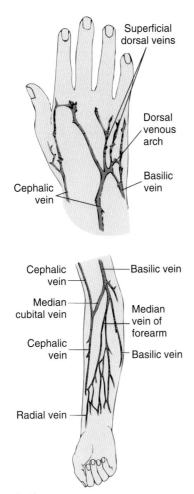

FIGURE 8-10 Veins easily accessible for venipuncture.

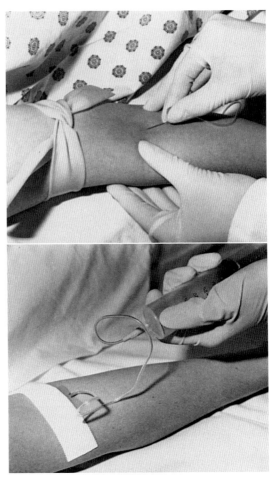

FIGURE 8-11 Butterfly set facilitates direct IV injection.

blood onto the patient's skin Remove the stylet/needle from the catheter and attach the adapter or syringe (Figure 8-12).

Extravasation Precautions

Extravasation or **infiltration** occurs when fluid leaks from the venous system into the tissues. The following precautions should be taken to prevent extravasation or infiltration:

1. Check for backflow or flashback to determine needle placement.
2. Immobilize the needle or catheter at the injection site.
3. Stop the injection immediately if the patient complains of discomfort at the injection site, if any resistance to the injection is felt, or if swelling around the site is observed.

If infiltration does occur, maintain pressure on the vein until bleeding has stopped completely. This procedure may help to prevent a painful hematoma.

Document in the medical record that the infiltration occurred, the potential volume, and the location of the infiltration.

Needle Disposal

Dispose of all needles and syringes directly into a puncture-proof container without recapping, if possible. Containers are labeled according to the type of contamination: biohazard, radioactive, or both. Radioactive syringes sometimes will require recapping before disposal to avoid radioactive contamination. If it is necessary to recap a used needle, use a needle cap holder or place the needle cover on a firm surface and insert the needle using one-handed technique. Safety syringes designed to prevent accidental needle sticks are now available and should be used when possible.

Withdrawal of Nonradioactive Materials from a Vial

Nonradioactive materials may be dispensed in liquid form or as a lyophilized (freeze-dried) material that has

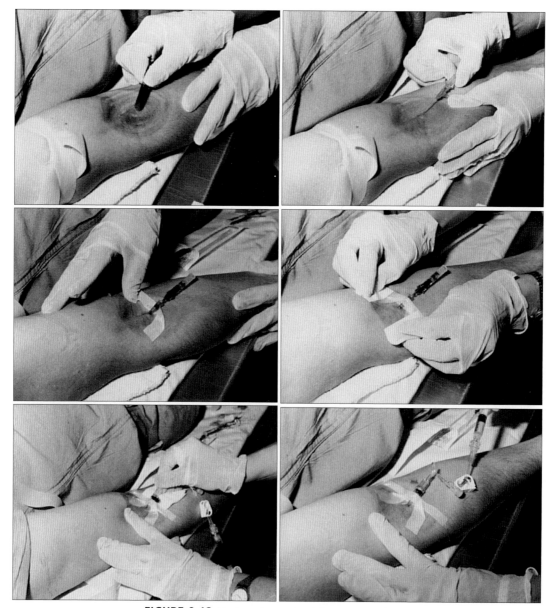

FIGURE 8-12 Venipuncture using intravenous catheter.

to be reconstituted. If lyophilized, a diluent will need to be added, according to the package insert, to bring contents into solution. According to USP Chapter 797,* the septum cannot be punctured more than two times and

*The United States Pharmacopeial Convention (USP Convention) is a nongovernmental, not-for-profit organization. This scientific body is responsible for setting standards for drug quality and related practices. USP also refers to the book of drug standards published by this organization. Much of the USP is devoted to drug standards, which are organized as drug monographs that provide specific information on drug strength, quality, purity, packaging, storage, and other requirements. The current version of USP (i.e., *United States Pharmacopeia*, 31st revision, and *National Formulary*, 26th edition; USP 31-NF 26) contains more than 4200 monographs for drug products. Chapter <797> of the USP describes standards for preparation of sterile drugs including radiopharmaceuticals.

the medication must be used within 1 hour of preparation. Assemble the syringe and needle. Read the label to verify the correct medication, concentration, and expiration date. If the drug is supplied in solution in a single dose ampule, a small file may be needed to score the neck of ampule. Snap off the top by using a 2 × 2 inch gauze to protect fingers (Figure 8-13). A filter needle may be used to draw up the medication and eliminate possible glass particles from being drawn into the syringe. If the drug is supplied in a vial, a metal or plastic cap will need to be removed. When withdrawing nonradioactive substances, a volume of air equal to the dose may be inserted into the vial before withdrawing the dose. Remove the needle cover, taking care not to contaminate the needle. Insert the needle into the rubber septum at a 45-degree angle, straighten the needle when puncturing the septum, and withdraw the desired amount while checking for any air bubbles. Air bubbles may be removed by tapping the sides of the syringe (Figure 8-14).

Withdrawal of Radioactive Materials from a Vial

A radioactive dose may be withdrawn from a shielded vial or supplied from the nuclear pharmacy as a unit dose. When handling radioactive materials, gloves must always be worn. Lead glass syringe shields are available to accommodate several syringe sizes to decrease the exposure when withdrawing and injecting radioactivity. Assemble the syringe and needle, and lock them securely into the syringe shield. Remove the needle cover, taking care not to contaminate the needle. Sanitize the rubber septum of the shielded vial with alcohol and insert needle at a 45-degree angle, straightening the needle when

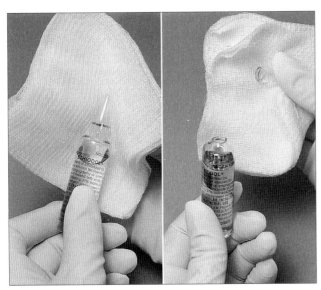

FIGURE 8-13 Preparing medication from an ampule.

puncturing the septum. This will prevent breaking off pieces of the rubber septum and introducing them into the vial. Turn the vial upside down and withdraw the desired volume while checking for air bubbles. Do not inject air into the vial when withdrawing radiopharmaceuticals.

Syringe Infusion Pumps

The syringe infusion pump is designed to deliver a small volume of medications over several minutes. In nuclear medicine, **the syringe infusion pump** is often used to administer nonradioactive pharmaceuticals such as adenosine, the pharmacological stressing agent used in association with myocardial perfusion imaging. The pump allows medications that should be pushed slowly over several minutes to be administered safely, reducing errors and potential adverse side effects.

The selection of a syringe infusion pump for a particular nuclear medicine department should be based on which pump best meets the requirements of the protocol. This selection often depends on the pharmaceutical used and the specific dosage requirements. It is important that the technologist ensures that the pump is compatible with the type of syringes used in the department and that the pump is capable of delivering the correct dosage based on protocol. The technologist must also be able to correctly calibrate the infusion pump and perform maintenance on the pump to ensure it is functioning properly. Training of staff that will use the infusion pump will help to eliminate potential medication errors and ensure the technologist is familiar with proper operation of the pump. Box 8-1 describes the protocol for administering medications through the use of a syringe infusion pump.

Intravenous Drip Infusion

The drip infusion set should always be positioned approximately 18 to 20 inches above the vein. If the set

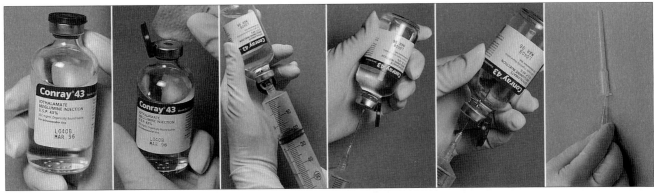

FIGURE 8-14 Drawing up medication from a vial.

BOX 8-1	Syringe Infusion Pump Administration

1. Connect prefilled syringe to tubing designed for use with the syringe infusion pump.
2. Slowly apply pressure to syringe plunger, filling the tubing to avoid injecting air.
3. Attach syringe to infusion pump.
4. Attach infusion pump tubing to main IV line.
   a. Stopcock: Cleanse stopcock port with alcohol and connect tubing. Turn stopcock to the open position.
   b. Needleless system: Cleanse needleless port with alcohol and connect infusion tubing.
5. Ensure infusion pump is secure by either attaching the pump to an IV pole or placing the pump safely next to patient, ensuring infusion pump will not fall from bed.
6. Set pump to deliver medication based on department protocol and manufacturer's recommendations. Press "start" button on pump to begin infusion.

BOX 8-2	Administering Nonradioactive Medication to an IV Solution Bag

1. Dilute the medication with the recommended diluents according to the package insert of the medication to be administered.
2. Calculate the amount of medication to be added to the intravenous solution bag.
3. Remove protective cover from the solution bag and inspect the solution bag for leaks, damage, or particulate matter in the solution. Do not use if such findings exists. Check the expiration date of solution.
4. Using appropriate technique, draw up the calculated dosage required for the procedure in a syringe.
5. Sanitize the injection port on the bag using alcohol.
6. Carefully remove cap from the syringe and insert the needle or needleless access device into the injection port of the solution bag.
7. Inject medication using aseptic technique.
8. Mix the solution bag by gently inverting container from end to end.
9. Properly label bag and document medication in patient's record.

is placed too low, fluid may flow back into the tubing, causing it to coagulate and form a clot. Infusion sets placed too high above the vein may cause infiltration due to increased pressure.

The drip rate on an IV drip infusion set is controlled by a clamp below the drip chamber. This clamp can be opened or closed to control the rate of flow (Figure 8-15). This is especially important for patients who must have their fluid intake closely monitored. Most patients are able to tolerate a flow rate of 15 to 20 drips per minute, which results in the patient receiving approximately 60 ml per hour. Box 8-2 describes the method of adding a nonradioactive medication to an IV solution bag. According USP 797 (see footnote) the medication must be used within 1 hour of preparation. Box 8-3 describes the steps to take when preparing for an IV drip infusion procedure.

Intravenous Drip Infusion Pump

Intravenous drip infusion pumps are used to infuse fluids or medications into a patient's circulatory system in a more precise method, allowing for monitoring of the amount of fluids to be infused in a certain time frame (Figure 8-16). Patients may arrive at a nuclear medicine department with an infusion pump already in use, receiving medications or fluid ordered by their physician. Some nuclear medicine protocols recommend the use of an infusion pump, for example, administering CCK to determine ejection fraction during a hepatobiliary study. It is critical that there is training for the technologist on the proper use of an infusion pump. The technologist needs to know how to set up an infusion pump and troubleshoot for problems that may occur during

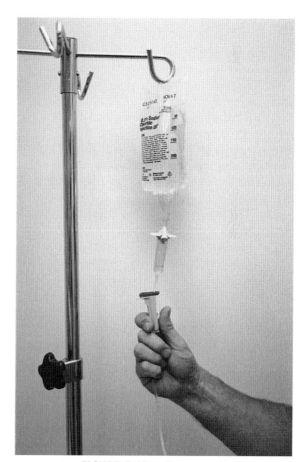

FIGURE 8-15 IV flow control.

the infusion, such as pump malfunction or infiltration of the IV fluid. With several different types of infusion pumps, the technologist must refer to the manufacturer's recommendations for the correct operation of the equipment.

BOX 8-3	Setup for an IV Drip Infusion Procedure

1. Obtain solution bag to be administered. Check expiration date. Remove the protective cap from the tubing insertion port and sanitize the port with alcohol.
2. Obtain infusion set. Straighten the tubing while checking for any defects.
3. Close the tubing with the clamp.
4. Remove the protective cover from spike on the drip chamber of the tubing. Care should be taken to keep the spike sterile. Insert the spike into the insertion port on the plastic bag.
5. Hang solution on IV pole and squeeze drip chamber until it is half full.
6. Prime tubing before using the IV set by removing the protective cap at the end of the tubing. Be careful to maintain sterility of the cap and the end of the tubing. Hold end of tubing over a waste basket or sink and slowly release clamp, allowing solution to run freely through tubing, removing air bubbles.
7. Reclamp tubing and replace cap on the end of the tubing using sterile technique. The drip infusion set is now ready for use.

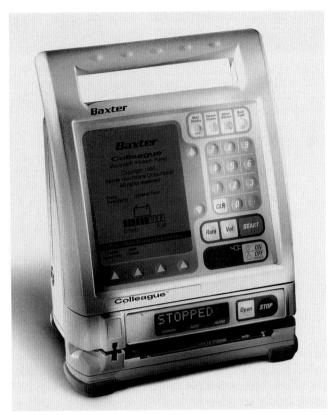

FIGURE 8-16 IV pumps regulate and permit self-administration of IV medications.

An infusion pump can be programmed to deliver medications or fluid continuously, intermittently, or on demand. The continuous infusion setting is programmed to administer flow rates of 1 to 999 ml/hr. Using this setting, the infusion pump administers fluids in small pulses, usually between 500 nl and 10,000 µl. The intermittent setting is programmed to administer high infusion rates alternating with low infusion rates to maintain patency. This setting is often used to administer medications that may irritate blood vessels at a continuous high flow rate. The on-demand setting is used to administer mediation as requested by the patient, such as pain medication. A maximum amount allowed during a time period is programmed to prevent overmedication of the patient.

The infusion pump comes with a built-in battery power, which allows the patient to be transported from their room to other areas within the hospital. Fully charged, most batteries will last for 6 hours at 125 ml/hr delivery rate. When the patient arrives in a nuclear medicine department with a pump already in use, the technologist should connect the power cord on the infusion pump to an electrical outlet. This ensures sufficient battery life during transport of the patient back to their room after a long procedure.

An audible alarm will sound if there is a problem with the infusion pump. The technologist can temporarily stop the audible alarm by pressing "silence" on most systems. Once the alarm is silenced, the technologist should identify the cause of the alarm and correct the condition. If the alarm is the result of a low battery charge, this can be corrected by immediately plugging in the battery into an electrical outlet. Often the cause of an alarm is the result of an occlusion in the IV line due to a crimp in the tubing caused by the patient's arm being bent. This problem can easily be corrected by straightening the patients arm and resetting the infusion pump. If there are signs of infiltration, such as discomfort, pain, or swelling at the site of IV insertion, the infusion should be stopped immediately. Before the procedure the patient's nurse should be informed if the procedure will be lengthy to ensure that the patient's prescribed medication can be continued. During the procedure the patient's nurse must be notified immediately if the infusion is stopped for any reason or if the IV fluid could possibly become exhausted before the nuclear procedure is complete.

Medication Administration through Established Intravenous Lines

Patients coming to the nuclear medicine department may arrive with an intravenous catheter, a standard IV set, or intravenous drip infusion in place. Often these established lines may be suitable for dose administration relating to a nuclear medicine procedure. The technologist should always look for signs of infiltration around the entry site before use. If signs of infiltration are present, the IV infusion should be discontinued and the patient's nurse should be notified. If the intravenous catheter or intravenous line is patent, the technologist may decide to use the site for dose administration, depending on

<table>
<tr><td>

BOX 8-4 | **Administering Medication through Primary IV Line**

1. Determine the flow rate (bolus or push) of the dose to be administered.
2. Wash hands and put on gloves.
3. Properly prepare the pharmaceutical and/or radiopharmaceutical according to package insert using aseptic and radiation safety techniques.
4. Sanitize the injection port closest to the patient using alcohol.
5. Pinch or clamp IV tubing between the IV bag and the port. This will prevent the medication from flowing back into the IV bag.
6. Flush the port with a minimum 10 ml saline. If resistance is experienced, confirm patency.
7. Sanitize the injection port and insert prepared syringe into the injection port. Never insert a needle directly into IV tubing.
8. Administer the medication following the proper procedure.
9. Flush the port with a minimum 10 ml saline. Unclamp tubing.
10. Monitor for signs of infiltration. If infiltration is suspected, do not use the IV line and notify the patient's nurse.

</td><td>

BOX 8-5 | **Administering Medication through an Intravenous Catheter with No Tubing Attached**

1. Wash hands and put on gloves.
2. Properly prepare the pharmaceutical and/or radiopharmaceutical using aseptic technique and radiation safety techniques for radiopharmaceuticals.
3. Sanitize injection port using alcohol.
4. Hold injection port and insert a saline flush syringe. Gently push saline, checking on ease of administration and signs of infiltration. If there is a question concerning the patency of the IV site, discontinue use of the IV site.
5. Remove saline flush syringe. Sanitize the injection port using alcohol. While holding the injection port, attach the medication syringe.
6. Administer the medication as indicated and flush with a minimum of 10 ml saline.

</td></tr>
</table>

hospital protocol. Procedures for administering a medication through established IV lines are described in Boxes 8-4 and 8-5.

Charting Medications

Notation that the study was completed and documentation of any medications given must be recorded in the patient's medical records. The records may be in hard copy form or documented electronically. The notation should include the time of day, the name of the drug, the dosage, and the route of administration. These four key elements are necessary for **compliance** and appropriate billing. Lack of documentation can result in loss of dollars, as coders need this valuable information to select the most accurate code and number of units for billing a payer. The entry must include the identification and credentials of the person who charted it. For legal purposes, the technologist who charts medications must follow the procedure and protocol established by the institution.

CONTRAST MEDIA

Positron emission tomography acquired with computed tomography (PET-CT) and magnetic resonance (PET-MR) are modalities that merge anatomical and physiological information into a single procedure. The merging of these modalities allow for attenuation correction and more accurate anatomical localization for the PET procedure while providing a CT or MR of diagnostic quality for physician interpretation. Often to produce a diagnostic CT or MR image, contrast media is used.

Pharmacology of CT Contrast Media

Radiopaque contrast media (ROCM) are often used in CT procedures to visualize low-contrast tissues in the body. Contrast media are composed of elements with high atomic numbers such as iodine. The element iodine is responsible for attenuating photons, causing a density difference between low contrast tissues. This allows structures containing the ROCM to be differentiated from the surrounding tissues, increasing the visualization of these structures. Types of low contrast tissues that can be visualized using contrast media are the kidneys, gastrointestinal tract, blood vessels, and biliary tree. The functional units of these organ systems are not actually visualized because the contrast media does not cross the cellular membranes. The organ systems are visualized because the contrast media are evenly dispersed throughout the vascular system of these organs and organ systems.

Intravenous ROCM are classified according to their chemical structure, **osmolality,** iodine content and ionization in solution.[6] Contrast media are currently only available in ionic or nonionic forms with either low osmolality. The osmolality of a solution is proportional to the number of particles in that solution. Thus, an ionic agent that dissociates into two particles forming an anion and cation will have a higher osmolality than a nonionic agent that does not dissociate in solution. Osmolality effects the distribution and movement of water between body compartments separated by permeable or semipermeable membranes such as blood vessels and extravascular spaces. **High-osmolality contrast media (HOCM)** demonstrates a greater attraction for water in order to equilibrate the pressure between the compartments. This imbalance leads to a greater incidence of adverse effects resulting in the infrequent clinical use of IV HOCM.[1]

TABLE 8-3	Radiopaque CT Contrast Media		
Category of ROCM	**Chemical Name of ROCM**	**Trade Name and Manufacturer**	**Ratio of Iodine to Osmotically Active Particles**
Low-osmolar nonionic agents	Iodixanol	Visipaque GE Healthcare	3:1 (3 iodine atoms per molecule and does not dissociate in solution)
	Iohexol	Omnipaque GE Healthcare	
	Iopamidol	Isovue Bracco Diagnostics Inc.	
	Iopromide	Ultravist Bayer Healthcare	
	Ioversol	Optiray Covidien	
Low-osmolar ionic agents	Ioxaglate meglumine	Hexabrix Covidien	3:1 (6 iodine atoms per molecule and dissociates into 2 osmotically active particles in solution)

ROCM, Radiopaque contrast media.
American College of Radiology: *Manual on contrast media*, Version 7, Reston, Va., American College of Radiology, 2010. Available on Internet: http://www.acr.org/SecondaryMainMenuCategories/quality_safety/contrast_manual.aspx. Accessed August 2010.

Intravascular ROCM have three main categories: high osmolar ionic agents, low osmolar ionic agents, and low osmolar nonionic agents. **Low osmolality contrast media (LOCM)** vary from having two to three times the osmolality of blood to having the same osmolality as blood.[6] Agents with the same osmolality of blood are referred to as an **isomolar** or an isotonic contrast agent. LOCM has lower incidence of adverse effects as compared to **HOCM**, which have five to eight times the osmolality of blood.[6] Examples of the currently used ROCM are listed in Table 8-3.

The iodine concentration of the intravenous ROCM used in CT imaging can be lower than the concentration needed in conventional x-ray imaging. Intravascular ROCM are water soluble and can be diluted so that they can be administered in lower concentrations. The serum iodine concentration for CT studies needs to be between 2 mg/ml and 8 mg/ml.

Pharmacology of MR Contrast Media

Effective contrast agents for MR possess magnetic properties and are called paramagnetic substances. Examples of **paramagnetic metals** are Gd(III), Mn(II), Mn(III), and Fe(III). These metals have unpaired electrons resulting in an overall positive or negative charge and are complexed with a chelating agent. Chelates are substances that have the ability to bind a metal with a ligand. The local magnetic field produced by the paramagnetic substances increase the rate of relaxation of hydrogen protons found in the tissue. This process is called proton relaxation enhancement and shortens both T1 and T2 relaxation times. The relaxation process is discussed in Chapter 12.

Metal ion chelate complexes may be administered intravenously or orally. The majority of contrast media are administered intravenously.

Contrast media may be either a positive or negative agent depending on whether the agent produces positive or negative contrast on the image. Positive contrast is used in the majority of procedures. The metal gadolinium has seven unpaired electrons and is an example of a positive paramagnetic contrast agent. Gadolinium is bound to an organic ligand by a chelate, for example diethylenetriaminepentaacetic acid (DTPA), and it forms a metal chelate complex. When comparing the metal chelate complex to the metal alone, the complex results in lower toxicity to the patient. Gadolinium is a positive contrast agent because it enhances the signal as it interacts with the hydrogen atoms within the patient's tissue. As the tissues accumulate this agent, the signal is enhanced by shortening the T1 relaxation time while leaving the T2 undisturbed. This results in a stronger signal emitted in the T1-weighted images, which is visualized as a bright region on the image.[5]

An example of a negative contrast agents used in MR is iron oxide. It is composed of particles and is called a superparamagnetic substance because it has very strong paramagnetic properties. This agent creates a local magnetic field that shortens the T2 relaxation time to a greater extent than the T1 relaxation time, resulting in negative contrast. Negative contrast results in a decreased signal. As the agent accumulates, the area will appear as a dark region on the image.

Gadolinium-based contrast media (GBCM) is the most common contrast media used in MR and may be ionic or nonionic with high or low osmolality. Examples of common GBCM used in MR are listed in Table 8-4.

TABLE 8-4	Gadolinium-Based MRI Contrast Media	
Category	**Chemical Name**	**Trade Name and Manufacturer**
Ionic with high osmolality	Gadopentatate dimeglumine (Gd-DTPA)	Magnevist Bayer Healthcare
	Gadobenate dimeglumine (Gd-BOPTA)	MultiHance Bracco Diagnostics Inc
Nonionic with low osmolality	Gadodiamide (DTPA-BMA)	Omniscan GE Helathcare
	Gadoteridol (Gd-HP-DOTA)	ProHance Bracco Diagnostics Inc
	Gadoversetide	Optimark
	Gd-DTPA-BMEA	Covidien
	Gadofosveset trisodium	Ablavar* Lantheus
	Gadoxetate disodium	Eovist Bayer Healthcare

*Please refer to: http://www.accessdata.fda.gov/scripts/cder/drugsatfda/index.cfm?fuseaction=Search.DrugDetails
American College of Radiology: *Manual on contrast media*, Version 7, Reston, Va., American College of Radiology, 2010. Available on Internet: http://www.acr.org/SecondaryMainMenuCategories/quality_safety/contrast_manual.aspx. Accessed August 2010.

Adverse Effects of Contrast Media

The American College of Radiology (ACR) has not noted any significant difference in the diagnostic quality of CT images obtained using any of the before mentioned categories of ROCM. The primary consideration in determining the type of ROCM to be used in a particular study is to decrease the probability of producing adverse effects.[1] To determine the appropriate contrast media to be used, the individual patient's pathology and history must be considered. A thorough patient history including any prior reactions to contrast injections is imperative before administering the ROCM. The technologist should always ask the patient to describe any food allergies or prior reactions to contrast media to determine the type and severity of the reaction. The physician should review the patient's history before any contrast media is administered.

Adverse effects are categorized as mild, moderate, or severe. The majority of adverse effects are not life threatening and are categorized as mild or moderate. Mild side effects are self-limiting and do not require medical treatment but do require monitoring. Examples of mild side effects are nausea, vomiting, flushing with a generalized feeling of warmth, headache, metallic taste, chills, rapid pulse, skin rash, itching, dizziness, and anxiety. The technologists should respond by stopping the infusion while reassuring the patient, notify the physician, and monitor the patient for at least 20 minutes. Mild adverse effects are reported to occur in 5% to 12% of all patients receiving HOCM.[1] This incidence rate has been decreased to 1% to 3% with the use of LOCM.[1,6] Moderate adverse effects take longer to resolve and may require medical treatment. Symptoms include **tachycardia, bradycardia, hypertension**, hypotension, **dyspnea**, mild bronchospasms, facial or laryngeal edema, and urticaria (hives). In addition to stopping the infusion, reassuring the patient, and notifying the physician, the technologist should also be prepared to administer oxygen and intravenous medications. The emergency team should be called if symptoms progress rapidly. Patients exhibiting any symptoms should be monitored to ensure that the adverse effects do not progress. Life-threatening effects usually occur within the first 20 minutes after administration of the agent.[1] Treatment of moderate adverse effects includes elevating the extremities in the case of hypotension and administering diphenhydramine for hives, a β-agonist for brochospasm, and epinephrine for hives or laryngeal edema. Severe adverse effects are life threatening and include vasovagal reactions, dyspnea related to laryngeal edema, moderate to severe bronchospasms, seizures, hypotension, cardiac arrhythmias, cardiopulmonary arrest, and lack of patient response. Prompt medical treatment is needed if the patient experiences any severe side effects. The technologist should call the emergency team and then notify the physician. Medical treatment begins with assessing the patient's airway, breathing, and circulation (ABCs) followed by the appropriate advanced cardiac life support (ACLS) treatment.

There are multiple mechanisms involved in producing adverse effects from the administration of ROCM, but the exact pathogenesis is not completely understood. The immune system sometimes responds to the administration of the ROCM with the release of pharmacologically active agents such as histamine, which may cause side effects ranging from a mild side effect, such as urticaria, up to a more systemic and life-threatening response referred to as an **anaphylactic reaction.** Anaphylaxis requires a first-time exposure to the antigen (foreign substance) that sensitizes the immune system to respond by producing antibodies that induce systemic hypersensitivity. Radiopaque contrast media may also induce an **anaphylactoid reaction** that requires no prior exposure to sensitize the immune system to produce an immunological response. This reaction is similar to anaphylaxis and can be just as lethal. Therefore, a "pretest" injection or history of a previous reaction will not always be beneficial in predicting an adverse reaction. Symptoms associated with anaphylaxis or an anaphylactoid reaction can range from mild to severe or may include a combination of adverse effects. Immediate treatment of life-threatening symptoms is crucial.

The osmolality of the ROCM is also responsible for adverse effects by causing the extracellular fluids to diffuse into the vascular compartments in an attempt to dilute the osmotically active particles. During this process, vasodilation occurs and flushing is experienced by most patients. The extravascular space becomes hyperosmolar because of dehydration, causing another fluid shift, which may be partially responsible for adverse renal side effects. It is imperative to know the patient's serum creatinine level before administering any type of ROCM. There is a direct relationship between the dose of ROCM and the adverse renal side effects in patients with an elevated serum creatinine level. Generally patients at risk are those with preexisting dehydration, renal disease, or diabetes. Adequate hydration is important in patients with renal dysfunction or patients who could be compromised by dehydration. Hydration of the patient before the study is not always possible and depends upon the patient's condition.

Contrast media may be contraindicated or premedication may be indicated in patients that are categorized as "at risk" for developing adverse reactions. At-risk patients include those with a history of asthma, allergies, renal disease, diabetes mellitus, cardiac disease, anxiety, pheochromocytoma, hyperthyroidism, or carcinoma of the thyroid. **Contrast-induced nephropathy (CIN)** is defined as an absolute rise in serum creatinine following administration of ROCM. The baseline **blood urea nitrogen (BUN)** and creatinine levels or an estimated **glomerular filtration rate (GFR)** is needed in patients suspected of renal disease. In general, at-risk patients should be given only LOCM because there is a decreased incidence of adverse side effects using this form of contrast media. A combination of LOCM and premedication has been noted to reduce reaction rates in patients who have previously experienced adverse effects from ROCM. Frequently used regimens for premedicating patients before administering ROCM can be found in Table 8-5.[1]

Before administering an IV iodinated contrast media, the patient's medications need to be reconciled to deter-

TABLE 8-5	Premedication Regimens	
Pharmaceutical	**Dosage Regimen**
Corticosteroid/Antihistamine Regimen	
Prednisone	50 mg by mouth at 13 hr, 7 hr, and 1 hr before
Plus	
Diphenhydramine (Benadryl)	50 mg intravenously, intramuscularly, or by mouth 1 hr before the administration of ROCM
Corticosteroid Regimen	
Methylprednisone (Medrol)	32 mg by mouth 12 hr and 2 hr before the administration of ROCM
Antihistamine such as Benadryl can be added	See Corticosteroid/Antihistamine Regimen

ROCM, Radiopaque contrast media.
American College of Radiology: *Manual on contrast media*, Version 7, Reston, Va., American College of Radiology, 2010. Available on Internet: http://www.acr.org/SecondaryMainMenuCategories/quality_safety/contrast_manual.aspx. Accessed August 2010.

mine if the patient is currently taking any medication that contains metformin. Metformin is an oral antihyperglycemic medication used to treat non–insulin dependent diabetes mellitus. The FDA has determined that metformin should be temporarily discontinued if a patient is undergoing a procedure requiring IV iodinated contrast media because of an the increased potential of developing lactic acidosis.[1] The patients at risk are those with renal dysfunction. The ACR recommends the discontinuation of metformin for 48 hours or until follow-up renal function is determined adequate before reinstitution of the medication. Other conditions causing decreased metabolism of lactate, such as liver dysfunction, or increased anaerobic metabolism such as cardiac failure or severe infections, can also put the patient at risk. GBCM used in MR does not need to be discontinued in the usual dosage range of 0.1 to 0.3 mmol per kg of body weight.[1]

The contrast media used in MR is administered in low doses resulting in a decreased occurrence of adverse effects as compared with the administration of CT contrast media.[1,3,4] Even though less frequent, the adverse effects are similar to those encountered when using nonionic iodinated contrast media. The GBCM are **osmotoxic,** which means that these agents have the ability to disturb the osmotic balance of the blood. The hyperosmotic side effects include low blood sodium and high blood potassium levels that can lead to dehydration. Acute mild side effects include events such as flushing, headache, nausea, and facial swelling and skin conditions including rashes, itching, and hives. A severe adverse renal side effect caused by GBCM is **nephrogenic** systemic fibrosis (NSF). NSF is a disease causing fibrosis of the skin and connective tissues. GBCM increases the risk of NSF in patients with renal insufficiency (GFR < 30 ml/min/1.73^2) or acute renal insufficiency of any severity due to hepatorenal syndrome.

Administration of Contrast Media

When performing CT and MR, bolus injections are superior to slower infusions for distinguishing between normal and abnormal structures. The recommended method for injection is to use a **power or pressure injector** capable of administering flow rates ranging from 1.0 to 10.0 ml/sec. The flow rate depends on the protocol of the study to be performed and the injection site. A large-gauge, flexible, plastic cannula is needed to deliver the bolus injection. A 20-gauge cannula is needed for flow rates of 3 ml/sec or higher.[1]

Preparation of the power injector includes clearing the syringe and tubing of any air. Air embolism is potentially fatal but extremely rare. Adverse effects caused by the injection of large amounts of air include air hunger, dyspnea, cough, chest pain, or expiratory wheezing. The incidence of air embolism is decreased with the use of power injectors as compared to administering the bolus by hand.[1] Treatment of air embolism includes administering 100% oxygen and placing the patient in the left lateral **decubitus** (left side down) position.[6] The position of the catheter tip should always be assessed by obtaining venous backflow before injecting the agent. If there is backflow, the technologist should palpate the injection site during the first 15 seconds of administration. If no backflow is observed or if the site is tender or infiltrated, an alternative site should be used. Always check the power injector and tubing for positioning to ensure that the IV line will allow maximum table movement, before exiting the imaging room and starting the procedure.

Power injectors may be used with **central venous lines** providing certain safety measures are practiced.[1] The position of the catheter tip needs to be confirmed by a scout scan or a recent chest radiograph. Venous backflow is assessed and if backflow is not obtained, the technologist may try administering saline to determine patency. Occasionally the bevel of the needle may be against the wall of the vein, preventing venous backflow. If there is no resistance when administering saline, the central line should be patent. Injection into venous catheters with large-bore needles have been obtained with flow rates up to 2.5 ml/sec. Peripheral central venous catheters with small-bore needles should not be used unless permitted by manufacturer's specifications.

Power injectors can also be used to deliver contrast media using **peripherally inserted central catheters (PICC)**. Studies indicate that contrast media can be administered using PICC lines at flow rates up to 2 ml/sec. Specifically designed PICC lines may tolerate flow rates up to 5 ml/sec.[1] The manufacturer's guidelines should be reviewed and followed.

Extravasation of Contrast Media

Extravasation or infiltration of high-osmolar media is particularly toxic to tissues. Patients at high risk for extravasation should have low-osmolar contrast media (LOCM) to lessen the toxicity to the surrounding tissues, if infiltrated. Patients at increased risk are those having difficulty communicating specific symptoms, such as pediatric and geriatric patients, severely ill patients, and patients with altered circulation.[2] Other risk factors for extravasation include chronic illness, fragile or damaged veins, multiple punctures of the same vein, arterial insufficiency and compromised lymphatic and/or venous drainage. Extravasation produces an acute inflammatory response that peaks in 24 to 48 hours and may proceed to more adverse events such as tissue ulceration and necrosis. A chronic inflammatory response may follow and can be associated with fibrosis and muscle atrophy.[1]

The method of treatment of extravasation of contrast media is not agreed upon by all radiologists, so there is a need for controlled studies to be conducted to determine the efficacy of the various treatments.[1] The most common treatment is to elevate the affected limb above the level of the heart. The injury produced in response to the extravasated media is mainly due to the hyperosmolality of the contrast media. Elevation induces a decrease in the capillary hydrostatic pressure promoting the resorption of the contrast media into the bloodstream. Warm or cold compresses may also be used. Cold compresses are thought to relieve the pain whereas warm compresses have been found to improve blood flow to the area, thus facilitating absorption of the extravasated contrast media.[1] If extravasation is significant, surgical consultation is recommended. The patient should be monitored and if the patient experiences increased swelling or pain after 2 to 4 hours, altered tissue perfusion, change in sensation, or skin ulceration or blistering, surgical consultation should be considered.[1] Patients should not be released until the radiologist has determined that the symptoms have improved or that new symptoms have not developed. Extravasation and any associated treatment should be documented in the patient's medical record and the referring physician notified.

INFECTION CONTROL

Medical asepsis is the technique used to prevent the spread of infection or disease by reducing the number of infectious microorganisms or pathogens. Microorganisms include bacteria, viruses, protozoans, and fungi.

Cycle of Infection

The cycle of infection involves a pathogenic organism, reservoir of infection, means of transmission, and a susceptible host (Figure 8-17). The reservoir of infection can be any place that microorganisms can find nutrients, moisture, and warmth. The human body provides this type of medium. Some microorganisms live on or within the body as part of normal flora and aid in digestion and skin preservation. These organisms are nonpathogenic as long as they are confined to their usual environment but can assume a pathogenic role outside their environment. Pathogens can also live in the bodies of healthy individuals without causing apparent disease. These persons are called *carriers* and may be a reservoir for infection without realizing it.

Although the human body is the most common reservoir of infection, any environment that will support growth of the microorganisms has the potential to be a secondary source. Such sources may include contaminated food or water or any damp, warm place that is not cleaned regularly.

Compromised immune systems of patients make them susceptible hosts. They may develop a secondary problem or nosocomial (hospital-acquired) infection. The annual incidence rate of nosocomial infections is approximately 5% of patients admitted to hospitals yearly. Most of these infections are not life threatening. The most common nosocomial infection is a urinary tract infection. However, statistics indicate that 20,000 patients a year die of hospital-acquired infections and that more than half of the infections leading to death are preventable.

The most direct way to intervene in the cycle of infection is to prevent transmission of the pathogen from the reservoir to a susceptible host. The most effective system to prevent transmission of disease is by practicing standard precautions, which are aimed at reducing risk of transmission of microorganisms from both recognized and unrecognized sources. Universal precautions were designed to reduce the risk of transmission of blood-borne pathogens. Body substance isolation was designed to reduce the risk of transmission of pathogens from moist body substances. The new term *standard precautions* combines the major features of *universal precautions* and *body substance isolation* into one standard. This standard applies to all patients, regardless of their diagnosis or presumed infection status, and is based on the use of protective barriers for contact with all body substances rather than on the isolation of a patient with a particular diagnosis. All patients are treated as potential reservoirs of infection. The Centers for Disease Control and Prevention (CDC) recommends a two-tiered system for health-care workers that implements standard precautions and transmission-based precautions, designed for persons with suspected or known infections.

The four main routes of transmission of disease are as follows:

Contact Transmission—Most frequent mode of transmission of nosocomial infections; it is divided into two subgroups: direct and indirect contact.

- Direct Contact: Involves body surface–to–body surface contact and occurs when the pathogens are placed in direct contact with a susceptible host. For example, skin infections can be transmitted by direct contact.
- Indirect Contact: Involves transport of the pathogen by a secondary source. An object that has been in contact with a pathogen is called a *fomite*. Examples of fomites are gloves, a contaminated urinary catheter, or the surface of the gamma camera.

Droplet Transmission—Occurs when droplets containing pathogens are propelled through the air by coughing, sneezing, or talking and are deposited on the host's conjunctivae, nasal mucosa, or mouth. Droplets do not remain suspended in the air and are therefore considered separate from airborne transmission. Special ventilation is not needed to prevent transmission.

Airborne Transmission—Circulation of droplet nuclei (5 μm or smaller) or evaporated droplets containing pathogens suspended in the air for long periods of time or dust particles containing pathogens. Special ventilation is required to prevent transmission. Examples of pathogens transmitted by the air would include *Mycobacterium tuberculosis* and the varicella virus.

Vectorborne Transmission—Occurs in mammals or insects in which pathogens develop and multiply before transmission to a new host. Examples of vectors are mosquitoes, flies, rats, and other vermin that transmit disease through bites.

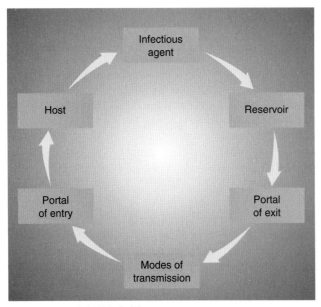

FIGURE 8-17 The cycle of infection.

Standard Precautions

The OSHA published regulations requiring health care employers to provide **hepatitis B virus (HBV)** immunizations to employees, as well as procedures and equipment to prevent transmission of **human immunodeficiency virus (HIV)** and other blood-borne diseases. Most hospital-acquired HBV or HIV infections are the result of percutaneous exposure. Individuals immunized for HBV are at virtually no risk for contracting the disease. The risk for nonvaccinated individuals acquiring HBV after an exposure ranges from 6% to 30% compared to 0.3% with HIV. There has been a 95% decrease in hospital-acquired HBV infections because of the practice of standard precautions and the availability of vaccines directed against the virus. Individual judgment must be used in determining when protective barriers or **personal protective equipment (PPE)** are needed.

- Consider all patient specimens and body fluids as potentially infectious.
- Wear gloves when it is likely that there will be contact with any body fluids, mucous membranes, nonintact skin, or any item or surface contaminated with body fluids (e.g., blood, urine, feces, wound drainage, oral scratches, sputum, vomitus).
- Wear masks and/or protective eyewear when it is likely that there will be exposure of the mucous membranes of the mouth, nose, or eyes with body fluids.
- Wear protective clothing when it is likely that clothing will be soiled with body substances.
- Wash hands before and after patient contact. Wash hands and other skin surfaces immediately and thoroughly after contamination with body fluids.
- Discard uncapped needle/syringe units and "sharps" in puncture-resistant biohazard containers.
- Clean blood and body fluid spills promptly with a 1:10 solution of bleach and water (prepared daily) or a CDC-approved disinfectant.
- Immediately report all needlesticks or incidents involving contamination by blood, body fluids, or tissues.

Handwashing Technique

Hands should always be washed before and after each patient contact and before and after glove use. Friction produced by good handwashing technique is the most effective means of eliminating microorganisms (Figure 8-18).

- If there are no foot or knee levers, use paper towels to turn the faucet on and off.
- Wet hands with continuously running water, keeping hands lower than elbows.
- Apply liquid soap and lather.
- Rub hands front and back and between fingers for at least 15 seconds.
- Rinse and dry thoroughly.
- OSHA also promotes waterless hand cleansing using an antibacterial solution.

Housekeeping

The technologist is responsible for maintaining a clean environment. These responsibilities include changing linens between patients and disinfecting the imaging area on a daily basis. Use a cloth moistened with disinfectant. The CDC recommends sodium hypochlorite bleach (e.g., Clorox) as the preferred disinfectant for preventing the spread of HIV and HBV, especially because HBV can survive in dried blood for up to 7 days. Bleach may used

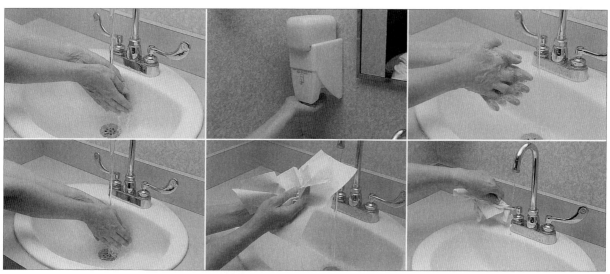

FIGURE 8-18 Handwashing techniques.

to disinfect and should be prepared daily in a 1:100 solution (2.5 tablespoons per gallon) because its effectiveness declines rapidly after preparation. When preparing and using this solution, the technologist should use PPE. The bleach solution should remain in contact with the contaminated source for at least 10 minutes to be effective.

VITAL SIGNS AND PATIENT ASSESSMENT

Good evaluation skills play a role in meeting the needs of patients while they are under the care of the technologist. Several aids are available to assist in assessing patients. Review the medical chart before starting the procedure and ask how the patient feels. Observe the patient closely while preparing him or her for the procedure. One of the easiest signs to recognize is skin color. Individual complexions vary, but if the patient becomes pale or cyanotic, quickly begin assessing the change. *Cyanosis* is a term that describes a bluish coloration in the skin and indicates lack of oxygen to the tissues. The patient that becomes cyanotic needs immediate medical attention. Touching the patient allows the technologist to further assess the patient as well as reassure the patient. The acutely ill patient may be pale, cool, and diaphoretic. If these signs are present, ask if they are new.

In addition to using observation to assess the patient, measurements such as vital signs are also used. Vital signs consist of the following:

- Temperature
- Pulse rate
- Respiration rate
- Blood pressure

Pulse-Rate Assessment

A pulse is the advancing pressure wave in any artery caused by expulsion of blood when the left ventricle of the heart contracts. Normal adult rate is 60 to 90 beats per minute (bpm). A rapid pulse is called *tachycardia*. A slow pulse rate is *bradycardia*.

- Normal rate: 60 to 90 bpm
- Tachycardia: >100 bpm
- Bradycardia: <60 bpm

Common pulse points are as follows (Figure 8-19):

- Radial artery
- Brachial artery
- Femoral artery
- Carotid artery

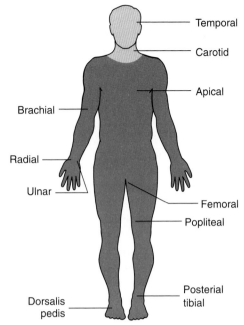

FIGURE 8-19 Location of peripheral pulses.

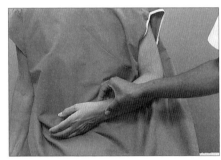

FIGURE 8-20 Measuring the radial pulse.

If the pulse is weak distally, then palpate more proximally. If pulse points are slow or irregular, the apical pulse can be assessed by placing the stethoscope between the left fifth and sixth ribs and listening for the heart sound, "lubb-dubb," which equals one beat.

The most convenient site for taking the pulse is the radial artery, located on the thumb side of the patient's wrist. The pulse is felt by gently compressing the artery with the fingertips. The technologist should never feel the pulse with his or her own thumb because it has a pulse of its own that interferes with obtaining an accurate reading. If a regular rhythm is noted, count the beats of the pulse for 30 seconds and multiply by two to obtain beats per minute. For irregular rhythms, a complete cycle of 1 minute is required (Figure 8-20).

Respiration-Rate Assessment

The normal adult respiratory rate is 12 to 16 breaths per minute. Notify the physician of any change in the

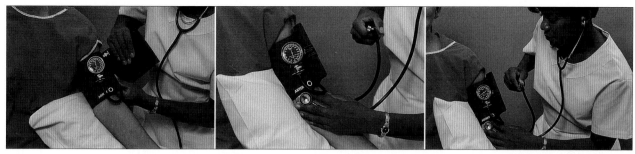

FIGURE 8-21 Assessing blood pressure.

patient's breathing pattern. Difficult or labored respiration is called *dyspnea*. Rapid breathing is tachypnea or hyperventilation. Oxygen is a prescribed drug and may only be administered to the patient with a physician's order. It may be difficult for the patient with lung disease to lie flat for even a short period. Many times, a change in position will alleviate the dyspnea.

Count the respirations without the patient being aware and count one breathing cycle (in and out) as one respiration. Count for 30 seconds and multiply by two to obtain respirations per minute.

Blood-Pressure Assessment

Blood pressure is the lateral pressure exerted on the walls of the arteries by blood flowing through the arteries. It reflects the contractile strength of the heartbeat and is a measure of the volume of blood pushed into the vessels by the heart. The pressure of blood within the arteries is highest whenever the heart contracts and is called **systolic pressure.** Between beats, when the ventricles are at rest, arterial pressure is at its lowest and is called **diastolic pressure.**

Blood pressure is measured in millimeters of mercury (mm Hg). Normal blood pressure varies, depending on age, weight, and physical status, but blood pressures of 100/60 to 140/90 mm Hg are considered to be within the acceptable range. The top number, systolic (*s* for "squeezing of the heart muscle") is a measure of the pumping action of the heart muscle itself. The diastolic pressure (*d* for "down" or "dilation of the heart muscle") indicates the ability of the arterial system to accept the pulse of blood that is forced into the system by the contraction of the left ventricle. Elevated blood pressure is called *hypertension;* low blood pressure is hypotension and may indicate shock. In a changing or emergency situation, the physician will need accurate readings to be able to make a valid evaluation of the patient's status.

The most common site for taking blood pressure is the brachial artery of the upper arm, but arteries of the lower arm, thigh, and calf may also be used. When the arm is used, the patient should either sit or lie down with the arm and blood pressure cuff at the level of the heart.

Equipment used to measure blood pressure includes a sphygmomanometer, a cuff, and a stethoscope. The procedure is begun by inflating the cuff to 180 to 200 mm Hg. The cuff contains an inflatable rubber bladder that should be centered over the brachial artery, 1 to 2 inches above the elbow. Cuffs should be wrapped snugly but not tightly. If the cuff is too loose, systolic and diastolic readings will both be falsely elevated (Figure 8-21).

A stethoscope with a flat diaphragm is best for taking blood pressure measurements. After locating the brachial artery by palpation, place the diaphragm of the stethoscope over the artery without touching the cuff or patient's clothing. Gentle application of the stethoscope should be used, because too much pressure can cause abnormally low diastolic sound (Figure 8-21). Please review the description of the procedure for obtaining blood pressure found in Box 8-6.

If there is difficulty hearing the diastolic sounds, completely deflate the cuff. Wait 15 seconds, have the patient raise his or her arm for a few seconds, and then retake the blood pressure. The diastolic sounds may become muffled before stopping or may remain muffled down to zero. In this case, record the diastolic pressure at the point the change is distinguished from clear to muffled, as well as when the sound ends completely (e.g., 120/80/62 mm Hg).

EMERGENCY CARE

Patient assessment is critical in determining the action to be taken when a patient experiences difficulty in breathing. Obstructed airways, heart attacks, strokes, seizures, and **syncope** are common causes of medical emergencies.

Cardiopulmonary Resuscitation

Cardiopulmonary resuscitation (CPR) is the basic life support system used to ventilate the lungs and circulate the blood in the event of cardiac and respiratory arrest. Part of the professional education of the technologist should include CPR training. Technologists are responsible for updating their certification in basic life

BOX 8-6	Blood Pressure Procedure

1. Explain the procedure to the patient and make him or her comfortable in a sitting or recumbent position.
2. The patient should be resting for 5 minutes before the blood pressure is taken.
3. Select the site and use the same site consistently because of variations in blood pressure taken in different locations. Blood pressure should also be taken with the patient in the same position each time.
4. Expose the site and position the patient's arm on a supporting structure at heart level.
5. Place the cuff so that its lower edge is 1 to 2 inches above the elbow, leaving space over the brachial artery free.
6. Using the middle and index fingers, palpate the brachial artery, which is located on the medial aspect of the arm at the level of the elbow.
7. Place the diaphragm of the stethoscope directly over the point of strongest pulsation.
8. Holding the rubber bulb in the palm of one hand, close the valve on the bulb with thumb and finger, then rapidly inflate the cuff by pumping the bulb.
9. Inflate the cuff to about 20 to 30 mm Hg above the expected systolic reading, or approximately 180 mm Hg. Inflation of the cuff should take 7 seconds or less.
10. Slowly open the valve on the bulb, releasing the pressure on the cuff steadily. Listen carefully for sounds of the first heartbeat and note the reading on the sphygmomanometer. This reading represents the systolic pressure.
11. After the first sound, the pulsing will get louder as the pressure is released slowly from the cuff (approximately 2 to 3 mm Hg per heartbeat). Continue deflation until all sound stops or the intensity of the sound suddenly decreases and seems muffled. This reading represents the diastolic pressure.
12. Open the valve to deflate cuff rapidly.
13. Remove the cuff and record values as systolic/diastolic (e.g., 120/80).
14. If a reading must be repeated, let all the air out of the cuff and wait 15 seconds before inflating the cuff again. Do not reinflate the cuff during the reading.
15. Wipe the eartips and diaphragm of the stethoscope with alcohol before storing.

support on a regular basis. Refer to Table 8-6 for basic life-support guidelines for the health care provider, published by the American Heart Association.

Syncope

Syncope, or fainting, is a mild form of neurogenic shock. The blood pressure falls as the blood vessels dilate, and the heart rate slows, resulting in a decreased supply of oxygen reaching the brain. The technologist needs to be responsive to any change in the patient's condition. There may be a noticeable change in the patient's coloring, and the skin may feel cool and clammy to the touch. Weakness or change in mental acuity may accompany this condition. Protecting the patient's head is the primary concern while easing the patient to the floor or any flat surface. Place the patient in the dorsal recumbent position, and elevate the patient's feet (Figure 8-22).

Seizures

The technologist's first duty is to protect the patient from injury. Assist the patient to the floor or any flat surface, remembering to protect the patient's head. Do not attempt to restrain the patient. There are different types of seizures, which may or may not result in loss of consciousness. Intense motor seizures (grand mal) usually result in loss of consciousness, followed by severe muscle spasms. Less intense motor seizures without loss of consciousness may be described as uncontrollable tremors that cause hyperventilation. Another type of seizure is characterized by a brief loss of consciousness during which the patient stares and is nonresponsive. Ask someone to call for a physician immediately, and observe the symptoms of the seizure as accurately as possible. Note when the seizure began and how long it lasted. Are both sides of the body involved equally? Where did the motor contractions begin, and did the contractions progress from one area to another? This information can be very helpful in treating the patient.

Myocardial Infarction

Sudden onset of chest pain or angina is assumed to be a myocardial infarction until proven otherwise. The technologist should prevent further damage by limiting the patient's movement and any exertion. The patient may become diaphoretic and pale, and may experience some nausea or heartburn. Assist the patient to a comfortable position, and ask someone to call for a physician. The technologist needs to be prepared to administer CPR, if necessary.

Diabetes

A patient with diabetes cannot metabolize glucose because of the lack of insulin production by the pancreas. These patients may be on some form of insulin, which has the potential to cause problems when they have taken their insulin and can have nothing by mouth (NPO). These patients may develop hypoglycemia (low blood sugar). The onset of symptoms may be sudden and include the following:

- General weakness
- Sweating, clammy, cold skin
- Tremors, nervousness, and irritability
- Hunger

TABLE 8-6	**Summary of American Heart Association Health Care Provider "CAB" Guidelines for Adults, Children, and Infants**		
	Recommendations		
Component	**Adults**	**Children**	**Infants**
Recognition	Unresponsive (for all ages) No breathing, not breathing normally (e.g., only gasping) No pulse palpated within 10 seconds	Not breathing or only gasping	
CPR sequence	CAB	CAB	CAB
Compression rate	At least 100/min		
Compression depth	At least 2 inches (5 cm)	At least ⅓ AP depth about 2 inches (5 cm)	At least ⅓ AP depth about 1½ inches (4 cm)
Chest wall recoil	Allow complete recoil between compressions; HCPs rotate compression every 2 minutes		
Compression interruptions	Minimize interruptions in chest compressions; attempt to limit interruptions to less than 10 seconds		
Airway	Head tilt-chin lift; if suspected trauma: jaw thrust		
Compression to ventilation ratio (until advanced airway placed)	30:2 (1 or 2 rescuers)	30:2 single rescuer 15:2 two HCP rescuers	30:2 single rescuer 15:2 two HCP rescuers
Ventilations: Trained and not proficient	Compression only		
Ventilation with advanced airway (HCP)	One breath every 6 to 8 seconds (8 to 10 breaths/min); asynchronous with chest compressions; about 1 second per breath; visible chest rise		
Defibrillation	Attach and use AED as soon as available; minimize interruptions in chest compressions before and after shock; resume CPR beginning with compressions immediately after each shock		

AED, Automated external defibrillator; *CAB,* chest compression, airway, breathing; *CPR,* cardiopulmonary resuscitation; *HCP,* health care provider.
Modified from Travers AH, Rea TD, Bobrow BJ, et al: Part 4: CPR overview: 2010 American Heart Association guidelines for cardiopulmonary resuscitation and emergency cardiovascular care, *Circulation* 122(supp 3):S676-S684, 2010.

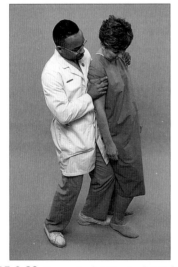

FIGURE 8-22 Support of patient who is fainting.

- Blurred vision
- Loss of consciousness

The condition can be quickly remedied by the administration of sugar (three pieces of candy or fruit juice). Report the occurrence of such symptoms to a physician. Protect the patient from falling by laying the patient down until the sugar takes effect. People can have hypoglycemia without diabetes; the treatment is the same.

Asthma

Bronchospasms cause difficulty in breathing or dyspnea in asthmatic patients. Stress or anxiety, such as having a nuclear medicine procedure, can precipitate this condition. The treatment of choice is to relieve the bronchospasm without the administration of oxygen. If the patient has a nebulizer that contains bronchodilating medication, this usually relieves the symptoms. An injection of epinephrine will relieve the symptoms of an acute episode and must be ordered and administered by a physician.

Emergency Code Carts

Emergency code carts contain essential items that could be needed during an emergency. The carts are located throughout the facility and should be easily accessible to all areas. The items may vary slightly, but most carts contain artificial ventilation equipment, emergency medications, bags of intravenous solutions, a defibrillator, blood pressure cuff, and stethoscope. These carts are inventoried and locked to keep them ready for use. To be able to assist if needed, the technologist should become familiar with the location of the cart and its components.

ANCILLARY EQUIPMENT

Glucometer

A **glucometer** is used to monitor peripheral blood glucose levels in patients. The glucometer gives valuable information about whether the blood glucose level is in the proper range. Most glucometers have a measurable range up to 500 mg/dl. A lab critical standard for blood glucose readings is less than 40 mg/dl or greater than 400 mg/dl. If the glucometer indicates the blood glucose level is outside the critical range, the blood glucose measurement should be repeated immediately using a fresh blood specimen. If the repeat test confirms a critical HIGH (>500 mg/dl), this indicates severe hyperglycemia and the physician should be notified immediately and a laboratory blood glucose test would be ordered to obtain quantitative results. If the test confirms the reading is critically low, the physician should be notified to determine if the patient needs to be treated for **hypoglycemia**. Refer to Box 8-7 for general instructions on how to use a glucometer to determine blood glucose levels.

In nuclear medicine, a glucometer is used to monitor blood glucose levels of patients before the administration of 2-deoxy-2-[^{18}F]fluoro-D-glucose (^{18}F-FDG) used in PET procedures. The patient's blood glucose should be determined because localization of ^{18}F-FDG is affected by blood glucose levels.

Nasogastric Tubes

A nasogastric (NG) tube is inserted through a nostril and terminates in the stomach. It is used for feeding, to obtain specimens of gastric fluids, or to drain fluids from the stomach. Nasoenteric tubes go farther into the intestinal tract to remove fluid and gas that may cause distention. Precautions should be taken to make sure the tubes are not pulled or tugged on when moving or positioning patients. The technologist needs to be aware that the

BOX 8-7	Glucometer Procedure

1. Verify timing and frequency of test according to physician's order.
2. Cleanse patient's hand.
3. Turn on glucometer. Calibrate according to manufacturer's instructions.
4. Check expiration date of reagent strips. Confirm type of strip is correct for the monitor.
5. Wearing gloves, select a puncture site on the lateral aspect of a finger.
6. Promote blood flow by massaging finger toward tip of finger.
7. Cleanse site with alcohol pad or other antiseptic. Allow area to dry thoroughly.
8. Engage the sterile lancet and remove cover. Secure patient's hand or finger so that it does not move.
9. Position sterile lancet firmly against the skin, perpendicular to the puncture site.
10. For lancets with an injector switch, push the release switch, allowing the lancet to pierce the skin. For lancets without an injector switch, use a darting motion to prick the site with the lancet.
11. Lightly squeeze the patient's finger above the puncture site until a drop of blood is collected. Wipe away first drop and squeeze again to form another drop.
12. Allow contact between the reagent strip test patch and the drop of blood until blood covers the entire patch. Do not smear the blood on the reagent strip.
13. Using a gauze, gently apply pressure to the puncture site.
14. Wait appropriate time as indicated by the manufacturer of the glucometer. After specified time, place the reagent strip into the glucometer as directed by the manufacturer.
15. The glucometer will signal when the reading is ready. After reading the digital display, turn the monitor off and properly dispose of supplies, including lancet, in the proper containers.
16. Properly document reading.

patient should not lie flat for 30 minutes after completing a feeding. The technologist should report any leakage in the tube or suction system. If appropriate, suction or feeding can be discontinued if the patient needs to be transferred for a study.

Oxygen Administration

In caring for a patient receiving oxygen, always note the flow rate in the medical chart or physician's orders. Oxygen can be administered by high–flow rate or low–flow rate devices. The low–flow rate devices most often used are the nasal cannula or simple oxygen masks. The nasal cannula is inserted into the patient's nostrils, providing a direct source of oxygen at a minimum flow rate of 0.5 and a maximum rate of 6 L/min (Figure 8-23). Simple masks must be set at an oxygen flow rate of no less than 6 L/min to prevent the buildup of exhaled carbon dioxide. Masks with reservoir bags should be set

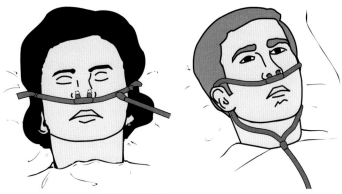

FIGURE 8-23 Nasal cannula.

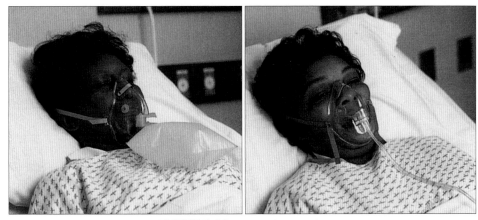

FIGURE 8-24 Oxygen face masks.

with a liter flow rate high enough to ensure that the bag never completely deflates during patient breathing. The mask fits over the mouth, nose, and chin of the patient (Figures 8-24).

During patient transport, portable oxygen is delivered through a gas or liquid storage container. Gas can be transported in cylinders made of steel or aluminium (Figure 8-25). For the safety of the patient and the practitioner, steel cylinders must not be used in the presence of a magnetic field (e.g., magnetic resonance imaging [MRI]). The stem valve on the top of the cylinder must be opened at least one to two turns to allow oxygen to flow into the regulator. The regulator has a pressure gauge that will give an indication of how much oxygen is in the cylinder. A knob on the regulator allows for flow adjustment to the patient in liters per minute. Both valves must be turned on for the patient to receive oxygen. A common oxygen rate is 3 to 5 L/min. Trauma (in shock) patients may require a higher rate of oxygen administration. Patients with **chronic obstructive pulmonary disease (COPD)** receive oxygen at a lower rate, usually less than 3 L/min. The carbon dioxide level controls the respiratory rate in these patients, and if too much oxygen is delivered, the respiratory rate may slow down to the extent that ventilation is insufficient.

Currently most health-care facilities use bulk liquid oxygen systems rather than oxygen supplied in gaseous form because of two factors: (1) gases shipped in bulk

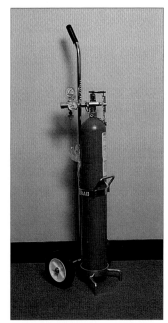

FIGURE 8-25 Oxygen tank.

are less expensive than gases shipped in cylinders, and (2) liquid oxygen takes up less space than gaseous oxygen. Portable liquid oxygen systems are available for patient transport. The portable device is filled from the bulk liquid oxygen system and provides an 8- to

12-hour supply of oxygen. Care must be taken to avoid spillage when filling the portable unit. Because of the extremely low temperature of liquid oxygen, direct contact can cause frostbite to the skin or eye injury. Avoid placing the portable unit in direct contact with the patient.

Precautions when using oxygen cylinders or liquid oxygen units include the following:

- Cylinders should be secured at all times and never allowed to stand free. Always use liquid oxygen units in the upright position.
- Care must be taken to prevent fire when oxygen is in use. Never place cylinders or liquid units near a heat source.
- Always determine the amount of oxygen in the cylinder or liquid unit before transporting the patient. Liquid oxygen units will vent gas when not in use.
- When transporting, secure cylinders in the cylinder cart and liquid oxygen units by straps. Never use the patient's stretcher to transport oxygen.

Catheters

The most common type of catheter is the urinary catheter. Flexible plastic tubing is inserted up the patient's urethra and into the bladder. Urine is drained from the bladder and flows through the tubing into the urine bag. To prevent backflow of urine, the bag must be kept below the level of the bladder. Catheterization is a sterile technique and needs to remain a closed system to prevent urinary infections. The catheter bag can be attached to the bed, stretcher, or wheelchair, but should never be placed directly on the floor.

Surgical Drains

Colostomies (surgical opening into the colon) and ileostomies (surgical opening into the ileum) allow for drainage of feces. The opening (**stoma**) is covered by plastic disposable bags or pouches (appliances), which must be changed frequently. Clean rather than sterile technique is needed when changing these appliances.

Dressings should be maintained, and any signs of fresh bleeding should be reported immediately. If hemorrhaging occurs, apply direct pressure to the site while calling for assistance.

QUALITY IMPROVEMENT

The chapter began by stating that it is the responsibility of the NMT to provide quality care to the patients. Quality care includes a myriad of aspects all toward the goal of having the patient's experience be efficient, appropriate, and handled with superior care and competence. To ensure quality care, various mechanisms are put into place to monitor current practices and to implement changes when needed.

In the present health-care environment, imaging departments must maintain reliable quality outcomes, a cost-efficient operation, easy access, and superior customer service to remain competitive in the marketplace. Compliance to all applicable regulations, laws, and standards must also be given special attention. One way for a department to differentiate itself from others is to provide consistent, superior service to patients, their families, and the referring physician, all the while giving the referring physician the accurate and timely answers needed to manage the patient's care. Instituting a quality plan to meet the department's needs will not only eliminate waste and redundancy while improving the services provided, but also decrease costs and enhance productivity. In years past, quality programs were voluntary. Payers now require facility accreditation by an approved agency for all advanced imaging services (MRI, CT, Nuclear Medicine and PET.) These accreditation programs all contain requirements for formalized ongoing quality improvement plans, where all employees participate. Therefore the days of voluntary programs are over; if providers wish to be paid for the services they perform they must implement these programs. While developing or sustaining a quality plan, the department will need to continually assess its needs, the needs of its stakeholders, and its known weaknesses. Throughout the process, the department will better understand internal and external processes and have an opportunity to systematically improve those processes. At this time, it is also crucial to assess the department's compliance with state and federal law and regulations, as well as professional standards and appropriateness criteria. Ultimately, a comprehensive quality program can highlight the barriers to providing superior service, identify the gaps within day-to-day processes, and provide appropriate documentation to satisfy accreditation demands.

DEFINING QUALITY

Before quality can be discussed, the definition of quality must be determined. To some, providing good quality service means meeting customer expectations with minimum effort and waste. How good is good enough? At a 99.9% confidence interval, which most would agree is very good, it can be estimated that at least 20,000 incorrect drug prescriptions are filled each year and that 15,000 newborn babies are accidentally dropped by medical staff numbers each year. After hearing this, most would agree that this is unacceptable. Going back to the aforementioned definition of quality, each department must establish its own criteria for defining quality. This definition should be customized for the department's unique contexts, processes, and expectations.

Quality management (QM) grew out of attempts to improve manufacturing processes using statistical theories to eliminate variances, revolutionizing the field of manufacturing. Defining quality within the manufacturing sector is concrete and objective; either the manufactured part is the correct shape and size or it is rejected. Individual parts must meet strict specifications in order to be included in the final product. Since "garbage in" equals "garbage out," it can be expected that by eliminating the variances within the manufacturing process of individual parts, a superior product will be produced. This concept revolutionized manufacturing and can also revolutionize health care, if adapted properly and embraced by the medical community. Imagine how this premise could impact health care. Visualize a single process and look at each step within that process. If each step within that process meets some guideline or standard, then the overall process will be maximized. But, defining quality in health care is much more subjective than in manufacturing, as *process and perception* play integral roles in defining quality in medicine. QM principles can lay the foundation for process improvement within medical imaging but must be adapted to the environment. As health care is revamped, redesigned, and retooled, it makes sense to use the principles and models that the field of QM has to offer.

QUALITY ACRONYMS

Various levels of monitoring must be used to provide quality care.

Within medical imaging, there are three levels of monitoring:

1. **Quality control (QC)**
2. **Quality assurance (QA)**
3. **Quality improvement (QI)**

Any comprehensive quality improvement plan requires components at each of these three levels to be effective in ensuring patient safety, providing quality care throughout the continuum, and improving the patient experience, ultimately enhancing the management of the care given.

Most NMTs are familiar with the term *quality control* as it relates to daily, weekly, monthly, or quarterly checks on cameras and other radiation detection equipment. QC also includes equipment calibration, acceptance testing, preventative equipment maintenance, film-badge monitoring, and providing standardized imaging protocols. QC can be defined as the aggregate of activities such as design analysis and inspection of defects to ensure adequate quality.

Quality assurance, which takes the monitoring one level higher, is most effective when it follows a comprehensive plan with delineated quality, technical, operational, and clinical indicators. These indicators of quality ascertain information about a specific process or service provided. Examples of midlevel quality indicators include

timely accessibility of clinical findings; timeliness of scheduling, procedure, and report turnaround; accessibility of previous studies, appropriate clinical indication, documentation, and patient history; and overall study appropriateness. This midlevel of monitoring and improvements to these quality indicators begin to truly impact the quality of patient care provided. QA assesses compliance to standards, policies, and protocols, and it provides documentation on such things as camera and procedure utilization studies, patient pregnancy testing and notification, patient and physician satisfaction surveys, and peer-review outcomes assessment. A peer-review assessment compares procedure results with current gold standards, such as comparing ejection fraction (EF) values with the results of cardiac catheterization studies. This midlevel of monitoring also begins to provide crucial documentation of compliance to regulatory or professional standards as well as outcomes assessment. QA can be defined as a departmental and systematic approach monitoring and evaluating the various aspects of a project, service, or facility to ensure that standards of quality are being met. QA traditionally involves only a few individuals; data are reviewed to solve "special" problems, emphasizing the identification of outliers and then taking steps to bring these outliers in line with the norm.

One way to comprehensively assess structure, process, and patient outcomes is to use the next level of monitoring. Several terms are often used interchangeably to describe this next level of monitoring in present-day health care but warrant some consideration of their differences: QI, performance improvement (PI), QM, and **total quality management (TQM)**. QI is a systematic, organization-wide approach for improving the overall quality of care, one that emphasizes performance improvement as well as the standard of care. Here, the focus is on identifying common causes and on processes rather than on outliers and clinical outcomes, as with QA. The QI approach tends to be proactive rather than reactive, again as in the case of QA. QM, on the other hand, is an all encompassing philosophy that permeates the organization's management infrastructure, policies, and practices. QI is another evolutionary philosophy that incorporates leadership concepts from TQM. QI emphasizes continuously making improvements, as well as the prevention of errors and empowerment of employees. Improving communication is key to any process, and most structure, process, and patient outcome issues can be addressed by improving communication at every point within that process. QI techniques can often identify current gaps within interdepartmental and intradepartmental communication. The term *QI* is used to identify this third level of monitoring. Each one of these phrases describes designs to improve the processes of the work performed by targeting the improvement of the standard of care and reducing the variability on the implementation of that standard. In other words, this third level of monitoring shapes current practice to provide the best level of service possible. This entire level of monitoring needs to be initiated by the leaders within the organization but must be ingrained in the culture of the organization to be effective.

PIONEERS OF QUALITY MANAGEMENT

Joseph M. Juran and W. Edwards Deming are often considered the "fathers" of QM, because they both independently made significant contributions to spawn the field of QM by promoting theories that effectively deploy best practices. The original theories and principles developed by Juran and Deming are evident in common day-to-day quality management tools and practices.

Juran was the first to publish a step-by-step sequence for "breakthrough" improvement. This process has evolved into Six Sigma* and today is the basis for quality initiatives worldwide. Juran is also recognized for adding human dimension to quality by broadening it from its statistical origins. He is probably most known for conceptualizing the Pareto Principle, a universal principle he called the "vital few and trivial many." Most will recognize this principle as the 80:20 rule, meaning that few (20%) are vital and many (80%) are trivial. To this day, many use the concept of 80:20 to assist in solving problems and issues, recalling that focusing 80% of time and energy on the 20% of work that is really important will help to manage time wisely.

Deming was a statistician with postgraduate training in mathematical physics. While working for the U.S. Government Services, he became immersed in the theories of measuring quality statistically, using the work of fellow statistician Walter A. Shewhart. He believed that Shewhart's principles could be applied to nonmanufacturing processes. Using Stewhart's early methods of statistical process control (SPC), Deming was able to document how to eliminate variability in manufacturing processes. Both Deming and Shewhart are credited for developing a consistent scientific approach to the management of processes. This process is known today as the *Plan, Do, Check, Act (PDCA) cycle*. See the section Problem-Solving Models, later in this chapter, for more information on the PDCA cycle.

---

*Six Sigma is a highly disciplined process that helps the user focus on developing and delivering near-perfect products and services. Why "Sigma"? The word is a statistical term that measures how far a given process deviates from perfection. The central idea behind Six Sigma is that if you can measure how many "defects" you have in a process, you can systematically figure out how to eliminate them and get as close to "zero defects" as possible. To achieve Six Sigma Quality, a process must produce no more than 3.4 defects per million opportunities. An "opportunity" is defined as a chance for nonconformance, or not meeting the required specifications. This means we need to be nearly flawless in executing our key processes.

ROLE OF QUALITY MANAGEMENT IN MEDICAL IMAGING

For decades, the manufacturing and retail sectors have used aggressive quality management methods to make their processes leaner, more accurate, and more productive. These sectors have benefited nicely from this overhaul. Though hospital systems have used quality management theories for years, they tend to choose less aggressive techniques, yielding far less impressive benefits. Today, the hospital systems that are ramping up their QM initiatives are seeking more aggressive QM theories and are seeing larger dividends and much better results, and are driving major changes in the delivery of patient care. As these theories and methods have become ingrained in the hospital culture, a new understanding and adoption of these methods has blossomed at the department level. QM programs can provide departments with the necessary tools to make substantial improvements in day-to-day processes within the department while focusing on key components of providing quality service.

UNDERSTANDING QUALITY DESIGNS

It is important to realize there is no right or wrong way to creating a QI plan, as long as components from each level of monitoring are included in the plan: QC, QA, and QI. It is also important to realize that there are many ways to collect data; there is so much more to QM than just time studies. Technologists may not be aware of the many higher-level quality improvement initiatives within their own workplace, because much of this work happens behind the scenes and without much fanfare. Quality initiatives do tend to gain attention just before accreditation or state surveys; however, these initiatives should be part of the daily operations. Some hospitals may have senior technologists coordinate these higher levels of monitoring, and others may even have a dedicated staff member who coordinates the QI initiatives for the entire imaging department.

There are many stakeholders to any successful QI plan, and successful programs require the full support and attention of everyone within that institution: administration, management, technical and support staff members, and physicians. Departments such as Quality Management, Risk Management, Infection Control, and Corporate Compliance play a significant role in developing and shaping institutional QI initiatives and may provide invaluable guidance when developing or implementing department level quality initiatives.

Hospital-based QM initiatives of the past focused on business and productivity models as the health care industry faced huge financial obstacles to integrate its services into various managed care models. Fifteen years later, a new focus within health care has prompted a shift in the pendulum. Enhancing overall patient safety, providing quality care throughout the continuum, enhancing the patient experience, and instituting better documentation at all levels have evolved as primary goals of current QM programs.

KEY FOCUS POINTS

Ensuring Patient Safety

Health care has certainly changed over the past 20 years. Whereas technologists once had the luxury of being assigned one scanner to operate for the day, technologists are now expected to perform multiple tasks simultaneously. Improved technology has also shortened imaging time, forcing the pace within the nuclear medicine department to increase. The elevated acuity of patients, increased procedure volumes, and a shortage of qualified and competent NMTs and full-time nuclear medicine–dedicated physicians has definitely played a major role in how nuclear medicine technology is practiced throughout the country today. This shift in how services are delivered has prompted a new focus on ensuring patient safety. In assessing patient safety within the department, technologists and physicians can monitor incident reports, observe entire processes from the time a patient enters the department until the time the study is fully completed, and fully review all policies to ensure that professional standards and regulations are addressed appropriately within department or hospital policies. Ultimately there should be milestones or verification points in place to ensure the right patient gets the appropriate study, the necessary documentation is readily accessible, and the correct physician gets the study results in a timely manner. The full continuum of care of a nuclear medicine patient also includes ensuring that the study is correlated with previous imaging procedures and that the nuclear medicine study does not interfere with the future care of the patient.

Providing Quality Care throughout the Continuum

Leading to this next focus point, as medicine continues to utilize technology, such as **electronic medical records (EMR)**, ordering prescription (e-prescribing) and procedures electronically, teleradiography, patient archival computer systems, automated laboratory testing, and robotic surgery, there is less opportunity for human monitoring and intervention. As these new technologies are implemented, processes must be adjusted to add proper documentation as well as steps and processes to monitor patients to determine that they receive the proper care. Whereas patients once were instructed to bring all previous films for correlation to their nuclear medicine study, today studies are transmitted electronically. If the patient's name or medical records number was not correctly entered into the computer system,

these past studies will not be accessible or available for review. This could lead to a potentially negative outcome in the medical management of the patient. Patient privacy laws have added another layer in the accessibility of previous studies. Access and correlation of current studies to previous studies can be addressed with updated computer hardware and software programs, education of staff members and physicians, and proper monitoring of the system. Providing consistency can also provide great benefits in offering quality services and can be assessed by comparing one department's services to the same department at a another hospital or similar department within the same hospital or physician office.

Enhancing the Patient Experience

It is easy to get caught up in the rushed, harried, and sometimes impersonal environment that today's health care breeds. Institutions that have recognized that this pace is negatively impacting the patient's experience have taken steps to focus on the patient. Patients who are well informed, understand what is happening to them, and feel they can ask questions are much more likely to hold still, be less anxious, and follow directions, which results in yielding a higher quality imaging study. Studies show that patients perceive better care when the caregiver sits while collecting a medical history or giving instructions versus standing with one hand on the door while performing these tasks. As boutique imaging centers cater to patient's needs by offering a salonlike atmosphere, same-day scanning appointments, immediate results, and designer gowns and robes, it is crucial for hospital-based imaging departments to pay significant attention to the patient's experience as well. Patients that have a positive medical experience, no matter what the diagnosis, are much more likely to return for future studies, as well as speak highly of the care they received within a department.

KEY COMPONENTS TO DEVELOPING A COMPREHENSIVE QUALITY-IMPROVEMENT PLAN

While building the components within the QI model (third level of monitoring) of a comprehensive QI plan, focus on the following components: planning, customer requirements, process management, analysis and management of data, and problem-solving models.

Planning

Any QI or performance improvement plan must relate to the overall strategic plan of the nuclear medicine facility. This is a continuation of the institutional plan if nuclear medicine is part of a larger organization. Short-term plans are usually developed for 1 year or less, and long-term planning normally extends to 3 years. Planning should take into account customers' needs and expectations, fiscal restraints, known barriers, environmental influences, state and federal regulations, accreditation, and professional standards, all of which impact the department.

There are a number of environmental factors to consider in planning. The type of market will have a direct effect on the nuclear medicine facility. In a capitated market with heavy managed care contracts, there will be more restrictions on the types of nuclear medicine procedures performed and the amount of reimbursement. A good understanding of the actual case mix is important in any planning. The competition must be considered. This includes other nuclear medicine facilities as well as other modalities. As algorithms are developed for patient care by new utilization management groups called **radiology benefit management (RBM),** nuclear medicine may or may not play a role in the diagnostic care of a patient or group of patients.

Fiscal restraints must be considered, especially in the area of human resources and facilities. The most efficient use of staff members may mean addressing issues of cross-training, productivity, threats of downsizing, and staff recruitment and retention. Equipment must be operationally sound, and replacement plans must be developed. Routine suppliers should be evaluated, and, when feasible, partnerships must be established.

Customer Service

It is imperative for a nuclear medicine facility to identify its customers and assess their needs and expectations. A customer is anyone to whom a service, product, or information is provided. Nuclear medicine facilities routinely identify the referring physician as an important customer. The referring physician's staff members may be direct contacts in scheduling and providing important information about the patient. In many instances nuclear medicine must depend upon a unique customer/supplier relationship for patients. Third-party payers, such as insurance companies, and RBMs, may actually be the primary customers because they dictate where the patient may go for services. Clinical outcomes become an important factor in assessing the quality of ancillary services. Third-party payers are interested in clinical outcomes, accessibility, and overall satisfaction of their clients when they select nuclear medicine suppliers. Several major third-party payers are now requiring accreditation through either the Intersocietal Commission for the Accreditation of Nuclear Medicine Laboratories (ICANL) or ACR to be reimbursed for nuclear medicine studies performed on their patients. As this trend spreads throughout the country, it is imperative that imaging departments obtain and maintain accreditation to remain compliant with payers standards. More information on lab accreditation for medical imaging modalities can be found on the ICANL website at www.icanl.org and the ACR website at www.acr.org.

The patients' needs and expectations must be considered in developing QI and performance improvement plans. The primary type of patient will influence perceptions of good customer service. For example, a geriatric population and a pediatric population will not view exceptional service in exactly the same manner.

Not to be forgotten is the internal customer, both within the department and the institution. Many of the deficiencies within a process occur when accountability moves from one party to the next. Many times the NMT's contact with other customers or suppliers can affect the success or failure of the total process, as in, for example, scheduling the patient, ordering or preparing the radiopharmaceutical, performing the procedure, generating the report, correlating with other modalities, and appropriately billing.

Understanding the customers' needs and expectations will involve asking the right questions. This is normally done using a survey format and in focus group settings. Only by asking these questions and addressing the issues can the nuclear medicine department provide viable services that address individual patient's needs.

Process Management

The greatest improvements can be seen in a nuclear medicine facility through efficient process management. One of the most effective ways of evaluating a process is to develop a flowchart. By using a flowchart, the technologist can identify those "bottlenecks" that cause delays or confusion. Time becomes an important factor in customer satisfaction, as well as cost-effectiveness. When turnaround time is decreased, quality, productivity, and cost-effectiveness improve. Once the time deficiencies have been identified, various problem-solving techniques can be used to address the root cause of the problem.

It may be of value to identify "best practices" through benchmarking. Once a process has been determined and fully understood, it may be necessary to network with other nuclear medicine facilities to determine which facility has the most efficient process management, for example, who has the shortest turnaround time, lowest expense, and most accurate results. Studying another type of business may also be of value when looking at processes. For example, bank billing practices may be related to nuclear medicine billing practices; delivering a package on time may be related to transporting a patient on time; and the patient check-in process may be related to the hotel check-in process.

Analysis and Management of Data

It has been said that a person can manage only that which they can measure. Within any system, measurements must be reliable and accurate. The decisions as to what data to collect should be based on relative importance, examples include measuring high volume or high cost procedures. Measuring must be selective and meaningful and should support process management, planning, and customer satisfaction. Measurement outcomes can benefit patient care.

Problem-Solving Models

Understanding and properly using problem-solving tools and techniques can help the NMT to improve a process. **Plan, Do, Check, Act.** The Shewhart cycle, or a similar model, is commonly considered the format for problem solving. It begins with the "plan" phase, determining the problem or what needs to be changed or improved. The "do" phase involves data collection and analysis in which the root cause of the problem is determined. Based on the data, possible solutions are determined and controls are established. A change is initiated in the "check" phase. In the "act" phase, results of the change are reviewed and modified as necessary, and continuous monitoring is established. Modifications of the Shewhart cycle include the 10-step JCAHO model (The Joint Commission, formerly the Joint Commission on Accreditation of Healthcare Organizations) and other methods that use a number of steps but follow the same principle. Table 8-7 provides a template for a PDCA cycle.

Problem-Solving Techniques

Many problem-solving techniques or tools may be used in combination or alone to improve a process:

- Brainstorming
- Affinity diagram
- Cause-and-effect (fishbone) diagram
- Force field analysis
- Flowchart
- Contingency diagram
- Interrelationship digraph

Brainstorming is a technique used to generate ideas from several people. Strive for quantity of ideas. The more ideas generated, the better the quality of the final idea chosen. Specific rules to obtain the most positive outcomes may include the following:

- Select a topic.
- Record *all* ideas.
- Record one idea at a time in the sequence given.
- Pass over participants who have no spontaneous ideas.
- Do not criticize, evaluate, or judge any of the ideas listed.
- Continue brainstorming until all ideas are listed or the time limit is reached.
- Clarify all ideas listed.
- Combining and improving on ideas is encouraged.

TABLE 8-7	PDCA Cycle Template

Improving Organizational Performance
Summary Report
PDCA Cycle
Date: 2009
Area: Nuclear Medicine
Project Name: Improving patient identification
Description of Project/Goals and Objectives: To resolve patient identification issues
Background Information: Various issues with patient identification were documented through incident reports and near misses.

Current Knowledge	Plan	Do	Check	Act
Benchmark data	Plan for improvement	Implement the plan and collect the data	Summarize what has been learned from analysis of the data	Recommended
Gap analysis				Action: Hold the gains or make changes and repeat the PDCA Cycle
Flowcharts Measures				
Review all incident reports, data and flowchart	Identify the gaps/ weaknesses: and plan how to resolve	Initiate educational component, strengthen policies where needed and review incident reports	Identify if education was sufficient to resolve issue	If improvements were made, review at a later date or if no improvements were made, repeat PDCA cycle

PDCA, Plan, do, check, act.

The affinity diagram is another brainstorming method that is effective with large groups. It is most often used with groups who do not work together, when full participation is required, in political environments, or when "group think" should be avoided. It is also an effective method when the topic under consideration is sensitive, there is a need to break from traditional ideas, thinking is chaotic, or many creative ideas are needed. This method brings understanding from chaos by quickly organizing a large number of ideas into groups whose ideas (issues) are naturally related and building consensus. The procedure includes the following steps:

- Select a broad topic.
- Write each clear and concise idea on a separate piece of paper.
- Mix responses together randomly.
- Group similar cards together without discussing the ideas.
- When notes belong to more than one group, make a duplicate note.
- Select a heading (main topic) for each group of ideas.
- Decide what to do with this information.

The cause-and-effect diagram (also referred to as the *fishbone diagram*) is a method that is used to determine the possible causes of a problem in a structured format. Unlike other QM-based tools, cause-and-effect diagrams do not analyze data; they help organize ideas and theories about potential causes of a problem. These theories will need to be verified later with data. See Figure 8-26 for an example of a cause-and-effect diagram.

- The focused problem under investigation is described in a box at the head of the diagram.
- A long spine with an arrow pointing toward the head forms the backbone of the "fish."

- A few large "bones" feed into the spine, representing main categories of potential causes of the problem.
- The smaller "bones" represent deeper causes of the larger bones to which they are attached.

Causes are most commonly grouped under the following categories:

- Methods
- Machines
- People
- Materials
- Measurements
- Procedures
- Policies

Force-field analysis is used to identify the forces that drive a situation and those that restrain it. Box 8-8 provides an example of a force-field analysis. The procedure for using the method is as follows:

- Identify the current situation.
- Identify the desired (ideal) situation.
- Identify the driving forces (those that make the desired situation achievable).
- Identify the restraining forces (those that prevent the current situation from becoming the desired situation).
- Determine which factors can be altered to achieve the desired situation.

The flowchart is one of the most useful tools to identify and improve a process. By listing process steps in a symbolic format, areas that are "bottlenecks" can be more easily identified and removed or changed. Typical symbols are used in Figure 8-1. In Figure 8-1, the rectangle indicates a step in the process, the diamond

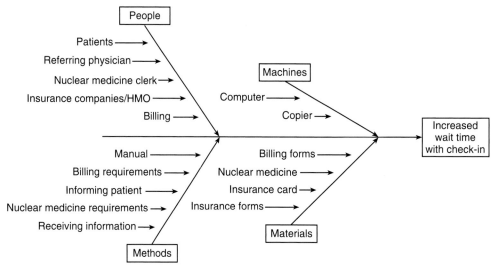

FIGURE 8-26 Cause-and-effect (fishbone) diagram.

BOX 8-8 | Force-Field Analysis

CURRENT SITUATION: Wait time for outpatients is too long during check-in.
 DESIRED SITUATION: Decrease waiting time for outpatient check-in to improve patient satisfaction.

Driving Forces
- Require less information on patients.
- Get information before patient's arrival.
- Electronically communicate with referring physicians' offices.
- Electronically communicate with HMOs and insurance companies.
- Cross-train others to help obtain information.

Restraining Forces
- Billing department requires too much information.
- Patient is not told of information needed before arrival.
- Lack of communication with referring sources.
- Only one person in the nuclear medicine department is trained to obtain information.
- Patient's perception that waiting time is too long.
- Process has too many steps.

BOX 8-9 | Contingency Diagram

QUESTION: How can it be ensured that outpatient satisfaction for timeliness of staff members continues to be low?
- Do not change the current process.
- Wait until patients arrive to tell them what information is needed.
- Schedule all patients for same arrival time.
- Eliminate the job position of nuclear medicine clerk.
- Keep the old, unreliable copier.
- Do not service the copier.
- Increase the information required of patients.
- Do not communicate with insurance companies.
- Do not provide information to referring physicians' offices.

---

indicates a decision point, the curved rectangle indicates a document, and arrows indicate a connector to the next step.

The contingency diagram is an effective method for looking at the negative parts of a problem and then reversing them to take positive action steps. Box 8-9 provides an example of a contingency diagram. The usual format to complete a contingency diagram is as follows:

- Identify the problem.
- Brainstorm for ideas to ensure that the problem will continue and possibly worsen.
- Review each idea to determine if the opposite can occur.
- Develop an action plan.

An interrelationship digraph is a method of linking related ideas. It involves the following procedure:

- Randomly space the ideas/issues.
- Select the first idea and relate it to the nearest idea/issue.
- Ask the question: does this idea/issue cause or influence the idea/issue to which it is being related?
- If the answer is "yes," draw an arrow from the first idea to this idea.
- Return to the original idea/issue and relate it to the next idea/issue.
- Continue to ask the question and draw arrows.
- When the first idea/issue has been related to all the other ideas/issues, follow the same sequence for each of the other ideas/issues.
- Identify the idea/issue that has the greatest influence on the others (the one with the most arrows pointing away from it).
- Identify the idea/issue that is most influenced by the others (the one with the most arrows pointing to it).

This method will help determine which ideas/issues to work on for the greatest possibility of altering a situation.

Measurements. Most problem solving involves some type of measurement, which may be in any phase of the PDCA cycle but is most important during the analysis (check) phase. The more common types of measurement include the following:

- A Pareto chart consists of a bar graph representing the frequency (from highest to lowest) of a problem and is used to help determine which area to work on first.
- A check sheet is used to collect data to identify patterns.
- A run chart is used to measure trends.
- A control chart is a run chart with upper and lower acceptable limits.
- A histogram is a bar graph of the distribution of data, which demonstrates variation.
- A scatter diagram is used to correlate two variables to look for cause and effect.

HOSPITAL-BASED QUALITY MANAGEMENT TOOLS

For years, hospital QM departments have utilized various tools in assessing quality developing quality initiatives and collecting data for demonstrating quality documentation. The following tools can also be used at the department level and can easily become incorporated into any department QI plan.

- *Open- or closed-chart reviews*—Review of active or past patient's medical records, ensuring that necessary documentation is present and filled in completely. These reviews are useful in assessing paper flow within department and medical records department. State and hospital accreditation survey-ors often choose this tool to assess overall compliance to hospital policies and professional standards.

- *Quality indicators*—Identified indicators that make up specific components of a department's QI plan. These indicators track, monitor, assess, or reassess specific processes within the department. Examples include tracking of incident reports, pregnancy compliance, medication documentation, and compliance to specific The Joint Commission's National Patient Safety Goals (NPSGs) or other professional standards.
- *Benchmarking*—Data to which to compare outcomes, cost, productivity, satisfaction, or results.
- *Policy review*—Ensures that the actual practice is reflected in the policy and that the policy reflects the actual practice. Sometimes these two items are not the same.
- *Form compliance*—Compliance to mandated processes, such as medication documentation, pregnancy compliance, medication event reporting, and contrast extravasation reporting. This monitoring is a great first step in building a QM program.
- *Performance improvement focus groups*—Engage staff members by allowing them to direct the project and solve the issue.
- *Satisfaction surveys: patient, employee, physician*—Quantify perception of others and identify issues to improve.
- *Time studies*—Tools to determine report or procedure turnaround times, which can identify where improvements can be made to shorten turnaround times and improve productivity.
- *Billing compliance*—Compliance with coding and billing guidelines established by the medical specialties or payers. Verification of procedure, radiopharmaceutical and other medication documentation compared to the bill and codes sent to the payer.

QUALITY DRIVERS

To be eligible to receive payment from Medicare, hospitals must be certified to meet certain conditions. Hospitals may gain such credentials by choosing to be reviewed by a state certification agency under contract to the Centers for Medicare & Medicaid Services or to be accredited by either JCAHO or the American Osteopathic Association.

—*National Health Policy Forum Issue Brief, No. 802, May 6, 2005*

The Joint Commission

The Joint Commission, formerly known as the Joint Commission on Accreditation of Healthcare Organiza-tions or JCAHO, is the nation's predominant standards-setting and accrediting body in health care. It is an independent, not-for-profit organization that evaluates and accredits more than 15,000 health care organizations. Since 1951, The Joint Commission has maintained state-of-the-art standards that focus on improving the quality and safety of care provided by health-care organizations. The Joint Commission's comprehensive accreditation process evaluates an organization's compliance with these standards and other accreditation requirements. This accreditation is recognized nationwide as a symbol of quality that reflects an organization's commitment to meeting certain performance standards. To earn and maintain The Joint Commission's Gold Seal of Approval, an organization must undergo an on-site survey at least every 3 years. Laboratories must be surveyed every 2 years.

As health care evolves, so do professional and accreditation standards. The Joint Commission has followed suit with several initiatives to address and solve many of the issues facing health care today. In capturing issues that happen throughout the continuum of a patient's care, The Joint Commission focuses on how individual departments provide services within the entire hospital system, identifying how nuclear medicine departments relate to other functions within the total care of a patient. This is evident in the recently implemented tracer methodology that The Joint Commission now uses in its accreditation surveys. This methodology traces the actual pathway that a patient has followed from the time of admitting to discharge through the hospital system. Instead of reviewing individual departments with its individual policies and practice, The Joint Commission is now assessing entire institutions and systems and focusing on the transition of care from one area to another along with the level of interdepartmental collaboration to provide quality patient care.

National Patient Safety Goals

In February 2002, The Joint Commission formed the Sentinel Event Advisory Group to advise The Joint Commission on the development of national standards to improve patient safety by reviewing documented medical events, which are reported to The Joint Commission through the sentinel event reporting process. The National Patient Safety Goals (NPSGs) became effective in January 2003. Each year, new goals are released and over the years several goals have been retired. Current NPSGs focus on general concepts that positively impact patient safety such as:

- Improving the effectiveness of communication among caregivers
- Improving the accuracy of patient identification
- Improving the safety of using medications

- Reducing the risk of health care–associated infections
- Accurately and completely reconciling medications across the continuum of care
- Reducing the risk of patient harm resulting from falls

Understanding Regulatory Changes That Impact Medical Imaging

While once considered biologicals, radiopharmaceuticals and contrast agent are now reclassified as "drugs" by the FDA. This shift in classification requires that the compounding, dispensing, and administration of radiopharmaceuticals and contrast media be performed under the same standards as the compounding, dispensing, and administration of any medication. The Joint Commission has followed suit and recently defined medications as prescriptions; sample medications; herbal remedies; vitamins; nutraceuticals; over-the-counter drugs; vaccines; diagnostic and contrast agents used on or administered to persons to diagnose, treat, or prevent disease or other abnormal conditions; radiopharmaceuticals; respiratory therapy treatments; parenteral nutrition; blood derivatives; IV solution (plain with electrolytes and/or drugs); and any product designated by the FDA as a drug. This reclassification necessitates that every department assess its current policies and practice regarding the storage, ordering, administration, monitoring, and documentation of radiopharmaceuticals, pharmaceuticals, and contrast material.

Nuclear medicine enhancing (interventional) pharmaceuticals can be defined as any medication (drug) that is administered for the sole purpose of enhancing the nuclear medicine study. The procedure for administering these medications and monitoring the patient following administration should be included in the department procedure manual. The NMT should have training on the pharmacological effects, recognizing adverse effects and steps to take. Examples of two nuclear medicine enhancing pharmaceuticals are captopril, when administered in conjunction with a renogram procedure; or CCK, when given as part of a hepatobiliary procedure. It is important for each practicing nuclear medicine technologist to fully understand the tasks that are within the scope of practice for a nuclear medicine technologist. Acting outside of the defined scope of practice can put the individual technologist and employer at great liability risk.

Understanding Professional Standards

The scope of practice for a NMT is defined in the *Scope of Practice for Nuclear Medicine Technologists,* a document developed and endorsed by the Society of Nuclear Medicine Technologist Section (SNMTS), and Nuclear Medicine Practice Standards, developed and endorsed by the American Society of Radiologic Technologists

(ASRT). These documents complement each other and in conjunction with other key documents, provide a portfolio of documents to aid in defining the profession of nuclear medicine technology.

RESOURCES FOR STANDARDS, GUIDELINES, AND REGULATIONS

Professional, practice, accreditation or clinical standards and guidelines include the following:

- ACR at www.acr.org
- ASRT at www.asrt.org
- ICANL at www.icanl.org
- SNM at www.snm.org
- The Joint Commission at www.jointcommission.org

BREAKING DOWN THE PROCESS

Issues of any size often seem overwhelming. Most people get caught up in the details or complexities of tangential issues. Few people can instinctively visualize the root of a complex issue. Breaking down the process and assessing where the breakdown of that process occurred can make for easier resolution and more effective improvements to fully address the initial issue. To most people, issues can be better understood and addressed if each step is broken down to manageable steps. Once the gaps and weaknesses have been identified, then the tools mentioned in this chapter can help to rectify the issue. Table 8-8 provides an example of breaking down the process.

PRACTICAL APPLICATION OF PROBLEM-SOLVING TECHNIQUES

The following examples illustrate how a team could use several of the problem-solving tools and measurements discussed in this chapter to improve a process.

Example 1:
Patient wait time has been identified as the greatest source of dissatisfaction for patients scheduled for nuclear medicine procedures.

A team is formed to develop a solution that will ensure the best outcome. During the planning phase, the team analyzes data already available (Figures 8-27 and 8-28). Of the patients studied in nuclear medicine, 65% are outpatients and 35% are inpatients. The team develops a flowchart of the process of scheduling patients through the department and discovers that the "bottleneck" causing longer waiting times for outpatients is during the check-in phase; for inpatients it is waiting for transportation to return to the nursing units after the procedure has been completed. Based on the data, the team determines that improving the process of checking in outpatients will have the greatest impact on outpatient

TABLE 8-8	Breaking Down the Process
Problem: Identification Issues	
Potential Steps to the Process	**Examples at Each Step of the Process**
Identify potential issue	Issues with patient identification: wrong patient gets wrong study or patient gets wrong radiopharmaceutical
Gather information, understand full scope of issue	Determine if caused by a process issue, or just one person; review any collected data, such as incident reports
Design data collection tools	Determine if further data needs to be collected
Collect data	Review policies on patient identification/ misadministration and compare with actual practice.
Interpret data	Determine if policies are sufficient or if clarification to current policies is warranted
Revise policies, adapt practice	Ensure that policy and practice are same, or at least complimentary
Present data to appropriate stakeholders, getting buy in	Present this data to managers, supervisors, leads, physicians, staff members
Educate on process improvement results and new practice/policy	Educate the staff members through staff meetings, e-mail, posting, and sign-off, and make policy accessible to all
Document process cycles are a convenient and easy way to document	Use *plan, do, check, act* cycle to document the issue, and steps to resolve the issue
Follow-up with monitoring	Monitor until compliant
Make adjustments as necessary	Reeducate staff members, or adapt policy if necessary

satisfaction because they make up the greatest number of patients and are most dissatisfied with patient waiting time.

The team can use a number of tools to find solutions to the problem. The cause-and-effect (fishbone) diagram can be used to brainstorm for root causes (Figure 8-26). Once causes have been identified, the team can develop measures to determine which causes can be changed to bring about the greatest impact on outpatient satisfaction. The contingency diagram can be used to identify those factors that will cause the problem to continue or worsen (Box 8-9). The force-field analysis can be used to identify the desired situation, (i.e., that outpatient waiting time for nuclear medicine procedures be decreased) and then identify the forces that would drive the desired outcome and those that are currently preventing it (Box 8-8).

Once the team has determined what they believe to be the major causes of the problem, measurements must be taken to prove the hypothesis. The check sheet is commonly used to measure multiple variables. It may be necessary to divide the measurements, such as for different days, times of the day, and sources of patient referrals. It is important to determine all the parameters that may be important when solving the problem before measurements begin in order to prevent having to take additional measurements later. Examples of possible check sheets for this particular problem are presented in Tables 8-9 and 8-10.

To analyze the data, the information is usually plotted on a Pareto chart, which identifies the cause having the greatest impact on the problem. This is sometimes referred to as the 80:20 rule, which means that 20% of the factors cause 80% of the problem; if the 20% are fixed, 80% of the "headaches" will disappear. Unfortunately, those 20% are usually the hardest factors to fix.

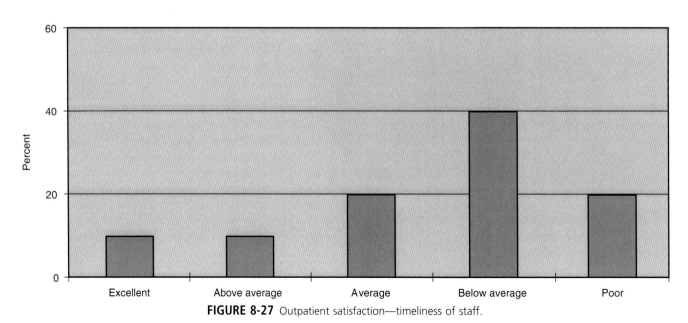

FIGURE 8-27 Outpatient satisfaction—timeliness of staff.

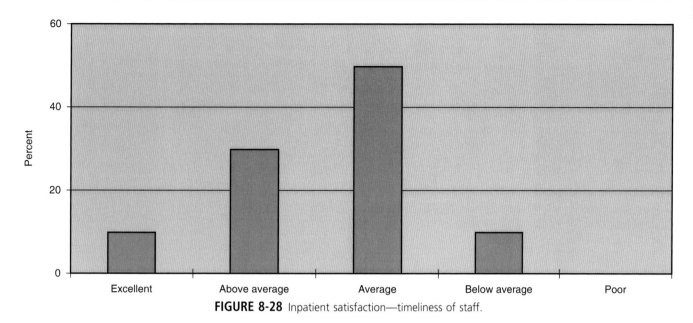

FIGURE 8-28 Inpatient satisfaction—timeliness of staff.

TABLE 8-9	Check Sheet				
Reason for Wait	**Mon**	**Tue**	**Wed**	**Thur**	**Fri**
Copier broken					
Clerk not available					
Patient arrives with no information					
Patient arrives late					
Patient arrives early					
Patient unable to fill out form					
Other					

Another chart that is helpful is the run chart, which is used to identify trends over time. If the team analyzed the data charted in Figure 8-29, it would conclude that something was causing greater delays on Wednesday and would look for causes such as the clerk's scheduled days off and more patients being scheduled from a particular referring physician on that day.

Based on the data analysis, the team might develop the following action plan:

• Work with the billing department to evaluate the amount of information required of outpatients and eliminate what is unnecessary.
• Develop a checklist of patient demographics and insurance requirements, and distribute this to referring physicians' offices to give to patients before their arrival in the nuclear medicine department.
• Determine what information can be provided by the referring physicians' offices before the patient's arrival.
• Work more closely with referring physicians' offices whose patients were least informed to better educate their staff members regarding the information that will be required from patients.

TABLE 8-10	Check Sheet		
Patients Arriving Without Billing Information			
Referral Source	**Week 1**	**Week 2**	**Week 3**
Payer A, B, or C			
Medicare			
RBM			
Dr. Jones			
Dr. Smith			
Dr. Johns			
Neurology group			
Cardiology group			
Pulmonary group			

• Reschedule the clerk's off time to better cover Wednesday mornings.

When the action plans are in place, the team must continue to monitor for improvements and alter the actions accordingly. Once the outpatient satisfaction starts improving, the team should begin to tackle causes of the "bottleneck" identified for inpatients using similar techniques.

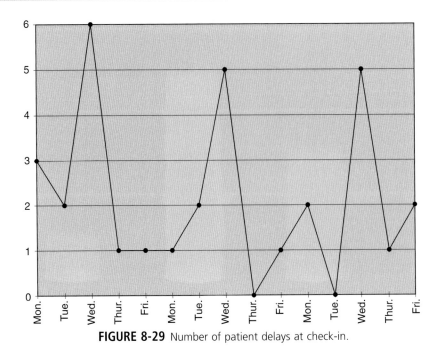

FIGURE 8-29 Number of patient delays at check-in.

Example 2:

Example of a QI initiative within the nuclear medicine department.

TOPIC: Documentation of pregnancy compliance

ISSUE: Pregnancy status of female patients of childbearing age must be documented before the administration of radiopharmaceuticals. If the patient is pregnant, the physician must determine if the nuclear medicine study is appropriate, and the risks, benefits, and potential complications must be discussed with the patient before the patient gives consent.

When building a QM program, choose a process that puts the department at risk. Take documentation of pregnancy in women of childbearing age as an example. Determine the minimum criteria that must be documented, such as name of patient, date, and date of last menstrual period. Some departments choose to also document signature of patient and acknowledgment of the technologist who gathered this documentation. Verify with state law, as well as state or federal radiation requirements, to ensure compliance to these laws. Consider current practice and determine if current practice limits liability.

To track the compliance of collecting pregnancy data, run a report of every nuclear medicine study performed on a female of childbearing age within the chosen month. Randomly select the names of 30 patients within that month, giving a decent sample size. Collect the files, chart, jacket, or database seeking the necessary documentation. Track the success at finding the necessary information. Generate documentation of findings in a written report or track in an Excel spreadsheet. Report these findings to necessary parties. Educate those involved with the findings and establish written communication and perhaps policies defining the new expectations. Implement a new process or policy, and then monitor this process for several months. Once the department has met compliance for three consecutive samplings, this monitoring can shift to periodic (quarterly) sampling until continual compliance has been documented.

BASICS OF CODING SYSTEMS

All procedures performed must be translated from the documentation provided in the medical record or procedure report into one or more standardized coding systems for billing payers. These coding systems are used universally by payers via standardized billing claim forms submitted to payers. The coding systems are numeric or alpha and numeric combinations associated with specific descriptions of procedures that are the basis for payment for procedures and products. Without the process of documentation and coding, providers do not receive payment (reimbursement) for the services and products. There are three key components of reimbursement: coding, coverage, and payment.

CODING SYSTEMS

Current Procedural Terminology

The **current procedural terminology (CPT)** is owned by the AMA and is the accepted medical nomenclature used to report medical procedures and services under public and private health insurance programs. CPT is also used for administrative management purposes such as claims processing and developing medical guidelines. There are three categories in CPT: Category I, II, and III. In general a physician or other health-care provider selects the CPT code with the name of the procedure or service that accurately identifies the services performed. They are further instructed not to select a CPT code that merely approximates a service. If no CPT exists, the service must be reported using an appropriate unlisted procedure or service code, usually identified with the last two digits 99.

Category I CPT codes are used to describe procedures in nuclear medicine. They are five-digit numerical codes that have descriptive terms to identify the majority of the procedures we perform in nuclear medicine. Most of the CPT Category I codes used by nuclear medicine professionals are located in the Radiology section, under the subsection of nuclear medicine. Diagnostic nuclear medicine CPT Category I codes begin with a 78 and are followed by three more numbers. Therapeutic nuclear medicine Category I codes begin with a 79, again followed by three numbers. CPT Category I codes are updated annually for implementation every year on January 1. More information regarding CPT, can be found on the AMA website at www.ama-assn.org. Additionally, there are comprehensive nuclear medicine specific coding guides published by the American College of Radiology at www.acr.org, or through the Society of Nuclear Medicine *Nuclear Medicine & PET Coder* published by MedLearn at www.snm.org or www.store.medlearn.com.

Category II CPT codes are supplemental tracking codes that are used for quality or performance measurements. Historically, these codes are not often used by nuclear medicine professionals. However, with the implementation of bonuses or penalties by payers for reimbursement, these codes are being used more for measuring quality and identifying if a provider qualifies for either a bonus or a penalty. It is easy to identify a Category II CPT code because it has four numbers followed by the letter "F."

Category III CPT codes are developed and used for emerging technology, services, and procedures. These codes are intended for temporary use (3 to 5 years) and not for permanent use by providers. Unlisted Category I CPT codes do not always offer the opportunity for specific data collection. Therefore Category III CPT codes can be developed to bridge this gap before a procedure being ready for widespread use. It is easy to identify a Category III CPT code because it is four numbers followed by the letter "T." Category III CPT codes are implemented twice a year, in January along with the CPT Category I and II CPT codes, and later in July.

Healthcare Common Procedure Coding Systems

HCPCS stands for Healthcare Common Procedure Coding System and is pronounced "hicks picks." There are two levels of HCPCS codes, level I and II. Payers have generally adopted the AMA CPT Category I codes as the HCPCS Level I codes. The Medicare **Centers for Medicare and Medicaid Services** (CMS) owns and establishes HCPCS Level II codes. HCPCS codes are updated annually with revised, new, and deleted codes available for implementation and use on January 1 of each year.

The HCPCS Level II codes are four-digit alphanumeric codes (e.g., AXXXX, CXXXX, JXXXX, or GXXXX) with unit descriptions used to identify drugs, radiopharmaceuticals, contrast agents, supplies, and services not already described in CPT Category I codes. Important for nuclear medicine procedures, the CPT Category I procedure codes do not include the drugs or radiopharmaceuticals. Therefore it is important to add the appropriate HCPCS Level II code and appropriate unit, along with the CPT Category I CPT code when drugs or radiopharmaceuticals are administered during a procedure. Radiopharmaceuticals and contrast agents are usually assigned in the "A" series of HCPCS Level II codes followed by four numbers. The "C" series of codes are temporary and are for hospital outpatient use only. Drugs and biologicals are traditionally represented by a "J" series code followed by four numbers. The "G" series codes are typically reserved for temporary use, or services and drugs packaged or bundled together. It is important to remember that these codes are only reported if administered to the patient, followed by the description of the code and the appropriate number of units. For example if you administered 3 mCi of thallium, report[3] units, A9505 *Thallium Tl-201 thallous chloride, diagnostic, per millicurie*. These codes are reported on the claim regardless of payment status; this means if there is no separate additional payment, correct coding principles instructs providers to report the codes that were administered.

International Classification of Diseases

The **International Classification of Diseases (ICD)**, Ninth Revision, Clinical Modifications (ICD-9-CM) is used to report injury or diseases. So far this chapter describes coding that reports *what* has been done (CPT) or *what* has been administered (HCPCS Level II). ICD-9 codes tell the story (to the payer) of "why" the procedure was ordered and necessary. In the next few years ICD-9 will be replaced by ICD-10 (same name, only tenth revision) for two reasons:

1. Descriptions of diseases are typically universal.
2. The ICD-9 system is outdated and has run out of numbers for many sections, making any future additions difficult. Several European countries have already made the switch to ICD-10.

The ICD-9 codes are three numbers, a period, and one/two numbers long (e.g., acute and chronic choleystitis [575.12]). The period is not used on the claim forms submitted to payers. ICD-10 codes are six digits, a combination of alpha and numeric codes, used to describe in detail diseases and procedures by organ system, equipment, drugs, and radiopharmaceuticals. ICD-9 and some ICD-10 codes describe the reason that the patient presents for a visit, the established disease, or the procedure or service. ICD-9 or ICD-10 codes could include the signs, symptoms, or established diseases for a patient. ICD-9 codes are discussed in more detail later. ICD-9 and ICD-10 codes are updated annually with revised, new, and deleted codes available for use each October 1.

Hospital Revenue Codes

Hospital revenue codes are four-digit numeric codes used only by hospitals for inpatient and outpatient claims. These codes are owned by the American Hospital Association and are updated periodically by the **National Uniform Billing Committee (NUBC)**. The purpose of these codes is for internal hospital finance tracking. Hospital revenue codes are primarily used to identify where in a facility the procedure or services was performed. They are also used by Medicare for the payment calculations to hospitals.

MEDICAL COVERAGE

Coverage is the term used by payers to assess if the reason for the procedure (ICD-9) is an adequate indication by medical practice standards, whereby the payer would believe it was medically necessary and therefore pay for the visit or procedure. ICD-9 codes are for tracking diseases and primarily used today by payers to determine if a claim should be paid. Payers do not simply pay for all procedures or visits. Payers are discriminating in that they pay only for those procedures they believe are medically necessary. Therefore, medical necessity is established by payers based on standards of care established by medical specialties and the peer reviewed scientific literature.

PAYMENT

Payment rates are individually established by each payer based on their medical policy described earlier and related to the procedure (CPT or HCPCS) or service performed. Providers of services should check with each payer for their established rates regarding the procedures and services they provide to the community. Typically, payment rates are adjusted to account for geographic locality variations. Additionally, large payers like Medicare have different payment systems based on the setting of care, and therefore payments are not universal. Most payment systems today are prospective payment systems. Providers know in advance the set payment rate established by CPT or HCPCS procedure codes. There still remain a few providers in rural areas that are paid based on retrospective systems. In these types of systems, reconciliations are performed at the end of a fiscal year and adjustments are made based on provider costs. Since third party payers are large in numbers and vary in payment policy, the Medicare payment systems important only to nuclear medicine will be described.

For hospital inpatient stays, Medicare payments for procedures are based on the patient's discharge diagnosis; a system called the diagnosis related group (DRG). The DRG system is the most extreme packaging and bundling system that we have today for payments. A single payment is given to the hospital based on the patient's episode of care during their entire hospital stay. Another packaging system is the Medicare **Hospital Outpatient Prospective Payment System (HOPPS)**. In this system, procedures are paid individually; however payment rates are in groupings of **Ambulatory Payment Classifications (APC)** categories/groups that result in averaging of payments based on clinical similarities and resource data from hospitals. The result of HOPPS is an averaged payment; therefore some rates may seem higher than expected, whereas others would appear low. The theory is that total payment rates will average out over time for the facility. This type of payment system is intended to incentivize providers to reduce costs.

The **Medicare Physician Fee Schedule (MPFS)** payment system is used for Medicare payments to physicians, physician offices, and **Independent Diagnostic Testing Facilities (IDTF)**. The MPFS, as it relates to nuclear medicine procedures, breaks down each code into the professional rate or component (physician work), the technical rate or component (equipment, technologist, medical supplies, etc.), and the global rate (combining professional and technical).

The MPFS is a prospective payment system based on an established relative value scale or unit (RVU) for each CPT code. The AMA recommends RVUs based on the physician work and practice expense to the CMS for establishing Medicare's RVUs for each CPT code. For more information about the Medicare payment system go to www.cms.hhs.gov.

BILLING COMPLIANCE

Billing compliance means that the provider has policies in place to ensure they are monitoring and following all the applicable coding guidelines including federal and state regulations. As noted above, each of the coding systems have guidelines established by the entity owning the system (also by medical specialties or by the payer) for appropriate selection and use of the code. In addition to guidelines, there are federal and state regulations that must be adhered to, as selecting codes outside the guidance and guidelines can result in serious consequences for the provider.

Important federal regulations that affect billing compliance include the Stark Law (Physician Self-Referral Law), which prohibits referring a Medicare patient for any health service to an entity that the provider (or an immediate family member) has a financial interest in unless an exception applies; the *False Claims Act* 31 U.S.C. §3729-3722, protects the federal government against fraud and abuse. Anyone who knowingly submits or causes another person or entity to submit, or knowingly makes, uses or causes to be made or used a false record or statement to get a false or fraudulent claim paid or approval of government funds are liable for three times the government's damages plus civil penalties of $5,000 to $11,000 per false claim. The term "knowingly" means that a person has (1) has actual knowledge of the information, (2) acts in deliberate ignorance of the truth or falsity of the information, or (3) acts in reckless disregard of the truth or falsity of the information with no proof of specific intent to defraud being required.

There are whistleblower provisions that allow anyone with evidence of fraud to sue on behalf of the government, to recover overpayment of federally funded health-care programs. The whistleblower may be awarded a percentage of the recovered funds. The federal Anti-Kickback Statute is a law to protect patient and the federal health-care programs from fraud and abuse. The law states that anyone who knowingly and wilfully received or pays anything of value to influence the referral of federal healthcare business, including Medicare and Medicaid, can be held accountable for a felony. The legal branch of the federal government, the Office of Inspector General (OIG), has a list of compliance program resources for hospitals, physician practices, pharmaceuticals, third-party billing located at www.oig.hhs.gov.

SUMMARY

- A request for a procedure, "an order," should include the patient's name, identification number, referring physician's name, and clinical indications for the procedure.
- Most patients have limited knowledge of nuclear medicine procedures and the term *nuclear* may initiate fear.
- The technologist must ensure that the correct procedure is scheduled and that there are no contraindications for the study.
- The technologist must determine the extent of the patient's physical ability and have an understanding of the different developmental stages from infant to older adult in order to understand and communicate with the patient effectively.
- Technologists are required to be competent in the administration of all procedure enhancing (interventional) medications.

- It is the responsibility and duty of the technologist to be familiar with the routes of administration, pharmacology, side effects, and adverse effects of all medications used in nuclear medicine procedures.
- Six rights associated with medications (including radiopharmaceuticals) and their administration: right dose, right medication, right patient, right time, route of administration, and right documentation.
- Routes of administration include topical, sublingual, oral, and parenteral.
- Parenteral routes of administration include subcutaneous, intramuscular, intradermal, intravenous, and intrathecal.
- When withdrawing a nonradioactive substance from a vial, a volume of air equal to the dose may be inserted into the vial before withdrawing the dose. However, do not inject air into a vial when withdrawing radiopharmaceuticals.
- Gloves must always be worn when handling radioactivity.
- One should dispose of all needles and syringes directly into a puncture-proof container without recapping if possible.
- The most direct way to intervene in the cycle of infection is to prevent transmission of the pathogen from the reservoir to a susceptible host.
- The most effective system to prevent the transmission of disease is by practicing standard precautions.
- Consider all patient specimens and body fluids as potentially infectious.
- Vital signs include temperature, pulse rate, respiration rate, and blood pressure. A technologist should know how to assess each of the vital signs and know the normal values for each.
- There are three levels of monitoring care: quality control (QC), quality assurance (QA), and continuous quality improvement (CQI).
- Quality or performance improvement plans must relate to the overall strategic plan of the nuclear medicine facility.

REFERENCES

1. American College of Radiology: Manual on contrast media, Version 7, Reston, Va., American College of Radiology, 2010. Available on Internet: http://www.acr.org/SecondaryMainMenuCategories/quality_safety/contrast_manual.aspx. Accessed August 2010.
2. Bellin M-F, Jacobsen JA, Tomassin I, et al: Contrast medium extravasation injury: guidelines for prevention and management, *Eur Radiol* 12:2807-2812, 2002.
3. Murphy KJP, Szopinski KT, Cohan RH, et al: Occurrence of adverse reactions to gadolinium-based contrast material and management of patients at risk: a survey of the American Society of Neuroradiology fellowship directors, *Acad Radiol* 6:656-664, 1999.
4. Runge VM: Safety of approved MR contrast media for intravenous injection, *J Magn Reson Imaging* 12:205-213, 2000.

5. Runge VM, Juroff LR, Jinkins JR: Central nervous system: review of clinical use of contrast media, *Top Magn Res Imaging* 12: 231-263, 2001.

6. Singh J, Daftary A: Iodinated contrast media and their adverse reactions, *J Nucl Med Technol* 36:69-74, 2008.

SUGGESTED READING

Brassard M: *The memory jogger plus+*, Methuen, Mass, 1989, GOAL/QPC.

Chantler C: The role of doctors in the delivery of heath care, *Lancet* 353:1178-1181, 1999.

Ehrlich RA, Daly JA, McCloskey ED: *Patient care in radiography with an introduction to medical imaging*, ed 6, St Louis, 2004, Mosby.

Jensen SC, Peppers MP: *Pharmacology and drug administration for imaging technologists*, St Louis, 1998, Mosby.

Kowalczyk N, Donnett K: *Integrated patient care for the imaging professional*, St Louis, 1996, Mosby.

Majchrzak J, Merlino D, Richmond D: *Nuclear medicine & PET coder 2010*, St. Paul, Minn., 2010, Medical Learning Incorporated.

Patch, GG, Morton KA, Arias JM, et al: Naloxone reverses pattern of obstruction of the distal common bile duct induced by analgesic narcotic in hepatobiliary imaging, *J Nucl Med* 32:1270-1272, 1991.

Scholtes PR: *The team handbook*, Madison, Wis., 1988, Joiner Associates.

Wilkinson JM, Van Leuven K: *Fundamentals of nursing: thinking and doing*, Philadelphia, 2007, FA Davis.

Principles of SPECT and SPECT/CT

James R. Galt, Tracy L. Faber

OUTLINE

OBJECTIVES

After completing this chapter, the reader will be able to:

- Discuss advantages of SPECT compared with planar imaging.
- Describe characteristics of the SPECT gantry.
- Discuss issues relative to multiple detector SPECT systems.
- Describe collimators used in SPECT.

- List SPECT acquisition modes.
- Compare circular and body-contour orbits.
- Describe principles of tomographic reconstruction.
- Discuss reconstruction algorithms, including their respective advantages and computational requirements.
- Describe frequency space filtering.

KEY TERMS

attenuation correction
body-contour orbit
circumferential profile
contrast
cutoff frequency
emission computed tomography (ECT)
filtered back-projection (FBP)

horizontal long-axis slices
iterative reconstruction
low-pass filter
maximum intensity projection (MIP)
Nyquist frequency
ordered subset expectation maximization (OSEM)
polar map

projection
resolution
short-axis slices
step-and-shoot
surface rendering
vertical long-axis slices
volume rendering

SINGLE PHOTON EMISSION COMPUTED TOMOGRAPHY

Clinicians use planar images in the diagnosis of many types of disease. X-ray images show the distribution of materials of different densities in the body by imaging the attenuation of photons passing through the body. Scintigrams, produced by a scintillation camera, are planar images of the distribution of a photon-emitting radioactive tracer administered to a patient. An inherent difficulty in the interpretation of planar images is the fact that they represent a **projection** through the body. Each point, or pixel, in the image represents the superimposition of all the material (in the case of an x-ray) or activity (in the case of a scintigram) in front of and behind it. In addition, the two-dimensional (2D) aspect of projection images means that objects perpendicular to the imaging plane appear to be shortened or are difficult to view at all. Determining the shape of the distribution requires that the physician assimilate the information in several views. Computed tomography (CT) helps overcome this problem by using several planar images to reconstruct tomographic images in which each pixel represents a single point within the subject (Figure 9-1). The pixels actually represent a small volume, often called a *voxel*, for volume element. Unlike planar images, tomographic images do not suffer from the overlap of structures in front of or behind the organ of interest.

In medical terminology, **emission computed tomography (ECT)** is distinguished from x-ray CT in that the photons used in ECT originate within the subject instead of from an external source. Consequently, ECT is a process-oriented measurement that records where the tracer is located within the patient. Single photon emission computed tomography (SPECT) produces images of gamma rays (or sometimes x-rays) emitted by a radioactive tracer. Positron emission tomography (PET) images the two 511-keV photons produced when a positron comes into contact with an electron. Computed tomography, however, measures the attenuation of photons as they pass through the patient and thus provides a measurement of anatomy in the form of attenuation coefficients.

Computed tomography excels in producing high-contrast, high-resolution images of a patient's anatomy and provides a means of identifying structural details but often cannot provide functional information about organs or tumors. Emission computed tomography excels at providing that functional information but it is often difficult to determine the exact location of tracer uptake. In addition, ECT images suffer from comparatively poor resolution and sensitivity compared to CT images. Although analysis of separate images with mental integration can be helpful, co-registration of CT and ECT images can give the clinician added confidence

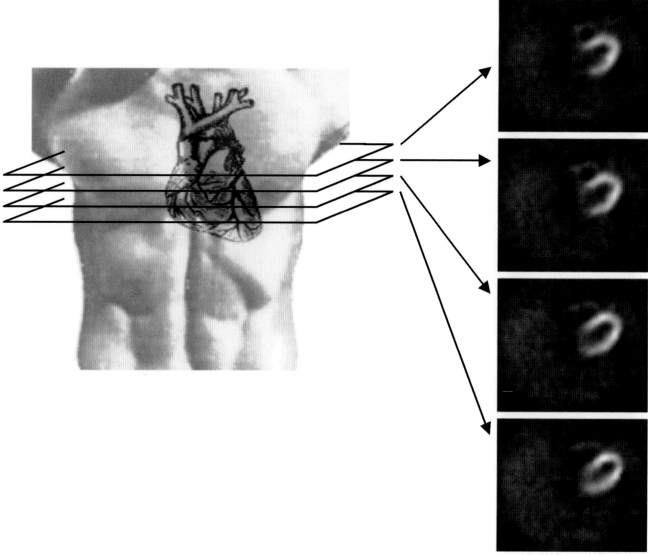

FIGURE 9-1 Tomography creates a stack of slices through the axis of the body; the slices show the distribution of radionuclide at each point. Here, myocardial perfusion images that slice through the chest are displayed.

in making a diagnosis.[60] Software methods to co-register ECT and CT images made independently are available,[59] but often the logistics of obtaining both sets of images, differences in body position between the scans, and lack of identifiable landmarks make accurate registration impractical. Hybrid PET/CT and SPECT/CT systems combine both modalities into one device. This allows CT and ECT images to be collected in one session, and after automated registration, to be displayed with precise registration as shown in Figure 9-2 and the corresponding color plate. When CT is available that is already registered with the ECT, it can also be used to replace sealed radioactive source transmission systems used for **attenuation correction.**

The clinical introduction of PET/CT systems has helped propel PET into the forefront of radiology, and PET/CT systems dominate the PET market. SPECT/CT has been slower to catch on, but as more systems enter into use, new applications are being identified and the demand may increase.[97] Applications for SPECT/CT include cutting-edge procedures for tumor imaging where tracer uptake may be very specific to the tumor, as in the ^{99m}Tc-labeled folate images[87] of Figure 9-2, or to finding added value and increased diagnostic confidence in standard procedures like bone SPECT.[117] The value SPECT/CT has been reported for number of SPECT applications.[28,91,95] Others have noted that adding CT to SPECT increases the complexity of the procedure and radiation dose to the patient and should be avoided when it does not provide additional information.[43]

Image Properties

The most common measurements of image quality are resolution, contrast, and noise. No matter which kind of image is produced, resolution refers to how well objects

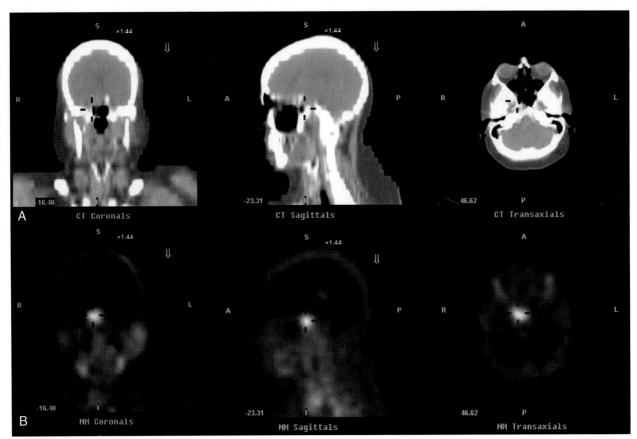

FIGURE 9-2 CT **(A)** and attenuation corrected SPECT **(B)** images of ^{99m}Tc-labeled folate (EC-20) showing tracer concentration in a nonfunctioning pituitary adenoma. SPECT/CT hybrid systems excel in imaging situations where anatomical location of the uptake is critical for interpretation but the emission image shows little anatomical detail. See Plate 1, which shows this figure with a color SPECT image fused onto the CT study.

can be separated in space (as opposed to blurring them together); contrast to how well different levels of brightness can be seen (brightness representing density for x-rays and radionuclide concentration in scintigrams); and noise to random additions to the image that interfere with the viewer's perception. In a scintigraphic image, resolution allows two objects that are close together to be separated. Contrast allows the determination of whether two objects have different activity concentrations. Noise is primarily due to counting statistics, giving planar images a speckled appearance and producing more complex problems in tomographic images.

Contrast in scintigraphic images can be defined as the measure of counts (or intensity) in the target (the object to be imaged) compared with the intensity in a background region. It is measured as:

$$\text{Contrast} = (C_o - C_b)/C_b$$

where C_o is the organ count and C_b is the background count. The higher the contrast, the more visible the target organ. Low contrast can make the target organ fade into the background. Contrast is most easily measured by graphing a count profile (the counts encountered along a line drawn through a region of interest in the image). The peak counts in the graph are taken to be C_o, and the minimum count level is taken to be C_b. Figure 9-3 shows profiles taken through the left ventricle in both planar and tomographic images from a myocardial perfusion study. The decreased background count level in the tomographic image causes increased contrast compared with the planar image.

Resolution in scintigraphic images is the measure of how close two point sources of activity can get and still be distinguished as separate. Because no medical imaging modality is perfect, a point source never appears as a single bright pixel but rather always as a blurred distribution. Two blurry points eventually smear together into a single spot when they are moved close enough to each other. Resolution is measured by taking a profile though a point source and analyzing the resulting curve. A profile through a perfect point source would look like a sharp single spike rising above the flat background. A profile through a real point source appears as a Gaussian-shaped curve. Resolution is the width of the Gaussian curve at a level of half of its maximum, or the full width at half maximum (FWHM).

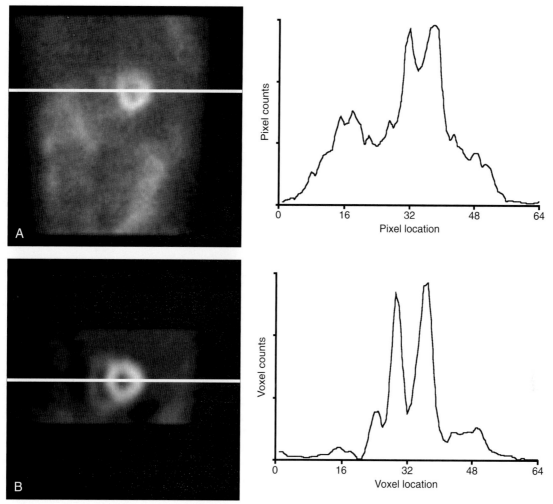

FIGURE 9-3 Profiles taken through the myocardium in a planar image **(A)** and a tomographic image **(B)** from a myocardial perfusion study show properties related to image quality. The lower background count level of the tomographic image results in improved image contrast. A profile of an image is a graph of counts versus location.

Noise in scintigraphic images is primarily the result of the random nature of counting statistics. Each pixel in a planar scintigram is assigned a number (or pixel value) that represents the number of photons detected in a small area of the camera's crystal. The random nature of nuclear decay produces random fluctuations in the number of counts detected in adjacent pixels. Noise can be thought of as a measure of irrelevant information in the image. Noise appears as a speckle in nuclear medicine planar images and is particularly noticeable in background regions. Noise is measured relative to the useful image information, called the *signal*. In planar scintigrams, the signal is proportional to the counts *(N)*, and the noise is proportional to the square root of *N*. Because the signal *(N)* increases faster than its square root, noise is a more serious problem for low-count images. As image counts increase, noise becomes less evident. Therefore, in low-count images, image quality can be improved greatly by even a small increase in the number of acquired counts. If count rates are high, the images will not be improved even by acquiring twice as many counts.

The effect of noise on tomographic images can be difficult to predict because each voxel is the product of the projection of that point in space from several different angles. In that sense, each voxel represents the summation of several projections and has better noise characteristics than individual projections. Tomographic reconstruction techniques, however, tend to increase noise.

SPECT images are superior to planar images in contrast but at some cost to resolution. Because each image represents a slice through the patient, much of the background activity is eliminated, increasing the contrast. Resolution decreases with distance from a scintillation camera. Because the camera must view the patient from all angles, it cannot be close to the organ of interest in all views. Practically, however, occlusion and superimposition of structures tend to reduce apparent resolution in planar images. For example, two point sources can be feet apart but still be seen as only one point in a planar image if one is in front of the other. Tomography, which eliminates these effects, often appears to provide higher resolution than planar imaging. This apparent increase in resolution can be seen in Figure 9-3. If the widths of the profiles taken through the myocardium are compared, the steeper slope of the profiles in the tomographic image implies a higher resolution.

INSTRUMENTATION

The main components of SPECT systems are the scintillation camera, the gantry (the frame that supports and moves the heads), and the computer systems (hardware and software). These components work together to acquire and reconstruct the tomographic images.

Scintillation Cameras

The basic components of a scintillation camera are a collimator, a sodium iodide (NaI[Tl]) crystal, photomultiplier tubes (PMTs), pulse height analyzers (PHAs), and spatial positioning circuitry. Gamma rays (photons) pass through the collimator and cause a scintillation event (a short burst of visible light) in the crystal. The glow of the scintillation is converted into electrical signals by the PMTs. The location of the scintillation event is determined by the positioning circuitry based on the relative signals from the different PMTs. The brightness of the scintillation is proportional to the energy of the photon, which is measured by the PHAs. Scintillation cameras as described here were developed by Hal Anger of the University of California at Berkley in the late 1950s and early 1960s and are still the most widely used cameras.[1] Early cameras were completely analog devices in which the output was sent to an oscilloscope, creating a flash on the screen. A lens focused the screen on a piece of x-ray film that was exposed one flash at a time. This allowed for planar imaging, but for SPECT the images must be made available to the computer digitally.

A *digital scintillation camera* may be defined as a camera system in which the computer is an integral part of system and is used for processing the scintillation event. Digital cameras provide a digital output, or images in the form of a computer matrix, rather than strictly analog signals sent to an oscilloscope. In reality, no commercial system is totally analog or totally digital. Most camera systems convert the position and pulse-height signals generated from analog circuitry in the camera to digital signals, which may then be further corrected for energy and position through digital processing. Camera designs that allow the output of each PMT to be converted to a digital signal have become common. Separation of the processing for each PMT leads to the ability to image at higher count rates. Digitization of each PMT's signal allows computer software to replace the complicated analog circuitry for positioning and pulse-height analysis. This allows greater processing flexibility, resulting in improved energy and spatial resolution. The evolution of scintillation cameras from analog to digital devices is shown in Figure 9-4.

Gantry

The frame that supports the scintillation camera used for SPECT must be able to rotate and position the camera precisely, making size and stability important factors. Size is a practical issue because the gantry is the largest part of the SPECT system, and its size determines the amount of room space needed. The gantry must be able to rotate the scintillation camera with its heavy collimator and lead shielding. This makes the gantry/camera combination very heavy (floor loading must be considered when positioning a camera within a department).

SPECT Systems

SPECT cameras consisting of a single scintillation camera mounted on a ring gantry formed the backbone of tomographic nuclear medicine for years, and their utility and flexibility maintain their importance today. Circular cameras are more easily manufactured and dominated through the 1980s. Most scintillation cameras manufactured today have a rectangular head shape because a rectangular field of view (the usable imaging area of the camera) is more efficient for SPECT and whole-body imaging. Rectangular heads do not give a significant advantage in cardiac imaging, however, and the patient's arms may interfere with the corners of the camera during SPECT.

Multiple detector SPECT systems are systems with more than one scintillation camera (Figure 9-5). They are more commonly sold today than single detector systems. The most obvious benefit of adding more detectors to a scintillation camera system is the increase in sensitivity. It seems obvious that doubling the number of heads doubles the number of photons that may be acquired in the same amount of time. The user may take advantage of the increase in sensitivity by acquiring more counts, by adding higher-resolution collimation, or by increasing throughput.

When two large field-of-view rectangular cameras are mounted opposite each other (180 degrees), they may speed whole-body bone imaging by allowing simultaneous acquisition of anterior and posterior images. A dual detector SPECT system capability can also increase throughput for 360-degree SPECT imaging by halving imaging time while collecting the same number of counts. A full 360 degrees of projections can be acquired by rotating the gantry 180 degrees. The gain in sensitivity may be traded off to achieve more precise images by allowing the use of higher resolution collimators.

However, these improvements may mean very little for cardiac SPECT, in which a 180-degree orbit is recommended. The addition of a second head does not result in doubled sensitivity for cardiac imaging because counts

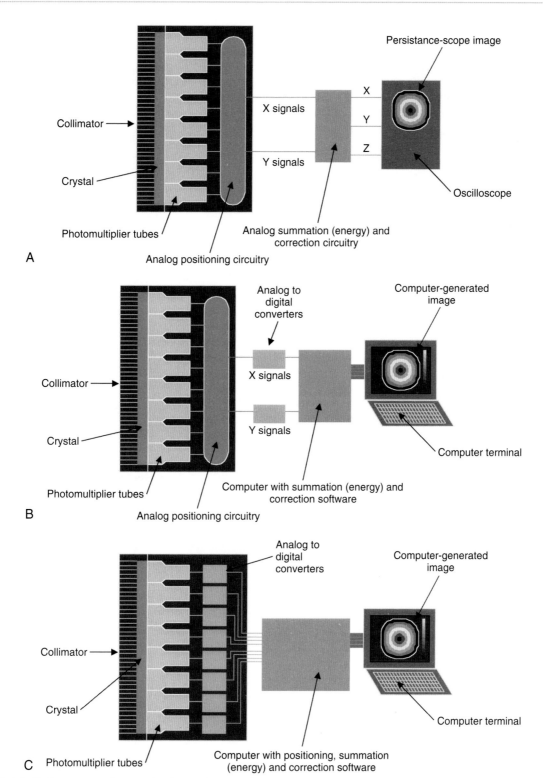

FIGURE 9-4 Scintillation cameras have evolved over the years from strictly analog devices in the early 1960s **(A)** to devices that produce computerized images **(B)**. Many cameras today digitize the output of the photomultiplier tubes **(C)**, which allows most of the signal processing to be done in software.

in posterior planar images are much more severely attenuated than those of the anterior projections. In systems designed for cardiac SPECT, the two detectors are mounted next to each other (at 90 degrees) on the gantry. This allows a full 180-degree orbit to be acquired while rotating the gantry only through 90 degrees.

The drawbacks of double-headed cameras include the increase in quality control (QC) required by the addition of the second head and some loss of flexibility. Double detector systems do not allow the same flexibility of movement that is enjoyed with many single-headed systems. This may prevent them from being easily used

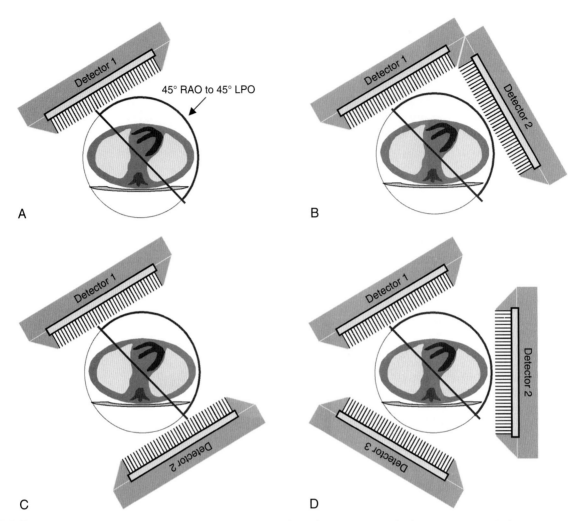

FIGURE 9-5 SPECT cameras may be configured with one, two, or three detectors. **A,** Single detector camera. An important consideration is that for ^{201}Tl myocardial SPECT, more than 66% of the counts are collected in the 180 degrees between 45 degrees right anterior oblique (RAO) and 45 degrees left posterior oblique (LPO). **B,** Addition of a second detector at 90 degrees doubles the sensitivity for both 180-degree and 360-degree orbits and is preferred for cardiac imaging. Flexibility may be lost, however, where simultaneous anterior and posterior images are desired. **C,** Addition of a second detector at 180 degrees doubles the sensitivity for 360-degree SPECT, but no increase in sensitivity is seen if a 180-degree orbit is recommended. **D,** A three-detector system, with detectors mounted at 120-degree intervals, increases the sensitivity for 180-degree SPECT by only 50% but triples the sensitivity for 360-degree orbits.

for some types of planar imaging (e.g., gated blood pool) in which it is often difficult to position the camera correctly. There is a great deal of variation between manufacturers in the camera movement allowed for planar imaging. Most manufacturers market dual detector systems that allow the cameras to be rotated to 180 degrees for general SPECT or 90 degrees for cardiac SPECT.

Triple detector cameras are usually dedicated to SPECT imaging. The three heads, as discussed for double-headed systems, result in increased sensitivity that may be used to increase throughput, counts, or resolution. However, if the three detectors are mounted rigidly at 120 degrees from one another, the system cannot perform simultaneous anterior/posterior imaging, which greatly reduces its utility for planar imaging. These systems also do not have a great impact on cardiac

imaging with 180-degree orbits, for the reasons discussed previously. Triple-headed SPECT systems are best suited for clinics that do a great deal of 360-degree SPECT imaging and can afford to have a camera dedicated solely to that task.

SPECT/CT Systems

The need for the correlation of SPECT's functional images with CT's anatomical images has been recognized for many years, and though software methods have shown promise, they have failed to gain clinical acceptance. Hybrid systems overcome the obstacles of bringing together images made on two different systems at two different times by combining both scanners into one gantry. A prototype SPECT/CT system, capable of performing simultaneous SPECT and CT scans of

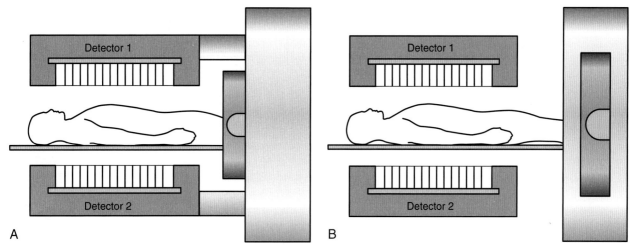

FIGURE 9-6 SPECT/CT scanners have been introduced with two different designs. **A,** CT has been incorporated directly into the SPECT gantry in one system where a low power x-ray tube and detector are mounted on the same ring that moves the cameras. **B,** Other systems have matched a standard CT unit with a SPECT system, sharing one imaging table (and maybe the same housing). This allows the use of a higher quality CT unit (at much higher expense). SPECT and CT images must be acquired sequentially in both systems since the two units are separated along the table.

phantoms, was reported in 1992.[72] Today's clinical SPECT/CT scanners use two different designs (Figure 9-6).

The first SPECT/CT design incorporated CT directly into the SPECT gantry with a low power x-ray tube and detector mounted on the same ring that rotates the cameras (limiting the speed of CT acquisition to the rotational speed of the SPECT gantry). The first SPECT/CT system introduced utilized this design and was capable of producing 1-cm CT slices of the full camera field of view in slightly under 10 minutes.[89] This system has been updated to a four-slice version that cuts the CT imaging time in half and produces approximately 5-mm slices. An evaluation of this system against a standard CT showed that it gave a much lower radiation dose to the patient at some loss of CT resolution (though contrast was better than a diagnostic CT system operating at the same radiation dose to the patient).[55] A second design (by a different manufacturer) utilizes cone beam CT with a flat-panel detector, allowing 14 cm of 1-mm thick CT slices to be acquired in one 360-degree gantry rotation.[107] The large CT field of view in the axial direction is designed to include the entire myocardium in one CT rotation of 12 seconds, enabling the possibility of a breath-hold acquisition. The advantages of these systems, compared to use of a standard, or diagnostic, CT scanner are greatly reduced cost, a somewhat smaller footprint, lower shielding requirements, and reduced radiation dose to the patient.

SPECT/CT current designs mount a standard CT scanner and a SPECT system so that one imaging table passes through both units. This design allows the use of a higher quality CT scanner (at much higher expense). SPECT and CT images are acquired sequentially, without repositioning the patient, in both systems as the table moves the patient between the two units. The advantage of these systems, compared to use a low dose CT built into the SPECT camera gantry, is the quality and speed of the diagnostic CT scanner.

SPECT/CT systems tend to be larger, heavier, and require more shielding than rooms prepared for traditional SPECT systems. During the CT scan, scatter can be a major source of radiation exposure to the technologist and a shielded control area is recommended and may be required.

A number of factors must be taken into account when acquiring SPECT/CT images. If a high-quality CT scan is not needed, the CT scan should be configured to minimize the patient's radiation dose. The patient must be encouraged to stay still through both procedures because if the patient moves, the images will not match. Even then, imaging the breathing chest may present a problem. Computed tomography images are acquired in much less time than SPECT images. A single CT slice represents a snapshot of the chest at one instant while SPECT images are acquired over several minutes. If standard CT procedures are followed and the patient is asked to hold their breath through the entire acquisition, it will almost guarantee that the two image sets do not match. Shallow breathing throughout the scan is recommended to minimize this source of image mismatch.

Collimators

The collimator is the focusing device of a SPECT camera. Gamma rays have too much energy to be focused by a lens in the same way that visible light photons are in a film or digital camera. Instead, collimators are made up of an array of long, narrow (usually) parallel holes that exclude all photons except those travelling parallel to the

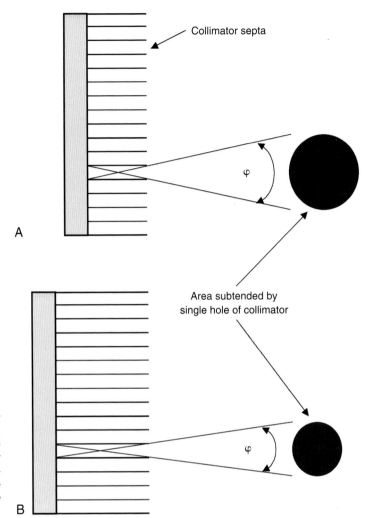

FIGURE 9-7 The resolution and sensitivity of parallel hole collimators depend on the shape, length, and size of the holes. **A,** Each hole in the collimator restricts the photons that may strike the crystal to those that originate within the arc φ. **B,** Lengthening the holes of the collimator reduces φ and the area exposed through each hole at a given distance. The longer the holes, the greater the resolution and the lower the sensitivity. It should also be noted that regardless of the length of the hole, the resolution degrades with the distance from the collimator.

direction of the hole (Figure 9-7). Collimators are rated by their sensitivity and resolution. In general, the sensitivity and resolution of a collimator are inversely related: a very high-sensitivity collimator has low resolution, and a very high-resolution collimator has low sensitivity. These properties are determined by the area, length, and shape of the collimator's holes.

Low-energy all-purpose (LEAP) and general purpose (GAP) collimators have relatively short, wide holes that accept more photons than high-resolution (HRES) collimators with long, narrow holes. This can be seen in the example in Figure 9-7. Increasing the length of the hole increases resolution by decreasing the angle subtended by the hole. This increase in resolution comes at the expense of sensitivity. In general, images with better resolution do not need as many counts to achieve the same image quality. Unless the images are very count poor or must be acquired very quickly, HRES collimation is generally preferred to LEAP collimation, particularly when multiple detector SPECT systems are used.

Collimators must be made of material that cannot be easily penetrated by photons of the range used in nuclear medicine (70 to 364 keV). This limits the selection to dense metals such as lead, silver, gold, and tungsten. Most collimators are made of lead, but some tungsten collimators are available at great expense. LEAP, GAP, and HRES collimators are all low-energy collimators and are suitable for imaging thallium-201 (^{201}Tl) (~72 keV), technetium-99m (^{99m}Tc) (140 keV), and iodine-123 (^{123}I) (159 keV). If higher energy radionuclides are used, the collimator septa (the walls that form the holes) must be thicker for the collimator to be effective. Thickening the septa reduces sensitivity for the simple reason that more of the crystal is covered by lead. Collimators designed for indium-111 (^{111}In) (171 and 245 keV) and gallium-67 (^{67}Ga) (93, 185, and 300 keV) are medium-energy collimators. Collimators designed for iodine-131 (^{131}I) (364 keV) are high-energy collimators. Ultra–high-energy collimators have been designed for SPECT imaging of the 511 keV annihilation photons of positron-emitting radionuclides, but their use has been accepted

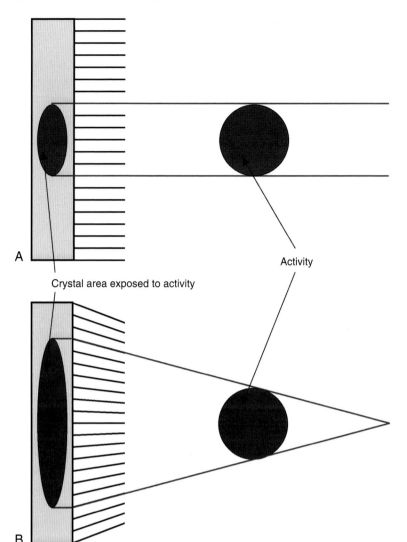

Crystal area exposed to activity

Activity

FIGURE 9-8 Converging collimators improve sensitivity at the expense of field of view. **A,** Parallel hole collimators expose the crystal only to photons that originate directly in front of the collimator. The image formed is a projection of the radionuclide distribution the same size as the distribution. **B,** Fan beam collimators have holes that are directed toward a line at a fixed distance in front of the collimator (parallel to the imaging table). The projection is magnified, more of the crystal is used, and sensitivity is increased. Objects at differing distances from the collimator are magnified by different amounts, resulting in a distorted image. Cone beam collimators are similar but converge to a point instead of a line.

only for myocardial imaging with fluorodeoxyglucose ^{18}F-FDG. These collimators are extremely heavy, and their weight may put a strain on the SPECT gantry. To recapture some of the sensitivity lost by thicker septa, most medium- and high-energy collimators are designed for lower resolution than low-energy collimators.

Parallel hole collimators are most commonly used for SPECT, but increased sensitivity can be obtained with converging collimators in which the holes converge on a line (fan beam) or a point (cone beam). Converging collimators require more complex setup procedures than do parallel hole collimators if used for SPECT, and once the images have been acquired, they require special image reconstruction software that may result in much longer reconstruction times. Converging collimators allow more of the crystal to be used, which increases sensitivity, as shown in Figure 9-8. This increase in sensitivity is realized with a decrease in the size of the field of view. In practice this usually limits the clinical use of converging collimation to brain imaging.

Converging collimators pose a problem for cardiac SPECT because the field of view does not necessarily cover the entire thorax. This truncation of data can lead to artifacts in the reconstruction. Currently, the best compromises have been either to use fan beam collimators with a very slight angle to improve resolution slightly with no truncation or to create a collimator with holes that change the pitch of their angles according to their location in the field of view. The latter type of collimator has holes that get closer to parallel toward their sides, which means that objects in the center of the field of view are imaged with higher resolution than those at the edges, but there is no truncation.

TOMOGRAPHIC ACQUISITIONS

SPECT images are created by mathematically combining many planar scintigrams (called *projections*) that have been collected at many angles around the body. The theory of SPECT requires that the scintillation camera

TABLE 9-1	Time to Complete a SPECT Study Using Step-and-Shoot and Continuous Acquisitions			
		Acquisition Time in Minutes		
Number of Frames	**Seconds/Frame**	**Continuous**	**Step-and-Shoot**	**Lost Time***
Long Acquisition				
16	60	16	16.8	5%
32	30	16	17.6	9%
64	15	16	19.2	17%
Short Acquisition				
16	12	3.2	4	20%
32	6	3.2	4.8	33%
64	3	3.2	6.4	50%

*Assuming lost time per frame due to camera motion: 3 seconds.

acquire enough images of the patient at different angles to obtain a complete description of the distribution of the radioactive tracer. Several projections over a 180-degree orbit would be satisfactory if there were no scatter or attenuation. Because this is not often the case, 360-degree orbits are used for most SPECT studies (the exception is cardiac SPECT). Numerous parameters define exactly how the rotating gamma camera travels around the patient in the process of collecting these images. These acquisition parameters help determine the quality of the final tomographic image.

SPECT Data Acquisition Modes

Most SPECT systems move in a fashion called **step-and-shoot** as they orbit the patient. The camera moves, stops, acquires an image, moves again, stops, and acquires another image. The optimum number of stops is determined by the system resolution and the pixel size (the better the resolution and the smaller the pixels, the more stops are required). The time during which the camera is moving and turned off is called *dead time;* it typically is 3 to 5 seconds per projection but may be as high as 8 seconds per projection. Long dead times increase acquisition time, reducing patient comfort, without benefit to image quality.

Continuous orbit cameras try to resolve this problem by acquiring counts at all times, even while the camera moves. Traditionally, continuous motion cameras move slowly and smoothly while counts from designated arcs are collected to form the planar projections. The smaller the arc used for each projection, the less the blurring from the camera's motion.

A final acquisition mode combines step-and-shoot with continuous acquisition; it therefore is termed *continuous step-and-shoot.* The camera is stopped at discrete projection angles but is not turned off during rotation. This minimizes the blur seen with continuous-rotation acquisition but maximizes the number of collected counts in a given time.

Table 9-1 shows the lost time resulting from step-and-shoot motion for both long acquisition (16 minutes, typical of most cardiac SPECT) and short acquisition (3 to 5 minutes), assuming that the lost time per frame is 3 seconds. Most cardiac SPECT studies use 32 or 64 total frames, whereas most general SPECT studies use 64 or 128 total frames. The 16-frame entry in the table assumes a 90-degree dual detector SPECT system and an acquisition with 32 total projections (16 per detector).

180-Degree versus 360-Degree Data Acquisition

As noted previously, the exception to the rule that 360-degree orbits are preferred is cardiac SPECT. The heart is located forward and to one side of the center of the thorax, resulting in a great deal of attenuation when the camera is behind the patient. The angles chosen for the 180 degrees are those closest to the heart, from 45 degrees right anterior oblique (RAO) to 45 degrees left posterior oblique (LPO). These projections are affected least by attenuation, scatter, and detector response because they are the closest to the heart. Reconstructions from 180-degree acquisitions have higher resolution and contrast than those from 360-degree acquisitions, particularly with ^{201}Tl images.[57,78] However, because 180-degree reconstructions are not truly complete (i.e., additional information is available from the other 180 degrees of projection), occasional artifacts are seen with 180-degree reconstructions that can be avoided with 360-degree reconstructions.[24,51,69]

Circular versus Body-Contour Orbits

Most SPECT systems offer a choice of circular or **body-contour orbits.** In the simple motion of circular orbits, the gamma camera is limited to rotating in a circle. The position of the detector is fixed at a given radius with respect to the center of rotation (COR). A minimal radius is chosen that allows the camera to clear the body

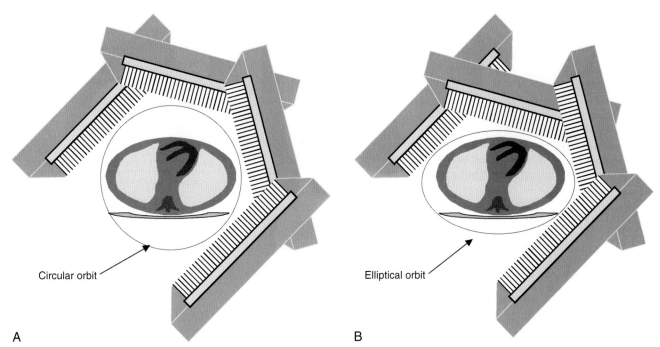

A   B

FIGURE 9-9 Elliptical and body-contour orbits keep the camera close to the patient during the entire SPECT acquisition. **A,** When a circular orbit is used, the camera is close to the body in some projections but far away in others. **B,** Elliptical and body-contour orbits try to maximize resolution by keeping the camera as close to the body as possible during the entire orbit. In cardiac imaging the asymmetric position of the heart in the body may lead to a widely varying heart-to-camera distance (and thus widely varying resolution) during the orbit, resulting in reconstruction artifacts.

at every angle. However, forcing the camera to stay at a fixed radius at one angle may result in it being very far from the body at another angle (after all, most people are not circular in cross section).

Body-contour orbits seek to keep the camera as close to the body as possible throughout the tomographic acquisition, thereby maximizing resolution.[53] The radius is changed angle by angle to minimize the distance while maintaining the same angles used in a circular orbit. The simplest body-contour orbits assume the shape of an ellipse, although some manufactures offer sophisticated sensors that minimize the camera-body distance in real time at each angle. Body-contour orbits are illustrated in Figure 9-9.

For general SPECT images, the results of body-contour orbits are superior to those of circular orbits. Some manufacturers' complicated setup procedures have made the body-contour technique prohibitively complex for use in the clinical setting. Use of body-contour orbits for cardiac SPECT is not as widely accepted. Because the resolution varies from angle to angle, the resulting reconstruction may be different from one created with a circular orbit. In cardiac SPECT, the heart is often put at or near the center of rotation when a circular orbit is used, which ensures that the heart is imaged with approximately the same resolution for all angles. Use of a noncircular orbit changes the distance from the detector to the center of rotation, or the heart, at each angle. This has been reported to cause apical defects,[42] or the base and septum

of the heart to appear as having slightly decreased counts, because these regions are relatively farther from the detector during a body-contour orbit.[75] These "artifacts" may be related to exactly how the noncircular orbit is effected, that is, how the gantry, camera heads, and patient table are moved during the acquisition. Others have found no significant difference in perfusion quantification applied to acquisitions performed with circular and noncircular orbits.[66,120]

Other Factors

Three important variables are the size of the image pixels, the average number of counts collected for each pixel, and the number of views obtained. In general, the pixel size should be less than one third the system resolution (measured as FWHM). The number of counts in each pixel is also related to the system resolution; the higher the resolution, the lower the number of counts obtained per pixel. In most cases the number of counts should be maximized without exceeding radiation dose limits or the patient's ability to remain immobile. The number of views depends on the resolution and the pixel size. If too few views are taken, resolution is lost and artifacts may be introduced.

SPECT imaging of the thorax, abdomen, or pelvis usually uses the camera's full field of view. A 128×128 pixel matrix is preferred for most low-energy studies because this gives a pixel size of about 4 mm for a typical

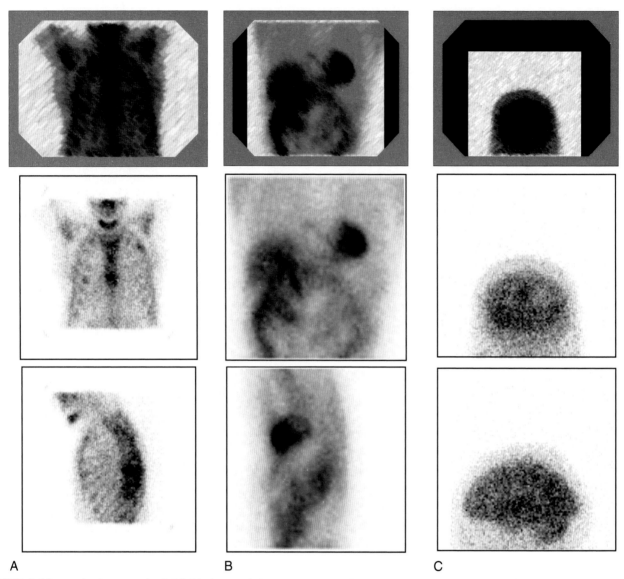

A   B   C

FIGURE 9-10 A, In body SPECT the full field of view of the camera is typically used, with a 128 × 128 matrix for a 51-cm camera giving 4 mm/pixel. **B,** Myocardial SPECT does not require the full field of view, which may be reduced by zooming the image. A zoom factor of 1.3 reduces the field of view to 38 cm and gives a pixel size of 6 mm for a 64 × 64 matrix. **C,** The brain is relatively small compared to the camera, and a zoom factor of 1.6 reduces the field of view to 32 cm, with 2.5 mm/pixel for a 128 × 128 matrix. Note that the zoomed area is shifted to the bottom of the camera, reducing the distance from the edge of the image to the edge of the camera. This helps the operator bring the camera closer than the patient's shoulder during setup.

51-cm wide large-field-of-view camera. For the study, 128 views should be acquired over 360 degrees. In some cases using medium- or high-energy collimation in which the pixel counts are low, a 64 × 64 pixel matrix may be satisfactory.

Pixels 6 to 6.5 mm in size have proved to be adequate for cardiac SPECT. This size is obtained by using a 64 × 64 pixel matrix for systems with a field of view of 38 to 40 cm. In these studies, 64 projections over 180 degrees are preferred (an image approximately every 3 degrees), but 32 projections are often used with satisfactory results. To achieve a field of view of this size in a large–field-of-view camera, some of the scintillation crystal area can be discarded through a process known as *zoom.* When a zoom factor is used, the field of view is reduced and the pixels of the image are used more efficiently (more of the image is occupied by the organ of interest, in this case the heart). A zoom factor of 1.3 reduces the field of view of a 51-cm camera to 38 cm. Camera zooms are described in Figure 9-10.

The scintillation camera should remain as close to the head as possible for brain SPECT. This allows for excellent resolution compared with body SPECT (remember that resolution decreases as the distance from the collimator increases). A zoom factor of 1.5 reduces the pixel size to less than 3 mm with a 128 × 128 pixel matrix. For the study, 128 views should be acquired over 360 degrees. An important consideration in choosing a camera for brain SPECT is the brain reach, or the distance from the edge of the camera to the usable field of view. If this distance is too great, it becomes difficult to position the camera close to the head (over the shoulder) without cutting the lower portion of the cerebellum out of the field of view.

Specific guidelines for the setup of different SPECT procedures can be found in *Procedure Guidelines Manual,* published by the Society of Nuclear Medicine.[104] The American Society of Nuclear Cardiology has published *Guidelines for Nuclear Cardiology Procedures,*[22] which has the recommended procedures for nuclear cardiology.

SPECT RECONSTRUCTION

Methods of reconstructing the radionuclide distribution from planar projections have been the subject of investigation since the possibility was proven by Johann Radon in 1917. The advent of computers accelerated research into different methods of image reconstruction, and many have been proposed. These reconstruction algorithms fall into two categories: iterative methods and analytic methods. Analytic methods are based on exact mathematical solutions to the image reconstruction problem, whereas iterative methods estimate the distribution through successive approximations. Accurate corrections for attenuation and other degradations require more complex iterative reconstruction techniques.

Filtered Back-Projection Reconstruction

Filtered back-projection (FBP) has been the most frequently used method of image reconstruction[6] and is an analytic reconstruction algorithm. As its name implies, FBP is a combination of filtering and back-projection. When a projection image is acquired, each row of the projection contains counts that emanate from the entire transverse plane. When projection images are obtained from many angles about the body, enough information is available in each row of the set of angular projections to reconstruct the original corresponding transverse slice. Figure 9-11 shows projections acquired from a phantom over many angles. The projections can be reordered such that single lines from each of the projection angles are stacked on top of each other. This type of image is called a *sinogram,* because a point source in this image traces out a sine wave (see Figure 9-11, *C*). A sinogram has all the projection data necessary to reconstruct a single slice of the original activity distribution.

Back-projection assigns the values in the projection to all points along the line of acquisition through the image plane from which they were acquired. This is shown in Figure 9-12. This operation is repeated for all pixels and all angles; the new values are added to the previous ones in what is known as a *superposition operation.*

As the number of angles increases, the back-projection improves.

Although simple back-projection is useful for illustrative purposes, it is never used in practice without the step of filtering. Note that the back-projection in Figure 9-12, *D,* is quite blurred compared with the original distribution from which it was created. Also, Figure 9-12, *B* and *C,* shows instances of the star artifact, which consists of radial lines near the edges of the object. This artifact is a natural result of back-projection applied without filtering. In clinical practice, a ramp filter is applied to each projection before back-projection (ramp filters are discussed in more detail later in the chapter). The ramp-filtered projections are characterized by enhancement of edge information and the introduction of negative values (or lobes) into the filtered projections. During superposition in the back-projection process, these negative values cancel portions of the other angular contributions and in effect help eliminate the star artifact (Figure 9-13). However, enough projections must be acquired to ensure that proper cancellation is obtained. Radial blurring or streaking toward the periphery of the image often indicates that too few projections were acquired. Finally, a noise-reducing filter, such as a Butterworth or Hanning filter, usually is applied before, during, or after the back-projection operation. These filters are discussed in more detail in following sections.

Iterative Reconstruction

Iterative reconstruction techniques require many more calculations and thus much more computer time to create a transaxial image than does FBP. As computers have progressed in speed and memory, they have made the transition from a research tool to routine clinical use. Their primary importance is their ability to incorporate corrections for the factors that degrade SPECT images. Iterative techniques use the original projections and models of the acquisition process to predict a reconstruction. The predicted reconstruction is then used again with the models to create new predicted projections. If the predicted projections are different from the actual projections, these differences are used to modify the reconstruction. This process is continued until the reconstruction is such that the predicted projections match the actual projections. The primary differences between various iterative methods are the ways the predicted reconstructions and projections are created and the ways they are modified at each step. Practically speaking, the more theoretically accurate the iterative technique, the more time-consuming the process. Maximum likelihood methods allow noise to be modelled, whereas least squares techniques, such as the conjugate gradient method, generally ignore noise.[7,100,115] Iterative filtered back-projection (IFBP) methods create the new reconstruction at every iteration by using FBP.[39,125]

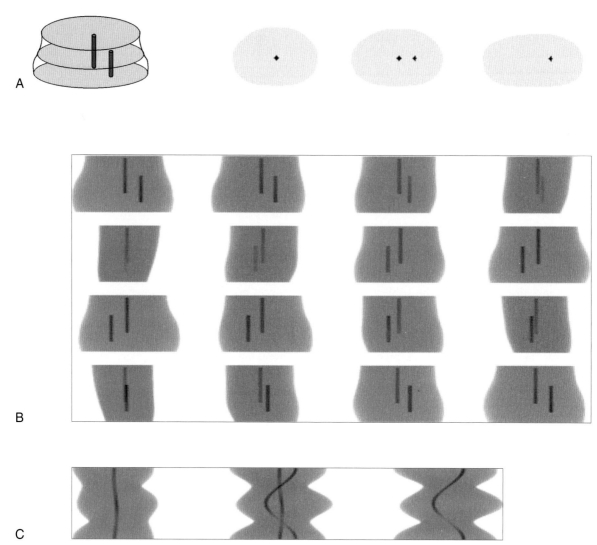

FIGURE 9-11 Projections and sinograms. **A,** Original 3D activity distribution is a tapered part of an ellipsoid, with two hot lines offset in two directions. Three slices through the original distribution are shown. **B,** Sixteen original projections created from the activity distribution. From top left to bottom right, these projections were acquired from the rear of the object, rotating around to the left, to the front, to the right, and then returning to the rear. **C,** Three sinograms created from the projections. Each sinogram contains a single horizontal line taken from each of the 16 projections, so that a single sinogram contains all of the information necessary to reconstruct a single slice of the original image. The left-most sinogram was taken from near the top of the projections shown in **B,** so that the outer background of the object is relatively small and the single hot spot is near the center. The right-most sinogram was created using a line taken from near the bottom of the projection set. Note that in this sinogram, the outer boundary of the background of the object is larger and the hot spot, which is offset from the center, traces a sine wave within the sinogram. The center sinogram was created using a line taken from near the center of the projection.

Based on the maximum likelihood criteria commonly used in statistical analysis, the most widely used iterative reconstruction method is maximum likelihood expectation maximization (MLEM).[100,113] The MLEM algorithm attempts to determine the tracer distribution that would "most likely" yield the measured projections given the imaging model and a map of attenuation coefficients if available. MLEM is simple to understand in theory. At each iteration, an estimate or "guess" of the correct reconstruction is generated. This may be a blank or uniform image at the first iteration. Projections based on this image are generated; these may include for example the known attenuation map created using a transmission scan or the known geometric response function based on the properties of the collimator. The estimated projections are compared to the actual acquired projections. If the estimated projections match the a projections, then the guess reconstruction may be considered correct. However, if they do not, the ratio between the two is created, reconstructed, and used to correct the current guess image. An important issue is how best to decide when the estimated and collected projections match well enough to stop the iterations. The MLEM algorithm converges slowly, requiring many more iterations than

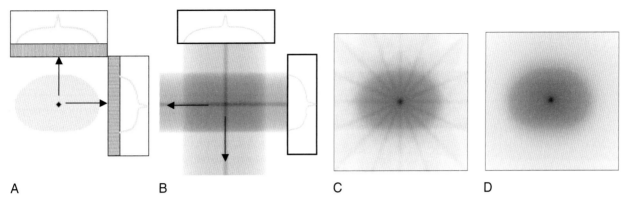

FIGURE 9-12 Simple back-projection. **A,** Two projections are acquired from a single slice. The original activity distribution is shown in the center, with the two projections to the top and right. Profiles through the projections are shown within each. **B,** Counts from the two projections are spread back out over the reconstruction, with counts from each projection being added to, or superposed on, the previous one. **C,** More projections added to the back-projection process start to make the reconstruction recognizable as the original transverse slice. **D,** Use of many projections gives a blurry representation of the original object. Note the rays from the back-projection process in the background of this image and in **C,** demonstrating the star artifact inherent in simple back-projection.

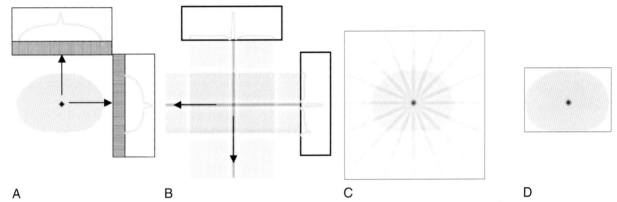

FIGURE 9-13 Filtered back-projection. **A,** Two projections are acquired from a single slice. The original activity distribution is shown in the center, with the two projections to the top and right. Profiles through the projections are shown within each. **B,** A ramp filter is applied to the projections, changing the profiles through each. Note that now the background of the object is reduced, and the point source has higher contrast. These two effects are the direct result of ramp filtering. Counts from the two filtered projections are spread back out over the reconstruction, with counts from each projection being added to, or superposed on, the previous one. **C,** More projections added to the filtered back-projection process start to make the reconstruction recognizable as the original transverse slice. **D,** Use of many projections gives a sharp, accurate reconstruction of the original object. Note that the star artifact is also reduced in both this reconstruction and the one shown in **C.**

IFBP algorithms; however, the slowly converging characteristics of this algorithm yield greater control over image noise.[71,113]

The point of convergence of this algorithm and the related number of iterations for clinical use are a source of debate.[102] There is no common rule for stopping the algorithms after a number of iterations on clinical data, and protocols describing the optimum number of iterations are largely empirically based. In practice the number of iterations chosen depends on the nature and complexity of the activity distribution. Brain SPECT, acquired in a 128 × 128 matrix, will require many more iterations than myocardial SPECT acquired in a 64 × 64 matrix. An example of the reconstruction of the myocardium with the MLEM algorithm is shown in Figure 9-14.

Another approach to the MLEM algorithm for iterative reconstruction is the **ordered subset expectation maximization (OSEM)** method,[58] in which the projection data are ordered into subsets, which are used in the iterative steps of the reconstruction to greatly speed up the process. The operation of OSEM is illustrated in Figure 9-15. Creation of the guess images are based on a subset of the projections, with different subsets being used to update the guess as the iterations continue. For example, if a SPECT acquisition utilized 64 projections and 16 subsets were chosen for OSEM reconstruction, each subset would contain 4 projections spaced equally through the projection set. In each OSEM iteration, the MLEM process is carried out on each subset (a very quick operation with only 4 projections) and the result

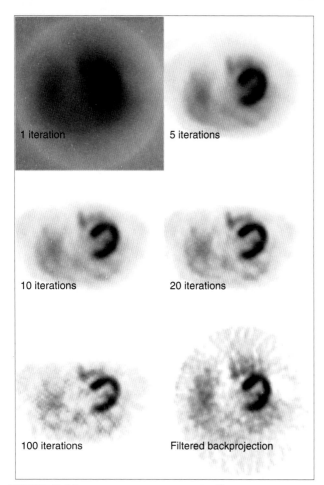

FIGURE 9-14 Iterative reconstruction of a ^{99m}Tc-sestamibi patient study (transaxial slices). The quality of images reconstructed with the maximum likelihood algorithm (beginning with a uniform image) improves with successive iterations. After a point, however, image noise begins to degrade the image, as can be seen in image produced by 100 iterations.

used as the guess image for the next subset until all subsets have been used. As with MLEM, the optimum number of iterations is usually determined empirically. The advantage of OSEM is that many fewer iterations are needed to reach a satisfactory result. MLEM and OSEM may be compared for brain SPECT in Figure 9-16.

In clinical use the key factors that must be chosen with OSEM reconstruction are the number of iterations and the number of subsets must be chosen. The product these two factors (number of iterations and number of subsets) gives the EM equivalent (roughly the number of MLEM iterations needed to get the same result). OSEM with a choice of 1 subset becomes the MLEM algorithm. The choice of 16 subsets and 2 iterations would give the equivalent of 32 MLEM iterations (in approximately $\frac{1}{16}$ the computational time). Likewise, 2 subsets and 16 iterations would give a similar result but take longer (approximately $\frac{1}{2}$ the computational time of MLEM). The more subsets used, the shorter the time required to

reconstruct; but care must be taken in low count studies to ensure that there are adequate counts in each subset for adequate reconstruction.

FILTERING OF SPECT IMAGES

In SPECT, filters are used either to enhance or to remove the high-frequency components of the image.[41] High-frequency components are sharp changes in image intensity, such as those seen at edges between the heart and the background or in noise points. Low frequencies contain information about slowly changing or constant intensities of the image, such as uniform regions of perfusion. Filters that remove high frequencies are called **low-pass filters** because they preserve (pass) only the low frequencies. This reduces noise but blurs edges. Filters that enhance high frequencies are called *high-pass filters*. They operate in the opposite manner; they pass only the high frequencies while attenuating low frequencies. This sharpens organ boundaries but increases noise.

A Fourier transform (implemented on the computer as a fast Fourier transform, or FFT) decomposes an image into its various frequency components. The frequency components are the spatial frequencies that make up the image. These frequencies are expressed in terms of cycles per distance (usually cycles/cm or cycles/pixel).

Low frequencies reflect the overall shapes of an image. High frequencies are the result of areas with sharp changes in pixel counts, such as edges (and image noise). The highest frequency in a digital image is 0.5 cycles/pixel, representing alternating bright and dark pixels. This frequency is called the **Nyquist frequency**. Because filters are defined in terms of spatial frequencies, it is important that careful attention be given to the units of the frequency. Some manufacturers define filters in terms of cycles/pixel, others use cycles/cm, and still others use a percentage of the Nyquist frequency; the difference is as important as the difference between inches, centimeters, and miles.

Ramp Filter

A ramp filter, which is a high-pass filter, is the most important filter for SPECT because the ramp filter erases the blurring of simple back-projection. Filtered back-projection refers to the ramp filter. It is important to note that the ramp filter is applied only in the transaxial plane because this is the only plane that experiences blurring in simple back-projection. The formula for the ramp filter is given by:

$$w(f) = |f|$$

where *w(f)* is the filter function, and *f* represents the spatial frequencies of the image. When graphed, the filter has the shape of a ramp (Figure 9-17).

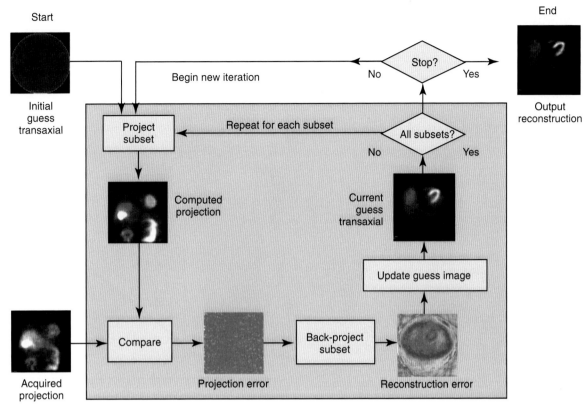

FIGURE 9-15 Basic operations of Iterative Reconstruction with Ordered Subset Expectation Maximization. The shaded box represents the calculation loop for subset calculations within each iteration. An initial guess at the transaxial distribution that created the measured projections is generated. New estimated projections are created based on that guess, but only for a small subset of angles. These computed projections are compared to the measured projections. A ratio of the projections is reconstructed and used to correct the current guess of the transaxial count distribution. This loop is repeated for each subset of projection angles until all have been used. At that point, the projection error is evaluated to see if it is low enough to stop the iterations. If so, the current guess of the transaxial is output. Otherwise, the iteration is repeated starting again with the first subset.

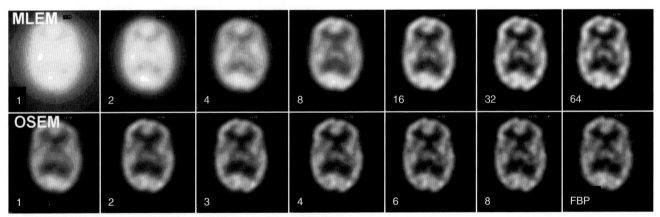

FIGURE 9-16 Iterative reconstruction of Tc-99m ECD brain SPECT (transaxial slices) with MLEM and OSEM. The images were acquired in a 128 × 128 matrix with 128 projections. Reconstruction was with MLEM (top) and OSEM (bottom), with the number of iterations of each algorithm in the lower left corner of each image. OSEM reconstruction used 8 subsets (each with 16 projections). All of the images were filtered with the same 3-dimensional Butterworth filter post-reconstruction. Note that OSEM produces an acceptable image with man fewer iterations than MLEM. After 8 iterations, the OSEM image is roughly equivalent to the 64 iteration MLEM image but required only ⅛ the time to reconstruct.

Hanning Filters

Hann (or Hanning) filters (Figure 9-18) are among the most commonly used smoothing (or noise reduction) filters for SPECT. The formula for a Hann filter is given by the following:

$$\text{if } |f| < f_m,$$
$$w(f) = 0.5 + 0.5\cos\left(\frac{\pi f}{f_m}\right)$$
$$\text{or if } |f| > f_m,$$
$$w(f) = 0$$

where $w(f)$ is the filter function, f represents the spatial frequencies of the image, and f_m is the maximum frequency, or **cutoff frequency,** of the filter. The Hann filter has a value of 1 at 0 frequency ($\cos(0) = 1$) and decreases to 0 at the cutoff frequency. Thus the cutoff frequency is the parameter used to define the Hann filter. The lower the cutoff frequency, the more high frequencies are removed from the image and the smoother the filtered image.

Butterworth Filters

Another common filter is the Butterworth filter (Figures 9-19 and 9-20), which is more versatile (and more complicated) than the Hann filter. The Butterworth filter is given by the equation:

$$w(f) = \frac{1}{\sqrt{1 + \left(\dfrac{f}{f_c}\right)^P}}$$

where $w(f)$ is the filter function; f represents the spatial frequencies of the image; f_c is the maximum frequency,

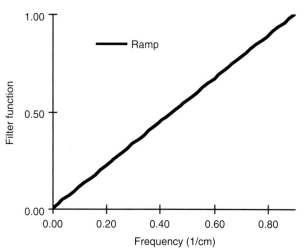

FIGURE 9-17 The ramp filter, the filter referred to in filtered back-projection, is used to remove the blurring given by simple back-projection. Note that the filter ends at a little greater than 0.8 cm⁻¹, or the Nyquist frequency for 0.6-cm pixels. Also note that the ramp filter allows more high frequencies than low frequencies and is considered to be a high-pass filter.

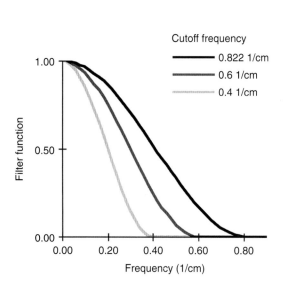

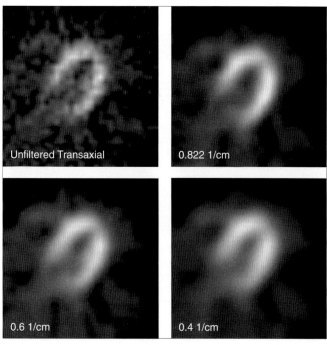

FIGURE 9-18 Results with three Hanning filters, applied to ^{201}Tl myocardial perfusion SPECT and using different cutoff frequencies, are plotted. The lower the cutoff frequency, the smoother the image after the filter is applied. When no smoothing filter is applied, the image might be considered too noisy for clinical use. A cutoff frequency of 0.4 cm⁻¹ smoothes most of the details out of the image.

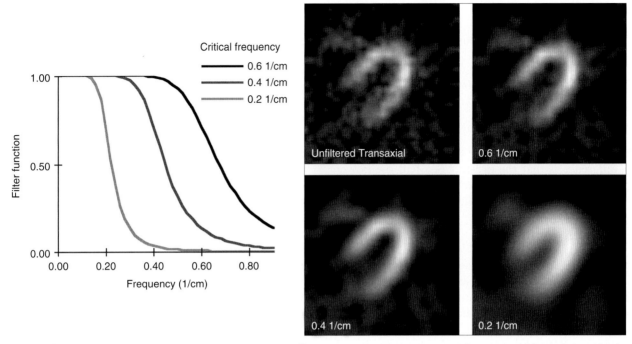

FIGURE 9-19 Results with three Butterworth filters, applied to ^{99m}Tc-sestamibi SPECT and using different critical frequencies, are plotted. The lower the critical frequency, the smoother the image after the filter is applied. The same power factor (10) is used for each of the filters. The higher the critical frequency, the more high frequencies are retained in the filtered image and the less smooth it appears.

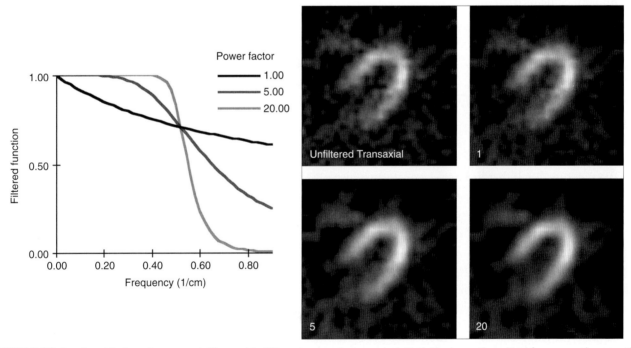

FIGURE 9-20 Results with three Butterworth filters with different power factors are plotted. The lower the critical frequency, the smoother the image after the filter is applied. The same critical frequency (0.52 l/cm^{-1}) is used for each of the filters. The effect of changing the power factor is less apparent than that of the critical frequency. Lower power factors retain more high frequencies but at the expense of middle and low frequencies.

or critical frequency, of the filter; and p is the power factor of the filter. The Butterworth filter has a value of 1 at 0 frequency and decreases to (but never quite reaches) 0. The Butterworth filter is characterized by a level plateau and a drop-off defined by the critical frequency. The power factor defines the steepness of this drop-off. It is important to note that the critical frequency of the Butterworth filter differs from the cutoff frequency of the Hanning filter. At $f = f_c$ the Butterworth filter equals $\frac{1}{\sqrt{2}}$, not 0. Some manufacturers refer to the critical frequency as a cutoff frequency in an attempt to avoid confusion.

Alternate definitions of the Butterworth filter are

$$w(f) = \frac{1}{\sqrt{1 + \left(\dfrac{f}{f_c}\right)2n}} \quad \text{and} \quad w(f) = \frac{1}{1 + \left(\dfrac{f}{f_c}\right)2n}$$

In the first example, n is the order of the filter. The only difference is that the order is one half the power factor. The second example removes the square root and at $f = f_c$, the Butterworth filter equals one half.

Gaussian Filters

Gaussian filters are preferred by some for noise reduction in SPECT because the Gaussian shape is often used modelling the SPECT system resolution. Gaussian filters may be implemented on nuclear medicine computer systems as a convolution filter, applied directly to the three-dimensional (3D) voxel matrix (as described for Image Smoothing in Chapter 4) or through the Fourier techniques described earlier.

Mathematically, the Gaussian function in the spatial domain may be defined as:

$$W(x) = e^{-ax^2}$$

where

$$a = \frac{4\ln(2)}{(FWMH)^2}$$

And as noted earlier, FWHM is the width of the function in the x axis at the value $\frac{1}{2}$. A unique property of the Gaussian function is that its Fourier transform is also a Gaussian function:

$$w(f) = \sqrt{\frac{\pi}{a}} e^{-\frac{\pi}{a}f^2}$$

Where a is the same as stated earlier.

Figure 9-21 illustrates Gaussian filters in frequency space *(A)* and in the spatial domain *(B)*. Unlike the Hanning and Butterworth filters, the Gaussian filter is not defined by a parameter in frequency space but by its FWHM in pixel space (more accurately called the spatial domain). As can be seen in the figure, increasing the FWHM of the filter broadens the curve in the spatial domain and forces it to decrease more rapidly in frequency space. The effect of the Gaussian filter on the image is the same whether the filter is implemented as a spatial convolution or in frequency space; the Gaussian shape is used as a blurring function to smooth the image. Thus, a Gaussian filter with a larger FWHM results in a smoother image with less noise.

When to Filter—Filtered Back-Projection

Smoothing filters can be applied before, after, or during back-projection. There are advantages and disadvantages to each method, but filtering in three dimensions is generally preferred to filtering in two dimensions (Figure 9-22).

Before Back-Projection. A 2D filter applied to each of the planar projections before back-projection actually filters in all three dimensions. After image reconstruction, the image will have the same resolution in all three dimensions. This offers an advantage if sagittal, coronal, or oblique images are needed. This is sometimes called a *prefilter* because it precedes the ramp filter, which is applied only in the transverse direction (perpendicular to the axis of the table). A 2D prefilter is the preferred method of soothing and noise reduction for SPECT images.

During Back-Projection. A one-dimensional (1D) smoothing filter is sometimes combined with the ramp filter and applied during the back-projection process. The advantage is that only one filter must the applied (i.e., a ramp-Butterworth, the combination of a ramp and a Butterworth filter), and computations are reduced. The disadvantage is that no smoothing has been done in the axial dimension. If sagittal, coronal, or oblique images are cut from the resulting image set, they will not have been equally smoothed in all directions and will appear to have horizontal streaks.

After Back-Projection. Filters may also be applied after image reconstruction, but they should be applied in all three dimensions. If a 2D filter is applied to the transaxial images, however, the same problems will occur as with filtering during back-projection. The images will not have been smoothed in the axial dimension. Another filter must then be applied (sometimes called a *y filter*) to compensate before images at other orientations are extracted. This leads to more computations (and longer processing times) than are required when filtering is performed before back-projection. This increase in time, however, is usually insignificant with today's computers.

When to Filter—Iterative Reconstruction

Three-dimensional postreconstruction filtering is the most widely used noise reduction method with MLEM or OSEM reconstruction. A number of iterations is chosen so that the reconstructed image begins to degrade the image (as shown in Figure 9-14) and a filter applied to reduce this noise. Prefiltering is usually avoided because the MLEM and OSEM algorithms are based on the assumption that the noise in each pixel follows the Poisson distribution, an assumption invalidated by prefiltering the image. An alternate approach is not using any noise reduction filtering but to set the number of

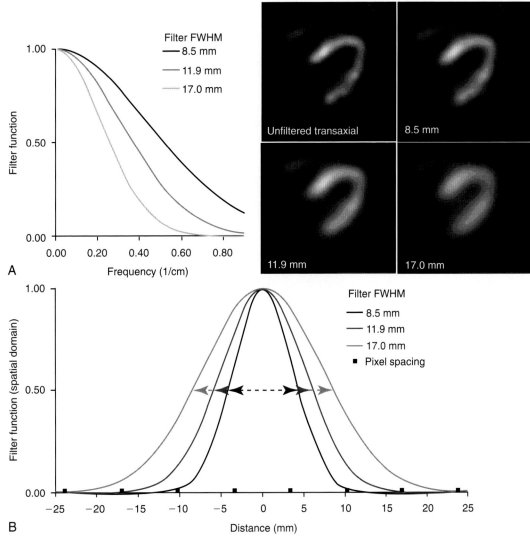

FIGURE 9-21 A, Three Gaussian filters, with different FWHM, are plotted in frequency space and in the spatial domain **(B)** and are applied to ^{99m}Tc-sestamibi SPECT images. Gaussian filters may be implemented by Fourier methods as described for the Hanning or Butterworth filters or as a convolution of the spatial domain curves **(B)** with the 3D voxel matrix. As the Gaussian filter's FWHM (defined in pixel space) is increased the function becomes wider in the spatial domain and narrower in frequency space (removing more high spatial frequencies), giving a smoother image. Square blocks denote the spacing of the 6.8-mm pixels of the example images. The FWHMs used to define the filters are 1.25, 1.75, and 2.5 times the pixel size.

iterations and subsets so that the iterative reconstruction stops before the image begins to appear noisy.

Units

The implementation of filters varies widely among manufacturers of nuclear medicine computers. In addition to the alternate definitions of the Butterworth filters and the choices of when to apply smoothing filters mentioned above, manufacturers specify cutoff and critical frequency values using different units, including cycles/cm, cycles/pixel, and Nyquist, which is equivalent to cycles/2 pixels. Table 9-2 is presented as an aid to conversion of the various units. The FWHM parameter used to define

TABLE 9-2	Conversion of Units of Frequency (Multiply by Column to Get Row)		
	From Nyquist	From Cycles/cm	From Cycles/Pixel
To get Nyquist	1	2* pixel size	2
To get cycles/cm	1/(2* pixel size)	1	1/pixel size
To get cycles/pixel	1/2	pixel size	1

*Pixel sizes are assumed to be centimeters (cm).

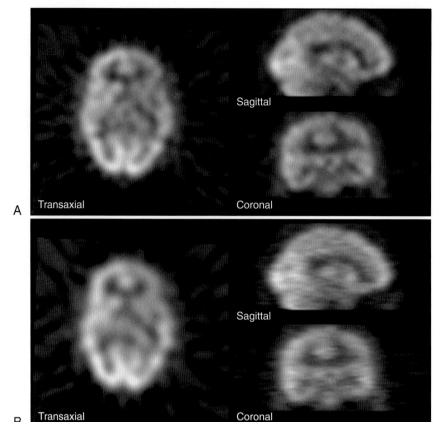

FIGURE 9-22 Filtering during back-projection leads to uneven resolution or smoothness in different directions. **A,** These SPECT brain images have been smoothed in three dimensions, either by prefiltering or by using a 3D filter after reconstruction. **B,** These images were smoothed with a ramp-Butterworth filter during reconstruction. The smoothing filter was applied only in the transaxial plane (as is the ramp filter). Horizontal streaks are evident in the sagittal and coronal images.

Gaussian filters may also be defined differently on different systems with some manufacturer's using mm and others using a factor that is multiplied by the pixel size.

SPECT IMAGE DISPLAY

Color versus Gray Scale

Different color scales may be used to highlight different features in SPECT images. Certain color scales may help distinguish normal from abnormal regions in some studies. Conversely, gray scale is actually better for highlighting very dim objects. Because color scales can be used to enhance or diminish various features, the same image can be made to look very different simply by changing the color table. SPECT images, therefore, should always be scaled and displayed in a reproducible and standardized manner to ensure reproducibility in qualitative analysis. In the past few years some automatic techniques for performing this task have been described.

Image Reorientation

Transaxial Images. The natural products of rotational tomography are images that represent cross-sectional slices of the body perpendicular to the imaging table (or long axis of the body). These images are called *transverse* or *transaxial slices* (Figure 9-23, *A*).

Longitudinal Images. SPECT images can be reconstructed so that the image slices are contiguous and the slice thickness is equal to the pixel size (defined as the length of one side of the square pixels). Once it is recognized that the pixels have depth as well as width, the terminology must be altered, and the pixels are more aptly called *voxels* (volume elements; pixel stands for picture element). The images may then be thought of as a 3D matrix of information about the patient. Using the computer, this 3D matrix can be resliced to give images at different orientations. Coronal slices are parallel to the surface of the imaging table. Sagittal slices are perpendicular to both transaxial and coronal slices. Sagittal and coronal slices are shown in Figure 9-23, *B* and *C*, respectively.

Oblique Images. The extraction of images is not limited to the natural *x*, *y*, and *z* directions, however. The computer may be used to extract images at any orientation, and these images are called *oblique images*. The short- and long-axis images commonly used in myocardial tomography are examples of oblique images. Oblique images may also be used to retrospectively obtain a desired image orientation for brain imaging. The important oblique sections used for viewing cardiac

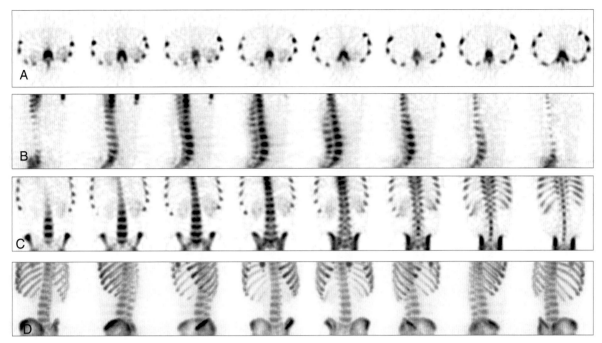

FIGURE 9-23 A, Original transaxial slices taken from a normal bone SPECT study. Transaxial slices are oriented such that the patient's right side is on the left side of the image. The patient's anterior is to the top of the image. Consecutive slices are displayed from the patient's superior to his inferior. **B,** Consecutive sagittal slices of the same study. Sagittal slices are oriented such that posterior structures are on the left and anterior structures are on the right. Consecutive slices are displayed from the patient's right to his left. **C,** Coronal slices taken from the same study. Coronal images are oriented such that the left side of the patient is shown on the right side of the image. Consecutive slices are displayed from the patient's anterior to his posterior. **D,** Volume-rendered maximum activity projection images displayed from different angles. Note that the whole "hot" skeleton can be seen, with bones closer to the viewing point more intense than those farther away.

images are described in the "Cardiac Quantification" section.

Three-Dimensional Displays

Interest in 3D displays for SPECT data has increased over the past several years. Currently the most common display mode is a 2D interactive slicing program that allows a user to view a 3D data set one slice at a time. Such displays are limited when the examiner is trying to gain an accurate idea of the size and shape of an organ or tumor or the extent and severity of disease. For these reasons, efforts have been underway to generate true 3D displays.[16,30,122] These displays generally fall into two categories: **volume rendering** and **surface rendering.**

Volume Rendering. Volume rendering offers the advantage of visualizing an object in 3D without having to explicitly identify the surface. The most common type of volume rendering in SPECT is the technique of **maximum intensity projection (MIP)** developed by Wallis and Miller.[123] In this approach, the reconstructed transaxial slices are first stacked to form a 3D tomographic volume. Maximum intensity projection involves rotating this 3D tomographic volume into a desired viewing angle and extracting the maximum pixel along each row and column of the rotated volume onto a 2D image plane. To enhance the 3D effect of the image, the volume can

be depth-weighted to emphasize structures in the front of the volume and deemphasize structures in the rear of the volume before the maximum pixel is extracted. Because the maximum pixel is always extracted, this type of volume rendering emphasizes hot spots and is very useful in blood pool and tumor imaging procedures. Maximum intensity projections of the normal bone scan shown in Figure 9-23 can be viewed in the final row. A similar example of both longitudinal slices and a MIP rendering of an abnormal bone scan is shown in Figure 9-24.

Wallis and Miller[122,123] and Miller, Wallis, and Sampathkumaran[81] have noted several advantages of volume-rendered gated cardiac blood pool studies using MIP. The most noticeable advantage of MIP is the enhanced contrast over standard planar imaging. Also, a volume-rendered display can be generated for any desirable viewing angle, allowing a clinician to view each structure of the myocardium from the best possible angle, even those views that cannot be routinely acquired during a planar study. The disadvantage of MIP is that it is essentially a modified planar technique with improved contrast but increased processing time. As such, it is well suited for hot-spot imaging procedures but has limited application in demonstrating cold lesions.

Surface Rendering. Surface rendering refers to methods that display an organ or region based on explicitly

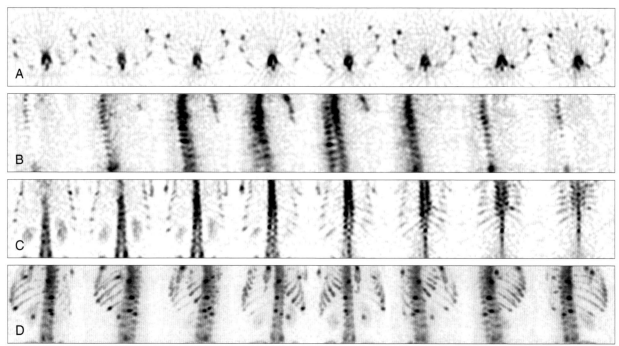

FIGURE 9-24 A, Original transaxial slices taken from an abnormal bone SPECT study. This patient has hot metastases at numerous locations in the spine and rib cage. **B,** Consecutive sagittal slices of the same study. **C,** Coronal slices taken from the same study. **D,** Volume-rendered maximum intensity projection images displayed from different angles. Note that the whole skeleton can be seen, but the hotter metastases are also obvious, and their locations are more effectively visualized than with serial slices.

detected boundaries. Generation of a surface-rendered display, therefore, requires segmentation. Segmentation is the process of separating the organ from the background or nearby structures. It can be accomplished using various methods, such as hand-tracing the volume of interest, using a thresholding technique in which pixels with values greater than the threshold are assumed to be part of the organ and all other pixels are assumed to be background, or complicated boundary detection algorithms. Usually, a thresholding segmentation process produces a binary data set in which myocardial voxels have a value of one and background voxels have a value of zero. A boundary tracking algorithm is then used to identify the surface of the myocardium as the boundary between 1s and 0s and convert it into geometric primitives, such as squares or triangles. In contrast, hand tracing and boundary detection methods usually result in a set of discrete surface points, which are then connected into geometric primitives, usually triangles.

Surface-rendered models are generally displayed using standard computer graphics packages, which allows rotation and translation of the "model," positioning of one or more light sources, and adjustment of the model's opacity (the amount of light shining through the model) or reflectance (the amount of light reflecting off the model). The speed of a 3D surface rendering depends greatly on the type and number of individual elements from which the model is composed. In general, however, surface-rendered displays are quite fast and often can be rotated and translated interactively. The accuracy of

such displays depends primarily on the surface detection and the mapping of function onto the surface, when this is performed. Figure 9-25 shows the surface renderings of two SPECT brain studies of the same patient, a baseline study and a Diamox challenge. The surfaces of these two brains were defined using a single threshold for segmentation.

The advantage of this kind of display is that it is often fast and easy to implement and with the proper segmentation can give useful results. The disadvantage of this technique is that many SPECT studies contain both physiological and anatomical information. Segmentation of a SPECT study into a binary data set using thresholding techniques often ignores some of the important physiological information present in the scan. In fact, improper segmentation from use of an incorrect threshold can give erroneous results. Unfortunately, because single thresholds are used for segmentation in most commercial packages, improper segmentation is a common finding. However, when this technique is applied with appropriate boundary detection algorithms, it is the most realistic way to view the results of quantitation.

SPECT PHYSICS AND IMAGE ARTIFACTS

Artifacts in SPECT images arise from the combined effects of photon absorption, Compton scatter, and the degradation in resolution with distance from the collimator. Each of these interrelated factors produces inconsistent information in the planar projections, in violation of the assumptions behind FBP, the most widely used tomographic reconstruction algorithm. The effect of these factors on SPECT images is quite complex and each is discussed separately.

Attenuation

An example of the attenuation process in myocardial SPECT is shown in Figure 9-26, *A*. Photons emitted from the heart and picked up by the detector in an anterior view have traversed a relatively small amount of tissue (soft tissue and bone). In a lateral view, photons must traverse a greater distance but through different materials (including lung) to reach the detector. As the detector moves about the patient, the projection profile varies with the attenuation along the projection ray and the distance to the collimator.

Attenuation is described quantitatively by the linear attenuation coefficient (commonly depicted by the Greek letter mu [μ]). For example, the value of μ for ^{99m}Tc in soft tissue is approximately equal to that of water: 0.154 cm^{-1}. The process of attenuation is described by:

$$A_x = A_0 e^{-\mu x}$$

where A_x is the activity measured after attenuation through a thickness of tissue x, and A_0 is the true activity at a point in the body.[106] Thus the term $e^{-\mu x}$ represents the fraction of photons that are attenuated over a distance x.

The probability of absorption increases as photon energy decreases; thus attenuation artifacts are reported to be more severe with ^{201}Tl agents than with ^{99m}Tc.[18,42] The most frequently noted effects of attenuation in myocardial SPECT are artifacts associated with breast attenuation in women and diaphragmatic attenuation in men.[18,21,42] Breast attenuation artifacts are commonly identified as a region of decreased count density over the anterior myocardial wall. If the breast position is the same between scans, the appearance of a "fixed" perfusion defect may result and may be interpreted as scar or partial reversibility (ischemia). A breast that is not in the same position between rest and stress scans may masquerade as a reversible defect. Similar changes in apparent perfusion patterns in the inferior myocardial wall can

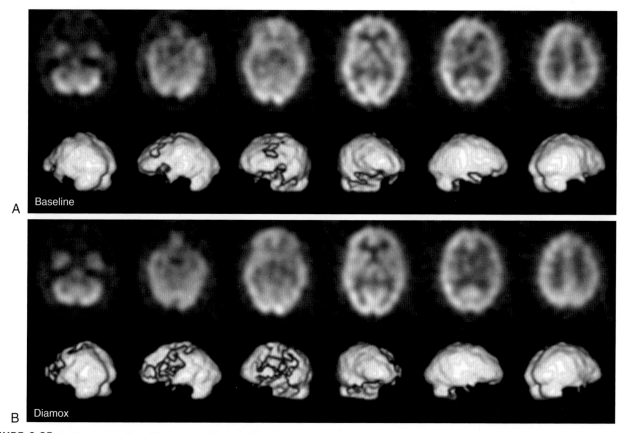

A   Baseline

B   Diamox

FIGURE 9-25 A, Transaxial slices *(top)* and surface-rendered views *(bottom)* of a baseline brain blood flow study. A threshold has been applied to the original images, and the resulting pixels have been connected into a single polygonal object that is then displayed from different angles using surface rendering. Note the "hole" in the left superior part of the brain, an effect created because of the pixels that did not survive the chosen threshold. The part of the brain corresponding to this "hole" may have decreased blood flow. **B,** The same serial slices and 3D views as seen in **A** from the same patient after a Diamox challenge. Diamox should increase brain blood flow in regions where the arterial blood supply is normal and thereby show relative decreases in blood flow distal to constricted or otherwise abnormal vessels. In this case, a relative decrease is seen in the same left superior region as in **A**, but with this pharmaceutical challenge, the abnormality is more profound. This can also be seen on the 3D image, because the "hole" in the brain surface is much larger in these views.

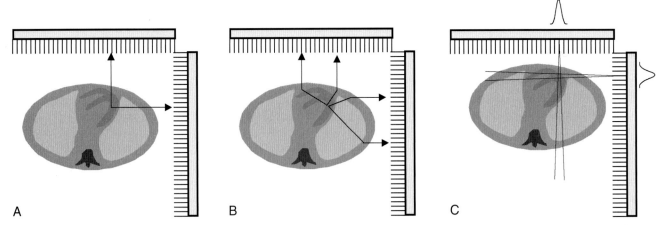

FIGURE 9-26 Physical factors that compromise SPECT include **(A)** nonuniform attenuation (photons emitted from a single point in the heart pass through different materials in different planar projections), **(B)** Compton scatter (photons emitted from that point no longer appear to originate there), and **(C)** varying resolution (the farther the distance from the point to the camera in each projection, the poorer the resolution).

result from differences in diaphragmatic attenuation between resting and stress scans.

Compton Scatter

When a photon undergoes Compton scattering though interactions with an electron, it changes direction and loses energy (see Figure 9-26, *B*). If detected in the photopeak energy window, Compton-scattered photons are likely to be mispositioned in the transverse image, leading to reduced image contrast and reduced lesion detection. Just as with attenuation, scatter can be a more severe problem with ^{201}Tl than with ^{99m}Tc, particularly in myocardial SPECT.

In myocardial SPECT, scatter affects the apparent extent and severity of the hypoperfused regions detected with ^{201}Tl or ^{99m}Tc. In some patients the scatter from high concentrations of activity in abdominal organs (primarily liver and bowel) may artifactually increase the counts in the inferior wall of the myocardium.[44,67,86]

Detector Response

The most important factors in the spatial resolution of images made with a conventional scintillation camera are the geometry of the collimator and the distance from the camera face. The resolution of both fan beam and parallel hole collimators degrades with distance. This effect is shown with a parallel hole collimator in Figure 9-26, *C*. As the camera orbits the patient for a circular acquisition, the only point in the patient that maintains the same distance from the collimator in all the views is at the COR. Because the spatial resolution at any given point in a SPECT image is a result of the resolution in each of the planar projections, the COR is the only point in the reconstructed image with symmetric resolution. This spatially varying resolution can lead to significant distortion in the reconstructed images, particularly for

180-degree acquisitions.[24,69] Although combining the two opposing views of a 360-degree acquisition degrades spatial resolution, it also minimizes its variation across the transverse plane.[7]

ATTENUATION CORRECTION, SCATTER CORRECTION, AND RESOLUTION RECOVERY

Methods exist to correct for attenuation, scatter, and variable resolution effects in SPECT. Some are straightforward and easily implemented; however, the trend is toward applying physical models of each of the effects within an iterative reconstruction technique.

The American Society of Nuclear Cardiology and the Society of Nuclear Medicine have issued a position statement on "the value and practice of attenuation correction for myocardial perfusion SPECT imaging."[56] This statement concludes that "attenuation correction should be regarded as a rapidly evolving standard for SPECT myocardial perfusion imaging" and that "the adjunctive technique of attenuation correction has become a method for which the weight of evidence and opinion is in favor of its usefulness."

Attenuation Correction

Although artifacts caused by attenuation, Compton scatter, and varying resolution present a problem for all SPECT imaging, the most commonly cited complications (and the most difficult to correct because of the variable media of the thorax) are attenuation artifacts in myocardial perfusion SPECT. These artifacts are often cited as the most significant factors limiting interpretative accuracy.[18,21,42] They reduce the specificity of cardiac SPECT by causing variations in normal tracer patterns that may overlap known coronary territories and resemble patterns associated with coronary artery disease.

Attenuation correction is the compensation for the effects of radiation attenuation in computed tomography, which may use mathematical estimate or measured transmission data.

Procedures for Minimizing the Clinical Impact of Attenuation. One method of handling attenuation artifacts is simply to reduce their clinical impact through scanning techniques and knowledge of their location and severity when they occur. For example, the effect of attenuation can often be detected in the rotating planar projection images where a "shadow" moves laterally across the body profile relative to the cardiac uptake. Compared with true hypoperfusion, attenuation artifacts can move "independently" of the heart and attenuate background activity in some of the projection images. The existence of such artifacts, when supplied to a physician, can reduce false positives. In addition, SPECT imaging in the prone position has been reported to minimize attenuation artifacts in myocardial perfusion studies in which the inferior wall may be involved.[26] When the patient is positioned this way, the heart, diaphragm, and subphrenic structures shift to reduce inferior wall attenuation while potentially increasing anterior wall attenuation.

Conventional Correction Methods. The most common correction methods used in commercial systems until recently have been a prereconstruction method based on work by Sorenson[105] and a postreconstruction method developed by Chang.[10] Both of these methods assume that the attenuation within the body is homogeneous, and both have been used effectively for SPECT applications in which the attenuation is approximately homogeneous, such as liver imaging. These methods have been shown to be inadequate for myocardial perfusion SPECT imaging because the attenuating material in a patient's thorax is too varied for a constant attenuation coefficient approximation to be effective.[113]

Sealed Source Transmission Scan–Based Correction Methods. The concept of using transmission scanning with radionuclide imaging was suggested early in the days of nuclear medicine.[70] After acquisition, the transmission projections are reconstructed using either FBP or statistical-based reconstruction algorithms.[128] Once a map of the attenuation values has been reconstructed, a physical model of the attenuation process can be incorporated into an iterative reconstruction technique to correct the degradation of attenuation. During MLEM or OSEM, for example, attenuation correction can be achieved by using the known attenuation coefficients to attenuate the counts in the guess image. By including this model of attenuation into the estimation of the projections in each iteration, a more accurate reconstruction can be achieved.

Currently, the most widely disseminated configuration for transmission imaging is the scanning line source approach with gadolinium-153 (^{153}Gd) as the external source.[108] It was initially commercialized on triple and dual 90-degree detector systems but can also be used on single detector systems. Scanning line source systems (Figure 9-27) use an electronic window that moves

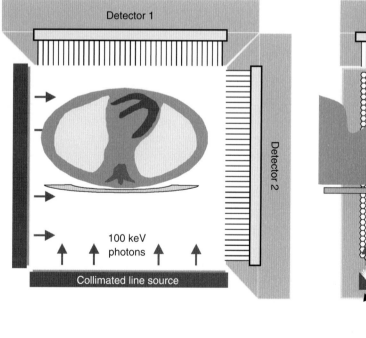

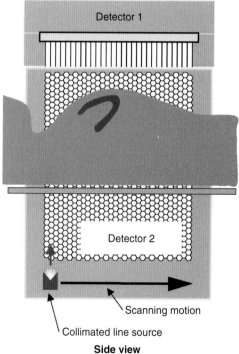

End view   **Side view**

FIGURE 9-27 The most commonly implemented method of acquiring transmission scans for attenuation correction uses line source scanning. During each projection of a step-and-shoot acquisition, a line source (usually filled with ^{153}Gd) scans across the camera's field of view. An electronic window opposite the line source acquires only counts with an energy that matches the line source.

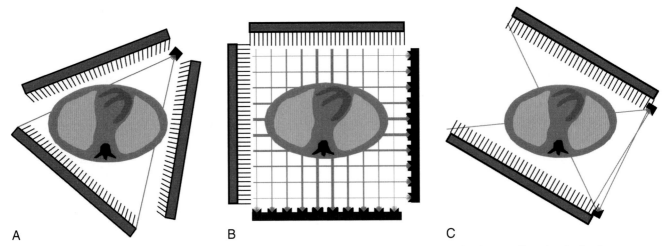

FIGURE 9-28 Other SPECT-based transmission hardware configurations include line source and fan beam collimation for fan beam systems **(A)**, arrays of line sources mounted opposite both cameras of a dual 90-degree camera system **(B)**, and asymmetric fan beam geometry using high-energy photons that penetrate the septa of a low-energy collimator **(C)**. Note that this system can also be used with a 90- or 180-degree camera configuration.

simultaneously and opposite the external source to separate transmission and emission data. Other methods of acquiring transmission scans are shown in Figure 9-28.[9,33,116]

Many transmission-based SPECT systems use simultaneous acquisition of emission and transmission data. This provides efficient acquisition and essential alignment of transmission and emission scans. However, it is very important that the technologist recognize that artifacts in the transmission scan can have a detrimental effect on the attenuation-corrected images. Careful and thorough quality control procedures, therefore, must be used with the transmission scan.[27] Many of the QC concepts used for conventional SPECT imaging extend to systems that perform transmission imaging. For example, COR alignment, which limits reconstruction accuracy in SPECT, can also affect transmission projection data alignment. The transmission projections and tomograms should be reviewed by the technologist to identify technical problems such as motion, missing frames or counts, and gating artifacts. Other problems that degrade transmission scans include excessive noise due to old line sources that have decayed beyond their useful lifetime and truncation of body from the transmission scan as shown in Figure 9-29. Transmission scan truncation can be a particular problem with small-field-of-view dedicated cardiac SPECT systems.[12]

SPECT/CT Correction Methods. The use of SPECT/CT has the benefit of providing an attenuation map of much higher quality than can be obtained with a sealed transmission source. In order for a CT scan to be used for attenuation correction, the pixel values must be scaled to match attenuation coefficients appropriate for the radionuclide being imaged and the CT and SPECT images must be precisely aligned. Patient motion between the two scans, or even heavy breathing as shown in

Figure 9-30, can result in a spatial mismatch and introduce artifacts into the attenuation corrected SPECT scan. The images should always be checked for alignment and if necessary realigned before reconstruction with attenuation correction as shown in Figure 9-31.[11,65]

It should also be noted that any artifacts in the CT scan can result in artifacts in the emission scan. Metal objects (whether inside or outside of the patient) can produce very severe artifacts in the CT scan. These artifacts (and the streaks that emanate from them) appear in the attenuation map as dense areas with a great deal of attenuation and they may cause over-correction in the SPECT image (Figure 9-32).

The initial experience with the use of SPECT/CT for attenuation correction of myocardial perfusion SPECT has been very promising.[38,76,109,118] The availability of the CT scan has also prompted many clinics to routinely utilize attenuation correction for general SPECT studies, improving the quantitative nature of the images and improving the visibility of focal hot spots as was seen in Figure 9-2.

Scatter Correction

Scatter correction methods for SPECT require estimation of the number of scattered photons in each pixel of the image. This is a complex matter because the scatter component of the image depends on the energy of the photon, the energy window used, and the composition and location of the source and the scattering medium.[34,37]

Energy Window–Based Methods. One of the most widely used scatter correction methods is the dual window scatter subtraction method suggested by Jaszczak and colleagues[62] for ^{99m}Tc. This method requires a second energy window at a lower energy (127 to 153 keV) than the photopeak window (89 to 123 keV).

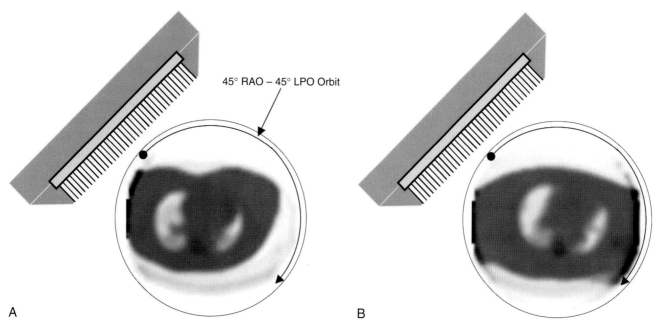

FIGURE 9-29 Truncation of the transmission scan can degrade the accuracy of attenuation correction and should be avoided. When a 180-degree orbit is used for cardiac SPECT, some truncation can be accepted as long the truncated area does not lie between the heart and the camera in any projections. Truncation of the right side of the body **(A)** would not significantly impact on the quality of cardiac attenuation correction using this map. Truncation of the left side of the body **(B)** would have an impact because it does fall between the heart and the camera in several projections. When truncation cannot be avoided, the attenuation corrected images must be carefully evaluated.

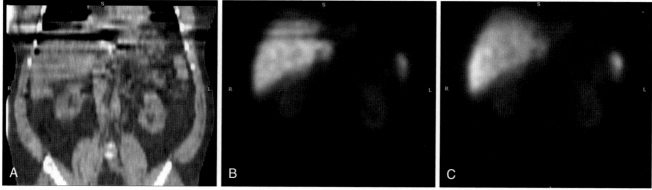

FIGURE 9-30 Coronal CT **(A)** and attenuation corrected ^{99m}Tc–sulfur colloid liver/spleen **(B)** images showing artifacts caused by heavy respiration during the CT acquisition. CT images are acquired much more quickly than SPECT images and represent snapshots in time compared to the SPECT image, which takes several minutes. In this case, the motion of the diaphragm resulted in the liver appearing in one slice but not the slice below it. Care should be taken to note this type of artifact and when present, reconstruction without AC is recommended **(C)**.

A fraction of this window is subtracted from the photopeak window. The dual window technique makes the assumption that the scattered photons in the scatter window are linearly proportional to the scattered photons in the photopeak window. The triple energy window (TEW) technique uses scatter windows on either side of the photopeak window. The contribution of scattered photons to the photopeak window is estimated as the average counts in the two scatter windows normalized to the photopeak window.[61] At best, energy window–based methods can provide only approximate scatter correction, and they may increase image noise.[8]

Iterative Correction Techniques. Reconstruction-based methods incorporate compensation for Compton scatter directly into the iterative reconstruction.[2,35,36] The physics of photon interactions provides a relationship between image scatter and the attenuation distribution in patients, suggesting that a measured attenuation map (from a transmission scan) can be used in conjunction with the source distribution provided by the emission scan to provide a study-specific correction.[82] Reconstruction-based techniques use this information to incorporate a physical model of the scattering process into the iterative reconstruction algorithm information.[3,63,79,124]

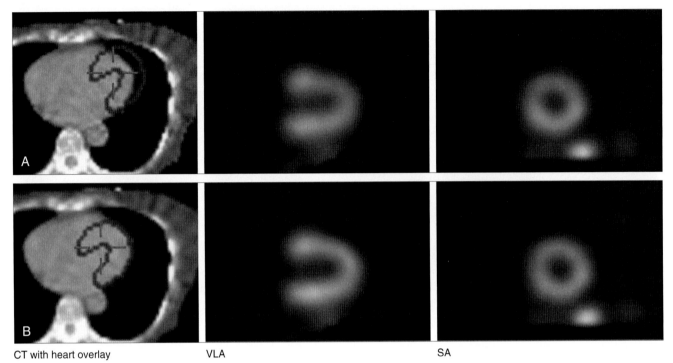

CT with heart overlay   VLA   SA

FIGURE 9-31 SPECT/CT images are acquired sequentially (first SPECT, then CT or vice versa). If the patient moves between the two scans, the spatial mismatch can result in artifactual defects. **A,** Patient movement between the SPECT and the CT acquisitions resulted in a mismatch between the location of the heart in the two modalities. This results in undercorrection of the anterior wall of the heart and an anterior wall defect. Correction software was used to realign the SPECT and CT before reconstruction and the heart reconstructs as normal **(B)**.

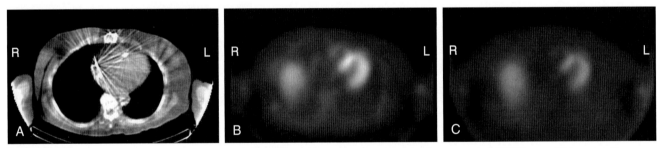

FIGURE 9-32 Metal artifacts in a CT **(A)** can result in artifactual hot spots in an attenuation corrected SPECT scan **(B)** because the reconstruction algorithm treats them as if they were very dense (with a lot of attenuation). When metal artifacts are noted, reconstruction without AC is recommended **(C)**.

Resolution Recovery

Several approaches have been proposed to compensate for the loss of resolution with distance from the collimator and the resulting distortions produced in SPECT images. Analytical approaches to the problem of distance varying resolution model the shape of the collimator response to remove the effects from the image.[88,103] Another approach is to use the frequency distance principle (FDP),[50,73] which states that points at a specific source-to-detector distance correspond to specific regions in the frequency space of the sinogram's Fourier transform. Applying a spatially variant inverse filter to the sinograms performs the resolution recovery. This inverse filtering is relatively fast but may also amplify noise in the image.

Resolution recovery may also be included in iterative reconstruction methods. It is possible to include resolution recovery in both IFBP[93,127] and maximum likelihood reconstruction techniques.[114,129] These methods take considerably more computations to implement than the frequency distance principle but have the potential to compensate more accurately for the resolution response.[111]

Current state of the art methods include a model of the known physical properties of the camera detectors and collimators within MLEM type methods. This approach was first presented in the 1980s,[114] but its computational intensity made it clinically infeasible until recently. The concept of resolution recovery within iterative reconstruction is very similar to that of attenuation correction.

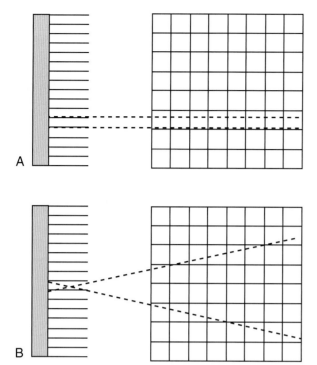

FIGURE 9-33 Standard projection and back-projection assumes that the counts detected in a single projection bin are parallel to and in line with the collimator hole **(A)**. In fact, counts from a cone-shaped area are detected within each collimator hole **(B)**. Using this model to project and back-project within an iterative reconstruction technique allows correction for detector response.

Conventional reconstruction, including projection and back-projection as implemented within EM algorithms, assumes that the photons counted in a projection bin placed over a collimator's parallel hole emanated in a straight line from a radioactive source perpendicular to the detector surface and aligned with the hole (Figure 9-29, *A*). It assumes that all other photons counted from this source are either image noise or counts from other sources positioned in a very narrow line parallel to and directly in front of the hole. However, it is well understood that events not directly in that parallel line may also pass through the collimator hole. In fact, counts from a cone-shaped region in front of a collimator hole actually are collected (Figure 9-29, *B*). When projecting within the iterative reconstruction algorithm, detector response can be accounted for by including the counts from the cone-shaped region as in Figure 9-33 and when back-projecting, by spreading the counts back out over the same region.

The shape and size of the cone-shaped region depends upon geometric collimator and detector properties. For example, Metz[80] and Tsui[112] showed how these detector response functions can be derived analytically for parallel hole as well as fan and cone beam collimators. These functions only need to be computed once and then stored for each collimator; during iterative reconstruction; the correct function is determined by accessing the type of collimator used for acquisition, which may be stored in

the DICOM* header or elsewhere in the patient database.

Note that the intersection of the cone with the image planes of the cone is dependent upon the distance between the collimator and the patient. This information may also be obtained from the database; in some cases, the actual distance of the camera from the center of rotation may be stored for every angle. In others, the radius and shape of the orbit may be enough to derive the needed distances to perform the resolution recovery.

Though all major manufacturers have available iterative resolution recovery software, each one is implemented differently. In fact, resolution recovery is very time consuming, and some commercial products may use different simplifying assumptions to accelerate them. In addition, some type of smoothing, or filtering, is generally incorporated into the iterative reconstruction. In some cases, the filter may be applied after the reconstruction is completed, or may be applied to the images during each iteration. These differences in filtering also imply that not all implementations will behave similarly.

Nevertheless, early work demonstrated that superior image quality can be obtained using resolution recovery algorithms. Kamphuis and associates,[64] showed that contrast is increased and noise is decreased with resolution recovery. Narayanan and colleagues[84] showed that adding resolution recovery to attenuation and scatter correction within an iterative reconstruction algorithm adds diagnostic value to cardiac images. Although currently more interest is being given to these algorithms for their potential to reduce scan times.

This reduction in scan times is achieved without sacrificing image quality because the noisier images produced by shorter, high resolution acquisitions can be smoothed to obtain the same noise and resolution as a filtered back-projection image. In addition resolution recovery algorithms actually reduce noise levels because their ability to accurately localize events leads to higher signal with less noise.[64] Numerous papers assessing the use of resolution recovery with shorter acquisitions in cardiac imaging seem to have borne out this premise.[4,20,74,121] Overall, using resolution recovery with shorter scan times generally provides images that have similar quality to those reconstructed with filtered back-projection or OSEM without resolution recovery. The sole exception may be for low count rest gated images, as reported by Venero and co-workers,[121] suggesting that there is a limit to how few counts may be collected and still provide a good quality image. However, DePuey and colleagues[19] did not see this degradation in quality even when scan times were reduced to one quarter.

Qualitative perfusion analysis also provides similar diagnoses with resolution recovery as with filtered

---

*Digital Imaging and Communications in Medicine (DICOM) is the industry standard for handling, storing, printing, and transmitting medical images and associated information.

back-projection, and quantitative functional parameters correlate highly. There does appear to be a slight reduction in end systolic volume with resolution recovery; however this does not appear to be the case with all algorithms. Again, differences in implementations may make it difficult to generalize their behavior.

Combining Attenuation Correction, Scatter Correction, and Resolution Recovery

As described in the literature, optimum accuracy of SPECT image reconstruction requires correction for Compton scatter, attenuation, distance-dependent spatial resolution, and image noise.[110,111,126] For example, it has been demonstrated that attenuation compensation without scatter compensation can result in an artificial increase in inferior wall counts.[67,77] Other reports demonstrate that scatter compensation is essential for accurate attenuation compensation.[39,110] An example of the application of both attenuation correction and scatter compensation to a myocardial perfusion scan is shown in Figure 9-34. In this example, the original emission and transmission projections are shown for a myocardial perfusion study. Transaxial slices of the emission and transmission studies after reconstruction with filtered back-projection are shown in Figure 9-34, *B*. Figure 9-30, *C*, shows **short-axis slices** reconstructed with filtered back-projection and an iterative technique that corrects for both attenuation and scatter. Corresponding **vertical long-axis slices** are shown in Figure 9-34, *D*. In the FBP reconstruction, breast attenuation artifactually decreases the counts in the anterior wall of the heart, but the attenuation and scatter corrections resolve this problem.

Iterative reconstruction algorithms provide the opportunity to investigate complete compensation of cardiac SPECT images for the effects of the patient's anatomy as described by the attenuation map and the limited, spatially varying resolution of SPECT. As noted above, adding resolution recovery to an iterative reconstruction algorithm improves diagnostic ability over using just attenuation correction or attenuation and scatter correction. It is anticipated that further improvements in the accuracy of cardiac SPECT reconstruction and diagnostic accuracy will result as these methods evolve.

CARDIAC SPECT QUANTIFICATION

Cardiac Reorientation

Most cardiac images are viewed in a standard format consisting of short-axis, **horizontal long-axis,** and vertical long-axis slices. Short-axis slices are also necessary for some automatic perfusion quantification algorithms. Generation of these standard sections from the original transaxial images has been performed interactively, requiring the user to mark the location of the left ventricular axis. The following sections describe the process of interactively creating these standard sections, along with their definitions.

Vertical Long-Axis Slices. Using a display of a transaxial slice through the middle of the left ventricle, the position of the long axis is denoted with a line drawn by the user. The 3D set of transaxial sections (some of which are shown in Figure 9-35, *A*) is resliced parallel to the long axis and perpendicular to the transaxial slices. Each of the resulting oblique images is called a *vertical long-axis slice* (Figure 9-35, *B*). The slices are displayed with the base of the left ventricle toward the left side of the image and the apex toward the right. Serial slices are displayed from medial to lateral, left to right.

Horizontal Long-Axis Slices. Using a display of a midventricular vertical long-axis image, the user once again denotes the left ventricular long axis. The 3D block of vertical long-axis slices is recut parallel to the denoted long axis and perpendicular to the stack. The resulting oblique cuts are called *horizontal long-axis slices* (Figure 9-35, *C*). They contain the left ventricle with its base toward the bottom of the image and its apex toward the top. The right ventricle appears on the left side of the image. Serial horizontal long-axis slices are displayed from inferior to anterior, left to right.

Short-Axis Slices. Slices perpendicular to the denoted long axis and perpendicular to the vertical long-axis slices are also cut from the stack. These are called *short-axis slices* (Figure 9-35, *D*); they contain the left ventricle with its anterior wall toward the top, its inferior wall toward the bottom, and its septal wall toward the left. Serial short-axis slices are displayed from apex to base, left to right.

Automatic Reorientation. Two approaches[46,83] start by identifying the left ventricular region in the transaxial images, using a threshold-based approach that includes knowledge of the expected position, size, and shape of the left ventricle (LV). Once this region has been isolated, the approach described by Germano and colleagues[46] uses the original data to refine the estimate of the myocardial surface. Lines at 90 degrees (vectors) to an ellipsoid fit to the LV region are used to resample the myocardium; a Gaussian function is fitted to the profiles obtained at each sample. The best-fit Gaussian function is used to estimate the myocardial center for each profile, and after further refinement based on image intensities and myocardial smoothness, the resulting midmyocardial points are fitted to an ellipsoid, the long axis of which is used as the final LV long axis. This method was tested on 400 patient images and the results compared with interactively denoted long axes. Failure of the method was described as either not localizing the LV, presence of significant hepatic or intestinal activity in the LV region of the image, or greater than 45 degrees difference between automatically and interactively

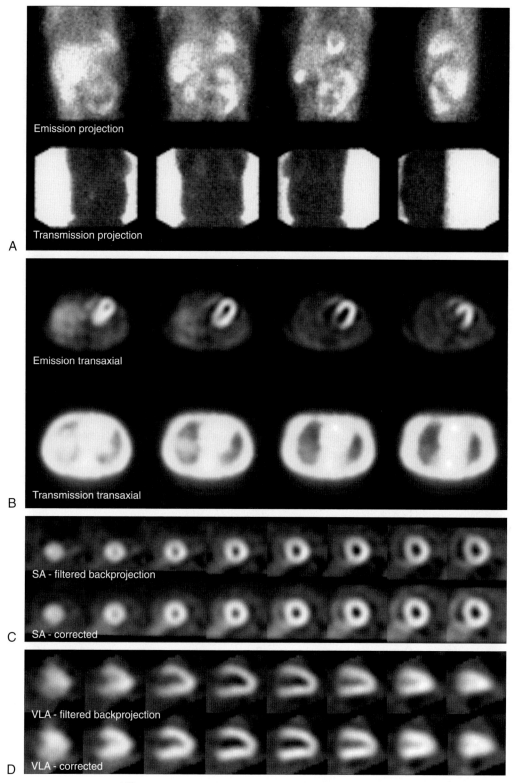

FIGURE 9-34 Attenuation correction of ⁹⁹ᵐTc SPECT of a normal female. **A,** Emission and transmission projections from a SPECT system equipped with scanning line sources. **B,** Emission and transmission transaxial slices through the heart. **C,** Short-axis (SA) slices reconstructed with filtered back-projection, which may be compared with those produced with corrections for attenuation and Compton scatter. **D,** Corresponding vertical long-axis (VLA) images. Breast attenuation artifactually decreases the counts in the anterior wall of the heart, a problem that is resolved when the corrections are applied.

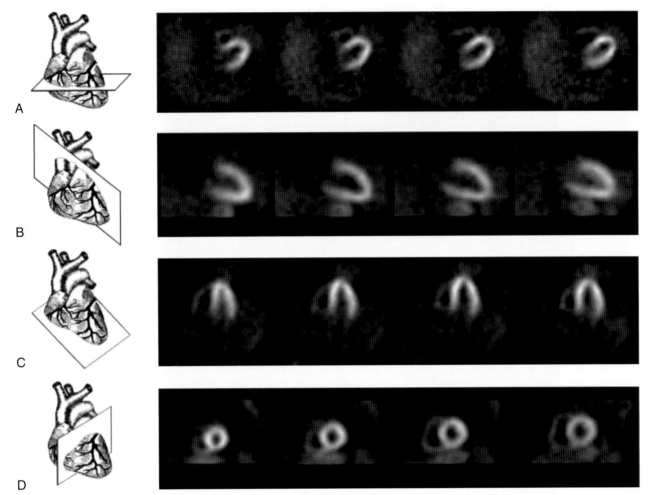

FIGURE 9-35 Standard oblique sections for viewing cardiac data. **A,** Original transaxial slices. The left side of the body is to the right in each slice, with the anterior side at the top. Slices are displayed from inferior to superior, left to right. **B,** Vertical long-axis slices. The base of the left ventricle is toward the left side of the image, and the apex is toward the right. Slices are displayed from medial to lateral, left to right. **C,** Horizontal long-axis slices. The base of the left ventricle is toward the bottom of the image, and its apex is toward the top. The right ventricle appears on the left side of the image. Serial slices are displayed from inferior to anterior, left to right. **D,** Short-axis slices. The anterior wall of the left ventricle is toward the top, the inferior wall is toward the bottom, and the septal wall is toward the left. Slices are displayed from apex to base, left to right.

determined axes. Using these criteria, the method was successful in 394 of the 400 cases.

Mullick and Ezquerra[83] use a more complex heuristic technique to determine the optimal LV threshold and isolate it from other structures. After this has been accomplished, they use the segmented data directly to determine the long axis. The binary image is tessellated into triangular plates, and the normal of each plate on the endocardial surface is used to "point to" the LV long axis. The intersection of these normal vectors (or near-intersections) are collected and fitted to a 3D straight line, which is then returned as the LV long axis. This method was tested on 124 patient data sets, and the automated long-axis orientation was compared with interactively determined angles. Failure was described as a failure to isolate the left ventricle; this method succeeded in 116 of 124 cases.

Slomka and associates[101] take a different approach entirely to automated reorientation. Their method registers the original image data to a "template" image in which the orientation of the LV is known and standardized. The template is created by averaging a large number of registered, normal patient data sets, and separate templates are created for males and females. The registration is done by first translating and scaling the image based on principal axes; the match is refined by minimizing the sum of the absolute differences between the template and the image being registered. This method was not compared with interactively reoriented images but was evaluated visually for 38 normal and 10 abnormal subjects and found to be successful for all.

Perfusion Quantification

All commercially available quantification methods for myocardial perfusion in SPECT are based on the idea that sampled counts in the myocardium of a patient's image can be compared with similar counts sampled

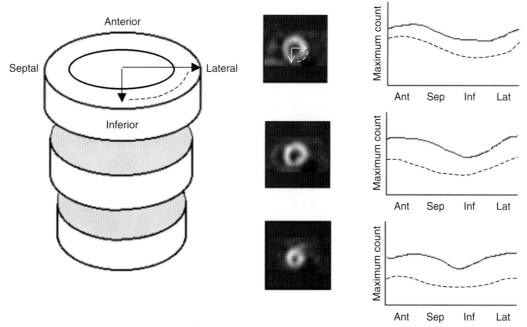

FIGURE 9-36 Creation of circumferential profiles for perfusion quantification. Short-axis slices are sampled at numerous angles about the center of the left ventricle; the maximum count in the myocardium at each angle is graphed against the angle. The result is a circumferential profile for each short-axis slice, seen as the solid line in the graphs at the right. Normal limits are created for each profile by studying normal subjects; these normal limits are shown as dotted lines in the graphs. Whenever a part of the circumferential profile falls below the normal limit, that portion of the patient's myocardium is considered to have a perfusion defect. The subject shown here is normal. *Ant,* Anterior; *Sep,* septal; *Inf,* inferior; *Lat,* lateral.

from a set of normal subjects. In its basic form, the quantitation algorithm samples the left ventricular myocardium in short-axis slices to determine the maximum count values within the myocardium at evenly spaced angles about the left ventricular long axis. For each short-axis slice, the resulting maximum count values are graphed against the angle at which they were encountered; such a graph is called a **circumferential profile.**

Circumferential profiles are amassed for a large number of normal subjects. The profiles are generally normalized for each person so that the maximum count value in each study is rescaled to a standard value, such as 100. This accounts for variations in uptake, dose, and overall perfusion rates. For each angle on each slice, both a mean normal value and its standard deviation are computed over the set of normal subjects. Normal boundaries or normal limits for each point in each profile are created based on these statistical values; for example, they may be set at 2 or 2.5 standard deviations below the mean normal value. By comparing a patient's circumferential profile angle by angle and slice by slice to the normal limits, perfusion defects can be pointed out automatically. Figure 9-36 shows the creation and use of circumferential profiles.

Generally, analysis is performed and normal limits are created for the stress study and for a normalized difference between the stress and rest studies. (If ^{201}Tl washout images are being quantitated, the percentage change between the stress and the washout images is analyzed

instead of the normalized difference between the two.) Separate normal limits must be created for males and females because normal differences in body shape cause different normal attenuation and scatter artifacts in the reconstructions. Abnormal areas or defects seen in the stress images that persist on the rest study are considered fixed. Abnormal regions in the stress study that improve or normalize in the rest study are considered reversible.

Methods vary primarily in the way in which the myocardium is sampled. For example, the previous description of short-axis circumferential profiles has been extended to a hybrid cylindrical/spherical coordinate system[42] and to ellipsoid sampling.[47] Another difference is the way in which the normal limits are generated; one approach uses receiver-operator curves to generate an optimum threshold for each myocardial region.[119] All the methods are similar, however, in that they sample the counts at discrete points in the myocardium and compare those values to some known "normal" values to localize perfusion defects.

Because few studies have compared these various approaches to perfusion quantification, it is not a simple matter to choose one based on its comparative accuracy. More practical issues, therefore, may be the most useful guide to choosing which of the methods may be best for clinical use. Certainly it is important to make sure that the approach has been validated and the results published. The manufacturer should have U.S. Food and Drug Administration (FDA) approval to market it for

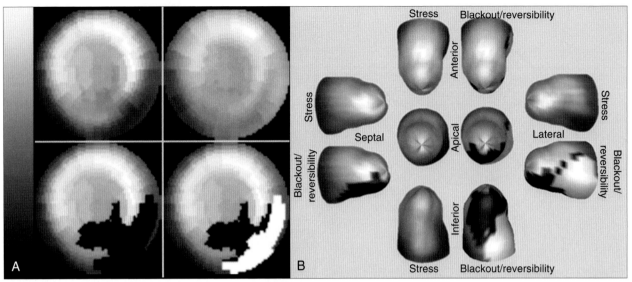

FIGURE 9-37 Polar (bull's-eye) maps and 3D displays of perfusion, quantified from a stress ^{99m}Tc-sestamibi/rest ^{201}Tl study. **A,** Polar plots of stress perfusion *(top left)*, rest perfusion *(top right)*, stress blackout *(bottom left)*, and reversibility whiteout *(bottom right)*. In polar plots, the anterior wall is toward the top, the septal side is toward the left, the lateral wall is toward the right, and the inferior wall is toward the bottom. For each plot, colors are scaled from 0% to 100% of the maximum myocardial counts. The blackout plot shows in black all abnormal regions in the stress image, determined from comparison with normal limits. The regions that normalize at rest are shown in white in the whiteout map. **B,** 3D displays of the same data as in **A.** Here, only stress and blackout/reversibility whiteout data are shown. Five different views of the left ventricle are provided; clockwise from top, they are anterior, lateral, inferior, and septal, with an apical view in the center. Note that the size and shape of the left ventricle can be better appreciated in this 3D display. Also, the size, shape, and location of the defects are immediately obvious.

clinical use. It is also important that the methodologies be kept up-to-date. New normal files are often required for new protocols, and a program that is no longer in active development will not be applicable to the latest technologies. For instance, some programs may not have normal files for dual isotope perfusion analysis. Others that were developed for use with all-purpose collimators may never provide normal limits for use with high-resolution collimators. In any case, the most important thing to keep in mind when using quantitative programs is to follow the acquisition and processing protocols developed for the technique exactly. Even small changes in reconstruction filtering or acquisition time can compromise the accuracy of the quantitation.

CARDIAC DISPLAY

Polar Maps

Polar maps, or bull's-eye displays, are another way to view circumferential profiles. They give a quick, comprehensive overview of the circumferential samples from all slices by combining them into a color-coded image. The points of each circumferential profile are assigned a color based on normalized count values, and the colored profiles are shaped into concentric rings. The most apical slice processed with circumferential profiles forms the center of the polar map, and each successive profile from each successive short-axis slice is displayed as a new ring

surrounding the previous. The most basal slice of the left ventricle makes up the outermost ring of the polar map. Figure 9-37, *A*, shows polar maps created by applying the CEqual quantification method to a ^{99m}Tc-sestamibi study. This kind of display allows immediate and comprehensive viewing of the quantitative results of the entire myocardium.

The use of color also can aid the identification of abnormal areas at a glance. Abnormal regions from the stress study are often assigned a black color, thus creating a blackout map. Blacked-out areas that normalize at rest are color-coded white, thus creating a whiteout reversibility map.[68] This can be seen in Figure 9-37, *A*. Additional maps, such as a standard deviation map that shows the number of standard deviations below normal of each point in each circumferential profile, can aid in evaluation of the study by indicating the severity of any abnormality.

Although they offer a comprehensive view of the quantitation results, polar maps distort the size and shape of the myocardium and any defects. Numerous improvements in the basic polar map display have helped to overcome some of these problems.[42] For instance, "distance-weighted" maps are created so that each ring is the same thickness. These maps have been shown to be useful for accurate localization of abnormalities. "Volume-weighted" maps are constructed such that the area of each ring is proportional to the volume of the corresponding slice. This type of map has been shown to be best for estimating defect size. However, more realistic displays have been introduced that do not have the distortions of polar maps.

Three-Dimensional Cardiac Displays

Three-dimensional graphics techniques can be used to overlay results of perfusion quantification onto a representation of a specific patient's left ventricle.[15,31] In the most basic form of such techniques, the pixel locations of the maximum-count myocardial points sampled during quantitation are used to estimate the myocardial surface. These points can be connected into triangles, which are then color-coded in a way similar to a polar map. Figure 9-37, *B*, displays the same information seen in the polar maps of Figure 9-37, *A*, using a 3D representation. Such displays routinely can be rotated in real time and viewed from any angle with current computer power. They have the advantage of showing the actual size and shape of the left ventricle and the extent and location of any defect in a very realistic manner. Some studies have shown that the 3D models are more accurate for evaluating the size and location of perfusion defects than polar maps[92] or slice-by-slice displays.[92,96]

The biggest disadvantage of 3D displays is that they require more computer screen space (and therefore more film or paper for hard copies) than polar maps. The entire left ventricle can be visualized in a single circular polar map but only one side of the left ventricle can be seen when it is displayed using 3D graphics.

CARDIAC GATING

Standard cardiac SPECT images suffer from motion blur, because the heart is always in motion. These images can show only a picture of the average position of the heart. It is well known that because the heart is moving, contracting and relaxing, perfusion defects can be missed or underestimated; they are, in a sense, "averaged" with normal myocardium that may move into the location previously occupied by the defect earlier in the cardiac cycle. In addition, it is well understood that the intensity of the myocardium in nuclear medicine images is related not only to radiotracer uptake but also to relative myocardial thickness.[40] As the heart contracts, the myocardium appears brighter in the reconstructed image. This effect also is "averaged" into a standard static (ungated) acquisition and may result in impaired diagnostic accuracy.[25]

Cardiac gating allows heart motion and contraction to be resolved by dividing the projections into discrete time parts coupled with the cardiac cycle. The electrocardiogram (ECG) is used to determine the heart rate and the onset of contraction at the QRS complex. The cardiac cycle is divided into a set number of predetermined time intervals, called *frames*, and counts collected during each frame are directed to a different projection set. Counts are directed into the first frame during the initial T/N seconds after the QRS complex is detected, where N is the number of frames and T is the length in seconds of the cardiac cycle. Then, counts are directed into the second frame for the second T/N seconds, and so on. This is repeated for each heartbeat during the acquisition, at every angle. At the end of the acquisition, there are N sets of complete projection images. When these are reconstructed, the result is N 3D sets of slices showing the heart at N points during the cardiac cycle. These four-dimensional data allow 3D analysis of motion and myocardial thickening,[14,30,48] as well as perhaps enabling better discrimination of the extent and location of perfusion abnormalities.[17] It has even been proposed that exercise ejection fraction can be measured using gated tomographic perfusion imaging by acquiring gated projections rapidly (in about 6 minutes) during stress. Although the resulting images are of poor quality and probably not useful for perfusion analysis, the endocardial surfaces may be detected with enough accuracy to compute end-diastolic and end-systolic volumes for ejection fraction calculation.[49]

There are a number of practical considerations for cardiac gating. First, each projection set and reconstruction will be reduced in counts by a factor equal to the number of collected frames. This precludes gating studies, which are normally low count, because image quality becomes too poor. Also, gating software should be able to deal with abnormal heartbeats and "reject" or ignore counts from these contractions. Similarly, the acquisition should be able to adjust to changing heart rates and direct counts to the projection frames accordingly. One commonly seen result of a change in heart rate is late frame drop-off. If the heart rate speeds up but the software fails to adjust, the heartbeat ends before counts have been directed into the last few frames. When the next contraction begins, counts are directed back into the first frames. Therefore, relatively fewer counts are seen in the late end-diastolic frame. Motion blur is also reintroduced, because for some early projections, the cardiac cycle is divided into eight frames, but for late projections, it is divided into six frames. Finally, the size of a gated data set increases proportionally to the number of frames collected. This raises both processing time and storage space for gated studies.

Quantifying Function

It is possible to obtain quantitative functional information from gated perfusion SPECT images. Global variables such as left ventricular volumes, mass, and ejection fraction can be calculated. Local properties of wall motion and myocardial thickening are also obtainable; these can then be displayed using either polar maps or 3D graphics. Most commercially available programs for quantifying cardiac function are fully 3D approaches, which start by detecting endocardial and epicardial surface points through the cardiac cycle. For instance, the Quantitative Gated SPECT (QGS) program determines the locations of the surface points through fitting of count activity profiles across the myocardium to asymmetric Gaussian curves.[48] Other methods seek definition of the same points by analysis of percent systolic count increases resulting from partial volume effect[29] analysis of count gradients followed by iterative relaxation labeling[30,32] or analysis of moments of the count distribution.[52]

Global Variables. Once the left ventricular endocardial (inner wall) and epicardial (outer wall) boundaries have been determined, the number of pixels within the chamber or left ventricular wall can be determined. Because the pixel sizes are known, the total volume in the chamber or myocardium can be computed. Myocardial mass is calculated by multiplying the myocardial volume by an assumed density, usually 1.05 g/ml. The end-diastolic volume is determined to be the largest chamber volume found in the gated set of images; the end-systolic volume is the smallest. The ejection fraction is computed using these values.

Endocardial Wall Motion. If the endocardial surface is detected at each point in the cardiac cycle, regional endocardial wall motion can be assessed by computing how each surface point moves. Wall motion is difficult to compute with much accuracy because it is impossible to say with certainty that a particular point in one time frame moves to a particular location in the next. In addition, there is a global translational component to left ventricular motion, which is difficult to assess and/or remove. In fact, most analyses of left ventricular wall motion rely heavily on simplified models of motion originally developed for 2D contrast ventriculograms or radionuclide ventriculograms. These models may assume, for example, that every point moves radially toward the left ventricular center of mass; regional motion is therefore forced to be "radial." Two approaches[29,45] use a 3D extension of the centerline method originally developed for contrast ventriculograms.[99] In this method, each left ventricular surface point is assumed to move in a direction perpendicular to the surface at that point. Note that no method for modeling endocardial motion is completely accurate in every case; therefore, quantitated left ventricular wall motion should be considered in conjunction with perfusion information.

Myocardial Thickening. Myocardial thickening is known to be a better indicator of myocardial viability than endocardial wall motion; therefore the ability to quantify this variable accurately from perfusion tomograms would be very valuable. The most promising methods use the fact that, as a result of detector response, myocardial thickness is linearly related to image intensity in perfusion images when the myocardial thickness is less than two times the resolution of the reconstructed images.[40] Because current SPECT systems provide resolution on the order of 1 cm, this thickness/intensity relationship should hold true for the vast majority of cases, in which the range of myocardial thickness is 0.5 to 2.0 cm. Note that there is no way to tell absolute thickness with this method; instead, only the change in thickness over the cardiac cycle can be assessed. For example, if the peak counts at one point of the myocardium double from end-diastole to end-systole, it can be postulated that the wall has doubled in thickness during contraction at that point.

One approach to quantification of wall thickening using this theory samples the myocardial counts at numerous locations (more than 4000) for every gated frame.[14] Then a time/intensity curve is created for each of the myocardial points. The curve is "smoothed" by fitting a cosine function to its values. The amplitude of the fitted cosine wave is used as a measure of the change in thickness from end-diastole to end-systole at the point in question. Thickening polar plots or 3D displays can be created to show the resulting "percent thickening" computed around the left ventricle. This method has proved to be very robust with respect to noise in simulation studies. However, quantification of myocardial thickening from perfusion SPECT images has not at this writing been truly tested in the clinic.

QUALITY CONTROL

Quality assurance (QA) is the approach taken to ensure that a quality product is provided. Suboptimal images can make diagnosis difficult or even lead to misdiagnosis. The phrase *quality control* (QC) encompasses the specific tests needed to achieve quality assurance. Several tests must be performed on scintillation cameras to verify that they meet performance specifications.[54] Although at one time these tests were performed using similar methods on almost any manufacturer's camera, today methods of testing and calibrating cameras vary widely from manufacturer to manufacturer.

Although the methods for performing QC procedures for multiple detector systems vary widely among manufacturers, the same procedures required of single detector systems apply. The additional QC calibrations and procedures required of multiple detector SPECT systems primarily deal with the registration of images between the two heads. All of the detectors may have excellent spatial resolution independently, but if images produced by the different detectors do not fall precisely on top of one another, this resolution will be lost.

Planar Gamma Camera Quality Control

Quality control for SPECT cameras must include the QC procedures common to all scintillation cameras. The camera energy peaks should be checked daily, and a uniformity test should be done. The camera's resolution and linearity should be checked weekly.[22,85] It is important to note that not only do these tests need to be done, but the results also need to be analyzed with a critical eye. It does no good to perform the tests if action is not taken when warranted.

SPECT Quality Control

SPECT reconstruction techniques depend on the consistency of the images from different views. Imperfections that go unnoticed in planar imaging can be amplified in the reconstruction process, resulting in severe artifacts in the transaxial images. Two calibrations uniquely important to SPECT are uniformity corrections and COR calibrations. These must be part of any clinic's routine QC procedures and must be performed weekly or monthly, depending on the manufacturer's recommendations and the user's experience with the equipment. Multiple-camera systems require additional tests to ensure that the two systems are adequately aligned.[85] Patient motion is a concern and should be monitored during the acquisition and checked after the acquisition. After acquisition, it is also important to maintain consistency in the processing of SPECT images. Standard protocols should be developed for reconstruction, filtering, and display.

Uniformity Correction. All scintillation cameras must correct for differences in energy responses from different PMTs. Although these corrections are important for reducing uniformity errors in planar projections, uniformity requirements for SPECT are more stringent and require further correction. Next to PMTs, the greatest sources of image nonuniformities are imperfect collimators. A local nonuniformity is propagated in the reconstructed transaxial slice in the form of a circular, or *ring*, artifact because the same nonuniformity is back-projected at each of the angles of acquisition (Figure 9-38). The higher the acquired counts for that slice, the more prominent the artifact, because it rides above the random noise

error. Also, the closer the local nonuniformity to the axis of rotation, the higher the amplitude of the artifact, because the back-projected lines are closer together (more overlapping of count values).

Uniformity defects are most easily seen in flood tests and in phantom acquisitions in which a large area of uniform activity is present (Figure 9-39). Artifacts can be much more difficult to detect in multihead SPECT because the uniformity defect does not usually complete the ring artefact. Clinical radiotracer distributions usually have low count rates in most of the image, making uniformity defects difficult to detect (Figure 9-40).

Center of Rotation. Artifacts caused by errors in the COR are unique to SPECT. The COR is the axis about which the camera rotates (Figure 9-41). The COR measurement determines the offset between the center of the camera matrix and projection of the COR of the camera face (they do not automatically correspond). If this offset is very large (more than two pixels), the reconstruction of a point source looks like a bright ring (Figure 9-42). Center-of-rotation errors too small to create a ring (as small as 0.5 pixel in a 64×64 matrix) can blur the image by spreading out the counts and possibly creating artifacts. Also, 180-degree reconstructions of a point source do not produce a full ring but rather a shape similar to a tuning fork (Figure 9-43). This can be much easier to detect than the simple blurring of 360-degree orbits.

Patient Motion. Patient motion is one of the more significant causes of artifacts in SPECT images, because motion as small as 0.5 pixel can yield significant artifacts.[5,23] The technologist should warn the patient not to move, should make sure the patient is comfortable so that movement is less likely, and should monitor the patient during acquisition. Images should be viewed after the procedure to check for patient motion, attenuation,

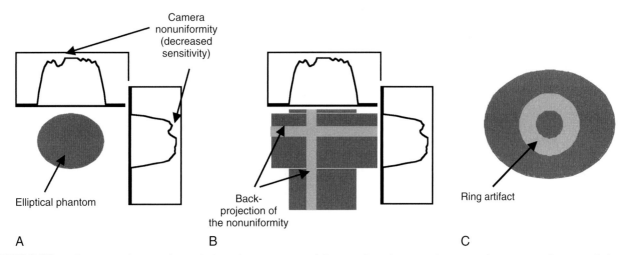

FIGURE 9-38 Uniformity artifacts are formed when there is an area of decreased sensitivity on the camera face. **A,** A quality control phantom is filled with uniform tracer solution. An area of decreased sensitivity resulted in a uniformity defect in the activity profiles of the two planar projections shown. **B,** When back-projected, these areas originate from the same pixels in each projection. **C,** The intersections of the uniformity defects from each of the projections scribes a circular defect in the transaxial image.

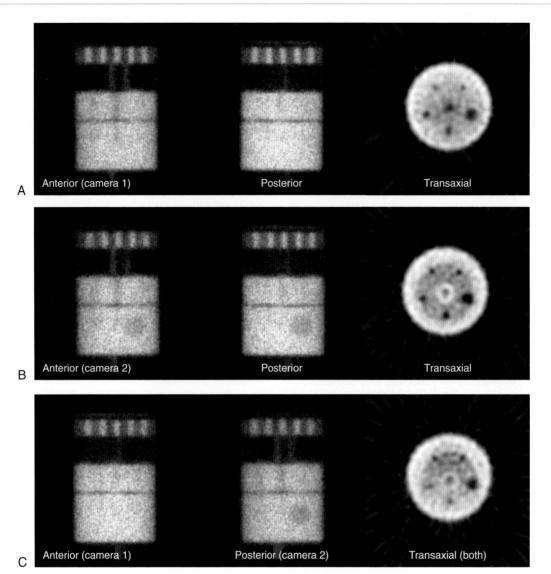

FIGURE 9-39 A SPECT phantom should be imaged quarterly as part of a clinic's routine quality control procedure. The resulting images should be compared with previous images to ensure that image quality has not degraded. Each camera of a multiple detector SPECT system should undergo quality control independently, and the system should be tested as a whole. In this example, camera 2 of a dual detector system has a uniformity defect (created by a clay mask approximately the size of a photomultiplier tube). **A,** Anterior and posterior projections from a 360-degree acquisition. Low count rates in SPECT acquisition with camera 1 are shown, along with a transaxial slice. The slice is uniform, except for the effects of attenuation, and defects *(solid plastic spheres)* are clearly seen. **B,** An identical acquisition using only camera 2 clearly shows the uniformity defect and the resulting ring artifact in the transaxial image. **C,** When the two cameras are used as a unit, the 360-degree acquisition is accomplished by rotating each camera through 180 degrees. The uniformity artifact in the transaxial slice is still significant but more difficult to diagnose.

or other factors that may reduce the accuracy of the reconstructed images. Patient motion can be detected by summed projections, sinograms, or cine displays (see Figure 9-44).

Summed projections are formed by adding all the planar projections for the SPECT acquisition. The heart can be seen as a blurry horizontal line across the center of the summed images of Figure 9-44. To evaluate motion, the technologist should look for a change in the height of the heart (in this example) that would indicate movement during acquisition. This works best for vertical motion (i.e., along the table).

The heart can be seen as a bright stripe from the top right to the lower left in the sinograms in Figure 9-44. The technologist should look for a break in this stripe that would represent the patient moving left to right. Sinograms, therefore, are best for detecting horizontal motion (i.e., across the table). Sinograms also show vertical motion but not as well as horizontal motion.

Cine displays of the planar projections are the simplest and most effective way of detecting patient motion. The playback of the acquisition can be watched as a movie to detect all types of motion, and this should be a routine part of the reconstruction process. The

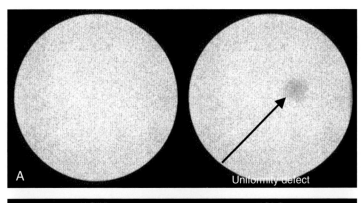

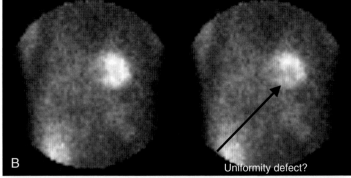

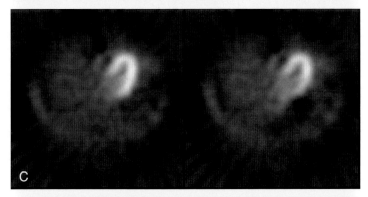

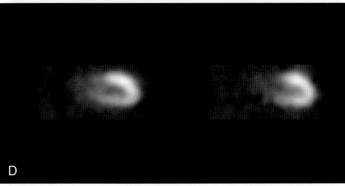

FIGURE 9-40 Uniformity artifacts are more difficult to detect in clinical images. **A,** Daily flood images from a system working correctly on the left and with a simulated uniformity defect on the right (similar to that of a faulty photomultiplier tube). **B,** This same uniformity was applied to clinical ^{201}Tl SPECT. Although it was easy to identify the defect in the flood image, it was very difficult to identify the defect in the clinical image, even when rotating the projections in cine mode. **C,** No ring artifact is evident in the transaxial images. The ring is incompletely formed because of the 180-degree camera orbit and the low background counts. **D,** Note the decreased counts in the inferior wall of the left ventricle resulting from the uniformity artifact. This could easily be mistaken for a perfusion abnormality. Clinical diagnoses could be further complicated if the patient is positioned differently between the stress and rest acquisitions and the defect appears in different areas of the body in the two scans, giving the appearance of a reversing defect.

technologist should watch the movie of the planar projections at a fairly rapid rate and observe the images for up and down motion. It should be noted that the best way to detect and correct motion is for the technologist to observe the patient and repeat the scan if motion occurs. Immediately repeating the scan might prevent the patient from having to return to the clinic on another

day for a repeat scan if the motion renders the scan uninterpretable.

Motion is much more easily detected with multihead systems (see Figure 9-44, C) because of the transition between detectors seen during cine of the projections. Sudden motion will be seen twice for each detector in cines: once when the motion occurs and once when the

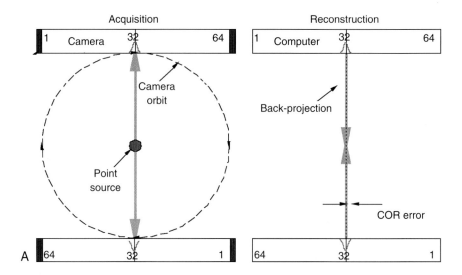

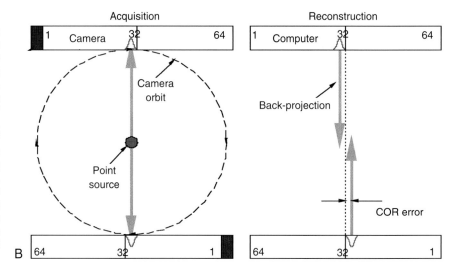

FIGURE 9-41 When properly calibrated, the digital image matrix is perfectly centered on the camera face and the central pixels always align with the imaginary line around which the camera rotates (center of rotation [COR]). **A,** When properly calibrated, a point source placed at the COR projects to the center of the pixel matrix (pixel 32 in this example). Upon reconstruction, the back-projection of opposing views overlay exactly. **B,** When improperly calibrated (illustrated by shifting the pixel matrix to one side of the camera), the point source projects to one side of the center of the matrix. Upon reconstruction, the projections do not meet in the center but are shifted to either side of the center of the matrix. The COR calibration measures and corrects for this shift (COR error).

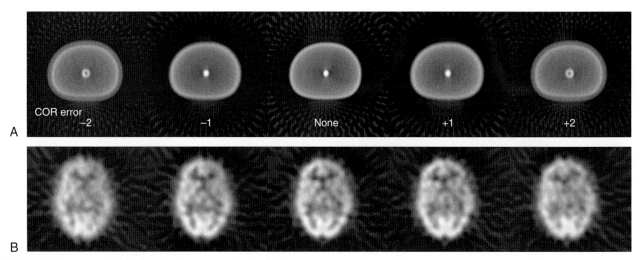

FIGURE 9-42 Center-of-rotation (COR) errors are most easily identified using a line or point source; they can be difficult to detect in clinical images. **A,** A simulated quality control phantom containing a line source is imaged using a 360-degree acquisition with COR errors of −2, −1, 0, +1, and +2 pixels. Extreme errors convert the single point of the line to a ring, but typical clinical errors (on the order of 1 pixel or less) severely degrade resolution. **B,** The same errors in brain SPECT produce loss of resolution and distortions that can be difficult to identify as COR problems.

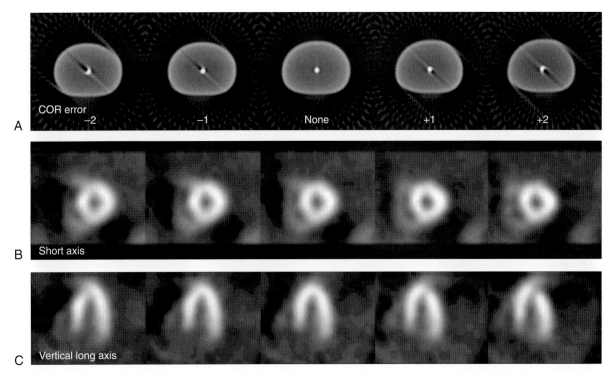

FIGURE 9-43 Center-of-rotation (COR) artifacts in 180-degree acquisitions have a different appearance from those in 360-degree acquisitions. **A,** The simulated quality control phantom from Figure 9-34 is imaged using a 180-degree acquisition with COR errors of −2, −1, 0, +1, and +2 pixels. Even small COR errors produce an artifact typically described as the shape of a tuning fork. **B,** The same errors in cardiac SPECT produce an apparent mismatch between the septal and lateral walls of the heart. **C,** The mismatch is most easily seen in the horizontal long-axis images, as is a characteristic defect near the apex of the heart.

cine makes the transition from one camera to the next. The observer should remember that, unlike a cine produced on a single-head camera, the sequence in projections does not correspond directly to time. For example, if a dual-headed camera is used to acquire 64 projections over 180 degrees, 32 projections will be acquired by each camera head. If patient motion occurs halfway through a scan, the motion will be visible in frame 16 (acquired by camera 1) and in frame 48 (acquired by camera 2). In addition, if the patient does not return to the original position, apparent motion will be visible between frame 32 (acquired by camera 1 at the end of the scan) and frame 33 (acquired by camera 2 at the beginning of the scan). The fact that motion is more easily detected by multihead systems does not mean that it will more severely affect the reconstructed images. Overall, the effects of the motion should be reduced when compared with a single-head system because the patient has less time to move. If significant motion is detected, however, the scan should be repeated.

Most manufacturers offer some sort of motion-correction software. Manual corrections require the operator to shift projections (either by dragging the image with the computer mouse or by specifying the motion by pixels) based on visual analysis. Automated methods perform the operation based on a number of different algorithms. Regardless of the implementation, these methods should be used with great care and the results of the correction should be evaluated by observing rotating cines of the corrected and uncorrected projections, as well as the reconstructed images.

Standards and Procedures

The National Electrical Manufacturers Association (NEMA) is a trade association for manufacturers of electrical products. The Nuclear Section of the Diagnostic Imaging and Therapy Systems Division developed the *NEMA Standards Publication for Performance Measurements of Scintillation Cameras.*[90] This document defines standards by which scintillation cameras may be measured. No performance standards have been set by NEMA; rather, the intent of the published standards is to define methods by which scintillation camera performance can be measured so that a comparison can be made between performance claims by different manufacturers. The American Association of Physicists in Medicine has published several pamphlets on scintillation camera QC and acceptance testing that can provide additional guidance in designing QC procedures.[13,94,98] The American Society of Nuclear Cardiology has released guidelines for instrumentation quality assurance and performance and quality control procedures for transmission-emission tomographic systems to be used for attenuation correction.[22]

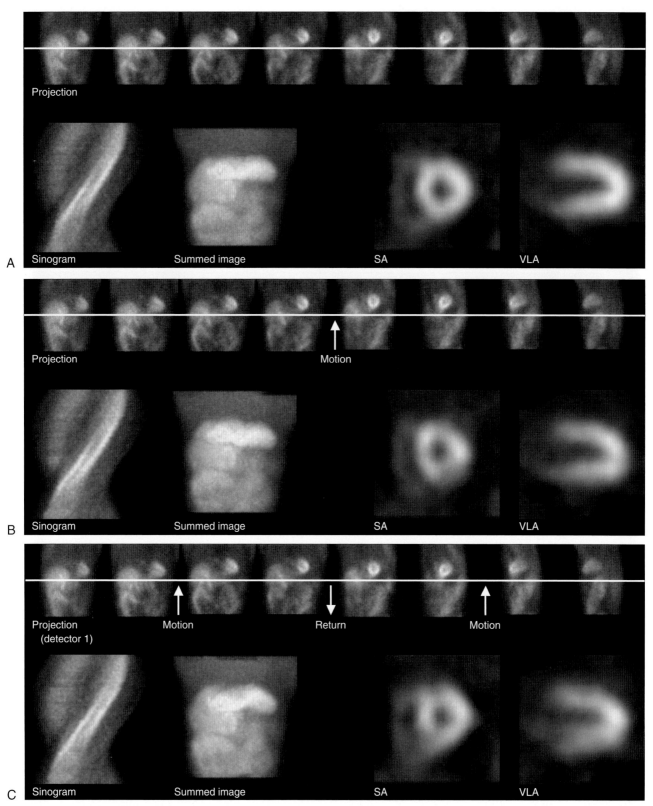

FIGURE 9-44 The projections in these diagrams illustrate how patient motion might be detected in a cine display in a normal ^{99m}Tc-sestamibi cardiac SPECT scan. If the distance between the heart and the horizontal line is compared in each panel, a 2-pixel vertical movement can be detected in the second two panels. This motion, easily detectable in the cine display, is difficult to detect using the sinogram and summed images. **A,** The heart maintains a uniform height above the line, and the resulting short-axis (SA) and vertical long-axis (VLA) images are fairly uniform. **B,** Shifting the projection up 2 pixels in the second half of the study simulates motion in a single detector system. Significant artifacts are evident in the SA and VLA images. **C,** Shifting the projection up 2 pixels in the second half of the study simulates motion in a 90-degree dual detector system. The motion appears one fourth of the way through the study because each detector simultaneously acquires one half of the projections. The heart appears to return to the original position at the midpoint of the cine (the first projection for detector 2). Significant artifacts are again evident in the SA and VLA images but do not appear to be as great as in the example above.

SUMMARY

- SPECT images are created from 2D projection images taken from around the patient.
- The principles of CT, SPECT, and PET are similar.
- SPECT images have poorer resolution than planar images but have improved contrast by removing overlying and underlying areas of activity.
- Dual detector systems are the most common SPECT scanners and most may have the detectors positioned at either 180 or 90 degrees apart to have flexibility to a variety of clinical needs.
- SPECT imaging is usually performed over 360 degrees with the exception of myocardial perfusion imaging, which is most commonly performed over 180 degrees.
- Triple detector systems usually have detectors placed at 120 degrees from one another.
- SPECT/CT systems have the advantage of performing rapid attenuation correction to the SPECT study and provide anatomical images for correlation with the SPECT.
- High-resolution collimators are generally preferred over all-purpose collimators because they have higher resolution at depth.
- SPECT data may be acquired in step-and-shoot or continuous-motion orbits. Step-and-shoot adds 3 to 5 seconds per projection.
- Body-contour orbits maximize camera resolution by keeping the collimator closer to the patient.
- SPECT body scans are most often performed with a 128 × 128-pixel matrix and 120 projections over 360 degrees using a body-contouring orbit.
- Myocardial perfusion SPECT studies are most often acquired using a 64 × 64-pixel matrix and zoom to magnify the heart in 60 to 64 projections over 180 degrees.
- SPECT images may be reconstructed using filtered back-projection (FBP). These images are noisy and are most commonly filtered with a low-pass frequency space filter to reduce noise.
- Iterative reconstruction algorithms require more time to process than FBP but produce images with less noise.
- The ramp filter has the highest resolution but it also produces high noise. Low-pass filters remove noise by use of a cutoff frequency. Butterworth filters use a critical frequency (like a cutoff frequency) and an order to create desired filtering.
- SPECT images may be reoriented to create axial, sagittal, and coronal slices. Myocardial studies are reoriented to create vertical long-axis, horizontal long-axis, and short-axis slices.
- Noncardiac SPECT studies are often displayed using maximum intensity projection (MIP) images that are shown in a cinematic loop.
- SPECT studies may be corrected for attenuation, scatter, and detector response.
- Attenuation correction by mathematical techniques may be applied only when there is uniform attenuation by the body. In the chest a method of measuring by a transmission beam must be used to map the tissue density over each slice. External radioactive sources or CT provides these measurements to attain accurate measured attenuation correction.
- Quality-control procedures for SPECT include extrinsic flood field uniformity correction to prevent ring artifacts and center-of-rotation (COR) offset correction.

REFERENCES

1. Anger HO: Scintillation camera with multichannel collimators, *J Nucl Med* 5:515-531, 1964.
2. Beekman F, Eijkman E, Viergever M, et al: Object shape–dependent PSF model for SPECT imaging, *IEEE Trans Nucl Sci* NS-40:31-39, 1993.
3. Beekman FJ, den Harder JM, Viergever MA, et al: SPECT modeling in nonuniform attenuating objects, *Phys Med Biol* 42:1133-1142, 1997.
4. Borges-Neto S, Pagnanelli RA, Shaw LK, et al: Clinical results of a novel wide beam reconstruction method for shortening scan time of Tc-99m cardiac SPECT perfusion studies, *J Nucl Cardiol* 14(4):555-565, 2007.
5. Botvinick EH, Zhu YY, O'Connell WJ, et al: A quantitative assessment of patient motion and its effect on myocardial perfusion SPECT images, *J Nucl Med* 34:303-310, 1993.
6. Brooks RA, DiChiro G: Principles of computer assisted tomography (CAT) in radiographic and radioisotopic imaging, *Phys Med Biol* 21:689-732, 1976.
7. Budinger TF, Gullberg GT: Three-dimensional reconstruction in nuclear medicine emission imaging, *IEEE Trans Nucl Sci* 21:2-20, 1974.
8. Buvat I, Rodriguez-Villafuerte M, Todd-Pokropek A, et al: Comparative assessment of nine scatter correction methods based on spectral analysis using Monte Carlo simulations, *J Nucl Med* 36:1476-1488, 1995.
9. Cellar A, Sitek A, Stoub E, et al: Multiple line source array for SPECT transmission scans: simulation, phantom, and patient studies, *J Nucl Med* 39:2183-2189, 1998.
10. Chang LT: A method for attenuation correction in radionuclide computed tomography, *IEEE Trans Nucl Sci* 1:638-643, 1978.
11. Chen J, Caputlu-Wilson SF, Shi H, et al: Automated quality control of emission-transmission misalignment for attenuation correction in myocardial perfusion imaging with SPECT-CT systems, *J Nucl Cardiol* 13(1):43-49, 2006.
12. Chen J, Galt JR, Case JA, et al: Transmission scan truncation with small-field-of-view dedicated cardiac SPECT systems: impact and automated quality control, *J Nucl Cardiol* 12(5):567-573, Sep-Oct 2005.
13. Computer-aided scintillation camera acceptance testing, AAPM Report No. 9, New York, 1981, American Association of Physicists in Medicine, American Institute of Physics.
14. Cooke CD, Garcia EV, Cullom SJ, et al: Determining the accuracy of calculating systolic wall thickening using a fast Fourier transform approximation: a simulation study based on canine and patient data, *J Nucl Med* 35:1185-1192, 1994.
15. Cooke CD, Garcia EV, Folks RD: Three-dimensional visualization of cardiac single photon emission computed tomography studies. In Robb RA, editor: *Visualization in biomedical computing 1992*, SPIE 1808:671-675, 1992.

16. Cooke CD, Garcia EV, Folks RD, et al: Visualization of cardiovascular nuclear medicine tomographic perfusion studies. In *Proceedings of the first conference on visualization in biomedical computing*, Atlanta, 1990, IEEE Press.

17. Corbett JR, McGhie AI, Faber TL: Perfusion defect size and severity using gated SPECT sestamibi: comparison to ungated imaging, *J Nucl Med* 35:115P, 1994 (abstract).

18. DePuey EG: How to detect and avoid myocardial perfusion SPECT artifacts, *J Nucl Med* 35:699-702, 1994.

19. DePuey EG, Bommireddipalli S, Clark J, et al: Wide beam reconstruction "quarter-time" gated myocardial perfusion SPECT functional imaging: a comparison to "full-time" ordered subset expectation maximum, *J Nucl Cardiol* 16(5):736-752, 2009.

20. Depuey EG, Gadiraji R, Clark J, et al: Ordered subset expectation maximization and wide beam reconstruction "half-time" gated myocardial perfusion SPECT imaging: a comparison to "full-time" filtered backprojection, *J Nucl Cardiol* 15:547-563, 2008.

21. DePuey EG, Garcia EV: Optimal specificity of thallium-201 SPECT through recognition of imaging artifacts, *J Nucl Med* 30:441-449, 1989.

22. DePuey EG, Garcia EV, editors: Updated guidelines for nuclear cardiology procedures, part 1, *J Nucl Cardiol* 8:G1-G58, 2001.

23. Eisner R, Churchwell A, Noever T, et al: Quantitative analysis of the thallium-201 myocardial bull's-eye display: critical role of correcting for patient motion, *J Nucl Med* 29:91-97, 1988.

24. Eisner RL, Nowak DJ, Pettigrew RI, et al: Fundamentals of 180° reconstruction in SPECT imaging, *J Nucl Med* 27:1717-1728, 1986.

25. Eisner RL, Schmarkey S, Martin SE, et al: Defects on SPECT "perfusion" images can occur due to abnormal segmental contraction, *J Nucl Med* 35:638-643, 1994.

26. Esquerre JP, Coca FJ, Martinez SJ, et al: Prone decubitus: a solution to inferior wall attenuation in thallium-201 myocardial tomography, *J Nucl Med* 30:398-401, 1989.

27. Evans SG, Hutton BF: Variation in scanning line source sensitivity: a significant source of error in simultaneous emission-transmission tomography, *Eur J Nucl Med Mol Imaging* 31:703-709, 2004.

28. Even-Sapir E, Lerman H, Lievshitz G, et al: Lymphoscintigraphy for sentinel node mapping using a hybrid SPECT/CT system, *J Nucl Med* 44:1413-1420, Sep 2003.

29. Faber T, Cooke C, Folks R, et al: Left ventricular function and perfusion from gated SPECT perfusion images: an integrated method, *J Nucl Med* 40:650-659, 1999.

30. Faber TL, Akers MS, Peshock RM, et al: Three-dimensional motion and perfusion quantification in gated single-photon emission computed tomograms, *J Nucl Med* 32(12):2311-2317, 1991.

31. Faber TL, Cooke CD, Pettigrew RI, et al: Three-dimensional displays of left ventricular epicardial surface from standard cardiac SPECT perfusion quantification techniques, *J Nucl Med* 36:697-703, 1995.

32. Faber TL, Stokely EM, Peshock RM, et al: A model-based four-dimensional left ventricular surface detector, *IEEE Trans Med Imaging* 10:321-329, 1991.

33. Ficaro EP, Fessler JA, Ackermann RJ, et al: Simultaneous transmission-emission thallium-201 cardiac SPECT: effect of attenuation correction on myocardial tracer distribution, *J Nucl Med* 36:921-931, 1995.

34. Floyd CE, Jaszczak RJ, Coleman RE: Scatter detection in SPECT imaging: dependence on source depth, energy, and energy window, *Phys Med Biol* 33:1075-1081, 1988.

35. Frey EC, Ju ZW, Tsui BMW: A fast projector/backprojector pair modeling the asymmetric, spatially varying scatter response function in SPECT imaging, *IEEE Trans Nucl Sci* NS-40:1192-1197, 1993.

36. Frey EC, Tsui BMW: A practical method for incorporating scatter in a projector/backprojector for accurate scatter compensation in SPECT, *IEEE Trans Nucl Sci* NS-40:1007-1016, 1993.

37. Frey EC, Tsui BMW: Modeling the scatter response function in inhomogeneous scattering media for SPECT, *IEEE Trans Nucl Sci* 41:1585-1593, 1994.

38. Fricke E, Fricke H, Weise R, et al: Attenuation correction of myocardial SPECT perfusion images with low-dose CT: evaluation of the method by comparison with perfusion PET, *J Nucl Med* 46(5):736-744, May 2005.

39. Galt JR, Cullom SJ, Garcia EV: SPECT quantification: a simplified method for attenuation correction for cardiac imaging, *J Nucl Med* 33:2232-2237, 1992.

40. Galt JR, Garcia EV, Robbins WL: Effects of myocardial wall thickness on SPECT quantification, *IEEE Trans Med Imaging* 9:144-150, 1990.

41. Galt JR, Hise LH, Garcia EF, et al: Filtering in frequency space, *J Nucl Med Technol* 14:152-162, 1986.

42. Garcia EV, Cooke CD, Van Train KF, et al: Technical aspects of myocardial perfusion SPECT imaging with Tc-99m sestamibi, *Am J Cardiol* 66:23-31E, 1990.

43. Gayed IW, Kim EE, Broussard WF, et al: The value of 99mTc-sestamibi SPECT/CT over conventional SPECT in the evaluation of parathyroid adenomas or hyperplasia, *J Nucl Med* 46:248-252, Feb 2005.

44. Germano G, Chua T, Kiat H, et al: A quantitative phantom analysis of artifacts due to hepatic activity in technetium-99m myocardial perfusion SPECT studies, *J Nucl Med* 35:356-359, 1994.

45. Germano G, Kavanagh PB, Kiat H, et al: Automatic analysis of gated myocardial SPECT: development and initial validation of a method, *J Nucl Med* 35:116P, 1994 (abstract).

46. Germano G, Kavanagh PB, Su HT, et al: Automatic reorientation of three-dimensional transaxial myocardial perfusion SPECT images, *J Nucl Med* 36:1107-1114, 1995.

47. Germano G, Kavanaugh PB, Waechter P, et al: A new algorithm for the quantitation of myocardial perfusion SPECT. I. Technical principles and reproducibility, *J Nucl Med* 41:712-719, 2000.

48. Germano G, Kiat H, Kavanagh PB, et al: Automatic quantification of ejection fraction from gated myocardial perfusion SPECT, *J Nucl Med* 36:2138-2147, 1995.

49. Germano G, Kiat H, Mazzant M, et al: Stress perfusion/stress wall motion with fast (6.7 min) Tc sestamibi myocardial SPECT, *J Nucl Med* 35:81P, 1994 (abstract).

50. Glick SJ, Penney BC, King MA, et al: Noniterative compensation for the distance-dependent detector response and photon attenuation in SPECT imaging, *IEEE Trans Med Imaging* 7:135-148, 1988.

51. Go RT, MacIntyre WJ, Houser TS, et al: Clinical evaluation of 360° and 180° data sampling techniques for transaxial SPECT thallium-201 myocardial perfusion imaging, *J Nucl Med* 26:695-706, 1985.

52. Goris ML, Thompson C, Malone LJ, et al: Modeling the integration of myocardial regional perfusion and function, *Nucl Med Commun* 15:9-20, 1994.

53. Gottschalk SC, Salem D, Lim CB, et al: SPECT resolution and uniformity improvements by noncircular orbit, *J Nucl Med* 24:822-828, 1983.

54. Graham LS: Quality control for SPECT systems, *Radiographics* 15:1471-1481, 1995.

55. Hamann M, Aldridge M, Dickson J, et al: Evaluation of a low-dose/slow-rotating SPECT-CT system, *Phys Med Biol* 53(10):2495-2508, 2008.

56. Hendel RC, Corbett JR, Cullom SJ, et al: The value and practice of attenuation correction for myocardial SPECT imaging: a joint position statement for the American Society of Nuclear Cardiology and the Society of Nuclear Medicine, *J Nucl Cardiol* 9:135-143, 2002.

57. Hoffman EJ: 180° compared to 360° sampling in SPECT, *J Nucl Med* 23:745-746, 1982.

58. Hudson HM, Larkin RS: Accelerated image reconstruction using ordered subsets of projection data, *IEEE Trans Med Imaging* MI-13:601-609, 1994.

59. Hutton BF, Braun M: Software for image registration: algorithms, accuracy, efficacy, *Semin Nucl Med* 33:180-192, July 2003.

60. Hutton BF, Braun M, Thurfjell L, et al: Image registration: an essential tool for nuclear medicine, *Eur J Nucl Med Mol Imaging* 29:559-577, 2002.

61. Ichihara T, Ogawa K, Motomura N, et al: Compton scatter compensation using the triple energy window method for single- and dual-isotope SPECT, *J Nucl Med* 34:2216-2221, 1993.

62. Jaszczak RJ, Greer KL, Floyd CE Jr, et al: Improved SPECT quantification using compensation for scattered photons, *J Nucl Med* 25:893-900, 1984.

63. Kadrmas DJ, Frey EC, Karimi SS, et al: Fast implementations of reconstruction-based scatter compensation in fully 3D SPECT image reconstruction, *Phys Med Biol* 43:857-873, 1998.

64. Kamphuis C, Beekman FJ, Viergever MA: Evaluation of OS-EM vs. ML-EM for LD, 2D and fully 3D SPECT reconstruction, *IEEE Trans Nucl Sci* 43:2018, 1996.

65. Kennedy JA, Israel O, Frenkel A: Directions and magnitudes of misregistration of CT attenuation-corrected myocardial perfusion studies: incidence, impact on image quality, and guidance for reregistration, *J Nucl Med* 50(9):1471-1478, 2009.

66. Keyes JW: SPECT and artifacts: in search of the imaginary lesion, *J Nucl Med* 32:875-877, 1991.

67. King MA, Xia W, DeVries DJ, et al: A Monte Carlo investigation of artifacts caused by liver uptake in single-photon emission computed tomography perfusion imaging with Tc-99m-labeled agents, *J Nucl Cardiol* 3:18-29, 1996.

68. Klein JL, Garcia EV, DePuey EG, et al: Reversibility bull's-eye: a new polar bull's-eye map to quantify reversibility of stress-induced SPECT Tl-201 myocardial perfusion defects, *J Nucl Med* 31:1240-1246, 1990.

69. Knesaurek K, King MA, Glick SJ, et al: Investigation of causes of geometric distortion in 180° and 360° angular sampling in SPECT, *J Nucl Med* 30:1666-1675, 1989.

70. Kuhl DE, Hale J, Eaton WL: Transmission scanning: a useful adjunct to conventional emission scanning for accurately keying isotope deposition to radiographic anatomy, *Radiology* 7:278, 1966.

71. Lalush DS, Tsui BMW: Improving the convergence of iterative filtered backprojection algorithms, *Med Phys* 21:1283-1285, 1994.

72. Lang TF, Hasegawa BH, Liew SC, et al: Description of a prototype emission-transmission computed tomography imaging system, *J Nucl Med* 33:1881-1887, Oct 1992.

73. Lewitt RM, Edholm PR, Xia W: Fourier method for correction of depth-dependent collimator blurring. In SPIE, vol 1092, *Medical Imaging III: image processing*, Newport Beach, Calif, 1989, Society for Photo-optical Instrumental.

74. Maddahi J, Mendez R, Mahmarian JJ, et al: Prospective multicenter evaluation of rapid, gated SPECT myocardial perfusion upright imaging, *J Nucl Cardiol* 16:351-357, 2009.

75. Maniawski PJ, Morgan HT, Wackers FJT: Orbit-related variation in spatial resolution as a source of artifactual defects in thallium-201 SPECT, *J Nucl Med* 32:871-875, 1991.

76. Masood Y, Liu YH, Depuey G, et al: Clinical validation of SPECT attenuation correction using x-ray computed tomography-derived attenuation maps: multicenter clinical trial with angiographic correlation, *J Nucl Cardiol* 12:676-686, 2005.

77. Matsunari I, Boning G, Ziegler SI, et al: Effects of misalignment between transmission and emission scans on attenuation-corrected cardiac SPECT, *J Nucl Med* 39:411-416, 1998.

78. Maublant JC, Peycelon P, Kwiatkowski F, et al: Comparison between 180° and 360° data collection in technetium-99m MIBI SPECT of the myocardium, *J Nucl Med* 30:295-300, 1989.

79. Meikle SR, Hutton BF, Bailey DL: A transmission-dependent method for scatter correction in SPECT, *J Nucl Med* 35:360-367, 1994.

80. Metz CE, Atkins FB, Beck RN: The geometric transfer function component for scintillation camera collimators with straight parallel holes, *Phys Med Biol* 25(6):1059-1070, 1980.

81. Miller TR, Wallis JW, Sampathkumaran KS: Three-dimensional display of gated cardiac blood-pool studies, *J Nucl Med* 30:2036-2041, 1989.

82. Mukai T, Links JM, Douglass KH, et al: Scatter correction in SPECT using nonuniform attenuation data, *Phys Med Biol* 33:1129-1140, 1988.

83. Mullick R, Ezquerra NF: Automatic determination of left ventricular orientation from SPECT data, *IEEE Trans Med Imaging* 14:88-99, 1995.

84. Narayanan MV, King MA, Pretorius H, et al: Human-observer receiver-operating-characteristic evaluation of attenuation, scatter, and resolution compensation strategies for 99mTc myocardial perfusion imaging, *J Nucl Med* 44:1725-1734, 2003.

85. Nichols KJ, Galt JR: Quality control for SPECT imaging. In DePuey EG, Garcia EV, Berman DS, editors: *Cardiac SPECT imaging*, Philadelphia, 2001, Lippincott Williams & Wilkins.

86. Nuyts J, DuPont P, Van den Maegdenbergh V, et al: A study of the liver-heart artifact in emission tomography, *J Nucl Med* 36:133-139, 1995.

87. Oykesiku NM, Halkar RK, Galt JR, et al: SPECT/CT of folatescan (Tc-99m EC20) in pituitary tumors: a novel imaging tracer and technique, *J Nucl Med* 45:368P, 2004.

88. Pan X, Metz CE, Chen CT: Noniterative methods and their noise characteristics in 2D SPECT image reconstruction, *IEEE Trans Nucl Sci* 44:1388-1397, 1997.

89. Patton JA, Delbeke D, Sandler MP: Image fusion using an integrated, dual-head coincidence camera with x-ray tube–based attenuation maps, *J Nucl Med* 41:1364-1368, 2000.

90. Performance measurements of scintillation cameras, NEMA Standards Publication NU1–1994, Washington, DC, 2001, National Electrical Manufacturers Association.

91. Pfannenberg AC, Eschmann SM, Horger M, et al: Benefit of anatomical-functional image fusion in the diagnostic work-up of neuroendocrine neoplasms, *Eur J Nucl Med Mol Imaging* 30:835-843, 2003.

92. Quaife RA, Faber TL, Corbett JR: Visual assessment of quantitative three-dimensional displays of stress thallium-201 tomograms: comparison with visual multislice analysis, *J Nucl Med* 32:1006, 1991.

93. Rigo P, Van Boxem PH, Safi JF, et al: Quantitative evaluation of a comprehensive motion, resolution, and attenuation correction program: initial experience, *J Nucl Cardiol* 5:458-468, 1998.

94. Rotating scintillation camera SPECT acceptance testing and quality control, AAPM Report No. 22, New York, 1987,

American Association of Physicists in Medicine, American Institute of Physics.

95. Ruf J, Lehmkuhl L, Bertram H, et al: Impact of SPECT and integrated low-dose CT after radioiodine therapy on the management of patients with thyroid carcinoma, *Nucl Med Commun* 25:1177-1182, 2004.

96. Santana CA, Garcia EV, Vansant JP, et al: Three-dimensional color-modulated display of myocardial SPECT perfusion distributions accurately assesses coronary artery disease, *J Nucl Med* 41:1941-1946, 2000.

97. Schillaci O, Danieli R, Manni C, et al: Is SPECT/CT with a hybrid camera useful to improve scintigraphic imaging interpretation? *Nucl Med Commun* 25:705-710, 2004.

98. Scintillation camera acceptance testing and performance evaluation, AAPM Report No. 6, New York, 1980, American Association of Physicists in Medicine, American Institute of Physics.

99. Sheehan FH, Bolson EL, Dodge HT, et al: Advantages and applications of the centerline method for characterizing region ventricular function, *Circulation* 74:293-305, 1986.

100. Shepp LA, Vardi Y: Maximum likelihood reconstruction for emission tomography, *IEEE Trans Med Imaging* 1:113-122, 1982.

101. Slomka PJ, Hurwitz GA, Stephenson J, et al: Automated alignment and sizing of myocardial stress and rest scans to three-dimensional normal templates using an image registration algorithm, *J Nucl Med* 36:1115-1122, 1995.

102. Snyder DL, Miller MI, Thomas LJ Jr, et al: Noise and edge artifacts in maximum-likelihood reconstructions for emission tomography, *IEEE Trans Med Imaging* MI-6:228-238, 1987.

103. Soares EJ, Byrne CL, Glick SJ, et al: Implementation and evaluation of an analytical solution to the photon attenuation and nonstationary resolution reconstruction problem in SPECT, *IEEE Trans Nucl Sci* NS-40:1231-1237, 1993.

104. *Society of Nuclear Medicine procedure guidelines manual 2001*, Reston, Va, 2001, Society of Nuclear Medicine.

105. Sorenson JA: Quantitative measurement of radioactivity in vivo by whole body counting. In Hine JH, Sorenson JA, editors: *Instrumentation in nuclear medicine*, ed 2, New York, 1974, Academic Press.

106. Sorenson SA, Phelps ME: *Physics in nuclear medicine*, ed 3, Philadelphia, 1987, Saunders.

107. Sowards-Emmerd D, Vesel J, Shao L, et al: Flat panel X-ray detector based SPECT/CT, *J Nucl Med* 50(Suppl 2):415, 2009 (abstract).

108. Tan P, Bailey DL, Meikle SR, et al: A scanning line source for simultaneous emission and transmission measurements in SPECT, *J Nucl Med* 34:1752-1760, 1993.

109. Tonge CM, Manoharan M, Lawson RS, et al: Attenuation correction of myocardial SPECT studies using low resolution computed tomography images, *Nucl Med Commun* 26:231-237, March 2005.

110. Tsui BMW, Frey EC, LaCroix KJ, et al: Quantitative myocardial perfusion SPECT, *J Nucl Cardiol* 5:507-522, 1998.

111. Tsui BMW, Frey EC, Zhao X, et al: The importance and implementation of accurate 3D methods for quantitative SPECT, *Phys Med Biol* 39:509-530, 1994.

112. Tsui BMW, Gullberg GT: The geometric transfer function for cone and fan beam collimators, *Phys Med Biol* 35(1):81-93, 1990.

113. Tsui BMW, Gullberg GT, Edgerton ER, et al: Correction of nonuniform attenuation in cardiac SPECT imaging, *J Nucl Med* 30:497-507, 1989.

114. Tsui BMW, Hu GB, Gilland DR: Implementation of simultaneous attenuation and detector response correction in SPECT, *IEEE Trans Nucl Sci* 35:778-783, 1988.

115. Tsui BMW, Zhao X, Frey E, et al: Comparison between ML-EM and WLS-CG algorithms for SPECT image reconstruction, *IEEE Trans Med Imaging* 38:1766-1772, 1991.

116. Tung CH, Gullberg GT, Zeng GL, et al: Nonuniform attenuation correction using simultaneous transmission and emission converging tomography, *IEEE Trans Nucl Sci* 39:1134-1143, 1992.

117. Utsunomiya D, Shiraishi S, Imuta M, et al: Added value of SPECT/CT fusion in assessing suspected bone metastasis: comparison with scintigraphy alone and nonfused scintigraphy and CT, *Radiology* 238:264-271, 2006.

118. Utsunomiya D, Tomiguchi S, Shiraishi S, et al: Initial experience with X-ray CT based attenuation correction in myocardial perfusion SPECT imaging using a combined SPECT/CT system, *Ann Nucl Med* 19:485-489, 2005.

119. Van Train KF, Areeda J, Garcia EV, et al: Quantitative same-day rest-stress technetium-99m sestamibi SPECT: definition and validation of stress normal limits and criteria for abnormality, *J Nucl Med* 34:1494-1502, 1993.

120. Van Train KF, Silagan G, Germano G, et al: Noncircular versus circular orbits in quantitative analysis of myocardial perfusion SPECT, *J Nucl Med* 36:46P, 1995 (abstract).

121. Venero CV, Heller GV, Bateman TM, et al: A multicenter evaluation of a new post-processing method with depth-dependent collimator resolution applied to full-time and half-time acquisitions without and with simultaneously acquired attenuation correction, *J Nucl Cardiol* 16(5):714-725, 2009.

122. Wallis JW, Miller TR: Three-dimensional display in nuclear medicine and radiology, *J Nucl Med* 32:534-546, 1991.

123. Wallis JW, Miller TR: Volume rendering in three-dimensional display of SPECT images, *J Nucl Med* 31:1421-1430, 1990.

124. Welch A, Gullberg GT, Christian PE, et al: A transmission map–based scatter correction technique for SPECT in inhomogeneous media, *Med Phys* 22:1627-1635, 1995.

125. Ye J, Cullom SJ, Kearfott KK, et al: Simultaneous attenuation and depth-dependent resolution compensation for 180° myocardial perfusion SPECT. Proceedings of the Medical Imaging Conference, *IEEE Trans Nucl Sci* 39:1056-1058, 1992.

126. Ye J, Liang Z, Harrington DP: Quantitative reconstruction for myocardial perfusion SPECT: an efficient approach by depth-dependent deconvolution and matrix rotation, *Phys Med Biol* 39:1263-1279, 1994.

127. Younes RB, Mas J, Pousse A, et al: Introducing simultaneous spatial resolution and attenuation correction after scatter removal in SPECT imaging, *Nucl Med Commun* 12:1031-1043, 1991.

128. Zaidi H, Hasegawa B: Determination of the attenuation map in emission tomography, *J Nucl Med* 44:291-315, 2003.

129. Zeng GL, Gullberg GT, Tsui BMW, et al: Three-dimensional iterative reconstruction with attenuation and geometric point response correction, *IEEE Trans Nucl Sci* 38:693-702, 1991.

PET Instrumentation

Paul E. Christian

OBJECTIVES

After completing this chapter, the reader will be able to:
- Describe positron decay and the production of annihilation photons.
- List positron-emitting radionuclides and their properties.
- List detector crystals that can be used for PET imaging and describe their properties.
- Explain the fundamental operation of dedicated PET scanners and their design.
- Discuss the advantages of a PET/CT scanning as a multimodality study.
- Describe the detection of true, scatter, and random events.
- Describe transmission imaging and its need and use in attenuation-correcting PET images.
- Characterize the visual presentation of nonattenuated and attenuation-corrected images.
- Define SUV and explain how it is calculated and used; discuss critical elements in generating quantitative measurements.

- Describe the process of storing reconstructed data in sinograms and reconstruction methods.
- List calibrations required of dedicated PET scanners.
- Discuss 2D and 3D imaging and the advantages and disadvantages of each.
- Describe how PET scanners acquire and store data.
- Describe the principles of time of flight.
- Discuss the advantages and disadvantages of time of flight PET.
- Discuss reconstruction of PET images.
- Describe attenuation correction techniques in PET.
- Discuss the implications of image fusion of PET with CT or MRI.
- Discuss the safe handling of PET radiopharmaceuticals to maintain ALARA principles.

Positron emission tomography (PET) is a powerful technique to image biochemical or physiological processes within the body. The metabolic and biological activity of disease always precedes any anatomic evidence of the illness. PET as a biological imaging technique does not replace anatomical imaging but adds the characterization of simple molecular processes that are taking place in normal or diseased tissues within the body. X-ray, computed tomography (CT), or magnetic resonance imaging (MRI) may see the anatomical defect, but PET as a molecular analysis adds information about the chemical activity of normal and abnormal tissue. Very short-lived positron-emitting forms of some of the most common organic elements (^{11}C, ^{13}N, and ^{15}O) can be used to study the most basic and fundamental biochemical reactions. These radionuclides, along with fluorine-18, represent the core of PET tracers that can be used to study the interaction of elementary chemical processes of all life, such as $^{15}O_2$, $H_2^{15}O$, $C^{15}O_2$, and ^{18}F-labeled glucose (sugar) (Table 10-1). More than 4000 different chemical compounds have already been radiolabeled with PET tracers and have been used to image molecular processes.

About 10 years ago, PET moved rapidly from a well-established research tool into routine clinical practice. Payment approval by Medicare and private insurance companies for PET imaging in some diseases relating to oncology, cardiology, and brain imaging has cleared the way for the expanded use of this powerful modality and made it more available to physicians and patients. The availability of PET radiotracers through commercial distribution networks has also allowed hospitals and clinics to add PET as a new service and has promoted the expansion of independent outpatient imaging centers and mobile PET imaging services.

The basic scientific principles of PET (i.e., physics, radiochemistry, scintillation detectors) have been discussed in earlier chapters. This chapter focuses on how these science fundamentals are brought together specifically for imaging positron-emitting radionuclides. Clinical applications of PET to brain and heart imaging are discussed in the respective organ system chapters. The application of PET in oncology is discussed in Chapter 13.

PHYSICS OF POSITRONS

In 1927, P.A.M. Dirac theorized the existence of the **positron** (positively charged electron) as an antiparticle of the negatron (negatively charged electron). The existence of the positron was later confirmed experimentally by Carl D. Anderson in 1932. Proton-rich nuclei decay by either electron capture or positron emission. These alternative decay pathways may exist in the same nuclei and be alternate forms of decay in some atoms, such as in naturally occurring potassium-40. In many of the radionuclides used for PET imaging, most decay pathways are predominantly positron emission.

When a positron is expelled from the nucleus of an atom, it travels only a short distance. During this travel across several millimeters, adjacent atoms are ionized and the positron loses energy and slows down. The positron then pairs up with an electron, and these two particles spiral in toward each other, forming a two-particle atom called a *positronium* for a tiny fraction of a second (Figure 10-1). When the antiparticle positron/electron pair interact, they annihilate each other, and the rest mass of each particle is completely converted into energy according to Albert Einstein's equation $E = mc^2$. Because the rest masses of the positron and the electron are exactly the same, the **annihilation** process converts the mass of each particle into pure electromagnetic energy

TABLE 10-1	Positron Radionuclides for PET		
Radionuclide	Half-Life	Maximum Range (mm)	Mean Range (mm)
^{11}C	20.38 min	5.0	0.3
^{13}N	9.96 min	5.4	1.4
^{15}O	2.03 min	8.2	1.5
^{18}F	109.75 min	2.4	0.2
^{82}Rb	75 sec	15.6	2.6

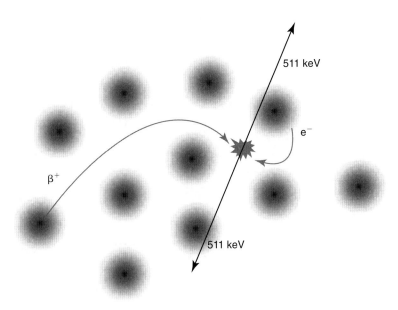

FIGURE 10-1 When the positron is emitted from the nucleus, it travels a few millimeters and ionizes many atoms before pairing with an electron and undergoing an annihilation interaction, which produces a pair of 511-keV annihilation photons that travel in opposite directions.

(511 keV from each particle). Therefore a pair of 511-keV **annihilation photons** is produced, with the photons being emitted in nearly opposite directions, 180 ± ~0.3 degrees apart. The minor variation from exactly 180 degrees apart is due to the motion of the particles at the time when the annihilation event occurs. Because the annihilation photons are not absolutely linear in their opposing directions this small angular variation is referred to as **non-colinearity.**

Each PET radionuclide emits its positron with a different energy, higher-energy particles having greater path lengths and greater mean ranges for the travel of the positron. Table 10-1 lists the maximum and the mean ranges of some of the most useful PET radionuclides, along with the half-life of each. In those PET radionuclides that have very large mean ranges, the positron may travel a distance of a few millimeters before the annihilation event occurs. This large particle range results in a slight mispositioning of the annihilation event from the actual location of the positron-emitting atom. Therefore a scan performed with ^{18}F (2.4-mm maximum and 0.2-mm average range) will produce a higher-resolution image than ^{82}Rb, which has a 15.6-mm maximum and 2.6-mm mean range in tissue.

PRODUCTION OF PET RADIOTRACERS

Positrons are emitted by proton-rich nuclei, therefore to manufacture positron-emitting radionuclides requires a device that can add protons to the nucleus. Small linear accelerators or cyclotrons provide a source of positively charged protons or deuterons of an appropriate energy to create these nuclei. Small medical cyclotrons are typically used for producing PET radiopharmaceuticals. Chapter 6 discusses both cyclotrons and the production

of PET radiopharmaceuticals (see Figures 6-3 and 6-4 for a diagram and photograph of a cyclotron). A cyclotron costs about $2 million to $3 million and must be accompanied by a radiochemistry laboratory that can manufacture the short-lived positron emitters such as ^{18}F, ^{11}C, ^{13}N, and ^{15}O. Fluorine-18 is the only one of these that has a half-life long enough (109.75 minutes) to be transported any substantial distance from the cyclotron. Therefore radiotracers ^{11}C, ^{13}N, and ^{15}O must be imaged using a scanner that is in the same facility where the cyclotron is located. At this time there are only two fluorine-18–labeled compounds approved for general distribution by the U.S. Food and Drug Administration (FDA), ^{18}F-fluorodeoxyglucose (^{18}F-FDG) and ^{18}F–sodium fluoride for bone imaging (however, ^{18}F–sodium fluoride scans are not reimbursed by Medicare or most other insurance providers at the time of this publication). ^{18}F-FDG can be shipped by ground or air transportation within a distance of a few hundred miles. Most oncology studies are performed using ^{18}F-FDG.

Generator-produced rubidium-82 is FDA approved, and is used by several dozen centers in the United States. Rubidium-82, which has a 75-second half-life, is an analog of potassium and is therefore a myocardial perfusion imaging agent. These generators are rather expensive and can only be afforded by those sites that can guarantee several myocardial perfusion studies every day. Since PET scanners have higher sensitivity and resolution than SPECT and therefore PET myocardial images provide substantially better quality with increased sensitivity and specificity for detecting coronary artery disease.

PET radiotracers that are produced on-site and those obtained from commercial PET radiopharmaceutical companies must be produced according to pharmaceutical current Good Manufacturing Practices (GMP) and

TABLE 10-2	Scintillation Detector Properties				
	NaI(Tl)	BGO	GSO	LSO	LYSO
Density (g/cm³)	3.7	7.1	6.7	7.4	7.4
Effective atomic number	51	75	59	71	66
Emission intensity (relative to NaI[Tl])	100	15	25	75	80
Decay time (ns)	230	300	30-45	40	40
Hygroscopic	Yes	No	No	No	No

BGO, Bismuth germinate; *GSO,* gadolinium orthosilicate; *LSO,* lutetium orthosilicate; *LYSO,* cerium doped lutetium yttrium orthosilicate; *NaI(Tl),* thallium-doped sodium iodide.

according to FDA and *United States Pharmacopeia (USP)* standards. Quality control (QC) of these radiotracers must be performed as with any radiopharmaceutical. The production of a single PET radiopharmaceutical requires very expensive equipment, including the cyclotron, target, automated synthesis module, hot cell (to contain the synthesis module), and any additional radiopharmaceutical QC and precursor preparation equipment.

PET RADIATION DETECTORS

Detecting 511-keV coincidence photons in PET would be most ideal if the scintillation material had a high density to stop the high-energy photons. Ideally, the material should also be a very efficient scintillator and create a large amount of light that would be released from the crystal very quickly. Most scintillation crystals lack at least one of these ideal attributes at 511 keV. However, several materials are efficient at high photon energy, some of which are listed in Table 10-2. The critical issue is to stop the annihilation photons and thus detect the radiation. Many PET scanners produced in the 1980s and 1990s and some still being produced today use **bismuth germinate** ($Bi_4Ge_3O_{12}$) or, as it is commonly known, **BGO.** Bismuth has a high atomic number and is therefore very good at stopping the 511-keV photons. Bismuth germinate is unfortunately a relatively slow scintillator and also yields a relatively small amount of light compared with NaI(Tl). In addition, BGO has poor energy resolution that requires energy windows that span from about 350 to 650 keV. The high stopping power of BGO compensates for its other deficiencies and is still a good scintillator for two-dimensional (2D) dedicated PET scanners.

Some dedicated PET scanners use other scintillation crystal materials. **Lutetium orthosilicate** (Lu_2SiO_5 [Ce] or **LSO**), cerium doped **lutetium yttrium orthosilicate** (**LYSO**), and **gadolinium orthosilicate** (Gd_2SiO_5 [Ce] or **GSO**) are used in some commercial PET systems. These crystals have slightly lower stopping power than BGO (see Table 10-2) but produce much more light per keV of detected photon energy than BGO. However, the main reason that these materials are used is that they are faster scintillators (see Table 10-2). Because the positron is identified by the coincidence detection of the photons on opposite detectors, faster materials are desired. Scanners using the fast scintillators—LSO, LYSO, or GSO—have been designed to operate only in three-dimensional (3D) acquisition mode in order to provide higher system sensitivity.

A 511-keV photon travels across the detector ring in about 3 ns. Slow scintillator materials will not allow the precise temporal measurement of simultaneous event detection. Thus very fast, light-emitting crystals provide more exact time measurements of simultaneous event detection.

PET SCANNER DESIGN

PET imaging requires the placement of detectors on opposite sides of the patient in order to simultaneously detect the coincidence photons produced by the annihilation process. PET scanners therefore have "electronic collimation" to determine the location of the annihilation event. The detectors used for coincidence detection identify an annihilation photon pair and determine a **line of response** (**LOR**) path representing the path of the photon pair (Figure 10-2).

PET scanners use detector materials made of BGO, LSO, LYSO, and GSO, which are configured as rectangular cube-shaped crystals about 4 mm in width and 10 to 30 mm in length. PET scanners have 10,000 to 28,000 or more of these crystals, which are laid out to form several rings of detectors. Each crystal is too small to have its own photomultiplier tube (PMT); therefore a group of crystals is put together in a detector block. Most commonly, four PMTs are used on a block to collect the light from all the crystals, measure the photon energy, and identify which crystal in the block was struck by the photon. These multicrystal blocks are typically constructed in one of two ways: as a "cut block" or as a reflective block of crystals. A cut block design is created from one larger crystal as shown in Figure 10-3, *A*, with cuts that are made at different depths through the crystal that allow the reflected scintillation photons to be distributed in a specified pattern over the four PMTs. The PMTs' signal outputs can then determine which of the

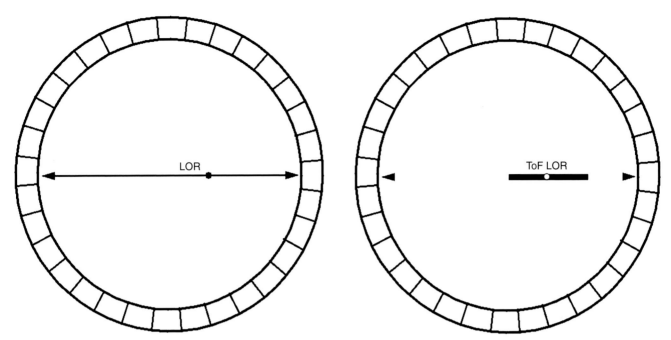

FIGURE 10-2 Detection of the annihilation photon pair in a ring of detectors defines the line of response (LOR), which defines a line through the decay event location. The exact location of the event along the line is not known; however, reconstruction of many LORs from different detectors will determine the location. Time of flight (ToF) timing resolution is available on some commercially available scanners. New fast scintillation detectors allow a region between two detectors to identify that the decay event occurred within a several centimeter segment of an LOR, which improves system performance.

crystal elements in the block detected the radiation. The alternative reflective block approach is to create a block from a group of small individual crystals (see Figure 10-3, *B*); each crystal is surrounded by a carefully designed amount of reflective material that spreads the light in a designated pattern onto the PMTs. Therefore both the cut block and reflective block designs do the same thing, namely, use reflective surfaces on the sides of individual crystals to distribute the scintillation photons to the PMTs.

The four PMTs are used to detect the scintillation light, and the output signals identify which crystal has detected the event using pulse strength information, similar to the Anger camera positioning circuitry. The output from the array of four PMTs—*A, B, C,* and *D* (Figure 10-4)—is used to calculate the transverse location *x*- and *z*-axis location of the event within the detector block by $x = (B + D)/(A + B + C + D)$ and $z = (C + D)/(A + B + C + D)$. The output from a 6×6 crystal detector block is shown in Figure 10-5. Crystal centers are shown by the curved contour lines for 36 crystals in this example of a reflective design detector block, and straight lines show the edges of the regions that define the effective crystal boundaries. Software can be used to adjust these boundaries that define each crystal. Several detector blocks are combined to form detector "buckets" or "modules." Dozens of these modules or buckets form rings of detectors around the patient (Figure 10-6). Each block of crystal/PMT assemblies forms this series of rings

of detectors, and each ring acquires one image slice from the patient.

PET scanners (Figure 10-7) typically have 18 to 40 or more consecutive rings of crystals and create a **field of view (FOV)** along the long axis of the patient for about 15-20 cm. Images of small organs, such as the heart or brain, may be acquired with a single bed position of the patient within the scanner. However, the possibility of distant metastases in cancer patients requires that a large area of the body be imaged. Whole-body PET scans are used in most oncology studies, which actually only cover from the hips up through the base of the brain (approximately 100 cm) or about eight or more bed positions. Total-body (nearly head to toe) scans are required with certain types of cancer where malignant tissue may grow in any area of the body, as with melanoma. In this case the number of bed positions will be increased to cover the total body area—10 or more bed positions. Scans of the whole body or total body are obtained by moving the imaging table many times to cover the desired length over the body, and the total time for data acquisition is 30 to 60 minutes.

One drawback with BGO systems is the relatively poor energy resolution of this crystal compared with NaI(Tl), LSO, LYSO, or GSO. With poorer energy resolution, the energy window when using BGO must be set somewhat wide. With most scintillation materials, a narrow energy window is effective at rejecting scattered photons, which will have a lower energy. The wide energy window employed with BGO is thereby not very efficient at rejecting scattered photons, and a method for scatter correction will be used during reconstruction.

PET scanners that use several adjacent detector blocks to create many rings have an FOV of only about 15-20 cm of active detectors that must be used over a single area of the body. One FOV must be large enough that the brain or heart may be completely viewed at one time. Whole-body studies require that the table move the patient many times to acquire data that is adjacent or overlapping in the case of 3D whole-body imaging in order to cover the entire area of interest in one study.

COINCIDENCE DETECTION: TRUE, SCATTER, AND RANDOM EVENTS

PET imaging is based on the detection of the annihilation pair of 511-keV photons. These photons are detected virtually simultaneously from scintillation detectors that are positioned on opposing sides of the patient. The 511-keV photons should arrive within a very short time of one another, which in theory should ensure that the photons are from the same annihilation event. A coincidence timing window allows the detection of the PMT electrical signals from the photon pair within the preset timing window, typically between 4 and 12 ns. Faster scintillators use the shorter timing windows, which may be required in full 3D whole-body acquisition. Using a shorter timing window allows the acceptance of random events to be reduced, thus improving the quality of the acquired raw data.

Electromagnetic radiation travels 30 cm/ns, so the coincidence timing window setting must allow time for the light to be released from the crystal, for the electronic pulse to build up in the PMT, for the pulse to reach the electronic circuits, and for the circuit to respond. Some systems are able to use the characteristics of new, faster crystals (LSO, LYSO, and GSO) or other scintillators yet to be developed that will have subnanosecond processing times.

A pair of annihilation photons striking two detectors at the same time is termed a **true count** or *true coincidence* annihilation event (Figure 10-8, *A* and *D*). When two atoms decay at nearly the same time, photons from two different annihilation events may be detected within the timing window. When this happens, a false event, referred to as a *"random"* event, is recorded (see Figure 10-8, *C* and *F*), and its false LOR is shown as a dotted line on the diagram. Because many atoms are decaying at nearly the same time, random events cannot be avoided. Processing software estimates these false events

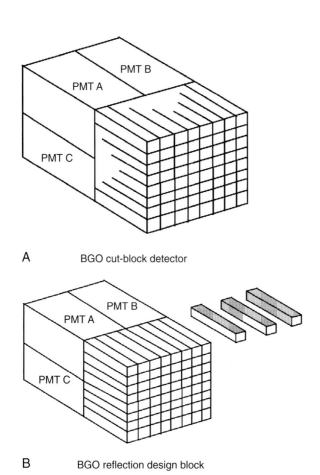

A   BGO cut-block detector

B   BGO reflection design block

FIGURE 10-3 A, A cut-block detector formed from one crystal with partial cuts to create the effect of many small crystals. The cuts form reflective surfaces to reflect light to four photomultiplier tubes (PMTs). **B,** A reflection design block is made from small individual crystals, each wrapped with a certain amount of light reflector to distribute the light to the four PMTs. Both block designs accomplish the same reflective distribution of light to four PMTs that can then determine which crystal element within the block detected the scintillation event. *BGO,* Bismuth germinate.

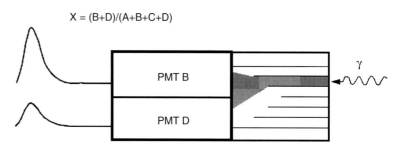

FIGURE 10-4 Light from a scintillation event in a single crystal element is distributed by the reflective surfaces onto the photomultiplier tubes (PMTs) in a specific pattern. Analysis of the pulse strength from each PMT is used to determine the *x* or *y* location of the photon.

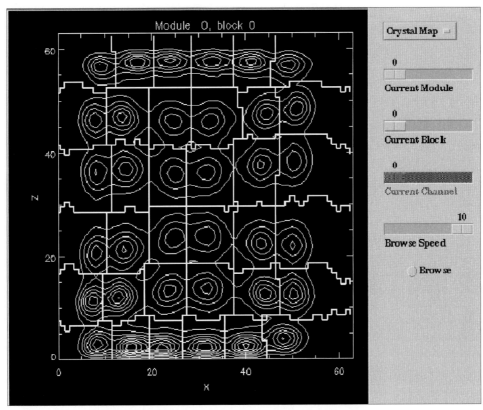

FIGURE 10-5 The output map from each crystal in a block is shown on the computer display as circular patterns of light intensity from each crystal in the detector block. Automated computer software shows the overlying linear pattern that defines the effective location of each crystal and balances the sensitivity of each crystal element.

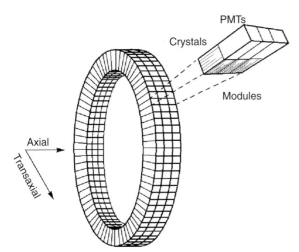

FIGURE 10-6 Detector blocks, or modules, are used to construct a ring of detectors around the patient. Hundreds of blocks are used to create 18 to 40 consecutive rings of detectors that form a cylindrical field of view about 5 cm long and that can acquire many slices of coincidence data at one time.

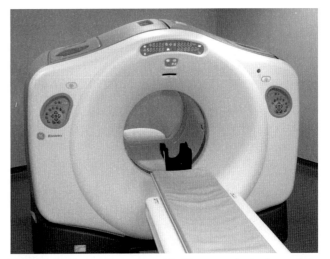

FIGURE 10-7 PET/CT scanner with CT scanner in the front of the gantry and PET scanner behind allow anatomical (CT) and metabolic PET images to be acquired in a study without repositioning the patient. The CT scan is performed first followed by the PET acquisition.

and applies corrections during reconstruction. **Random count** rates are also higher when there is more activity present or when the scanner is in 3D mode. In certain clinical situations, such as where there is a hot source of radioactivity just outside the scanner FOV (e.g., brain,

bladder, tumor, injection site), the random events may be 50% of all coincidence events detected. Without correction the image will have very low contrast of true hot lesions, and some tumors may be missed. A common way to estimate the random events' contribution is to

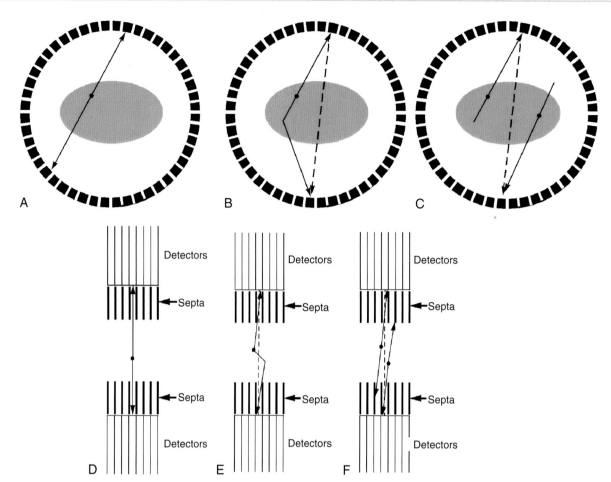

FIGURE 10-8 True coincidence detections are depicted in the left diagrams (**A** shows transaxial event, whereas **D** shows axial interactions). Scattered photons (**B, E**) also create a false location of the coincidence *(dotted line)* by misdirecting photons to a false location. Random events (**C, F**) occur when two disintegrations happen within the timing window and one photon from each creates a false coincidence.

collect and subtract data from a "delayed event" timing window (>12 ns) and to use this information as a measure for random events correction. Using data from the long timing window ensures that all events with this delay are random events, and a fairly accurate correction may be made. Additional techniques may also be available on some systems.

Another mispositioning error of PET data comes from the scatter of annihilation photons between their origin and the detectors (see Figure 10-8, *B* and *E*). Normally, nuclear medicine imaging reduces scatter in the image by selecting a relatively narrow energy window, which eliminates the detection of the scattered photons. However, BGO has relatively poor energy resolution, and the energy window is rather wide; therefore a narrow energy window technique is impractical. Scatter is always present in clinical imaging, representing about 15% of data in 2D mode, and reconstructed images will require correction. The original 2D scanner design used septa between detector rings to aid in reducing both the scatter and random events fraction of events. Scanner manufacturers provide various techniques that are employed in factory-set reconstruction algorithms to either estimate

or mathematically model scatter and correct for it during image reconstruction. Scatter correction is very important in 3D imaging, particularly when hot organs are nearby or just outside the FOV of the detectors. Approximately 50% of photons scatter within the body. Therefore scatter correction and accurate **attenuation correction** are imperative when quantitative information is needed.

Scatter is affected by the distribution of radioactivity, size, and density of the object or objects and their locations relative to the detectors. Scatter cannot be measured directly, but various estimates and mathematical models may be used for estimated corrections, with various techniques for 2D or 3D mode acquisition. The most accurate techniques may look at the pair of emission and transmission slices and adjust the model to the size and activity distribution within the patient. Complex scatter corrections are based on estimating the scattering physics within the emission and transmission images but may be computationally intense and require a longer time to reconstruct slices. However, reasonable estimates for scatter correction are provided in the manufacturer's reconstruction software.

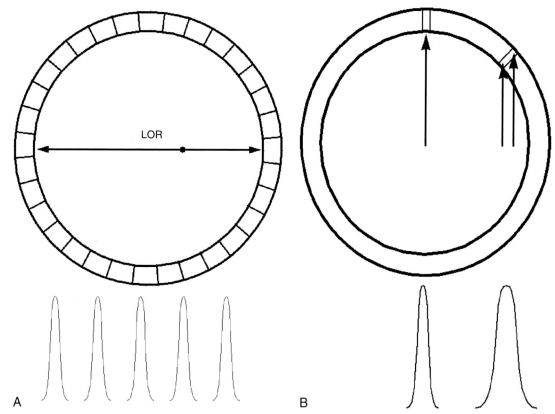

FIGURE 10-9 A, Pair of gamma rays creates a coincidence detection that represents a line of response (LOR). Resolution is limited only by the size of the detectors, as shown by the equal full width at half maximum (FWHM) curves below. **B,** Axial resolution degrades at the edges of the field of view because of variations in the depth of interactions that can occur. Therefore sources of radioactivity near the edge of the gantry ring have poorer resolution (wider FWHM) than sources at the center.

Correction techniques may also be employed for the dead time loss, particularly in 3D mode where accurate compensation for count rate losses is important because count rates are very high, and dead time losses become a measurable and significant fraction of all counts. It is important to remember that scatter and random events are a 3D effect as demonstrated in the lower diagrams of Figure 10-8, *D* to *F*. Random events, scatter, and dead time corrections should be a routine part of the image correction and reconstruction process.

DATA ACQUISITION

The detection of an annihilation photon pair by opposing crystals creates one event or LOR between two detectors. Millions of these LORs will be acquired and stored for use in the reconstruction of the 3D distribution of radiotracer. If two photons are from the same annihilation interaction, they should be detected by opposing crystals at about the same instant. As mentioned previously, the coincidence circuit sets a narrow timing window to ensure that accepted pulse pairs are detected within about 4 to 12 ns or less. Data acquisition may also include acquisition of delayed events (those that are definitely random events), using the delayed timing window. Faster scintillating crystals may allow the use of shorter coincidence timing windows, which will reduce the random events fraction.

Spatial resolution of PET scanners is determined primarily by the size of the crystals and their separation. The spatial resolution of PET images will therefore be very close to the size of the crystal, typically 3 to 5 mm. Thus since all of the crystals are identical the full width at half maximum (FWHM) will be about the same resolution over the diameter of the ring (Figure 10-9, *A*), and therefore the resolution of dedicated PET is significantly better than that of SPECT (about 4 mm reconstructed resolution for PET and >12 mm for SPECT). With a large number of crystals and hundreds of independently operating PMTs, the count rate capability of the PET scanner is significantly higher than that of scintillation cameras. On gamma cameras, collimators have an efficiency that is a tiny fraction of 1%, that is, only a very few photons are detected for thousands of atoms decaying in the patient. Ring PET systems are not limited by multihole collimators, and about 1.5% to 2% of all photons produced in the patient are detected by the PET scanner. The PET scanner is therefore about 50 to 100 times more sensitive than the gamma camera, which produces higher quality than SPECT. In addition, the higher sensitivity for detecting events, much higher count-rate capability, better resolution (independent of depth), and many more counts in the study give PET the highest-resolution and highest–count density images in all of tracer imaging. PET scans are produced from many dozens of millions of events. The higher–spatial resolution images will be possible only when very high data density is obtained. Some new scanner systems may have software options that correct for depth of interaction blurring by applying a point spread function correction. Some vendors refer to these corrections has high definition (HD) imaging.

As previously mentioned, PET information is acquired by recording LORs between two individual crystals as coincidence photons are detected. As shown in Figure 10-9, *A*, the spatial resolution measured in FWHM will have about the same value as the dimension of an individual pixel and will have similar resolution all the way across the detector ring. However, as shown in Figure 10-9, *B*, the resolution near the edge of the ring will be slightly worse because of the thickness of the crystal and the possibility for the event to be detected at different depths within that crystal.

The crystals in a ring scanner detect coincidence LORs over a wide angle of almost 90 degrees, so meaningful information is obtained over a fan-shaped region of the ring (Figure 10-10, *A*). The top crystal of the ring therefore has a 90-degree angle of sensitivity for radiation detection. Each crystal around the ring creates a different fan-shaped sensitivity pattern of LORs (see Figure 10-10, *B* and *C*). Therefore angular sampling around the gantry takes data from the patient from many very small angles to produce high-resolution and high–data density images. Line-of-response data acquired from the thousands of crystals are sorted into lines of response that are parallel and thus form projection information as shown in Figure 10-11. Once the raw LOR data are reformatted to form projection data from each angle, the result can be thought of as being similar to SPECT raw projection count profiles.

For each slice the count profiles may be taken from each projection angle and laid out to form a **sinogram** (Figure 10-12). Each horizontal row in the sinogram represents the count profile (or projection) across the distance of the gantry as seen from each angle. The vertical axis of the sinogram is the angle from which the projection is taken over 180 degrees. Projection information from the next 180 degrees around the object is not needed, because it is a repeat of the information from the first 180 degrees. The sinogram will therefore contain all the data that will be needed to reconstruct one transaxial slice; hence a sinogram is needed for each slice in the image volume. Reconstruction of a transaxial slice will therefore be somewhat similar to reconstructing SPECT; both are projections at various angles. Viewing sinogram data is sometimes helpful in identifying that data were adequately received from all detectors.

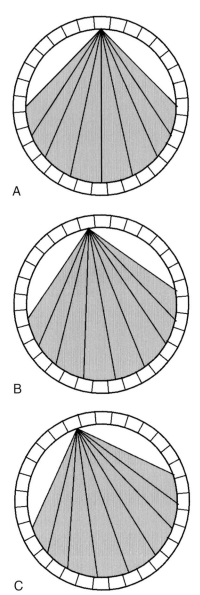

FIGURE 10-10 Each detector is limited to having coincidence detection over about 90 degrees, which creates a fan pattern of possible coincidence detection lines of response (LORs). Each crystal has a different orientation of its sensitivity pattern so that all crystals are used to provide a complete set of LORs from around the patient.

Figure 10-13 depicts how a sinogram may be formed during 2D data acquisition. A point source in the scanner emits an annihilation pair, and one module—module 5, for instance—may have coincidence detection with any of the modules on the opposite side of the ring. On the sinogram, module 5 interactions occur along a downward angle toward the right. Module 37 on the opposite side of the ring uses a downward left angle to represent the possible LORs for this module. When a coincidence event occurs between modules 5 and 37, the pixel value at the intersection of those detectors is incremented by one event. If another annihilation pair is emitted from the same point, but on a different angle, a different pair of detectors (19 and 46, for example) will have the LOR

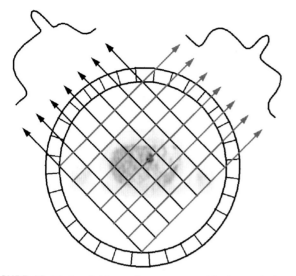

FIGURE 10-11 Parallel lines of response provide the equivalent of projection information from all angles around the patient.

data stored as a pixel count at the intersection of those modules. As can be observed in Figure 10-13 *(right)*, all counts from this fixed point source will create a sine curve–shaped pattern down the sinogram, as shown by the white curve. All possible detector pairs that may observe this interaction will have LOR data stored on this curve. The reconstruction process will calculate the activity represented at each projection (the horizontal line of the sinogram matrix) as observed from all angles, represented by the vertical sinogram axis.

Acquisition software allows a wide variety of operational modes. Scans may be simple one–bed-position static images; dynamic; cardiac gated; respiratory gated; 2D or 3D; or whole-body, multiple–bed-position studies or may acquire all information in list mode and allow the other acquisition mode data to be extracted from the list mode data. PET-only scanners may also include the acquisition of emission data alone, transmission data

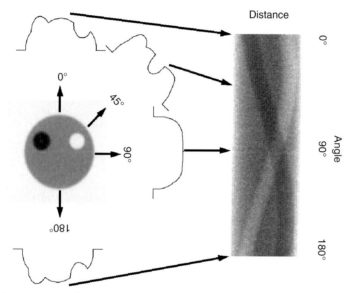

FIGURE 10-12 For each slice, the projections from each angle are placed in a horizontal row of a matrix called a *sinogram*. The sinogram plot is represented as the distance across the field of view of the scanner plotted against the angle from which the projection is taken. Each projection through 180 degrees is used to form a complete set of projection information. Hot and cold objects within a cylinder filled with radioactivity each create a sine wave pattern on the sinogram *(right)*. Only 180 degrees of data are needed to form a complete set of projection information, because the next 180 degrees would be a repeat. One sinogram represents the data from which only one slice in the data will be formed; therefore one sinogram must be acquired per slice.

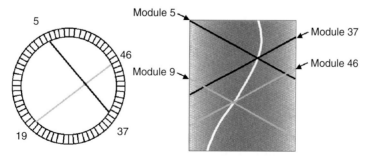

FIGURE 10-13 Sinogram information is also represented by the intersection of two detectors. Each detector module creates a line of possible detection with opposing detectors as represented by an angular dark line. Module 5 on one side of the ring detects a photon at the same time as module 37. The intersection of these two detector lines represents the line of response (LOR) at which this event was detected. The intersection of another detector pair, modules 19 and 46, also demonstrates this. Because these two LORs were obtained from the same point in space, a sinusoidal pattern *(right)* that represents the pattern is seen on the sinogram from that point in space.

alone, or a combination of emission and transmission images acquired in various orders (acquisition of all emission data and then all transmission data, all transmission data and then all emission data, or interlacing a transmission/emission study at each bed position). However, PET/CT scanners require that the CT scan be performed first so that the reconstructed attenuation correction map from the CT scan can be used for PET reconstruction with attenuation correction. PET data acquisition is most commonly terminated by a specified amount of time for the acquisition at each bed position. A standard patient radiopharmaceutical dose will produce good-quality images because standard protocols are used that provide predefined times for emission and transmission data. Deviations from the department standard protocol will therefore require the technologist to modify the acquisition times or processing parameters to provide optimal quality images.

An acquisition interface program is available on all systems and allows the technologist to use predefined acquisition protocols. The program also allows changes to any parameters necessary. The time of acquisition, orientation of the patient on the table, and mode of acquisition may all be changed as needed to accommodate tailoring the study to the individual patient. Likewise, processing protocols with override options are available on all commercial systems to facilitate easy transitions between customized and standardized operation.

2D AND 3D SCANNER CONFIGURATION

PET is by the nature of its physics is a 3D imaging technique. The use of septa for 2D imaging may be helpful to reduce scatter and random events and to limit the count rate. Recent improvements in detector materials, electronics, correction techniques, and algorithms have facilitated the application of 3D imaging to routine clinical use. Such 3D techniques are principally desired to increase the sensitivity of the scanner, but they may create additional challenges or problems, resulting in count rate limitations, less accurate random and scatter correction at very high count rates, and biased quantitative measurements, and may therefore limit the quantity of radioactivity that may be injected into the patient. The increase in sensitivity may allow for more accurate data and result in a more precise observation of the true distribution of radiotracer. PET scanners that operate only in 3D mode rely solely on electronic collimation and often employ narrow coincidence timing windows to reduce the random fraction. The elimination of the septa may enlarge the gantry opening and thus reduce claustrophobia, accommodate larger patients, and allow some positioning variation so that the patient position is similar to radiation treatment planning positions.

Ring-design dedicated PET 2D scanners may have tungsten or lead septa that sit inside the ring of crystal

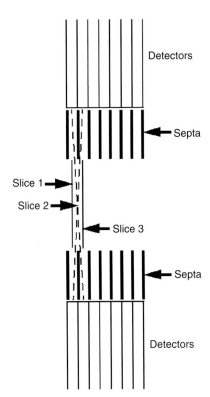

FIGURE 10-14 With septa in place, photons are limited to striking mostly one ring. However, one photon may strike one ring, and another photon may strike an adjacent second ring, creating a virtual slice in between that is called an *interplane slice*. The interplane slices provide improved resolution and nearly double the number of image slices beyond the actual number of detector rings.

detectors and are positioned between detector rings (Figure 10-14). The septa are 1 to 3 mm thick and project about 8 to 10 cm into the axis of the gantry. These septa serve two purposes: (1) to limit the FOV of events to those within the same detector ring, or events with contiguous planes, and (2) to reduce the number of scatter and random events from outside the plane. With the septa in place, the scanner operates in what is termed *2D mode*; that is, coincidence photon detection events are, for the most part, limited by the septa to a single detector ring. Thus a single slice of information from one 2D plane is acquired. The detector electronics and septa also allow the detection of an additional slice between the crystal rings (see the *dotted lines* in Figure 10-14). These virtual planes are termed *interplane slices* and allow for the creation of nearly twice the number of image slices as there are rings of crystals. For example, a scanner with 18 rings of crystals will generate an additional 17 interplane slices for a total of 35 slices. An interplane slice is created by the coincidence events of ring 1 with ring 2 and of ring 2 with ring 1; therefore the interplane slices may have a different sensitivity than the direct (same ring) slices. As a point of interest, the resolution of the scanner may not be the same in all directions. The resolution along the z-axis (axis along the center of the rings) may have slightly different

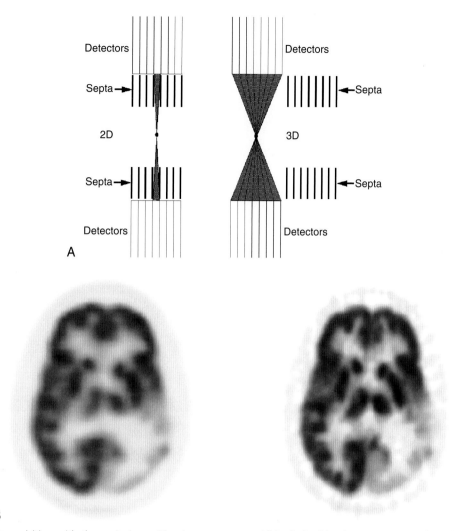

FIGURE 10-15 A, 2D acquisition with the septa in position has scanner sensitivity limited by the septa. 3D mode with the septa retracted from the gantry significantly increases the sensitivity. **B,** Brain images demonstrate a 2D image *(left)* and a higher-quality 3D image *(right)*.

resolution than the resolution in the *x*- or *y*-axis across a slice.

Retracting the septa creates the ability to place the scanner in 3D detection mode, where annihilation photon pairs can now be detected through a wide angle across the detector rings, thereby significantly increasing the sensitivity of the scanner (Figure 10-15). The retraction of the septa increases the sensitivity by a factor of 4 to 10, depending on the individual scanner design and on the organ and distribution of radiotracer being imaged. Without the septa, the number of possible LORs between a given crystal and opposing crystals increases significantly, thus dramatically increasing the number of LOR events detected and increasing the data density in the image.

Although 3D imaging demonstrates a theoretical improvement in imaging, the lack of septa results in a significant increase in both scattered photons and random coincidence events. Good correction techniques for both those factors must be made to minimize image artifacts

when performing 3D imaging. The comparative 2D and 3D brain images shown at the bottom of Figure 10-15 demonstrate the advantages of using 3D mode for brain imaging. There is a significant improvement in the resolution and contrast because noise is reduced as the number of detected events is dramatically increased. In 3D mode, high amounts of activity just outside the detector FOV may create a significant increase in random events. Inadequate correction for random events will reduce image contrast, which may mask subtle lesions adjacent to these sites of high activity, such as around the brain, bladder, or myocardium. Most scanners with LSO or GSO crystals have no septa and therefore operate only in 3D mode.

Although 3D mode acquires significantly more events (4 to 10 times more), reconstruction algorithms are more complex and require more elegant corrections for 3D random events and scatter than for 2D imaging. With much more data and the added complexity of corrections, there is a significant increase in the reconstruction time needed for 3D data. Data sets for 3D mode will be

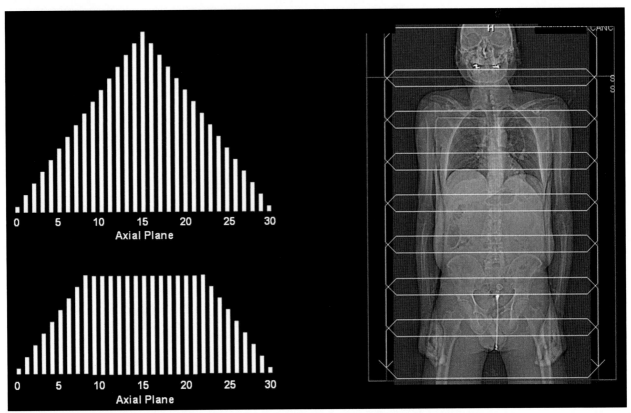

FIGURE 10-16 In 3D mode each detector may be allowed to have coincidence with all opposing detectors in all rings, creating a pyramidal sensitivity curve along the long central axis of the scanner *(upper left)*. If the number of rings for coincidence is limited from the possible maximum of 15 *(upper left)* for the example shown to a ring difference of 11, the sensitivity curve flattens *(lower left)*. An overlap by several rings (2 to 3 cm) will compensate for the very low sensitivity of the end rings of the scanner. The topogram *(right)* shows the overlap of about 2 cm of each bed position (total of eight bed positions).

8 to 12 times larger than 2D data sets, and their typical reconstruction times are 6 to 8 times longer than those of 2D data sets. The disk space and archival storage space for 3D data sets also slow down processing, transferring, and archiving of 3D data.

Whole-body imaging with the scanner in 3D mode improves patient throughput because it provides an increase in scanner sensitivity and may allow a decrease in the time required for emission imaging. One consideration when applying the 3D mode to whole-body imaging is the reduced sensitivity at the ends of the FOV as compared with the sensitivity at the center of the scanner. In 3D mode the wide acceptance angle (Figure 10-15, *right*) creates high sensitivity in the center that diminishes at the edges, creating a pyramidal sensitivity distribution (Figure 10-16, *left, upper*). Extremely large acceptance angles by the scanner contribute only a small amount to the global sensitivity; therefore it is advantageous to reduce the dramatic shape of the sensitivity curve by limiting the number of ring differences that are allowed. Figure 10-16 (*left, lower*) demonstrates a change in the sensitivity curve when the ring difference is limited to 11 rings instead of 15 in this example of a 31-ring scanner. To compensate for the PET reduced sensitivity at the FOV ends, a significant overlap of scanned area with two

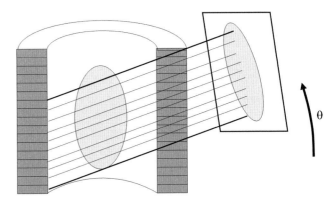

FIGURE 10-17 In 3D mode projection planes are acquired not just laterally, as in 2D, but also at oblique angles. These oblique projection plane data are processed back into axial 2D planes using single-slice rebinning or Fourier rebinning and then using an iterative reconstruction algorithm.

adjacent bed positions is performed (see Figure 10-16, *right*). An overlap of several centimeters is used to ensure adequate data density over the entire scanned area.

As there are no septa in 3D mode, the LOR events are allowed to take place over several rings to increase sensitivity. Parallel events from off-axis rays create projections at many angles (Figure 10-17), not just from rays that traveled perpendicularly to the axis of the scanner as in 2D systems. The data from these 3D projection planes significantly increase the amount of projection information that must be stored for reconstruction. Special processing techniques must be used to reconstruct the image volume from these 3D projection planes.

Whole-body imaging in 3D mode may provide very high count rates, and some data may be lost because of dead time limitations of the system. Technologists must carefully consider the injected dose of activity, patient uptake time before imaging, and count rate measured by the scanner to ensure that there is no compromised imaging due to the effects of high count rate on the performance of the scanner. In addition, dead time correction techniques must be employed for 3D data. With no septa, the random and scatter fractions are increased as compared to 2D mode. Therefore accurate random events and scatter correction are more crucial in 3D mode than in 2D mode.

Whole-body imaging in 3D mode presents some challenges and has disadvantages. The advantage of higher sensitivity creates problems with dead time and count rate limitations and may require the use of lower amounts of radiotracer. There is a significant increase in the size of 3D data sets that must be stored, accessed, reconstructed, and archived. These steps take a much longer time because of the increased volume of data. In particular, the reconstruction of complex 3D data must be rebinned correctly before more advanced algorithms produce the slices. The 3D mode also creates a significant increase in the number of random events that are detected, which then requires the application of accurate correction techniques during reconstruction.

PET/CT SCANNERS

Dedicated whole body PET scanners without a CT scanner are no longer commercially available because of the overwhelming advantages of having both scans performed in a single study. The PET/CT scanner (Figure 10-7) is designed with a high-performance dedicated ring PET scanner along with a high-performance CT scanner in the same gantry. The patient is positioned on the scanner table and a CT scan of the desired body area is quickly acquired (usually in less than 1 minute for a whole-body scan). Afterward, the PET emission scan data are acquired. The CT scan serves two purposes: (1) it provides a perfectly aligned anatomical image that matches the exact location of the functional image of the PET scan, and (2) the CT scan is transformed into an attenuation map for correcting the PET images. The PET/CT scanner therefore solves many of the problems that may cause misalignment if separate CT and PET scans alone were fused with software. PET/CT viewing software allows the display of the PET scan, CT scan, and color-overlaid PET on the CT scan (Figure 10-18).

(See the color plates for examples of color-overlaid PET images on black-and-white CT scans.) Cursor reference lines help to identify the slice locations on 3D projections from the transaxial, coronal, and sagittal views simultaneously displayed on the computer screen. PET scans are most commonly viewed directly on the computer instead of on film so that the physician may virtually move around within the body and correlate lesion location in other projections.

An excellent example of the clinical utility of PET/CT is when cancer invades lymph nodes. On CT, lymph nodes are considered normal as long as they are smaller than 10 mm, and abnormal once they are 10 mm or larger. On the other hand, PET shows the metabolic function of the tissue within the lymph node and can detect disease earlier than the anatomical manifestation occurs (even if the node is normal based on size).

As previously discussed, the axial CT slices from the PET/CT scanner may be converted into a transmission map to be used for attenuation correction of the corresponding PET emission slices. Cancer patients who are referred for PET or PET/CT scans often have other imaging studies, which sometimes include the use of x-ray contrast material. If contrast is present, the CT image pixel values will be very high in the location of the contrast and, when converted into 511-keV attenuation values, will cause an overestimation of activity in the corrected emission image. Figure 10-19 (top) demonstrates increased FDG activity in the bowel on attenuation-corrected coronal slices. However, the coronal CT images generated from the PET/CT study demonstrate a significant amount of barium in the large intestine, creating overcorrection for attenuation correction values (Figure 10-19, middle). The non–attenuation-corrected images (see Figure 10-19, bottom) show no increased FDG uptake; therefore the barium caused falsely high attenuation values that overcorrected bowel activity, which may have been erroneously interpreted as colitis.

RECONSTRUCTION ALGORITHMS

The LORs are stored during data acquisition, and this raw data must first be reformatted into sinograms, each sinogram representing one image slice. **Filtered back-projection (FBP)** techniques are the simplest and quickest way to create the image slice from the projection information stored in a sinogram. However, FBP creates severe streak or star artifacts, increasing image noise and thus reducing contrast, which may mask lesions (Figure 10-20, left). Faster computers and computational capacity now allow more sophisticated algorithms to be routinely used. Iterative methods are techniques that sequentially refine estimated pixel values and provide a more accurate reconstruction of the radiotracer's distribution in the body. Iterative algorithms significantly reduce streak artifacts compared with FBP

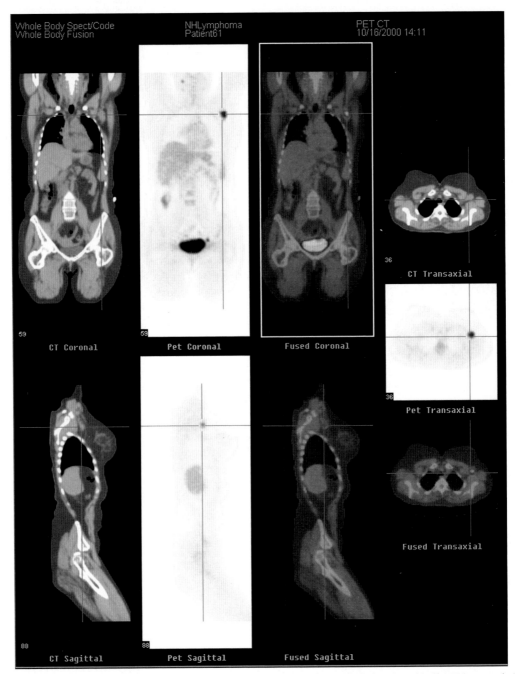

FIGURE 10-18 The display of the combined PET/CT study shows reference cursors on CT *(left column)* and PET images *(middle, left)* at the same time, in addition to the overlay image *(middle, right)*. The transaxial images are shown in the right column. The advantage of the combined PET/CT is to have exact location correlation between the two modalities, CT showing high-resolution anatomy and PET demonstrating molecular function of the tissue at that site.

reconstruction techniques but provide images with a lower signal-to-noise ratio (see Figure 10-21, *right*).

There are a number of reconstruction algorithms that are termed *iterative methods*. **Iterative reconstruction algorithms** are those that estimate the image values and serially update those estimates by repeated calculations. As diagrammed in Figure 10-21, the acquired original sinogram is compared to an estimated calculated sinogram. The calculated sinogram is compared to the

estimate, which may originally start out with the same value in all pixels, and the difference (or error in the estimate) is used to update the estimated values. The estimated sinogram is then back-projected to create a new estimated image; the estimated image is then forward-projected into a new updated estimate sinogram, and the comparison and update loop is performed sequentially for a predefined number of iterations or until the difference reaches a mathematical convergence

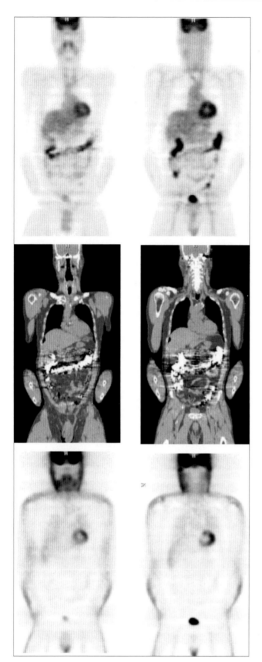

FIGURE 10-19 A patient who received barium before a PET/CT scan shows falsely increased uptake in the colon because of over-compensation of attenuation correction due to the barium in that location *(top)*. The CT portion of the study demonstrates the location of the barium *(middle)*. The non–attenuation-corrected images show no FDG uptake in the colon. Careful patient screening is needed to avoid false-positive studies.

(i.e., the difference between the original and estimated sinograms is below a certain value). The final image is the result of refined estimations and has significantly less noise and artifacts than FBP reconstruction.

Iterative algorithms are computationally intense and therefore are somewhat time-consuming. Maximum likelihood expectation maximization (MLEM) was one of the first iterative algorithms available for SPECT reconstruction and eventually found application in PET. MLEM typically requires 20 to 30 iterations or more using the entire set of data, which requires a long time to reconstruct. There are other techniques for performing these calculations; however, the most common of these is a faster and more efficient version called **ordered subset expectation maximization (OSEM).** Instead of using all of the data in each iteration (required by MLEM), OSEM uses selected subsets of the projection data, which can then be used with fewer iterations. PET reconstruction using OSEM may use a small number of iterations (2 to 4 iterations) but several subsets (4 to 14 or more), and thus the reconstruction time is substantially reduced. Figure 10-22 shows MLEM reconstruction with a limited number of iterations: 1, 2, 4, and 8. The image improvement with each iteration is very subtle, and a good clinical image will require 20 to 30 or more iterations. Figure 10-23 shows the same data reconstructed with only one iteration but using a different number of subsets to improve the image quickly. A quality image may be available with only two to four iterations but using a large number of subsets (14 to 50). Very high quality, high-resolution images are generated using a balance of iterations and a high number of subsets, such as perhaps 4 iterations and 24 subsets, when there is a high data density in the acquired study. One commercial vendor uses another algorithm called *row-action maximum likelihood algorithm (RAMLA)*, which provides similar results to OSEM.

As previously mentioned, 3D mode imaging significantly increases scanner sensitivity by collecting projection plane data as was shown in Figure 10-17. Current 3D techniques rebin the 3D information into 2D projection information (sinograms) and then use usual 2D iterative reconstruction algorithms. Therefore most current techniques to reconstruct 3D PET data use a two-step process: rebin the data from 3D to 2D and then use an iterative reconstruction algorithm. The 3D LOR information is rebinned into 2D projection sinograms using algorithms such as single-slice rebinning (SSRB) or Fourier rebinning (FORE). Iterative reconstruction of a large number of these 3D projection sinograms takes significantly longer than 2D reconstruction. SSRB blurs 3D projection information into a 3D stack of slices. FORE uses a frequency-distance principle in Fourier space and places information more accurately into the appropriate 2D slice location. The details of these techniques are highly mathematical and beyond the scope of this text.

As previously discussed, the reconstruction of 3D data requires that the raw data, 3D sinograms, be either rebinned into 2D information or reconstructed completely as a full 3D volume. Full 3D reconstruction techniques are extremely computationally intense and at this writing are not commercially available. These advanced, 3D reconstruction algorithms, with more accurate corrections, will become available in the near future when

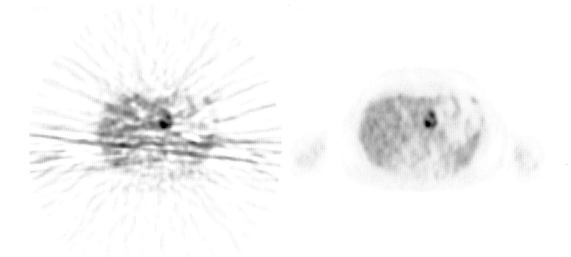

FIGURE 10-20 The filtered back-projection (FBP) reconstruction algorithm *(left)* leaves significant streak artifacts on reconstructed slices, and lesion contrast may lower because of a higher background in the image. More advanced iterative reconstruction algorithms *(right)*, such as ordered subset expectation maximization (OSEM), improves the overall quality of this image of a tumor within the liver.

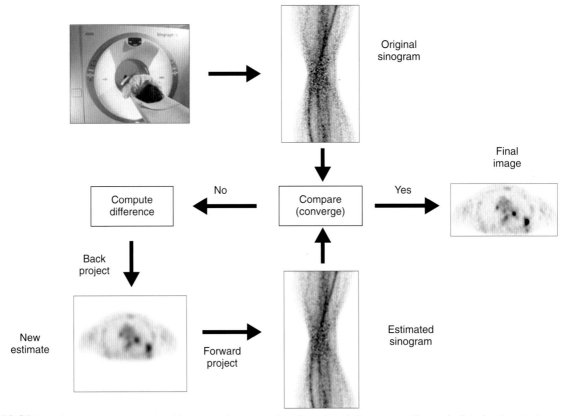

FIGURE 10-21 Iterative reconstruction algorithms start by comparing the original sinogram with a calculated estimate sinogram *(center bottom)*. The difference between the two sinograms is used to update the data and back-project an estimated image slice; that updated slice is forward-projected to update the estimated sinogram. A series of updates or iterations is completed in each loop until the difference is very small (convergence) or until the prescribed number of iterations has been completed and the final reconstructed image *(right)* is completed.

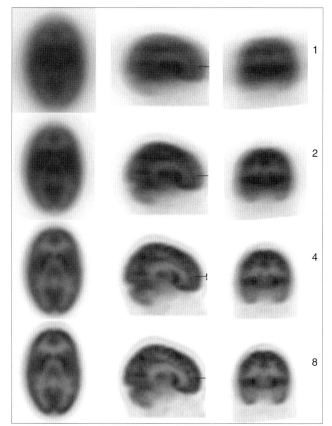

FIGURE 10-22 Using the fundamental maximum likelihood expectation maximization (MLEM) algorithm, which requires several dozen iterations to obtain high-resolution images. Shown are axial, sagittal, and coronal images from *1, 2, 4,* and *8* iterations.

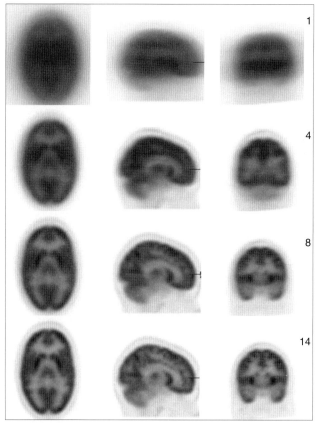

FIGURE 10-23 Using the ordered subset expectation maximization (OSEM) algorithm; the number of subsets is indicated, with *1, 4, 8,* and *14* subsets within one iteration showing more rapid image improvement compared with maximum likelihood expectation maximization (MLEM) (see Figure 10-20). OSEM is a significantly faster reconstruction than MLEM to achieve a high-quality image.

the reconstruction time can be decreased as larger computer memory, faster data transfer technology, and more advanced computers become available.

ATTENUATION CORRECTION BY TRANSMISSION IMAGING

Early attenuation correction was approximated using the Chang attenuation method, which created an elliptical outline of the body and mathematically estimated the attenuation value at each pixel. This technique required all pixel attenuation values to be the same and therefore large errors occurred where tissue density changes significantly, such as in regions of the lung and in bones. The only area where this is valid is the head.

The correct distribution of radiotracer can be represented in the images only when accurately measured attenuation correction values have been applied during image reconstruction. The reason attenuation correction is so important in the high-energy photon imaging in PET, is because the annihilation photon pair must travel the full width of the body, which produces a significant amount of attenuation, even at 511 keV (Figure 10-24). In addition, the body has a complex mixture of tissues, each with a different effect on photon attenuation. In the

chest, for example, lung tissue is filled mostly with air, both muscle and fat have similar attenuation, and bone tissue has higher photon energy absorption. The only way to accurately compensate for this variable attenuation is to pass a beam of radiation through the body and measure or "map" the attenuation. On PET-only instruments the measured attenuation data for each slice are obtained by rotating a line source of radioactivity, as shown in Figure 10-25, around the patient at each bed position. These radioactive line sources are usually 5 to 20 mCi of ^{68}Ge. The radioactive line source is held in a shielded housing within the gantry, and a robotic system loads the source into a rotating ring that moves around the patient while the scanner operates in transmission scanning mode. The transmission scan usually takes 1 to 3 minutes per bed position and may be performed before or after the emission data have been acquired, preferably at each bed position. Most scanners use an interlaced acquisition of emission-transmission-transmission-emission (ETTE) mode during whole-body imaging. Transmission scan data are reconstructed into attenuation correction maps for each slice. Figure 10-26, *A,* shows the transaxial, coronal, and sagittal reconstructed

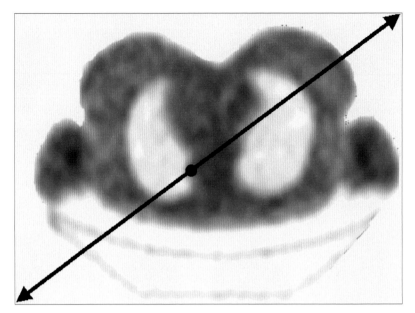

FIGURE 10-24 The pair of annihilation photons must traverse the entire width of the body as shown *(arrows)* on this transmission scan. Although the photons are of high energy, the attenuation across the full width of the body is significant. Because of the complexity of tissues along this path (muscle, fat, lung, bone, and the imaging table), a measurement of radiation attenuation must be obtained.

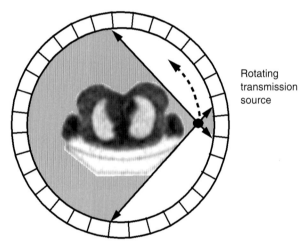

Rotating transmission source

FIGURE 10-25 A transmission image is obtained by acquiring data from a rotating transmission rod source of a long-lived positron-emitting radionuclide, usually ^{68}Ge. The transmission data may be acquired before, after, or interleaved into the emission PET scan. The low-resolution transmission scan shown here and in Figure 10-22 is replaced by a high-resolution transaxial CT scan on PET/CT scanners.

images without attenuation correction. Note that the lungs (low-attenuation areas) appear falsely filled with radiotracer, while areas deep in the body show up falsely void of tracer. The reconstructed attenuation map (see Figure 10-26, *B*) from the transmission scan shows dramatic attenuation differences between lung, soft tissues, and bone. Attenuation-corrected images (see Figure 10-26, *C*) show the corrected amounts of radioactivity in the lungs, which have no uptake of tracer, while deep structures such as the spine and internal organs are now appropriately brighter. Note that without attenuation correction the body appears to have radiotracer uptake in the skin, demonstrated as a bright outline, which disappears with attenuation correction. This artifact is due to a lack of any attenuation for annihilation photon pairs that travel transaxially to the detectors without passing through the patient and is thereby misrepresented as a high-activity area.

Figure 10-27, *A*, shows the transaxial, coronal, sagittal, and maximum intensity projection (MIP) anterior image on a patient study when no attenuation correction has been applied. Again the body appears to have increased tracer uptake in the skin, the lungs appear to take up the radiotracer, and deep organs are artifactually faint (e.g., "cold"). The transaxial, coronal, and sagittal slices are all positioned through small lesions in the right lobe of the liver that are only very faintly seen and could easily be overlooked. It is not apparent that there is more than one lesion in this location. With the application of measured transmission attenuation correction (see Figure 10-27, *B*), there is a dramatic change in the appearance of all images. The lesions in the right lobe of the liver are now much more evident, and the definition of at least two lesions becomes clear.

The invention of the combined PET and CT scanner not only created the advantage of having a perfectly aligned high-resolution anatomical study for comparison with the physiological PET image but also provided the use of the CT scan to create the attenuation correction map for the PET study. Multislice CT scanners, which will be discussed in Chapter 11, provide high-resolution studies that can be performed on a large area of the body in less than 30 seconds. This has the advantage of reducing the procedure imaging time significantly as the slow process of using a radioactive transmission source for imaging is replaced by the much faster CT process. When the CT component of the combined examination is performed, it can be done in several ways: CT for

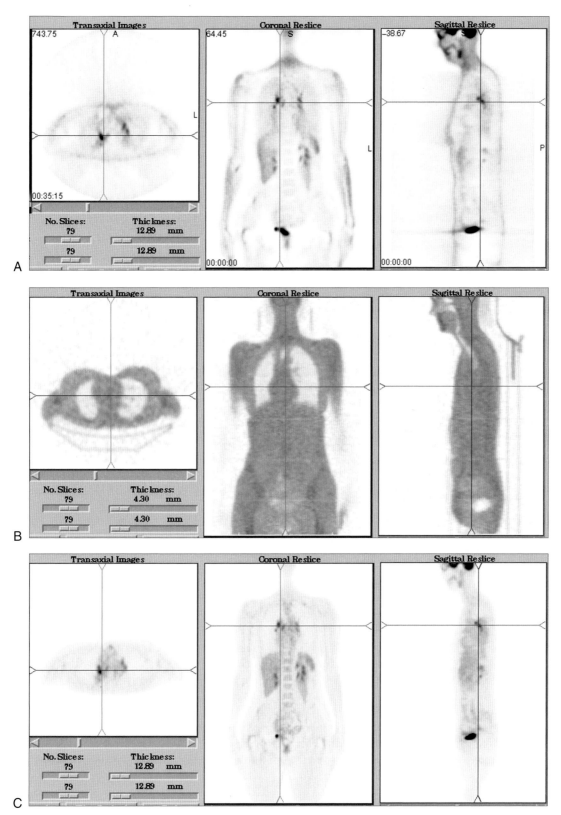

FIGURE 10-26 Without attenuation correction **(A)**, transaxial, coronal, and sagittal images demonstrate falsely hot activity on the body surface and falsely low activity within deep structures. The lungs, an area of low attenuation, appear falsely hot. **B,** Transmission images at the same planes as **A** in all three projections. Areas of the lungs, nasopharyngeal area, trachea, and other sites where attenuation is low are seen in white. **C,** The same planes with attenuation correction. The hot skin artifact has been removed, and the lungs now appear appropriately void of radioactivity. Deep structures within the body are more easily seen because the images now demonstrate a correct relationship of activity.

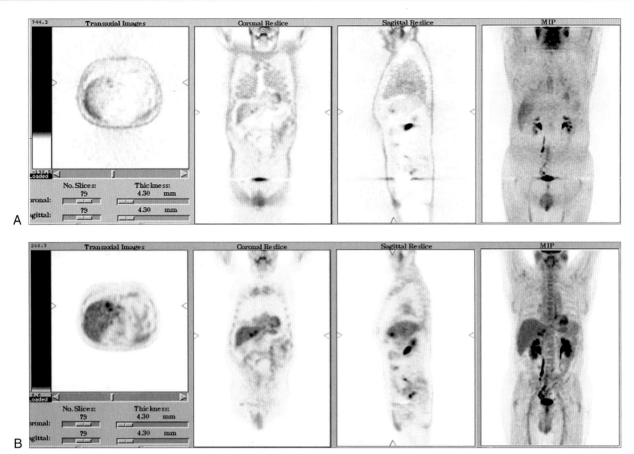

FIGURE 10-27 A, Images without attenuation correction are shown in the transaxial, coronal, sagittal, and maximum intensity projections. **B,** Attenuation correction allows two lesions in the liver that may have been missed without attenuation correction to be seen easily.

attenuation correction only, diagnostic CT, or diagnostic CT with CT contrast material.

Computed tomography scans for attenuation correction only are sometimes referred to as *low-dose CT* when talking about PET/CT procedures. In these studies the CT controls for both x-ray beam energy, peak kilovoltage (kVp) and beam current, milliamps (mA) are set low to minimize radiation exposure to the patient. This CT scan will demonstrate poor to moderate resolution of anatomy because it will have high statistical noise in the image that will mask fine resolution. Diagnostic CT with moderate to high kVp and mA is associated with significantly higher radiation exposure but produces high-quality detailed anatomical images for correlation with the PET study. The interpreting physician should select the specific protocols and application to different diseases that dictates the level of CT to be performed. For example, a PET brain study would likely require only a low-exposure CT because there may be little advantage in having a high-resolution anatomical correlation when the CT is used solely to provide attenuation correction. On the other hand, a PET/CT looking for small pulmonary nodules may require a high-quality CT with thin slices to provide anatomical images that have excellent resolution.

The transmission scan, whether by external rotating radioactive source or by CT, needs special processing before being used in the PET reconstruction process for attenuation correction. The transmission image, or map, may need two processes to take place before applying PET reconstruction. The first step is the transcription of the map from the acquired energy to the energy of 511 keV for PET attenuation correction application. If a source of ^{68}Ge was used for the transmission study, then the energy is already at 511 keV and this step may be skipped. However, the CT scan is generally obtained at 70 to 140 kVp, meaning that the average x-ray energy is substantially lower. The attenuation coefficients are vastly different for different tissues at various energies. Lung, muscle, fat, and bone tissues in the CT scan will all require different amounts of compensation to reflect what the attenuation coefficients would be at 511 keV.

The second step before applying the transmission map for attenuation correction is to reduce pixel noise in the transmission image. Radioactive ^{68}Ge source transmission scans are exceptionally noisy, but even high-quality CT studies require noise reduction to prevent transmission scan noise from changing the noise structure within the PET scan. A process known as *image segmentation* is commonly applied. Segmentation refers to selecting image regions for various types of tissues or organs that are identified in smoothed image slices. For example, the area of each lung can be automatically identified and all lung pixel values are replaced with known linear attenuation coefficients for lung. Likewise regions of muscle, fat, bone, and so on will be replaced with known attenuation coefficients for these tissues. The resulting segmented images have less noise because they have been smoothed and tissue values reassigned to all pixels. On some commercial systems the attenuation correction CT (CT-AC) file may be saved and viewed for quality control purposes. This file will look like a very smooth CT because the CT has often been blurred to the same spatial resolution as the PET study and the CT-AC map is applied during the PET image reconstruction process.

When the CT scan is used to create an attenuation correction map there are several steps in this process. The CT study may first be segmented by separating out image regions that have the same CT attenuation coefficients, such as the imaging table, dense bone, soft tissue, and lung. Because the CT scan was performed at a low energy (80 to 140 keV), the attenuation coefficients for each type of tissue in the image must be transcribed to the attenuation coefficients at 511 keV to properly correct attenuation at the PET energy.

TIME OF FLIGHT PET

The idea for using **time of flight (ToF)** difference measurements between detectors to determine the position of the site of an annihilation interaction is not new. ToF PET has been around for several decades and was first demonstrated as feasible using ultra fast detectors such as BaF_2, which has a light decay time of less than 1 ns. ToF PET has not been viable as a commercial product until the last few years as technical challenges have been overcome using ultrafast electronics and computer data storage and processing techniques have made it feasible in the clinic. All primary medical imaging equipment vendors now offer ToF PET scanners in their line of PET/CT products.

Time of flight PET is accomplished by using detector materials such as LSO or LYSO that have very short light decay times. The arrival time of scintillation events in each detector is recorded and when an annihilation photon pair is detected within the required timing window (usually about 5 ns in ToF scanners) the time difference $\Delta\tau$ between the photon arrival time is computed (Figure 10-28, *upper*). The following equation is then used to calculate the distance **d** from the center of the gantry at which the annihilation event took place (where **c** is the velocity of light).

$$d = \frac{\Delta\tau \times c}{2}$$

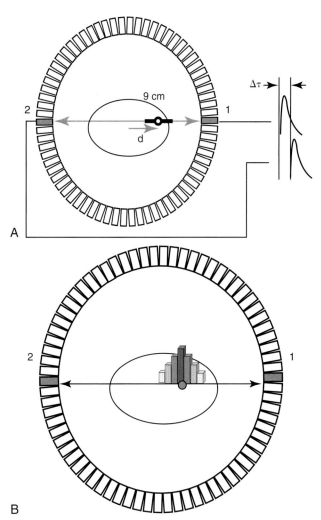

FIGURE 10-28 A, The pulse arrival time difference (Dt) between detector 1 and detector 2 is computed and this time difference is used to calculate the offset distance d from the center of the gantry to identify the location of the annihilation event to within about 9 cm. The 9 cm long LOR is used in the reconstruction of the ToF image instead of an LOR that would reach all the way across the image. The short LOR results in an improvement in contrast. **B,** On some PET systems the ToF LOR is coded as a probability of the location as show by the plot along the LOR. This probability allows more accurate estimate of the annihilation event location.

The light decay time of currently used scintillation detector materials and time response of the PMT is not accurate enough to determine the exact point of the annihilation event, however, it can be identified to within about 9 cm. You can think of the scanner as recording this event not as an LOR between detectors but as a short LOR bar instead of a line (see Figure 10-28, *upper*). Another way to determine the position information is to record a probability LOR (see Figure 10-28, *lower*) to record the most likely location of the annihilation event. The distinct advantage of ToF is that there is not a full LOR across the FOV of the scanner but only a short line in which the annihilation event took place. This affects the image contrast and signal-to-noise ratio of detecting

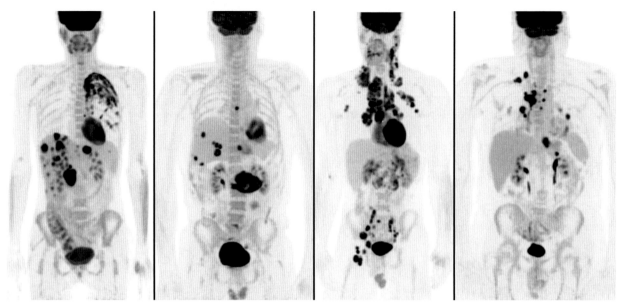

FIGURE 10-29 MIP images with ToF PET from four patients have improved lesion-to-background contrast and a larger signal-to-noise ratio as compared to standard PET acquisition and reconstruction techniques. Note the excellent resolution and contrast of small lesions. This improvement allows slightly faster acquisition to achieve a certain level of lesion detection and has an advantage in large patients *(right image)* where the random events fraction causes image contrast loss and difficulty in lesion identification.

increased areas of radiotracer uptake. The effect on the signal-to-noise ratio of a small lesion is the same effect as acquiring at least 2.5 times the number of events to improve lesion detection. Figure 10-29 shows ToF PET scans with improved lesion detection and lesion contrast improvement. ToF scanners thus can produce high quality images using a slightly shorter acquisition time. With the use of a shorter coincidence timing window in ToF imaging there is image improvement as the likelihood of detecting random events is reduced. In routine PET techniques large patients have a higher random events fraction than smaller patients. Therefore the reduction in the randoms fraction with ToF means that there is more improvement in image quality in the larger patient than normal weight or smaller patients.

Most ToF scanners record the incoming data from the detectors in list mode so that events and timing markers are accurately recorded; then this list mode information is reformatted to identify coincidence events and compute the ToF LOR information. Images are then reconstructed from this reformatted list mode data. In the near future most PET scanners will be of ToF design as this technology continues to mature and provides a substantial improvement in image resolution.

SCANNER CALIBRATION AND QUALITY CONTROL

PET scanners differ significantly from nuclear medicine gamma cameras in image quality control issues. In general, PET scanner quality control is more often

updating and refining calibration values more than viewing test images, as is done with gamma cameras. Therefore PET requires a meticulous program of calibrations and verification of image quality. This program should be built around the manufacturer's recommendations as a minimum set of calibrations and tests and then expanded or modified to meet the specific needs of the institution as experience is increased and after instrument performance has been monitored. The terminology of the calibrations and tests discussed in this chapter may differ from the terminology used by various vendors and from the way in which the calibrations and tests are performed; however, all these calibrations are used with every type of scanner.

Calibrations may be separated into two general types: characterization (or operation) calibrations and correction calibrations. Characterization calibrations are those that are fundamental to the operation of the PET scanner, such as energy, position, PMT gain, and coincidence timing window. Correction calibrations are those that compensate for inherent variations in the scanner and perform meaningful scaling of the image, such as normalization, **blank scan,** and absolute activity (well counter) calibrations.

Characterization and Correction Calibrations

Energy Window Calibration. Energy window calibration is typically performed only after repair, during quarterly preventive maintenance (PM) service, or just before a **normalization calibration** is done. The energy resolution of BGO is relatively poor, and the energy window may be set as wide as 300 to 650 keV; because the PET scanner operates at only one radionuclide energy (511 keV), a check of the energy window is not required frequently. Scanners using other types of detector materials may need additional checks and calibrations for the energy setting. Energy calibration is usually performed by a service engineer, but on some systems, calibration may be performed by the technologist.

Gain Settings. The calibration and adjustment of amplifier gains from PMTs are fundamental to ensure that a uniform sensitivity response from the individual detectors and modules is maintained. Frequent sensitivity drift may occur if gains are not updated at recommended intervals, or even more frequently. Gain settings should be adjusted to compensate for temperature changes that affect the performance and stability of the electronics. This calibration is typically performed using the radioactive rod sources used for **transmission imaging.** Calibrations require a high number of events for fine-tuning gain adjustments; therefore the procedure usually takes many minutes to acquire sufficient data. Depending on the manufacturer, these data may also be used to update crystal maps (see Figure 10-5), PMT gain, and energy window definition (the crystal maps may be adjusted by service engineers to match the sensitivity of individual detectors to the other detectors in a module). Gain updating compensates for variations in the changes in detector module gain over time. Gain update calibration procedures should be run at least weekly or even daily to keep systems in top performance and to prevent sensitivity drift. The more frequently they are run, the more uniform the performance of the scanner will be.

Crystal map calibration and PMT gains may be strongly linked on some systems. Therefore significant changes in the crystal maps will affect the PMT gain. If a map is distorted, attempts at further calibration may fail. The update gains program balances the gain characteristics of the four PMT channels on a specific block by aligning the photopeak to a specific histogram channel. PMT gain will drift with temperature changes and age. An increase in temperature is likely to affect the whole system, resulting in a change in system sensitivity but usually little change in spatial resolution. This results in quantitative image value errors, so quantitative information requires stable performance and frequent system calibration. A temperature shift of as little as 2° C may change the overall sensitivity of the scanner.

Coincidence Timing Calibration. Timing windows are significantly longer than the time it takes for photons to traverse the distance across the detector ring. The coincidence timing calibration adjusts for the timing differences in the event detection circuitry. Timing information is used to generate a histogram (a plot of time versus the number of events at each time) and analyzed to determine timing differences from various detector circuits.

Blank Scan. Blank scans are performed daily to provide accurate transmission scan data for the attenuation correction of images. Radioactive decay of the transmission sources, dead time corrections, and detector sensitivity may vary frequently; therefore a blank scan must be obtained each morning before clinical use of the scanner. Blank scans are used as a reference uniformity measure for the transmission scan used in attenuation correction. It is very important to acquire and evaluate blank scans daily, because attenuation correction made with poor or outdated blank scans will have artifacts that will show up in the emission patient images. Patient data that are archived should have the results of that day's blank scan stored for reference in case future image reconstruction is required. Blank scans are typically viewed by reconstructing the sinogram for each slice (Figure 10-30, *A*). A sinogram is a plot of projection angle versus distance

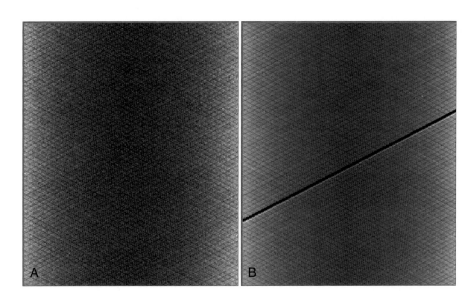

FIGURE 10-30 A, Normal blank scan with appropriate sensitivity response of all detectors. **B,** One detector module is displaying an inappropriate sensitivity as demonstrated by the dark diagonal line. Dark or white diagonal lines may be seen when one or more detector modules are malfunctioning or out of calibration.

across the detector of the source location. Each point on the sinogram represents a specific location between two detectors operating in coincidence. Blank scans should be evaluated visually for any abnormal streaks (see Figure 10-30, *B*) that show specific crystal or module variations and changes in regional sensitivity. Broad diagonal bands will be seen on the sinogram when PMT problems arise or signal is lost from a module. Some systems may use an algorithm to analyze the blank scan to evaluate daily variations statistically and report a quantitative parameter of detector uniformity performance.

In some respects, the blank scan may be thought of as viewing a daily uniformity flood image on a scintillation camera, providing an overall indicator of scanner performance. The blank scan, however, is data that represent the sensitivity response to the transmission source without any attenuating material (or patient) being present in the gantry ring. Any significant artifacts in the daily blank scan are an indication that there are problems with the system that should be investigated and resolved before injecting and imaging any patients.

Normalization Calibration. The 2D normalization calibrations are done to measure the efficiency for all LORs. Normalization calibration is performed by rotating radioactive rod sources, which contain a low activity source of radioactivity, and acquiring data that will be used to balance the efficiency of all detectors in the scanner. The normalization calibration is used much like a high-count uniformity correction in the scintillation gamma camera. Very high statistics are therefore required, and the normalization scan takes at least 6 to 24 hours, depending on the strength of the radioactive source. It is done at low count rates to simulate the count rate of patient data and approximate the level of dead time losses seen during patient acquisition. A normalization scan for 3D mode may need to be acquired separately. The normalization calibration table is used to correct for sensitivity from all detectors; therefore it is essentially a uniformity correction used in the reconstruction. Normalization calibrations are performed quarterly or after major service.

Absolute Activity Calibration (Well Counter Calibration). Well counter calibration is an historical term for a calibration more appropriately referred to as **absolute activity calibration**. Absolute activity calibration factors are used to convert pixel values into a measure of absolute activity per voxel. This calibration is performed by taking a precisely known amount of activity and loading a water-filled phantom whose volume is accurately known. The phantom is imaged, reconstructed, and processed into a set of correction factors that allows the conversion of a patient scan into a representation of the percentage of injected dose per volume or gram of tissue. This conversion creates an image that represents a quantitative image for the measurement of **standard uptake values (SUVs)** of tissue or tumors. Separate acquisition

and processing of data are required for 2D and 3D well counter calibration factors. Absolute activity calibrations are performed only after all other calibrations have been performed, and they should be done quarterly or after major service.

Quality Control

Quality control of any imaging device, including PET scanners, is a test or series of tests that verify proper operation of the scanner and allow checks that the calibrations are appropriate and working properly. The QC tests must be sensitive enough to detect changes in the scanner performance and ensure that clinical images will be an accurate representation of the radiotracer distribution and that no artifacts are present. A list of problems that may occur with PET scanners is listed in Box 10-1. Daily tests must be performed and images reviewed to attempt to identify any variation in the performance of the scanner.

Daily QC must be done to measure the output of each detector and ensure that calibrations are properly applied. A blank scan that may be applied to attenuation-correct patient studies for that day may be reconstructed as sinograms prior to being reformatted into a calibration table. The blank scan (see Figure 10-30) will show artifacts if there are any problems with detector modules, signal cables, high-voltage drift, gain changes, and so on. An alternative daily test may be to image a uniform cylinder of radioactivity, which can have a transmission scan applied to verify that the attenuation correction components are all working. A regular schedule of calibrations will optimize image quality by ensuring that the instrument is working correctly for all studies.

Detailed PET scanner acceptance testing and performance testing procedures are described by the National Electrical Manufacturers Association (NEMA), in its publication *NU-2*. In addition, there should be a budget, plan, and schedule for replacing the calibration and transmission radioactive sources in the gantry. As radioactive sources decay, the transmission beam through the patient will become weaker and limited in statistical

---

BOX 10-1 | **PET Scanner Failures**

- Detector malfunction
- High-voltage drift
- Energy drift
- Gain drift
- Cable breakage
- Power supply drift or failure
- Temperature drift or cooling system failure
- Coincidence timing malfunction
- Transmission source or robotics malfunction
- Septa mispositioning or misalignment
- Imaging table failure

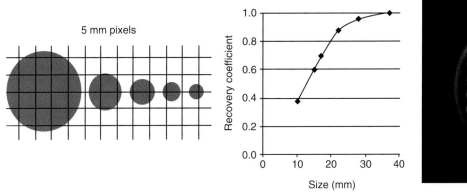

FIGURE 10-31 The partial volume effect occurs when voxels fail to contain all tissue that contains the same concentration of radioactivity. When objects (lesions) are smaller they are accurately sampled by fewer voxels *(left)* and therefore record less radioactivity and are quantitatively low and dimmer. *Middle,* The resolution recovery curve demonstrates the qualitative inaccuracy because lesions are smaller in size. The quantitative measurement is reduced and smaller objects are more difficult to see. *Right,* The PET scan of a Jaszczak phantom (Data Spectrum Corporation) with hot rods shows the reduced intensity of small rods.

accuracy, particularly when applied to larger patients. Because months can go by before a source is replaced, it is helpful to slightly extend the transmission acquisition time to ensure that a sufficient data density is being achieved. Otherwise image noise and horizontal line artifacts on coronal and sagittal images may appear, caused by high noise in the transmission data that will limit the accuracy of attenuation correction in the reconstruction algorithms.

A quality control program must be established for PET scanners and should include daily, weekly, and quarterly tests in addition to a regular schedule of PM service. An aggressive, comprehensive QC program is needed to reduce artifacts, increase uptime, produce higher-quality images, and thus ensure diagnostic accuracy.

PARTIAL VOLUME EFFECT

In any volumetric imaging, CT, MRI, SPECT, or PET, the ability to accurately resolve and quantify small objects becomes challenging. The **partial volume effect** is caused when the size of an object begins to approach the resolution limits of an imaging system. The problem occurs when a voxel contains more than one type of tissue, which in the case of PET contains a different concentration of radioactivity. For example, Figure 10-31, *left,* demonstrates that as spherical objects get smaller there are an insufficient number of voxels that are completely within the sphere, and thus the voxels do not contain the correct concentration of radioactivity that is in the object. As objects get to about two times the voxel size there are almost no voxels that accurately sample the correct concentration and the object becomes very dim and can no longer be detected. Also the quantitative accuracy of the radioactive concentration is falsely lower in small objects. The partial volume effect is measurable when the size of the object is less than

about 25 to 30 mm and, as mentioned, objects smaller than this are dimmer and measure a falsely lower quantity of radioactivity. The curve in the middle of Figure 10-31 shows the decreasing measured concentration of radioactivity with object size. This curve is known as the resolution recovery curve and as shown, objects below 30 mm in diameter will loose quantitative accuracy as they get smaller in size.

Figure 10-31, *right,* shows an ^{18}F PET scan of a Jaszczak deluxe phantom (Data Spectrum Corporation, Hillsborough, N.C.) with a hot rod insert. The phantom is uniformly filled with ^{18}F and the concentration in all of the rod sections is the same; however, the image demonstrates that the visual intensity of the rods diminishes dramatically between the six sizes of rods from 12.7 mm to 4.8 mm in diameter.

PET scanners typically have a field of view that is about 700 mm in diameter and images are sometimes reconstructed into a 128 × 128 matrix. This means that the pixel size is about 5.4 mm (700 mm/128), which is actually larger than the spatial resolution of the scanner, about 4.5 mm FWHM. To resolve small lesions a finer pixel size may need to be used and some scanners offer reconstruction into a 168 × 168 or larger matrix size. Using a larger matrix size does require that there is sufficient data density in the images to truly improve resolution without degrading quality because of statistical noise.

QUANTITATIVE IMAGE INFORMATION

The absolute quantitative uptake of the radiotracer in tumors can be measured in an effort to differentiate between malignant and benign tissue. The SUV can be useful in measuring tumor metabolic function. PET scanner calibration of absolute activity (well counter calibration) allows the conversion of image data into an activity measure of radiotracer uptake per pixel or voxel in the image. Standard uptake value measurements are based on either the injected activity per patient weight in kilograms or the injected activity per body surface area (BSA) in square meters. The injected activity (minus residual in the syringe) must be accurately known and the time of injection recorded. Activity measurements may be in microcuries or megabecquerels. Body surface area is usually calculated in the following manner:

$$BSA\,(m^2) = (weight\,in\,kg)^{0.425} \times (height\,in\,cm)^{0.725} \times 0.007184$$

Tumor SUV is determined by placing a region of interest (ROI) over the tumor and using computer programs to automatically calculate the value. The computer operator can select whether the calculation is to be done per weight or per BSA. Calculations are based on the following formula:

$$SUV_{BW} = (ROI\,activity, mCi/ml)(injected\,activity, mCi/patient\,weight, g)$$

or

$$SUV_{BSA} = (ROI\,activity\,units)/(injected\,activity/BSA)$$

Accurate information is needed for the exact time of dose measurement, activity administered, injection time, patient height and weight, and the time at which the images were acquired at each bed position. Standard uptake values change with time, so it is critical to specify the time at which the SUV image was obtained. If follow-up quantitative measurements are obtained for comparison, the precise time between injection and imaging must be replicated.

SUV values may be reported in different ways. The most common way to use SUV is reported by body weight (BW) and to report the maximum pixel value within the ROI (SUV_{max}). In addition, the SUV may be normalized to not only body weight but also body surface area or lean body mass. Besides SUV_{max}, SUVs may be reported using the ROI average pixel value, peak pixel value, or other methods to report the data; however, SUV_{max} based on body weight is most frequently used.

Figure 10-32 shows ROIs drawn on two tumors in the liver on an FDG PET scan. The normal SUV of the liver is around 1.5 to 2.5. The tumor with the large ROI has a maximum SUV_{bw} value of 14.6 and the smaller tumor has a maximum SUV_{bw} value of 6.2. The most common use of SUVs is to track the progression or remission of disease on PET scans following therapy. It is also difficult to compare SUV values from different PET scanners or institutions because of the variation in the use of factors such as glucose concentration, tracer uptake time before imaging, ROI size, resolution capabilities, and calibrations.

The usefulness of the absolute SUVs remains controversial. It is widely recognized that accuracy in calculating these values is difficult and that rigorous QC and

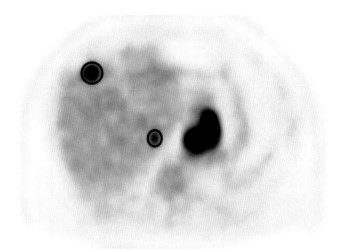

FIGURE 10-32 This FDG PET/CT transaxial image shows two ROIs positioned over lesions within the liver. The maximum pixel value SUV_{bw} over the large circular ROI is 14.6 and the maximum SUV_{bw} over the small ROI is 6.2.

calibration are required. The technologist must also pay particular attention to the details of administering the radioactivity and to recording the time of injection and the time of imaging. Image reconstruction and filtering techniques may also affect the result of the SUV value. Moreover, small lesions are affected by the partial volume effect, where small sources of radioactivity have their activity distributed artificially among too many voxels, resulting in false resolution and contrast, and an underestimation of radioactivity. Accurate SUVs can be obtained only when the size of the lesion is two to four times the pixel size. SUVs may be of significant value when they are applied to serial studies on one patient to evaluate the effectiveness of cancer therapy; however, the exact uptake time to scan time must be exactly the same for each study.

The partial volume effect has a large influence on the SUVs of small lesions. It is common practice to not apply a correction for the partial volume effect but for physicians to simply report the SUV for a tumor and then on follow-up studies again report the SUV without correction. SUVs may measure slightly differently from scanner to scanner because of calibration factors. Therefore the best practice is to perform follow-up studies on the same scanner.

Investigations have shown value in measuring lesion uptake at two different points in time (often called dual time point imaging), for example, at 1 hour and 3 hours postinjection. Malignant tumors continue to accumulate FDG with time, whereas inflammatory processes decrease in activity with time. Therefore false-positive studies with PET are avoided by characterizing the FDG kinetics by this dual point measuring technique. By doing this, the sensitivity and specificity of PET in lung cancer and identification of solitary pulmonary nodules are each increased.

DISPLAYING PET DATA

The PET computer system creates image data of a volume within the patient that is represented by a series of adjacent slices. The small crystal size creates 3- to 5-mm slices across the long axis of the body. The challenge facing the physician and technologist is how to organize or reformat this large volume of information into the most meaningful display that (1) aids in rapidly identifying abnormalities, and (2) provides the best spatial relationship to normal landmarks (organs) within the patient to provide an accurate location of any abnormalities. It is difficult to look through 200 to 300 transaxial slices of a whole-body PET study and be able to identify abnormalities and relate their location to structures that may be outside the axial plane that is being viewed. Even observing more than a dozen axial slices on the computer screen at one time does not clearly show the best relationship of a source of radiotracer to structures in other slices. Therefore the 3D volume should be reformatted to create planes through the volume that provide the most information about normal and abnormal structures. Whole-body transaxial slices are reformatted to create a series of coronal and sagittal slices. The coronal slices are the most commonly viewed set of images because the symmetric view of the body allows the best comparison of right and left structures in addition to providing the view of the largest axial plane through the body. Coronal slices represent the view that most people think of the distribution of organs within the body and also produce a convenient display to view the entire body using the fewest number of images.

Viewing all projections and all transaxial, coronal, and sagittal slices at one time has significant advantages in providing the spatial relationship of lesions or questionable areas in each of the different projections. This is most convenient when reference lines appear on the images to identify the location of each plane through the volume (see Figure 10-26, C).

Three-dimensional studies may be most dramatically displayed using the reprojection of the volume information back into a series of projections from around the body. This display technique is called the *MIP*. The reconstructed volume of the body is projected back into 2D projection images at equally spaced angles around the body. A ray passing through each plane is used to project the maximum pixel value along that ray onto the 2D projection image (Figure 10-33). Therefore the pixel with the most counts, or brightest intensity, is placed into the image. In Figure 10-33 the tumor pixel intensity is highest and is therefore projected on each image. The 2D projection images are then displayed on the computer in a continuous-loop cinematic mode to present the whole volume on one projection. The viewer's eyes and brain sort out the 3D relationship of various structures as the image position changes in the movie display.

IMAGE FUSION AND PET/MRI

In the early 1990s the fusion of SPECT brain scans with MRI or CT was shown to be very useful in the correlation of the exact site of anatomical (CT or MRI) and physiological (PET or SPECT) information. Although radiology's anatomical images have high resolution, the anatomical images demonstrate disease only when it has progressed to create a change in tissue density (as seen on CT) or has changed in its proton density (as shown with MRI). Disease is therefore seen only when the structure of tissue has degraded because of the illness. PET, as a biological chemistry image, commonly shows disease changes at the molecular level, and so problems may show up with PET before they are evident on CT or MRI. The PET 3D radiotracer information can be aligned or fused with a high-resolution CT or MRI image of anatomy. Tumor uptake of FDG or other PET radiotracer is often very high compared with surrounding normal tissues, but the exact location of the increased uptake may be difficult to determine.

Image fusion software is widely available that can import DICOM slice information from CT, MRI, SPECT, or PET and allows two image sets to be aligned by identifying anatomic points on each modality that can be matched up between two different modalities. The problem with using anatomical points is that the radiotracer modalities do not have sufficient spatial resolution to be precise (within a very few millimeters) in location. This problem can be resolved in part by placing external skin-surface markers (called fiducial markers) on the patient that can be seen on both imaging modalities. These markers can contain a small amount of ^{18}F in addition to a material that will show up on CT or MRI. These points can then be aligned, which in theory should align the organs within the body. However, this technique has a few logistical problems. An MRI is usually performed before the PET scan is ordered, and the images therefore do not have the external markers present.

The invention of PET/CT and its common availability has typically reduced the need to perform image fusion of the PET/CT with another CT scan unless that CT study performed at the time of the PET/CT was a low-dose CT for attenuation correction only. Most fusion studies are now performed between PET and MRI. PET brain studies are the most commonly performed body region where the fusion of PET is required. The fixed nature of the brain within the skull makes the fusion process relatively simple and extremely fast because commercial fusion software is very flexible and has many fusion options available. Mutual information processing is often used for brain PET and MRI fusion and in the brain is extremely accurate. Fully automated, semiautomated or manual fusion techniques are also available for the computer user. If the patient is in a slightly different position, two rigid images may not align satisfactorily

Maximum intensity projection

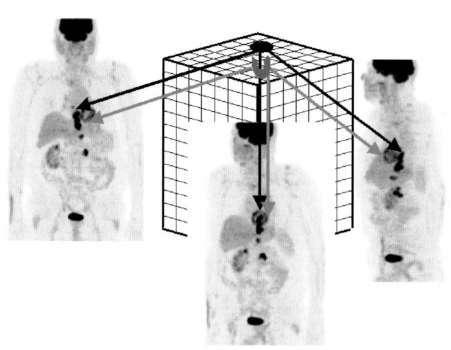

FIGURE 10-33 When the volume of the scan has been reconstructed as shown by the 3D voxels, data may be reprojected along rays through the volume to show the volume projected at various angles around the patient. Each ray through the volume projects the maximum count onto images called the maximum intensity projection (MIP). A set of MIP images created at equal angles from around the patient volume may be displayed in a closed-loop cinematic display to create a movie of the entire patient volume. The MIP images are a convenient media to quickly observe the whole patient.

and deformable or nonrigid techniques may be required to stretch or rotate one of the images sets (usually the PET) to conform to the anatomical image volume.

Several of the color plates found within the pages of Chapter 13 demonstrate combined PET/CT studies and displays.

PET/CT scanners have substantially improved the sensitivity and specificity of each modality for detecting disease as these two modalities have been combined. At this time there is substantial development work in making combined PET/MRI scanners. There are several important advantages of combining these two modalities, principally that there is no radiation exposure from the MRI (unlike CT, which has very high exposure), the MRI study differentiates soft tissue differences much better than CT and therefore the combined studies in neurology and oncology have much more potential for providing physiological and molecular imaging information than with PET/CT. There are many technical challenges that must be overcome to make PET detectors work within the high magnetic field within an MRI scanner, but employing new scintillation light detection devices such as avalanche photodiodes may overcome these problems. In addition techniques to create an attenuation correction map at 511 keV for the PET study must be calculated from the MRI scan. Also, the best time advantage

will come from acquiring the MRI and PET images simultaneously to improved patient throughput.

Will PET/MRI eventually replace all PET/CT scanners? This is not likely (at this writing), because the initial cost of these systems will be very high and the initial applications may focus on unique disease problems. In addition, CT remains the most common imaging procedure for following oncology studies. This textbook has added an entry level chapter on MRI to introduce the technical concepts to understand the physics of MRI image and the means for producing different types of MRI images that may be used in fusion studies.

RADIATION SAFETY IN PET

Chapter 7 discusses some of the issues relative to the use and handling of PET radionuclides. Several comments are worth reviewing here because the specifics of PET fundamentals are discussed. Technologists performing PET procedures commonly have higher radiation exposure than when working in general nuclear medicine. This increased exposure is principally from two sources: handling millicurie quantities of high-energy photon emitters and being in proximity to patients that have been injected with high-energy gamma radiation. The energy spectrum from the patient is not as high as might be expected. The patient emits many Compton-scattered–photons, and the mean energy is in the range of 200 to 300 keV.

An additional small source of radiation exposure for patients and staff members comes from the long-lived radioactive sources in the gantry that are used for transmission imaging and for scanner calibration. As with all nuclear medicine, PET uses the application of time, distance, and shielding to maintain *as low as reasonable achievable* (ALARA) radiation safety practices.

The 511-keV annihilation photons have a half-value layer of 4 mm of lead. This requires special syringe shields, typically made from tungsten, which has about 1.4 times the effectiveness as the same thickness of lead. Waste containers should also be of thicker shielding material, and the laboratory bench for handling PET radionuclides should have a 1- to 2-inch–thick L-block of lead with a 4-inch–thick lead glass viewing window. Tongs and remote manipulators should be employed whenever possible when handling vials, syringes, and sources. Reducing the time of handling radioactive materials has significant advantages when working with high-energy radionuclides. Time reduction and increased distance are particularly helpful during injection and uptake periods and when positioning the patient for imaging.

The exposure rate from a patient receiving 10 mCi of FDG will exceed 1 mR/hr at 1 m. It would therefore be unwise to allow injected patients to return immediately to public waiting areas during the FDG uptake period before scanning. A dedicated injection/uptake room is ideal; it may require $\frac{1}{8}$ to $\frac{3}{8}$ inch or more of lead in the walls of the room if this space is adjacent to unrestricted and heavily occupied areas. It may also be beneficial for the wall between the PET scanner and the control room to contain lead shielding in particularly busy laboratories. These details should be worked out with the radiation safety officer of the institution.

REQUIREMENTS FOR GATING AND RADIATION THERAPY TREATMENT PLANNING

PET/CT fused images provide an important tool for radiation therapy treatment planning. This is particularly useful in 3D conformal beam radiation therapy. Intensity-modulated radiation therapy (IMRT) uses a multileaf collimator system to conform the shape of the therapy beam to the tumor. Computed tomography scans are normally used in IMRT treatment planning; however, the PET scan fused with the anatomical CT scan may allow the IMRT beam to be further refined to deliver more radiation to the most metabolically active areas of the tumor. Precise IMRT delivers more radiation to exactly where it is needed and less radiation to surrounding areas, thus reducing side effects and complications.

There are several additional requirements for hardware and software for certain clinical applications of PET/CT. Cardiac or respiratory gating may be occasionally required with PET studies for cardiology or oncology applications. ECG gating of cardiac studies is quite straightforward and requires only the interface of the ECG hardware and software similar to what would be used for planar or SPECT cardiac nuclear medicine studies.

Respiratory gated radiation therapy treatment is performed at some facilities and is particularly important for lesions in the lung or near the diaphragm, therefore respiratory gated CT treatment planning is required. Respiratory gating of PET images may be done in a different way by each scanner vendor. Respiratory gating may be done either by a physiological trigger from electrodes positioned on the chest or by monitoring the respiratory cycle with an external video camera. The external respirator camera system monitors the position of a lightweight reflective marker that sits on the patients chest during imaging to measure the respiratory phase and amplitude of chest movement in real time. The respiratory signals are combined with the PET acquisition data to provide respiratory gated images. Respiratory gated PET creates some advantages in lesion visualization because there is no blurring due to respiratory motion and lesions will visually be more intense. Also the SUV value of respiratory blurred lesions will be lower and respiratory gated quantitative SUVs will be slightly higher and more accurate.

PET scans performed for radiation therapy treatment planning must be performed with the patient in the position that is identical to their position during treatment planning and therapeutic irradiation. An external beam laser alignment system may be desirable in the PET suite but is not required. A flatbed pallet for the PET scanner is required that can accommodate the attachment of patient positioning devices such as a patient molds and immobilization masks. The most accurate positioning is to have the radiation therapy technologist come to the PET suite with the patient and devices and position the patient before the PET scan.

SUMMARY

- A PET image is based on detecting a pair of annihilation photons that creates a line of response (LOR) between two of the detectors in the gantry.
- Scintillation detector crystals of BGO, LSO, GSO, or LYSO are used on commercial PET systems.
- Detector modules group dozens of small rectangular crystals (3 to 6 mm wide and 20 to 30 mm long) with four PMTs. Hundreds of modules are used to create a ring around the patient.
- The sensitivity of PET scanners is about 1% to 2%.

- PET technology uses electronic collimation and produces reconstructed spatial resolution of about 4 to 5 mm at all locations within the image slice.
- The resolution of PET is about four times better than that of SPECT.
- The annihilation photon pair must be detected within a timing window of 4 to 12 ns.
- Annihilation photons are detected as coincidence events that are classified as true events if there is no scanner, random events if the photons are not from a single annihilation, or scatter events if a Compton interaction deflects one of the photons.
- PET data acquisition stores events as LORs within sinograms.
- PET scanners may be designed to operate in 2D or 3D configurations or both.
- The 2D systems have lead septa between rings of detectors to reduce scatter and random events.
- The 3D configurations have no septa; this increases sensitivity but results in a higher number of random events and scatter, which must be very accurately corrected during reconstruction.
- PET reconstruction is similar to SPECT reconstruction in that the acquired data are stored in sinograms (2D or 3D), which contain projection information.
- If data are 3D, then they must be put into 2D form before reconstruction; this can be done using single-slice rebinning (SSRB) or more commonly using Fourier rebinning (FORE). Then typical 2D reconstruction techniques can be applied.
- PET reconstruction can be performed with a variety of algorithms: filtered back-projection (FBP), ordered subset expectation maximization (OSEM), or row-action maximum likelihood algorithm (RAMLA) on commercial systems.
- OSEM and RAMLA are the most commonly used because they reduce streak artifacts and image noise compared with FBP.
- Attenuation correction is performed in PET.
- Mathematical attenuation correction techniques (Chang method) may be used if the tissue attenuation is the same at all areas within a transaxial slice.
- Measured attenuation correction may be performed by two techniques: by performing a transmission scan using a radioactive source rotated around the patient or by performing a CT scan to measure tissue density.
- Because annihilation photons must completely traverse the entire width of the human body, there is significant attenuation even though the radiation is of high energy.
- Transmission scans are slow but provide accurate attenuation correction measurements because the radioactive sources are of high energy (^{68}Ge [511 keV]).
- CT scans are obtained at low energies (70 to 140 keV maximum energy of a broad range). Therefore tissue attenuation measurements must be adjusted to 511 keV before attenuation correction may be applied.
- Segmentation techniques are used to replace tissue values in transmission scans or CT scans with known tissue values for areas of lung, air, soft tissue, and bone in order to reduce noise in the transmission attenuation correction maps (images).
- PET scanner calibrations are important to keep the system operating optimally. Blank scans or other calibration scans must be performed daily to measure the performance of each detector.
- Quality control in PET consists of ensuring that calibrations are up-to-date, and a test image from the scanner must be reviewed before scanning patients. An aggressive program of calibrations and test imaging will ensure scanner uptime and image quality.
- PET images may give quantitative measurements of radiotracer uptake if calibrations are accurately performed. Standard uptake values (SUV) provide a measure of the percentage of injected dose uptake in tumors. The absolute activity calibration (often called the *well counter calibration* for strictly historical reasons) calibrates the PET scanner to the dose calibrator measurement.
- The partial volume effect falsely lowers SUV measurements
- Radiation safety is very important with PET radionuclides because the high-energy, short-lived tracers emit more radiation than traditional nuclear medicine radionuclides.
- Distance is most effective in occupational protection from PET radionuclides.
- The half-value layer of lead is 4.1-mm thick. Lead shields, L-blocks, and dose calibrator shields should be 1 to 2 inches thick. Tungsten has a smaller half-value layer than lead, and therefore syringe shields made of tungsten are more effective.

SUGGESTED READING

Cherry SR, Sorenson JA, Phelps ME: *Physics in nuclear medicine*, ed 3, Philadelphia, 2003, Saunders.

Christian PE, Swanston NM: *PET Study Guide*, Reston, VA, 2010, Society of Nuclear Medicine.

Phelps ME, editor: *PET: molecular imaging and its biological applications*, New York, 2004, Springer-Verlag.

Valk PE, Bailey DL, Townsend DW, et al: *Positron emission tomography*, London, 2003, Springer-Verlag.

von Schultess GK, editor: *Clinical positron emission tomography*, Philadelphia, 2000, Lippincott Williams & Wilkins.

Wahl RL, editor: *Principles and practice of positron emission tomography*, Philadelphia, 2002, Lippincott Williams & Wilkins.

Wernick MN, Aarsvold JN, editors: *Emission tomography: the fundamentals of PET and SPECT*, London, 2004, Elsevier Academic Press.

CT Physics and Instrumentation

Paul E. Christian

OUTLINE

OBJECTIVES

After completing this chapter, the reader will be able to:
- Describe the physics processes involved in the production of x-rays.
- Describe the role of each component in the x-ray tube and its operation.
- Discuss the proper adjustment of x-ray tube voltage and current in CT.
- Name the principal parts of a CT scanner.
- Discuss the function of each CT scanner component.
- Describe how a helical CT scanner operates and the component changes that made this technology possible.
- Discuss how CT image data are acquired and processed.
- Describe the calculation process of Hounsfield units.
- Discuss the advantages of multislice CT.
- Describe CT number values assigned to various tissues and how these values are assigned into meaningful display windowing.

- List parameters set by the operator for CT use and describe the effect of each on the images.
- Discuss CT image quality issues.
- List the origin of CT image artifacts and describe their prevention.
- Discuss appropriate parameters for the acquisition of low-dose CT for PET attenuation correction.
- Describe the parameters and image characteristics required for a diagnostic-quality CT scan.
- Discuss the integration of CT procedures into the combined PET/CT examination.
- Discuss occupational radiation exposure from operating a CT scanner.
- Discuss patient radiation exposure from a CT scanner.
- Describe a program of CT quality control.
- Discuss the importance of CT quality control.

KEY TERMS

adaptive detector array
beam hardening
Bremsstrahlung radiation
CT collimation
CT dose index (CTDI)
CT number (Hounsfield unit [HU])
helical (spiral) CT

high-contrast resolution
increment
isotropic pixel
low-contrast resolution
milliampere-seconds (mAs)
multislice CT (MSCT)
peak kilovoltage (kVp)

pitch
reconstruction field of view (FOV)
rotation speed
slice thickness
x-ray filter

This chapter is intended to provide an introduction to the principles and operation of a computed tomography (CT) scanner. The chapter is not intended to be comprehensive in discussing all aspects of this technology but is presented to describe the critical physics processes, instrumentation components, image acquisition/reconstruction parameters, and display techniques used in CT imaging. The material contained in this chapter should provide the reader with enough information to allow the reader to understand the technical parameters and processes to use the CT scanner in performing combined SPECT/CT and PET/CT studies. The CT component of a combined nuclear medicine and PET/CT procedure requires a working understanding of CT instead of a thorough and comprehensive understanding of the wide variety of clinical CT-alone procedures. The goal of this concise chapter is to acquaint readers with a fundamental understanding of these systems in order to later attain mastery needed for the particular requirements of their application of PET/CT. This chapter, combined with the PET/CT medical applications discussed in Chapter 13, provides an overview of the PET/CT systems and the selection of appropriate procedural applications to a variety of diseases.

X-rays were discovered by Wilhelm Conrad Roentgen on November 8, 1895, as he worked with light emission from electric current that was applied to electrodes of a glass vacuum chamber. He immediately recognized that these newly discovered invisible rays could penetrate human tissue and could distinguish between tissue densities, principally soft tissue and bone. This amazing development was the first opportunity to view the anatomy of the human body non-invasively. Within a few years systems were developed both for taking x-ray images on film and for performing fluoroscopic procedures. However, at that time there was no understanding of the health hazards of radiation, and the exposure levels for both patients and health-care workers were very high. By the mid-1930s, x-ray systems were widespread, and x-ray procedures and studies with contrast materials were being performed.

PHYSICS OF X-RAYS

The electromagnetic spectrum, as described in Chapter 2, demonstrated that high-energy photons, described as x-rays and gamma rays, overlap in their respective energy regions and therefore have identical properties. The difference between the two is their origin; x-rays are produced in the electron shell structure of the atom, whereas gamma rays are created by the nuclear forces at the center of the atom. In x-ray tubes there are two different types of reactions that produce x-rays: **Bremsstrahlung radiation** and characteristic x-rays.

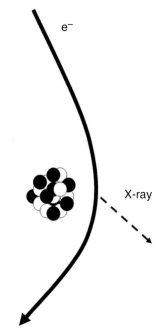

FIGURE 11-1 Bremsstrahlung radiation is produced when an electron passes in close proximity to the nucleus, causing the electron to slow significantly, lose energy, and deviate from its path. The kinetic energy lost due to the lower velocity of the electron is released as electromagnetic radiation in the form of an x-ray.

Bremsstrahlung Radiation

Bremsstrahlung is a German word meaning *braking radiation*. Bremsstrahlung radiation occurs when energetic electrons pass very near the nucleus of an atom. The strong force of the positively charged atom causes the negatively charged electron to rapidly decelerate; the path of the electron is significantly changed, and some of the kinetic energy of the electron is lost and is converted through the Bremsstrahlung process into electromagnetic energy (Figure 11-1). The continuous energy spectrum of these x-rays is caused by the randomness of the distance between the electron and its proximity to the nucleus. The closer the distance between the electron and the nucleus, the greater the deceleration of the electron and the higher the x-ray energy emitted. As the atom is about 10^{-8} cm in diameter and the nucleus is only 10^{-12} cm, the likelihood of the electron coming close to the nucleus is low and therefore the efficiency of the production of x-rays is rather low; only about 1% of the electrons produce an x-ray.

Characteristic X-Rays

Characteristic x-rays are produced following the ionization of an atom that leaves an inner shell, typically the K shell, with an electron vacancy. Outer-shell electrons that drop in to fill the inner-shell vacancy must lose energy, which is released as electromagnetic radiation (x-ray) with a specific or *characteristic* energy determined by the energy difference between the two shells (see Figure 2-24).

X-RAY TUBE AND THE PRODUCTION OF X-RAYS

X-Ray Tube Design

The x-ray tube is a glass envelope that contains a high vacuum so that accelerated electrons from the internal electrodes may move with ease. Power between the electrodes is supplied from a generator typically as rectified three-phase power at approximately 50,000 to 150,000 V and several hundred milliamperes. Within the x-ray tube is a cathode (Figure 11-2, *A*) that has a very small filament (coil of wire), which is several millimeters in length. The housing around the filament forms the focusing cup of the cathode. When a current is applied to heat the filament, electrons are boiled off and are generously available for acceleration to the anode by the rectified high voltage. X-ray tubes for CT scanners have an anode that rotates thousands of revolutions per minute in order to prevent the beam of electrons from the cathode from burning the anode and to remove heat from the anode. The rotating anode disk (see Figure 11-2, *A*) is often constructed using several layers of materials with the underlying layer composed of materials such as titanium/zirconium/molybdenum (TZM) or graphite. The electron beam strikes the surface layer of the anode where the x-rays are produced via Bremsstrahlung radiation and characteristic x-rays. The x-ray beam exits the tube from a window in the side of the tube. X-ray tubes in CT scanners may use standard, high-resolution, and sometimes ultrahigh-resolution focal spot sizes and secondary collimation to improve image resolution. These settings change the line-pair-per-centimeter resolution in the final images.

Rotating anode tubes are required to remove the vast amount of heat that is generated by modern CT scanners. Often the tube may be surrounded by an oil bath to efficiently remove heat, and chilled water or cooled air may also be required to remove heat quickly so that the tube does not require a long cooldown time between uses. Only about 1% of the energy applied to the system is converted into x-rays that exit the tube window; the remaining 99% of energy creates heat.

The voltage applied to the electrodes of an x-ray tube is typically in the range of 30 to 150 **kVp (peak kilovoltage)** for a wide range of x-ray applications. A low-kVp potential difference on the electrodes will accelerate the electrons from the cathode with very little force and the Bremsstrahlung x-rays that are produced will have low energy. Thus for higher peak kilovoltage applied to the anode there will be a proportional increase in the energy (keV) of the x-rays that are produced (see Figure 11-2, *B*). The x-rays needed for imaging an extremity will

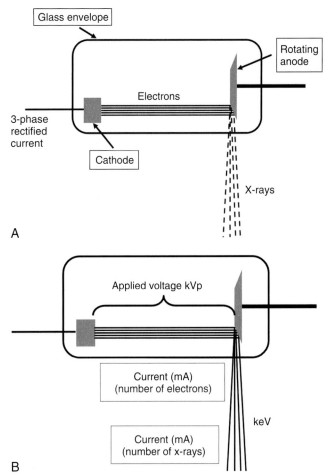

FIGURE 11-2 A, The x-ray tube is an evacuated glass envelope with a cathode that emits electrons and high voltage potential applied to the anode. The anode is rapidly rotating to dissipate heat and prevent the anode from being burned by the electron beam within the tube. X-rays are emitted through a window in the side of the tube. **B,** The higher the kilovolts peak (kVp) applied to the electrodes, the faster the electrons are accelerated and thus produce higher-energy x-rays. When more current (mA) is applied, there is a proportional increase in the number of electrons produced and the resulting number of x-rays that are emitted by the tube.

require little penetrating power, and low voltages need only be applied to the x-ray tube. However, when it is necessary to penetrate the abdomen, higher-energy x-rays must be produced and therefore higher kVp will need to be applied to the x-ray tube.

The x-ray energy distribution that is produced by Bremsstrahlung radiation is manifested as a continuous energy spectrum (Figure 11-3). The continuous energy distribution comes from the wide variation in the distance between the braking electron and the nucleus, in addition to the amount of deceleration (or braking) of the electron as it comes into the electromagnetic field of the nucleus. Extremely low energy x-rays may not have enough energy to exit the glass window of the x-ray tube. In addition to Bremsstrahlung radiation, the electrons cause some ionization of the lower-energy shells of the atoms in the anode tungsten target. Subsequently K-shell

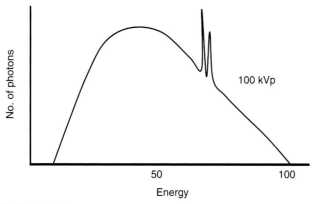

FIGURE 11-3 The x-ray spectrum produced from the tube is a continuous spectrum with the maximum energy set by the kVp applied to the tube and the total number of x-rays determined by the current (mA) that is applied. The Bremsstrahlung radiation creates the continuous spectrum of x-rays while ionized atoms in the anode emit characteristic x-rays superimposed as discrete peaks on the continuous curve. Extremely low energy x-rays are not emitted from the tube, because they are internally absorbed by the glass window of the tube.

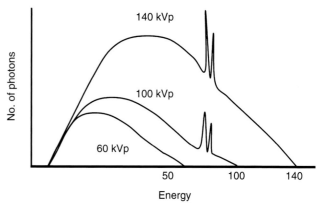

FIGURE 11-4 The variation of the applied voltage (kVp) changes the maximum x-ray energy and stretches the x-ray spectrum to higher keV energies as shown by the two upper curves at 140 and 100 kVp, respectively. When the kVp setting is below the characteristic x-rays for tungsten (60 kVp as demonstrated in the lower curve), the characteristic peaks do not appear because the electron energy within the tube was not high enough to cause ionization of the anode tungsten atoms.

x-rays are produced at 69.5 keV and the M-L shell transition is at 57.0 keV. These characteristic x-rays are seen as discrete energy peaks on the continuous Bremsstrahlung spectrum in Figure 11-3.

Voltage Variation

An increase in the high voltage applied to the x-ray tube will result in a corresponding increase in the maximum energy of x-rays that are produced. In addition there is also an increase in the amplitude of the spectrum as more x-rays are produced by the higher velocity of the electrons that have been accelerated to the anode (Figure 11-4). Note that not only the amplitude of overall spectrum is increased, but there is also a significant change in the contribution of characteristic tungsten x-rays with higher kVp settings (see Figure 11-4). When the kVp is lower than the characteristic tungsten x-ray peaks, the x-rays are produced solely by Bremsstrahlung radiation. The spectrum will be continuous in nature, because the electrons that were incident upon the anode did not have sufficient energy to remove any K-shell electrons and thus produce ionization of the anode atoms. The energies required for typical PET/CT studies of the body will be in the range of 80 to 140 kVp, depending on the size of the patient and the detail that is required for the clinical application. The energies that can be selected on a CT scanner are usually defined by a limited set of energies such as 80, 100, 120, and 140 kVp, so there is no continuous energy option available to the operator. A general rule is that an increase of approximately 15% in kVp is roughly equivalent to doubling the **milliampere-seconds (mAs).**

The kVp setting selects the maximum possible energy of the x-ray beam. Higher-energy x-ray photons are

needed to penetrate large bones of the shoulder, hip, vertebrae, and so forth; therefore a higher kVp setting will be required. The kVp setting also defines the fraction of photons that will successfully reach the detectors of the scanner, because higher-energy photons are less attenuated by the body. More photons reaching the detectors will result in lower quantum noise in the images; however, the radiation exposure to the patient will increase.

When the spectrum of x-rays passes through the body, the lower-energy (softer) x-rays are most easily absorbed; as the beam passes through, there is a shift in energy distribution so that a larger fraction of the remaining photons have a higher energy. This spectral shift is referred to as **beam hardening.** Beam hardening will create artifacts seen as dark streaks that radiate from the outside toward the inner part of the body. These artifacts may appear to radiate from dense bone where there was a significant absorption of low-energy photons, but higher-energy x-rays continue through the body.

Advantages to using a higher kVp:

- Greater penetration through the body
- Decrease in quantum noise
- A reduction in beam hardening artifacts

Compromises:

- Higher dose to patient
- Reduces differences in tissue densities

Current Variation

The applied current is the other primary setting that can be adjusted in the x-ray tube. Figure 11-5 shows that there is a proportional increase in the number of x-rays, at all energies, when the current in milliamperes (mA) is increased. Both the Bremsstrahlung and characteristic x-rays that are produced increase proportionally with the current. The current setting in radiography is often referred to as *mAs*, which for planar x-rays is the mA multiplied by the exposure time in seconds. In CT the time will be the rotation time in seconds. The range of currents that may be used in a CT scanner is commonly very wide, about 50 to 400 mA; it is continuously

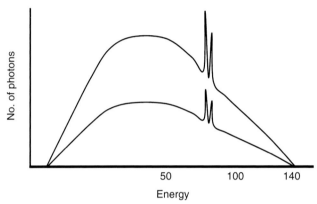

FIGURE 11-5 The variation of the current increases the total number of x-rays, and the curve rises without a change in the maximum energy of the x-rays: high current *(upper curve)*, low current *(lower curve)*. The number of characteristic x-rays produced also changes proportionally to the current.

variable and typically does not limit the operator to a few preset values. This wide range of current settings is required to adjust the scanning parameter to the patient and clinical application of the body area being studied, the patient, and the procedure. For example, a pediatric study on a 5-year-old child would not require the same photon density in the image as would a study of the bones in the spine of a heavy adult.

The mA is a direct defining parameter of the number of photons generated by the x-ray tube. The higher the number of x-rays reaching the detector, the lower the quantum noise in the image. However, the mA and the time are the dominant parameters that determine the radiation dose to the patient.

Advantages to using higher mA:

* Decrease in image noise
* Increase in contrast resolution

Compromise:

* Higher mA increases dose to the patient

The effects of adjusting both kVp and mA are shown in Figure 11-6. Figure 11-6, *A*, shows a patient scan using 80 kVp and an mA setting of 200. Although the mA is moderately high, the low kVp produces an image with relatively moderate image noise. If the kVp is increased to 140 as shown in Figure 11-6, *B*, there is a

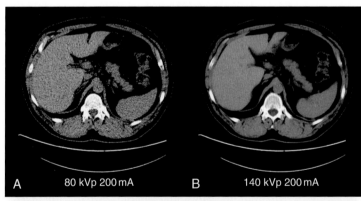
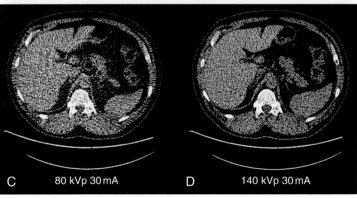

FIGURE 11-6 Peak kilovoltage (kVp) and mA have a significant influence on image quality, as shown in these images from single-patient study acquired with different parameters. **A,** At 80 kVp and 200 mA the low x-ray energy penetrating power compromises the number of photons, creating a noisy image. Note that the low energy does not provide high-quality visualization of the vertebrae. **B,** When both the energy and the current are high (140 kVp and 200 mA), the image noise is low and a high-quality diagnostic image is formed. Note that the 140-kVp energy creates detail within the vertebrae. **C,** When both the energy and the current are low (80 kVp and 30 mA), the image quality suffers; the image is extremely noisy, and concentric ring artifacts are created because the detectors in the array do not perform the same. **D,** If the energy is increased to 140 kVp, the instrument artifacts are no longer present.

significant reduction in quantum noise as even more x-rays are produced due to the increased voltage. Fine detail of the organs, edges of regions of density changes, and so forth, are all superior with the kVp change. Also note the improved resolution within the vertebral body due to the availability of more high-energy photons.

To understand the impact of the current setting on the clinical quality of the images, compare image *A* in Figure 11-6 with image *C*. Image *A* was acquired using 80 kVp and 200 mA, whereas image *C* used the same 80 kVp but only 30 mA. The image quality is very poor in image *C* due to the very low number of photons, because both the voltage and current settings were at the lowest values that can be set on this CT scanner. Image *C* is extremely "noisy" to the point of not resolving the edges of organ structures. Image *C* also has ring artifacts because the data density on the CT detectors is too low to give accurate measurements of attenuation. Because these scans were performed on a 240-lb patient, the low-dose CT study required for PET attenuation correction could be performed with minimal voltage and currents for this size of patient. Image *D* of Figure 11-6 demonstrates that raising the energy to 140 kVp but leaving the current at 30 mA recovers the unacceptable low beam intensity so that the ring artifacts are removed. The minimal kVp and current for this size of patient should be about 120 kVp and 50 mA. All CT systems have some settings that may be below what would be clinically acceptable for low-dose PET attenuation-correction parameters. If a diagnostic CT study were needed for this size patient, the parameters of 140 kVp and 200 mA (see Figure 11-6, *B*) would be appropriate settings for this size of patient. The image quality demonstrates low noise and high resolution of fine structures in addition to differentiating structures.

X-Ray Filter

Both planar x-ray and CT imaging system position an absorbing **x-ray filter** into the x-ray beam. Figure 11-7 shows the location of the x-ray beam filter in the general design of the CT scanner. The beam-modifying filter has two purposes:

1. Filtering absorbs the very low energy x-rays that would not have sufficient energy to transmit through the body tissue and would thus only increase patient exposure without adding information to the imaging process. By removing the low-energy x-rays, the beam is *hardened* so that the broad energy distribution has been somewhat removed, and the result is a somewhat more uniform average energy of the beam. The filter may reduce patient radiation exposure by as much as 50%.
2. Filtering aids in shaping the energy distribution of the beam. A filter somewhat in the shape of a bow tie is often used to prevent the edges of the beam from

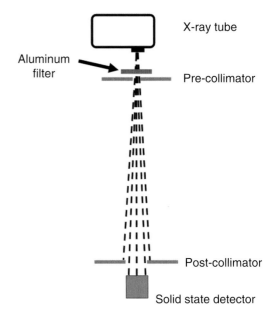

FIGURE 11-7 The configuration of the x-ray tube and solid-state x-ray detectors uses the placement of an aluminum filter in the beam to remove low-energy x-rays that could not pass completely through the patient, and the filter also shapes the beam. Precollimators and postcollimators before and after the patient reduce scatter radiation.

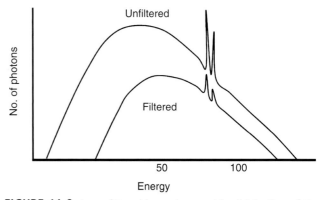

FIGURE 11-8 An unfiltered beam has a wide distribution of the continuous Bremsstrahlung spectrum. The filter absorbs the low-energy portion, creating a spectrum that is more beneficial to imaging the patient with reduced radiation exposure.

hardening; therefore the energy distribution across the field of the detectors is more uniform.

The filter on a CT scanner is not interchangeable with other filters; it is a permanent installation for modifying the beam as mentioned and reduces the unused low-energy radiation, which adds nothing to the image formation. Figure 11-8 demonstrates the change in the x-ray spectrum as the filter absorbs a sizable fraction of the x-rays. The result is that the very low energy x-rays, which would be completely absorbed in the body and not pass through to the detectors, are completely removed, thereby reducing the patient exposure. The lower spectrum in Figure 11-8 demonstrates the reduction of both the Bremsstrahlung and characteristic x-ray components of the spectrum.

PRINCIPLES OF COMPUTED TOMOGRAPHY

Although x-ray images are of high resolution, there are many superimposed structures that create difficulty in viewing a particular organ or area of interest. *Tomography* (from the Greek word *tomos* meaning "section") is a term that refers to the ability to view an anatomic section or slice through the body. Anatomical cross sections are most commonly referred to as *transverse axial tomography* in reference to section images created as though the body had been sliced through in a manner akin to slicing bread. Computed tomography images achieve not only minimal superimposition of tissues but also improved contrast differences of tissues over planar x-ray techniques.

The CT scanner was developed by Godfrey Hounsfield in the very late 1960s. This x-ray–based system created projection information of x-ray beams passed through the object from many points across the object and from many angles (projections). The first studies in humans were performed by Hounsfield and James Ambrose at Atkinson-Morley's Hospital in England in 1971. To deal with the reconstruction of the projection information, Allan M. Cormack, a mathematician, applied the mathematical reconstruction techniques to convert CT data into image slices. Early CT scanners were limited to use in the brain; however, in 1974 Robert Ledley introduced techniques that led to the development of the first CT scanner that could perform whole-body imaging of patients. By the late 1970s many hospitals had installed CT body scanners, and this new x-ray technology came into widespread use in clinical practice. Computed tomography not only produces cross-sectional images but also has the ability to differentiate tissue densities, which creates an improvement in contrast resolution. Hounsfield and Cormack were awarded the 1979 Nobel Prize in Medicine for their development of the CT scanner.

CT SCANNER DESIGN

The basic technology employed in the CT scanner is designed to provide a source of x-rays to be transmitted through the patient. Early CT scanners used an x-ray tube and scintillation crystal detector that moved laterally across the patient; the gantry would rotate a few degrees, and then the detector would move again. This acquisition process would take several minutes to acquire 180 degrees of projection data. Images were reconstructed into relatively coarse resolution images (80×80 pixels) and required about 5 minutes to reconstruct each slice.

The CT system consists of a computer workstation for operation of the scanner, image processing computers, electronics cabinets, the gantry, and the patient imaging table. The gantry (Figure 11-9) houses the key components of the scanner; many components associated with the production of the x-ray beam and detection and acquisition of the beam must be located within the

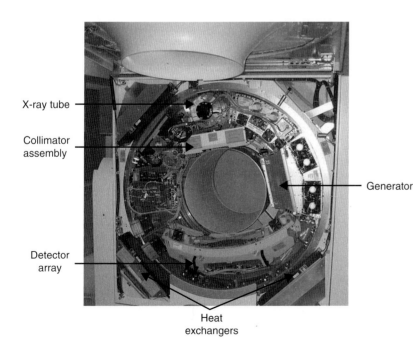

X-ray tube

Collimator assembly

Detector array

Generator

Heat exchangers

FIGURE 11-9 The multislice helical CT gantry has nearly all components on the slip-ring rotating gantry. The x-ray tube sits opposite the detector array. The collimator array and power generator for the x-ray tube are also on the rotating gantry, while heat exchangers that remove heat from the gantry are on the fixed portion of the gantry. Power and signals from the gantry may be passed through the slip-ring contacts.

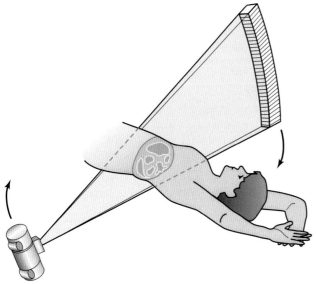

FIGURE 11-10 The x-ray tube generates a fan-shaped beam of x-rays that traverse through the patient to irradiate the detector array. The rotating gantry provides transmission measurements through the patient from many projection angles.

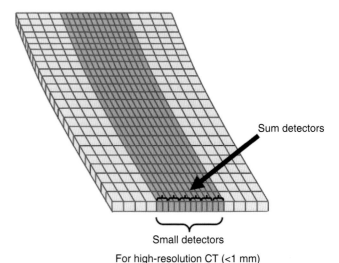

FIGURE 11-11 The CT detector array may have more than 800 detectors across the lateral portion of the patient and at least as many detectors that image each slice. The small detectors in the center of the array may be summed for lower-resolution scans that use the full detector array.

rotating portion of the gantry. The fan-beam x-ray tube sits opposite the detector array within the rotating gantry. The three-phase power generator is also within the gantry module. X-ray detectors and the data acquisition system are also on board the rotating gantry. Heat from the generator, x-ray tube, and other components must be removed efficiently; therefore two or more heat exchangers are typically found on the system. As seen in Figure 11-10, the x-ray tube in a CT scanner is designed to produce a fan beam of x-rays that is approximately as wide as the body. Thus tissue attenuation is measured over a large region from one position of the x-ray tube. The x-ray tube on a CT scanner is a much more heavy-duty unit than the tubes used for standard x-ray imaging, because the tube must stay on for extended periods of time to complete large-area imaging and often requires that the gantry be cooled with chilled water in order to remove the high quantity of heat that this tube produces. On the opposite side of the patient (see Figure 11-10) is the detector array that measures the strength of the x-ray beam at various points laterally across the body.

The x-ray detectors used in CT scanners have changed dramatically since the advent of the early systems that used a single highly collimated beam of x-rays that was measured by a single sodium iodide scintillation detector; the beam moved laterally across the patient and then rotated and scanned another projection. Later generations of scanners used arrays of scintillation detectors or migrated toward arrays of xenon-filled gas detector arrays once fan-beam x-ray tubes were employed. Today all CT scanners use solid-state detectors that have very high efficiency at the low energy of x-rays produced by

CT scanners. Solid-state detectors may be made of a variety of materials that create a semiconductor junction similar to a transistor. Ultrafast ceramic detectors use rare earth elements such as silicon, germanium, cadmium, yttrium, or gadolinium, which create a semiconducting *p-n* junction. The *p-n* junction creates an interface where an electronic signal is easily generated when radiation is detected by the junction. The more radiation that is detected, the larger the electrical signal that is produced; therefore the solid-state detector signal is proportional to the amount of radiation that is detected. Ceramic solid-state detectors are very fast, can be extremely stable, and are produced to form an array of very small, efficient detectors that can cover a large area.

Detector systems in **multislice CT** scanners use detectors that are no longer in a single transverse line across the patient but are in a two-dimensional (2D) array. The size and sophistication of the detector arrays depend on how many slices can be performed simultaneously by the scanner. The array size for a 16-slice CT (Figure 11-11) may have more than 800 detector elements laterally across the gantry by 16 or more detectors across the central gantry axis. The size of the individual detector elements is less than 1 mm on each side. Some manufacturers have detectors of smaller size in the center with detectors twice this size on the outer edges. Utilizing this configuration, the signal from pairs of small inner detectors may be added together to effectively produce larger detectors when high resolution is not required.

The solid-state CT detector arrays may be constructed in a variety of configurations, which vary significantly between commercial systems and periodically change

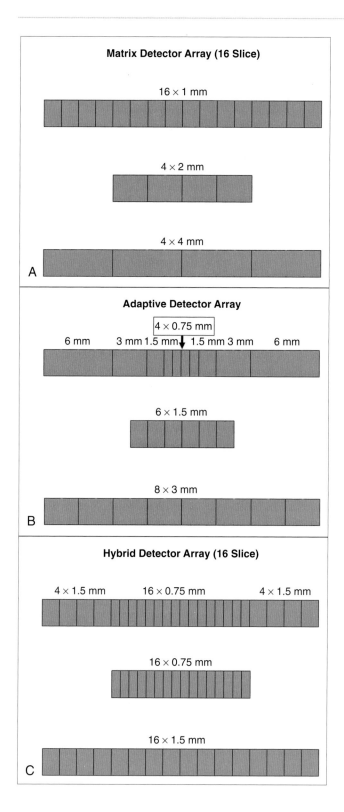

A, Detector arrays with equal-sized detectors allow imaging at the finest resolution (16 1.0-mm detectors) set by the detector size; alternatively the output from pairs of detectors may be summed to effectively create eight 2.0-mm detectors (second row of **A**), or four detectors outputs may be summed to create four 4.0-mm detectors. **B**, Adaptive arrays have smaller detectors in the center with larger detector elements of different sizes at the edges of the array (smallest 0.75 mm to 6.0 mm). Summing the center 0.75-mm elements with the adjacent 1.5-mm elements can create the equivalent of six 1.5-mm detectors (middle row of **B**), or a different summing scheme may create an array of eight 3.0-mm detectors. **C**, A hybrid detector array has only two detector element sizes but may create a large number of high-resolution slices (16 0.75-mm slices—middle row of **C**) or sum detectors in a variety of detector sizes while maintaining a large number of slices.

1.0-mm detectors, which may be used individually for the highest resolution on the system. Adjacent detectors may be summed to effectively create detectors that are twice the size. In the second row of Figure 11-12, *A*, the central detectors have been summed to form the equivalent of four 2.0-mm detectors; eight 2.0-mm detectors may also have been effectively defined. If even less *z*-axis spatial resolution is allowed, the detector matrix could have four 1.0-mm detectors summed to create the equivalent of four 4.0-mm detectors (Figure 11-12, *A, bottom row*).

An example of an **adaptive detector array** is shown in Figure 11-12, *B*, where several different size detectors—0.75, 1.5, 3.0, and 6.0 mm—are positioned to create an array in the *z*-axis direction. If high-resolution imaging in 0.75-mm detectors is required, then only the central four detectors of that size would be used. If 1.5-mm equivalent size detectors are selected, the system may sum pairs of the small 0.75-mm detectors. The larger 3.0-mm detectors may be partially irradiated by the tube, and the result would be as shown in Figure 11-12, *B (middle row)*, to create the equivalent of six 1.5-mm detectors. Further, the bottom row demonstrates that this adaptive system may also create an eight-slice system with the equivalence of 3.0-mm detectors. The advantage of adaptive detector arrays is that they permit great flexibility.

A hybrid adaptive type of design usually has only two detector sizes, some of which are double the size of the smallest detectors (see Figure 11-12, *C*). This design allows the use of only the smallest detectors to acquire in the highest resolution possible (see Figure 11-12, *C, middle row*) 16 slices with 0.75 mm. The bottom row of Figure 11-12, *C*, demonstrates adding the output of the 0.75-mm detectors to effectively create 16 1.5-mm detectors. Other combinations using partial detector irradiation and summing may create additional options.

with models of CT systems within a vendor's line of products. The simplest of these array designs is the matrix detector design as demonstrated in Figure 11-12, *A*. The *z*-axis of the detector array is composed of an array of elements that are equal in their dimensions (**isotropic pixel**). In this simple example there are 16

FIGURE 11-12

Collimation

In routine radiographic studies, radiation of the body with x-rays must be restricted to the region being examined to limit radiation exposure to the patient and reduce scatter radiation. Computed tomography scanners therefore use collimators to protect the patient and limit the beam to the size of the detector array that is active during data acquisition. The configuration of **CT collimation** is shown in Figure 11-7. Adjacent to the x-ray tube is a set of prepatient collimators that restrict the width and shape the beam to the area of interest for a single rotation of the tube and detectors around the patient. The collimator must be in perfect alignment with the tube and detector array to optimize the beam location. In addition, the collimators shape the beam and, along with the focal spot size on the anode, influence the penumbra (or spreading) of the x-ray beam. The **slice thickness** that may be reconstructed can never be thinner than the collimator width. Collimator options on a system might be similar to 0.6, 0.75, 1.0, 1.5, 2.0, 3.0, 4.0, 5.0, 6.0, 7.0, 8.0, and 10.0 mm, although most diagnostic studies will be acquired using collimators less than 4.0 mm in most PET/CT and CT-alone applications.

In addition to the prepatient collimators, CT gantries usually employ a set of postpatient collimators (see Figure 11-7) that are positioned just before the x-ray beam reaches the detector array. The postpatient collimators, if present, reduce the scattered x-rays from entering the detector array, which would reduce the image contrast. These detector collimators also define the slice thickness, which can range from 0.3 mm to several millimeters, depending on the system.

Beam collimation sets the actual thickness of the x-ray beam and therefore defines the thinnest slice thickness that may be obtained. However, in multislice CT the beam collimation does not equal the slice thickness. Choosing the slice thickness is one of the first parameters defined in setting up a CT protocol, because it sets the resolution that may be obtained. Selecting an appropriate collimation thickness will prevent small lesions from being missed if a thicker slice would fail to sufficiently resolve the lesion. Examples of using sufficiently thin collimation in PET/CT might be selecting a 0.75-mm or thinner collimation for identifying small lesions and structures in the lungs or defining the appropriate resolution required for head and neck disease. Abdominal disease may not require this same thin collimation.

Thinner collimation produces less streaking of high-density objects (e.g., metal, bone). If collimation that is too thin is used to cover large body areas, there will be additional scanning time and therefore a higher likelihood of patient motion. Collimation should be sufficiently thinner than the lesions to be detected.

Very thin collimation may limit the number of photons reaching the detectors and subsequently generate noisier images. Collimation is closely associated with reconstructed slice thickness in determining the level of quantum noise (or quantum mottle) that is produced in the slice images. Slice thickness therefore becomes important because it defines the volumetric dimension of the image voxels. For example, a slice thickness of 10 mm may completely miss a 6-mm lung lesion. A 3-mm slice thickness would definitely locate the lesion but would have only about one third of the photons and therefore have significantly more quantum mottle. Visually this produces an image with lower contrast resolution.

Advantages of thinner collimation:

- Less volume averaging
- Better resolution on reformatted sagittal and coronal images
- Increased spatial resolution
- Fewer streaking artifacts from high-density objects

Compromises of thinner collimation:

- Increased quantum mottle
- Increased scanning time
- May result in an increased number of slices as defined by the reconstruction slice thickness

Rotation Speed

In **helical (spiral) CT** (sometimes referred to as *spiral CT*), the gantry rotates continuously in one direction on the slip-ring system while the patient table moves at a constant speed through the gantry to quickly perform the scan of a relatively large body area (Figure 11-13). The **rotation speed** is the time required for the gantry to make one complete revolution. A typical low-performance

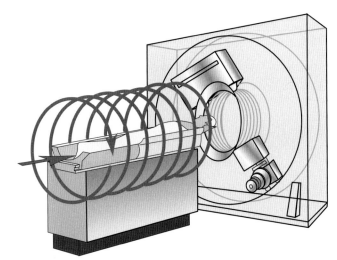

FIGURE 11-13 Multislice helical CT detector motion creates a spiral pattern along the patient as both the gantry and imaging table move during image acquisition to cover a large area of the body. The more slices obtained by the scanner, the faster the imaging table motion.

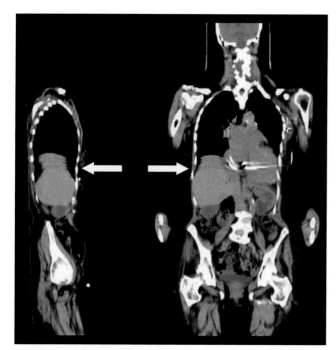

FIGURE 11-14 Multislice, helical CT reduces the need for patient breath holding; however, if a patient does take in a breath, or cough, during the acquisition, an artifact will appear due to the shifting position of the liver and spleen during this scan on a 16-slice scanner.

CT system with two to eight rows of detectors will primarily be used for general CT procedures and may also have a rotation speed that will not exceed one rotation per second. In order to prevent motion, breath holding by the patient will be required in studies where the CT acquisition of the chest or upper abdomen will take more than a couple of seconds. Commonly a diagnostic CT scan of the chest is performed with the patient holding his or her breath at end inspiration. The scanner may use automated verbal prompts to instruct the patient to take in a deep breath and hold it during the acquisition. These deep inspiration–breath hold CT scans will not line up with the PET scan and will cause misalignment of the CT scan that may be used for attenuation correction; therefore shallow breathing or breath holding mid-inspiration may provide CT images that are more closely aligned with the position of the lungs, liver, and diaphragm during the PET study. Even with a state-of-the-art, multislice CT system, motion artifacts may occur if the patient moves. Figure 11-14 demonstrates a motion artifact caused by the patient taking a deep breath when instructed to shallow-breathe during a 16-slice, whole-body PET/CT acquisition.

State-of-the-art (high-performance), multislice CT systems have very fast rotation times. Faster CT rotation speeds may be desirable for reducing the likelihood of patient motion artifacts or may be necessary for high-throughput CT applications or for cardiac procedures. Sixteen-slice, 40-slice, 64-slice, and higher-resolution systems will have rotation speeds that are a

small fraction of a second in order to capture very fast physiological changes in the body such as CT angiographic studies, cardiac calcification measurements, and respiratory or cardiac gated studies. Common gantry rotation speeds of 0.3 to 1.0 second with a table motion of about 10 to 20 mm/sec are used in oncological PET/CT acquisitions. The patient dose is in proportion to the rotation time when all other parameters are held constant, and short rotation times may reduce both exposure and patient motion artifacts. The one benefit to longer rotation times is that the x-ray tube can deliver a higher mAs, which leads to increased contrast resolution in the images. A clinical application of this in a large patient would be to change the tube rotation time from 0.5 second per rotation to 1.0 second per rotation so that the mA may be increased appropriately for the patient size.

Pitch. The continuous motion of the CT x-ray tube and detectors in the gantry as well as the imaging table creates the need to coordinate the speed of each motion to provide the desired spacing of images. Images conceivably could be overlapping or adjacent to one another, or spaces could be created between images. In helical CT, *pitch* is the ratio of the patient's movement through the gantry during one 360-degree beam rotation relative to the beam collimation.

For single-slice CT:

$$\text{Pitch} = \text{table movement per rotation/slice collimation}$$

or

$$\text{Volume Pitch} = \text{table movement per rotation/total slice volume}$$

For a 5-mm table movement and collimation of 5 mm, the pitch would be 1.0. In multislice CT the definition and calculation of pitch is not as clear because technology and vendor terminology may differ slightly. As an example, on Siemens systems the term *volume pitch* is used along with *pitch factor*. These terms may be calculated as follows:

$$\text{Volume pitch} = \text{table movement per rotation/total slice volume}$$

For a table speed per rotation of 24 mm and a slice volume of 12 mm, the volume pitch is calculated as 2.0. This term may be clarified by calculating the pitch factor:

$$\text{Pitch factor} = \text{table movement per rotation/detector row collimation}$$

The collimation, in this case, for a 16-slice CT system equals 16 times 1.5 mm, or 24.0 mm; for a 24-mm table movement per rotation, the pitch factor equals 1.0.

On most CT and PET/CT systems the pitch is entered as a parameter that is set in defining the procedure for the acquisition of patient data. On other vendor systems the fundamental parameters of table speed and collimation are defined and the system computes and sets the pitch. The operator should become familiar with his or her own systems and understand the impact of selecting these parameters and how they impact the image set that is generated. Multislice CT systems allow very narrow collimation (0.6 to 2.0 mm) compared with that typically used in combined PET/CT acquisitions. If diagnostic CT images are being acquired as a part of the combined procedure, it is common for the pitch to be 0.75 to 2.0. When the pitch is greater than 1.0, there are interspaces created and some portion of the body is being missed; therefore a diagnostic CT would not use a pitch greater than 2.0 where a significant area would be missed.

To understand the clinical impact of pitch, review the images in Figure 11-15. The area of beam coverage (see Figure 11-15, *top*) when the pitch is equal to 2.0 shows spaces equal to the width of the beam. When the pitch is 1.0 (see Figure 11-15, *middle*), there is no space between the slices. Slices now are adjacent to one another and body areas are not missed. When the pitch is less than 1.0, as in Figure 11-15 *(bottom)* where the pitch is 0.75, there is an overlap of the slices and no small disease would be missed. For high-resolution CT the pitch is often set at a small value (often less than 1.0).

One good analogy to pitch is a toy Slinky or a coiled telephone cord. The coil may be stretched by various extents so that there may be a different space between each rotation of the spring. In its normal position the cord is tightly pulled together so that in each 360-degree rotation of the cord it is touching the adjacent rotation, like a pitch of 1.0. If the slices are too thin, then there may be a significant number of images to review. In addition, very thin slices may increase the radiation exposure to the patient without any benefit of enhanced diagnostic capability. If the pitch is set too thick, then small areas of disease may be missed because the lesion is between the slices. A large pitch and thick slices may also provide low-contrast images, because lesions may have overlying or underlying normal tissue within the slice thickness.

Increment. Computed tomography data are acquired as projection information along the helical path, and therefore slices may be reconstructed at various positions along the helix, although the slice thickness is limited (primarily) by the collimation thickness and pitch. One additional important factor in defining the slices and their positional relationship to one another is the distance between the reconstructed axial slices in the z direction. The **increment** is the distance between the slices. Following data acquisition the user may define how much the slices should overlap or if space should be allocated between images. For example, if a 100-mm area of the body were covered with 5-mm-thick slices and no overlap between slices was desired, the increment would be 5 mm and 20 images would appear adjacent to one another. However, if the increment were 2.5 mm, then each slice would have a 50% overlap with the adjacent slice and there would be a total of 40 slices (Figure 11-16).

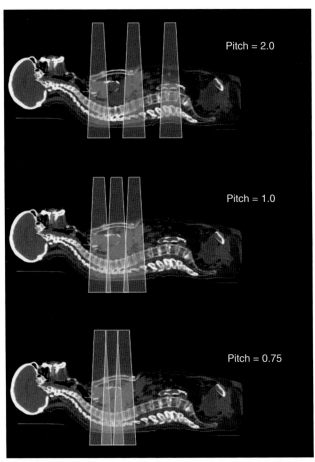

FIGURE 11-15 The x-ray beam is depicted by the shaded area from the top position on these sagittal CT slices. A pitch of 2.0 separates the slices from one another by a distance equal to the beam width *(top)*. When the pitch is 1.0, the beam position is adjacent to the prior and following rotation *(middle)*. A pitch of 0.75 *(bottom)* demonstrates that the beam position overlaps the prior and following area to overlap body regions.

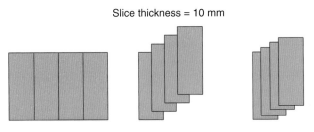

FIGURE 11-16 The increment sets the distance between slices independent of the slice thickness. In this diagrammatic example for a 10-mm slice an increment of 10 mm places the slices adjacent *(left diagram)* to one another without an area missed between slices. An increment of 5 mm for these 10-mm-thick slices creates an overlap of 50% for each slice *(middle)*. An increment of 3 mm creates significant overlap of slices *(right)*. To ensure that no tiny lesions are missed, the slice thickness and increment should be carefully selected.

Advantages:

- Greater overlap of body areas to generate smooth, three-dimensional (3D) reformatted images
- A reduction in the possibility of missing small lesions

Compromise:

- Increased number of images and subsequent reconstruction time

The following information demonstrates the important relationships between scan length, collimation, increment, and the number of slices generated.

Scan Length	Collimation	Increment	No. of Slices
100 mm	5 mm	5 mm	20
100 mm	5 mm	2.5 mm	40
100 mm	2.5 mm	1.25 mm	50
100 mm	1 mm	1 mm	100

Since multislice, helical CT data can be reconstructed at any point along the volume, slices may be reconstructed at almost any desired thickness. The increment is set to determine if there will be spacing between adjacent slices or if there will be overlapped slices. Overlap may prevent small lesions from being missed. Overlapping slices is of significant help when the CT slices are used to generate 3D or maximum-intensity projections. The overlap helps to smooth out the data, and jagged edges in the sagittal, coronal, and any other reformatted planes are significantly reduced.

Objects that are of similar size, or smaller, than the thickness of a single CT slice may be difficult to detect. Figure 11-17 *(left)* demonstrates an irregular lesion that is about 3 mm in size as it may be positioned with 5 mm slices with an increment of 5 mm, such that slices abut. If the lesion if centered so that it is completely contained

within the 5 mm slice then it may be seen. However if it is only partially within a slice then it may not be visualized because most of the other tissue in that thickness may provide only a low contrast view of this lesion and it may be missed. If the increment is changed to 3 mm but the slice thickness is retained at 5 mm (see Figure 11-17, *middle*) then there will be some overlap of the slices and the 3-mm lesion has a more likely chance of being visualized. When the slice thickness and increment are both set to 3 mm as shown in Figure 11-17, *right*, the lesion now occupies most of the thickness of the slice and the contrast for this lesion will be higher and the likelihood of detection improves. This example demonstrates how slice thickness and increment must be critically set for the detection of small lesions, such as when small (3 mm) pulmonary nodules need to be detected.

MULTISLICE HELICAL CT SYSTEMS

Multislice CT technology was developed in the early 1990s to address patient throughput. Helical CT was developed soon thereafter not only to aid in patient throughput, but also to reduce patient motion artifacts. Although the terms *helical* and *spiral* are used interchangeably to describe this new technology, this text will use the term *helical* because it more accurately describes the 3D path of the gantry around the patient.

There are four important technical developments that define current helical CT systems:

1. Continuous radiation of the x-ray tube
2. Continuous-motion gantry using slip-ring technology
3. Continuous motion of the imaging table
4. Continuous data transfer from the detector array

The ability to feed continuous power to the x-ray tube is an important factor in helical CT. The provision of

Slice thickness 5 mm   Slice thickness 5 mm   Slice thickness 3 mm
Increment 5 mm   Increment 3 mm   Increment 3 mm

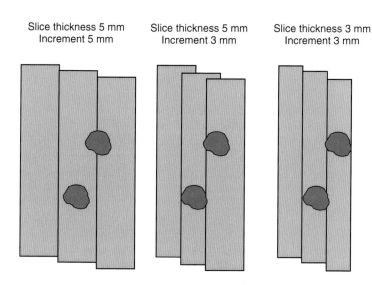

FIGURE 11-17 CT slices of thickness 5 mm and 5-mm increment (left) will show low contrast of a 3-mm lesion. When the increment is set at 3 mm there is less chance of missing the 3-mm lesion *(middle)*. When the slice thickness is set at 3 mm and increment is also at 3 mm the contrast of the lesion will be better and the lesion will be easier to visualize and not missed by thick slices.

power to the tube requires the removal of large amounts of heat from the tube. Early CT systems had large power and signal cables that wound around within the gantry as the x-ray tube and detectors moved around the patient. With each rotation they had to unwind, which significantly limited the gantry rotation speed. On current systems a series of conductive rings allows power and signals to be transferred to and from the rotating gantry. More recently scanners transmit the digital data from the detectors back to the computer system using high-speed radiofrequency signals. Computers synchronize the motion of the gantry and coordinate the table motion to properly acquire data from known positions of the gantry rotation and the imaging table position, allowing very high speed data acquisition. At the time of this writing, multislice scanners have rotation speeds of a fraction of a second with 64-slice detector arrays in common use for dedicated CT scanners, and higher-speed and higher-resolution systems on the horizon. These higher-speed and higher-resolution CT systems are required for fast-contrast CT angiography and gated cardiac CT but are not required for routine oncology work in PET/CT imaging in its current practice.

IMAGE DATA ACQUISITION

The high performance of CT scanners creates a volume of reconstructed data instead of a group of slices. The data acquired from the helical motion of the gantry are obtained as projection information, as in both SPECT and PET. The projections in this case represent the attenuated beam of radiation from which the algorithm will eventually determine the attenuation coefficient at each pixel in the image matrix. Once the patient volume has been scanned, the raw data from the scan may be reconstructed with various parameters to provide images with optimal diagnostic information. The raw data may be used to create several image sets to reveal different information from just the one set of raw data. For example, the raw data may be used to generate one set of data to be used for attenuation correction of SPECT or PET. Another reconstruction set of images may be high-resolution thin slices, whereas another may be smoother, thicker slices.

The beam width as set by the detector size and collimator determines the maximum resolution that may be obtained in the study. Data acquisition may sample over 2000 projections in each rotation of the tube, and the detector array size sets the number of slices that are obtained in each rotation. Thus a typical CT acquisition for combined SPECT/CT or PET/CT may take less than 1 minute.

CT scanners, at this writing, come as 8, 16, 40, 64, 128, or more multislice systems. How many slice CT scanner is needed for a PET/CT system? The answer to this question depends heavily on the PET/CT clinical applications that are to be performed with this scanner.

For instance if the PET/CT will be used primarily for oncology applications, a 16- or 40-slice scanner may be extremely suitable for performing a wide variety of PET/CT scans and the CT scans will be able to provide high resolution diagnostic scans in a very short amount of time. However, if PET/CT cardiac studies will be performed and some of those studies will be gated CT and gated PET then the minimum configuration should likely be a 64 slice CT. This would allow gated CT studies of the heart and very fast speeds of gantry rotation for improved cardiac calcification scoring, CT coronary angiography, and other applications in addition to viewing combined high performance CT studies with overlying PET color scans.

CT IMAGE RECONSTRUCTION

The reconstruction of multislice CT images will be computed from the helical projection data. Since the x-ray beam is either fan-shaped or cone-shaped in a helical pattern, special reconstruction algorithms are used to account for this unique beam geometry. Image reconstruction may use different reconstruction algorithms that will calculate the attenuation at each pixel in the slice. It is common for the voxels that are produced to be isotropic (same dimensions in all three axes), as shown in Figure 11-18. The calculated voxel values from CT are not attenuation values or linear attenuation coefficients but rather are represented by other unique units.

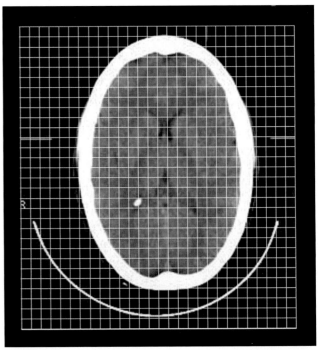

FIGURE 11-18 CT images are composed of arrays of pixels that have each been assigned the calculated CT number for that region. To best reformat CT slices into coronal, sagittal, and volumetric images, the pixels should be isotropic (same dimension on each axis).

Since CT measures the attenuation of the x-ray beam in each projection, the fundamental calculation could be calculation of the linear attenuation coefficient using Lambert's equation of x-ray absorption:

$$I/I_0 = e^{-\mu x}$$

where I_0 equals the original intensity of the unattenuated x-ray beam, I equals the measured intensity of the beam at the detector, e is Euler's number, μ equals the linear attenuation coefficient, and x is the thickness of the attenuator. However, since the thickness of the material along the path of the x-ray beam passes through many pixels, the attenuation measurement represents the summation of the individual attenuating pixels. It is not meaningful to assign the pixel values in the image to the attenuation coefficients, and therefore a more meaningful value is assigned. The pixel values assigned in the image are called **CT numbers (Hounsfield units [HU])**. They are computed by calculating the relative difference between the linear attenuation coefficient of tissue and that of water. The equation used is:

$$CT_{tissue} = (\mu_{tissue} - \mu_{water})/\mu_{water} \times 1000$$

where μ_{tissue} is the attenuation coefficient of the area examined and μ_{water} is the known value for the attenuation coefficient of water. The CT number for water has a value of 0 because:

$$(\mu_{water} - \mu_{water})/\mu_{water} = 0$$

The CT value for air would be −1000, and the CT value for dense bone is about +1000. Various CT tissue values are listed in Box 11-1. Note that there are ranges for each type of tissue because the density of the tissue may vary substantially. Also note that many soft tissues have overlapping ranges of CT values. Therefore CT does not discriminate well between different soft tissues types; this makes sense considering that the attenuation of x-rays at these low energies is actually dependent on Compton and photoelectric interactions, which are primarily a measure of atomic density, and all soft tissues are similar in that respect. Magnetic resonance imaging (MRI) is much better at soft-tissue differentiation.

A variety of algorithms have been used to reconstruct CT images. Filtered back-projection (FBP) and iterative algorithms may be available on commercial CT systems; however, there are usually proprietary algorithms on each type of commercial system that have been tailored for that specific type of system by the manufacturer. The manufacturer may typically have algorithms that are designed to generate images for a variety of imaging situations. These may be for specific types of clinical applications. For example, a standard algorithm for soft tissue would be different from an algorithm to visualize details of the bones where the CT numbers have substantially different values and there is more need for visualizing fine resolution and better defining the edges between tissue types.

After the scan data have been acquired several parameters must be defined before reconstructing the images. The reconstruction diameter, which acts like a software zoom on the data, may be defined. The full field of view (FOV) on a system may be 700 mm, for example, which would include the imaging table and patient extremities and leave plenty of space around the patient. This full **reconstruction field of view** may be needed if this reconstructed data set is to be used to attenuation-correct a SPECT or PET study. Smaller FOVs may be used for diagnostic CT studies or studies where the CT will be simultaneously displayed with SPECT or PET. A reconstruction diameter of about 500 mm is commonly used for whole-body PET/CT studies; a reconstruction diameter of 300 mm or smaller may be desired if only the head or neck region is to be viewed. The reconstruction FOV will be set into a matrix size, and therefore the smaller the reconstruction FOV, the greater the magnification of the image and the finer the detail that may be seen. Reconstruction matrices might be 340 × 340, 512 × 512, 768 × 768, or 1024 × 1024 for very high resolution CT procedures. Most often a 512 × 512 matrix size will be used, and if the slice thickness and the increment for body studies are around 5 mm each, then the PET/CT body study will generate about 200 to 300 slices. The pixel size within the image may be calculated by

$$Pixel\ size\,(mm) = FOV\,(mm)/(matrix \times zoom)$$

For example, an FOV of 500 mm into a 512 × 512 matrix with a zoom of 1.0 will have a pixel size of 0.97 mm. The advantage of adjusting the matrix size is that the optimal spatial resolution for the type of study being performed and the detail required to best visualize

BOX 11-1	CT Numbers for Various Tissues in Hounsfield Units (HU) or CT Numbers
Air	−1000
Lung	−850 to −200
Fat	−30 to −250
Water	0
Heart	10 to 60
Brain	20 to 40
Blood	20 to 80
Liver	20 to 80
Muscle	35 to 50
Spleen	40 to 60
Bone	150 to 500
Bone (dense)	350 to 1000
Metal	>2000

the area being evaluated may be selected. However, very large matrix sizes require more storage and data transfer time to migrate the studies to an archive, viewing computer, or picture archiving and communication system (PACS).

Another important parameter that is set before CT reconstruction is the reconstruction kernel. The kernel is an algorithm that, in the case of CT reconstruction, defines the clinical application and amount of smoothing that will be applied in the reconstruction process. Each vendor's CT scanner will have a variety of kernels that optimize the image quality to a particular body area or tissue type. Bone images will require an algorithm that maintains sharpened edges or bone margins. For example, on a Siemens system the kernels are defined by a letter (or letters) followed by a number. The letter identifies the body area or clinical application (e.g., *H,* head; *B,* body; *U,* ultrahigh resolution; *C,* child head), and the number typically ranges from 10 to 90. Most clinically useful filters use numbers in the range of 30 to 40. The higher the kernel number, the sharper the image; conversely the lower the number, the smoother the image. A reconstruction protocol may allow the predefining of several reconstructions, each using a different kernel, which will be automatically executed upon completion of data acquisition.

Advantages of tailoring algorithms and kernels:

- Desired image detail is obtained.
- Filters may sharpen or smooth reconstructed images.
- Raw data may be reconstructed post-acquisition with a variety of filters.

Compromise:

- Multiple reconstructions may be required if significant detail is required from areas of the study that contain bone and soft tissue.

Additional postprocessing filters are often available on CT systems to further augment image quality. A postprocessing filter such as a low-contrast enhancement (LCE) filter will improve **low-contrast resolution** while it decreases image noise. These filters may also have several options that perform various levels of enhancement and noise reduction, giving the user more subtle options. A high-contrast enhancement (HCE) filter will produce sharpening of high-contrast differences as in the head imaging and brain imaging. An additional filter might optimize the filtering to enhance viewing of the posterior fossa region by reducing beam-hardening artifacts.

Since CT reconstruction is very computationally intense, the rapid reconstruction of slices is performed using a cluster of high-performance computers, which have often been especially designed to perform efficient image reconstruction.

CT DISPLAY

Digital image display of CT information creates unique challenges due to the wide variation in CT numbers in the image. For instance, the chest area contains lung tissue (CT numbers in the range of −850 to −200), fat (CT numbers −250 to −30), soft tissue (CT numbers 10 to 80), and bone (CT numbers 150 to 500 or more). Thus the range of CT numbers in the image is from −850 to 500, or 1350 numbers. The human eye is thought to be able to discern only 30 to 100 different shades of gray; therefore because of the wide range of CT values, only a limited range of values are displayed in the image. It is also important to remember that digital imaging often is limited to 8 bits of data, and therefore only 256 intensity values are assigned over the entire gray scale from black to white.

A grayscale window is assigned to some limited range in the CT numbers, and within this window the full black-to-white gray scale is reassigned to 256 shades of gray. Figure 11-19 demonstrates the assignment of a window width on the Hounsfield unit (or CT number) scale. A window centerline and window width may be placed at any desired location on the CT number scale. This flexible window centerline and width allow the desired tissue to be displayed while allowing CT values below or above the window to be out of the viewable intensity range. Figure 11-20 demonstrates on one patient—using two different body regions, the chest and the abdomen—how various tissues may be viewed using different window centerlines and window widths. The top row demonstrates a slice through the chest assigned to three different window settings. A bone window may be set with CT values selected from 400 to 1000 to view details of the dense bone in the vertebrae. Windowing from CT number 0 to −1200 allows the lung tissue to be viewed, while windowing from −85 to 165 creates a scale to better evaluate soft tissue. The lower row of images shows these same windows on an abdominal slice where the high-CT window (400 to 1000) demonstrates the bone detail well. The window for viewing the details of lung tissue (0 to −1200) makes all soft tissues appear white and is therefore not useful for viewing the abdomen. Soft tissues are displayed with a window of −85 to 165. As was labeled on the images in Figure 11-20, predefined window values may be assigned to frequently used windows. Bone window, lung window, abdomen window, head window, neck window, and other windows may be preassigned on viewing systems. The viewing software also allows the operator to assign and save his or her own viewing windows.

DISPLAY OF VOLUMETRIC IMAGE DATA

For many years, viewing CT data was limited to viewing one or just a few slices of the study on film. Display computers that are fast, have sufficient memory, and are

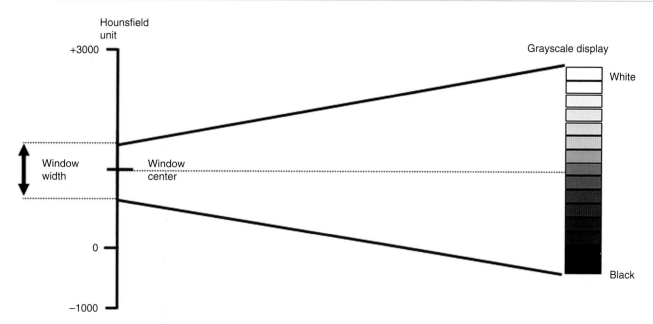

FIGURE 11-19 CT numbers have a wide range of values as shown on the vertical scale, −1000 to +3000. The fraction of the CT scale that is of use in viewing a patient study can be selected using a window centerline and window width. This selected range of values is then stretched from black to white to increase the dynamic range of viewing. The wide variation in CT numbers for various tissues—lung, tissue, and bone—requires changing the window center and width.

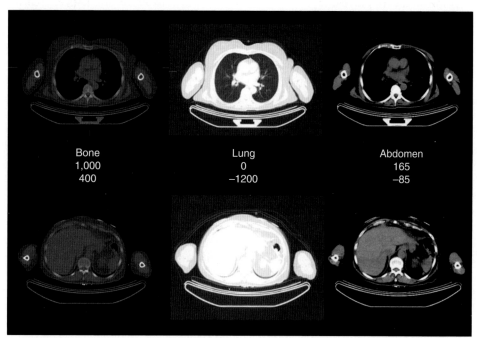

FIGURE 11-20 Some preset CT viewing windows are compared in two different areas—chest and abdomen—in a patient. The top row shows images of the same slice displayed with three different windows: bone window (400 to 1000) for detailed visualization of dense bones such as the vertebrae *(left)*, while lung tissue is not visible and soft tissue is very light gray; lung window (−1200 to 0) for viewing the very low densities of lung tissue and air *(middle)*, while soft tissue is white; and abdomen window (−85 to 165), where the soft tissues are displayed with shades of gray but lungs and bone are not seen. The bottom row shows the same abdominal slice with the bone window suppressing soft tissue *(left)*. The lung window has no use because all soft tissues are white *(middle)*. Appropriate shades of gray are used for the soft tissues *(right)*, with bone and lung not scaled for visualization.

powerful allow the CT slice data to be reformatted into a variety of displays. Some of the most dramatic display options are those that allow the CT data to be depicted as though the true anatomy of the patient were being visualized. Maximum intensity projection (MIP) images are generated by taking a stack of image slices and projecting back the maximum intensity of the brightest pixel along that path. This technique uses the same principles as MIP imaging for SPECT and PET, which has been described in previous chapters. Although these displays are interesting, the true anatomic representation is not as natural as images created by shaded surface displays (SSDs).

Shaded surface display images are shaded and have artificial light sources to create the illusion of viewing real anatomy. Software control of the CT windowing of the CT numbers may allow certain anatomical structures and organs to be displayed with false coloration applied to mimic real anatomy. Although these images are attention-grabbing they typically have little use to the radiologist in interpreting the examination but can have usefulness in surgical planning and marketing radiology studies. The creation of SSD images is typically done in three steps: (1) reconstruct the CT data from the 2D slices using thin overlapping slices, (2) segment out unwanted data using thresholding of the CT numbers or cropping or segmenting out overlying structures, (3) render or shade the projected images to provide depth perception and illumination of the patient. Virtual colonoscopy uses SSD images from within the colon and does have practical application to the radiologist for interpretation of these studies. The SSD images from within the colon are generated and the observer moves along or "flies through" the colon to locate polyps.

Computed tomography images are also the standard display used in radiation therapy treatment planning. Computed tomography scanners in the radiotherapy department are integrated with precision laser alignment systems to provide an exact location of disease relative to the body and external anatomic markers and to align the therapy beams. Treatment planning software is used to create the CT treatment volume for the radiotherapy beam. PET/CT studies are increasingly being used for radiation therapy treatment planning, because the PET physiological information may be as important as the anatomic location of disease from the CT scan in determining the treatment volume.

IMAGE QUALITY

Although CT images are relatively simple displays, the generation of the images is based on the settings and parameters discussed in this chapter, as well as some others that are beyond the scope of this introductory material. Each parameter setting that is selected before data acquisition or those parameters chosen in the reconstruction and display will have an effect on the appearance of the final images and their subsequent diagnostic reliability. This section will discuss some of the issues relative to the quality of CT images.

Contrast Resolution

Contrast resolution in general is the ability to differentiate between different tissue densities in the image. Contrast resolution relates to two different terms in CT that describe the ability to discriminate between objects that have either high or low contrast compared with the background. **High-contrast resolution** is the ability to see small objects and details that have a high density difference compared with the background in which those objects or organs reside. An example would be the ability to see a small, dense lesion in the lung tissue or to see objects where bone and soft tissues are adjacent. In high-contrast resolution the objects have a very high density difference from one another. *Low-contrast resolution* is another term used to describe image quality. Low-contrast resolution is the ability to visualize objects that have very little difference in density from one another. Examples of low-contrast resolution would be visualizing soft-tissue lesions within the liver where the lesion density is about the same as that of the liver or trying to differentiate gray matter from white matter in the brain. Low-contrast resolution will always be better when there is very low image noise, the confidence in seeing the edges of tissue areas is improved, and the uniformity of soft tissues is clear on the images.

Contrast resolution describes the ability to visualize objects and should not be confused with spatial resolution. Spatial resolution in CT has changed with the implementation of multislice, helical systems. Spatial resolution must no longer be discussed in terms of x and y resolution of a slice, and the slice thickness having a different spatial resolution. Systems can now create isotropic voxels, that is, a voxel with the same dimensions in all directions (in other words, a *cubic voxel*). High-performance CT scanners can now generate images that have a resolution of much less than 1 mm. The clinical application for this resolution is somewhat limited to certain CT procedures because the number of images is very high and patient exposure is also high. In combined SPECT/CT and PET/CT studies the resolution of the CT needs to be significantly higher than in the radionuclide study; therefore at this writing the finest resolution of a combined study need not go below about 3 mm, as would be the case in looking for small lung nodules and trying to determine if they are metabolically active. Computed tomography resolution depends on many factors including focal spot size, detector element size, collimation, pitch, slice thickness, increment, reconstruction algorithm and kernel, matrix size, and the reconstruction FOV.

Image Noise

Image noise is generated by random statistical variations in the pixel values that are used to create the image. A noisy image is typically one in which areas that should have uniform appearance are seen as grainy or mottled (see Figure 11-6, *D*). The reduction of noise in CT is more complicated than just increasing the number of photons (mAs) that penetrate the patient. Noise can be reduced by adjusting the kernel filter to be smoother or may be changed by selecting a different matrix size, slice thickness, beam energy, current, or most typically a combination of these. Large patients produce more scatter and attenuate a greater number of x-rays, which results in noisy images. Written criteria for tailoring the procedure parameter to compensate for variations in patient size should be developed so that acquisition protocols can be selected or modified to create the most desirable quality of images with the least patient radiation exposure. It is important to remember that image noise is related to patient radiation exposure by the equation:

$$\text{Noise} \sim \sqrt{1/\text{dose}}$$

Therefore the dose must be increased four times to reduce the noise by half.

Slice thickness will also have an effect on image noise. Thin-slice studies are generated with few x-rays and will therefore have more noise. Thin slices have poorer low-contrast resolution but better high-contrast resolution and better edge definition. Thick-slice CT does have lower noise and better low-contrast resolution but lacks edge definition. In clinical practice most abdomen and pelvis CT studies are viewed with a 5.0-mm slice thickness and increments of 5.0 mm. Current practice with state-of-the-art equipment does not recommend any thicker slices. Thinner slices are commonly used for imaging the brain (<4.0 mm), neck (1.0 to 3.0 mm), and lungs (1.0 to 4.0 mm), because these procedures may be looking for smaller disease sites. Specialized high-resolution CT studies for viewing fine bone detail, CT angiographic studies, coronary calcification studies, and so on, will require very thin slice images (1.0 mm or less).

CT PROTOCOLS

All CT scans begin by performing a scout scan (topogram) so that the region of the body to be covered by the CT scan can be defined. Scanning parameters may be set up before the scout scan or, as is most often the case, may be determined after the scout scan, which is sometimes called a *topogram*. For the scout scan the CT tube and detector of the gantry are not rotating about the patient but are placed in a fixed position to create an anterior or posterior planar whole-body "x-ray," as seen in the right side of Figure 10-16. The scout scan is most commonly performed in the anterior-posterior (AP) orientation (beam passing from the anterior to the posterior) to provide the operator with a coronal image; however, posterior-anterior and lateral scout scan options are available. The lateral scout scan is helpful for defining scanning regions for the brain or head/neck CT studies, whereas the AP scout scan is most commonly used in body CT studies or PET/CT oncology whole-body studies.

Scout scan parameters are fairly simple and are not critical to the CT study itself since the scout scan is for general localization only and is not used by the physician in making a diagnosis; therefore the operator should limit the radiation exposure to the patient from the scout scan. Scout scans are built into imaging protocols, and the imaging parameters are typically preset. Low settings for the kVp and mA are used and a reasonable scan speed is set. The length of the scout scan should be appropriate to ensure that the desired region for imaging will be well covered by the scout scan. When the planar image is displayed on the monitor, the operator will select with cursors the area for the CT acquisition.

Computed tomography scans performed in conjunction with SPECT and PET studies will usually fall into one of two categories: low-dose CT for attenuation correction of a radionuclide study or high-quality CT, commonly referred to as a *diagnostic CT study*. Diagnostic CT studies produce high-quality images to identify disease and are optimized to the area of the body imaged and the timing of contrast material localization. Diagnostic CT procedures performed as independent studies without a radionuclide examination most often use contrast media.

Low-Dose CT for PET Attenuation Correction

If high-quality CT images are not required with a SPECT/CT or PET/CT study, the CT parameters may be significantly altered to reduce the radiation exposure to the patient. All CT procedures will begin with a scout scan to define the area of the body to be scanned. As outlined at the beginning of this chapter, key parameters include rotation time, kVp, and mA. Some general recommendations for a normal size adult might be a kVp of 80, mA of 50 to 120 (depending on the manufacturer), collimator thickness of 1.5 mm, pitch of 1.0, slice thickness of 4.0 to 5.0 mm (set the increment the same), rotation time of 0.5 second (or fastest available), reconstruction FOV as large as possible, and a kernel that is smooth as recommended by the manufacturer for CT attenuation-correction scanning. Before the parameters for low-dose CT attenuation-correction protocols are determined, it is recommended that the vendor be consulted regarding their recommendations; any modifications from those parameters should then be made. This is to ensure that low-dose parameters will not create any artifacts from instrumentation or software causes as seen in Figure 11-6, C. Attenuation-correction CT studies will need to be adjusted for patient size and thickness, and special adjustments will be needed for pediatric patients. The reconstruction diameter of low-dose CT for SPECT or PET attenuation correction must include the full body width so that the CT is generated over the full width of the patient; it is often set to the maximum diameter of the gantry bore to ensure that there is no truncation of any part of the body, which may cause an artifact on the corrected SPECT or PET image.

Diagnostic CT

The term *diagnostic CT* may not clearly define the exact procedure that is being performed. To some radiologists *diagnostic CT* may mean that the image quality is excellent with low noise by using optimal slice thickness along with sufficient kVp and mAs settings to appropriately detect disease. To other radiologists *diagnostic CT* may also mean that contrast media have been administered to the patient and that the CT scan is performed following an appropriate timing sequence following the administration of contrast material. Oncology patients often have chest, abdomen, and pelvis diagnostic CT examinations performed one after another using different scanning parameters to optimize imaging in each body area. Performing attenuation-correction CT studies in combined SPECT/CT or PET/CT procedures requires one continuous scan of the body region using only one set of CT parameter settings, in which case the ideal diagnostic CT study has been compromised in some way (e.g., time since contrast administration, breath holding, slice thickness). Combined PET/CT and contrast diagnostic CT studies cannot be performed in the same manner.

CT parameters will vary from vendor to vendor; however, consider as an example a CT image of the abdomen and consider for now that contrast is not injected. The examples will be for a 16-slice Siemens helical CT system, although systems that have more slices or fewer slices are in use.

Abdomen CT. The beam energy must be appropriate to penetrate the abdomen without beam hardening; therefore 120 kVp may be selected (increase for large patients and decrease for very slender patients). The current needs to provide a sufficient number of photons to produce a high-quality image; therefore 200 to 350 mA will be used. Collimation should not be thicker than 1.5 mm. The rotation speed should be relatively fast (0.5 to 1.0 second) to reduce motion and breathing artifacts. Routine CT-alone procedures may require the patient to hold their breath during the scan. The table speed should be sufficient (about 25 mm/rotation) to have a pitch near 1.0, and this table speed should perform the scan over the selected body region in less than about 45 seconds (or faster depending on the system). For reconstruction the slice thickness should be set at about 3.0 to 5.0 mm, and the increment should be set at the same value. A body kernel with a mid-range number, such as a B30f, should provide appropriate image quality. The reconstruction FOV may be set at about 300 mm or adjusted depending on the size of the patient.

If an intravenous (IV) contrast medium were to be used with this study, parameters might be selected as follows. Using an automatic injection system, administer 100 ml of Omnipaque 350 at 3.0 ml/sec and begin the scan at about 60 seconds following the completion of the injection. Multiphase scans may be obtained from a single injection by performing sequential scans by capturing the arterial phase with a scan at 20 to 25 seconds and the venous phase at 60 to 75 seconds postinjection. CT imaging of the liver is normally performed with this procedure (check vendor recommendations).

Chest CT. A CT of the chest for oncology applications will use a thinner slice than the abdomen and, because there is less attenuation, will require fewer mA. Typically the kVp is set at 120 kVp, and the fastest rotation speed (0.5 second) should be selected to minimize patient motion. The beam current should be 100 to 120 mA, collimation should be set to the minimum thickness (<0.75 mm), and the pitch should be 1.0. The scan is normally obtained with breath holding and the table speed set at about 12 cm/sec or greater so that the whole region of the chest is easily covered during the breath-holding period. The reconstructed FOV is set to exclude the body outside of the lungs. The slice thickness is selected to be thin (1.0 mm) and the increment is set at 1.0 mm in order to visualize very small lesions. A kernel with a high resolution, such as a B50f, is used. The final image quality should be very high (low noise) with thin slices in order to detect small lesions.

Neck CT. To detect a mass in the neck, IV contrast media must be used to aid in the identification of vascular structures. The CT acquisition would be started 45 seconds after the IV administration of 100 ml of contrast material injected at 3 ml/sec. The small structures to be identified in the neck will require very high quality images with thin slices. A beam energy of 120 kVp with current of 150 to 200 mA should be used with a fast tube rotation time (less than 0.5 seconds). The collimation should be as thin as possible (less than 0.75 mm) and the pitch selected at 1.0. The reconstructed images should use a FOV to zoom the images, which should have a slice thickness of 3 to 4 mm with the increment set at the same value so that the slices are adjacent to one another. The kernel should be of medium resolution, B31s. It is common to have a second reconstruction with very thin slices (1 mm) and an increment that creates an overlap (increment 0.7 mm).

Contrast Media. Previously this chapter described the difficulty that CT has with differentiating various soft tissues, because they have very similar attenuating densities. To enhance the detection of lesions and to aid in defining normal structures, a contrast agent is frequently used. In oncology patients, contrast media is used in about 95% of patient studies. Contrast may be administered by oral, rectal, or IV methods. The use of oral contrast media is essential to distinguish regions of bowel from abnormal fluid collections or masses in the abdomen. Figure 10-32 demonstrates artifacts that can be created on PET studies from the use of barium sulfate in the bowel. To reduce these artifacts, a negative contrast agent or water should be used. Patients who cannot drink the oral contrast may require a nasogastric tube. Rectal contrast is required to delineate the rectosigmoid colon if a lower pelvic mass is suspected.

The use of IV contrast media in helical CT improves the detection of vessels as well as the detection and characterization of lesions. Diagnostic CT requires that the scan be timed exactly after the contrast administration to have the contrast media in the desired vascular location: arterial, venous, and equilibrium phases. Good-quality contrast studies will be obtained only when the contrast media concentration, circulation time, total volume of contrast, injection rate, and delay time are optimal. Because these contrast applications require rapid and time-critical scans of a limited body area, they may need to be performed separately from the combined PET/CT examination; otherwise the timing and region scanned need to be altered in order to use a contrast diagnostic CT as the CT for PET or SPECT attenuation correction.

Chapter 8 described the use and treatment of adverse reactions to radiopaque contrast media. The American College of Radiology manual on contrast media should be consulted as a resource for developing departmental protocols for the use of contrast. When CT contrast studies are used for attenuating PET or SPECT procedures, the emission images must be reviewed to determine if areas of high CT contrast concentration have created artifacts on the emission study.

Integrated PET/CT Protocols

Diagnostic CT procedures are defined to study individual organs or limited body regions. The technical acquisition settings and reconstruction parameters must be optimized along with the administration and optimally timed post-administration to maximize diagnostic information. The principal modification of CT procedures as they are performed as a component of the combined PET/CT procedure is that some of the parameters will be compromised in the combined procedure. Gantry tilt is not available on PET/CT systems, contrast media may cause artifacts on the attenuation-corrected PET images, and a larger body area must be covered in whole-body oncology applications.

The biggest impact on CT is the reduced optimized use of IV contrast media. CT procedures are performed by optimizing the delay time from contrast injection to the time that it enters the organ system in the manner that is most advantageous to characterize the arterial, venous, or delayed tumor blush phase of contrast flow and localization. Because of this delay time, CT procedures are performed individually (neck, chest, abdomen, and pelvis) and whole-body imaging is not commonly performed as a CT study. However, the need to have exact body position between the CT and PET images requires the performance of both studies sequentially with the patient in identical positions. The CT acquisition therefore cannot be timed optimally for any IV contrast media that may be administered. Intravenous contrast use with whole-body CT is more commonly

done to demonstrate the vascular phase of contrast location and the arterial cannot be captured.

In the combined PET/CT procedure the topogram, or scout scan, is always performed first, most commonly from the AP projection. The scout scan is used to define the body area to be covered by the CT and PET scans. The CT is performed next because the CT reconstruction for PET attenuation correction is required before PET reconstruction. Since exactly the same body alignment and position is required, the patient is not instructed to take in a deep breath for the CT. Depending on the speed of the CT scan, the patient may be allowed to continue normal breathing or may be instructed to take a breath, breathe out half the breath, and hold that position during the CT acquisition. The PET acquisition is performed last, and the patient should not be allowed to move during the entire combined scan procedure. Since most PET reconstructions are completed after each bed position is acquired, the CT scan is reconstructed for PET attenuation correction so that these attenuation maps are available at each bed and slice position. Additional CT reconstructions are usually performed following the acquisition of PET data. These additional CT reconstructions are performed to optimize different scan characteristics in providing the optimal images for viewing different tissue components such as soft tissue, lung, or bone. The reconstructions may be performed within the automated protocol or may be reconstructed later from the raw CT data.

CT ARTIFACTS

A CT image artifact is anything that causes a discrepancy in the pixel values measured in the study. Although there are a variety of reasons for generating artifacts, there are three primary sources of artifacts common to computed tomography:

1. Operator
2. Scanner
3. Patient

Artifacts may be qualitative or quantitative because there may be more visual artifacts instead of significant variation of the CT numbers assigned into the image, or vice versa. Operator-generated artifacts are those that are a result of the parameters and settings that have been selected by the operator for the patient study. Examples of operator-caused artifacts include those from inappropriate settings of kVp, mA, slice width, increment, kernel, and so forth. Scanner artifacts are those that are generated by the electrical or mechanical operation of the scanner. They may include ring artifacts from mismatched detector performance (see Figure 11-6, C), streaks, incorrect mechanical motion (which may vary rotation of gantry or table speed), image distortion, partial volume, and so on. Patient-generated artifacts

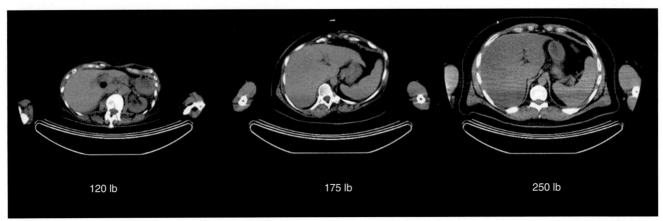

FIGURE 11-21 A standard CT protocol does not work for all sizes of patients. Three adults were all scanned with the same protocol, and all images were acquired with the arms down. The 120-lb patient has no artifacts from the moderate CT settings of 100 kVp and 180 mA. However, in a 175-lb patient beam-hardening artifacts appear in the posterior aspect of the liver. When these settings are applied to a 250-lb patient, there are many streak artifacts in the mid-to-posterior portion of both the liver and the spleen in addition to noise throughout the slice. Proper image quality can come only from adjusting the imaging parameters to the body size.

commonly come from patient motion, beam hardening (which can be reduced by increasing kVp and/or mA before acquisition), or metallic objects (commonly generate streak artifacts).

In PET/CT studies, metal, patient motion, and contrast media may cause a variety of artifacts. Metal and IV contrast often cause focal uptake sites of FDG due to false HU values placed into the CT image and then generate inappropriate overcorrection of the attenuation-corrected PET images. Breathing causes mismatches between the CT attenuation-correction map and the PET studies, which commonly cause either overcorrection or undercorrection of the PET images. Instructions to the patient to control breathing and the use of faster multislice CT scanners reduce breathing artifacts. Truncation artifacts (from using a small FOV for CT reconstruction) may cause false edges of the CT attenuation-correction map and create unusual artifacts of falsely increased activity. Figure 11-21 shows that one preset CT protocol will not produce acceptable diagnostic images for all sizes of patients. Larger patients have streak artifacts from beam-hardening artifacts. These artifacts are reduced by increasing kVp and mA in accordance with body size. Metallic implants cause false increased HU values in the CT attenuation-correction map, causing a false increase in radioactivity. The same is true for focal areas of contrast media. Viewing non–attenuation-corrected PET data usually eliminates the confusion.

CT RADIATION SAFETY

Occupational radiation safety considerations in CT are similar to those in radiography and fluoroscopy. The exposure levels from the scanner may be quite high; therefore imaging suites have lead-lined walls to shield hospital workers from exposure. Typically imaging

rooms for CT have $\frac{1}{16}$- to $\frac{1}{8}$-inch–thick lead in the ceiling, floor, walls, and doors. The thickness of shielding will depend on the distance from the scanner, occupancy factors of the adjacent areas, and scanner properties. Lead glass windows are also used between the control room and the scanner. Because the lead in the walls is most commonly on the back of the wallboard, any penetrations in the walls due to light switches, wall plugs, and so forth must have additional shielding so that there are no hot spots created from these areas. Health physicists should be consulted in planning CT imaging areas. Warning lights and signs are posted at entrances to the imaging room to prevent entry while the x-ray beam is turned on.

If personnel must absolutely be in the CT room with the patient during the procedure, lead aprons must be used. The exposure rate immediately adjacent to the scanner may exceed 300 μSv/1000 mAs. Several feet from the x-ray tube aperture the exposure rate will drop to less than 50 μSv/1000 mAs (the manufacturer information should be consulted for exposure rates at various locations around the scanner).

The radiation dose to the patient is of considerable concern with CT imaging because it is the highest exposure in medical imaging, with the possible exception of fluoroscopy. "As low as reasonably achievable" (ALARA) principles should apply when CT is integrated with SPECT and PET imaging. The CT parameters (particularly kVp and mAs) should conform to guidelines specified by the interpreting physician to yield the image quality needed for the study. For example, if the radiation exposure from CT is only to be used for attenuation-correction purposes, then the CT parameters may be very modest and the result will be a significantly lower exposure to the patient. If a diagnostic-quality CT is required for appropriate anatomic correlation with the SPECT or PET study, then the CT parameters will result

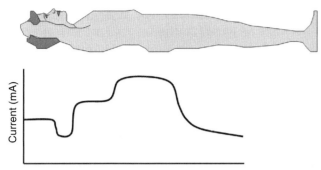

FIGURE 11-22 Automatic tube current modulation adjusts the current (mA) and often the kVp from the strength of beam received by the detector array. The current is adjusted to the body thickness as the patient moves through the scanner so that the radiation exposure is lowered over thin body areas such as the head, neck, extremities, and lung where there is less attenuating tissue; however, the current is high where needed in the abdomen.

in a significantly higher patient dose. Additional parameter adjustments may be required based on patient size and age if pediatric studies are performed.

Information on the estimated radiation exposure from an individual CT examination is available to the operator immediately before the scan is started. When patient information has been entered into the scanner computer, the protocol has been selected, and any parameters adjusted specifically for that patient have been changed, the screen will display the **CT dose index (CTDI)** measured in mGy. The CTDI sums the dose from each gantry revolution based on the parameters for kVp, mA, collimation, rotation speed, and so on. The dose may be further specified by the term $CTDI_w$ for the "weighted" measurement, or $CTDI_{vol}$ for the average dose over the total "volume" scanned.

Since the thickness of the patient and the amount of the beam that is transmitted through the body changes in different regions, the mA and possibly the kVp could be reduced in certain regions to reduce exposure as long as sufficient beam strength is being received by the detectors. All commercial systems have some type of automatic tube current modulation of the beam to reduce exposure in this manner. Each vendor has its own unique marketing name for this software, which can be activated or turned off by the CT operator. Figure 11-22 shows a diagram of the body along with a curve that represents the current that is modulated as the patient is moved through the scanner. In areas of low attenuation such as the neck, lungs, and lower extremities the current (and possibly the kVp) can be reduced on the fly to decrease the patient exposure. It is recommended that clinical protocols leave this automated current modulation turned on unless there is a need for the operator to turn it off for a specific examination. In this way the global patient population will receive reduced exposure.

CT QUALITY CONTROL

As with any instrumentation, CT scanners also need a program to periodically test the performance of the scanner and to compare that performance with some standard. This standard can be a set of predefined criteria, or it may also be the performance of this individual CT unit at the time of installation.

Who requires quality control (QC) of CT scanners? In the United States, The Joint Commission (TJC) requires certain quality criteria for radiology studies. Computed tomography scanners are licensed by states, and there are typically licensing agencies within each state that may have specific programs and schedules for performing QC and safety testing of CT scanners in order to maintain the license for the scanner. At this time, there are no federal guidelines for CT testing; however, some professional organizations publish recommended tests and testing programs. Since CT delivers high radiation exposure to the patient, there is an ethical obligation to ensure that systems are functioning properly and that the quantity of radiation being delivered to the patient is within acceptable limits.

As an example of a thorough testing program Box 11-2 lists the tests in the American College of Radiology (ACR) CT quality control program. A daily quality control program is recommended by vendors of the individual scanners. Hardware (e.g., phantoms, mounting brackets) and software for performing these tests are included on the system. Typically the daily tests will begin with an x-ray tube warm-up procedure in which the output of the tube is checked at various settings and the stability of the tube and detector array is checked. The results of this warm-up test are automatic on modern systems, and the computer screen will display a message that the system is acceptable for use or report results and possible service recommendations if warranted. At least one phantom is included to test the CT number values, noise level in a test scan, and perhaps resolution pattern testing with either visual or computer-generated analysis. Figure 11-23, *B*, demonstrates the results of the image of the water phantom. The image should appear uniform without any ring or streak artifacts. Figure 11-23, *C*, shows the low–contrast resolution phantom, which contains several circles within the center rectangle, which should be visible. High-contrast resolution (see Figure 11-23, *A*) is evaluated with patterns that should have constant visualization patterns from one day to the next to ensure image quality. These phantom tests will vary among vendors, although commercial phantoms are available for more thorough or alternative testing to the manufacturers' recommendations. These phantom studies take usually less than 5 minutes to perform and should be finished and evaluated before imaging any patients each day. Tube warm-up may need to be repeated during the day if the scanner has not been active for a period of 1 to 2 hours or more.

From American College of Radiology: *ACR technical standard for diagnostic medical physics performance monitoring of computed tomography (CT) equipment*, www.acr.org

A comprehensive quality control program for CT (or SPECT/CT or PET/CT) scanners should be written and strictly followed. This program must include daily testing procedures in detail and should also describe other periodic testing that will ensure compliance with licensing and accreditation agencies. On at least an annual schedule a complete calibration and safety testing procedure should be performed. The annual testing must include dosimetry testing to ensure that radiation exposure to the patient is within guidelines. Dosimetry tests must be performed by a certified health physicist or radiology physicist. The equipment for performing dosimetry measurements is shown in Figure 11-24. A pencil ionization chamber is positioned at the center of a standardized plastic phantom of specific dimensions and then near the edge of the phantom. Radiation measurements at specific settings are used to measure patient exposure.

The last item in the written QC program should indicate the actions to be taken if various quality control activities fail to provide measurements and image quality within prescribed parameters. These actions should be followed to prevent inappropriate irradiation of a patient, questionable image quality, or both.

SUMMARY

- The electromagnetic radiation produced by CT x-ray tubes consists of Bremsstrahlung and characteristic tungsten x-rays.
- The peak kilovoltage (kVp) applied to the x-ray tube determines the highest-energy photon that will be produced (in keV), and the current (mA) applied to the tube determines the number of x-rays produced.
- Higher kVp is needed to penetrate thicker body areas or larger patients.

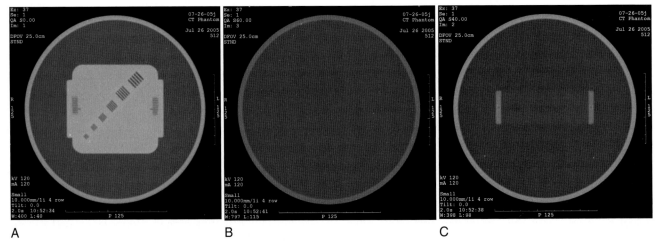

FIGURE 11-23 CT quality control images. **A,** A high-contrast section of a water-filled cylinder demonstrates visualization of spheres of different sizes in the center of the phantom. **B,** Image uniformity is measured daily using a water-filled cylinder to evaluate not just the image uniformity to visually inspect for ring artifacts but also a quantitative measure of the CT number for water in addition to a statistical analysis of image noise. **C,** A low-contrast image section of the phantom is used to visually assess CT image performance.

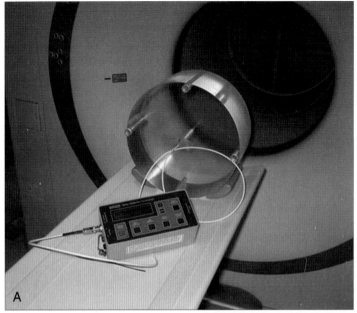
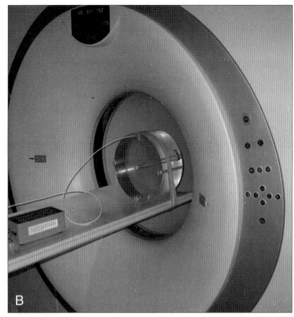

FIGURE 11-24 CT dose is measured annually to ensure that exposure of the patient is within guidelines. A pencil-sized detector is positioned at the center of a plastic phantom **(A)** and at the edges **(B)** of the phantom and irradiated with different mA and kVp to measure exposure at different parameters.

- High-density material such as large bones will create beam-hardening artifacts.
- Higher mA settings produce more x-rays to reduce image noise. High mA settings are used to obtain low-noise scans and for large body areas or large patients.
- Current multislice, helical CT scanners use a fan beam–pattern x-ray beam and ultrafast ceramic detector array to acquire CT data.
- Multislice, helical CT requires continuous radiation, continuous gantry motion, continuous imaging table motion, and continuous data transfer from the detector array.
- The beam thickness is set by the collimator (usually less than 1 mm to several millimeters), and the maximum spatial resolution is determined by the size of the individual detector elements, the reconstruction field of view (FOV), and the matrix size.
- The rotation speed of the gantry plays a role in determining the mAs. A fast rotation time helps reduce motion artifacts.
- Pitch is a parameter that is used to define the desired image spacing by coordinating the table speed and gantry rotation speed.

Pitch factor = table movement per rotation/detector row collimation

- The increment distance defines the distance between the reconstructed axial slices and allows spaces between slices (if the increment exceeds the slice thickness) or overlap of slices (if it is less than the slice thickness).

- CT numbers (the same as Hounsfield units) relate tissue density compared to water and are defined by the relationship $CT_{tissue} = (\mu_{tissue} - \mu_{water})/\mu_{water} \times 1000$.
- The CT number for water is 0, for air the CT number is −1000, the bone values are about 150 to as high as 1000 or more, and for most soft tissue and muscle the CT values are about 20 to 80.
- Computed tomographic reconstruction is defined for an FOV. A small FOV value for reconstruction magnifies (or zooms) the image and provides finer detail.
- CT reconstruction algorithms have letters and numbers associated with their application properties. High numbers indicate that a sharper image will be reconstructed.
- Display windows are used to view CT scans to limit the gray scale of the image to the tissues of interest. Window settings are modified to view different areas of interest with the image.
- High-contrast resolution is the ability to see small objects that have a high density difference. Low-contrast resolution is the ability to see small objects that have little density difference.
- Low-dose CT protocols are used for PET attenuation correction and do not present CT images that have high noise and are not useful for high-confidence CT interpretation.
- Diagnostic CT protocols use thin collimation, an appropriate kVp, and mAs to provide low-noise, high-resolution CT images.
- Integrated (combined) PET/CT protocols are performed by defining the area to be scanned using a scout CT scan, performing one CT acquisition over

the defined area, and then acquiring a PET study over the same area.

- Fused images are reviewed with a colorized PET study fused to the black-and-white CT volume.
- CT artifacts are generated from three sources: operator, scanner, or patient.
- Patient radiation exposure from CT is very high; ALARA principles should apply, and the most conservative parameters to obtain the necessary image quality should be used.
- CT quality control procedures must be performed on a regular basis. Daily x-ray tube warm-up and calibration are performed, and phantom images are acquired and analyzed.

SUGGESTED READING

Frank ED, Long BW, Smith BJ, editors: *Merrill's atlas of radiographic positioning & procedures*, ed 11, St Louis, 2007, Mosby.

Graham DT, Cloke P: *Principles of radiology physics*, ed 4, Edinburgh, 2003, Churchill Livingston.

Goldman LW: Principles of CT: radiation dose and image quality, *J Nucl Med Technol* 35:213-225, 2007.

Goldman LW: Principles of CT and CT technology, *J Nucl Med Technol* 35:115-128, 2007.

McQuattie S: Pediatric PET/CT imaging: tips and techniques, *J Nucl Med Technol* 36:171-178, 2008.

Seeram E: *Computed tomography: physical principles, clinical applications, and quality control*, ed 3, St Louis, 2008, Elsevier.

Principles of
Magnetic Resonance Imaging

Kenneth Fox, Mathew Dixon

OUTLINE

Introduction to Atomic Structure
and Basic Principles
The Hydrogen Nucleus
Alignment
Precession

Resonance
MR Signal and Free Induction
Decay
T1 and T2
    T1 Recovery

T2 Decay
T1 and T2 Contrast
Pulse Sequences
Artifacts
MRI Safety

OBJECTIVES

After completing this chapter, the reader will be able to:
- Discuss the history and background of MRI.
- Describe the basic principles behind MRI.
- Discuss hydrogen atoms and magnetic moments.
- Define spin-up and spin-down characteristics.
- Describe precession of atoms in an external magnetic field.
- Write the Larmor equation and discuss it.
- Discuss resonance in MRI.

- Discuss the MRI signal.
- Describe the difference between T1 and T2 brain images.
- Discuss pulse sequences.
- Discuss diffusion weighted imaging.
- List and describe some MRI artifacts.
- Explain MRI safety principles and their importance in occupational and patient safety.

KEY TERMS

diffusion weighted imaging (DWI)
flip angle
Larmor equation
magnetic moment

precession
pulse sequences
spin-down
spin-up

resonance
T1
T2
tesla (T)

Magnetic resonance imaging (MRI) is a powerful imaging modality that has become an integral component of our medical armamentarium. It has become most useful in the areas of musculoskeletal, body, and neurological imaging, and spectroscopy. The first successful nuclear magnetic resonance experiment (NMR, a precursor to MRI), was made in 1946 by two scientists in the United States, Felix Bloch, working at Stanford University, and Edward Purcell, from Harvard University. These two scientists found that when certain nuclei were placed in a magnetic field they absorbed energy in the

radiofrequency range of the electromagnetic spectrum, and re-emitted this energy when the nuclei transferred back to their original state. The strength of the magnetic field and the radiofrequency at which energy was absorbed matched each other as earlier demonstrated by Sir Joseph Larmor (Irish physicist, 1857-1942), and this is known as the Larmor relationship (discussed later in the chapter). Bloch and Purcell were ultimately awarded the Nobel Prize in Physics in 1952 for their discovery.

In the late 1960s and early 1970s Raymond Damadian, MD, an American physician at the State University of New York in Brooklyn, demonstrated that an NMR tissue parameter (termed *T1 relaxation time*) of tumor samples, measured in vitro, was significantly higher than normal tissue. In a 1971 paper in the journal *Science*, he suggested that these differences could be used to diagnose cancer. In 1974, he received the first patent in the field of MRI when he patented the concept of NMR for detecting cancer (U.S. Patent 3,789,832). It included the idea of using NMR to scan the human body to locate cancerous tissue but did not describe a method of how to generated images from a scan or how it would be done.

Damadian's theories were later expanded on by Paul Lauterbur who developed a way to generate the first MRI images by using gradients. Damadian subsequently built the first full-body MRI machine and produced the first MRI scan of the human body on July 3, 1977, and took nearly 5 hours to generate one image. Modern MRI scanners (Figure 12-1) can now produce images in a matter of minutes.

MRI is now used on a daily basis as a primary imaging modality or in combination with other imaging modalities to provide answers to a diagnostic question. There have been many advances in hardware, new magnet designs, coils, pulse sequences, and contrast agents that have allowed physicians to develop new techniques and implement them as important clinical tools. Clinically, MR systems are divided into high field and low field categories, which essentially denotes a magnet strength of 1.0 **tesla (T)** or greater for the former and less than 1.0 T for the latter. In clinical practice, the vast majority of MRI is performed at 1.5 T or below, with 3.0 T scanners becoming more popular. Even higher magnet field strengths exist, but these are mostly limited to research at this time as the potential affects of these stronger systems on the human body are investigated. In general, 1.5 T and 3.0 T scanners provide optimal clinical imaging quality and efficiency, with lower field systems generally providing inferior imaging quality and requiring more time to perform similar exams. Remember that with MRI, time and increasing magnet strength usually equates to better MR signal and improved image quality.

There are several important concepts that provide a foundation for understanding the basis of MRI acquisition that will be discussed herein.

INTRODUCTION TO ATOMIC STRUCTURE AND BASIC PRINCIPLES

The basic principles of MRI rely on the magnetic properties of the nucleus of the atom. Atoms are composed of protons, neutrons, and electrons with protons having a net positive charge, neutrons having no net charge, and electrons having a net negative charge. Protons and neutrons are within the nucleus, and electrons orbit around the nucleus. Protons and neutrons within the nucleus each with its own mass, charge, and spin influence its intrinsic magnetic properties. The **magnetic moment** represents a vector indicating magnitude and direction, and describes the magnetic field characteristics of the nucleus. The composition within a nucleus can either contain an even number of protons and neutrons (determined by the mass number), which will result in a magnetic moment of zero, or an odd number of protons and neutrons, which will generate a magnetic moment. Atoms with an odd number of protons plus neutrons have nuclei that spin randomly and can acquire a magnetic moment and align with a magnetic field.

Magnetism is generated by moving charges, usually electrons that will align in either a random or nonrandom orientation when placed in an external magnetic field (Figure 12-2). Magnetism is a fundamental property of matter and can either be diamagnetic, paramagnetic, or ferromagnetic. Outside a magnetic field, diamagnetic substances exhibit no magnetic properties outside of a magnetic field; however, when placed within an external magnetic field they are slightly repelled and have negative magnetic susceptibility.

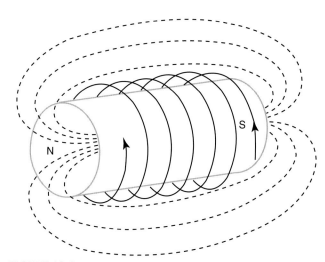

FIGURE 12-2 Main Magnetic Field. A large electric current in loops of wire at superconducting temperatures will produce a very large magnetic field. *N*, North, *S*, south.

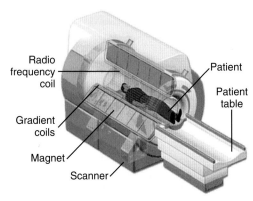

FIGURE 12-1 Diagram of an MRI scanner.

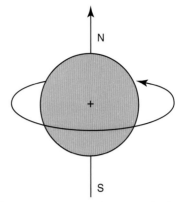

FIGURE 12-3 **Hydrogen Proton.** The positively charged hydrogen proton (+) spins about its axis and acts like a tiny magnet. *N*, North, *S*, south.

Paramagnetic substances also exhibit no magnetic properties outside of a magnetic field but when placed within an external magnetic field are slightly attracted, which increases with an increase in the external magnetic field. These substances have positive magnetic susceptibility.

Ferromagnetic substances exhibit very strong attraction when exposed to the external magnetic field and can act as projectiles. These substances are of extreme importance in the discussion of MRI safety which is discussed later in the chapter.

Examples of MR active nuclei include hydrogen, carbon, nitrogen, oxygen, fluorine, sodium, and phosphorus (Box 12-1). These nuclei will align with an external magnetic field as long as the mass number is odd. The strength of the total magnetic moment is specific to every nucleus and determines sensitivity to magnetic resonance.

THE HYDROGEN NUCLEUS

The hydrogen nucleus is the basis for clinical MRI. About two thirds of the body is composed of water, and each hydrogen atom in the water molecule contains one proton. There are differences in the composition of water in various tissues and organs, with pathological processes frequently creating a water composition that is different from that found in normal tissues. Because the composition is dissimilar and because hydrogen contains a single proton, it gives a large magnetic moment that spins about an axis like the spinning of a top (Figure 12-3). Thus, the hydrogen protons in our body act like innumerable tiny magnets.

ALIGNMENT

In the absence of an applied magnetic field, the magnetic moments of the hydrogen nuclei are randomly oriented. Upon placing the nuclei within a strong external magnetic field (B_0), the magnetic moments of the hydrogen nuclei align with the magnetic field. Some align parallel with the magnetic field (in the same direction) and some align antiparallel (in the opposite direction) (Figure 12-4).

Based on quantum mechanics, these hydrogen nuclei possess energy in two discrete quantities: low and high. Low-energy nuclei align their magnetic moments parallel

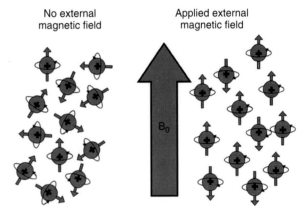

No external magnetic field

Applied external magnetic field

B_0

Net magnetization

FIGURE 12-4 **Alignment of Protons with the B_0 Field.** With no external magnetic field, hydrogen protons (+) are oriented randomly. When the protons are placed in a strong magnetic field (B_0), a net magnetization will be produced parallel to the main magnetic field.

to the external magnetic field and are termed *spin-up nuclei*. High-energy nuclei align their magnetic moments in the antiparallel direction and are termed *spin-down nuclei*.

The strength of the external magnetic field determines which nuclei will orient spin-up or spin-down. There are always fewer high-energy (spin-down) nuclei than low-energy nuclei, therefore the small number of **spin-down** nuclei will be cancelled out by the larger number of **spin-up** nuclei. In so doing, there will be a larger number of nuclei oriented parallel to the external magnetic field, which will produce a net magnetic moment that will precess about this external magnetic field.

PRECESSION

A spinning top spins on its axis at the same time it is being pulled down by gravitational force. Likewise, a hydrogen nucleus (proton) in the presence of a magnetic force (like the effect of gravity on the top) spins on its axis and is acted upon by the external magnetic field causing precession. The combined effect of spinning and falling creates **precession** when placed within a strong magnetic field (Figure 12-5).

This precession follows a circular path around the magnetic field, and the precessional frequency is determined by the **Larmor equation** (Figure 12-6).

The Larmor equation includes the main magnetic field strength multiplied by a constant. The constant is called the gyromagnetic ratio, which is a relationship between the angular momentum and magnetic moment of each MR active nucleus and is a characteristic of each type of nuclei. For hydrogen protons, the gyromagnetic ratio is equal to 42.6 MHz/T (megahertz per tesla). The main magnetic field strength, B_0, depends on the magnet design. For a typical superconducting MR system, the magnetic field strength may be 1.5 T. The frequency of precession then will equal 42.6 MHz/T × 1.5 T, or about 64 MHz (64 million times per second). In addition, hydrogen will have a different Larmor frequency at different field strengths (higher Tesla magnets).

For example:

At 1.5T: 42.6 MHz × 1.5 T = 63.9 MHz/T

At 1.0T: 42.6 MHz × 1.0 T = 42.6 MHz/T

At 0.5T: 42.6 MHz × 0.5 T = 21.3 MHz/T

The Larmor frequency is important because if energy is delivered to the hydrogen nuclei at a different frequency to that of the Larmor frequency of the nucleus, resonance (defined next) will not occur.

RESONANCE

MRI uses radiofrequency (RF) energy synchronized to the precessional frequency (Larmor frequency) of the protons, resulting in **resonance**. An example of resonance is one of a child on a swing, someone pushes the child and if the person pushing the child thrusts at the optimal time, the system will gain energy and the child will go higher and higher.

In our case, an RF pulse is generated that exactly matches the Larmor frequency of hydrogen (proton) causing the nucleus to gain energy and resonate. If an RF pulse is of a different frequency than that of the Larmor frequency of the nucleus, resonance does not occur.[4]

The resulting "gain" of energy will cause an increase in the number of spin-down (high-energy) nuclei because some of the spin-up (low-energy) nuclei have gained energy via resonance and become high-energy nuclei (flip). The energy difference between spin-up and spin-down nuclei will increase as the magnetic field strength increases and is termed *excitation*.

Remember earlier in our discussion that we described the magnetic moment as a vector. Vectors indicate both magnitude and direction and are important in MRI for determining the x, y, and z axes along the direction of the main magnetic field (Figure 12-7). The direction parallel to B_0 is the longitudinal direction (z direction) and corresponds in MRI to the head-to-foot (or foot-to-head) direction. The transverse plane (x, y) for a patient who is supine and head first is defined by x in the left-to-right

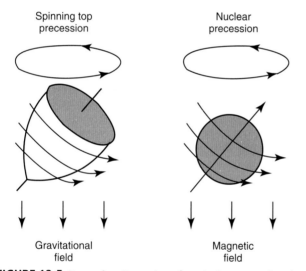

FIGURE 12-5 Precession. Precession of a spinning top and nuclear precession are similar in that an external force combined with the spinning motion causes precession.

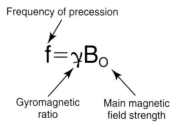

FIGURE 12-6 Larmor Equation. The Larmor equation allows us to determine the frequency of precession of a proton in a magnetic field.

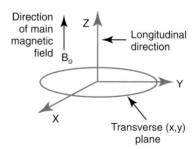

FIGURE 12-7 Coordinate System. For a typical 1.5-T cylindrical-bore imaging unit, the z axis (longitudinal direction) is often aligned with the main magnetic field; the plane perpendicular to this is called the *transverse plane*.

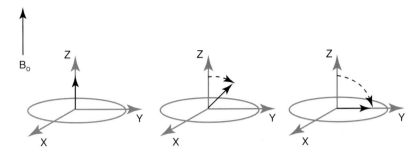

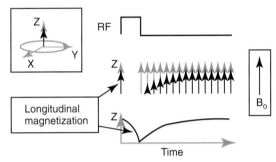

FIGURE 12-8 Absorption of RF Energy. *Left:* Prior to an RF pulse, the net magnetization *(small black arrow)* is aligned parallel to the main magnetic field and the *z*-axis. *Center and right:* An RF pulse at the Larmor frequency will allow energy to be absorbed by the protons, thus causing the net magnetization to rotate away from the *z*-axis.

direction, and *y* in the anterior-to-posterior direction. When protons are placed within a strong magnetic field, the magnetic fields from the protons combine and form a net magnetization vector that is parallel to the external magnetic field in the longitudinal direction. An RF pulse is then applied and its energy is absorbed, which results in the rotation of the net magnetization vector away from the longitudinal direction toward the transverse direction. This rotation of the magnetization vector is known as the **flip angle** and it depends upon the strength and duration of the RF pulse (Figure 12-8).

If the net magnetization vector rotates into the transverse plane it is termed a *90-degree RF pulse*. If it rotates 180 degrees into the *z* direction, it is termed a *180-degree RF pulse*. The degree of rotation will become important later in our discussion of pulse sequences and image acquisition. In summary, the result of resonance is magnetization in the transverse plane, which precesses at the Larmor frequency only if an RF pulse is applied at exactly the Larmor frequency of hydrogen.

MR SIGNAL AND FREE INDUCTION DECAY

Now that resonance has occurred at the Larmor frequency, we have precession in the transverse plane (*x, y*). If we place a receiver coil in the region of a moving magnetic field, a voltage will be created within this coil (Faraday's law). This voltage constitutes the MR signal with a frequency that is defined by the Larmor equation. When the RF pulse is turned off, the protons lose their energy and realign with the external magnetic field (relaxation). The high-energy protons will return to a low-energy position and realign in a spin-up orientation. Transverse magnetization gradually converts (decays) to longitudinal magnetization (recovery), and as transverse magnetization decays, so does the magnitude of the voltage induced in the receiver coil. This process in turn results in decreased MR signal and thus is termed *free induction decay (FID) signal*.

T1 AND T2

The RF pulse energy is absorbed, causing protons to flip from the longitudinal direction (longitudinal magnetization) and begin precessing in the transverse direction

FIGURE 12-9 Longitudinal (T1) Relaxation. Application of a 90-degree RF pulse causes longitudinal magnetization to become zero. Over time, the longitudinal magnetization will grow back in a direction parallel to the main magnetic field.

(transverse magnetization). Once the RF energy is switched off, the transverse magnetization decays and the longitudinal magnetization recovers with time and realigns with the main magnetic field, B_0 (Figure 12-9). This is the concept behind T1 and T2.

T1 refers to the recovery of longitudinal magnetization (T1 recovery), **T2** refers to the decay of transverse magnetization (T2 decay). Longitudinal magnetization is also referred to as M_Z, and transverse magnetization as M_{XY}.

T1 Recovery

T1 recovery results in the protons that had absorbed the RF energy and "flipped" to a higher energy state in the M_{XY} direction, losing energy and returning to the low-energy state. The nuclei do this by interacting with the surrounding environment or lattice, and this is referred to as spin-lattice relaxation. Energy releases to the surrounding lattice and causes the nuclear magnetic moments to recover their original longitudinal magnetization (M_Z). This rate of recovery is exponential and the time it takes to recover 63% of the final longitudinal magnetization is the definition of T1, which varies between different tissues (Figure 12-10).

The magnetization of tissues with different values of T1 will grow back in the longitudinal direction at different rates. These differing rates of T1 recovery and T2 decay allow us to take advantage of the individual vectors of various tissues such as fat, water, muscle,

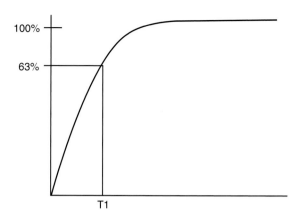

FIGURE 12-10 **Definition of T1.** T1 is a characteristic of tissue and is defined as the time that it takes the longitudinal magnetization to grow back to 63% of its final value.

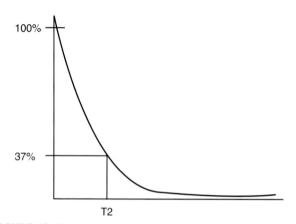

FIGURE 12-11 **Definition of T2.** T2 is a characteristic of tissue and is defined as the time that it takes the transverse magnetization to decrease to 37% of its starting value.

and cerebrospinal fluid (CSF), which will be discussed later.

T2 Decay

T2 decay results from the loss of transverse magnetization (M_{XY}) as the protons lose the energy absorbed by the RF pulse and decay from a high energy state to a lower energy state in the longitudinal direction. T2 decay loses its energy by exchanging its energy with the surrounding nuclei, which is called *spin-spin relaxation*. This is also an exponential process and is the time it takes the transverse magnetization to decrease to 37% of its starting value (Figure 12-11). Different tissues have different values of T2 and dephase at different rates.

T1 and T2 Contrast

As previously stated, different tissues will demonstrate different T1 and T2 characteristics. We can utilize these differences to obtain image contrast between differing tissues. As a review, initially there is a random array of protons precessing in either a spin-up or spin-down

BOX 12-2   **Causes of T2 Dephasing**

Spin-spin interactions
Magnetic field inhomogeneities
Magnetic susceptibility
Chemical shift effects

orientation. An external magnetic field is applied resulting in a majority of the protons aligning in the spin-up orientation parallel to the magnetic field with net magnetization in the *z* direction (longitudinal magnetization). A 90-degree RF pulse is applied, which rotates the net magnetization into the *x-y* plane (transverse magnetization), where the magnetic moments of hydrogen are in the same place on the precessional path around B_0 at any given time. These moments are in phase, whereas magnetic moments that are not in the same place on the precessional path around B_0 are out of phase. Immediately after the 90-degree RF pulse, transverse magnetization is maximized and then begins to dephase because of several processes (Box 12-2). The signal from the dephasing protons cancels out, and the MR signal decreases (Figure 12-12). Recall that transverse magnetization can be measured by a receiver coil, and the electric current in a wire will produce a magnetic field perpendicular to the loop of a wire. Measurement of the transverse magnetization, which is a magnetic field, is possible because it induces a current in a loop of wire (Figure 12-13). This induced electric current is then digitized and recorded in the computer of the MR system for later reconstruction as an MR image.

Decay and recovery times are used to produce images with specific contrast. For example, water has a long T1 and long T2, fat has a short T1 and short T2, cerebrospinal fluid has a long T1 and long T2, white matter has a short T1 and short T2, and gray matter has an intermediate T1 and intermediate T2 (Figure 12-14). If we were to create an image at a time when these curves were widely separated, we would produce an image that has high contrast between these tissues. Thus white matter contributes to the lighter pixels, CSF contributes to the darker pixels, and gray matter contributes to pixels with intermediate shades of gray, resulting in T1-weighted contrast.[2]

As stated earlier in the chapter, T2 is the time it takes for transverse magnetization to decay to 37% of its original value (see Figure 12-11). Recalling our different decay and recovery times we are able to take advantage of these differences and produce images based on this contrast mechanism, called T2-weighted contrast. We can see in Figure 12-15 that CSF is associated with lighter pixels, white matter is associated with darker pixels, and gray matter is associated with intermediate gray-level pixels.

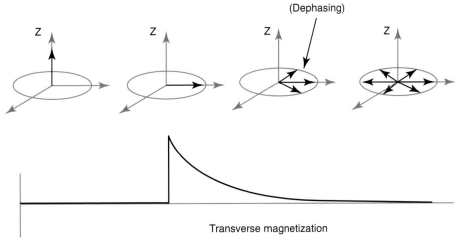

FIGURE 12-12 Immediately after application of a 90-degree RF pulse, transverse magnetization is maximized; it then begins to diphase.

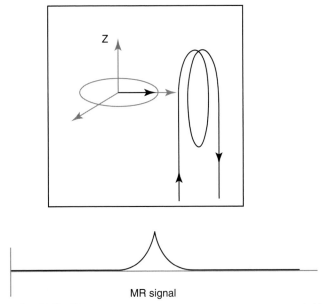

FIGURE 12-13 **Measurement of the MR Signal.** A magnetic field *(black arrow)* that is near and perpendicular to a loop of wire will produce an electric current in the loop. The current can be digitized and stored for later reconstruction into an MR image.

PULSE SEQUENCES

Our ultimate goal is the creation of images of varying contrast by obtaining images at specific decay and recovery times. Contrast is controlled by varying MR **pulse sequences** (Figure 12-16) to accentuate or diminish characteristics of certain diseases, normal tissues, or even foreign objects. The diagram that follows provides an explanation of a spin-echo pulse sequence.

Figure 12-16 is a pulse sequence for spin echo (SE) with TR (repetition time) representing the time between each 90-degree pulse for each slice, and TE (time to echo) representing the time between the 90-degree pulse and

the peak of the spin echo. The 180-degree pulse will rephase the spins, which will generate an echo (TE). If we use a short TE and short TR with a 90-degree pulse followed by a single 180-degree pulse, we can generate a T1-weighted image (Figures 12-17 and 12-18).

We can also use a pulse sequence that will produce a T2-weighted image by using a long TR and long TE, which will maximize T2 contrast (Figures 12-19 and 12-20).

Another type of pulse sequence can be used to suppress unwanted signals in MR images (e.g., signals from fat or fluid) by controlling TR and TE and using 180-degree pulses to "invert" the longitudinal magnetization.[2] The tissues will grow back at different rates, and when the tissue to be suppressed crosses the zero axis, application of a 90-degree pulse will rotate all other signals into the transverse plane, and the resulting signal from the tissue at the zero point is zero and therefore will not contribute any brightness to the resulting tissue. This sequence is termed *inversion recovery* (Figures 12-21 and 12-22).

A final sequence to be considered is one that has extreme utility for stroke evaluation and is termed **diffusion weighted imaging (DWI)**. Diffusion imaging depends on the random motion of water molecules in tissue. Water diffusion characteristics can be displayed by using DWI where foci of bright intensity suggests restricted motion of water (ischemia or infracted tissue) within that location, such as that seen with a cerebrovascular accident (Figure 12-23). Other sequences can also be employed to generate vessels but this topic is outside the scope of this chapter.

ARTIFACTS

Artifacts are present in to some degree in all MRI images. Therefore it is important that the causes of some artifacts are understood. Many are unavoidable or are irreversible

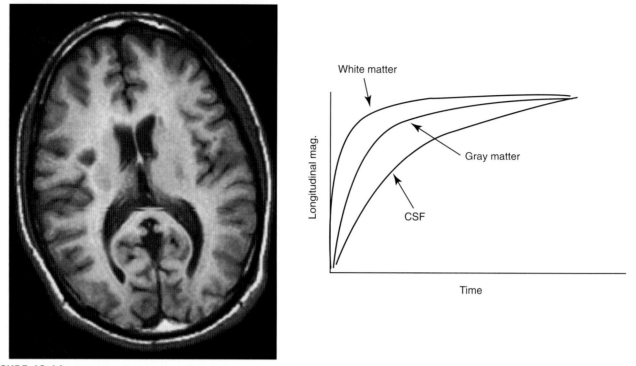

FIGURE 12-14 **T1-Weighted Contrast.** Different tissues have different rates of T1 relaxation. If an image is obtained at a time when the relaxation curves are widely separated, T1-weighted contrast will be maximized. *CSF*, Cerebrospinal fluid; *Mag*, magnetization.

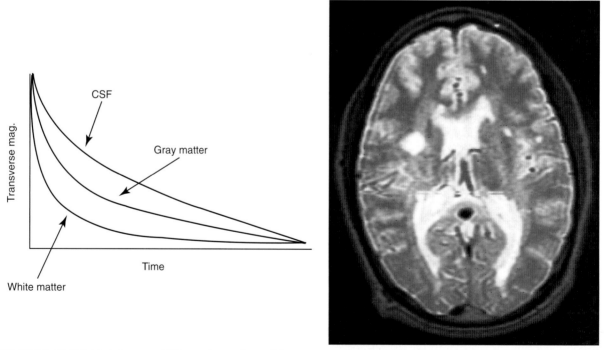

FIGURE 12-15 **T2-Weighted Contrast.** Different tissues have different rates of T2 relaxation. If an image is obtained at a time when the relaxation curves are widely separated, T2-weighted contrast will be maximized. *CSF*, Cerebrospinal fluid; *Mag*, magnetization.

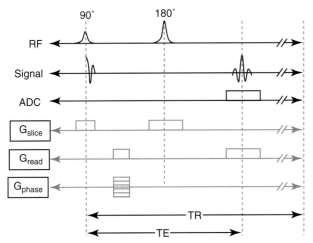

FIGURE 12-16 Pulse Sequence Diagram. A pulse sequence diagram can be used to show the relative timing of certain events during an MRI acquisition. The timing of RF pulses, the signal formed from these pulses, and the digitization of the signal is shown. TE is shown as the time to the echo, and the repetition time (TR) is shown as the time it takes to go through the pulse sequence once. This pulse sequence uses a 90-degree RF pulse with a 180-degree RF pulse to rephase spins to form an echo. T1- and T2-weighted images may be created with this pulse sequence. *ADC,* Analog-to-digital converter; in all pulse sequence diagrams; *Gslice,* slice select gradient; *Gread,* frequency encoding gradient; *Gphase,* phase encoding gradient.

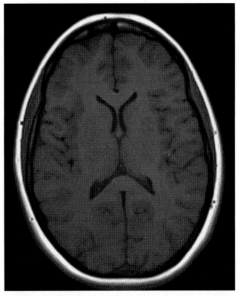

FIGURE 12-17 T1-weighted image using a pulse sequence with short TR and short TE.

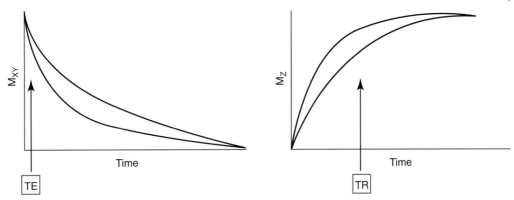

FIGURE 12-18 A short TR and short TE will result in a T1-weighted image. *TE,* Time to the echo; *TR,* repetition time.

and can only be reduced by applying correction algorithms to the acquired data, whereas others can be avoided. This section discusses the appearances, causes, and remedies of several common artifacts encountered in MRI.

One of the most common artifacts is motion artifact (Figures 12-24 and 12-25), which can be created by arterial or CSF pulsations, breathing, swallowing, or even eye movements. This artifact occurs when moving structures or fluids are imaged over time and are then placed into a single static image, moving in the phase encoding gradient during the pulse sequence (see Figure 12-16). Anatomy will move during the scan and get "misplaced" in the phase encoding direction as the

phase gradient changes during the image acquisition. In the examples that follow, one image is acquired during systole, another during diastole, and so on, resulting in a change in position between each phase encoding step. The anatomy "moves" between these steps and become mismapped into the field of view when the image is read out during the frequency encoding step (see Figure 12-16). This artifact can be remedied by changing the phase encoding direction, swapping phase and frequency encoding directions (x and y as discussed earlier). Many other techniques can also be used, such as presaturation pulses, respiratory compensation techniques, or gating, all of which are beyond the scope of this chapter.

Another common artifact is termed *aliasing* or *wrap-around*. This occurs when the anatomy you desire to image produces an image that lies outside the field of view (FOV). The anatomy will result in an image that wraps around onto the top or beside the anatomy inside the FOV (Figure 12-26).

Aliasing can occur in either the frequency or phase encoding direction and can be easily corrected by increasing the field of view.

The last artifact in this section that will be discussed is metallic susceptibility artifact, which includes dental amalgam or any ferromagnetic (discussed earlier) object (Figures 12-27 and 12-28). This artifact can cause large distortions in the image resulting in signal voids ("blackening"). The metal becomes magnetized by the external magnetic field (B_0) resulting in a change in the precessional frequency and phase resulting in signal loss. This artifact can be corrected by either removing the metal object, lowering TE, or using a different sequence of acquisition (spin echo rather than gradient echo). The

"cost" of lowering TE, or using a spin echo sequence for acquisition rather than gradient echo, can result in the loss of the ability to detect small hemorrhages, which uses the magnetic susceptibility artifact.

Not all artifacts are detrimental to MRI. One artifact that must be discussed further is called *chemical shift artifact*. This type of artifact uses the different precessional frequencies of fat and water. Although fat and water both contain hydrogen protons, fat also contains carbon and water contains oxygen; therefore fat will precess at a lower frequency than water. Remembering the Larmor equation (see Figure 12-6) allows us to calculate the different precessional frequencies between fat and water for a given main magnetic field strength. The advantage of this artifact can be utilized in clinical practice by physicians in the example for further evaluation of adrenal lesions (Figures 12-29 and 12-30). Pulsation sequences can be generated as either in phase or out of phase. In phase, fat and water signals add constructively, and out of phase, fat and water signals cancel each other out. Therefore in an example of an adrenal adenoma (a benign lesion), which is composed of fat, in-phase and out-of-phase MRI can be performed, and on out-of-phase imaging the adenoma will drop out (turn black). This is of significant importance to the radiologists and patients and can provide a conclusive diagnosis, eliminating the need for further evaluation.

MRI SAFETY

The key thing to remember with MRI is that the magnet is always ON. Because of this there are risks not only to the patient but also to physicians, technologists, nurses, housekeeping, security, and even family members. MRI safety takes this into account by publishing literature and guidelines for MRI safety and using labeling criteria established by the U.S. Food and Drug Administration, as shown in Figure 12-31.

Any metallic object can act as a projectile resulting in serious injury to a patient on the MRI table. The ways to avoid potential risks is to follow a list of current MRI safety policies established by the American College of

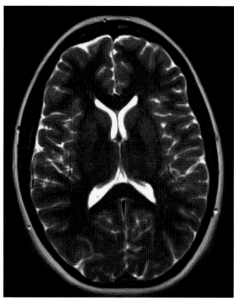

FIGURE 12-19 T2-weighted image using a pulse sequence with long TR and long TE.

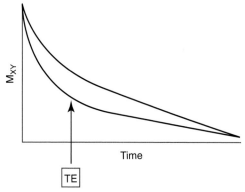

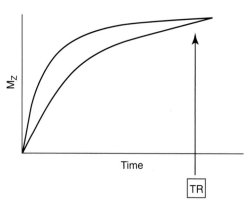

FIGURE 12-20 A long TE and long TR will result in a T2-weighted image. *TE,* Time to the echo; *TR,* repetition time.

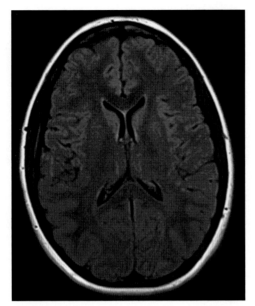

FIGURE 12-21 Inversion recovery with a fat nullification sequence.

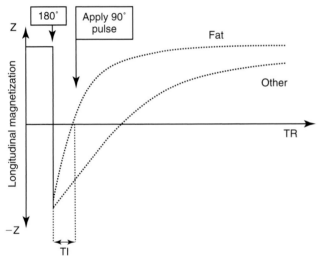

FIGURE 12-22 Inversion of the Signal in the Inversion-Recovery Sequence. After initial inversion of the longitudinal magnetization, T1 relaxation occurs and the signals from different tissues cross the zero axis at different times. When the signal to be suppressed crosses the zero axis, a 90-degree RF pulse will rotate all other signals into the transverse plane for image formation. *TI*, Inversion time.

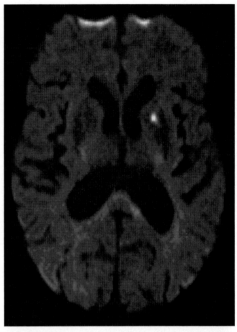

FIGURE 12-23 Diffusion weighted image showing acute infarct.

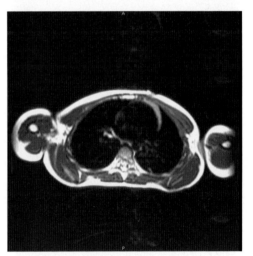

FIGURE 12-24 Respiratory motion artifact.

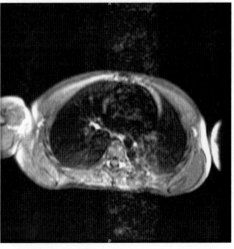

FIGURE 12-25 Cardiac pulsation artifact.

Radiology in 2007. Within this publication, there are sections for establishing Zones for Site Access Restriction due to the static magnetic field; MRI and non-MRI personnel safety education requirements; patient, MRI personnel, and non-MRI personnel screening; safety practices related to pregnant and pediatric patients; and safety practices related to induced voltages, auditory considerations, and thermal injury. Many other topics are discussed within this publication, which can be perused at your leisure at a later time. A few of the concepts mentioned earlier will be discussed further in the MRI safety policies document.

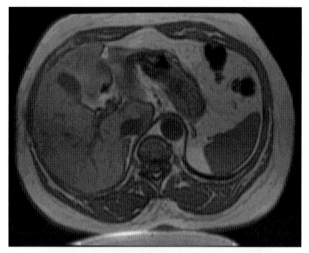

FIGURE 12-26 Aliasing.

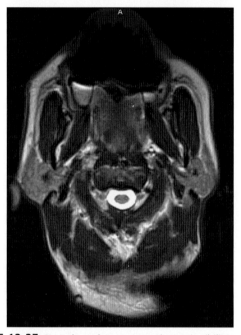

FIGURE 12-27 Dental amalgam magnetic susceptibility artifact.

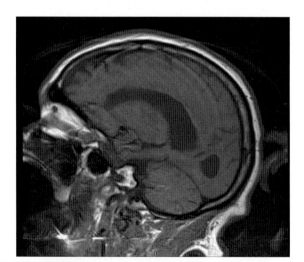

FIGURE 12-28 Dental amalgam magnetic susceptibility artifact. Also note the motion artifact.

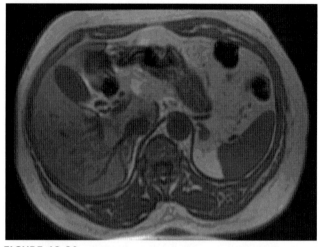

FIGURE 12-29 MRI in-phase image demonstrating a left adrenal gland nodule.

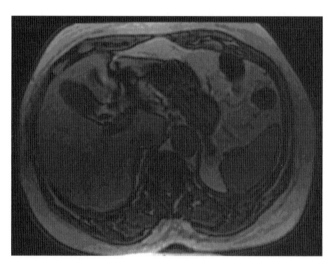

FIGURE 12-30 MRI out-of-phase image; notice the left adrenal nodule has dropped out (turned black).

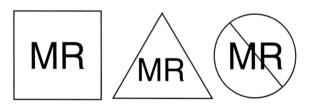

Green square
MRI safe

Yellow triangle
conditional

Red circle
not MRI safe

FIGURE 12-31 U.S. Food and Drug Administration labeling criteria (developed by ASTM [American Society for Testing and Materials] International) for portable objects taken into Zone 4. Square green "MR Safe" label is for wholly nonmetallic objects, triangular yellow label is for objects with "MR conditional" rating, and round red label is for "not MR safe" objects.

Any person undergoing an MRI procedure must take off all readily removable metallic personal belongings and devices on or in them (e.g., watches, jewelry, pagers, cell phones, body piercings (if removable), contraceptive diaphragms, metallic drug delivery patches, cosmetics containing metallic particles (such as eye makeup), and clothing items that may contain metallic fasteners, hooks, zippers, loose metallic components, or metallic threads. Before being permitted entrance, each patient with a history of potential ferromagnetic foreign object penetration must undergo further investigation with acceptable methods of screening, including patient history, plain x-ray films, prior computed tomography (CT) or MRI studies of the questioned anatomical area, or access to written documentation as to the type of implant or foreign object that may be present. If there are any questions that arise they must be brought to the attending radiologist for review.

Foreign bodies to be aware of include intravascular coils or clips, certain heart valves, cochlear implants, intraocular foreign bodies, bullets, or shrapnel, just to name a few.

All MRI personnel are screened as part of their employment process to ensure they are "MRI Safe," not only for their own protection but for the protection of patients and non-MRI personnel as well.

Protocols for imaging pregnant and pediatric patients are covered in detail within the ACR publication and will not be discussed. Three time-varying gradient magnetic field–related issues will be further discussed in this section: induced voltages, auditory considerations, and thermal injury.

Induced voltages are important in patients with implanted or retained wires in anatomically or functionally sensitive areas (e.g., myocardium, epicardium, or brain). These patients should be considered to be at higher risk especially from faster MRI sequences, such as echo planar imaging (which may be used in sequences such as DWI, functional imaging, or perfusion weighted imaging). Cardiac pacemakers or pacer wires left in the body from a previous pacemaker used to be considered absolute contraindications for MRI, because they could act as an "antenna" and cause cardiac fibrillation. However, today it could be acceptable to scan some patients with implanted wires (pacemaker has been removed) as long as the wires are cut close to the skin but not looped outside the chest. Modern pacemakers are being developed that are MRI compatible, but this, as with any implanted device, should be evaluated case by case.

Auditory considerations can be overcome by offering hearing protection to anyone undergoing an MRI scan. This protective device should be in place before initiation of imaging. Of much greater importance is the risk of thermal injury, because electric currents and voltages can be induced in electrically conductive materials when placed within the MRI scanner during the imaging

process. Examples of conductive materials include wires, electrocardiogram leads, or external metallic implants (skin staples and superficial metallic sutures are nonferromagnetic and "MR Safe"). When these conductive materials are introduced to the static magnetic field, resonance can be induced in the circuitry between the transmitted RF power and this material, resulting in rapid and clinically significant heating sufficient enough to result in tissue thermal injury or burns. Therefore, to avoid this complication, all visually evident leads or monitoring devices should be checked by the MRI technologist before scanning.

No topic on MRI safety would be complete without discussing the usage of gadolinium (an MRI contrast agent) in the renally impaired or a complication that can arise when using this contrast in the renally impaired known as nephrogenic systemic fibrosis (NSF). NSF was first observed in 1997 and formally described in 2000. If administering gadolinium to patients with renal impairment, collagen can be deposited into tissue, typically the distal extremities but can occur in other parts of the body, resulting in skin thickening and fibrosis. There is no definitive cure and the disease is progressive and can be fulminant in approximately 5% of cases. Patients that develop NSF are typically middle-aged, but this complication can also occur in elderly or pediatric patients. It is the role of radiologists, technologists, and ordering physicians to work as a team to avoid or modify the usage of gadolinium in patients with renal dysfunction.

SUMMARY

- MRI relies on the magnetic properties of atoms, which are composed of protons, neutrons, and electrons.
- The hydrogen nucleus is the basis for clinical MRI due to its single proton, which (because of its large magnetic moment) causes protons to align in either a parallel or antiparallel orientation with a discreet quantity of energy.
- When the hydrogen nucleus spins on its axis, it precesses at a frequency determined by the Larmor equation (frequency).
- MRI uses radiofrequency waves synchronized to the Larmor frequency to excite protons and result in a "gain" in energy.
- T1 refers to the recovery of longitudinal magnetization, and T2 refers to the decay of transverse magnetization.
- Differing rates of T1 recovery and T2 decay allow us to distinguish between various tissues such as fat, water, muscle, and cerebrospinal fluid.
- Image contrast is controlled by varying pulse sequences to accentuate or diminish characteristics of certain diseases, normal tissues, or foreign objects.

- Artifacts are encountered to some degree in all MRI images and are reduced by applying correction algorithms to the acquired data. The most common artifact is motion, which can be created by breathing, swallowing, eye movements, or pulsations from the heart or CSF.
- The MRI magnet is always ON, and any metallic object can act as a projectile. It is important to understand how to avoid potential risks by reviewing current MRI safety policies.

SUGGESTED READING

Bushberg JT, Seibert JA, Leidholdt EM, et al: *The essential physics of medical imaging*, ed 2, Philadelphia, 2002, Lippincott Williams & Wilkins.

Cowper SE, Robin HS, Steinberg SM, et al: Scleromyxoedema-like cutaneous diseases in renal dialysis patients, *Lancet* 356:1000-1001, 2000.

Damadian RV: Tumor detection by nuclear magnetic resonance, *Science* 171:1151-1153, 1971.

Jain SM, Wesson S, Hassanein A, et al: Nephrogenic fibrosing dermopathy in pediatric patients, *Pediatr Nephrol* 19:467-470, 2004.

Kanal E, Barkovich AJ, Bell C, et al: ACR guidance document for safe MR practices, *Am J Radiology* 188(6):1447-1474, 2007.

Pooley RA: Fundamentals physics of MR imaging, *Radiographics* 25:1087-1099, 2005.

Pusey E, Stark DD, Lufkin RB, et al: Magnetic resonance imaging artifacts: mechanism and clinical significance, *Radiographics* 6:891-911, 1986.

Steadman G: *Understanding magnetic resonance imaging* (website): www.elp.manchester.ac.uk/pub_projects/2003/MNATOGCS/index.htm. Accessed November 18, 2010.

Westbrook C, Roth C: *MRI in practice*, ed 3, Oxford, 2005, Blackwell Publishing.

Clinical PET/CT in Oncology

Nancy M. Swanston, Paul E. Christian

OBJECTIVES

After completing this chapter, the reader will be able to:
- Discuss the principles of PET/CT FDG oncology imaging.
- State the principal reasons for the recent rapid growth of PET oncology imaging.
- Recognize the normal biodistribution of FDG and list those organs with intense, moderate, or mild FDG activity.
- Compare the various patterns of normal FDG myocardial activity.
- Discuss the normal patterns of head and neck FDG activity.
- Discuss benign causes of increased FDG activity.
- Describe the variations in FDG biodistribution caused by improper patient preparation.

- Recite the steps in properly preparing a patient for an FDG PET scan.
- Explain the significance of peripheral blood glucose levels in FDG imaging.
- Recall the necessary historical information that should be obtained from each patient.
- List the various modes of PET and PET/CT acquisition and their uses.
- Discuss the advantages of dual point time imaging.
- Describe patient positioning and comfort issues that can hinder the acquisition of high-quality scans.
- Discuss the advantages of a longer uptake time for FDG PET imaging.
- Share the value of future PET oncology radiotracers.
- Identify potential future directions of PET/CT oncology.

KEY TERMS

2-[^{18}F]-fluoro-2-deoxy-D-glucose
   (^{18}F-FDG)
dual time point imaging
glucometer

glucose-6-phosphate (G-6-P)
glycolysis
hexokinase
mesothelioma

peripheral blood glucose
phosphorylate
radiopaque contrast media (ROCM)
solitary pulmonary nodules (SPNs)

Each year around 1.4 million new cases of cancer are diagnosed in the United States, along with another 1 million cases of basal cell and squamous cell skin cancers. Currently, approximately 11 million Americans have a history of cancer. Many of these people are living cancer-free lives because of more effective cancer treatments. Others may be newly diagnosed with the disease and are seeking information on their best course of action. Still there are many patients with recurrence of the disease who are receiving treatment. Considerable advances in oncology continue to occur in patient care, research, prevention, and education. Despite these advances, key questions persist regarding diagnosis, differentiation of malignant versus benign disease, cancer staging and grading, monitoring of response to therapy, and identification of those whose cancer has recurred. Positron emission tomography (PET) imaging in oncology is a rapidly emerging tool, and its availability is increasing. PET imaging represents one of the most effective diagnostic tools in nuclear medicine. When comparing nuclear medicine imaging devices, PET scanners have the best resolution. Now that almost all PET scanners have computed tomography (CT) for anatomical correlation, there has been an improvement in the confidence associated with identifying areas of hypermetabolism illustrated in PET. When comparing various nuclear medicine radiopharmaceuticals, positron-emitting radionuclides can be bound to the building blocks of life, the organic atoms in simple molecules. Utilizing these molecules allows the human body to be evaluated at the cellular level. PET is a powerful tool that can offer a sound mechanism to study fundamental biochemical processes.

During the initial PET development in the late 1970s, the principal clinical investigations involved the heart and brain. However, in the late 1980s, investigators began to show the value of PET technology in cancer detection. During the early 1990s, scholarly investigations continued to support this early experience, clearly demonstrating that the sensitivity and specificity of PET in cancer detection exceeded those of most routine medical tests and radiological imaging techniques. The continued proliferation of clinical investigations and scientific publications provided the necessary clinical validation of PET for certain types of cancer, and cost analyses demonstrated huge potential savings through the avoidance of unnecessary tests and needless surgery.

In 1998 the Centers for Medicare and Medicaid Services (CMS) announced that fluorodeoxyglucose (FDG) PET scans would be reimbursed for patients with solitary pulmonary nodules or non–small-cell lung carcinoma. This breakthrough in reimbursement opened the door for Medicare payments for other cancers in which experience had shown that PET was the most accurate imaging technique for identifying and staging the disease. Medicare coverage followed for melanoma, lymphoma, colorectal cancer, head and neck cancer, esophageal cancer, recurrent breast cancer, and thyroid carcinoma. Most third-party insurance companies now also cover FDG PET scans for a variety of cancer patients.

Payer reimbursement has been the driving force behind the rapid expansion in the number of PET facilities available to patients and referring physicians. However, to expand the number of locations offering PET services, it has also been necessary to simultaneously increase the number of cyclotron facilities that produce FDG. PET has expanded not only among academic institutions and large hospitals, but also among private business interests that have brought freestanding imaging centers and shared mobile scanners to community hospitals and rural areas. Similar worldwide growth is occurring as PET continues to establish its position as a powerful and valuable oncological imaging tool.

INTRACELLULAR ^{18}F-FDG METABOLISM

In PET cancer imaging, the most widely used radiopharmaceutical is 2-[^{18}F]-**fluoro-2-deoxy-D-glucose** (^{18}F-**FDG**). Biochemically, ^{18}F-FDG is a nonphysiological compound with a chemical structure very similar to that of naturally occurring glucose; it serves as an external marker of cellular glucose metabolism.

The ability to noninvasively image cellular glucose metabolism is important in oncological applications because many cancer cells use glucose at higher rates than normal cells. Current research also demonstrates that numerous malignant tumors express higher numbers of specific membrane transport proteins, with greater affinity for glucose than normal cells. This results in increased glucose flow into cancerous cells. Additionally, once glucose has entered the tumor cells, **hexokinase** (the first intracellular enzyme involved in glucose breakdown) is usually much more active than in normal cells. These factors increase the probability of being able to noninvasively visualize malignant tumors in the body.

Both glucose and FDG are absorbed by facilitated diffusion into cells with the assistance of certain specific membrane transport proteins. Once in the cell's cytosol, glucose is broken down by a series of enzymatic steps called **glycolysis**. The first step in this pathway occurs when hexokinase enzymatically adds a phosphate group to glucose (a process to **phosphorylate**), creating a new compound: **glucose-6-phosphate (G-6-P)**. FDG follows the same process in its transformation to FDG-6-phosphate (FDG-6-P).

The cell membrane is impermeable to both of these intermediate phosphorylated compounds, and neither can recross the cell membrane. Glucose-6-phosphate continues through the next glycolytic step with its transformation into fructose-6-phosphate by the action of phosphoglucoisomerase. However, because of its chemical structure, FDG cannot be enzymatically transformed into fructose-6-phosphate (Figure 13-1). Because FDG-6-P cannot be broken down or recross the cell

Normal cell FDG metabolism

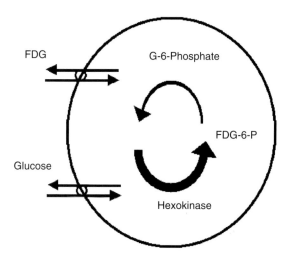

Cancer cell FDG metabolism

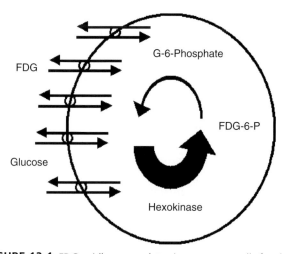

FIGURE 13-1 FDG avidly accumulates in cancerous cells for three main reasons: (1) cancer cells express more numerous specific membrane transport proteins with greater affinity for glucose than do normal cells (allowing for increased rates of facilitated diffusion into the cytosol), (2) the hexokinase enzymes in cancer cells transform FDG into FDG-6-P at higher rates than do normal cells, and (3) FDG-6-P cannot be further metabolized and therefore remains "trapped" in the cytosol.

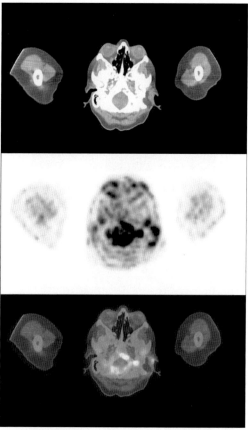

FIGURE 13-2 FDG PET/CT scan for a patient with breast cancer illustrating intense activity that has accumulated in the left ear because of chronic otitis media with a mixed infection of multiresistant *Staphylococcus aureus* and an *Aspergillus* species. The upper image is the CT, middle image is the PET scan, and the lower image demonstrates the fused PET scan on the CT. (See Color Plate 5.)

membrane, it remains trapped within the cell. As more FDG molecules enter the cell and are transformed into FDG-6-P, they continue to accumulate within the cellular cytosol.

Intracellular FDG activity varies with different types of cancer. Increased intracellular localization usually correlates with more aggressive tumors and greater numbers of viable tumor cells; however, this correlation is not perfect. FDG PET provides a marvelous, noninvasive imaging tool in a wide variety of cancers because these cancer cells demonstrate increased rates of

facilitated glucose diffusion across the cell membranes, have higher rates of glucose phosphorylation, and demonstrate greater FDG-6-P accumulation within the cytosol than most normal cells.

Because FDG acts as a visual marker of cellular glucose metabolism, it creates both advantages and problems. Because many different types of cancer demonstrate increased FDG utilization, FDG PET can serve as a powerful screening tool in the investigation of a wide variety of cancers; however, this power comes at a price. Many normal and noncancerous conditions, such as infection, inflammation, atelectasis, healing tissues, and muscular activity, also can increase intracellular FDG use (Figures 13-2, 13-3, and 13-4). Thus normal tissues or benign processes can masquerade as malignancies. Essentially, FDG PET cancer screening is a broad-based or shotgun approach. Cancers are detected, but so are other occasionally confounding and potentially misleading benign processes.

Of greater concern are those cancers that use FDG at the same rate as normal surrounding tissues. In these cases, tumors remain hidden within the normal imaging

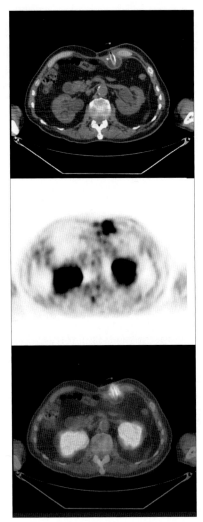

FIGURE 13-3 A gastrostomy tube is in place in the abdomen and is seen on the CT scan. The PET scan *(middle)* demonstrates elevated FDG activity along its insertion route and perimeter consistent with inflammation. The fused PET/CT scan is shown at the bottom. (See Color Plate 6.)

prevent muscle uptake, patients should not participate in strenuous exercise for 24 hours before the study.

Before any FDG injection, the technologist should confirm the patient's identity and obtain a brief history to ensure that a PET scan is appropriate. The history should include, at least, information about height, weight, fasting state, diabetes, pregnancy, breast-feeding, surgeries, prior chemotherapy or radiation therapy, and the results of any recent imaging procedures (detail in Box 13-1). The examination should be completely explained to the patient and any questions should be answered. After the intravenous (IV) line is started, the patient should be placed on a bed or in a reclining chair for 10 minutes and asked to relax and refrain from talking. If the brain is to be imaged, the patient should also close the eyes, and the room should be quiet and dark.

Barriers such as language, learning, and hearing should all be assessed before the patient's arrival to the PET center. For example, if the patient does not speak English or is hearing impaired, the facility may need to coordinate language assistance from an interpreter, a sign-language professional, or one of the patient's family members so that a thorough history can be obtained for the patient. Information may need to be repeated when dealing with language barriers, and speech should be slow, simple, and clear. In addition, with CT now being used as the method for attenuation correction, facilities may have different protocols for the breathing regimen during the CT acquisition. The patient needs to be educated and directed about this aspect of the procedure so that matching between the PET images and CT images is maximized. Communication becomes quite difficult if the patient is hearing impaired or speaks a different language from that of the operator.

background and go unnoticed and possibly untreated. The fact that FDG PET fails at times to distinguish the presence of cancer has stimulated many attempts to develop new methods of PET cancer detection. Several additional PET radiotracers are mentioned at the end of the chapter, but most of the chapter focuses on FDG as the predominant PET cancer imaging agent, with all its inherent advantages and problems.

PATIENT PREPARATION AND INJECTION

PET radiotracers provide images of fundamental metabolic processes within the body. These radiotracers, such as FDG, are extremely sensitive to small changes in tissue metabolism. It is critical, therefore, to ensure that the patient's baseline metabolic activity starts at appropriately low levels and that the patient remains at rest before, during, and after injection of the radiotracer. To

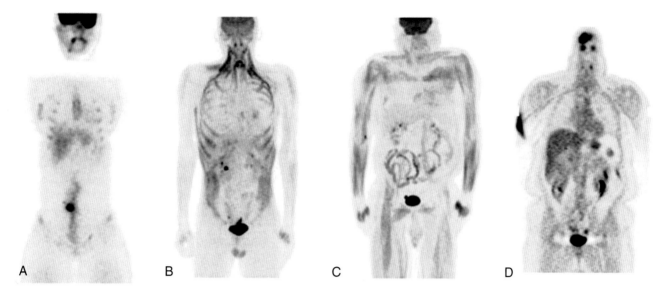

FIGURE 13-4 Mild to intense FDG uptake can be represented in healing surgical wounds (**A**), intense coughing (**B**), muscle from exercise (**C**), and as a result of a truncation artifact (**D**).

To reduce the pretest **peripheral blood glucose** level, patients arriving for an FDG PET scan should fast for 4 to 6 hours before the appointment. The peripheral blood glucose level can be measured with a **glucometer.** Ideally the value should be less than 120 mg/dl. Increased blood glucose levels can compete with FDG, resulting in little difference between tumor and normal soft-tissue uptake and in very-low–contrast images. Some laboratories inject patients with glucose as high as 200 mg/dl and have reported no degradation in image quality. However, there are no published, controlled scientific studies to adequately establish an upper limit for the measured peripheral blood glucose level.

Some laboratories contend that the peripheral blood glucose level should be measured in every patient. Other laboratories do not measure the glucose level, assuming that it will be sufficiently low (as long as the patient has been fasting and has no history of diabetes or of blood relatives with diabetes). Diabetic patients can be one of the more difficult populations to manage. More involved practices can be developed to ensure commitment to service can be achieved (Box 13-2). Patients with elevated peripheral blood glucose levels may sometimes be studied after their glucose level has been reduced, either by an additional time delay or after injection of fast-acting insulin formulations, as directed by a knowledgeable physician. However, insulin administration within 2 hours of FDG injections can also result in reduced tumor uptake of FDG, resulting in lower-contrast images.

FDG usually displays normally faint activity within the body, providing a general anatomical distribution of the solid organs. However, patients with diabetes and high peripheral blood glucose levels (>150 mg/dl) may demonstrate inhomogeneous or inadequate tissue activity because of the lack of insulin, insulin resistance, or

---

BOX 13-2 | Overview of Diabetic Patient Preparation

1. Patient should be consulted before appointment to determine nature of disease. In this way, the caregiver can identify important information related to management of diabetes, such as the mechanism of control (diet therapy, insulin administration, and/or use of oral hypoglycemics)
2. Ask direct questions during consultation.
   - Do you regularly perform fasting blood glucose measurements? If yes, what are your levels?
   - If the answer to the above question is "no," it might be advantageous to arrange a time for a preconsultation in which blood glucose level can be assessed.
   - Do you journal your condition? Are there periods in the day that trend high or low?
3. If the patient is a type I/insulin-dependent diabetes mellitus (IDDM) patient, schedule the patient as early in the day as possible. Instruct the patient to fast and present to clinic refraining from injecting insulin unless administration is necessary.
4. With type II/non–insulin-dependent diabetes mellitus (non-IDDM) patients may find it easier to have an appointment in the late morning or afternoon. In this way the patient can eat a light breakfast, take oral medications, begin the fast, and present at minimum 4 hours later for appointment.
5. Request that the patient bring all medications related to the management of their disease to the appointment.
6. After accurately and completely performing medication reconciliation, review list for all drugs used to manage diabetes.
7. Review the patient history record to see if any other medical conditions or hormonal abnormalities exist that could produce diabetic syndromes (pancreatic disease, therapies, infection, etc.)
8. Be alert for signs and symptoms of hypoglycemia.
9. Develop policies to manage patients with extremely low or high blood glucose levels.
10. Perform fasting blood glucose measurement. Serial measurements can be performed if there is potential for patient to reach desired range of serum glucose.

competition from the increased nonradioactive extracellular glucose. Patients with diabetes mellitus must continue their standard snacks between meals and have their insulin injections before FDG PET scans. Such patients may present serious difficulties in the acquisition of diagnostic FDG PET studies, and the close involvement of knowledgeable referring physicians or endocrinologists before the scan date is prudent to avoid problems and potential havoc to the daily schedule.

In hospital settings it is imperative to discern ahead of time whether the patient is an inpatient or outpatient. This determination will assist in eliminating problems that may be associated with transporting the patient throughout the hospital, understanding the patient's intake of fluids, understanding the patient's diet, or understanding the patient's condition. Timing is an element that needs to be managed when working with a radioisotope with a half-life of 109 minutes. Valuable time could be lost if personnel, a wheelchair, a stretcher, or an oxygen tank has to be found at the last minute to transport the patient. Another area to consider is the patient's caloric intake. If the patient is receiving dextrose solution or total parental nutrition, it should be discontinued 6 to 8 hours before the injection of the FDG. This is so that competition for binding sites does not occur between the radioactive sugar analog used in PET imaging and sugar compounds in these items. Inpatients should also be assessed to ensure that they can tolerate the procedure. PET imaging in oncology is generally not considered an emergency procedure, so if patients need some time to recover from other procedures or feel they could not remain motionless during imaging to achieve optimal results, the appointment can be rescheduled.

FDG should be administered while the patient is in a resting state; therefore it is less disruptive to place an intracatheter in a peripheral vein of the upper extremities 10 minutes or more before the time of administration. This IV line may be used to access a small amount of blood for peripheral glucose testing. It is essential to use fastidious technique and to ensure proper placement of the intracatheter before the FDG injection. Infiltration must be avoided. If a patient is going to have iodinated contrast along with the PET/CT exam, an 18- to 20-gauge intracatheter should be used for FDG injection and then kept for utilization with the contrast media. Residual measurements for FDG in the injecting apparatus will not be possible, so it is imperative that proper injection technique is utilized. A 20- to 30-ml saline flush after the FDG injection helps to reduce venous FDG uptake in the upper extremity. Port-a-caths or indwelling central catheters should not be used to inject FDG unless absolutely necessary. Retention in the reservoirs and the tips of the catheter lines can cause errors in the evaluation of the chest wall and, more importantly, the mediastinum.

The normal injected FDG dose ranges from 5 to 20 mCi. The most common adult dose, 10 mCi, is at the lower end of this range so as to reduce radiation exposure to the bladder. The pediatric dose is determined by body weight and is based on 150 µCi/kg. The injection is performed using a three-way stopcock attached to the IV line and to the dose syringe. Again, after injection, the IV should be slowly flushed with 20 to 30 ml of saline to help eliminate any activity in nearby veins. The patient should rest quietly following the injection for approximately 60 to 90 minutes. Tumor concentration of FDG continues to increase with time, whereas soft-tissue activity diminishes; therefore longer update times increase tumor to soft-tissue contrast and improve lesion detection. Before imaging, the IV may be discontinued if no contrast will be administered at the time of the scan. The patient should void immediately before the imaging sequence.

Radiopaque contrast media (ROCM) may be used to enhance radiographic visualization of low-contrast tissues within the body, such as the vessels and the gastrointestinal tract. The most common ROCMs used in facilities today are forms of iodine and barium. Enhancement is accomplished because of the photon-absorbing properties of the elements. The osmotic activities of ROCMs contribute to the adverse reactions in the heart and renal system associated with its use. Generally, 1000 to 1500 ml of oral contrast is administered incrementally to patients before imaging. Iodinated contrast can also be given and the amount is usually based on the anatomical location requiring contrast enhancement. Protocols can be developed to incorporate the use of contrast into the CT scanning used for attenuation correction or to add the procedure to the end of the PET/CT exam. If the latter is done, the patient's position and landmarks on the scanner should not be altered. The imaging professional must be knowledgeable about the various forms of contrast media, routes of administration, adverse effects and reactions, drug interactions, and so on, before incorporating the use of contrast media into protocols.

PET SCAN ACQUISITION

Selecting the Scan Type and Body Area

PET oncology imaging can be performed in several ways: limited-area scanning, dynamic imaging, whole-body imaging from the base of the skull to the mid-thigh, or total-body imaging. Limited-area imaging is used when the patient's history indicates the need to evaluate only a very specific area of the body, such as in those patients who have a solitary pulmonary nodule discovered on a screening CT examination and no known cancer. Scanning protocols with a limited number of bed positions (approximately three or four) over the chest can cover both lungs entirely. Dynamic imaging requires continuous imaging in a single bed position; it would be done only if the exact position of the lesion is known and the study is tailored especially to evaluate the possibility of a benign or malignant process in a single, well-defined lesion.

Patients in oncology studies most commonly receive a whole-body PET scan from the base of the skull to midthigh. This scan requires about five to eight bed positions, depending on the scanner's field of view (FOV) and the patient's height. Normally these scans are obtained just after the patient has voided. They can start from the pelvis and continue toward the head so that the bladder can be imaged while it is nearly empty, thus avoiding reconstruction artifacts created as the bladder fills with activity. If there is a concern that a patient may not be able to tolerate the procedure in its entirety, it may be advantageous to begin imaging at the vertex or base of skull, then proceed to the pelvis if the majority of disease and opportunity for spread are in the upper body.

Total-body imaging is performed if there is a question that a cancer might include the head or legs. These scans cover from the top of the head through the feet and require more than 10 bed positions. Total-body scans are most commonly used for patients with malignant melanomas or sarcomas. On some scanners the scanning protocol may be set up to start just above (or below) the bladder, scan the empty bladder first and continue in one direction along the body, then to return to the starting point and scan the remaining portions of the body in the opposite direction.

If cancer is suspected in the pelvis, it occasionally may be necessary to place a urinary catheter to reduce normal bladder activity. Some facilities use diuretics to enhance excretion of FDG, whereas others add a continuous saline flow through the urinary catheter to further reduce bladder activity. However, in most cases these interventions are highly irritating to the patient and may actually end up being counterproductive.

Another important aspect to note is if patients are not able to lie still or motionless throughout the imaging sequence. They may need to get medications prescribed by their referring physician to help manage pain. Also, alternate methods of imaging could be pursued, for example, positioning the patient prone versus supine to alleviate pressure on areas of the body where the pain originates. If the patient is a radiation therapy candidate and immobilization devices have been made that will be used during the PET/CT imaging sequence, fluctuations in position are not permitted, making pain management medications even more critical to manage the patient's comfort. This can take some time, further clarifying why it is important that all of these conversations occur before appointment time. Motion artifacts created by patient movement during the CT and PET acquisitions can be detrimental to the interpretation of the PET/CT images.

Benign and inflammatory processes often decrease FDG concentration with time, whereas malignant tissue continues to increase in FDG uptake. Therefore imaging at two time points (**dual time point imaging**) allows the differentiation between cancerous and benign tissue.[2,3,5]

Patient Positioning and Comfort

Before the imaging procedure, the patient should void. In addition, the patient should remove any metallic objects that might cause attenuation artifacts. The patient should be placed in a comfortable recumbent position with a support sponge or pillow under the knees and a support to help hold the arms still. The PET physician should establish the preferred patient arm position. Most PET scans are acquired with the arms raised above the head in order to compliment the CT. Acquiring images with the patient's arms to the sides would significantly increase beam hardening and truncate CT data. However, when dealing with melanoma or sarcomas where the disease process could be in the upper extremities, the arms may need to be left at the sides. Some large patients may need arms-up imaging or may place their arms on their abdomen to fit into the scanner. Most commonly, however, the average patient can place the arms at the sides, and the selected scanning protocol can be performed. The technologist may use a strap to support the patient's arms, cover the patient with a blanket, and encourage the patient to relax and hold still during the scanning procedure. Because PET scanners have much higher resolution than routine nuclear medicine imaging devices, the patient's cooperation and proper positioning are critical. Imaging from the base of the skull to midthigh may require 20 to 45 minutes or more, and total-body imaging may extend close to 1 hour.

The imaging tables on scanners have a weight limit and some tables sag significantly under the weight of a heavy patient even before the allowable weight limit is reached. The internal diameter of the scanner opening also limits the size of patients that can be imaged. Additionally, larger patients typically have greater attenuation and reduced image quality. For these reasons, acquisition time for emission scans and CT parameters should be increased appropriately for such patients. All patients should be weighed before injection of the radiopharmaceutical.

If there is a question of cancer involvement of the head or neck, it may be helpful to place the patient in a head holder fitted with a chin restraint to reduce possible motion. The examination could be acquired in two parts, adjusting the CT parameters, for example, to allow a zoom to be used on the head and neck region so that the small anatomical structures in that area are better visualized by the interpreting physician. In addition, the portion of the examination focusing on the head and neck can be acquired with the arms to the sides to eliminate the interference from the bones in the arms. Small lesions in the head and neck may be detected if the PET scan acquisition time is doubled to obtain a higher data density (see Plate 3). The chest, abdomen, and pelvis portion can be routinely imaged with arms above the head either before or after the head and neck portion. The patient should always be checked before the scanning protocol begins to ensure that the person is safe and that no body parts will be pinched as the table moves through the scanner. It also should be verified that the acquisition program is set for the desired orientation. Again, most PET scanners have significantly higher resolution than planar or SPECT cameras. The patient rotation and symmetry may be very important when the interpreting physician views the finished study.

The acquisition parameters should be properly set to acquire high-quality images. The acquisition mode, two-dimensional (2D) or three-dimensional (3D), depends on the technical capabilities of the individual scanner and its ability to appropriately correct for high random counts and an increased scatter fraction if used in 3D mode. PET scanners have about four times the spatial resolution of SPECT and the imaging matrix should be a minimum of 128 × 128 or higher. Most 2D scanners can overlap bed positions by at least one acquisition slice (or more) to help prevent sensitivity changes of the outer slices of each bed position, which may cause a "hot" or "cold" slice at the ends of each bed position. In large patients, overlapping data by three to seven slices may further aid in the reduction of these artifacts. In 3D, whole-body acquisition, the scanner's sensitivity is low at the end of the FOV and therefore an overlap of up to 30% with the next bed position may be required to provide sufficient sensitivity and prevent artifacts. Although 3D mode yields more total counts, the number of random and scatter events increases dramatically. The manufacturer's recommendations may be a useful guide in establishing acquisition protocols at individual institutions.

In facilities in which dedicated PET-only scanners are used, radioactive rod sources are installed in the scanner gantry for transmission attenuation-correction imaging. The scanner may allow for different acquisition ordering to acquire the transmission-emission images. Each technique should be selected to reduce the likelihood of patient motion, which can create misalignments between the acquired transmission and emission scans. The transmission and emission scans, therefore, should be interlaced so that both of these acquisitions are completed at each position before the table is shifted to the next position. The most time-effective protocol performs transmission scans at two different positions while the radioactive rods are exposed in the gantry. Thus the emission scan (E) and transmission scan (T) are interlaced as ETTE acquisitions; that is, emission, transmission, move the table, transmission, emission for adjacent bed positions, or TEET if the emission scans are between the transmission scans. Transmission scans using these radioactive rod sources typically require a 3-minute transmission scan at each bed position, which adds a

significant amount of time to the procedure. PET/CT scanners use the CT scan to generate the transmission scan, providing an attenuation-correction map that has lower statistical noise in the image. The CT scan may take only a few seconds, thus reducing the total procedure time as compared to transmission source techniques. PET/CT scanners do not typically have transmission sources, and the CT must be performed with all PET acquisitions in the combined procedure.

Evaluation of the patient should be continual throughout imaging so that all observations can be reported to the physician (e.g., patient movement, coughing, noncompliance with breathing protocol). The patient's ability to comply with necessary imaging parameters dictates the need for additional imaging, changes in protocol, or cessation of the exam. Box 13-3 gives an overview of the steps involved in a PET/CT procedure. If the patient is a radiation therapy candidate, the imaging sequence will be set up slightly different with the addition of a flat table top to the couch on the scanner. In addition, immobilization devices and lasers may need to be used during the patient's exam so that the positioning

---

BOX 13-3 Sample PET/CT Procedure for Oncology

1. Verify patient identification by two unique identifiers, and review order for PET/CT procedure.
2. Ask the patient to change into a gown or scrubs if necessary. All metal objects should be removed.
3. Measure patient height and weight.
4. Complete a patient history record, teaching/education document, and medication reconciliation.
5. Measure peripheral blood glucose. (Proceed if <160 mg/dl or consult PET MD if >160 mg/dl. If >200 mg/dl do not inject patient.)
6. Set a peripheral IV in appropriate site based on disease and condition of patient.
7. Administer anxiolytics if prescribed.
8. Inject 10-15 mCi of ^{18}F-FDG and slowly flush with 20 ml of normal saline. Record the time (clock time on scanner).
9. Discontinue IV if no longer necessary and assay residual radioactivity. Record the time of the assay.
10. Give the patient a warm blanket. Remind patient of localization time of 60-90 minutes.
11. Have patient void just before imaging sequence. Be cognizant of potential contamination.
12. Position the patient on the scanner in selected manner. Use devices to elevate legs, stabilize head, and eliminate potential for linen to obstruct translation of the bed.
13. Review selected breathing instructions.
14. Select appropriate PET/CT protocol.
15. Scout is typically anterior and posterior only with low mA.
16. Perform CT with optimized parameters per PET physician standing orders.
17. Perform PET acquisition for 3-5 min per bed position.
18. Reconstruct images and review before dismissing patient.

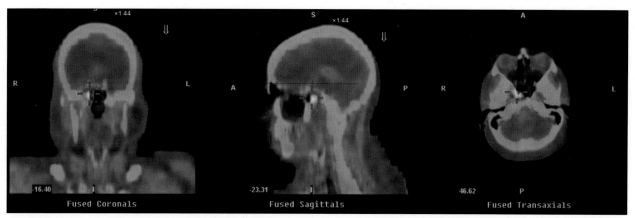

| Fused Coronals | Fused Sagittals | Fused Transaxials |

COLOR PLATE 1 Color SPECT image fused into a CT study showing tracer concentration (^{99m}Tc-labeled folate [EC-20]) in a nonfunctioning pituitary adenoma. SPECT/CT hybrid systems excel in imaging situations where anatomical location of the uptake is critical for interpretation but the emission image shows little anatomical detail.

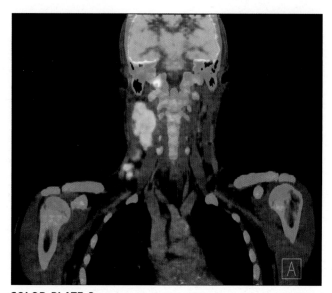

COLOR PLATE 2 Higher resolution PET images may be obtained using a zoom to change the pixels to a smaller size. When zoomed images, such as this image of neck cancer, are acquired, it is helpful to significantly increase the acquisition time so that more events populate the pixels to provide a high count density. Small lesions that approach the intrinsic resolution of the PET scanner may become detectable with sufficiently high counts.

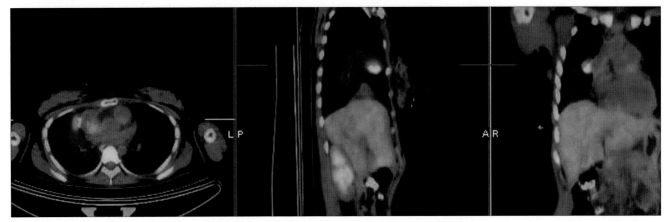

COLOR PLATE 3 Misalignment of the patient between the PET and CT studies may cause visual misregistration, and the attenuation correction map from the CT may cause PET artifacts or distort standard uptake values.

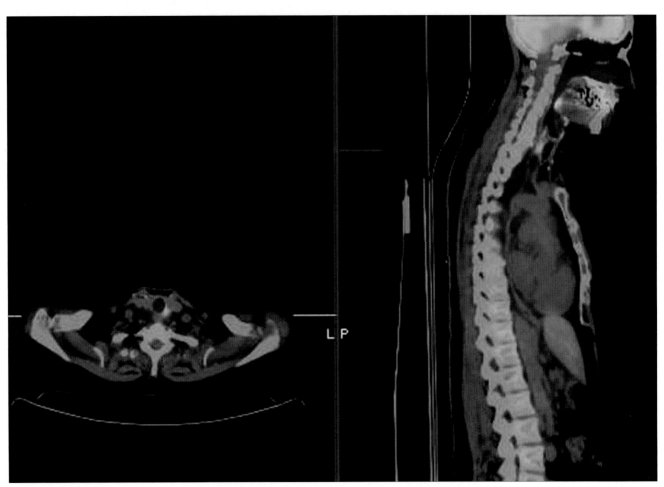

COLOR PLATE 4 Proper PET and CT alignment demonstrates the precise location of FDG uptake on the anatomic CT grayscale image in these small lesions near the esophagus and tongue.

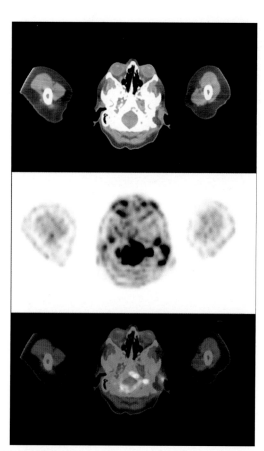

COLOR PLATE 5 FDG PET/CT scan for a patient with breast cancer illustrating intense activity that has accumulated in the left ear due to chronic otitis media with a mixed infection of multiresistant *Staphylococcus aureus* and an *Aspergillus* species. The *upper image* is the CT, *middle image* is the PET scan, and the *lower image* demonstrates the fused PET scan on the CT.

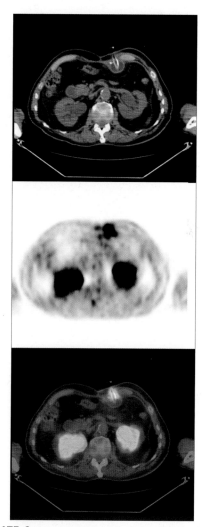

COLOR PLATE 6 A gastrostomy tube is in place in the abdomen and is seen on the CT scan. The PET scan *(middle)* demonstrates elevated FDG activity along its insertion route and perimeter consistent with inflammation. The fused PET/CT scan is shown at the *bottom.*

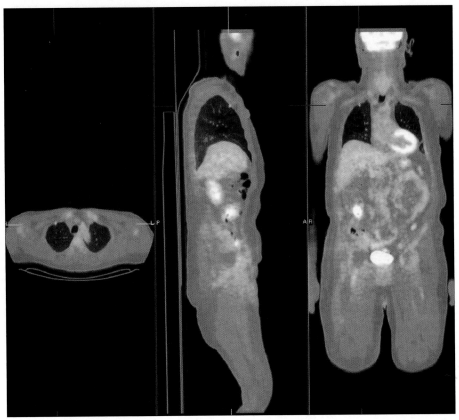

COLOR PLATE 7 High count density and proper alignment between the PET and CT images allows visualization of a very small lung lesion (4 mm as measured on CT).

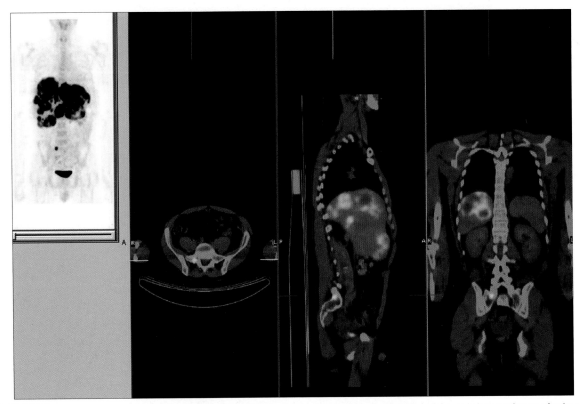

COLOR PLATE 8 A recent biopsy site on the right upper pelvis demonstrates intense focal FDG uptake. It is imperative to obtain a detailed patient history.

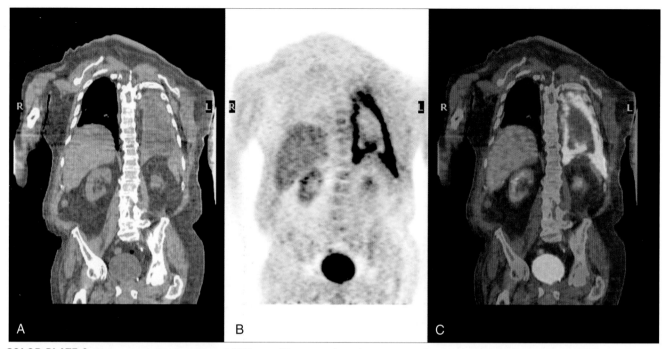

COLOR PLATE 9 The coronal CT scan **(A)** and FDG scan **(B)** on a patient that was experiencing fever, left chest pain, with known exposure to asbestos diagnosed with mesothelioma. The fused PET/CT scan **(C)** demonstrates the exact location of the intense FDG uptake on the anatomic CT scan.

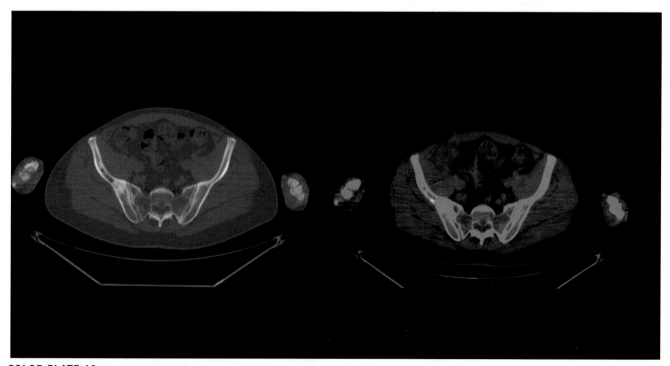

COLOR PLATE 10 The FDG PET/CT fused image *(right)* in a patient with a history of plasmacytoma post radiotherapy that illustrates recurrent disease within the right ileum. The CT scan is seen on the *left*.

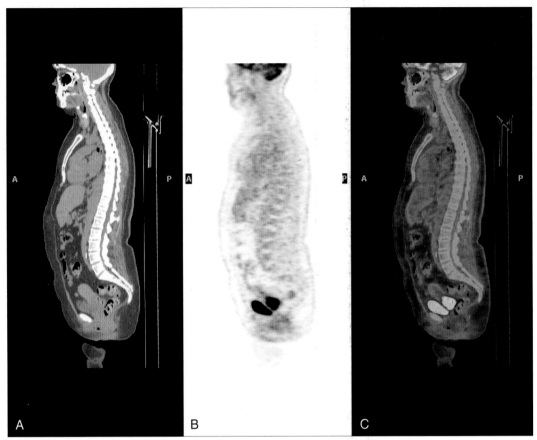

COLOR PLATE 11 An FDG PET/CT on a patient with squamous cell carcinoma of the cervix that shows FDG activity consistent with primary tumor. The PET sagittal scan **(B)** shows the region of tumor uptake above the bladder. The fused PET/CT image **(C)** allows correlation of sites of increased uptake with anatomy.

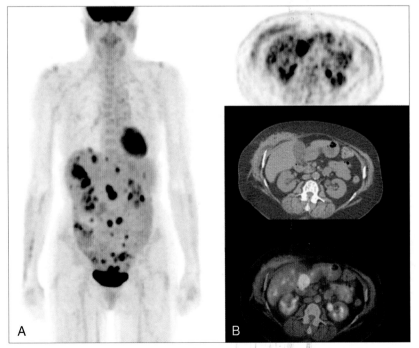

COLOR PLATE 12 An FDG scan in a patient with ovarian cancer demonstrates extensive hepatic, peritoneal, and pelvis metastatses **(A)** and another patient **(B)** with recurrent ovarian cancer with a soft-tissue mass in the pyloric region linked to serosal metastasis.

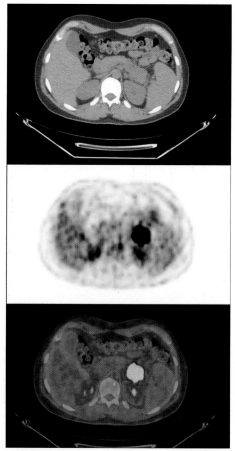

COLOR PLATE 13 FDG PET/CT scan on a patient with pancreatic carcinoma status post chemotherapy. The patient has recurrent disease in the tail of the pancreas and a new lesion in the inferior pancreatic tail. In addition, there were two nodes found to be FDG avid in the mediastinum.

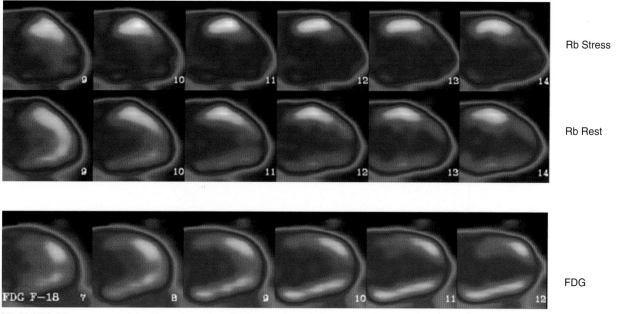

COLOR PLATE 14 A 69-year-old male with CAD, referred for preoperative risk stratification prior to lung cancer surgery. The vertical long axis Rb-82 images show severely dilated LV, medium-sized area of severe stress induced ischemia in the mid-distal anterior wall, large area of moderate ischemia in the inferior wall, medium-sized apical infarct, and LVEF of 20% to 25%. The FDG scan shows normal uptake in the inferior wall consistent with viable (hibernating) myocardium and infarct in the apex.

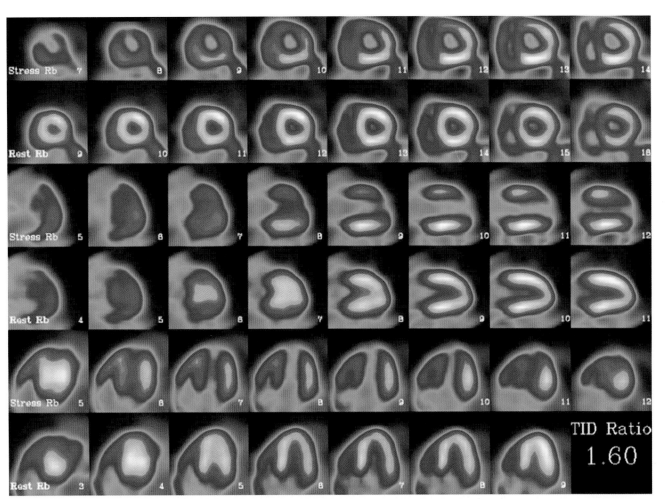

COLOR PLATE 15 A 70-year-old female with CAD, status post CABG X 2 in 2003 and stent placement with angina. The scan shows large-sized severe stress-induced ischemia of the septum, mid-distal anterior wall, anterolateral wall, and apex. Evidence of transient ischemic dilatation of LV.

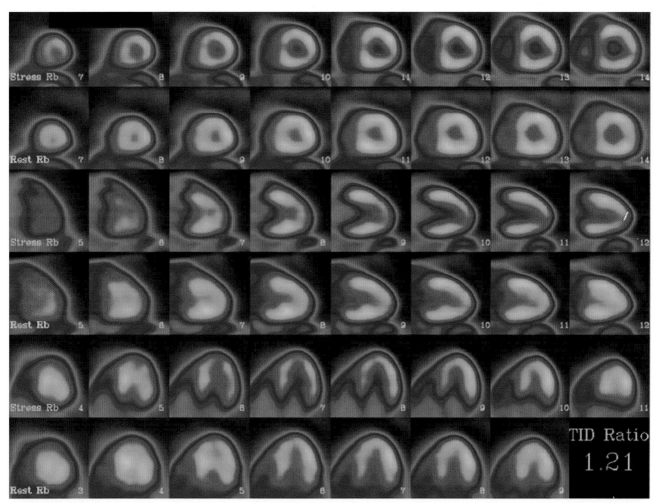

TID Ratio
1.21

COLOR PLATE 16 A 49-year-old male with diabetes referred for preoperative risk stratification prior to distal esophageal/post mediastinal mass surgery. The scan shows ischemia in the septum and apex. Dilatation of both RV and LV after stress suggests a more severe perfusion abnormality that may be related to diabetes or multivessel disease.

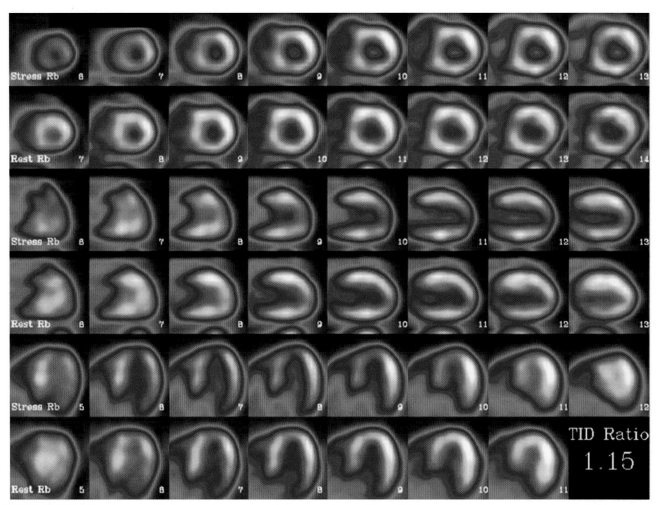

COLOR PLATE 17 A 84-year-old obese male smoker with hypertension and hyperlipidemia; referred for preoperative evaluation prior to retroperitoneal sarcoma surgery. The scan shows stress-induced ischemia in the apex and septum. LVEF of 58%.

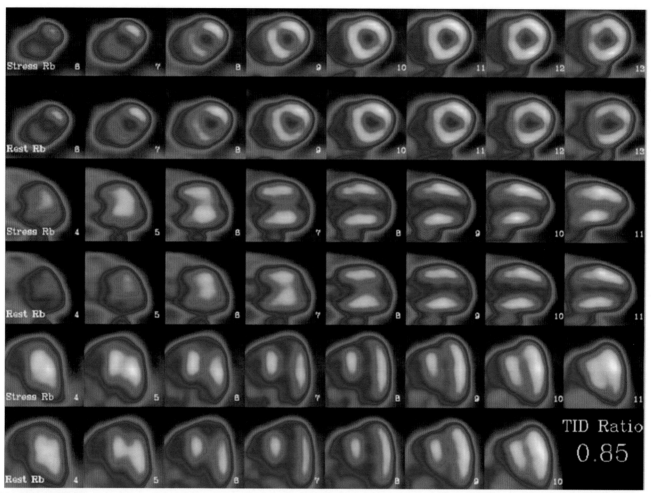

COLOR PLATE 18 A 69-year-old male with gastric cancer, hypertension, diabetes, and abnormal EKG; referred for preoperative evaluation prior to gastrectomy. The scan shows medium-sized infarct in the distal anteroseptum, apex, inferoapical/distal inferolateral walls with minimal ischemia in the infarct zone. LVEF of 64%.

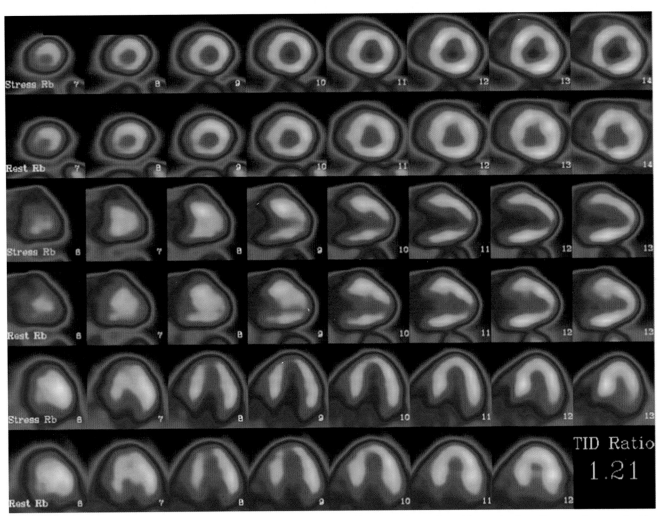

COLOR PLATE 19 A 73-year-old male with hyperlipidemia, diabetes, and hypertension; referred for evaluation. The scan is normal with no evidence of stress-induced ischemia or scar. LVEF of 55%.

of the patient mimics the treatment position. More and more patients are having PET imaging before radiation therapy to better anatomically delineate areas of disease. This allows for improvements in the delivery of dose to tumor and minimizes radiation burden to normal tissue.

NORMAL WHOLE-BODY FDG DISTRIBUTION

In PET oncology, a thorough knowledge of normal anatomy and normal FDG distribution in the body is required before any evaluation of pathological accumulations can be attempted.

Many organs and body structures accumulate FDG. The most common and constant sites of intense activity are:

- Brain
- Liver (moderate)
- Kidneys (especially the calyces and pelves)
- Bladder

Sites with variable activity include:

- Salivary glands
- Thyroid
- Heart and vascular structures
- Thymus (in children)
- Spleen
- Esophageal ampulla
- Stomach
- Bowel (especially the colon)
- Endometrium (during menses)
- Bone marrow
- Muscles
- Testicles

Although a completely normal FDG PET scan (Figure 13-5) can be easily recognized, it is necessary to evaluate several hundred FDG PET studies to feel comfortable with the many intriguing and sometimes quite disturbing normal variations in FDG localization.

Following the injection of FDG into the blood steam uptake begins in glucose avid tissues, such as the brain, inflammatory sites, and malignant tissue. Uptake in malignant tissues continues to increase for a period of many hours while body soft tissue concentration of FDG falls with time. Thus the best cancerous tumor to soft tissue ratio is achieved by waiting a long time interval, however, the short half-life of ^{18}F (109.75 min) limits imaging after a few hours of delay. Although imaging may begin at 60 minutes it is best to begin imaging at 90 to 120 minutes post injection. This time delay is also advantageous because the concentration of FDG in sites of inflammation will fall with time and prevent falsely increased uptake, masquerading as a malignancy.

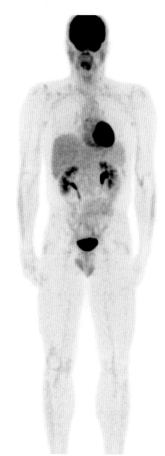

FIGURE 13-5 Normal total-body FDG PET scan. Intense activity accumulates in the brain, pharyngeal constrictors, salivary glands, left ventricular myocardium (variable), urinary collecting system, and bladder. Moderate activity appears in the liver, spleen, and testicles.

NORMAL VARIATIONS IN FDG LOCALIZATION

The purpose of this section is not to delineate all the possible variations in normal FDG PET studies but to demonstrate some common differences in normal subjects. Occasionally, only hard-earned experience, focused histories, physical examinations, additional imaging studies, biopsies, or surgery can accurately determine what is (or is not) a normal variation. The value of a pertinent and accurate history of pathology results (usually obtained by the PET technologist) and of correlative imaging studies (e.g., ultrasound [US], CT, magnetic resonance imaging [MRI]) cannot be overemphasized.

Myocardial activity is the most noticeable normal variation (Figure 13-6). Although most fasting patients demonstrate little or no left ventricular activity, which is an advantage in the search for tumors, especially in the left lung base, intense left ventricular activity can occur as a normal variant in fasting patients. Also, heterogeneous activity frequently appears in diabetic patients

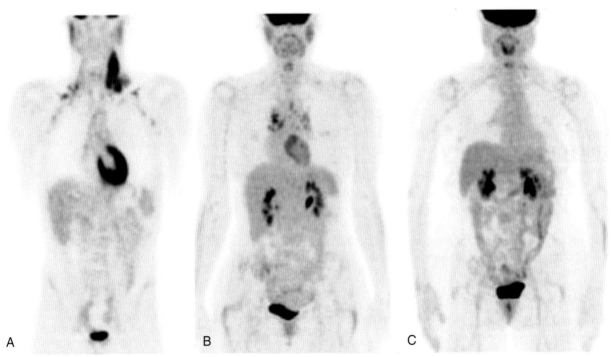

FIGURE 13-6 Normal myocardial left ventricular activity variations in patients with normal fasting peripheral blood glucose levels (<120 mg/dl) showing intense **(A)**, patchy **(B)**, and absent activity **(C)**.

even when their blood glucose level is less than 120 mg/ dl. Glucose clamp protocols (procedures to maintain a constant blood glucose level), therefore, are used when myocardial PET imaging is performed in these patients.

Evaluation of the thyroid can be difficult because normal activity varies from a complete absence to a faint nodular pattern to an intense diffuse uptake (Figure 13-7). Faint uptake is normal. However, upon investigation of intense symmetrical uptake, the presence of an autoimmune disorder such as Graves disease or Hashimoto disease generally is suspected. In addition to FDG, another positron emitter has been used in assessing thyroid carcinoma. Iodine-124 (^{124}I) with a half-life of 4.2 days can be used for volumetric measurements in patients presenting with Graves disease. An intense nodule in the thyroid bed usually requires further investigation, as this focal uptake is suspicious for malignancy.

Many different normal patterns occur around the mouth. FDG accumulates in the salivary glands (including the parotid, submandibular, and sublingual glands), the labial or buccal muscles, the laryngeal and anterior spinal muscles, and, frequently, the pharyngeal constrictors (Figure 13-8). If a patient grinds the teeth or chews, the muscles of mastication may appear very prominent (Figure 13-9).

Extraocular muscles frequently demonstrate diffusely increased activity. Occasionally only certain complementary muscle pairs or the muscles of a single eye appear (Figure 13-10).

Two sets of normal variations frequently cause diagnostic frustration and potentially important misdiagnoses: (1) muscular or brown fat activity in the neck and shoulders (especially near the trapezius, sternocleidomastoid, and subclavius muscle groups) and (2) gastrointestinal tract activity (especially in the colon).

Exercise, shivering, and muscular tension can lead to increased FDG use as a result of the metabolic demands of the muscles and possibly due to the brown fat in the neck (Figure 13-11). Most of the time, the diffuse activity throughout the stressed muscles presents little diagnostic difficulty. However, activity in the neck and supraclavicular regions can be quite nodular, mimicking metastatic disease in the lymph nodes in these areas. Occasionally, unilateral neck activity causes even more anxiety. Physical examination or additional imaging (US, CT, or MRI) may help, but sometimes only a biopsy can rule out possible tumor involvement.

Variable amounts of normal, increased activity frequently occur within the small and especially the large bowel. FDG can present as a diffuse, focal, or, commonly, scattered regional tubular pattern (e.g., ascending colon plus sigmoid colon) (Figure 13-12). The causes of these patterns are obscure but may be related to peristalsis or gas. The problem lies in the occasional difficulty of distinguishing normal from inflammatory processes or even tumors. Again, more invasive measures (colonoscopy or barium enema) may be necessary to further evaluate the possibility of pathology.

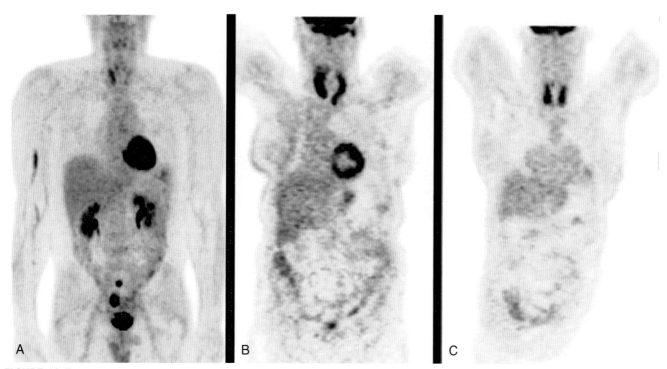

FIGURE 13-7 FDG thyroid activity can vary from normal patchy activity **(A)**, asymmetric intense activity associated with multinodular goiter from chronic autoimmune thyroiditis **(B)**, very symmetric uptake associated with lymphoma in the thyroid **(C)**, to completely absent activity.

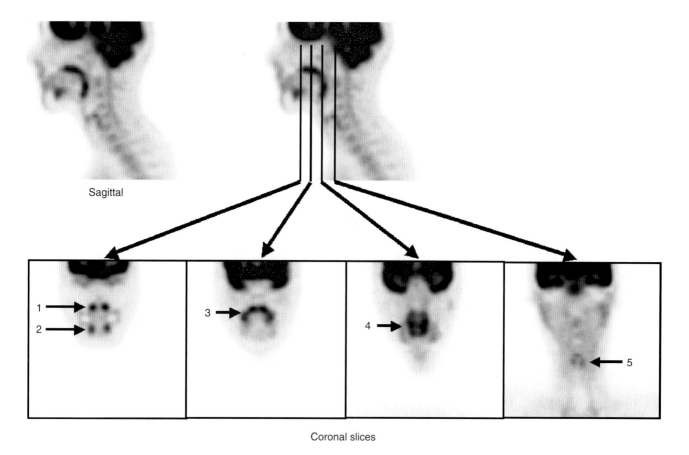

FIGURE 13-8 Normal physiological activity around the nasopharyngeal area. Various coronal images demonstrate *(1)* bilateral symmetric nasopharyngeal activity, *(2)* salivary gland activity, *(3)* oropharyngeal activity, *(4)* hypopharyngeal activity, and *(5)* laryngeal activity.

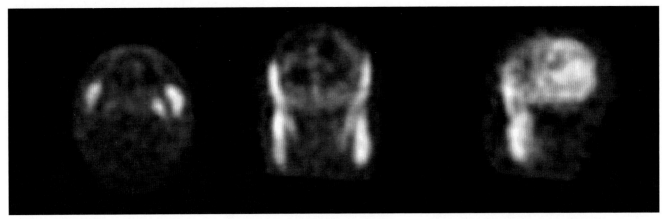

FIGURE 13-9 Normal activity in the muscles of mastication. This patient was chewing gum immediately after injection of FDG. Bilaterally increased muscle activity can be seen on the transaxial, coronal, and sagittal views.

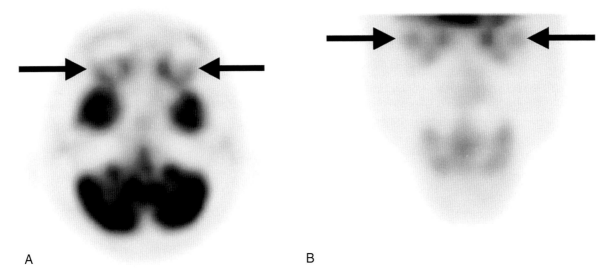

A   B

FIGURE 13-10 Normal extraocular muscle FDG activity present on transaxial **(A)** and coronal **(B)** slices. Activity normally occurs in the extraocular muscles *(arrows)* but can be variable. In this case, activity predominates in the medial rectus muscles. A relaxed patient with the eyes closed may demonstrate less activity.

Although not strictly normal variations, PET oncology examinations show FDG accumulations in a variety of commonly encountered locations. Activity may occur in recent surgical incisions, ostomy sites, recovering hematopoietic bone marrow, arthritic joints (especially the acromioclavicular joints), infections, focal or diffuse inflammation (particularly after recent radiation therapy), pleural effusions, biopsies, or injection sites (Figures 13-13 and 13-14). Color Plate 8 shows a pelvis biopsy site in a patient with hepatic cancer. The site of FDG activity in the pelvis could have been misinterpreted as metastases unless the biopsy site is noted on the history form by the technologist.

PET ONCOLOGY APPLICATIONS

Although FDG PET imaging has been documented in scientific literature to be effective in a wide variety of

cancers, at this time, the government and private insurance companies limit coverage to a select number of cancer groups. The following discussion focuses on these select primary indications for FDG PET oncology studies. In addition, examples of some other cancers for which patients might be referred for PET scans are also presented.

Solitary pulmonary nodules (SPNs) and non–small-cell lung carcinomas (NSCLCs) were the first FDG PET oncology studies covered by Medicare. Reimbursement coverage has now been extended to melanoma, lymphoma, colorectal, head/neck, esophageal, recurrent breast cancers, and thyroid carcinoma. Private insurance companies may cover FDG PET studies in other types of cancer, usually after a thorough review of individual patient needs and circumstances. However, insurance carriers usually require preauthorization for any PET examination.

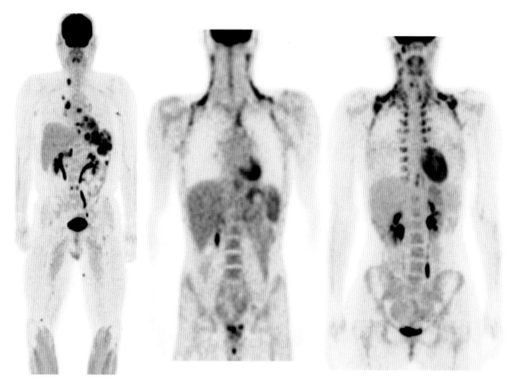

FIGURE 13-11 Lower leg activity *(left)* caused by the patient walking approximately 1 mile just before the FDG injection. In the middle image, the neck muscle activity is fairly smooth and symmetrical. However, in another patient *(right)*, the neck muscle activity occurs in a much more nodular and somewhat asymmetrical pattern, mimicking cancerous involvement of supraclavicular nodes. Neither patient had any adenopathy. Also, note the normal, fairly symmetrical activity along both sides of the spine at the costovertebral joints.

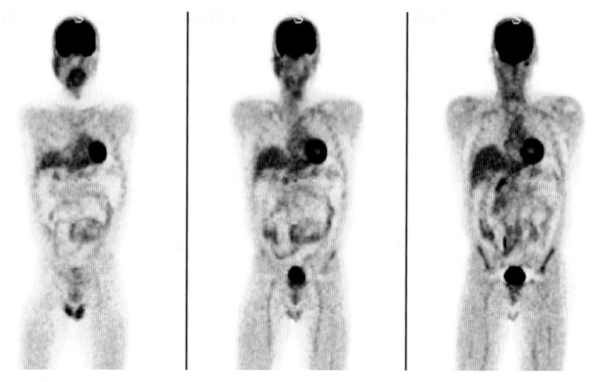

FIGURE 13-12 Normal gastrointestinal tract activity. These coronal slices demonstrate increased but normal tubular activity throughout large portions of both the small and large bowel.

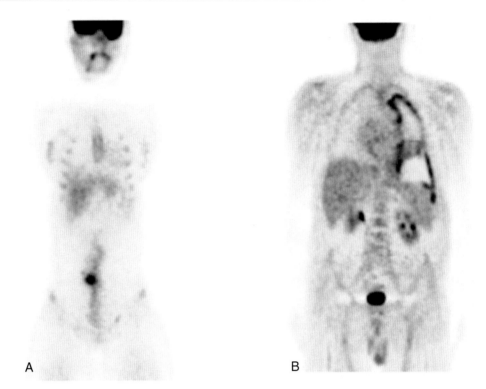

A   B

FIGURE 13-13 Mild to intense FDG activity commonly localizes in surgical wounds **(A)** and inflammatory conditions **(B)**. In the latter case, the FDG accumulates in a diffuse inflammation of the left pleura.

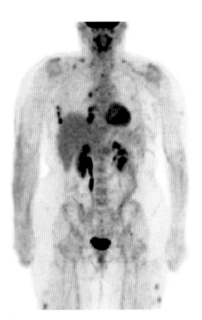

FIGURE 13-14 FDG localization at injection sites. The three areas of moderate activity in the thighs represent recent injection sites. Metastases are present in the thorax.

In the following discussion, the individual comparative statistical values (e.g., sensitivity, specificity) of FDG PET and complementary imaging modalities are not enumerated, because these values are very well presented in other sources.[1,4]

SOLITARY PULMONARY NODULE

In the United States, lung cancer is the leading cause of cancer death, having a high prevalence and a poor prognosis. The chances of survival depend on many factors but generally are related to the particular type of cancer and its spread (stage) in the body. Usually, the smaller the original tumor and the less that it has spread, the better the chance of survival. In patients with a high risk of developing lung cancer (e.g., cigarette smokers), screening protocols (chest radiographs and chest CT) increasingly are used in the hope of discovering lung cancer in its earlier and potentially more curative stages. With these screening examinations, many new single pulmonary nodules are discovered. However, both benign and malignant conditions can result in lung nodules. Biopsies of all these nodules in search of cancer would be extremely expensive and invasive and frequently would result in nondiagnostic findings.

Increased FDG use in an SPN suggests malignancy. However, benign processes (e.g., tuberculosis, fungal infection, pneumonia) can also demonstrate increased FDG metabolism, and biopsies are often still needed to determine the true nature of the nodule. On the other hand, lesions with no FDG activity are almost always benign. Occasionally, low-grade lung cancers can show little or no FDG uptake (Figure 13-15).

PET outperforms CT in determining whether an SPN is benign or malignant. Even though PET is an expensive

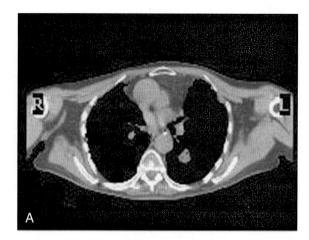

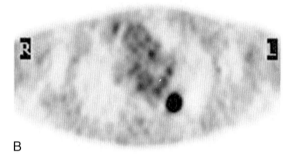

FIGURE 13-15 An FDG PET/CT scan in a patient with esophageal and bladder cancer now presenting with a new 2.9-cm spiculated mass as seen on the CT scan (**A**) in the left lung that is FDG avid (**B**). The solitary pulmonary nodule has a standard uptake value of 16.5 and was found to be a third primary of non–small-cell lung carcinoma.

tool, cost analysis demonstrates that including FDG PET studies in the evaluation of solitary pulmonary nodules saves millions of dollars a year in the United States alone. Dual time point PET imaging increases the sensitivity and specificity of the procedure because inflammatory disease may be differentiated from a benign process.[3,5]

NON–SMALL-CELL LUNG CARCINOMA

In evaluating newly diagnosed NSCLC, FDG PET is superior to CT and MRI in finding lymph node involvement and distant metastases, especially in the adrenal glands. This allows more accurate assessment of the tumor stage and a better determination of whether a patient should undergo an invasive biopsy, would benefit from a potentially curative surgery, or should receive only noninvasive therapies (radiation, chemotherapy, or both).

Many pulmonary lesions identified by CT or MRI cannot be definitely classified as either benign or malignant, because anatomical imaging cannot provide all the information necessary to evaluate the functional status of individual lesions. FDG PET provides complementary metabolic information that helps direct the proper clinical management of each patient. However, because FDG PET identifies any process that takes up more FDG than normal surrounding tissues, FDG imaging also demonstrates many infections (especially fungal infections) and inflammatory processes. Furthermore, low-grade malignancies, bronchoalveolar cell carcinoma (BAC) in particular (Figure 13-16), may use FDG at essentially the same level as normal surrounding tissues and may be hidden within this background.

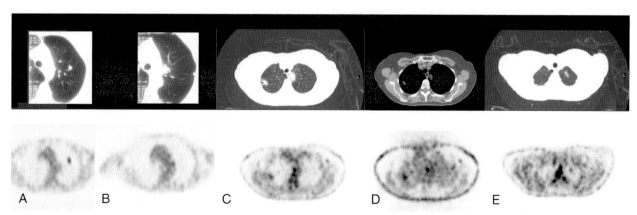

FIGURE 13-16 CT scans are positioned on the top row and PET scans on the bottom row for several patients with pulmonary nodules. The left upper and lower images (**A** and **B**) demonstrate images of two pulmonary nodules in the same patient both on CT and FDG PET. The CT and PET in images shown in **A** demonstrate prominent FDG uptake on the PET image corresponding to the nodule present on the CT image, suggesting cancer. On the CT scan of images shown in **B**, there is no PET activity along the pleural surface where the second nodule resides on the CT image, strongly suggesting a benign process. The three images on the right (**C, D,** and **E**) in the upper and lower rows represent PET/CT images from a patient with bronchoalveolar carcinoma. In the images in **C,** a right upper lobe lesion measuring 2 cm with a standard uptake value of 2.2 is represented first in a CT image with lung windows and PET. This low-grade FDG uptake can also be seen in the corresponding nonattenuated image (**D**). This patient also has a small focus measuring 1.8 × 1 cm (**E**) with an SUV of 1.5, which is seen as mildly FDG avid in the left upper lobe.

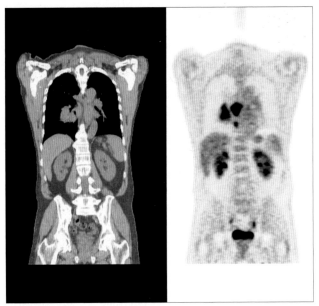

FIGURE 13-17 The coronal images of the CT and FDG scans in a patient with small cell lung carcinoma shows disease represented by a large accumulation of FDG in the right hilum and mediastinum. Note normal activity in the liver, spleen, kidneys, ureters, and bladder.

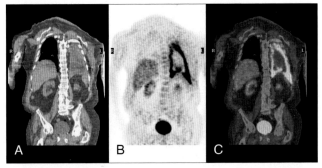

FIGURE 13-18 The coronal CT scan **(A)** and FDG scan **(B)** on a patient who was experiencing fever, left chest pain, with known exposure to asbestos diagnosed with mesothelioma. The fused PET/CT scan **(C)** demonstrates the exact location of the intense FDG uptake on the anatomical CT scan. (See Color Plate 9.)

Standard uptake values (SUVs) cannot distinguish between benign and malignant diseases with any helpful degree of accuracy because, as mentioned previously, common fungal and infectious processes can use FDG at very high rates, and BAC or other low-grade tumors can use FDG at background levels.

Dual time point imaging offers some hope that a more accurate differentiation between cancer and benign processes can be made by obtaining FDG utilization rates within a single region of interest (ROI) at various intervals, starting immediately after injection and extending up to 4 hours later. If the standard uptake values continuously rise, cancer appears to be much more likely. If the values plateau or decline after the initial rise, benign processes are suspected. It remains to be clearly established whether these time-activity curves can be used clinically, which would help avoid many invasive procedures.

OTHER CHEST MALIGNANCIES

Small Cell Lung Carcinoma

Small cell lung carcinoma (SCLC) accounts for 15% to 20% of all lung cancers. It is also known as oat cell carcinoma, small cell undifferentiated carcinoma, and poorly differentiated neuroendocrine carcinoma. SCLC (Figure 13-17) has been found to be one of the most rapidly increasing types of cancer in women. SCLC can be staged like NSCLC; however, most physicians use a two-stage system categorizing patients into limited stage versus extended stage. Limited stage is defined by the existence of disease in only one lung and all lymphadenopathy occurring on the same side of the chest. All other instances of this disease are labeled as extensive. The stage then defines the type of drug combinations used in chemotherapy. PET imaging can be a useful tool in assessing lymphatic involvement and metastatic spread; however, it is limited because it cannot differentiate SCLC from NSCLC.

Mesothelioma

Mesothelioma is a rare form of cancer that develops in the pleura—the lining of the chest. It is treated much differently from NSCLC and SCLC. It can also occur in the peritoneum or the pericardium. Most people that get this disease have had some exposure to asbestos during their lifetime (Figure 13-18). There is a long latency period associated with asbestos disease, so individuals may develop mesothelioma 30 to 40 years after exposure. Like most cancers, the prognosis of this disease is based on early diagnosis, accurate staging, and appropriate treatment prescriptions. There are currently three staging systems utilized in mesothelioma: the Brigham system, the Butchart system and the American Joint Commission on Cancer (AJCC) TNM system (T describes the extent of primary tumor, N details spread to nearby lymph nodes, and M indicates metastatic spread).

PET is a very sensitive technique that can be used to assist physicians in determining the stage of this disease so that patient outcomes are improved. Most mesothelioma patients will need a scan only from the base of the brain to the pelvis. Arms should be positioned over the head to minimize beam-hardening effects on the CT and improve the image quality of the overall PET/CT exam.

MELANOMA

The incidence of malignant melanoma has risen steadily over the past century. In the United States alone, the incidence rate has doubled just in the last 30 years.

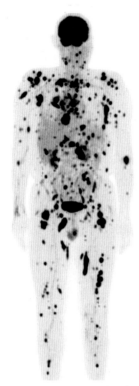

FIGURE 13-19 Very extensive metastases from malignant melanoma. Note the normal, intense brain activity that may hide metastases.

Currently, approximately 7700 people die each year from melanoma in the United States alone. Several factors help determine the chances of survival in patients with melanoma, including tumor thickness (Breslow index), depth of invasion (Clark index), tumor location, and the presence of metastases. The presence of metastases dramatically lowers the chance of survival.

Melanoma avidly uses FDG, allowing total-body PET to assess the presence of metastases much more accurately than other conventional techniques (US, CT, bone scintigraphy). PET stands out as the single best screening examination for high-risk melanoma patients and for patients in whom recurrence is suspected (Figure 13-19).

The search for possible metastases in the brain can be very difficult because the neurons also avidly use FDG. The normally intense neuronal activity can obscure metastases, which commonly occur at the gray-white junction. Also, with attenuation-correction algorithms, small surface skin metastases may be difficult to visualize because of slight misalignments of the CT and emission images. Some institutions use both attenuated and non-attenuated whole-body PET images to help evaluate for the possibility of faint skin lesions (Figure 13-20).

The skin is the body's largest organ. The two main layers of the skin are the epidermis and the inner dermis. The epidermis is mostly made up of squamous cells.

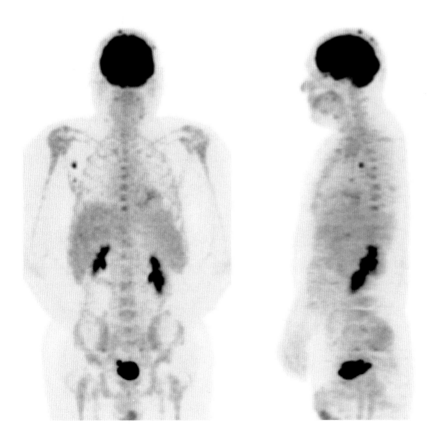

FIGURE 13-20 Faint scalp melanoma metastases present on both the coronal and sagittal views. There are also right axillary and posterior mediastinal metastases. Faint skin surface metastases may sometimes be missed with attenuation-correction protocols if there are slight misalignments between transmission and emission scans.

Then directly under these flat, scale-like cells are the round cells known as *basal cells*. Two other common but less serious forms of cancer are squamous cell and basal cell carcinomas. The lower part of the epidermis contains melanocytes. Melanoma occurs when these cells become malignant. It is important to note that when melanoma starts in the skin it is called *cutaneous melanoma*. It may also begin in the choroids of the eye and is then labeled *ocular* or *intraocular melanoma*. It can however occur in the digestive tract, vagina, or anywhere that melanocytes are found.

Again, it is important for the technologist to obtain a history, including previous surgery, on all patients. Any patient with a history of melanoma, even if referred for another indication, should have a total (head to toe) body scan. Care should be taken to ensure that the site of the original melanoma is clearly included in the scan. If using dedicated PET, the acquisition times for both the emission and transmission scans may be slightly reduced during imaging of the lower extremities from the times used for the rest of the body.

LYMPHOMA

Almost 5% of all cancers in the United States are lymphomas. They cover a wide variety of tumors of the immune system that are divided into two broad categories: Hodgkin disease (HD) and non-Hodgkin lymphoma (NHL). The presentations and therapies of these two groups differ. Hodgkin disease occurs less often than NHL. It usually involves the upper mediastinum and tends to spread from one lymph node station to contiguous nodes (Figure 13-21). The type of therapy (radiation, chemotherapy, or both) depends mostly on the stage of the disease. Hodgkin disease affects individuals primarily

between ages 15 and 34 years or those older than 55 years. The following information is considered when staging an individual with Hodgkin lymphoma: number and location of diseased lymph nodes, presence of disease on one or both sides of the diaphragm, and metastatic spread to bone marrow, spleen, liver, lung, or bones.

NHL covers a broader range of subtypes than HD and usually spreads more widely throughout the lymph nodes and other organs of the body. Therapy for NHL depends more on the histological subtype than the tumor stage. Unlike lung cancer, most cases of lymphoma are not preventable.

Lymphomas (with the occasional exceptions of low-grade NHL and mucosa-associated lymphatic tissue lymphomas [MALTomas]) tend to avidly accumulate FDG, which makes these tumors visible in almost all cases. FDG PET, therefore, is a valuable tool for accurately staging lymphomas and evaluating tumor response to therapy (see Figure 13-21). Pretherapy PET scans should be obtained to document the original state of FDG utilization (some low-grade tumors fail to accumulate FDG) and to allow accurate assessment of the response to therapy.

PET outshines all other anatomical imaging modalities in the evaluation of lymphomas (especially in the evaluation of the therapeutic response) because neither CT nor MRI can distinguish between scar tissue and residual tumor after therapy. Persistent FDG tumor activity after therapy strongly suggests residual or recurrent tumor. Lack of FDG activity essentially excludes persistent tumor, especially if FDG activity was present on the pretherapy examination.

Gallium-67 (^{67}Ga) scintigraphy has provided the standard for assessing the response of lymphomas to

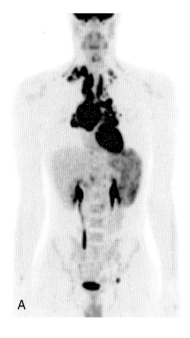
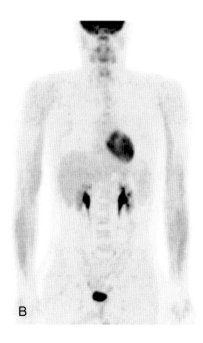

FIGURE 13-21 FDG evaluation of the response of lymphoma to chemotherapy. The pretherapy scan **(A)** shows intense activity in multiple mediastinal, supraclavicular, splenic, periportal, and left inguinal metastases. After 5 months of therapy **(B)**, the lymphoma is in complete remission.

A   B

treatment, with good results seen in the neck and thorax and poor results in the abdomen and pelvis. FDG PET detects significantly more disease (and smaller tumors) than ^{67}Ga scintigraphy because more lymphomas accumulate FDG than ^{67}Ga and because gallium scintigraphy has a lower resolution.

If the patient's history includes lymphoma of the head or neck, the patient should be placed in a head holder, and the head, neck, and shoulders should be carefully positioned to ensure anatomical symmetry in the coronal plane. The head holder also helps reduce patient motion. If the patient's history includes central nervous system lymphoma, the area imaged should extend to the top of the head.

At times, hormone therapy is used as a treatment in lymphoma. For example, high doses of synthetic hormones such as dexamethasone, methylprednisolone, and prednisone are used to try and kill malignant lymphocytes. This therapy has proven very effective for some patients and it is becoming more common to see individuals on these drugs presenting for PET. This can be problematic, because these medications have been known to elevate blood sugar. Most times, when blood sugar levels extend above 200 mg/dl, PET facilities cancel the FDG PET procedure so that localization of the radiotracer is not compromised.

Other Components of the Lymphatic System

Spleen	Stomach
Thymus	Intestines
Tonsils	Skin
Bone Marrow	Adenoids

MYELOMA

Myeloma is a disease that begins in the marrow, the spongy tissue found in the center of the bone. Myeloma occurs when B lymphocytes, called *plasma cells,* form a mass in the marrow. If a single mass or tumor is detected outside the marrow, the disease is typically classified as plasmacytoma (Figure 13-22). However, most myeloma patients present with more than one site of disease. It is estimated that around 55,000 patients live with this cancer in the United States. It is more common in men and rarely occurs in individuals younger than 50 years. The disease is classified into three stages. Staging depends on the levels of M protein in the blood, number of bony lesions, hemoglobin values, and blood calcium levels. There is currently no cure for the disease, so the goal is to slow progression down by prescribing the most appropriate form of treatment to more effectively limit symptoms.

PET can be an integral part of staging and determining the extent of disease in these patients. At times, if patients are asymptomatic, the best treatment decision may be to forego treatment as the risks and side effects of treatment might outweigh the benefits. The main form of treatment for myeloma is chemotherapy.

COLORECTAL CANCER

In the number of newly diagnosed cases each year, colorectal cancer ranks fourth behind skin, lung, and prostate cancers in men, and behind skin, breast, and lung cancers in women. This cancer is more prominent in individuals older than 50 years who have a personal or family history of the disease. These cancers frequently metastasize, particularly to the liver. Before potentially curative surgery is attempted, an intensive search for metastases should be undertaken, so that inappropriate surgery and exposure to possible surgical morbidity can be avoided.

CT is relatively good at evaluating for the presence of metastases in the liver but relatively poor at detecting extrahepatic sites of involvement. FDG PET more accurately assesses liver and, especially, extrahepatic tumor involvement, improving candidate selection for surgery (Figure 13-23). Although expensive, PET is a superb, cost-effective screening tool for colorectal cancers, mainly because it identifies more sites of tumor involvement and more accurately determines nonresectable disease, thereby avoiding unnecessary and more costly surgical procedures.

When necessary, FDG PET can be used to search for cancer when the patient's plasma tumor markers are rising and conventional anatomical imaging techniques have failed to detect any disease or to differentiate scar tissue from recurrent tumor.

Tumor tissue in the liver may not have a substantially different tissue density on a CT; and IV contrast may help identify tumors or metastases, but this is not guaranteed. FDG localization demonstrates the glucose metabolism of tissue, which may be positive in the case of colon cancer or colon metastases. In the case of colorectal cancer, a critical analysis must be undertaken to determine whether FDG PET should replace all other anatomical imaging modalities as the first-line screening method because of the serious problems inherent in these conventional diagnostic tools.

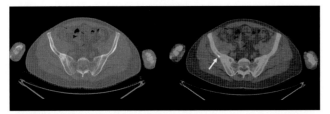

FIGURE 13-22 The FDG PET/CT fused image *(right)* in a patient with a history of plasmacytoma post radiotherapy that illustrates recurrent disease within the right ileum. The CT scan is seen on the left. (See Color Plate 10.)

HEAD AND NECK CANCER

Head and neck cancers are almost exclusively squamous cell carcinomas (95%). Fortunately, squamous cell carcinomas tend to use FDG avidly, making PET an excellent imaging choice with these cancers (Figure 13-24). Therapy and survival are mainly determined by the tumor location, its local or regional spread, and the presence (or absence) of lymph node metastases. Distant metastases occur fairly infrequently, but in about 15% of the cases, a second tumor develops in the esophagus or pulmonary bronchi.

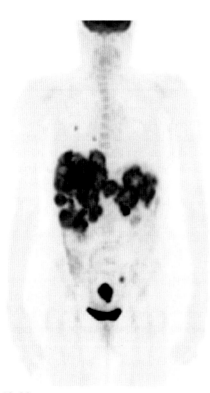

FIGURE 13-23 Extensive colorectal metastases, with disease occurring in the presacral, left iliac, hepatic, splenic, and right pulmonary locations.

It is critical that the physician understands the extent of the disease so that the best course of treatment is prescribed. Detection of lymph node involvement is very important when surgical dissection is contemplated because survival drops drastically when lymph node metastases are found. FDG PET distinguishes cancerous lymph node involvement better than CT or MRI. Head and neck carcinoma will also spread to the lung, so evaluating patients for recurrence is very important.

Many head and neck tumors recur locally, usually within the first 2 years after the original resection. In these cases, it can be very difficult to differentiate tumor recurrence from postoperative scarring or changes caused by radiation therapy. FDG PET accurately identifies tumor recurrences. When clinical evidence of local treatment failure exists, distant metastases can be identified in approximately 60% of these cases. Again, FDG PET can be effectively used to screen for distant metastases because of the greatly increased FDG utilization in these tumors. Radiation therapy can cause local reactive inflammatory changes and increased local FDG metabolism, leading to the possible erroneous conclusion that local treatment failed. For this reason, it is advisable to wait at least 1 month, and preferably longer (3 months), after the completion of radiation therapy to assess for tumor recurrence.

Normal variants, such as salivary gland uptake and lingual, buccal, pharyngeal, laryngeal, and neck muscle activity, can cause many diagnostic difficulties in the evaluation of head and neck tumors. Fortunately, correlation with complementary anatomical imaging and a physical examination can usually determine the true tumor status.

ESOPHAGEAL CANCER

The incidence of esophageal cancer has been rising over the last few years. The American Cancer Society predicts that there will be 16,500 new cases and 14,500 deaths annually. Esophageal cancer continues to typically be

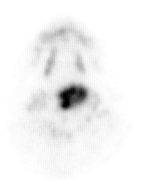

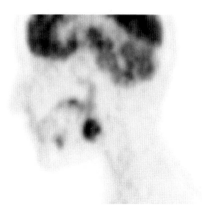

FIGURE 13-24 Head/neck cancer with tumor demonstrates intense activity, even more than the usual pharyngeal and salivary gland activity and equal to the activity in the brain.

TABLE 13-1	Esophageal Cancer by Stage
Stage	**Description**
0	Cancer is found only in the innermost section of the esophagus (carcinoma in situ).
I	Cancer only in the innermost layer of the esophagus to the next layer in the wall of the esophagus.
IIA	Cancer spread to the layer of esophageal muscle or to the outer wall of the esophagus.
IIB	Cancer involves any of the first three layers of the lining of the esophagus and spread to nearby lymph nodes.
III	Cancer has invaded more deeply to the outer lining of the esophagus and may have spread into the locoregional lymph nodes and tissues.
IVA	Cancer has spread to the nearby or distant lymph nodes.
IVB	Cancer illustrates distant metastatic spread in the lymphatic system and other parts of the body: liver, lungs, brain, and bones.

diagnosed in advanced stages, leading to a poor survival rate. It is most common for cancer patients to be categorized as either squamous cell carcinoma or adenocarcinoma if esophageal cancer is diagnosed as primary site of disease. The origin of the cancer is still not completely understood and for many families it becomes one of the most difficult things to deal with during their lifetime. Hopefully, with continued education, research, and improvements in technology, better mechanisms to eliminate cancer will become available to the public.

The esophagus is a 10-inch hollow muscular tube located behind the trachea that carries liquids and substances from the throat to the stomach. It is typically described in sections consisting of the upper third, middle third, and lower third. It consists of several layers of tissue, including mucous membranes, muscle, and connective tissue. Glands in the esophagus produce mucus that keeps the passageway moist and makes swallowing easier. When an individual develops esophageal cancer, normal function and anatomical structure become compromised.

In 2001 PET imaging was approved for esophageal cancer by the CMS. PET shows levels of hypermetabolism at the cellular level using FDG. The literature supports that the inclusion of PET imaging into the patient algorithm changed patient management in diagnosis and initial staging by 14%. In addition, when utilized for staging, a 20% change in patient management was illustrated (Table 13-1).

BREAST CANCER

Excluding skin cancer, breast cancer ranks as the number one malignant tumor in women. It is believed that about 40,170 people will die annually from the disease. A little

over 1% of those individuals will be men. About 1910 cases of male breast cancer are expected annually. The most important prognostic factors in the long-term survival of breast cancer patients are the number and extent of axillary and other lymph node metastases. The survival rate drops precipitously if malignant axillary lymph nodes are present, and the rate drops even more if distant metastases are found.

Appropriate therapy depends mostly on accurate staging (or on accurate restaging after initial therapy). Currently, no anatomical imaging modality can accurately assess the presence and extent of lymph node metastases. Therefore, axillary lymph node dissections are performed for prognosis and for determining the need of adjuvant chemotherapy and radiation therapy. Studies now under way are aimed at determining the value of sentinel node biopsies. If these studies demonstrate that sentinel node biopsies accurately determine prognosis and the presence of lymph node metastases, breast cancer patients could be spared the morbidity of axillary lymph node dissections.

FDG PET detects axillary and mediastinal lymph nodes quite well, although micrometastases are frequently missed, which diminishes the utility of PET in these instances. For patients who have had previous lumpectomies, mammographic assessment can be very difficult. Surgical scars can mimic recurrent tumors. PET demonstrates an excellent ability to detect local recurrences, which helps prevent unnecessary repeat biopsies and even further scarring. At the same time, PET can monitor for possible lymph node involvement and distant metastases, which would alter the planned therapies.

Finally, because FDG utilization is related to cellular metabolism, PET can help demonstrate responses to therapy. Figure 13-25 shows an example in which a significant reduction in FDG activity occurred in the metastatic nodes 3 months after therapy, and only very faint activity was seen after 5 months. Nonresponders demonstrate little or no decreased FDG use after therapy. With newer therapy regimens, FDG PET may offer an effective method of determining which of the available therapy options would have the greatest chance of success.

BRAIN CANCER

Tumors that begin in the brain are known as *primary brain tumors;* however, they are very rare. Most tumors in the brain are classified as secondary tumors because they are malignancies that develop from a different primary such as lung or breast. The pediatric population experiences more primary brain tumors, and adults typically experience secondary disease. Physicians typically classify brain tumors by grade. The rating of low-grade (I) to high-grade (IV) tumors reflects how atypical the cancer appears under the microscope. The high-grade tumors appear more abnormal and the cells typically

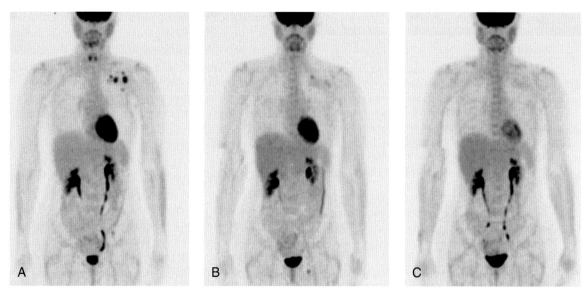

FIGURE 13-25 Serial FDG scans used to monitor breast cancer therapy. The left image **(A)** shows increased activity in several left axillary lymph nodes. After 3 months of chemotherapy **(B)**, the nodes are still slightly visible. After 5 months **(C)**, only very faint activity remains in the lymph nodes.

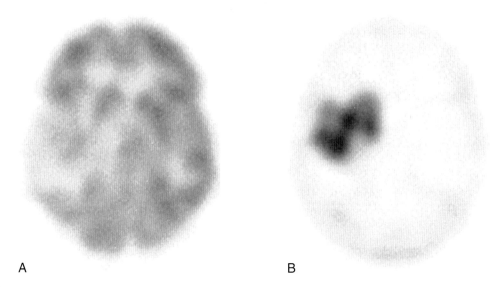

FIGURE 13-26 FDG PET imaging **(A)** of a low-grade brain cancer (grade II astrocytoma) demonstrates less glucose utilization than in normal brain. The FDG scan provides no information on the extent of the recurrent tumor. The ^{18}F-ACBC PET scan **(B)**, performed with a synthetic amino acid, shows limited utilization by normal brain tissue. The extent of the low-grade recurrent tumor is now clearly evident. This example dramatizes the value of imaging different metabolic processes with PET.

grow more rapidly. Gliomas are the most common brain tumors. There are several types of gliomas such as astrocytoma, ependymoma, oligodendroglioma, and brain stem gliomas.

Because the normal cerebral and cerebellar neurons use FDG avidly, primary and metastatic brain tumors can be, and are, missed. Figure 13-26 shows a brain tumor that cannot be identified with FDG imaging. FDG accumulation is comparable to that of normal cortical gray matter. However, after evaluation of the same patient using a synthetic amino acid (^{18}F-ACBC), a marker of protein synthesis, the tumor is easily

recognized. This case reinforces the point that imaging of different cellular processes may be necessary in different individuals or in different types of cancer to assess each patient accurately.

Currently, FDG PET generally is used as an adjunct imaging tool to help differentiate residual tumor from radiation necrosis and edema (Figure 13-27) and not as a screening tool for primary or metastatic brain tumors. MRI is especially adept in screening for and evaluating primary or metastatic brain tumors. In cases where MRI results are inconclusive, FDG PET can be a good tool to use.

PROSTATE CANCER

Apart from skin cancers, new cases of prostate cancer are diagnosed more frequently in men than any other form of cancer, and only lung cancer kills more often. Most cases of prostate cancer occur in men older than age 50 years and the incidence increases significantly for men older than 65 years. An effective screening and staging tool, therefore, would be valuable. Unfortunately, FDG PET does not detect the presence of local disease or distant metastases very well. This poor performance may be related to various factors but is probably due to the modest rate of FDG utilization in primary prostate tumors, involved lymph nodes, and bony metastases. Routine bone scintigraphy defines more lesions than FDG PET. In addition to a digital rectal exam (DRE), evaluating levels of prostate-specific antigen (PSA), a protein that is made by normal and prostate cancer cells, is routinely used to spur further examinations. For example, a PSA score of 4 ng or higher might prompt a physician to move to ordering a prostate biopsy. Adenocarcinoma represents over 95% of all histopathology in prostate carcinoma. The remaining tumors in cancer of the prostate consist of squamous cell carcinoma, transitional cell carcinomas, undifferentiated carcinomas, and sarcomas.

Because the prostate is situated just below the base of the bladder, the normally intense bladder activity may obscure small prostate tumors. However, primary tumors occasionally can be visualized (Figure 13-28). Although FDG PET poorly demonstrates primary and metastatic prostate cancers, an abnormal FDG PET scan in patients with prostate cancer almost always indicates the presence of local or metastatic disease. Prostate cancer tends to grow more slowly than other cancers. Therefore, the need for new PET radiopharmaceuticals in the future will allow this powerful imaging modality to become a much more effective tool in the evaluation of this common and deadly cancer.

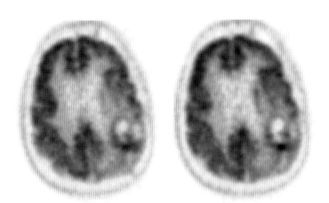

FIGURE 13-27 FDG PET imaging of a patient with glioblastoma multiforme, status post resection and chemotherapy, that finds FDG activity involving the posterior aspect of the reception cavity of the left parietal lobe compatible with viable tumor and not radiation necrosis.

CERVICAL CANCER

Trends in the 5-year survival rates for women with cervical cancer have been on the rise since the 1970s. This is

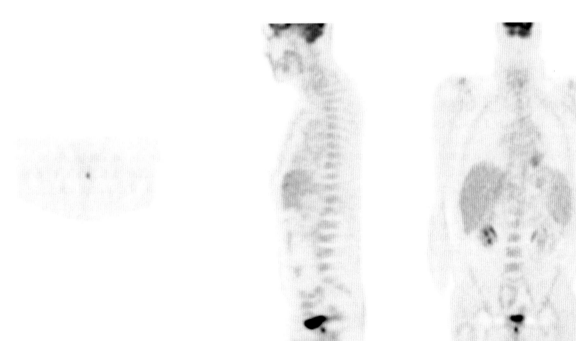

FIGURE 13-28 The increased FDG activity present on the transaxial, sagittal, and coronal images just below the bladder represents prostate cancer. However, normal activity in the bulbous urethra may appear in a similar manner.

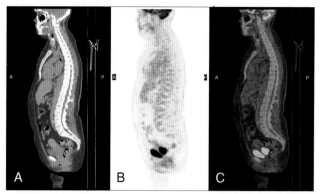

FIGURE 13-29 An FDG PET/CT on a patient with squamous cell carcinoma of the cervix that shows FDG activity consistent with primary tumor. The PET sagittal scan **(B)** shows the region of tumor uptake above the bladder. The fused PET/CT image **(C)** allows correlation of sites of increased uptake with anatomy. (See Color Plate 11.)

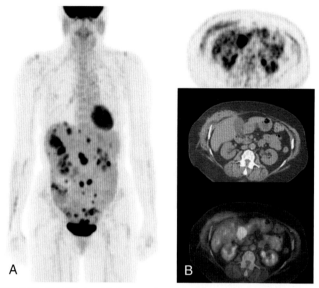

FIGURE 13-30 An FDG scan in a patient with ovarian cancer demonstrates extensive hepatic, peritoneal, and pelvis metastases **(A)** and another patient **(B)** with recurrent ovarian cancer with a soft-tissue mass in the pyloric region linked to serosal metastasis. (See Color Plate 12.)

a direct result of early detection, prevention, and education about the need to seek appropriate medical care. However, it is still estimated that close to 4070 women will die of the disease annually.

The distal, narrow area of the uterus is known as the *cervix*. It connects the uterus to the vagina. Physicians still cannot explain why some individuals get cancer and others do not; however, having certain risk factors yields a higher chance for having cervical malignancy. The human papillomavirus (HPV), for example, is one of the major risk factors associated with cervical cancer and is a very common viral infection. Women who do not have regular pap smears also tend to go on to develop cervical cancer because precancerous cells are not detected early and treated. The other risk factors include a weakened immune system, age, sexual history, smoking, use of oral contraceptives, and giving birth to multiple children. Another factor that may increase the likelihood of cervical carcinoma occurs in females or the natural daughters of women who took diethylstilbestrol (DES) during pregnancy.

Staging of cervical cancer is important to ensure that patients receive the most appropriate form of intervention. Cervical cancers are grouped into four stages. PET can be an important diagnostic tool in the initial staging of patients with cervical carcinoma (Figure 13-29). There are still limited data to reflect its usefulness in the management of recurrent cervical cancer. There are certain technical aspects of imaging this disease that must be considered when using FDG because of its excretion in the urine. Because the cervix is close to the bladder, different options for patient preparation (urinary catheterization) have been discussed to minimize bladder activity interference.

OVARIAN CANCER

Ovarian cancer is a fairly common and often deadly form of cancer in women. Approximately 22,000 new cases are diagnosed in the United States each year, accounting for about 15,000 deaths. Ovarian cancer usually strikes older women, and because the early symptoms are rather vague (and potentially misleading), the correct diagnosis is usually made when the disease is in an advanced stage. The most prominent sign or symptom is enlargement of the abdomen. However, there are no effective and proven methods for screening patients suspected of ovarian cancer that are similar to the use of mammography in breast cancer. If women have persistent symptoms or are considered high risk for ovarian carcinoma, they should have a combination of a pelvic exam, transvaginal ultrasound, and blood test for the tumor marker CA-125.

Proper staging leads to a more accurate prognosis. The most common form of treatment is surgical intervention and chemotherapy. Patients in whom the cancer is confined to the ovary have a 5-year survival rate greater than 90%. However, in one third of the cases, distant metastases are present at the time of the original diagnosis. Another one third develop metastases within the first year after surgery, accounting for the fairly dismal overall survival rates. Survival also varies with the age of the patient. This metastatic spread is due to a process called *shedding*. When ovarian cancer spreads, it tends to form new tumors on the peritoneum and the diaphragm. The cancer cells can then also enter the lymphatic system and travel to other parts of the body.

Fortunately, ovarian cancers usually originate from the epithelium and commonly demonstrate quite noticeable FDG uptake (Figure 13-30). Ovarian cancers usually spread superficially over local structures (e.g., fallopian tubes, uterus, bladder, opposite ovary) and throughout the peritoneum, as well as to nearby pelvic and periaortic lymph nodes. Although rare, ovarian cancer can also be described as *germ cell tumors* or *stromal tumors.*

Correct staging with conventional anatomical imaging can be very difficult in ovarian cancers, and extensive surgical exploration is usually required. FDG PET offers a screening tool with the potential to obviate some primary laparotomies (because of the presence of unsuspected peritoneal studs, involved lymph nodes, or distant metastases) or second-look laparotomies in cases of possible tumor recurrence. PET may also prove helpful in the evaluation of tumor response to therapy and in patient management.

Potential pitfalls in FDG PET evaluation of ovarian cancers are well-differentiated tumors whose FDG utilization rates are at background levels, or microscopic peritoneal metastases, which may also be indistinguishable from the normal surrounding background tissues, especially when adjacent to the liver, spleen, or colon. In addition, PET may fail to delineate small stage I cancers.

PET/CT imaging in the pelvis may occasionally require bladder catheterization, administration of a diuretic to reduce bladder activity, or administration of oral contrast media to better define the structures in the abdomen and pelvis.

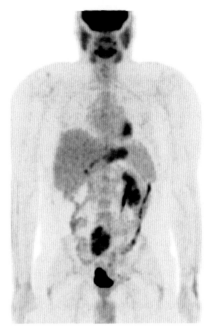

FIGURE 13-31 An FDG scan in a patient with testicular cancer shows a large collection above the bladder that represents a retroperitoneal metastasis. Note the commonly occurring, normally increased activity in the stomach and in the colon, especially in its descending portion.

TESTICULAR CANCER

Testicular cancers are divided into two major categories: seminomas (50%), and nonseminoma germ cell tumors (NSGCT) (50%). Although rare, these tumors are the most common solid tumors in young males (15 to 40 years of age) and their incidence is increasing. When first diagnosed, a large percentage of these tumors have already metastasized (approximately 30% of the seminomas and 70% of the nonseminomas). Metastases commonly occur in the periaortic, iliac, and inguinal lymph nodes. Distant metastases are seen commonly in the lungs, liver, pleura, and cerebrum.

These tumors are usually treated with a combination of surgery, radiation, and chemotherapy, depending on the histological diagnosis and the tumor stage. It is important to stage these tumors accurately to determine the most effective therapies. Modifications of the TNM staging system such as the Lugano staging system, which is a hybrid of the Boden/Gibb system, are typically used to describe this disease.

Testicular cancers, especially seminomas, avidly take up FDG (Figure 13-31). Although few large studies exist to support the use of FDG PET in testicular cancers, it may be beneficial in the staging or restaging of these tumors and in the evaluation of therapeutic response. This would allow more individualized therapies, with a possible reduction in the number of surgical interventions.

A substantial problem in the imaging of testicular tumors with PET is the varying degree of FDG use by the different subsets of testicular cancers. Mature teratomas offer a dramatic example. Mature teratomas (tumors consisting of more than one tissue type) demonstrate a benign histology but arise from malignant precursors and must be removed surgically. These particular tumors show very little FDG activity and cannot be distinguished from necrotic or fibrous tissues. This makes assessment of these tumors with FDG ineffective and reemphasizes the point that if tumors do not take up FDG more than the surrounding normal tissues, they are not identified, and a different metabolic process must be examined. Molecular imagers must be clearly advised about the clinical indications for each PET examination; in addition, they must know the particular tumors being evaluated and must understand the various PET presentations of these different tumors. For accurate assessment of each case, PET imaging requires meticulous attention to technical detail, to information gathering, and to scan interpretation. When a larger range of PET radiotracers and techniques becomes available, a much heavier burden will rest on the molecular imager to understand the unique characteristics of each delivery system and its interaction with the vast array of known cancers.

THYROID CANCER

An example of thyroid cancer is presented not to tout the strength of FDG PET in the evaluation of this particular type of cancer but to review the strengths and weaknesses of FDG PET imaging.

Thyroid cancers cover a wide range of histological types, ranging from the most well differentiated form (papillary) to the most deadly anaplastic form. They are divided in two main categories: follicular cell tumors and C-cell tumors. This division is based on the two kinds of cells in this gland. The follicular cells make thyroid hormone and the C cells form calcitonin. Metastases to the thyroid can occur from primary lung, breast, and kidney cancer, as well as melanoma. Imaging protocols and treatments are fairly well established, although some controversies still exist. Iodine-131 (^{131}I) whole-body imaging remains the diagnostic workhorse. Well-differentiated thyroid cancers usually continue to trap and organify iodine, allowing tumor detection with ^{131}I whole-body scanning. In addition, they retain the ability to secrete thyroglobulin (Tg). Poorly differentiated or anaplastic thyroid cancers do not normally organify iodine, rendering ^{131}I ineffective in the imaging or treatment of these cancers. Hurthle cell carcinoma has the same result typically on ^{131}I imaging. It is another thyroid carcinoma classified as of follicular origin that seldom traps iodine. The preferred treatment for thyroid carcinoma is principally complete or nearly total thyroidectomy with follow-up treatment with radioactive iodine or external radiation therapy. Some patients, however, may have a lobectomy instead of total thyroidectomy. The type of surgical intervention depends on the type, stage, and size of the nodule. The patient's age is also considered. If thyroid cancer metastasizes, it routinely spreads to nearby lymph nodes, nerves, or blood vessels. Once it reaches the lymph nodes, it can spread further into the lungs or bones.

FDG uptake in thyroid cancers tends to follow the proliferative potential and metabolic activity of these tumors, with the more aggressive and poorly differentiated tumors using FDG at a higher rate than the better differentiated forms. It would seem that the more common, well-differentiated forms of thyroid cancer would not utilize FDG to any noticeable degree and that the less common, more poorly differentiated forms would take up FDG at much higher rates. Although this tendency exists, the correlation is weak. Aggressive and anaplastic tumors can be FDG negative, and well-differentiated thyroid tumors can be FDG positive (Figure 13-32). Normal variants and benign thyroid processes cause further confusion. Many thyroid nodules avidly accumulate FDG, whereas other nodules use FDG moderately if at all. This makes FDG evaluation of the thyroid difficult and treacherous. It is important to always look at symmetry of this butterfly-shaped gland. A thin section called the isthmus separates the two lobes. Use this as an imaginary line to assess asymmetry in FDG PET imaging. In addition, the thyroid typically is around the size of a quarter. This can also be used as a reference point.

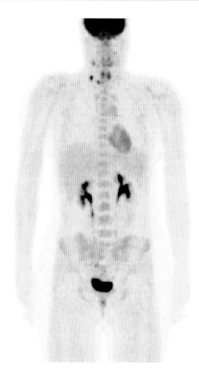

FIGURE 13-32 FDG accumulates in residual nests of the thyroid cancer on the right side of the neck. These lesions were not demonstrated on whole-body ^{131}I scans.

BOX 13-4	Major Types and Characteristics of Thyroid Cancer
Papillary and follicular	80% to 90% of all thyroid carcinomas. Both arise from follicular cells and are slow growing. Treatment is usually successful if detected early.
Medullary thyroid cancer	5% to 10% of thyroid cancer cases. Arises in C cells, not follicular cells, and is manageable and controllable if detected early, before spread.
Anaplastic thyroid cancer	1% to 2% of all cases. Least common, most aggressive, difficult to control, follicular cell origin.

Although imaging of the thyroid with FDG presents inherent diagnostic problems, the following two points should be emphasized:

1. In cases of recurrent thyroid cancer and negative ^{131}I whole-body scans, FDG PET imaging is a reasonable diagnostic approach to search for more poorly differentiated forms of thyroid cancer.
2. When unexplained abnormal findings occur in the thyroid bed on FDG PET examinations obtained for other indications, additional conventional tests (e.g., US, ^{123}I scintigraphy, biopsies) should be performed to exclude unsuspected thyroid cancers (Box 13-4) (which occasionally have been identified first on FDG PET imaging).

PANCREATIC CANCER

Around 35,000 people will die of pancreatic cancer annually. Even though incidence rates have declined in the last couple of decades, the disease remains a silent killer because of the difficulty of diagnosing the cancer in its early stages. The 5-year survival rate is about 4% for all stages combined.

The pancreas is located deep in the abdomen between the stomach and the backbone. It is responsible for making insulin, other hormones, and enzyme-containing pancreatic juices for digestion. This 6-inch gland comprises a head, body, and tail. Pancreatic cancer typically begins in the pancreatic ducts. About 60% to 70% of all tumors are found in the head of the pancreas. At times, the patient may present to the physician because they are experiencing bile duct obstruction. Tumors in the body and the tail of the pancreas most often go undetected (Figure 13-33).

PET has been shown to be helpful in differentiating chronic pancreatic masses from malignant disease, assessing for metastatic spread to the liver, and predicting response to chemotherapy. Delineating acute inflammation from disease can be a limitation in pancreatic imaging with FDG. However, one of the most prominent obstacles may be the high incidence of poorly controlled diabetic patients with pancreatic carcinoma. Elevated serum glucose levels will result in decreased uptake of FDG.

FUTURE TRENDS

PET is rapidly emerging in several venues: instrumentation is continually evolving; new reconstruction and processing algorithms are becoming more sophisticated and reliable; opportunities for the exploration of targeted gene therapy and monitored gene expression are on the forefront; and radiochemistry is becoming a more stable and reproducible environment. In addition, as PET becomes more affordable to a wider population, clinical applications will continue to thrive. Hopefully, the clinical examples detailed in this chapter demonstrate the nearly limitless future potential of PET imaging in oncology. More importantly, the inherent power and weakness of FDG PET are defined. The power of FDG PET lies in its ability to image a functional parameter (FDG utilization) rather than anatomical changes. Its weakness lies in the fact that FDG uptake does not necessarily distinguish between benign and malignant processes.

Functional imaging depends completely on effective delivery systems or radiopharmaceuticals to visualize the desired intracellular metabolic processes. Radioactive tracers arrive at their desired cellular locations through the actions of these delivery systems (e.g., FDG in the cellular cytosol by the increased facilitated diffusion and the increased hexokinase activity of cancerous cells). Because an enormous array of interesting and potentially

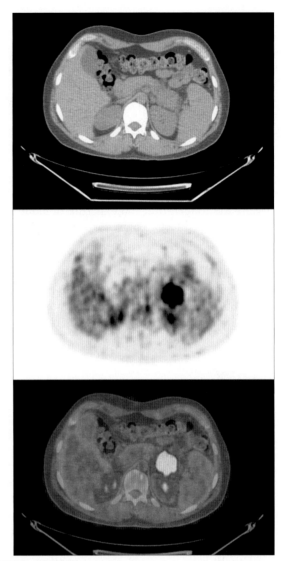

FIGURE 13-33 FDG PET/CT scan on a patient with pancreatic carcinoma status post chemotherapy. The patient has recurrent disease in the tail of the pancreas and a new lesion in the inferior pancreatic tail. In addition, there were two nodes found to be FDG avid in the mediastinum. (See Color Plate 13.)

useful metabolic pathways exists, the development of effective systems for delivering individualized PET radiotracers to targeted cells could transform PET into an even more powerful clinical and research tool.

New PET radiopharmaceuticals are becoming available to research institutions with PET scanners: ^{18}F-fluorothymidine (^{18}F-FLT) (cellular proliferation); ^{18}F-fluoromisonidazole (^{18}F-FMISO) (hypoxia); ^{18}F-fluorouracil (^{18}F-FU) (chemotherapy response); and ^{18}F-fluorodeoxyphenylalanine (^{18}F-FDOPA) (movement disorders and neuroendocrine tumors). Even more PET radiopharmaceuticals will be available to institutions with an on-site cyclotron: ^{11}C-thymidine (^{11}C-dThd) (cellular proliferation); ^{11}C-methionine (^{11}C-Met) (protein synthesis); ^{11}C-tyrosine (^{11}C-Tyr) (protein synthesis); ^{11}C-acetate (lipid synthesis, myocardial oxidation, and prostate cancer); ^{11}C-choline (phospholipid synthesis and prostate cancer); and ^{15}O-H$_2$O, and ^{13}N-ammonia (perfusion). On-site cyclotrons allow the production of positron emitters that have very short half-lives (^{11}C, 20 minutes; ^{13}N, 10 minutes; ^{15}O, 2 minutes) and that fortuitously are also the building blocks of organic molecules.

Many novel radiopharmaceuticals will become available in the future, emerging from the imaginative efforts and ingenuity of biochemists, molecular biologists, biochemical and molecular engineers, cellular physiologists, geneticists, pharmacologists, and physicists. Indeed, PET will require the cooperation and expertise of many basic scientists and skilled technologists to expand its present utility and secure its place in the future of molecular medicine. With the success of PET/CT, the boundaries between general radiology and nuclear medicine will continue to be blurred; however, by imaging both anatomy and function the information gained for the patient will improve.

SUMMARY

- In most types of tumor-forming cancers, PET imaging is the most sensitive imaging technique for diagnosing cancer and looking for metastases since it views physiology and not just anatomy.
- Combined PET/CT studies are more accurate than either modality alone because the sites of increased metabolic activity from PET may be correlated with anatomy.
- Biochemically, FDG behaves very similarly to natural glucose.
- Cancer cells have increased glucose uptake.
- Cancer cells have increased levels of hexokinase.
- FDG is phosphorylated by the action of hexokinase into glucose-6-phosphate (G-6-P), which cannot cross the cell membrane and the ^{18}F is therefore trapped within the cell.
- Patient preparation for PET imaging includes no strenuous exercise for 24 hours before the study, fasting for at least 4 to 6 hours, no insulin administration within 2 hours of the study, and desired level of hydration.
- Peripheral blood glucose levels should be measured and be ideally below 120 mg/dl.
- Diabetic patients may require special preparation before the PET scan.
- Patients should rest on a gurney or recliner chair for at least 10 minutes before FDG administration.
- Patients should be in the resting state during FDG administration and an 18- to 20-gauge IV line should be flushed with 20 to 30 ml of saline following FDG injection.
- Patients should remain resting for 60 to 90 minutes during the FDG uptake period.
- Patients should empty their bladder completely before imaging to reduce radiation exposure and to avoid artifacts in the images.
- The area to be imaged depends upon the disease and patient history.
- Patients should remove metal objects that may interfere with PET or CT images.
- The patient's arms should be down if head and neck disease is suspected.
- Most whole-body oncology PET scans are performed from the base of the skull to the thighs.
- PET imaging may begin to cover the bladder area first before significant accumulation of urine occurs in the bladder, especially if pelvic disease is suspected.
- The patient's head should be included in the whole-body scan when prior disease has been documented or suspected in that area.
- Patients with disease that may be present throughout the total body should be completely scanned from head to toe.
- Melanoma patients should be scanned to include the total body.
- The normal biodistribution of FDG includes intense uptake in the brain and moderately low uptake in liver and spleen that is greater than resting muscle.
- Myocardial uptake is highly variable in intensity.
- Benign diseases and physiological changes in organ function will affect FDG uptake in those organs.
- Sites of inflammation will show increased FDG uptake.
- Tumor activity continues to increase with time, and normal and inflammatory uptake diminishes with time; thus, tumor to background ratios increase with time. Therefore, uptake times of 90 minutes are preferred over the minimum uptake time of 60 minutes.

REFERENCES

1. Gambhir SS, Czernin J, Schwimmer J, et al: A tabulated summary of the FDG PET literature, *J Nucl Med* 42(suppl 5):1S-93S, 2001.
2. Kumar R, Loving VA, Chauhan A, et al: Potential of dual-time-point imaging to improve breast cancer diagnosis with 18F-FDG PET, *J Nucl Med* 46:1819-1824, 2005.
3. Matthies A, Hickeson M, Cuchiara A, et al: Dual time point 18F-FDG PET for the evaluation of pulmonary nodules, *J Nucl Med* 43:871-875, 2002.
4. Ruhlmann J, Oehr P, Biersack HJ, editors: *PET in oncology*, Berlin, 1999, Springer-Verlag.
5. Zhuang H, Pourdehnad M, Lambright ES, et al: Dual time point 18F-FDG PET imaging for differentiating malignant from inflammatory processes, *J Nucl Med* 42:1412-1417, 2001.

SUGGESTED READING

American Cancer Society (website): www.cancer.org. Accessed July 17, 2010.
Centers for Disease Control and Prevention (website): www.cdc.gov. Accessed July 17, 2010.

Centers for Medicare and Medicaid Services (website): www.cms.gov. Accessed July 17, 2010.

National Comprehensive Cancer Network (website): www.nccn.org. Accessed July 17, 2010.

Valk PE, Bailey DL, Townsend DW, Maisey MN: *Positron emission tomography: basic science and clinical practice*, London, 2003, Springer-Verlag.

von Schultess GK, editor: *Clinical positron emission tomography*, Philadelphia, 2000, Lippincott Williams & Wilkins.

Wieler HJ, Coleman RE, editors: *PET in clinical oncology*, Berlin, 2000, Steinkopff Verlag.

Central Nervous System

Katherine Zukotynski, David Gilmore, Edward Hsiao, Kevin Donohoe

OUTLINE

OBJECTIVES

After completing this chapter, the reader will be able to:
- Diagram and describe the anatomy of the central nervous system.
- Diagram and describe the circulation of cerebrospinal fluid.
- Discuss the properties of radiopharmaceuticals used in imaging the brain and spinal cord.

- Describe the technical parameters and instrumentation used for CSF studies.
- Describe the use, dose, administration, and procedures for SPECT and PET brain studies.
- List clinical indications for nuclear medicine studies of the brain and spinal cord.

KEY TERMS

blood-brain barrier (BBB)
carcinoma
cerebrospinal fluid (CSF)
cerebrospinal fluid shunt evaluation
digital imaging and communication
    in medicine (DICOM)

hormone receptors
lipophilicity
metastatic lesion
pledget
radioligand
radionuclide cisternogram

subarachnoid space
thecal sac

CHEMISTRY OF THE BRAIN

The human central nervous system (CNS) is that part of the nervous system that consists of the brain and spinal cord, a highly specialized processing center for transferring information between the body and the outside world.

The principal cells of the CNS are neurons, glia, and the cells that compose the blood vessels and meninges.

The neuron is the principal functional unit of the CNS, whereas the glial cells (such as astrocytes or oligodendrocytes) provide a supporting system for the neurons and their dendritic and axonal processes. It is estimated that there are 10^{11} neurons in the human brain. Beyond embryonic development neurons are incapable of cell division so that destruction of even a small number of neurons responsible for a certain function may result in severe clinical dysfunction.

Neurons may interact with one another in one of two ways: by means of electrical action potentials transferred directly from one cell to another, or through neurotransmitters that carry information across synapses in a process referred to as synaptic transmission. Neurons may have differing distributions of interconnections with other neurons and may use different neurotransmitters at different synaptic transmission sites.

Neurotransmitters are chemicals that include amines (e.g., norepinephrine, dopamine, and serotonin), amino acids (e.g., gamma-aminobutyric acid [GABA], glutamic acid, aspartic acid, and glycine), and peptides (e.g., endogenous enkephalins). Neurotransmitters are stored in membrane-bound sacs (vesicles) in the terminal axonal branches of neurons and may be released in varying amounts into the synaptic cleft where they can interact with neuroreceptors on the membrane of postsynaptic neuron.

Neuroreceptors are polymers found on a neuron membrane that are capable of recognizing specific neurotransmitters from the prosynaptic neuron or from the bloodstream. Neurotransmitters must have the correct shape, charge, and other physiochemical properties to bind to a specific neuroreceptor. Therefore a specific neuroreceptor will only respond to specific neurotransmitters while ignoring other molecules.

The interaction of neurotransmitters and neuroreceptors results in the translation of information to postsynaptic neurons by changing the state of ion channels on the postsynaptic neuron or by triggering cascades of intracellular reactions. Some neurotransmitters act within fractions of a second, whereas others have an effect over hours or even days. Thousands of synapses, connecting with a single postsynaptic neuron, are integrated to determine the final effect on the postsynaptic neuron. The availability of a large number of different neurotransmitters, neuroreceptors, and post-synaptic connections with other neurons means that a vast number of different combinations are possible and thus a tremendous amount of information can be encoded. Furthermore, similar arrangements exist between neurons and other organs, such as at neuromuscular junctions, the interface between neurons and muscles.

The effect of a neurotransmitter on the postsynaptic cell, may be classified as excitatory, inhibitory, or modulatory, depending on the properties of the neuroreceptor. For example, acetylcholine stimulates skeletal muscle cells to contract but causes cardiac muscle cells to relax. Thus muscarinic acetylcholine receptors are excitatory, but nicotinic acetylcholine receptors are inhibitory. Various drugs may mimic naturally occurring neurotransmitters and may bind to postsynaptic receptors to produce the same effects as the neurotransmitter or to competitively block the neurotransmitter. For example, antibodies can block acetylcholine neuroreceptors in patients with myasthenia gravis, preventing the muscle from contracting normally.

The maintenance of life in all organisms, including human beings, requires information processing, which in turn requires blood flow to cells and consumption of energy by cells. Blood flow can be monitored with single photon emission computed tomography (SPECT) using radioactive tracers labelled with iodine-123 (^{123}I) and technetium-99m (^{99m}Tc). The rate of glucose consumption, can be evaluated with positron emission tomography (PET) using positron-emitting radionuclides, particularly fluorine^{-18} (^{18}F). In many ways blood flow and glucose metabolism are linked. Therefore SPECT and PET often reflect a combination of the two processes and, currently, play an important role in imaging various CNS diseases.

In some CNS diseases, nuclear medicine imaging techniques used in combination with anatomical imaging techniques such as computed tomography (CT) or magnetic resonance imaging (MRI) can provide a powerful tool to assess the extent of disease, to document the effectiveness of therapy, and to monitor progression and/or regression. For example, measurement of the metabolic activity of a tumor may make it possible to detect residual or recurrent disease from damage to normal brain tissue resulting from radiation. Both ^{18}F-labeled fluorodeoxyglucose (used to evaluate glucose metabolism) or ^{11}C-methionine (used to evaluate increased amino acid transport and, in part, protein synthesis) may delineate the functional boundaries of a brain tumor and provide valuable information before and after therapy. This information may then be used to modify the treatment plan sooner than if only data regarding the patient's clinical status or lesion size is available. Treatment, therefore, need no longer be based solely on clinical response, gross morphology of the lesion, and histopathological examination.

In addition to measuring blood flow and glucose metabolism, PET and SPECT can be used to measure the number and affinity of **receptors,** such as neurotransmitter receptors associated with specific processes or **hormone receptors** that characterize certain tumors. Estrogen receptors are increased in many breast tumors in both the primary and metastatic sites. Fluorine-18-estradiol accumulation, as determined by PET, makes it possible to tailor treatment on the basis of the number of estrogen receptors in a **metastatic lesion** from **carcinoma** of the breast. A brain metastasis containing estrogen receptors is more likely to be treated successfully with estrogen-receptor blocking drugs, such as tamoxifen, than are cancers that do not contain estrogen receptors. Receptors are also found on pituitary tumors. Using the dopamine receptor binding agent ^{11}C-N-methylspiperone (NMSP), it is possible to classify pituitary adenomas according to whether they possess dopamine receptors. If the tumor contains dopamine receptors, administering a dopamine-receptor agonist such as bromocriptine can be used to treat the tumor chemically rather than surgically. If a tumor contains somatostatin receptors, on the other hand, it can be treated with somatostatin **analogs.**

ANATOMY AND PHYSIOLOGY

An understanding of anatomy is as important for appropriate image acquisition as it is for efficient image interpretation. The CNS consists of the brain and spinal cord. One of the body's largest organs, the brain is divided into four major parts: the cerebrum, cerebellum, diencephalon (thalamus and hypothalamus), and brain stem.

Cerebrum

The surface of the cerebrum is composed of gray matter (cerebral cortex), which primarily contains neurons with an underlying layer of white matter, which primarily contains nerve tracts. The two hemispheres of the cortex are connected by the corpus callosum. The cortex (Figure 14-1) is subdivided into four lobes, which are named similarly to the cranial bones that overlie them: the frontal lobe, the temporal lobe, the parietal lobe, and the occipital lobe. The frontal lobe extends from the forehead posteriorly to the central sulcus and inferiorly to the lateral fissure. It is involved in higher mental activities such as planning, judgment, and personality. The precentral gyrus of the frontal lobe is involved in motor function, including speech. The temporal lobe is located below the lateral fissure and extends posteriorly along the sides of the brain. It is involved in hearing, language, memory, and learning. The parietal lobe is separated from the frontal lobe by the central sulcus and from the temporal lobe by the lateral sulcus. The postcentral gyrus involves sensory function. The occipital lobe is located posteriorly and forms boundaries with the parietal and temporal lobes. It contains the principal cortical areas involving vision.

Deep within each cerebral hemisphere are paired structures of gray matter, called the *basal ganglia,* (or basal nuclei) which are responsible for the control of muscle tone and tremor, the initiation of movement, and emotions. Fibers extend from the basal ganglia to other parts of the cerebral cortex.

Cerebellum

The cerebellum is located in the inferior and posterior portion of the cranial cavity beneath the occipital and temporal lobes of the cerebrum. It is involved in the coordination of movement of skeletal muscle, or proprioception; however, other functions, such as memory, can also involve the cerebellum.

Diencephalon (Thalamus and Hypothalamus)

The diencephalon consists primarily of the thalamus and the hypothalamus. The thalamus is composed of paired ovoid masses of gray matter slightly posterior and medial to the basal ganglia, which are involved in the relay of sensory impulses from other parts of the CNS. The thalamus is also involved in the sensations of pain and temperature. The hypothalamus, also composed of gray matter, is located beneath the thalamus. It is involved in autonomic functions such as regulating body temperature, water balance, pituitary function, hunger, and emotional expression.

Brain Stem

The brain stem consists of the medulla, pons, and midbrain. Cardiac and respiratory centers necessary for survival are located here, as are pathways connecting the cerebrum, cerebellum, and spinal cord.

Spinal Cord

The spinal cord, which is composed of both gray and white matter, is a cylindrical structure that extends from the medulla and brain stem to the second lumbar vertebra. The spinal cord and its spinal tracts convey sensory impulses to the brain and motor impulses from the brain to the periphery. The spinal cord also contains reflex neuronal circuits.

Ventricular System and Cerebrospinal Fluid

Cavities within the brain, called *ventricles,* are filled with **cerebrospinal fluid (CSF),** a transudate of blood that is secreted from the choroid plexus located in the lateral, third, and fourth ventricles of the brain (Figure 14-2). CSF is a clear, colorless liquid that protects the brain from shocks, delivers nutritive substances, and removes waste from the brain and spinal cord. The total volume of CSF in an adult is approximately 125 to 150 ml. On average, the choroid plexus produce 500 ml of CSF every 24 hours, which means the CSF is completely replaced four times a day.

The dynamics of CSF flow are demonstrated in Figure 14-3. CSF produced by the choroid plexus of the lateral ventricles (first and second ventricle) enters the third ventricle through the interventricular foramen (foramen of Monro). It is then transported through the small tunnel, known as the *aqueduct of Sylvius* into the fourth ventricle, which lies between the cerebellum and the pons. CSF leaves the fourth ventricle through the lateral apertures (foramina of Luschka) and the median aperture (foramen of Magendie) to enter the subarachnoid (thecal) space surrounding the spinal cord. In this space, CSF descends along the posterior aspect of the spinal cord and then ascends along the anterior aspect of the cord to enter the **subarachnoid spaces** surrounding the skull base, composed of the basal, posterior, midline, and lateral cisterns.

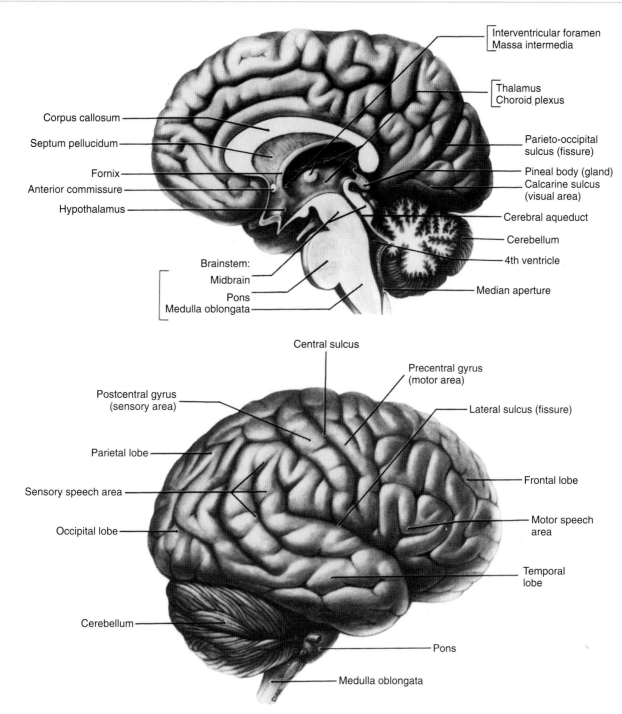

FIGURE 14-1 Topographic anatomy of major cortical regions.

The largest posterior cistern is the cisterna magna, which lies posterior to the cerebellum and may be punctured for injection of a radioactive tracer if more distal injections at the level of the lumbar spine are contraindicated or technically difficult. Finally, the CSF enters the outer convexities of the brain and is resorbed through the arachnoid granulations into the dural venous sinuses, which drain into internal jugular veins as part of the systemic venous system.

Blood Supply

The brain is metabolically very active and requires a continual supply of oxygen and glucose. The brain consumes about 20% of the oxygen used by the entire body. If deprived of oxygen for more than several minutes, the brain can suffer permanent damage. Although the brain represents only 2% of the total body weight, it requires 20% of the total cardiac output. The brain's total blood

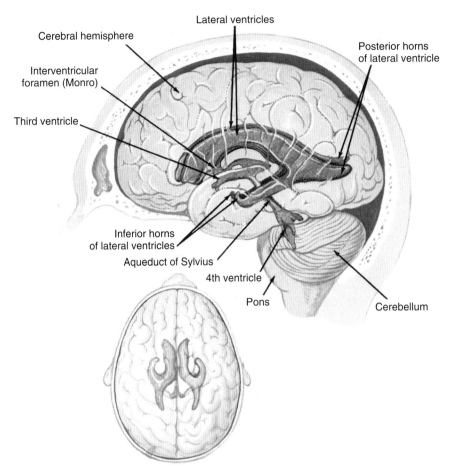

FIGURE 14-2 Cerebral ventricles projected on the lateral surface of the cerebrum. *Smaller drawing,* Ventricles viewed from above.

supply is replaced with fresh oxygenated blood six times a minute, which corresponds to a mean perfusion time of 10 seconds. Cerebral perfusion was previously measured with radionuclide angiography and currently is more commonly measured with CT or MRI contrast studies. Glucose is the principal source of energy for the brain. In fact, areas of the brain involved in mental functions show an increased utilization of glucose, as demonstrated with PET.

Typically, the right common carotid artery originates from the right subclavian artery, and the left common carotid artery originates from the aorta. At the level of the larynx, the common carotid arteries divide into the internal and external carotid arteries. Inside the cranium, the right and left internal carotid arteries and the basilar artery, supply blood to a circle of arteries called the *circle of Willis.* From this circle of blood vessels the anterior, posterior, and middle cerebral arteries (Figure 14-4) extend to supply blood to the cerebral cortex. The components of the circle of Willis include the two internal carotid arteries, the two anterior cerebral arteries, the anterior communicating artery, the two posterior communicating arteries, the basilar artery, and the two posterior cerebral arteries. The circle of Willis tends to equalize blood pressure to the brain and provides collateral blood flow.

After arterial blood is stripped of oxygen and other nutrients in the capillary bed, it collects in small venules, then into larger veins, and finally into the large dural sinuses (superior and inferior sagittal, straight, and transverse), which drain blood into the internal jugular veins that descend on either side of the neck, subsequently joining with the right and left subclavian veins. The joining of the internal jugular with the subclavian vein forms the right and left brachiocephalic veins, which deliver blood to the superior vena cava (Figure 14-5).

Blood-Brain Barrier

The **blood-brain barrier** (BBB) protects the brain from potentially toxic substances in the blood. The barrier is made up of tight endothelial junctions and continuous basement membranes found in the brain capillaries and prevents the movement of a variety of larger molecules into the brain. Movement of substances across the BBB is controlled by active transport or by the degree of **lipophilicity** of a substance (high lipophilicity enables a substance to cross the barrier).

Pathological processes including high-grade neoplasm, infarction, infection, trauma, or toxins often cause the BBB to lose its integrity, allowing normally

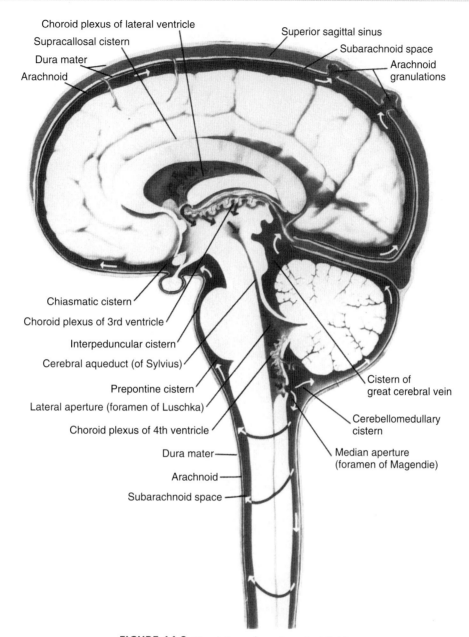

FIGURE 14-3 Circulation of cerebrospinal fluid.

restricted water-soluble substances to enter the brain. The water-soluble contrast agents used in CT or MRI can therefore cross the BBB to localize these pathological processes as enhancing lesions. In comparison, many of the radiopharmaceuticals used in nuclear imaging of the brain are lipophilic and can traverse the intact BBB (e.g., ^{99m}Tc-hexamethylpropyleneamine oxime [^{99m}Tc-HMPAO]). Other nuclear medicine agents may cross the intact BBB by specific transport processes (e.g., 2-deoxy-2-[^{18}F]fluoro-D-glucose [^{18}F-FDG]).

Neurons and Neuroglia (Glial Cells)

The nervous system consists of two major cell types: neurons and neuroglia. Neurons are highly specialized cells that carry either sensory impulses to the brain (afferent) or motor response impulses to the body (efferent). There are millions of sensory neurons, tens of millions of motor neurons, and tens of billions of interneurons that connect sensory and motor neurons, making complex human mental and motor function possible.

Neurons consist of three major parts: the cell body, the dendrite, and the axon (Figure 14-6). Dendrites conduct nerve impulses (action potentials) toward the cell body, which contains the cell nucleus. Axons conduct the nerve impulses away from the cell body to other neurons or tissue. The interface between one neuron and another is called a *synapse*. At the synapse, chemicals called *neurotransmitters* are secreted from membrane-enclosed sacs, called *vesicles,* at the distal end of each axon.

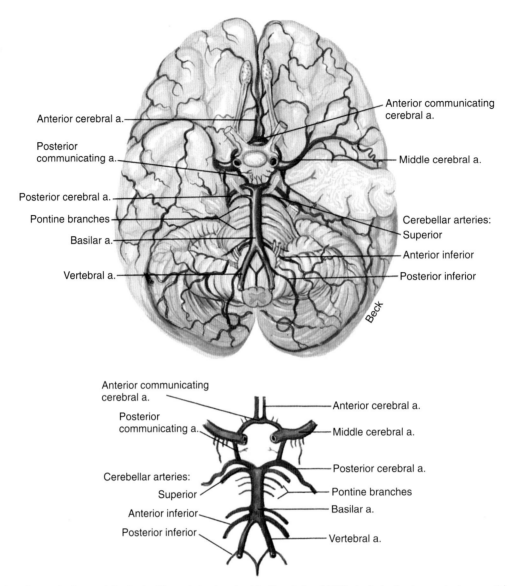

FIGURE 14-4 Arteries at the base of the brain. The arteries involved in the circle of Willis include the two anterior carotid arteries, the two anterior cerebral arteries, the anterior communicating artery, the two posterior communicating arteries, the basilar artery and the two posterior cerebral arteries.

As discussed at the beginning of this chapter, the actions of neurotransmitters impinging on a postsynaptic neuron are integrated to determine whether the postsynaptic electrical action potential will be passed to another neuron. Acetylcholine and the catecholamines, norepinephrine and dopamine, are examples of neurotransmitters. Each of these substances has a characteristic inhibitory, excitatory or modulatory effect on the postsynaptic neuron. The effect of acetylcholine is excitatory in the brain and inhibitory in the heart. The repolarization of neurons after transmission of action potentials consumes much of the energy of the brain and accounts for about half of the glucose utilization.

Neuroglial cells, such as astrocytes, are the supportive and protective cells in the CNS. These cells have no synapses and do not transmit electrical impulses. As opposed to neurons, glial cells can divide and reproduce in response to injury, a process known as *gliosis*.

RADIOPHARMACEUTICALS

There are several different radiopharmaceuticals that can be used to image the brain. Transient perfusion agents that do not cross the BBB are more commonly used in planar imaging and include ^{99m}Tc-diethylenetriamine pentaacetic acid (DTPA) and ^{99m}Tc-pertechnetate. Common perfusion agents that may be used for both planar imaging and SPECT include HMPAO and ^{99m}Tc-ethylene L-cysteinate dimer (ECD). ^{123}I-isopropyl iodoamphetamine (IMP) is a rarely encountered radiopharmaceutical used to study brain perfusion. An example of a radiopharmaceutical that may be used as metabolic imaging agent is ^{18}F-FDG (PET). Although

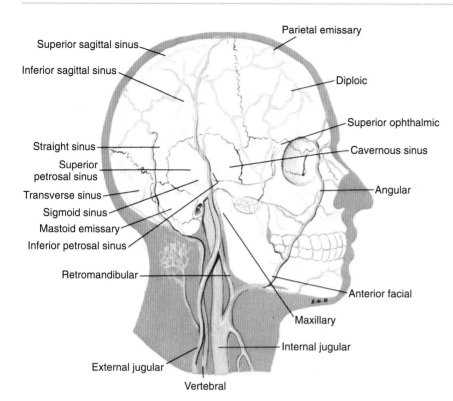

Superior sagittal sinus

Inferior sagittal sinus

Parietal emissary

Diploic

Superior ophthalmic

Cavernous sinus

Straight sinus

Superior petrosal sinus

Transverse sinus

Sigmoid sinus

Mastoid emissary

Inferior petrosal sinus

Angular

Retromandibular

Anterior facial

Maxillary

Internal jugular

External jugular

Vertebral

FIGURE 14-5 Semischematic projections of the large veins of the head. Deep veins and dural sinuses are projected on the skull. Note the connections (emissary veins) between the superficial and deep veins.

several PET agents are available for evaluating metabolism, blood flow, and the presence of receptors, most of these, such as ^{11}C, ^{13}N and ^{15}O, are still under investigation. CSF imaging may be done with either ^{111}In-DTPA or ^{99m}Tc-DTPA as permitted.

PLANAR AND SPECT IMAGING TRACERS

Before the development of contrast enhanced CT and MRI techniques for imaging the brain, planar gamma camera imaging was used to evaluate patients with suspected stroke or brain tumors through the detection of break down in the BBB. This was done with either transient perfusion agents such as ^{99m}Tc-DTPA and ^{99m}Tc-pertechnetate or first-pass extraction agents such as ^{99m}Tc-HMPAO and ^{99m}Tc-ECD.

Technetium-99m-DTPA and ^{99m}Tc-pertechnetate are hydrophilic agents that accumulate in the brain parenchyma as a result of leakage from the circulation through a compromised BBB (e.g., with stroke or tumor). ^{99m}Tc-pertechnetate also normally accumulates in the choroid plexus and salivary glands and demonstrates slow blood pool clearance occasionally making the distinction between normal choroid uptake and breakdown of the BBB difficult. ^{99m}Tc-DTPA does not have these difficulties. Both agents may be used for planar imaging but not for SPECT and are less commonly used since the advent of CT and MRI.

Technetium-99m-HMPAO and ^{99m}Tc-ECD are lipophilic agents that are extracted by the brain parenchyma during the first pass. The uptake is highest in the cortical

and subcortical gray matter with relative decreased uptake in white matter. Both agents have the superior imaging characteristics of ^{99m}Tc and may be used to acquire planar images as well as SPECT. Both agents slightly underestimate the true cerebral blood perfusion, especially with high flow states.

Technetium-99m-HMPAO is a neutral lipid-soluble radiopharmaceutical that crosses the BBB and then becomes a polar hydrophilic molecule that remains trapped in the brain in a distribution proportional to the cerebral blood flow. ^{99m}Tc-HMPAO accumulates slightly more in the frontal lobes, thalamus, and cerebellum. The first-pass extraction is thought to be 80% and the retention time is approximately 24 hours. Originally requiring rapid use following preparation (within 30 minutes), the addition of stabilizing agents now allows a shelf-life of up to 4 hours. SPECT image acquisition should be obtained within 15 to 120 minutes after radiopharmaceutical injection.

Technetium-99m-ECD is also a neutral lipid-soluble radiopharmaceutical that passively diffuses across the BBB. It accumulates slightly more in the parietal and occipital lobes. The first-pass extraction is estimated to be 60-70%. In vivo conversion of the neutral lipophilic agent into nondiffusible polar metabolites in the neuron occurs more slowly than for HMPAO with a slow washout of approximately 6% per hour. The blood clearance of ^{99m}Tc-ECD is more rapid than ^{99m}Tc-HMPAO resulting in superior brain-to-background ratio at 15 to 30 minutes after radiopharmaceutical injection. Images are suboptimal if delayed, because almost 25% of the brain activity is cleared after 4 hours.

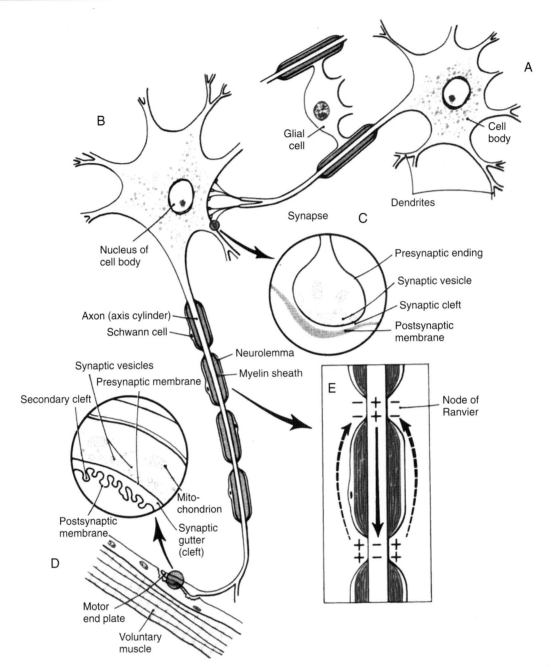

FIGURE 14-6 Neurons of the central nervous system (CNS). Neuron *A* is confined to the CNS and terminates on neuron *B* at a typical chemical synapse *C*. Neuron *B* is a ventral horn cell; its axon extends to a peripheral nerve and innervates a voluntary muscle at the myoneural junction *D*. In *E* the action potential is moving in the direction of the *solid arrow* inside the axon; the *dashed arrows* indicate the direction of flow of the action current.

Normally the angiographic images obtained with any of these agents demonstrate prompt symmetric perfusion with tracer defining the general intracranial flow and extending to the calvarial convexities bilaterally. Static planar images obtained using ^{99m}Tc-DTPA and ^{99m}Tc-pertechnetate show tracer activity in the vessels, in the face, and soft tissues of the scalp. Because the brain blood pool is relatively small, there is little tracer activity normally seen inside the skull with the non-specific, hydrophilic perfusion agents. Increased activity may be seen at sites of compromised BBB.

The more brain-specific lipophilic agents ^{99m}Tc-HMPAO and ^{99m}Tc-ECD show similar findings during the angiographic phase immediately following tracer injection because, as with the hydrophilic tracers, early flow images are simply recording delivery of tracer through the arterial system. Delayed static planar images using these agents, however, are different. In normal patients, ^{99m}Tc-HMPAO and ^{99m}Tc-ECD show clear activity in the brain parenchyma, primarily the gray matter. The lipophilic amine derivative ^{123}I-isopropyl iodoamphetamine (IMP) also localizes in brain tissue,

TABLE 14-1	Physical Characteristics of Radionuclides that are Used in Brain Imaging		
Radioisotope	Half-Life	Mode of Decay	Energy (Radiation)
^{99m}Tc	6 hours	Isomeric transition	140 keV (γ)
^{111}In	2.8 days	Electron capture	173 keV, 247 keV (γ)
^{201}Tl	73 hours	Electron capture	68 to 80 keV (Hg x-rays), 135 keV, 167 keV (γ)
^{67}Ga	78 hours	Electron capture	93 keV, 185 keV, 300 keV, 395 keV
^{11}C	20 minutes	Positron emission	511 keV (γ)
^{18}F	110 minutes	Positron emission	511 keV (γ)

but because the tracer usually washes out within 1 hour, imaging must be done soon after injection of the tracer.

Tumors of the brain are most often imaged either with fluorodeoxyglucose (FDG) PET or with SPECT tracers such as thallium-201 (^{201}Tl). Like many radiopharmaceuticals, ^{201}Tl does not cross the BBB in normal individuals, but it diffuses rapidly across an altered BBB. Thallium is most commonly imaged with SPECT and has been used to diagnose brain tumors, clarify the nature of lesions found with CT or MRI, and detect tumor recurrence. The positive predictive value is much better than the negative predictive value; however, thallium is usually not very helpful in determining the tumor type or predicting the clinical outcome.

In addition to ^{99m}Tc and ^{201}Tl, other radionuclides employed in single-photon imaging of the brain are indium-111 (^{111}In), which is used for imaging the CSF system, and gallium-67 (^{67}Ga) used in determining the extent of sarcoidosis in the CNS (Table 14-1).

CSF Imaging Tracers

Indium-111-DTPA is the only radiopharmaceutical approved in the United States for the assessment of CSF dynamics. It satisfies the following criteria: (1) it is physiologically governed by CSF flow, (2) it has an adequate physical half-life of 2.8 days for the study, (3) it has a desirable photon emission for imaging (173 and 247 keV), (4) it has a relatively low radiation dose to the patient, and (5) it has low chemical toxicity. To perform the procedure a physician administers 500 μCi of ^{111}In-DTPA intrathecally (into the subarachnoid space), usually via lumbar puncture between L3 and L4. Once injected into the subarachnoid space, the ^{111}In-DTPA

follows CSF flow up the spinal cord over the lateral convexities of the brain and is then absorbed by the arachnoid granulations in a manner similar to that of normal CSF. During the lumbar puncture, a 21- to 22-gauge spinal needle connected to a three-way stopcock is often used to monitor CSF pressure, sample the CSF for routine cell and chemical tests, and administer the radiopharmaceutical. The patient is often kept in a horizontal position for 2 hours after injection to minimize headaches caused by CSF leakage or changes in CSF pressure due to the lumbar puncture.

PET Tracers

Often the same information can be obtained with either SPECT or PET agents. For example, both PET and SPECT show reduced temporal and parietal tracer accumulation in Alzheimer's disease, and both methods can be used to assess the severity of the disease. In healthy controls, both PET and SPECT demonstrate high tracer accumulation in the cerebral cortex, basal ganglia, thalami, and cerebellar cortex.

PET radiotracers are being used increasingly for imaging brain blood flow and metabolic activity, particularly in patients with seizure disorders and dementia. The high metabolic demands of the normal brain result in high blood flow to the cerebral cortex. Studying blood flow and metabolic activity separately is difficult, as was mentioned earlier; however, in some diseases the separation of the two processes is not needed for diagnosis. For example, focally diminished metabolic activity and diminished blood flow is seen in patients with Alzheimer's disease. Because diminished blood flow also accompanies a number of other causes of diminished metabolism, tracers that are more specific for identifying changes seen in diseases such as Alzheimer's disease, are currently being sought. PET imaging has gained increasing popularity in recent years because of the better image quality of PET over planar and SPECT studies, the widespread availability of FDG, and the design of PET/CT scanners that merge PET information with high-resolution CT. More recently CNS PET has been fused with MRI.[19,21]

PET extends the technology to include biologically important radiotracers that can be synthesized using radioactive forms of carbon (^{11}C, half-life 20 minutes), oxygen (^{15}O, half-life 2 minutes), nitrogen (^{13}N, half-life 10 minutes), and fluorine (^{18}F, half-life 110 minutes). Many of the radiotracers are identical to substances normally found in the body and can be used to measure blood flow, blood volume, metabolism or the presence of receptors. For example, Alternatively, ^{15}O-labeled water may be used to measure blood flow. Alternatively, ^{15}O- and/or ^{11}C-labeled carboxyhemoglobin may be used to measure blood volume. ^{11}C-methionine may be used to assess amino acid metabolism, whereas ^{11}C-methylspiperone may be used to measure dopamine receptor activity. Depending on the molecule into which ^{11}C is incorporated, the resulting radiopharmaceutical may be used to monitor several types of receptor activity: ^{11}C-carfentanil demonstrates opiate receptor activity, ^{11}C-flunitrazepam demonstrates benzodiazepine receptor activity, and ^{11}C-scopalamine demonstrates muscarinic cholinergic receptor activity. Since these radionuclides are produced in a cyclotron and have short half-lives, they require rapid synthesis and rapid quality-assurance methods.

Fluorine-18-FDG is a glucose analogue that may be used to evaluate glucose metabolism by the brain. It crosses the BBB through a glucose transporter system and is then phosphorylated by hexokinase-1. Because the resulting metabolite FDG-6-phosphate cannot be further metabolized and cannot exit the cell, the tracer is trapped in the brain parenchyma. Approximately 4% of the administered dose localizes to the brain with peak uptake at 35 minutes following radiopharmaceutical injection. Radiopharmaceutical doses typically range from 5 to 20 mCi.

IMAGING TECHNIQUES AND PROTOCOLS

Brain Perfusion Imaging: Planar and SPECT

Whether an imaging modality is anatomical in orientation, as with CT, or metabolic, as with nuclear medicine, viewing the body from a ring of detectors surrounding it increases the contrast between lesions and normal tissues, which translates into improved diagnostic information.[18,19] Therefore, although certain diagnoses can be made with planar imaging, PET or SPECT is often better than planar imaging to solve clinical problems (e.g., locating the point of origin of an epileptic seizure).

The planar imaging technique may be used for imaging brain perfusion. Most often, a "blood-flow" study is performed where sequential 2- to 3-second images are taken for 1 to 2 minutes. Blood flow images can be obtained from any projection, depending on the site of the disease. Images are most often obtained from anterior or posterior projections to allow for the comparison of perfusion to both sides of the brain. Posterior blood-flow studies are often better tolerated by children because the large head of a gamma camera can be frightening when placed inches from a child's face. CNS blood flow studies can be performed in the supine or upright position. The former makes it easier to immobilize the head. Blood-flow images are often followed by immediate static blood-pool images in the anterior, posterior, and both lateral projections. A vertex view is also sometimes helpful. The delayed static views are normally taken from the same projections as the blood pool images.

SPECT of the brain provides higher contrast and better localization, but requires a longer time to complete compared with planar imaging. Using radiopharmaceuticals labelled with ^{99m}Tc, including patient preparation, SPECT requires approximately 1 to 2 hours. Once injected, the radiopharmaceutical distribution in the brain will reflect blood flow demands at the time of injection. If the patient is actively speaking or moving, for instance, the areas of the brain necessary for those actions will demonstrate more blood flow than other areas and therefore take up more of the radiotracer. To minimize changes in local metabolic demands within the brain, the patient should be instructed to rest quietly following tracer injection, and the imaging room should be quiet and dimly lit to minimize environmental stimuli. An intravenous (IV) line should be placed approximately 15 minutes before injection of the radiotracer so that the patient does not experience pain when the radiotracer is injected. Prior to injection, the patient should be placed in a comfortable, supine position with the head in a head holder and immobilized with a Velcro strap. The sagittal plane of the patient's head should be perpendicular to the table. The head should be flexed so that the cerebellum is included in the field of view. The detector must be positioned as close as possible to the patient's head to ensure acquisition of high-quality images. Care must be taken to monitor the patient for motion during the imaging procedure. Often patients with certain neurological disorders find it difficult to maintain a fixed position during the scanning procedure.

For ^{99m}Tc-labeled radiopharmaceuticals, the rotating gamma camera is typically equipped with a low-energy, high-resolution parallel hole collimator. Fan beam collimators may be used to improve the resolution of the images. Improved sensitivity can be obtained with three- and four-headed SPECT scanners, but the introduction of multiple heads complicates scanner design and quality control. Most facilities in the United States have two-headed gamma cameras which can be used for both SPECT of the brain and other diagnostic studies.

Image acquisition begins approximately 30 minutes to 4 hours after injection of the radiopharmaceutical. In general, SPECT acquisition should include 64 images acquired for 20 to 40 seconds each through a range of 360 degrees. The patient's ability to endure the acquisition should be considered in the selection of the acquisition time. When choosing the acquisition matrix size, a general rule is that each pixel should approximate half of the extrinsic full width at half maximum (FWHM). A 128×128 matrix, although providing good resolution, might not contain a statistically valid number of counts per pixel and requires longer reconstruction times and greater computer disk space. Magnification can be used to keep both the matrix and pixel size small. A 64×64 matrix with a magnification factor of 2.0 approximates a 128×128 matrix. This saves reconstruction time and reduces the amount of computer disk space used. Table 14-2 provides guidelines for brain SPECT acquisition on single-, dual-, and triple-head gamma cameras.

SPECT brain images may be obtained using a filtered back-projection or iterative reconstruction technique. To produce high-resolution, low-noise images, often

TABLE 14-2	SPECT Acquisition Parameters*			
Number of Detectors	Number of Images per Detector	Time per Image (sec)	Matrix Size	Collimator
1	60	30	64 × 64	High resolution
2	60	30	128 × 128	High resolution/ fan beam
3	40	45	64 × 64	High resolution/ fan beam

*30-minute acquisition.

TABLE 14-3	Processing Filters
Type of Filter	Use and Effect
Preprocessing	Two-dimensional filter applied to planar views before reconstruction, with resulting smoothing effect
Reconstruction	Simple back-projection technique of the ramp filter; range of filters used (high-frequency noise contribution to filters, which drastically smooth image)
Postprocessing	Filter applied in all three dimensions of reconstructed image; smoothing

a combination of preprocessing, back-projection, and postprocessing filters is used (Table 14-3). The selection of an appropriate SPECT processing protocol depends on the radiopharmaceutical, the imaging instrumentation, and the computer software being used. Knowledge of cross-sectional anatomy and familiarity with the expected resolution are essential for processing data accurately. System calibration such as center-of-rotation and field-uniformity corrections should be performed prior to the reconstruction in order to generate artifact-free SPECT images. Attenuation correction is also important in order to compensate for photon attenuation within the brain. Uniform attenuation correction is typically sufficient for brain SPECT and may be accomplished using a computer-generated model fitted to the brain image. In recent years, hybrid SPECT/CT devices have become increasingly popular. In this case, the CT portion of the study may be used for attenuation correction as well as for anatomic localization. The CT provides a more accurate map of the tissue attenuation within each slice of the brain and can be used for implementation of nun-uniform attenuation correction. Close attention must be paid to ensure accurate alignment of the SPECT and CT images, however, so that an artifact is not introduced.

SPECT brain images can be reoriented along the x-, y-, or z-axes or in a specific oblique plane; this allows for correction of positioning errors as well. The images can be quantitated using left-to-right hemisphere ratio programs or by placing individual regions of interest over specific structures located in the brain.

BOX 14-1   Brain Scan Protocol

Radiopharmaceutical
^{99m}Tc-ECD (Neurolite)

Dose
25 mCi IV

Radiation Dosimetry
Organ receiving the largest radiation dose = bladder wall = 0.27 rad/mCi
Effective dose = 0.041 rem/mCi

Patient Preparation
Preinjection: The most important aspect of patient preparation is to achieve a consistent environment at the time of injection and uptake. Ask the patient to empty their bladder before beginning. Dim the lights in the room. Have the patient lie down. Place the IV, then wait at least 10 minutes before injecting. Instruct the patient not to speak or to read. There should be no interaction with the patient before, during, or up to 5 minutes after injection. Note if the patient's eyes were open or closed during injection. If sedation is required, it should be given after injection of the radiopharmaceutical when possible.

Procedure
SPECT images 30 minutes to 4 hours after injection. Optimum scan time is 60 minutes postinjection. The patient's head should be lightly restrained to minimize motion. It is not possible to rigidly bind the head in place. Patient cooperation is necessary. Sedation may be required.

Instrumentation
360-degree rotation. 90 images. Angle step 4. 20 sec/frame, 128 × 128 matrix.

Analysis
Reconstruction in the transaxial, coronal, and sagittal slices with reprojections.

A common method of display of SPECT brain images includes sagittal, coronal, and transverse planes shown simultaneously. This allows the physician to correlate images on one view with the other two tomographic planes. Volume and surface rendering programs allow three-dimensional display of brain SPECT images, which can be useful in localizing and determining the extent of disease. Box 14-1 provides information on brain scan protocols.

Brain Death Study

An important application of planar brain imaging is in the diagnosis of brain death. Although there are clear-cut clinical criteria for establishing death, patients on cardiopulmonary support systems may be brain dead even though the circulatory and respiratory systems continue to function. Measurement of regional cerebral blood flow by means of planar or SPECT imaging can document the absence of blood flow through the distribution of the internal carotid arteries, which occurs when neuronal activity is insufficient to sustain life.[17]

Two types of radiopharmaceuticals can be used: those that distribute in the cerebral parenchyma according to the blood flow (HMPAO and ECD) and those that distribute in the blood vessels (^{99m}Tc-pertechnetate and ^{99m}Tc-DTPA).[20] Images are obtained during the blood-flow phase and immediately after the accumulation of the tracers. For the blood-flow phase, images are obtained at 3-second intervals for 1 to 2 minutes. These images demonstrate tracer present in the arteries and veins in individuals without brain death and the absence of such activity in individuals with brain death, because brain death is equivalent to a complete absence of cerebral perfusion. This portion of the study provides identical information with both the vascular and parenchymal tracers, but it requires careful execution and may be uninterruptible if the injection site is infiltrated, if the camera is not set to the right energy window, or if image acquisition on the computer is not started immediately. In such situations, delayed views are very helpful, because adequate time is available to correct the acquisition parameters (Table 14-2) and reposition the patient for this phase of the study. The characteristic pattern on delayed scans obtained with ^{99m}Tc-DTPA shows an absence of blood flow through the cerebral cortex; that is, no filling of the sagittal and transverse sinuses. Delayed views are particularly useful if tracers with parenchymal accumulation (HMPAO and ECD) were injected, because they clearly show accumulation in the brain if brain death is absent and no accumulation if brain death is present.[16] For information on brain death protocols, please refer to Box 14-2.

Cerebrospinal Fluid Dynamics

CSF dynamics may be investigated with ^{111}In-labeled DTPA. For example:

- **Radionuclide cisternogram** is used for the diagnosis of the cause of hydrocephalus, where hydrocephalus is abnormal enlargement of the CSF spaces due to abnormal production, absorption, or circulation of CSF. The tracer is injected into the subarachnoid space of the lumbar spine, and the head is imaged at 3 hours and 24 hours after injection.[1]

| BOX 14-2 | **Brain Death Study Protocol** |

Radiopharmaceutical
^{99m}Tc-ECD (Neurolite)

Dose
25 mCi IV

Radiation Dosimetry
Organ receiving the largest radiation dose = bladder wall = 0.27 rad/mCi
Effective dose = 0.041 rem/mCi

Patient Preparation
Place tourniquet tightly around patient's forehead to reduce scalp circulation.

Procedure
A flow study is performed in the anterior projection. Static blood pool images are then collected: anterior, left lateral, right lateral, and if possible posterior.

Instrumentation
High resolution collimator
Flow: 32 frames, 2 sec/frame, 64 × 64 matrix
Blood Pool: 128 × 128 matrix, 5 min/view

- **Cerebrospinal fluid shunt evaluation** is used for the evaluation of the patency of ventriculoperitoneal shunts. The tracer is injected into the shunt reservoir, and images of the head and abdomen are obtained immediately after injection, 3 hours after injection, and, if necessary, 24 hours after injection.[10]
- *Cerebrospinal fluid leak imaging* is used for the diagnosis of CSF leaks. The tracer is injected into the lumbar subarachnoid space, and images of the head are obtained 3 hours and 24 hours after injection.[4]

Radionuclide Cisternography

Following tracer injection using lumbar puncture, a normal cisternogram shows activity in the basal cisterns by 3 hours after injection, with flow over the convexities by 24 hours. Slight reflux into the ventricles can be normal at 24 hours but should not be seen after this time. Noncommunicating hydrocephalus shows a lack of ventricular reflux and slow or normal flow over the convexities. Normal-pressure hydrocephalus shows ventricular reflux that persists beyond 24 hours. Flow over the convexities is significantly delayed or absent. Imaging time frames differ for pediatric patients and are addressed in Chapter 23. Box 14-3 covers the cisternogram protocol.

Cerebrospinal Fluid Shunt Evaluation

In noncommunicating hydrocephalus, the constant production of CSF and its inability to escape flow through

Radiopharmaceutical
^{111}In-DTPA

Dose
500-μCi intrathecal injection into the subarachnoid space via a lumbar puncture by a physician.

Radiation Dosimetry
Organ receiving the highest radiation dose = spinal cord = 3.5 rad/mCi
  Effective dose = 0.52 rem/mCi

Patient Preparation
Patients with suspected CSF leak should have their nostrils packed with pledgets. These are left in place for 6-8 hours and during the scan. The pledgets are then removed and counted in the well counter. A 5-ml blood sample is also drawn at this time and counted in the well counter. The patient's nostrils are then repacked with gauze and left in place for 24 hours. Count gauze and 24-hr blood sample.

Procedure
Patient is imaged 4-6 hours, 2 days, and 3 days postinjection.
Place patient supine and image the head.
Views: Anterior, posterior, right lateral, left lateral. On day 1, also image the injection site. The first set of images is only to check that the radiopharmaceutical has been properly injected.
Patient must be imaged on the same camera every day because the activity is quantitated from day to day. Record counts for each image every day.
Special Note: Pledgets should be left in place when imaging.

Instrumentation
Dual head: Medium-energy collimator 128 × 128 matrix, 300 sec/view

the foramen of Monroe and the foramina of Luschka into the subarachnoid space results in the enlargement of the ventricles, which leads to compression and atrophy of the cerebral cortex and subsequent dementia. Ventriculoperitoneal (VP) shunts can be used to divert CSF from the ventricles to another site. VP shunts consist of proximal tubing leading from the ventricle, usually to a reservoir, then through a section of distal tubing from the reservoir to another site for absorption, usually the peritoneal cavity. Less frequently, shunts are placed that connect the reservoir with the pleural space or the cardiac atrium. Another type of shunt used in patients with increased intracranial pressure without hydrocephalus (also called *pseudotumor cerebri*) is the lumboperitoneal shunt.

There are two established tracer injection techniques for VP and ventriculoatrial (VA) shunts. With the more popular VP technique, a small volume of the tracer is injected into the shunt reservoir and the injection tube is not flushed. This technique results in visualization of the reservoir and the distal tubing within minutes as well as the appearance of activity in the abdomen within 1 hour, if both the proximal and the distal tubing are patent (Figure 14-7). Lack of tracer movement is seen with obstruction of either the proximal or the distal tubing. It is important to use a small volume of tracer and refrain from manually flushing it from the reservoir with a syringe. Manual flushing can result in tracer moving either forward into the peritoneal cavity or backward into the ventricles. Even if manual flushing does show movement of tracer into the peritoneal cavity, the pressures generated with manual flushing are not the same

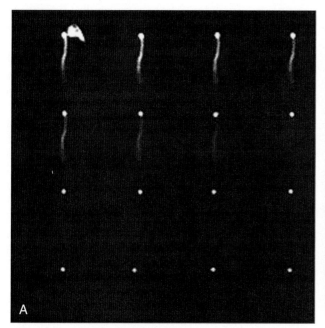

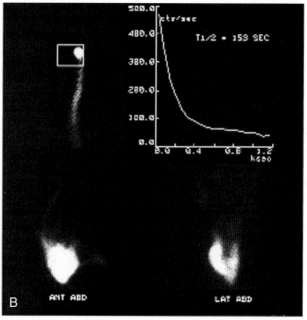

FIGURE 14-7 Patent ventriculoperitoneal shunt. **A,** Clearance of the radiopharmaceutical from the shunt bulb (reservoir) and the distal tubing is rapid *(sequence of 16 images)*. **B,** The time activity curve derived from the bulb *(upper right)* confirms rapid clearance. Anterior and lateral abdominal views demonstrate adequate peritoneal distribution of the radiopharmaceutical *(bottom)*.

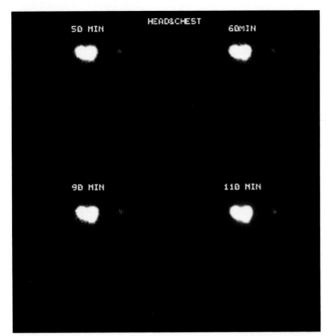

FIGURE 14-8 Obstructed ventriculoatrial shunt. There is accumulation of the radiopharmaceutical within the ventricles, indicating patency of the proximal tubing but no clearance and no visualization of the distal tubing and no accumulation in the abdominal cavity, which indicates distal obstruction.

BOX 14-4	**CSF Shunt Protocol**

Radiopharmaceutical and Dose
Determine dose activity and volume. Check with physician before administering dose. Volume may not exceed 0.2 ml.
1 mCi ^{99m}Tc-DTPA in 0.2 ml, prepared with preservative free saline.
Or
500 µCi ^{111}In-DTPA when extended imaging is required.

Patient Preparation
None

Injection
Injection is done by the physician.

Procedure
Immediate flow followed by immediate statics Ant/Post Head, R. Lat /L. Lat Head, Ant/Post Abdomen; repeat static images at 24 hours. Also 48 hours with ^{111}In-DTPA
Patient must be imaged on the same camera every day because the activity is quantitated from day to day. Record counts for each image every day.

Instrumentation
Dual head: Medium- or low-energy collimator. Immediate flow 10 sec/frame for 20 min. 64 × 64 matrix.
Statics 128 × 128 matrix, 300 sec/view

as physiologic pressures, and a false negative study can result. In certain cases, tracer may be injected into the shunt reservoir while the distal tubing is compressed with a finger so that the radioactivity flows retrograde into the ventricles. This manipulation demonstrates if the proximal tubing is patent (Figure 14-8). Subsequent spontaneous tracer clearance from the entire system may be monitored. For example, tracer in the abdomen at the distal tip of a VP shunt suggests patency of the rest of the shunt. Delayed views are needed to show tracer dispersion in the peritoneal cavity.

There are several different shunt types. For example, the Ommaya shunt is a system consisting of a reservoir and tubing used to deliver chemotherapeutic agents to the ventricles and the subarachnoid space. Nuclear medicine procedures are performed to evaluate the patency of the shunt and, in the case of the Ommaya shunt, to evaluate the distribution pattern of the radiotracer in the CSF to predict the distribution of chemotherapeutic agents. Refer to Box 14-4 for the CSF shunt protocol.

Cerebrospinal Fluid Leaks

Radionuclide studies are sensitive for the detection of a CSF leak. First, absorptive **pledgets** are placed in the nasal cavity close to the site of the suspected leak. Since the cribriform plate is the most common site of fracture leading to CSF rhinorrhea, pledgets are typically placed in the nasal cavity close to the cribriform plate. Following the placement of pledgets, tracer is injected into the

thecal sac via a lumbar puncture. The injection site is imaged immediately after radiopharmaceutical administration to rule out extravasation of the injected dose out of the subarachnoid space. Once imaging has confirmed proper placement of tracer in the thecal sac, subsequent images can monitor the movement of the tracer through the CSF adjacent to the spine up into the skull. Although images detecting the extravasation of tracer outside the normal confines of the subarachnoid space can sometimes confirm a leak, leaks are usually diagnosed by noting elevated and/or asymmetric counts on the pledgets (Figure 14-9).

Imaging is routinely performed when activity reaches the basal cisterns, typically at 1 to 4 hours after injection. Anterior, left lateral, right lateral, and posterior projections of the head and an anterior image of the abdomen are obtained 2 hours after injection for 200,000 counts. Positioning for these projections is the same as that used in planar brain imaging. Additional views of the head or spine may be indicated and additional delayed images (typically 6, 24, and 48 hours) may be helpful. Images should be obtained with the patient in a position that optimizes visualization of the suspected site of CSF leakage. If a wide, segmental appearance is seen initially with no activity in the basal cisterns at 2 to 3 hours, reinjection is required.

The quantitative diagnosis of CSF rhinorrhea is done after the intrathecal administration of ^{111}In-DTPA. The cotton pledgets (1 cm²) placed in both nostrils (typically by an otorhinolaryngologist) have a string attached—one string each pledget—to allow for retrieval and labeling of the anatomic location. A 5-ml heparinized blood sample is obtained from the patient when the pledgets are placed. The pledgets are removed approximately 6 hours after injection of the radiopharmaceutical, and a second 5-ml heparinized blood sample is obtained. The anterior-most pledgets should be removed before the more posterior pledgets are removed to help prevent cross-contamination of the different sites. Further, each pledget string should be labelled with the location of the pledget to assist in proper removal.

After centrifugation of both blood samples, 0.5 ml of plasma is withdrawn from each sample. A scintillation well counter with a 150- to 250-keV window is used to count each pledget and each blood sample. The results

are expressed as the ratio of pledget activity (cpm) divided by the average plasma activity (cpm). Normal pledget to plasma ratios are 1:1.3. Radiation safety and contamination precautions should be observed. Box 14-3 outlines the cisternogram and leak protocol.

Positron Emission Tomography

For FDG PET imaging, the patient is injected with 10 mCi ^{18}F-FDG. The patient is asked to sit quietly in an armchair with the legs and arms uncrossed for approximately 45 minutes and to refrain from talking and reading during this time. The room lights are kept low, the eyes are covered with a piece of black cloth, and the ears are plugged. The purpose of these preparations is to minimize sensory stimulation and activation of the brain, particularly the auditory and visual centers.

With new PET scanners, the entire brain can be covered with a single field of view. Two scans are acquired: an emission scan and an emission plus transmission scan. A transmission-emission subtraction scan is then calculated. Typically the 3D FDG emission scan is 20 minutes long, and the images are reconstructed in a 128 × 128 matrix, 25.6 cm in diameter, using a ramp transaxial filter with a cutoff of 4 mm and an axial filter width of 8.5 mm. The transmission scan is obtained in 2D and is 10 minutes long.

With hybrid PET/CT scanners, a CT scan is used for transmission imaging and attenuation correction instead of a germanium-68 source. Typical CT parameters are helical high-speed acquisition, 1 second per rotation, 5 mm slice thickness, 22.5 mm per rotation, 140 kVp, 90 mA, 7.7 seconds total time (with a four-detector scanner), single field of view, and 35 slices. This CT protocol results in an average radiation exposure of 7.71 mGy. Chapter 13 provides additional information on the acquisition protocol.

PET images of the brain demonstrate high glucose metabolism in the cerebral cortex, cerebellar cortex, basal ganglia, and thalami (Figure 14-10). Many things can affect tracer uptake including patient motion,

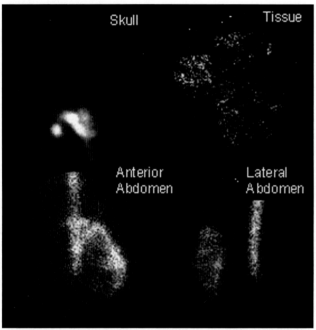

FIGURE 14-9 Positive cerebrospinal fluid leak in a 56-year-old female patient with a history of two previous head traumas, headache, and a spontaneous excess of fluid from the nose. Pledget to plasma count ratios were 0.76 to 8.53 on the right and 62 to 220 on the left (normal ≤1.3). Radioactivity is seen in the abdomen outside of the spinal column.

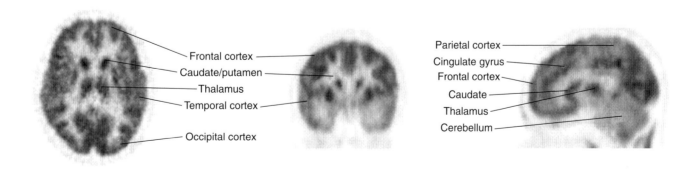

A Transaxial plane

Coronal plane B Sagittal plane

FIGURE 14-10 ^{18}F-fluorodeoxyglucose (FDG) PET scan of the brain of a healthy person.

dreams, intense thought processes such as problem solving, visual and auditory stimuli and drugs. For example, general anesthesia will reduce the uptake in the cerebral cortex whereas phenytoin (Dilantin) treatment will reduce the uptake in the cerebellum.

CLINICAL PET AND SPECT STUDIES

Normal Distribution of Cerebral Blood Flow and Metabolism

There are several radiopharmaceuticals used to image cerebral perfusion and metabolism. Typically, radiopharmaceutical activity is uniformly distributed between the lobes of the brain, however, the normal biodistribution may change with patient age or activity following the radiopharmaceutical injection. In particular, in very young children, there is intense tracer uptake in the sensorimotor cortex, thalamus, brain stem and cerebellar vermis with relatively decreased perfusion to the cerebral cortex particularly in the frontal lobes (Figure 14-11). This evolves over time so that the images of the brain resemble those seen in adults by approximately 2 years of age. In the elderly, there is often a decreased global activity that is most pronounced in the frontal lobes. Comparison of the study to be analyzed with large databases of age-matched normal subjects may improve detection of abnormalities and their interpretation.

Cerebrovascular Disease

Clinical symptoms and signs often suggest the sites of cortical or subcortical injury in patients with an acute stroke. However, lesions are not always found at the site suggested by clinical manifestations. The clinical picture may be the result of secondary effects, such as deafferentation (damage to nerve tracts rather than to the neuron itself) caused by lesions in an unexpected location. The degree of mental dysfunction may be far greater than that suggested by the anatomical lesions seen with noncontrast CT. Small subcortical lesions, such as lacunar infarctions, may result in extensive cortical dysfunction. The neurological examination cannot effectively predict what the patient's eventual neurological deficiency will be. Anatomical imaging with CT and MRI, although currently the mainstay for imaging cerebrovascular disease and stroke, may not immediately reveal the extent of involvement. Arteriography can show the status of large vessels but does not provide information about cerebral microcirculation and small collateral branches. SPECT and PET make it possible to delineate the severity and extent of the perfusion/metabolism abnormalities from the time of onset of the stroke. Distant neuronal activity change may also be identified. For example, crossed cerebellar diaschisis following a stroke, or in other words hypoperfusion of the contralateral cerebellum, may be clearly seen with functional imaging and yet be invisible on anatomical imaging.

PET and SPECT can measure cerebral blood flow, glucose and oxygen metabolism, and blood volume, thus providing a more functional assessment of the severity of cerebrovascular diseases. In the early hours of an acute stroke, cellular metabolism may be maintained while perfusion is reduced, a situation referred to as "misery perfusion." As time progresses, damaged vessels may result in excessive perfusion or "luxury perfusion." The area of lowest regional blood flow or metabolism usually predicts the region that will eventually develop hypodense change (gliosis) on noncontrast CT, although the perfusion and metabolic lesions are often larger, reflecting the surrounding area of ischemia. The blood flow or metabolic abnormalities seen with PET or SPECT correlate better with the neurological defects than do those seen with noncontrast CT. SPECT may also be used to demonstrate vascular reserve. The idea is that the administration of acetazolamide (Diamox), a carbonic anhydrase inhibitor, causes vasodilation, which leads to increased perfusion. Abnormal vessels unable to dilate to the same extent as normal vessels cause blood to be shunted toward tissue supplied by the normal vessels. Therefore, comparing pre– and post–Diamox infusion images causes perfusion abnormalities to be accentuated, improving diagnostic accuracy and underlining poor vascular reserve when present (Figure 14-12).

The nuclear medicine images reflect function, whereas conventional CT and MRI images reflect structure. Studies of the cerebral circulation are helpful in establishing a prognosis after acute cerebral ischemia. In stroke, metabolic abnormalities seen on PET are frequently more extensive than the corresponding conventional CT findings. The pattern of metabolic abnormalities in PET has been shown to correlate with the clinical syndrome and with the degree of eventual recovery.[2,7,8]

Tumors

The annual incidence of intracranial CNS tumors ranges from 10 to 17 per 100,000 and for intraspinal tumors up to 1 to 2 per 100,000. It is thought that approximately 50% of these tumors represent primary sites of disease, with the reminder being metastatic foci. CNS tumors rarely metastasize beyond the confines of the brain and spinal cord.

Although certain brain tumors may appear to be less aggressive (e.g., low-grade astrocytomas) than others (e.g., high-grade glioblastoma multiforme), the anatomical location of a lesion often has a critical impact on management and outcome. The four major classes of brain tumors are: gliomas, neuronal tumors, poorly differentiated neoplasms, and meningiomas.

Gliomas are derived from glial cells and include astrocytomas, oligodendrogliomas, and ependymomas. There

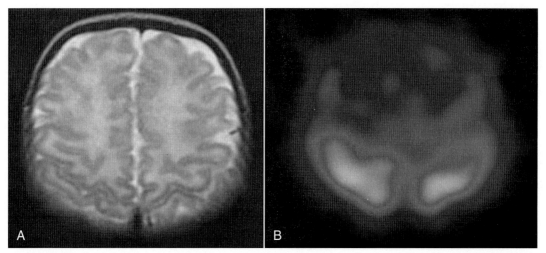

FIGURE 14-11 MRI **(A)** and SPECT **(B)** in a 7-week-old girl. SPECT shows decreased metabolic activity in the frontal cortex. *(Images courtesy of Children's Hospital Boston.)*

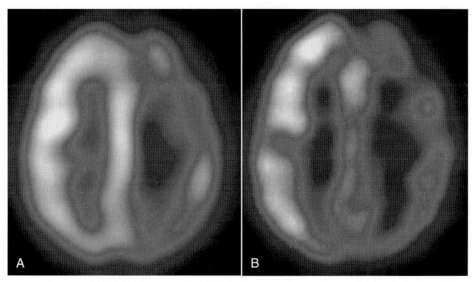

FIGURE 14-12 SPECT in a 13-year-old girl with headaches. **A,** Baseline SPECT showing relative decreased perfusion to the left cerebral hemisphere compared with the right cerebral hemisphere. **B,** SPECT following Diamox administration showing more pronounced reduction in perfusion to the left cerebral hemisphere. *(Images courtesy of Children's Hospital Boston.)*

are several different types of astrocytomas categorized by their histological features, anatomical distribution, and clinical picture. One type of highly aggressive astrocytoma is known as a glioblastoma multiforme. Thought to be responsible for 15% to 20% of all intracranial neoplasms, treatment includes surgical resection, external radiotherapy, and chemotherapy. At times, radiation necrosis of the brain occurs in patients who have received 5000 to 6000 rad of external radiation therapy.

Functional imaging may be used to evaluate neoplastic disease of the CNS. In particular, nuclear medicine studies may be particularly helpful in differentiating recurrent disease and radiation necrosis, or distinguishing neoplastic disease such as lymphoma from infection such as toxoplasmosis in an immunocompromised patient.

When neurological symptoms recur or change in patients treated with radiation, it is virtually impossible to distinguish radiation necrosis and gliosis from tumor recurrence by anatomical imaging techniques or by clinical examination. Nuclear procedures often eliminate the need for a second craniotomy and tissue biopsy. Cerebral blood flow and blood volume are not well correlated with the degree of malignancy; therefore metabolic studies are preferred.

Technetium-99m-labeled HMPAO or ECD are generally not sensitive for imaging brain tumors. SPECT images of brain tumors are performed either with ^{99m}Tc-sestamibi or ^{201}Tl. Although they have lower resolution, they have a higher target-to-nontarget contrast than does FDG PET. Accumulation of SPECT tracers is less specific than accumulation of FDG. For example, ^{201}Tl can

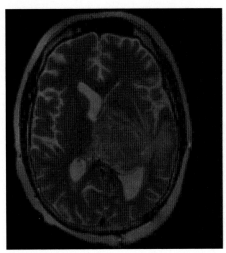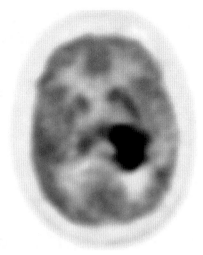

FIGURE 14-13 MRI and FDG-PET images in a 20-year-old man with a history of left thalamic astrocytoma demonstrate marked FDG avidity of the mass. *(Images courtesy of Children's Hospital Boston.)*

accumulate in stroke because of the damage to the BBB. FDG PET imaging has a high sensitivity for detection of higher grade tumors, such as glioblastoma multiforme, and is particularly useful for detection of tumor recurrence after surgery or radiation therapy. Interpretation of FDG PET images of brain tumors can be made difficult by relatively high uptake in the cerebral cortex. Fusion of PET and CT or MRI scans is readily obtained with hybrid scanners or fusion software (Figure 14-13). To make image fusion possible using software, the images from the two modalities have to be made available on a common image format platform, such as **digital imaging and communication in medicine (DICOM)**.[11]

Although FDG PET is probably the most commonly encountered radiopharmaceutical for imaging CNS tumors, other agents such as ^{18}F-thymidine and ^{11}C-methionine may demonstrate improved sensitivity and specificity in certain cases.

Epilepsy

Epilepsy is one of the most common pathologies of the brain. It is estimated that approximately 1% of the population suffers from epilepsy and that 800,000 Americans have focal seizures that do not progress to grand mal seizures (partial complex epilepsy). Seizures may be due to a spectrum of pathology including neoplastic disease, infection, trauma, and vascular abnormalities. For most patients with partial epilepsy, diagnosis is based on a multidisciplinary team evaluation consisting of clinical history and physical examination, the use of surface electroencephalography (EEG), and imaging with both anatomical and functional modalities. Approximately 20% of patients have intractable epilepsy and are not controlled with medication alone. These patients may benefit from surgical intervention. However, for surgery to be effective, additional information

concerning the precise localization of the epileptic focus is essential. Radiological techniques such as CT and MRI may show an anatomical abnormality. Functional imaging may provide additional information when localizing findings are identified. More importantly, functional imaging may demonstrate localizing abnormalities even in the face of normal CT or MRI. Typically, special localizing measures, such as intraoperative electrocorticography and direct recordings from stereotaxically implanted depth electrodes, are valuable for improved localization, but these techniques are invasive and may be complicated by significant risks.

In the ictal state (during a seizure), perfusion and metabolism are increased to the epileptogenic focus and at sites of seizure propagation.[3] In the interictal state (between seizures), both perfusion and metabolism are reduced in the area of prior seizure. With SPECT, increased cerebral blood flow can be measured immediately after the onset of a seizure (ictal imaging). This requires hospitalization of the patient and continuous video and EEG monitoring.[15] The ^{99m}Tc-labeled radiopharmaceuticals, either HMPAO or ECD, can be prepared and kept near the patient so that the injection can be made as soon as there is evidence of seizure activity, typically within seconds after seizure onset. In order to localize an epileptogenic focus or site of seizure origin, it is essential that the radiopharmaceutical be injected immediately and before seizure activity has spread to other parts of the brain. Since both ^{99m}Tc-HMPAO and ^{99m}Tc-ECD are extracted from the circulation and then trapped in the brain parenchyma for several hours, acquisition of images may be delayed to ensure patient stability before imaging. Ictal imaging with PET radiopharmaceuticals is not possible, because FDG is difficult to store near the patient given the relatively short half-life of ^{18}F and, more importantly, because FDG accumulates much more slowly in the brain than does ECD or HMPAO.

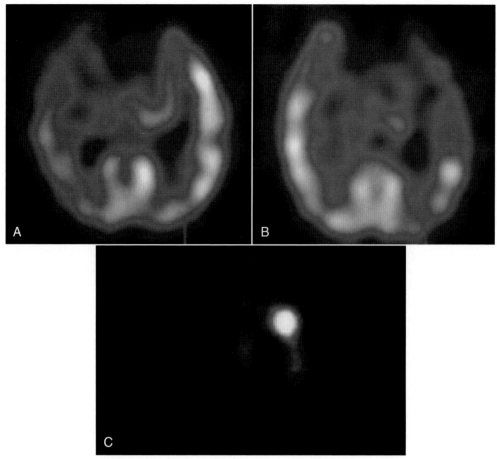

FIGURE 14-14 13-year-old girl with seizures. **A,** Ictal SPECT demonstrates increased tracer perfusion to the left temporal lobe compared with the contralateral side. **B,** Interictal SPECT demonstrates decreased tracer profusion to the left temporal lobe corresponding to the area of increased tracer perfusion on ictal SPECT. **C,** Subtraction image (ictal–interictal SPECT) illustrates the focus of perfusion abnormality in the left temporal lobe. *(Images courtesy of Children's Hospital Boston.)*

Overall, ictal SPECT is felt by many to be the most sensitive imaging technique for localizing an epileptogenic focus. In particular, sensitivity and specificity are high when both ictal and interictal SPECT are performed followed by the construction of subtraction images (Figure 14-14). Interictal PET is thought to be more sensitive than interictal SPECT but less sensitive than ictal SPECT in localizing an epileptogenic focus.

PET obtained during partial complex seizures (ictal scans) (see Figure 14-14) may show marked increases in local brain metabolism and perfusion in the general region of seizure onset, but because of propagated neuronal activity, the ictal scans are less useful in predicting epileptic origin than those made during the interictal state. PET scans made during nonfocal seizures show a generalized increase in brain metabolism and perfusion. Unlike the typical PET scans found in partial epilepsy, no focal changes are found during interictal or ictal scans of patients with petit mal seizures. A diffuse increase in metabolism is seen at the time of the petit mal seizure.

PET scans obtained during the interictal state are most valuable in the management of the patient with partial complex seizures (older terms: *temporal lobe*

epilepsy or *psychomotor epilepsy*) in which consciousness is impaired. PET and SPECT are less useful in generalized seizures. The results of interictal PET scans in patients with complex partial seizures have been compared with the results of CT and EEG in multiple reports. These studies showed that approximately 70% of the patients had zones of hypometabolism on interictal FDG scans in the involved regions.[9]

PET and EEG are complementary methods of localizing areas in the brain causing epileptic activity. Focal abnormalities can be identified with PET even if EEG data are unable to reveal the focus. The combined use of surface EEG and PET has eliminated the need for depth electrodes in some surgical candidates. PET can aid in the localization of the site when the EEG findings are inconsistent. Electroencephalography can verify the epileptogenic nature of a zone of hypometabolism determined by PET. An excellent correlation has been obtained between the site of hypometabolism, as determined by PET, and the presence of a pathological abnormality in the surgical specimen regions.[9]

In summary, for patients with intractable epilepsy, SPECT and PET provide information about local brain function that is quite different from the results of electrical measurements with EEG or structural assessments with CT/ MRI. The combination of functional imaging and EEG has been useful in the presurgical evaluation of these patients for determining the site of seizure onset. Either technique can give false-positive or false-negative results, but when used in combination, they yield more reliable localizing information.

Movement Disorders

There is a wide spectrum of movement disorders including disease with decreased movement, such as Parkinson disease or parkinsonian syndromes, and diseases with increased movement, such as Huntington disease.

Parkinsonism is an idiopathic neurodegenerative condition resulting in a clinical syndrome characterized by resting tremor, rigidity, and bradykinesia. Pathologically, there is loss of dopaminergic neurons in the substantia nigra. Many dopamine neurons have their cell bodies in the substantia nigra, from which neuronal fibers project into the caudate nucleus and putamen, where dopamine is released. The discovery of dopamine deficiency in the caudate nucleus and putamen of patients with Parkinson's disease whose brains were examined at autopsy was a major advance in neurobiology and paved the way for the development of an effective means of treating this debilitating disease: namely, the administration of L-dopa to increase the synthesis of dopamine.

Parkinson's disease is a primary example of the use of in vivo biochemical assessment of neuroreceptors. The technique not only provides accurate diagnosis, the ability to quantify the status of presynaptic and postsynaptic dopaminergic neurons, but also correlates with neuropsychological and clinical assessment.

Early in Parkinson's disease, there is a decrease in the number of presynaptic neurons that produce dopamine, with a subsequent decrease in the density of dopamine active transporter (DAT), the presynaptic membrane bound transporter that removes dopamine from the synaptic gap and delivers it back to the presynaptic neuron at the end of the stimulation phase. Postsynaptic D1 and D2 dopamine receptors, on the other hand, have demonstrated preservation or even an increase in number. Measurement of these presynaptic and postsynaptic sites with either a positron-emitting or a single photon–emitting radiotracer makes it possible to identify changes in the receptor populations in patients with Parkinson's disease even before symptoms occur.

The DAT–specific **radioligand** WIN-35,428 (also called *beta-CIT*) has been radiolabeled with ^{11}C or ^{18}F for PET[5] imaging and with ^{123}I or ^{99m}Tc for SPECT[6] imaging of patients with motor disorders. For example, TRODAT is a ^{99m}Tc-labeled compound that crosses the human BBB and binds to the dopamine transporter.[14] In healthy individuals a high concentration of this radioligand is observed in the basal ganglia (caudate

nuclei and putamen). In Parkinson disease, radioligand binding is reduced in both the caudate and the putamen, but the reduction is more prominent in the putamen (the posterior element), a finding that is consistent with the more pronounced loss of dopaminergic terminals in this brain structure. It is important to emphasize that PET changes can be observed in patients with relatively mild symptoms of Parkinson disease.

Huntington disease is a hereditary neurodegenerative disorder associated with gamma-aminobutyric acid (GABA) and glutamic acid decarboxylase deficiency in the caudate nucleus and putamen. Typically presenting between the ages of 35 and 50 years, the disease ultimately progresses to uncontrolled repetitive movement called chorea and dementia. Functional imaging demonstrates decreased perfusion and metabolism in the caudate nucleus, even with normal anatomical scans.

Dementia

The number of people suffering from dementia has increased with the increasing age of the population. It is estimated that almost 7 million people in the United States have dementia, and at least 2 million of those are severely affected.

Dementia is a clinical syndrome characterized by progressive cognitive decline beyond what might be expected with normal aging. Patients may display a constellation of clinical symptoms including memory loss, personality change, and difficulty with higher cortical function. Cognitive decline may be rapid or slow, occurring over days or over several years. Typically symptoms must be present for at least 6 months for the diagnosis of dementia to be made. Anatomical imaging with CT or MRI plays an important role in detecting focal cerebral disease such as tumor, infection, or infarction, in determining ventricular size, and in detecting neurodegenerative disease. Functional imaging with SPECT or PET may, however, show changes well before structural change is apparent. For example, FDG PET is thought to be close to 90% sensitive for the diagnosis of Alzheimer's disease, and metabolic changes may be identified well before structural changes are present. Further, an FDG PET scan may be more sensitive than a CT or MRI scan for detecting the extent of brain dysfunction. Advantages of FDG PET compared with SPECT include improved resolution as well as evaluation of glucose and oxygen metabolism in addition to regional cerebral blood flow.

Dementia is rarely due to diseases for which there is a cure, although acetylcholinesterase inhibitors, such as Donepezil, have shown an ability to delay the decline in cognitive and behavioral changes in some patients. However, if imaging shows no evidence of Alzheimer's or other irreversible disease, treatable diseases such as thyroid dysfunction, vitamin B_{12} deficiency, drug intoxication, and depression may be more actively pursued. Imaging with anatomical studies can also show treatable structural abnormalities that can lead to dementia such as subdural hematomas.

Certain patterns of radiopharmaceutical distribution have been recognized that suggest specific types of dementia. These include Alzheimer's disease, Lewy body disease, Parkinson's disease, Pick disease, primary progressive aphasia, vascular dementia, and normal pressure hydrocephalus. In particular, use of functional imaging may help identify those patients with mild cognitive impairment who are more likely to progress.

The diagnosis of Alzheimer's disease is usually made by the exclusion of the other causes. Because the disease is so progressive, the diagnosis must be made in the early stage for patients to benefit from the treatment. Alzheimer's disease can be diagnosed on the basis of clinical and psychological testing in only 50% of the patients who present with memory loss. Usually, the diagnosis is not made before thousands of dollars have been spent on tests.

Accounting for the cause of dementia in approximately 50% to 80% of patients, the disease is characterized by abnormally accelerated neuronal death, especially pronounced in the hippocampus and the parietal, temporal, and, to a lesser degree, frontal lobes. Diagnosis can be definitively made at autopsy by the identification of characteristic neurofibrillary tangles and amyloid plaques. As a result of the neuronal degeneration, a secondary decrease in blood flow and in oxygen and glucose metabolism occurs in the involved regions. These changes give rise to the characteristic pattern of regional cerebral blood flow and glucose metabolism on SPECT and PET imaging in patients with Alzheimer's disease[19] (Figure 14-15). The disease, manifested as hypoperfusion/hypometabolism, typically involves the parietotemporal cortex symmetrically, whereas during the early stages the pattern may be asymmetrical. It often extends into the adjacent occipital lobes. Frontal lobe involvement occurs to a lesser degree, and there is sparing of the basal ganglia, thalamus, sensorimotor cortex, occipital visual cortex and cerebellum. The distribution of disease is more symmetrical in the transaxial plane than that observed in patients with multi-infarct dementia, in which the defects are multifocal and show a high contrast between normal and abnormal areas of brain; often the defects correspond to the distribution of a major cerebral artery, such as the middle cerebral artery. Also in multi-infarct dementia, the sensorimotor cortex, basal ganglia, and cerebellum are often involved. So saying, the diagnosis of dementia can be complicated by the coexistence of Alzheimer's disease and multi-infarct dementia, which is found in about 30% of patients who come to autopsy.

Dementia with Lewy bodies is also an important cause of dementia to be accurately diagnosed because of its rapid progression, visual hallucinations, and potentially severe adverse reaction to neuroleptic agents. ^{18}F-FDG PET and SPECT show changes similar to Alzheimer's disease but tend to involve the occipital lobes and cerebellum with sparing of the hippocampus.

The frontotemporal dementias represent a diverse group of diseases with differential diagnosis including familial frontotemporal dementia, Pick disease, semantic dementia and primary progressive aphasia. Frontotemporal degeneration occurs in approximately 16% of early dementias and is clinically characterized by behavioral disturbances more than by losses of cognitive capacity and memory. SPECT shows hypoperfusion and FDG PET shows reduced glucose metabolism in the frontal and temporal lobes with sparing of the other parts of the cerebral cortex.[13] Pick disease is a form of frontotemporal degeneration that predominantly affects the frontal cortex. Progressive aphasia is another form of frontotemporal degeneration that is characterized by loss of speech ability, and degeneration predominantly affects the temporal lobe.[12] Other disease processes that may result in decreased perfusion and metabolism of the frontal and temporal lobes include depression (although often these patients have normal functional scans), amyotrophic lateral sclerosis, progressive supranuclear palsy, spinocerebellar atrophy, and cocaine abuse. In particular, AIDS dementia is associated with patchy, multifocal cortical and subcortical regions of hypoperfusion commonly in the frontal, temporal, and parietal lobes as well as in the basal ganglia. Focal areas of increased activity may also be seen in these patients.

It is expected that the number of clinical PET studies of patients with dementia will increase in the future. Early and accurate diagnosis of Alzheimer's disease can lead to prompt initiation of therapy. The most important reason for this is the increasing availability of therapies that have one or a combination of the following two effects: (1) enhancement of cognitive function and memory, and (2) slowing down of the processes that lead to neurodegeneration, such as inflammation and deposition of beta amyloid. At present the most important application of PET is differentiation of Alzheimer's disease from frontotemporal degeneration that does not benefit from the current treatment for Alzheimer's disease, an indication covered by Medicare.

Novel radioligands, such as ^{11}C-PIB, which can quantify amyloid burden in Alzheimer's disease are also under investigation. Other PET radiopharmaceuticals are being investigated that bind to muscarinic receptors, nicotinic receptors, and components of the cholinergic system.

SUMMARY

- Neurons are the fundamental units of the nervous system and communicate with each other by means of electrical action potentials and molecular messengers that carry information and modulate the electrical activity.
- Glucose is the principal source of energy for the brain and its consumption can be measured by PET.

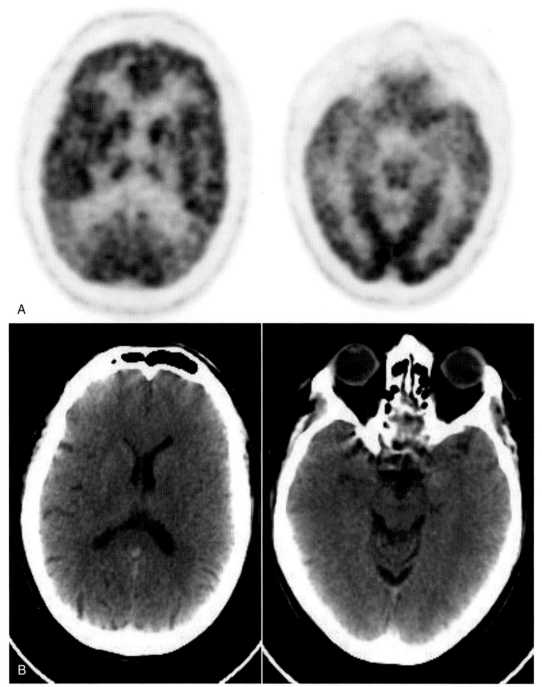

FIGURE 14-15 FDG-PET of the brain in a person with Alzheimer's disease. **A,** FDG-PET showing decreased metabolic activity in the parietal and temporal lobes. **B,** Corresponding CT images. *(Images courtesy of Beth Israel Deaconess Medical Center.)*

- Molecular messengers, called *neurotransmitters,* include amines, amino acids, and peptides.
- Radioactive tracers make it possible to detect and quantify molecular abnormalities including those involved in intercellular communication.
- In patients with diseases of the central and peripheral nervous system, nuclear medicine techniques can be used to assess the effectiveness of surgery or radiation

therapy, can document the extent of involvement of the brain by tumors, and can determine progression or regression of the lesions in response to treatment.
- If a tumor contains somatostatin receptors, it may be treatable with somatostatin analogs.
- To study the dynamics of CSF flow, the cisterna magna can be punctured for injection of a radioactive

tracer if more distal injections at the level of the lumbar spine are contraindicated or technically difficult.

- The brain consumes about 20% of the oxygen used by the body and requires 20% of the total cardiac output.
- The circle of Willis tends to equalize blood pressure to the brain and provides collateral blood flow.
- The BBB protects the brain from potentially toxic substances released by metabolic processes.
- Movement of substances across the BBB is controlled by active transport or by the degree of lipophilicity of a substance.
- The effect of acetylcholine is excitatory in the brain and inhibitory in the heart.
- In CNS imaging, the use of single photon–emitting radiopharmaceuticals is based on the detection of a compromised BBB.
- When measuring radioactivity in pledgets to determine the extent of a CSF leak, the results are expressed as the ratio of pledget activity (cpm) divided by the average plasma activity (cpm).
- In CNS SPECT imaging, patient preparation, including room preparation, is very important.
- SPECT or PET makes it possible to delineate the severity and extent of perfusion/metabolism abnormalities, define the precise localization and extent of tumors, confirm the site of epileptogenic lesions, identify the chemical abnormalities in the brains of patients with Parkinson's disease, and reveal characteristic patterns of different dementias.

REFERENCES

1. Bai J, Yokoyama K, Kinuya S, et al: Radionuclide cisternography in intracranial hypotension syndrome, *Ann Nucl Med* 16:75-78, 2002.
2. Baron JC: Clinical use of positron emission tomography in cerebrovascular diseases, *Neurosurg Clin N Am* 7:653-664, 1996.
3. Barrington SF, Koutroumanidis M, Agathonikou A, et al: Clinical value of "ictal" FDG-positron emission tomography and the routine use of simultaneous scalp EEG studies in patients with intractable partial epilepsies, *Epilepsia* 39:753-766, 1998.
4. Colletti PM, Siegel ME: Posttraumatic lumbar cerebrospinal fluid leak: detection by retrograde in-111-DTPA myeloscintography, *Clin Nucl Med* 6:403-404, 1981.
5. Frost JJ, Rosier AJ, Reich SG, et al: Positron emission tomographic imaging of the dopamine transporter with 11C-WIN 35,428 reveals marked declines in mild Parkinson's disease, *Ann Neurol* 34:423-431, 1993.
6. Haapaniemi TH, Ahonen A, Torniainen P, et al: [123I]beta-CIT SPECT demonstrates decreased brain dopamine and serotonin transporter levels in untreated parkinsonian patients, *Mov Disord* 16:124-130, 2001.
7. Hashimoto J, Sasaki T, Itoh Y, et al: Brain SPECT imaging using three different tracers in subacute cerebral infarction, *Clin Nucl Med* 23:275-277, 1998.
8. Heiss WD, Podreka I: Role of PET and SPECT in the assessment of ischemic cerebrovascular disease, *Cerebrovasc Brain Metab Rev* 5:235-263, 1993.
9. Henry TR, Votaw JR: The role of positron emission tomography with [18F]fluorodeoxyglucose in the evaluation of the epilepsies, *Neuroimaging Clin N Am* 14:517-535, ix, 2004.
10. Hidaka M, Matsumae M, Ito K, et al: Dynamic measurement of the flow rate in cerebrospinal fluid shunts in hydrocephalic patients, *Eur J Nucl Med* 28:888-893, 2001.
11. Hsiao CH, Kao T, Fang YH, et al: System integration and DICOM image creation for PET-MR fusion, *J Digit Imaging* 18:28-36, 2005.
12. Jauss M, Herholz K, Kracht L, et al: Frontotemporal dementia: clinical, neuroimaging, and molecular biological findings in 6 patients, *Eur Arch Psychiatry Clin Neurosci* 251:225-231, 2001.
13. Jeong Y, Cho SS, Park JM, et al: 18F-FDG PET findings in frontotemporal dementia: an SPM analysis of 29 patients, *J Nucl Med* 46:233-239, 2005.
14. Kung MP, Stevenson DA, Plossl K, et al: [99mTc]TRODAT-1: a novel technetium-99m complex as a dopamine transporter imaging agent, *Eur J Nucl Med* 24:372-380, 1997.
15. Kuzniecky R, Mountz JM, Thomas F: Ictal 99mTc HM-PAO brain single-photon emission computed tomography in electroencephalographic nonlocalizable partial seizures, *J Neuroimaging* 3:100-102, 1993.
16. Larar GN, Nagel JS: Technetium-99m-HMPAO cerebral perfusion scintigraphy: considerations for timely brain death declaration, *J Nucl Med* 33:2209-2213, 1992.
17. Laureys S, Owen AM, Schiff ND: Brain function in coma, vegetative state, and related disorders, *Lancet Neurol* 3:537-546, 2004.
18. Maria BL, Drane WE, Mastin ST, Jimenez LA: Comparative value of thallium and glucose SPECT imaging in childhood brain tumors, *Pediatr Neurol* 19:351-357, 1998.
19. Silverman DH: Brain 18F-FDG PET in the diagnosis of neurodegenerative dementias: comparison with perfusion SPECT and with clinical evaluations lacking nuclear imaging, *J Nucl Med* 45, 594-607, 2004.
20. Spieth ME, Ansari AN, Kawada TK, et al: Direct comparison of Tc-99m DTPA and Tc-99m HMPAO for evaluating brain death, *Clin Nucl Med* 19:867-872, 1994.
21. Townsend DW, Beyer T: A combined PET/CT scanner: the path to true image fusion, *Br J Radiol* 75 Spec No:S24-S30, 2002.

Endocrine System

Stanley J. Goldsmith

OBJECTIVES

After completing this chapter, the reader will be able to:
- List the organs that comprise the endocrine system, describe their anatomy and physiology, and explain the relationships of their hormonal functions.
- Discuss the radionuclides that may be used for thyroid uptake and imaging procedures relative to their advantages and disadvantages for imaging.
- Discuss the role of radioiodine uptake, thyroid scan, and whole-body imaging in the planning of radioiodine therapy.
- Discuss radionuclide therapy for the treatment of hyperthyroidism.

- Describe the role of nuclear medicine procedures in the management of thyroid carcinoma.
- Explain procedures for parathyroid imaging using dual-tracer ^{99m}Tc-sestamibi-pertechnetate subtraction and dual-phase ^{99m}Tc-sestamibi imaging.
- Discuss the role of somatostatin receptor imaging.
- Describe the use of radiopharmaceuticals for imaging the adrenergic tumors (pheochromocytoma and paraganglioma) and neuroendocrine tumors.

KEY TERMS

carcinoid tumor
endocrine system
hyperthyroidism
hypothyroidism
lingual thyroid
neuroendocrine system
neuroendocrine tumors

octreotide
pheochromocytoma
somatostatin
somatostatin analogs
somatostatin receptor (SSTR)
thyroglobulin
thyroid ablation

thyroid nodule
thyroid carcinoma
thyroid-stimulating hormone (TSH)
thyroid stunning
thyrotropin-releasing hormone
  (TRH)

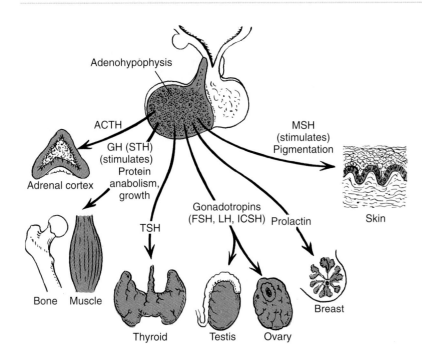

FIGURE 15-1 Anterior pituitary hormones and their target organs: adrenocorticotropic hormone (ACTH), thyroid-stimulating hormone (TSH), follicle-stimulating hormone (FSH), luteinizing hormone (LH), male analog of LH (ICSH), and melanocyte-stimulating hormone (MSH). Nuclear medicine procedures are essential elements in the evaluation of the function and structure of the thyroid gland, the parathyroid glands, the adrenal medulla, and tumors arising from the distributed neuroendocrine system. The parathyroid glands, the adrenal medulla, and neuroendocrine function are not under the direct influence of the anterior pituitary gland.

The term **endocrine system** applies to the several organs (the organs of internal secretion) whose principal function is the synthesis, storage, and secretion into the circulation of biologically active substances (hormones) that regulate diverse metabolic and biochemical processes throughout the body. The principal endocrine glands are the pituitary gland (anterior and posterior), the thyroid gland, the parathyroid glands, the islet cells of the pancreas, the adrenal glands (cortex and medulla), and the gonads (ovaries or testes) (Figure 15-1). In some instances, the secretory cells are clustered together and form distinct organs, specifically the pituitary, thyroid, and parathyroid glands, whereas in other organs the secretory cells are clustered as distinct morphological structures within organs such as the adrenal cortex or adrenal medulla within the adrenal gland, the islets of Langerhans within the exocrine pancreas, the C (parafollicular) cells within the thyroid, the Sertoli cells in the testes, and the theca interna and granulosa cells in the ovaries.

Biologically active substances are also synthesized and secreted by many cells scattered in other tissues throughout the body, such as the Kulchitsky cells distributed throughout the bowel. These cells are derived from the embryonic neural crest and are identified as neuroendocrine cells. Collectively, these cells are known as the *distributed endocrine system,* even though in normal physiology, the biologically active secretions from these cells act locally and these functions are known as *paracrine functions,* indicating local control of cell function. This includes synthesis of other biologically active molecules (peptides, amines, immunoglobulins) that influence many physiological processes nearby in contrast to the endocrine tissues that secrete hormones into the circulation.

Diagnostic nuclear medicine, both imaging and nonimaging applications, has played a significant role in the current understanding of the function and disorders of the endocrine glands, classically the thyroid, parathyroid, and adrenal glands, and more recently the distributed neuroendocrine cells. These procedures are used to monitor treatment of the disorders that affect these organs and cells, including tumors arising from them (Table 15-1).

Radioactive agents are useful also for the treatment of a number of endocrine disorders. The radionuclide iodine-131 (^{131}I) is used directly for treatment of patients with **hyperthyroidism** and **thyroid carcinoma.** ^{131}I-metaiodobenzylguanidine (^{131}I-MIBG) is used to treat metastatic **pheochromocytoma** and **paraganglioma.** Clinical trials are underway to assess the efficacy of radiolabeled peptide somatostatin receptor ligands to treat neuroendocrine tumors based on these compounds binding with high affinity to specific receptors.[17,49,81] These agents, although promising in clinical trials in the United States and Europe, are not yet available in clinical practice.

This chapter provides a review of the endocrine and distributed endocrine system: anatomy, physiology, clinical aspects, and diagnostic in vivo imaging and radionuclide therapy procedures used in clinical nuclear medicine departments. Accordingly, this chapter has been organized based on the volume and importance of nuclear medicine procedures in endocrine practice rather than the usual pituitary-to-gonad sequence used in the past. Many clinical investigations have been published that describe new positron emission tomography (PET) tracers to image endocrine organs and tumors as well as other radiolabeled molecules for targeted radionuclide therapy. These research applications are not part of

TABLE 15-1	Radiotracers Used for In Vivo Assessment of Organ Function, Clinical Diagnosis, Management, and Treatment of Endocrine Disorders		
Endocrine organ	**Diagnosis**		**Treatment**
Thyroid	^{99m}Tc-pertechnetate		^{131}I sodium iodide
	^{123}I sodium iodide		^{90}Y-DOTA TOC*
	^{131}I sodium iodide		^{90}Y-DOTA Lan*
	^{18}F-FDG		
	^{111}In-DTPA-pentetreotide		
Neuroendocrine	^{111}In-DTPA-pentetreotide		^{90}Y-DOTA TOC*
Gastroentric-pancretic NET	^{123}I-MIBG		^{90}Y-DOTA Lan*
Bronchial carcinoid	^{18}F-FDG		^{177}Lu-DOTA Tate*
	^{18}F-FDOPA*		^{111}In-DTPA-pentetreotide*
	^{11}C-hydoxytryptophan*		
	^{64}Cu-peptides*; ^{68}Ga-peptides		
Parathyroid	^{99m}Tc-MIBI		
	^{99m}Tc-MIBI and ^{99m}Tc-pertechnetate		
	^{99m}Tc-MIBI and ^{123}I		
Adrenal medulla	^{123}I-MIBG		^{131}I-MIBG*
	^{111}In-DTPA-pentetreotide		
Adrenal cortex	^{131}I-iodocholesterol (NP-59)*		
Pituitary	^{111}In-DTPA-pentetreotide		
	^{11}C-compounds*		
	^{18}F-compounds*		
Gonads	^{131}I-iodocholesterol (NP-59)*		

FDOPA, Fluro des oxy phenyl alanine; *Lan*, lanreotide; *Tate*, octreotate.
*Investigational or limited access.

current nuclear medicine practice and therefore will not be reviewed because they are beyond the scope of this chapter.

THYROID GLAND

Nuclear medicine procedures involving the thyroid are the most common procedures performed on the endocrine system organs.

Anatomy, Physiology, and Pathophysiology

The thyroid gland is located in the neck. It is usually somewhat butterfly shaped with a lobe of tissue on each side of the thyroid cartilage, joined to a variable degree in the lower portion by an isthmus of tissue (Figure 15-2). In the adult, each lobe weighs approximately 8 to 10 g. The embryonic origins of the thyroid gland involve evagination of tissue from the base of the tongue, which then migrates caudally (downward) into the neck and divides into two lobes positioned on each side of the thyroid cartilage. Occasionally, remnants of tissue remain along the migration path and are seen as an incidental finding during imaging. Asymmetrical development and a number of variations from the usual migratory path of the thyroid gland occur and are usually of no consequence. The most common evidence of the embryological descent is a small amount of midline tissue arising from the isthmus, the pyramidal lobe. The thyroid gland tissue can even develop without migrating

into the usual location in the neck, resulting in a **lingual thyroid,** a round mass of thyroid tissue at the base of the tongue (Figure 15-3). In these instances, the total amount of thyroid is usually too small to produce sufficient thyroid hormone. This results in increased secretion of **thyroid-stimulating hormone [TSH],** which promotes thyroid tissue growth and thyroid hormone secretion. The mass of tissue at the base of the tongue enlarges and may cause obstructive symptoms. Although the patient may have normal thyroid hormone levels and hence be clinically *euthyroid,* elevated serum TSH is an indication for treatment with supplemental thyroid hormone. This suppresses the elevated TSH and the tissue mass regresses. Another common but less frequently observed remnant of thyroid gland origin is the thyroglossal duct cyst, a midline cyst found superior to the thyroid, which evolves from a remnant of the embryonic duct that normally atrophies during fetal development. This remnant may or may not retain functioning thyroid tissue. If functional tissue is retained, it will be visualized on thyroid imaging.

The thyroid gland secretes the thyroid hormones thyroxine (T_4) and triiodothyronine (T_3) which regulate tissue metabolism and are essential for normal body development and maintenance of function. Thyroid hormone synthesis (Figure 15-4) depends on the trapping and organification of iodine ingested in food and water. Iodine or iodide is actively trapped by the thyroid gland by an active biochemical mechanism (the sodium-iodide transporter) and retained in the intrathyroidal iodine pool. This trapping mechanism maintains a gradient of

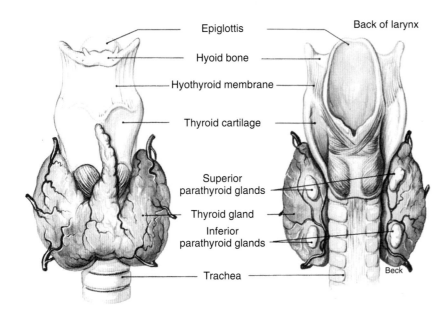

FIGURE 15-2 Thyroid and parathyroid glands in "normal" anatomical configuration. The thyroid is represented as a butterfly-shaped structure with a lobe of tissue on each side of the inferior portion of the thyroid cartilage. A prominent pyramidal lobe of the thyroid is depicted in the midline. Four parathyroid glands are illustrated in the classic superior and inferior symmetric distribution. In clinical nuclear medicine imaging of both the thyroid and parathyroid glands, considerable anatomical variation is encountered.

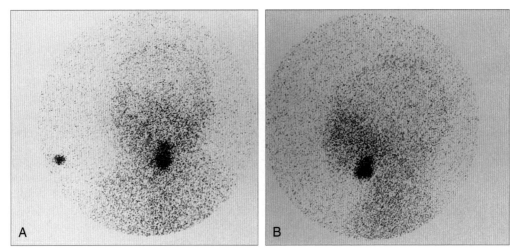

FIGURE 15-3 Lingual thyroid demonstrated in a 9-year-old child (2 mCi ^{99m}Tc-pertechnetate). Anterior view **(A)** and left lateral view **(B)** demonstrate outline of skull, facial activity, and neck. A solitary focus of radiotracer uptake is seen in the midline of the neck near the base of the tongue. No uptake is seen in the thyroid bed.

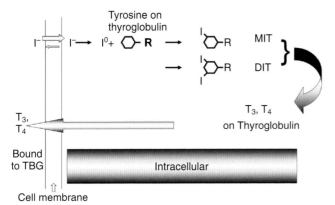

FIGURE 15-4 Schematic of iodine metabolism and synthesis of the thyroid hormones T_3 and T_4. T_3, Triiodothyronine; T_4, tetraiodothyronine; *MIT*, monoiodotyrosine; *DIT*, diiodotyrosine; *TBG*, thyroxine-binding globulin.

about 6:1 (ratio of intrathyroidal iodine to plasma iodine). In hyperthyroidism, the ratio may be as high as 10:1. Iodine in the intrathyroidal iodine pool is rapidly organified (another specific active biochemical process); that is, iodine is bound to tyrosine, which is an abundant component of the intrathyroidal protein **thyroglobulin**, forming monoiodotyrosine (MIT) and diiodotyrosine (DIT). Once iodine is bound to tyrosine, it is no longer a component of the intrathyroidal iodine pool and therefore more iodine is extracted from plasma, maintaining the gradient between the intrathyroidal iodine pool and the plasma. After organification of the iodine (by binding to the organic compound tyrosine; in essence, iodinating the tyrosine), the MIT and DIT molecules undergo an enzymatic step known as *coupling* to form triiodothyronine (T_3) and/or tetraiodothyronine (T_4). The T_3 and T_4 molecules synthesized on the protein thyroglobulin are stored until released into the circulation by proteolytic cleavage of thyroglobulin in response to TSH in the normal subject. In most instances of hyperthyroidism, T_3 and T_4 are released into the circulation without the pituitary-derived TSH stimulation. TSH-secreting tumors of the pituitary are very rare. Hence, a feature of hyperthyroidism is suppressed TSH levels. Thyroglobulin itself is a large protein that is not secreted into the circulation under normal conditions; it gains access to the circulation during inflammation of the thyroid, after interruption of vascular barriers by surgery, and in thyroid malignancies.

After secretion into the circulation, T_3 and T_4 are bound to the specific binding protein in the plasma, thyroxine-binding globulin (TBG). T_4 is bound to TBG with high affinity and only a small portion circulates as free T_4, whereas T_3 is more loosely bound. At the tissue level, the free T_4 is converted to T_3. Triiodothyronine has a direct effect on cellular metabolism, stimulating oxidation. An individual's overall metabolic status is determined by free T_4 and T_3. The total TBG and the fraction of TBG-binding sites available vary and influence the serum assays of T_4. In hyperthyroidism, T_4 and T_3 synthesis and secretion are increased, as are levels of TBG, resulting in increased plasma levels of total and free T_4 and T_3. Likewise, in **hypothyroidism** thyroid hormone secretion is decreased, as is the absolute amount of TBG, and the T_4 and T_3 levels are low.

At one time, serum total T_4 was the routine in vitro screening test of thyroid function and provided a convenient means to confirm the thyroid functional status and to identify patients with hyperfunctioning and hypofunctioning thyroids. Total T_4 is, however, only an indirect measure of thyroid function, representing predominantly the protein (TBG) bound serum T_4. Only a small fraction of the total T_4 is in the free form and the metabolic status of an individual is more directly a function of the free T_4 fraction and/or the T_3 level. Triiodothyronine is not usually described as total or free T_3, because T_3 is bound less avidly than T_4 and the overall measurement of T_3 is not influenced significantly by the amount of unsaturated TBG to the degree that T_4 levels are. The amount of TBG is regulated in part by the thyroid status of the individual so that hyperthyroid patients have increased total TBG and hypothyroid patients have decreased levels. In addition, in hyperthyroidism and hypothyroidism, the fraction of the TBG occupied by T_4 is increased or decreased consistent with the clinical state. There are occasional familial genetic factors resulting in decreased TBG even in the euthyroid state. In these situations, the subject will be euthyroid but the (total) T_4 will be low. Drugs such as estrogens increase the amount of TBG, whereas androgens decrease TBG levels. Salicylates and the anticonvulsant drug diphenylhydantoin (Dilantin) occupy binding sites on the TBG molecules, leaving fewer sites available for T_4 (or T_3) occupancy. In these instances of increased or decreased TBG binding sites, the measured T_4 value is not a reflection of the free T_4 and therefore it is not an accurate reflection of the clinical status. Free T_4 and T_3 determine the level of the body's metabolism; their values are consistent with the clinical status even if disturbances in TBG binding distort the serum total T_4 or T_3 levels.

The overall function of the thyroid gland is regulated by the hypothalamic-pituitary axis via TSH, which is secreted by the pituitary gland. The hypothalamus communicates with the pituitary via **thyrotropin-releasing hormone** (TRH). In fact, there is a servomechanism or feedback between the pituitary (and/or the hypothalamus) and the thyroid in which the pituitary has receptors for the thyroid hormones T_4 and T_3. When the pituitary and hypothalamus do not detect sufficient circulating and available thyroid hormone, TSH is secreted, maintaining and stimulating thyroid gland growth and promoting each step in thyroid hormone synthesis. When there is sufficient thyroid hormone feedback, the pituitary gland decreases the synthesis and release of TSH. Hence, low or undetectable levels of TSH suggest either pituitary gland failure (rare) or more commonly, excessive thyroid hormone production. High plasma TSH levels indicate hypothyroidism, that is, inadequate thyroid hormone levels with failure to suppress TSH. Rarely, of course, a TSH-producing pituitary tumor could secrete sufficient TSH to create the situation in which the patient has hyperthyroid symptoms, elevated serum T_4 and T_3, and elevated 24-hour thyroidal iodine uptake but with elevated TSH levels. Nevertheless, plasma TSH levels are considered to be the most sensitive means to determine thyroid gland function; regardless of serum T_4 and T_3, low TSH usually indicates excess thyroid gland function and high TSH levels indicate insufficient thyroid gland function. Direct measurement of TSH has become the procedure of choice for the diagnosis of hyperthyroidism (overfunctioning) and hypothyroidism (underfunctioning). In recent years, highly sensitive TSH assays with sensitivity as low as 0.01 mU/L have become available (so-called third-generation assays). This assay permits differentiation of low but still normal levels from thoroughly suppressed values. The TSH level is also useful to determine in patients who have undergone total thyroidectomy for thyroid carcinoma, if the dose of thyroid replacement hormone is appropriate.

A pharmacological block at the organification step of iodine metabolism provides the basis for therapy of hyperthyroidism with antithyroid drugs, such as the sulfonylureas, methimazole, and propylthiouracil. These drugs interfere also with proteolysis and release of the thyroid hormone. Organification defects occur also on a congenital basis (goitrous cretinism) as a result of enzyme deficiency, as well as after irradiation and inflammation.

Clinical Aspects

Diseases of the thyroid gland can be classified into two types: functional disorders (overactive or underactive)

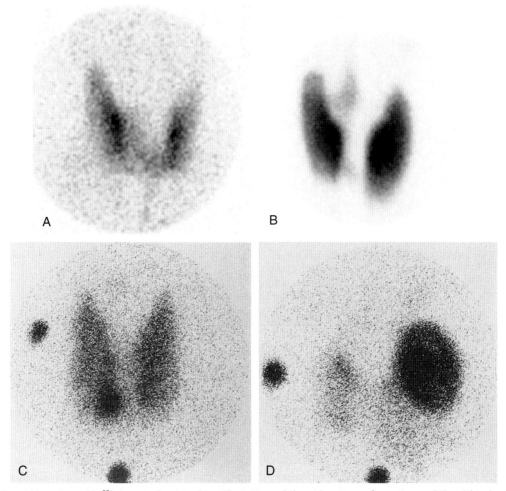

FIGURE 15-5 Thyroid imaging with ^{99m}Tc-pertechnetate (5 mCi). **A,** Normal thyroid; note configuration and thyroid-to-background activity. **B,** Hyperthyroid (Graves disease); diffuse enlargement and hyperactivity are seen. **C,** Nonsuppressed thyroid and an area of hyperfunction is seen overlying the medial aspect of the right thyroid lobe. The symmetrical right and left thyroid lobes are readily seen. **D,** Large, somewhat heterogeneous area of activity is seen on the left, representing the dominant functioning thyroid nodule, with only faint activity representing the suppressed thyroid gland.

and structural disorders (anatomical changes such as nodules). In many instances, both function and anatomy are involved; however, in other circumstances, derangement of only one or the other aspect exists. Thyroid enlargement may be associated with either an overactive or underactive thyroid. A patient with an overactive thyroid (hyperthyroidism) can have one of several anatomical findings: an enlarged thyroid, a normal-sized thyroid or a palpable nodule (Figure 15-5). A **thyroid nodule** may be associated with normal thyroid function or hyperthyroidism or it may be malignant. Changes in laboratory values also are actually nondiagnostic in many instances when viewed as an isolated result. A suppressed TSH is often indicative of hyperthyroidism providing that the clinical and other laboratory findings correlate with the diagnosis. Low to absent TSH is also indicative of hypothyroidism secondary to pituitary insufficiency, either panhypopituitarism or isolated TSH deficiency. Accordingly, for proper evaluation, it is necessary to integrate the findings from the clinical examination, laboratory results (including T_4, T_3, and TSH), and nuclear medicine procedures (uptake and scan) (Table 15-2).

The disorders of function are overactive thyroid (hyperthyroidism) and underactive thyroid (hypothyroidism). These clinical disorders have an impact on diverse body functions and may be associated with a variety of thyroid anatomical findings (gland size, presence or absence of nodules) and laboratory results (high or low TSH, 24-hour iodine uptake) (see Table 15-2). Hence, thyroid iodine uptake and function should be part of the overall assessment of the patient with known or suspected disturbed thyroid function.

HYPERTHYROIDISM

Hyperthyroidism, or thyrotoxicosis, is a clinical disorder characterized by an increase in metabolism and the effects of this increased metabolic rate on the entire body. The patient often has an increased appetite and food intake but nevertheless loses weight. Classically, patients sleep poorly, feel tired upon waking, complain

TABLE 15-2	Differential Diagnosis of Enlarged Thyroid	
Clinical Features of Hyperthyroidism	**Clinical Features of Euthyroidism (Normal)**	**Clinical Features of Hypothyroidism**
↓ TSH; T$_4$, T$_3$	Normal TSH	↑ TSH; ↓ T$_4$, T$_3$
↓ Iodine uptake	Normal T$_4$, T$_3$	↓ Iodine uptake
Diffuse increase size or hyper nodule	If ↑ T$_4$, consider estrogens, pregnancy, familial	Diffuse increase size or small; if large, congenital or acquired synthesis defect or antithyroid drugs (blocking synthesis); if small, consider chronic thyroiditis (Hashimoto), surgery, or radiation
If iodine uptake ↓, consider thyroiditis (subacute); T$_4$, T$_3$ intake; or true hyper + ↑ iodine intake	If ↓ T$_4$, consider androgens, familial, phenytoin (Dilantin), or salicylates	
If TSH is ↑, consider TSH-producing pituitary tumor	If ↑TSH, preclinical hypothyroidism If ↓ TSH, preclinical hyperthyroidism	If TSH is ↓, consider nonfunctioning pituitary (tumor)

TSH, Thyroid-stimulating hormone.

of muscle weakness and wasting, and gastrointestinal disturbances, including increased bowel frequency and diarrheal stools. They report feeling warm and having increased sweating, tremors, rapid pulse, palpitations (that may be associated with arrhythmias), and emotional outbursts. All these findings are related to increased thyroid hormone levels in the blood, which is the result of increased production and release of thyroid hormone by the thyroid gland. The most common etiology of hyperthyroidism is Graves disease, in which the thyroid is stimulated by an immunoglobulin (thyroid-stimulating immunoglobulin or TSI) that, in some instances, also stimulates receptors on the extraocular muscles, resulting in stare, lid lag, double vision, and other consequences known as *orbitopathy*. In extreme cases, vision may be threatened as a result of damage secondary to corneal dryness because the eyelids do not close properly when the patient is asleep.

Alternately, a solitary nodule (known as a *toxic nodule, toxic adenoma, solitary "hot" nodule,* or *Plummer disease*) or multiple thyroid nodules (toxic multinodular goiter [TMNG]) become autonomous and produce excessive thyroid hormones, independent of the usual TSH regulation by the pituitary (see Figure 15-5). These foci of autonomous hormone production are clinical examples of so-called G protein disease, in which the biochemical steps involved in hormone synthesis proceed without TSH receptor activation. Instead, the next step in the hormone synthesis sequence, usually stimulated by the second messenger G protein, is sustained without initial receptor stimulation by either TSH or a TSH-like immunoglobulin.[67] Specific chromosomal changes have been identified in adenomas and carcinomas, and there is incremental expression of a variety of oncogenes. At the present time, however, these observations have no clinical application.

Another basis for clinical hyperthyroidism may be subacute thyroiditis. In this instance, there is an outpouring of thyroid hormone from the inflamed thyroid into the vascular space as a result of damage to the follicular structures and increased capillary permeability. Serum T$_4$ (and T$_3$) levels are elevated but the 24-hour thyroidal iodine uptake and serum TSH are low. Other causes of clinical hyperthyroidism include extrathyroidal sources of thyroid hormone, such as surreptitious ingestion of thyroid hormone (the patient denies ingestion for complex psychological reasons) or the existence of struma ovarii, a gynecological tumor in which an ovarian tumor differentiates to form functioning thyroid tissue. In these instances, the thyroid gland is small and the thyroidal iodine uptake is low.

When the thyroid gland is the source of excessive thyroid hormone, the gland is usually diffusely enlarged, as in Graves disease, and homogeneously active. Alternatively, when hyperthyroidism is secondary to overproduction of thyroid hormone by a solitary nodule (Plummer disease) or multiple nodules (multinodular goiter), these nodules may be palpable and certainly are detected by ultrasound and seen on scintigraphy as focal areas of increased or decreased function.

HYPOTHYROIDISM

Hypothyroidism is a syndrome caused by thyroid hormone deficiency, usually as a result of failure of the thyroid gland to synthesize and release thyroid hormone. This is known as *primary hypothyroidism*. Occasionally the thyroid is intact, but TSH is deficient (so-called *secondary hypothyroidism*) either congenitally or more commonly secondary to a pituitary tumor that interferes with normal pituitary production and release of TSH.

Primary thyroid failure has a number of causes. When the thyroid gland functions inadequately, TSH rises to stimulate further production of the thyroid hormones. If the gland has been removed surgically or damaged by ^{131}I therapy or chronic inflammation, including the long-term outcome of Graves disease, there are no palpable findings. TSH is elevated but the patient does not have a goiter.

If, however, the thyroid gland TSH receptors are intact but the gland cannot efficiently produce thyroid hormone because of either a congenital or acquired defect such as an organification defect, serum TSH rises and further stimulates thyroid gland growth; the gland enlarges but the patient gradually develops hypothyroidism. Unless the TSH stimulation is suppressed by thyroid hormone replacement therapy, TSH elevation continues, and further growth of the inefficient thyroid occurs. When patients take an antithyroid drug (propylthiouracil [PTU], methimazole [Tapazole]) as therapy for hyperthyroidism, thyroid hormone synthesis is blocked. As the T_4 and T_3 levels are reduced, TSH secretion will occur in response to the normalized or low thyroid hormone levels. If excess antithyroid drugs are administered, TSH will rise above normal, stimulating thyroid tissue growth as well as synthesis of thyroid hormones. The thyroid will enlarge. Hence the term *goitrogenic drugs*.

Hypothyroidism with an enlarged thyroid may occur in children with inherited metabolic defects of thyroid hormone synthesis, the so-called goitrous cretins. More commonly an enlarged thyroid (goiter) and hypothyroidism are seen in older patients with acquired defects of the thyroid hormone synthesizing enzymes as a result of thyroiditis or subclinical autoimmune thyroiditis. Hence, an enlarged thyroid gland can be seen in hypothyroidism as well as in hyperthyroidism (Graves disease or toxic multinodular goiter), and hypothyroidism may occur in patients with an enlarged thyroid as well as those without thyroid tissue.

THYROID NODULES

The second category of thyroid disorders is structural: palpable masses in the region of the thyroid without (or with) clinical alterations of thyroid function due to thyroid hormone overproduction or underproduction. In this instance the concern is whether the palpable finding represents malignancy. In the past, nuclear imaging was used early in the evaluation to identify whether the mass was either functional (that is, the mass trapped tracer and therefore was designated as hot or warm versus nonfunctional as indicated by the absence of tracer, which was designated as cold). Functional nodules were invariably benign (usually a functioning adenoma or

a palpable nodule in a multinodular goiter) with an incidence of malignancy no greater than that found in the general population. In the event the patient has a thyroid scan to evaluate a palpable nodule instead of going directly to ultrasound and needle biopsy, a cold nodule is suspect for thyroid carcinoma until proven otherwise. Thyroid carcinoma is found in 25% to 35% of the cold nodules. The remainder are nonfunctioning adenomas, focal areas of thyroiditis (usually chronic) or cysts. At the present time, patients with palpable nodules are often referred for sonography and fine needle aspiration (FNA) without undergoing nuclear medicine imaging with either ^{123}I-iodide or ^{99m}Tc-pertechnetate. If malignancy is suspected based on cytological examination of the thin needle aspirate, the patient is referred for surgery. The patient is usually referred to nuclear medicine 6 weeks after subtotal or near total thyroidectomy either for ablation of the surgical remnant or imaging evaluation of residual thyroid tissue before ablation with ^{131}I.

THYROID CANCER

Thyroid carcinoma is the most common endocrine neoplasm, and mortality from thyroid carcinoma exceeds mortality from all other malignant endocrine tumors. The overall incidence of differentiated thyroid carcinoma has increased steadily in the United States and Western Europe. At autopsy it is a common finding, detected in 3% to 10% of the population. Nevertheless, thyroid cancer accounts for less than 1% of all deaths from malignancy. Differentiated thyroid carcinoma includes papillary carcinoma, follicular variant of papillary carcinoma, and follicular carcinoma. Papillary carcinoma accounts for approximately two thirds of the cases of differentiated thyroid carcinoma, follicular carcinoma for the other third. Together these two histopathological classifications account for 95% of the malignancies involving the thyroid, the remainder consisting of anaplastic carcinoma, medullary carcinoma (actually a malignancy of the thyroid C cells; see later section, Neuroendocrine System), lymphoma, and metastatic adenocarcinomas. The significance of differentiating between papillary and follicular carcinoma is that follicular carcinoma is more apt to spread by vascular invasion to distal sites including the skeleton, whereas papillary carcinoma is more apt to spread via lymphatics to regional and subsequently mediastinal lymph nodes and the lungs. These differences, however, are statistical and any individual patient may have an atypical clinical course. Accordingly, management often has to be individualized based upon patient-specific characteristics. It is useful to categorize patients at diagnosis as low risk, intermediate risk, or high risk based upon a number of clinical factors including age; gender; size of the primary tumor; histopathological findings, such as extrathyroidal extension; specific histological features, such as tall cell variant; lymph node involvement; and presence or

TABLE 15-3	Thyroid Cancer Management Based on Risk Assessment	
Low-Risk Patient	**Medium-High Risk Patient**	**Known Metastases**
^{123}I scan; Tg	^{123}I scan; Tg	^{131}I dosimetry → determine MTD
If no "surprise," treat ^{131}I, 50-75 mCi	If no "surprise," treat ^{131}I, 100-150 mCi	Prescribe MTD ^{131}I
WB scan, 1 week post-treatment	WB scan, 1 week post-treatment	WB scan, 1 week postprescription
Monitor Tg	Monitor Tg	Monitor Tg
At 1 year, follow-up with rTSH Tg, ^{123}I or ^{131}I scan	At 1 year, follow-up with rTSH Tg, ^{123}I or ^{131}I scan	At 6-12 months, ^{131}I WB scan and/or repeat dosimetry, MTD prescribe PRN
If negative, continue to monitor rTSH stimulated Tg q year; scan PRN	If negative, continue to monitor rTSH stimulated Tg q year; scan at increasing intervals	Reevaluate at 6-12 months Assess age, renal function if doses greater than 150 mCi are considered

Tg, Thyroglobulin; *MTD*, maximal tolerated dose; *WB*, whole body; *rTSH*, recombinant thyroid-stimulating hormone; *PRN*, as necessary.

absence of metastases.[32] Rather than propose a uniform protocol for all patients, it seems appropriate to outline a course of management based on the variation in clinical presentation and assessment of risk (Table 15-3).

Within the thyroid, thyroid carcinoma is seen as a cold area because even differentiated malignant tissue generally functions less efficiently (less iodine trapping) than normal thyroid tissue (Figure 15-6). After thyroidectomy, of course, the ability of differentiated thyroid carcinoma to trap and organify iodine provides the basis for identification of metastases, surveillance, and therapy. Other malignancies such as medullary carcinoma, undifferentiated carcinoma, lymphoma, and metastases to the thyroid are also identified as cold nodules, but after detection and removal, ^{131}I is not used in their management and therapy.

After appropriate preparation, the patient is referred to the nuclear medicine service for diagnostic imaging to determine the amount and location of residual thyroid tissue or tumor based on the ability of this tissue to concentrate radioiodine (see Table 15-3). For effective evaluation and identification of residual thyroid tissue or tumor, steps should be taken to raise the plasma TSH before administration of the diagnostic tracer. This is accomplished in one of several ways: by not replacing thyroid hormone after total thyroidectomy, by discontinuing replacement thyroid hormone if the patient has been receiving it, or by injection of recombinant human TSH (rhTSH) (Thyrogen, Genzyme, Cambridge, Mass.).

Thyroid carcinoma presents in a variety of ways:

- A suspicious nodule without evidence of local or distal spread
- A large nodule without additional evidence of disease
- With cervical lymph node involvement (clinical, surgical, or scan evidence)
- Vascular invasion (histopathological finding)

- Invasion of soft tissues adjacent to the thyroid (clinical, surgical, or scan finding)
- Finding of advanced disease on scanning with metastases to mediastinal lymph nodes, the lungs, or skeleton (x-ray or scan finding)
- Metastatic involvement as the reason for initial presentation (clinical or x-ray)
- Symptomatic metastases after a long interval following initial diagnosis and treatment

This variety of possible clinical and pathological scenarios is the basis for risk categorization.[69] Since there are so many management and treatment options involving nuclear medicine (and laboratory procedures), a patient-specific approach based largely on risk assessment is recommended in Table 15-3.

In Vitro Procedures

The first direct assays of T_4 and T_3 were performed by a competitive binding technique using thyroxine-binding globulin as the binding protein and radiolabeled T_4 and T_3. Subsequently, the thyroxine-binding globulin was replaced by specific monoclonal antibodies with greater sensitivity and specificity. This technique, radioimmunoassay, was often performed in nuclear medicine laboratories.[14,15] Over time alternatives to radiolabeled T_4 and T_3 as the signalling molecules were replaced by fluorometric and other techniques that were easier to automate. Currently, these procedures are performed in clinical chemistry laboratories and are no longer components of nuclear medicine technology.

Nuclear Medicine Procedures

In vivo function tests and imaging: In vivo tests for evaluating thyroid function are based on the usual association of the degree of iodine uptake and overall thyroid

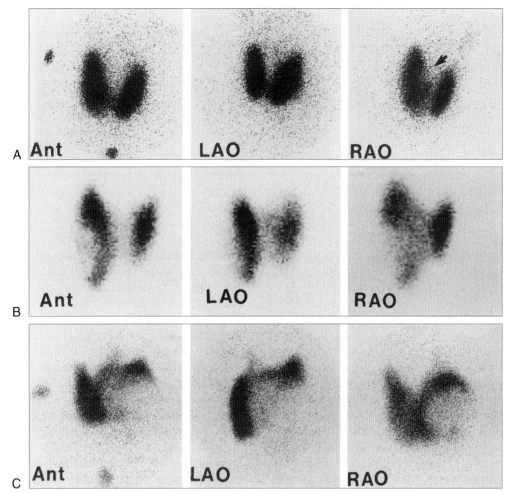

FIGURE 15-6 Three-view thyroid scintigraphy (^{99m}Tc-pertechnetate): anterior, left anterior oblique, and right anterior oblique views in three different patients demonstrating a solitary cold nodule of various sizes. **A,** Small defect (cold nodule) corresponding to a palpable nodule *(arrow)* is seen on the medial aspect of the right thyroid lobe in the right anterior oblique view. Oblique views increase the sensitivity of thyroid scintigraphy for the detection of small cold nodules, which might not be seen in the anterior projection alone. **B,** Moderately large (3 × 1 cm) cold nodule in the lower portion of the right lobe. **C,** Large (5 × 4 cm) cold nodule replacing most of the left thyroid lobe. *Ant,* Anterior; *LAO,* left anterior oblique; *RAO,* right anterior oblique.

function. The most common of these is the thyroid uptake test. Thyroid gland imaging is performed to determine the size, location, and function of the thyroid gland and to evaluate palpable findings near, on, or within the thyroid gland[8] (see Figures 15-5 and 15-6).

Radionuclides

Iodine-131 (^{131}I). The use of radioactive isotopes of iodine to perform in vivo thyroid function tests and thyroid imaging is based on the unique avidity of the thyroid gland for iodine. These procedures were initially performed with ^{131}I, an isotope of iodine that was readily available because it is produced either as a fission product or by neutron bombardment in nuclear reactors. With a physical half-life of 8.1 days, ^{131}I is practical for distribution and storage in nuclear medicine departments equipped with adequate shielding for the energetic 364-keV gamma emission. In addition to the radiation

safety concerns, currently there is increased emphasis on security of radioactive materials and renewed emphasis on the requirement that radioactive materials are to be securely stored. Practically, this requires a locked radiopharmacy or radioactive material storage room.

Iodine-131 decays by beta decay with the emission of a beta particle and several gamma rays, the most abundant of which is a 364-keV gamma emission. The 364-keV gamma emission is the signal detected in thyroid uptake studies. ^{131}I was used as a thyroid imaging agent for many years but it has been replaced for imaging the intact thyroid by ^{99m}Tc-pertechnetate and ^{123}I-iodine. It is no longer appropriate to use ^{131}I to image the thyroid gland although ^{131}I is the agent of choice for whole-body surveillance following thyroidectomy in patients with the diagnosis of differentiated thyroid carcinoma.

The beta particle emission from ^{131}I is the basis for radionuclide therapy of hyperthyroidism, for thyroid remnant ablation and thyroid cancer treatment but it is

TABLE 15-4	Physical Characteristics and Absorbed Doses of Radionuclides Used in Thyroid Imaging and Diagnostic Studies						

						centiGrey (rad)	
Nuclide	Dose Administered	$t_{1/2}$	Emission	Energy (keV)		Thyroid	Whole Body
[131]I	5 to 10 mCi	8.1 days	Gamma, beta	364		1.2*	0.05 to 0.1
	100 mCi					20*	1
[123]I	200 mCi	13 hours	Gamma	159		0.5 to 2.0	0.06
	400 mCi					1.0 to 4.0	0.12
[99m]Tc	4 mCi	6 hours	Gamma	140		<1	<0.1

*Assumes average body and thyroid weight, thyroid turnover, and 20% uptake.
Rad, Radiation absorbed dose.

no longer appropriate as a diagnostic tracer. In doses of 5 to 50 μCi, the radiation absorbed dose to the thyroid is acceptable for diagnostic uptake and turnover studies.

Iodine-123 (^{123}I). Iodine-123 decays by electron capture (EC) to tellurium-123 ([123]Te); two high-energy gamma photons are emitted with energies of 529 keV (abundance ~1.4%) and 505 keV (abundance ~0.32%). Subsequently, the [123]Te emits a 159-keV gamma photon with an abundance of 83.3%. This 159-keV gamma emission, therefore, is the principal emission. For thyroid imaging, a pinhole collimator is usually used. Pinhole collimators are relatively energy independent, although there is some loss of resolution when higher energy radionuclides are used. When whole body imaging is performed with a low-energy collimator, the high-energy photons degrade the images; better quality images are obtained with a medium-energy collimator. Nevertheless, it is common practice to use a low energy collimator when parallel hole collimator whole body imaging is performed.

[99m]Tc-Pertechnetate. Thyroid imaging is most often performed using ^{99m}Tc-pertechnetate.[1,3,7,33] The charge and size of the pertechnetate ion are sufficiently similar to the iodide ion to be recognized by the thyroidal iodine trap. Consequently, ^{99m}Tc-pertechnetate enters the intrathyroidal iodine pool. Technetium-99m-pertechnetate is not organically bound, however, and cannot be used to measure uptake in the traditional sense. ^{99m}Tc-pertechnetate uptakes have been performed but because it is not organified, the ^{99m}Tc-pertechnetate washes out of the thyroid after reaching peak intrathyroidal concentration at about 20 minutes. Approximately 5% of the administered intravenous dose is localized by that time. The technique is not widely used.

Technetium-99m-pertechnetate is an ideal choice for thyroid imaging because of its 6-hour half-life and 140-keV gamma emission. It is readily available either from a molybdenum generator or purchased daily in bulk.[3] ^{99m}Tc-pertechnetate has several advantages over ^{131}I and even ^{123}I as a thyroid imaging agent. The 140-keV gamma emission of ^{99m}Tc is more efficiently detected by the ⅜- to ½-inch scintillation camera crystal than is the 364-keV gamma photon of [131]I. The short physical half-life and isomeric transition mode of decay of ^{99m}Tc results in a more favorable patient radiation absorbed dose than [131]I. Combined with low cost, this permits routine use of several (4 to 10) mCi of ^{99m}Tc-pertechnetate for diagnostic studies that provide better image quality than possible with ^{131}I and often better than [123]I. A typical scanning dose of [131]I (100 μCi) results in an absorbed dose to the adult thyroid of 20 rad, assuming a 20% uptake and typical turnover rate, and a 1-rad whole-body dose, whereas a 4-mCi dose of ^{99m}Tc-pertechnetate yields an absorbed dose of less than 1 rad to the thyroid and a whole-body absorbed dose of 0.1 rad (Table 15-4).

In summary, ^{99m}Tc-pertechnetate provides excellent quality images at great convenience to the nuclear medicine service and the patient and is currently widely used for thyroid imaging. These images identify the size and location of thyroid tissue. Images are obtained 15 to 20 minutes after injection. The concern that because ^{99m}Tc-pertechnetate is trapped but not organified, it might provide misleading information about whether a nodule is hot or cold is not relevant because thyroid carcinoma characteristically traps poorly compared to normal thyroid. This is the basis for the cold nodule.

In patients with thyroid carcinoma, ^{99m}Tc-pertechnetate may be used to image the thyroid bed remnant after surgery, but it is not useful to detect metastatic disease because its short physical and biological half-life in the thyroid makes detection difficult when combined with the fact that trapping itself is often reduced in thyroid carcinoma compared to normal thyroid tissue.

^{99m}Tc-MIBI. ^{99m}Tc-sestamibi or ^{99m}Tc-MIBI (methoxyisobutyl isonitrile) is a lipid soluble radiotracer commonly used for myocardial perfusion scintigraphy. It distributes proportional to blood flow and is rapidly extracted (extraction efficiency approximately 0.65) and passes the cell membrane binding to mitochondrial proteins. Because the thyroid is a metabolically active organ, there is rapid and vigorous thyroid uptake of this tracer followed by slow washout over hours. [99m]Tc- MIBI is commonly used in parathyroid adenoma localization because it is vigorously extracted by both thyroid and parathyroid tissue. The tracer has been used also to further a cold nodule identified on ^{99m}Tc-pertechnetate or ^{123}I-iodide scintigraphy. Solid tumors that trap iodine (or pertechnetate) poorly will localize ^{99m}Tc-MIBI; hence the so-called flip-flop phenomenon. As thyroid ultrasound has become more readily available, ^{99m}Tc-MIBI thyroid scintigraphy is less commonly performed.

Fluorine-18 (^{18}F)-FDG. Fluorine-18-FDG PET is widely used in patients with neoplasms for the determination of the extent of disease, evaluation of response to therapy and surveillance following therapy. Hypermetabolic foci in the thyroid gland are observed as an incidental finding. Biopsy of these areas identifies thyroid carcinoma in 30% to 90% of these cases leading to the recommendation that hypermetabolic foci identified as an incidental finding should be further evaluated. It has also been shown that differentiated thyroid carcinoma increases anaerobic glucose metabolism as it dedifferentiates.[86,87]

Accordingly, ^{18}F-FDG is recommended as a diagnostic imaging tool in patients with proven thyroid carcinoma with elevated serum thyroglobulin and negative whole-body ^{131}I scans. If the metastatic foci are limited in number and surgically accessible, the observation makes surgical removal possible provided there is no other evidence of inoperable disease. The degree of ^{18}F-FDG uptake in metastatic thyroid carcinoma has prognostic significance. Increased anaerobic glucose metabolism (demonstrated by increased ^{18}F-FDG uptake) is indicative of more aggressive tumor and a poor prognosis.[86] It is likely that ^{18}F-FDG PET imaging will have a regular role in the management of patients with thyroid carcinoma, particularly in those with metastatic disease.

Indium-111 (^{111}In)-DTPA-Pentetreotide. This tracer identifies organs, tissues, and tumors that express **somatostatin receptor (SSTR)** and is used classically to identify the extent of disease and to localize **neuroendocrine tumors.** Diffuse activity may be seen in apparently clinically normal thyroid glands depending upon the imaging technique. At the present time, there are no explicit criteria to define normal versus diffusely increased activity. Nevertheless, diffuse increased activity is seen in thyroiditis, especially chronic Hashimoto type with lymphocytic infiltration because lymphocytes express SSTRs. Focal accumulation of ^{111}In-DTPA-pentetreotide is suspicious for the C-cell derived medullary carcinoma of the thyroid that also has increased expression of SSTRs. Differentiated papillary and follicular carcinomas, although not of neuroendocrine origin, have also been identified as expressing SSTRs.

Thyroid Iodine Uptake

Thyroidal iodine uptake (24-hour iodine uptake) is a frequently requested in vivo nuclear medicine procedure to assess or confirm thyroid function, particularly in patients suspected of having hyperthyroidism based upon either symptoms or confirmatory lab tests, particularly suppressed TSH. Availability of TSH assays in routine clinical screening examinations has identified more patients with abnormal values; either suppressed values representing hyperthyroidism or conversely, elevated TSH suggestive of hypothyroidism. Because of the sensitivity of the TSH assay, many patients have been identified with one or the other condition while their symptoms are quite mild. The entities subclinical hyperthyroidism and subclinical hypothyroidism are used in these circumstances where the presentation is based upon an abnormal TSH level rather than clinical symptoms. This has led to increased use of the 24-hour thyroidal iodine uptake to confirm suspected thyroid dysfunction based on screening TSH values. While useful for this purpose, the thyroidal iodine uptake is affected by dietary and other sources of increased iodine intake. Iodine deficiency will result in an elevated iodine uptake. It is unusual in the United States to observe iodine deficiency because iodine is readily available in foods. For many years, table salt has been supplemented with sodium iodide. Nevertheless, from time to time, iodine deficiency is observed because of bizarre dietary practices. Patients with elevated TSH values are usually treated with thyroid hormone replacement.

In patients thought to be hyperthyroid based on symptoms, elevated serum T_4, and suppressed TSH, the thyroidal iodine uptake is of value to differentiate between thyroiditis, in which case the thyroidal iodine uptake will be low compared to Graves disease, multinodular goiter, and autonomous adenomata. Even in hyperthyroid patients with Graves disease or multinodular goiter, dietary or medicinal iodine ingestion may lower the 24-hour uptake to a level that precludes ^{131}I therapy at that time. The patient should be placed on a low iodine diet and reevaluated after 2 to 3 weeks.

Careful technique is essential so that results accurately reflect patient variables rather than technical variables. Thyroid iodine uptake is, in fact, a nonspecific measure of thyroid function, because the value is influenced by factors other than intrinsic thyroid function, specifically total iodine intake. The 24-hour uptake is increased when there is inadequate daily dietary iodine; conversely, the 24-hour thyroidal iodine uptake is low when patients have increased their dietary iodine, taken supplements or medication containing iodine, or have recently undergone x-ray studies with iodinated contrast material.

Over the past 50 years, ingestion of dietary iodine in the United States has increased in general as a result of the use of iodized salt, improved availability and increased preference for saltwater fish, dietary fads and supplements, iodinated preservatives in food (e.g., white bread), and iodinated compounds in food dyes and medication. These phenomena have produced a decrease in 24-hour thyroid iodine uptake values independent of the level of thyroid function.

Dietary fads may also result in iodine-deficient diets resulting in markedly elevated 24-hour thyroidal iodine uptake. The wide regional variation in dietary iodine observed throughout the United States would seem to suggest that no single, published figure or range can be accepted for the normal 24-hour thyroid iodine uptake. Nevertheless, if there is no history of exposure to excess dietary iodine (e.g., kelp, mineral supplements) or iodinated organic compounds (contrast media), the thyroid iodine uptake is expected to be increased in hyperthyroidism, reflecting increased thyroid function, and decreased in hypothyroidism, reflecting decreased thyroid function. In general, values below 12% are considered low at this time and require explanation usually by correlation with history. Any 24-hour thyroid uptake values in excess of 25% should be considered suspicious and are certainly compatible with hyperthyroidism. In hyperthyroid patients, values of 35% to 95% are typically observed.

Occasionally, a patient presents with rapid onset of symptoms of hyperthyroidism, abnormal elevations of serum T_3 and T_4, and appropriate suppression of TSH but is found to have very low iodine uptake. In these instances, so-called subacute thyroiditis should be considered. It is not appropriate (or possible) to treat these patients with radioactive iodine.

Thyroidal iodine uptake is most commonly performed with 5 to 10 μCi of ^{131}I. The uptake can be measured at any time after administration of radioiodine but approximately 24 hours has evolved to be the most practical and reliable interval because it provides better discrimination between hyperthyroid, euthyroid, and hypothyroid populations than earlier time points.[8] In addition, 24 hours is usually long enough after oral administration to minimize differences caused by variations in the rate of gastrointestinal absorption. Uptake values do vary because of bioavailability depending on the type of radioiodine preparation used (e.g., liquid is absorbed more rapidly than capsules). There are variations in the degree of digestion, and the rate of absorption of capsules from different manufacturers is still observed.[51] In the euthyroid subject, orally administered radioiodine uptake has usually reached a plateau at 18 to 20 hours and is stable for several hours thereafter.

The thyroid uptake probe contains a 1- to 2-inch sodium iodide crystal with open-face collimation. Standards should be counted in an appropriate phantom. The Society of Nuclear Medicine has published consensus procedure guidelines on the issues involved in performing this procedure (Box 15-1).[8]

The thyroid uptake test is billable as a stand-alone procedure or in combination with a thyroid scan. Most frequently, physicians request a thyroid uptake and scan. In most instances, this is typically performed using 4.0 mCi of ^{99m}Tc-pertechnetate for imaging, followed by 5 μCi of ^{131}I given orally with the patient returning the next day for the 24-hour thyroid iodine uptake.

BOX 15-1 | **Thyroid Uptake (^{123}I or ^{131}I)**

1. Ask patient about the following: possible interfering medications, such as thyroid hormone, antithyroid medication, and vitamins or mineral supplements; recent x-rays with contrast; pregnancy or nursing; and other recent nuclear medicine procedures.
2. Count standard and record value.
3. Administer ^{131}I (5 to 10 μCi) or ^{123}I (200 to 300 μCi) orally
4. At 18-24 hr after administration, count standard for 1-2 min at fixed distance from crystal surface in uptake probe.
5. Count patients neck at same distance (25 to 30 cm) from crystal surface. Perform similar count over thigh.
6. Neck counts – Thigh counts/Standard counts × 100 = Thyroid uptake
7. Procedure can be performed at earlier or later time intervals as relevant to clinical situation.

Perchlorate Discharge and Thiocyanate Washout Tests

These procedures are infrequently performed in current practice. They are used to demonstrate a thyroidal organification defect that is now usually of academic interest. Patients with an organification defect have clinical features of thyroid enlargement and elevated TSH levels. They may or may not be clinically euthyroid but the organification defect renders the thyroid less efficient in thyroid hormone production.

Accordingly, the TSH level increases to maintain adequate synthesis of the thyroid hormones and clinical euthyroid status. Consequently, the thyroid gland enlarges. Treatment with thyroid hormone replacement therapy based on these findings is usual without the need to demonstrate an organification defect.

Nevertheless, if desirable to demonstrate the existence of an organification defect in a nodule, the perchlorate discharge test is performed with a small dose of radioactive iodine (usually 5 to 20 mCi ^{131}I; the procedure could also be performed with a small amount of ^{123}I) given orally (or intravenously if sterile, pyrogen-free tracer is available). Counts are recorded over the thyroid bed with a thyroid uptake probe. When the radioiodine is administered by mouth, counts are usually taken every 15 to 30 minutes for 1 to 2 minutes for approximately 2 hours. When sterile pyrogen-free material is available for IV administration, more frequent counting is performed: every minute if a dynamic recording device is available or at 5-minute intervals if interval counting is done. The 2-hour recording period allows sufficient time for thyroid uptake of the tracer iodine, which will take place based upon iodine trapping regardless of whether an organification defect is present. At 2 hours after ^{131}I has been administered, 600 to 1000 mg of potassium perchlorate is administered orally. The perchlorate ion competes with circulating iodide ion at the thyroid trap, blocking entry of additional ^{131}I (see Figures 15-4 and

15-7). In normal subjects the count rate remains stable over the next several measurements because the trapped iodine has been organified. If an organification defect exists, a significant decrease in the count rate (10% to 50% or more) is observed because the unbound ^{131}I washes out of the intrathyroidal iodine pool and is replaced by perchlorate ion (Figure 15-7). Because the perchlorate displaces the unbound radioiodine, the procedure is called the *perchlorate discharge test*. The thiocyanate washout test is based on the same principle as the perchlorate discharge test except that the thiocyanate is injected intravenously because it is available in sterile vials. The perchlorate washout test has been used also to demonstrate the degree of organification defect induced by antithyroid drugs such as PTU or methimazole.

Thyroid Imaging

Thyroid imaging is performed with a gamma camera and a pinhole collimator. It is most commonly performed at approximately 20 minutes after 5 mCi of ^{99m}Tc-pertechnetate is injected intravenously. Zoomed images obtained with a parallel-hole collimator should not be used to evaluate thyroid nodules because small (~1 cm) cold nodules may not be detected.

With pinhole collimation, image size varies with distance. The pinhole collimator should be used at a fixed distance from the surface so that some uniformity is established within a department (Figure 15-8). Physicians and technologists become accustomed to the usual image size and recognize enlarged lobes or glands to get an objective measure of size. It is useful to take additional images with a marker within the field of view. Regardless of the specific distance of the camera crystal surface to the thyroid, the marker provides an internal calibration by which estimates of organ dimensions and a calculation of area (or volume) can be made. In the author's department, a ruler with 1-cm alternating blocks of cobalt-57 (^{57}Co) and lead provide an objective means to assess thyroid size independent of the distance of the camera from the patient's skin surface, the only

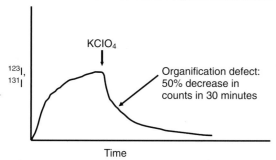

Perchlorate washout test for organification defect

^{123}I, ^{131}I

KClO$_4$

Organification defect: 50% decrease in counts in 30 minutes

Time

FIGURE 15-7 Perchlorate washout test: schematic drawing of data (counts versus time) following oral radioiodine. At 2 hours, potassium perchlorate is administered by mouth, blocking further iodine trapping (temporarily). In the normal situation, the counts remain stable as the trapped iodine has been rapidly organified. In the patient with an organification defect, the counts decrease as the nonorganified radioiodine is free to washout, that is, to exchange for nonradioactive iodine in the plasma as the plasma radioiodine is present in lower concentration at 2 hours because of excretion.

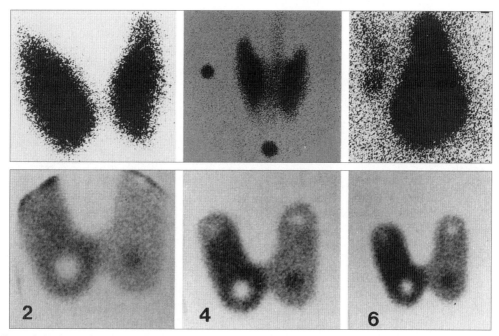

FIGURE 15-8 Effect of distance of pinhole collimator on scintigraphic thyroid gland size: Images are shown at 2, 4, and 6 cm from the surface of the thyroid phantom. As the pinhole collimator comes closer to the imaged object, the recorded image becomes larger. Accordingly, conclusions about gland size require simultaneous imaging of a source of known size or correlation with findings on palpation.

remaining variable being the distance of the thyroid below the neck surface.

A variety of pinhole inserts are available. The diameter of the aperture of the insert determines the spatial resolution of the system. As usual, there is a trade-off between sensitivity and resolution, with sensitivity decreasing as the aperture diameter decreases and the resolution improves.

Iodine-123 thyroid images are acquired for 10 minutes in the anterior, right anterior oblique, and left anterior oblique projections. In addition, it is a frequent practice to obtain a second anterior view with either a size marker or a sternal notch marker or both. Images with 100,000 counts suitable for thyroid gland scintigraphy are usually obtained in the euthyroid or hyperthyroid patient for 10 minutes at 20 hours after ^{123}I administration.[7,50] A typical adult scanning dose of 200 to 300 µCi results in a thyroid absorbed dose of 1 to 4 rad and a whole-body absorbed dose of 0.12 rad. Imaging of the thyroid can be performed as early as 2 to 4 hours but is best performed at 24 hours after oral administration. Quantification of uptake can also be performed at that time. There are difficulties, however, in using ^{123}I to measure uptake at 24 hours and many practitioners continue to use microcurie doses of ^{131}I for thyroid iodine uptake even when ^{123}I is used for thyroid imaging.

The Society of Nuclear Medicine has published a consensus procedure guideline on technical recommendations for thyroid scintigraphy (Box 15-2).[7] In addition to the anterior projection obtained with the pinhole at a consistent distance from the neck, additional anterior views should be obtained at greater distances if necessary to ensure inclusion of the entire gland. Alternately, the patient can be reimaged with a parallel-hole collimator after obtaining oblique pinhole views. Oblique views better define nodules that may be on the anterior or posterior surface of the gland and thus obscured by activity within the normal lobe. It is customary to obtain an anterior image and both right and left anterior (45-degree) oblique views (see Figure 15-6). The sternal notch should be identified, usually by obtaining an additional image with a marker at the notch. In addition, right-left orientation should be identified by placing an additional marker on the right side. The images should be reviewed by the nuclear medicine physician before the patient leaves. The image findings should be correlated with the palpable findings. Activity in palpable nodules is compared to the remainder of the gland characterized as either increased (warm or hot) or decreased (cold) in activity.

The principal reason to image a thyroid with palpable findings is to determine if a palpable nodule is cold, hot, or similar in function to the reminder of the thyroid. Of solitary cold nodules, 20% to 30% are malignant, most commonly differentiated thyroid carcinoma. Recently it was reported that even in multinodular goiters, 10% of the dominant cold nodules contained malignant cells. Accordingly, cold nodules should be biopsied and followed clinically even if the initial biopsy is benign. Depending on a number of factors, including age, gender, palpable findings, and patient anxiety, it is sometimes appropriate to have the nodule removed for thorough histological examination. If it is found to be malignant, the patient should undergo subtotal or total thyroidectomy, depending on other risk factors and local surgical practice and skill.

In some settings it may be desirable to observe these nodules, in which case the patient should receive exogenous thyroid hormone to therapeutically suppress the gland. This course can be chosen in chronic thyroiditis (if thyroid antibodies are found) on the premise that the nodule represents a focal area of organification defect secondary to Hashimoto involvement, as opposed to malignancy. Multiple nodules can be uniformly active or can vary in activity. In the clinically euthyroid patient, this usually represents a post–Hashimoto thyroiditis. These patients may have elevated TSH, a compensatory response to the inefficient handling of iodine and thyroid hormone synthesis. The differential diagnosis of a cold nodule includes adenoma, cyst, focal thyroiditis, and hemorrhage.

A solitary warm nodule is likely to represent a functioning adenoma (see Figure 15-5). The remainder of the thyroid gland may be visible, indicating that the adenoma is not functioning at a level sufficient to suppress TSH. Alternatively, the scan may reveal a warm nodule with suppression of the remainder of the gland even in the clinically euthyroid patient. The only evidence of hyperthyroidism may be a suppressed TSH. Of course, a solitary hot nodule may be found in a patient who is hyperthyroid. This is also called *toxic nodule* or *Plummer disease*. Alternatively, a solitary area of thyroid tissue can

---

BOX 15-2　Thyroid Scan (^{123}I or ^{99m}Tc-Pertechnetate)

1. Query patient about pregnancy, breast-feeding, thyroid medications, and recent nuclear medicine procedures.
2. Administer ^{123}I (200-500 µCi) orally or ^{99m}Tc-pertechnetate (4-6 mCi) intravenously.
3. ^{123}I imaging at 4 hr or 18-24 hr or both; ^{99m}Tc-pertechnetate imaging begins at 15-20 min after injection.
4. Use pinhole collimator positioned properly at distance to assure entire thyroid appears in field of view. If usual pattern or size is observed, consult with nuclear medicine physician.
5. ^{99m}Tc-pertechnetate acquisition: 100,000-200,000 count image in anterior position or 5-min acquisition (whichever is first).
6. ^{123}I acquisition: 50,000-100,000 or 10-min acquisition (whichever is first).
7. For both ^{99m}Tc-pertechnetate and ^{123}I: Repeat acquisition for similar time in right anterior oblique (RAO) and left anterior oblique (LAO) position. Some departments acquire an additional anterior view with a marker or ruler.

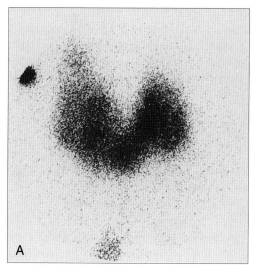 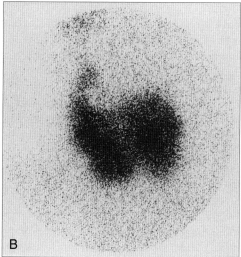

FIGURE 15-9 Multinodular goiter in a patient with Hashimoto disease. Pinhole collimator, anterior views in the same patient, 9 months apart. Occasionally discrepancies are seen in areas that trap pertechnetate but do not organify iodine. **A,** 400 mCi [123]I. **B,** 4 mCi ^{99m}Tc-pertechnetate.

represent a surgical remnant or an anatomical variant in which only one lobe or a portion of a lobe developed congenitally. After thyroidectomy for carcinoma, a solitary focus can represent residual thyroid tissue or tumor. For these reasons the patient history contributes to the scan interpretation and differential diagnosis.

Significant discrepancies in the focal findings of ^{99m}Tc-pertechnetate and radioiodine images have been observed in Hashimoto thyroiditis. Figure 15-9 shows multiple nodules in a patient with Hashimoto thyroiditis. Some nodules are perfused, trap pertechnetate, and appear warm on ^{99m}Tc-pertechnetate images. Because they do not organify iodine, they are cold on ^{123}I or ^{131}I imaging at 24 hours. The traditional view that ^{99m}Tc-pertechnetate might not identify cold nodules is not consistent with a study that compared blind readings of ^{99m}Tc-pertechnetate and ^{123}I scans in 316 patients and found agreement in 92% to 95%. In 12 patients with thyroid carcinoma, no discrepancy was found on images obtained with either radionuclide.[50]

Whole-Body Imaging. In thyroid carcinoma, the role of nuclear medicine, aside from identifying suspect nodules as cold, is primarily in the management and treatment of the patient after surgical removal of most if not all of the functioning thyroid and readily identifiable cervical lymph node involvement. This involves a wide variety of options including the choice of radionuclide (^{131}I versus ^{123}I) and dose used for imaging, the method of preparing the patient (thyroid hormone withdrawal versus use of rhTSH), the role of serum thyroglobulin determinations, and therapeutic dose selection. Since thyroid carcinoma patients present with a variety of clinical, pathological, and nuclear medicine findings, it is recommended that the selection of options be individualized based upon risk and disease burden (see Table 15-3).

The initial nuclear medicine therapy procedure involves ^{131}I ablation of remnant thyroid tissue. In the United States, until a decade ago, the regulatory limit for the use of ^{131}I in an outpatient setting was 30 mCi. Patients receiving more than 30 mCi had to be hospitalized for radiation isolation purposes. This accounted for many patients with no additional evidence of residual tumor being treated with 30 mCi of ^{131}I to ablate the surgical remnant. Results varied. In 1992, Harry Maxon and colleagues[55] demonstrated that successful ablation depended upon delivering a radiation absorbed dose of 30,000 cGy to the thyroid remnant. To accomplish this, the nuclear medicine physician had to determine (or estimate) the weight (mass) of the residual tissue, the fractional uptake, and the biological turnover rate (to determine the effective half-life). Although there remains a divergence of opinion about the management of many aspects of thyroid carcinoma, the removal of the restriction on the allowable administered dose of ^{131}I has made it more convenient to select a dose that results in successful ablation of normal tissue in virtually all cases, usually 50 to 75 mCi of [131]I. It is no longer necessary to determine the thyroid remnant radiation absorbed dose.

There have been two other recent advances that have had a substantial impact of management of patients with thyroid carcinoma: the more general availability of more reliable thyroglobulin (Tg) assays and the approval and clinical availability of recombinant human TSH (rhTSH [Thyrogen]) in place of thyroid hormone withdrawal to augment TSH levels to stimulate ^{131}I uptake by residual thyroid tissue. Recombinant human TSH has been demonstrated to be at least equivalent to thyroid hormone withdrawal in detection of remnant thyroid tissue and detection of thyroid metastases by [131]I (or ^{123}I) imaging or detection of a rise in serum Tg.[70] Although rhTSH was approved specifically for diagnostic purposes in the postsurgical follow-up of thyroid cancer patients to determine if there is residual thyroid tissue or residual or recurrent tumor, it is now approved to prepare patients for ^{131}I ablation of the postsurgical thyroid remnant.[70] Data has been reported that demonstrates a prolonged residence time of radioiodine in metastatic lesions and reduced whole body radiation in patients prepared for radioiodine therapy with rhTSH rather than thyroid hormone withdrawal. These observations are attributed to a more rapid decrease of plasma TSH levels and better renal function during the euthyroid state.[38]

To prepare for ^{131}I imaging in the management of thyroid carcinoma, the patient should follow a low-iodine diet for 1 to 2 weeks before ^{131}I administration and avoid iodinated contrast material during this interval. As stated, the use of rhTSH has changed the management of patients with thyroid carcinoma. Nevertheless, either because of expense (approximately $1000 for 2 vials, 0.9 mg) or the practitioner's reluctance to replace a traditional protocol, some patients continue to be prepared for imaging by withdrawing thyroid hormone replacement therapy. For thyroid hormone withdrawal, assuming that the patient had been on a long-acting preparation, either T_4 or a combination of T_4 and T_3, several weeks should elapse to allow TSH levels to rise before radioiodine imaging is performed. The patient gradually develops symptoms and signs of hypothyroidism, including lethargy, soft-tissue swelling, weight gain, constipation, coarsening of the skin, and bradycardia, as well as intolerance to cold. Serum T_4 and T_3 levels fall to the hypothyroid range. Often, it is possible to make a clinical assessment that the patient is hypothyroid and proceed without a serum TSH value, which may not be available for several days. Nevertheless, serum for the TSH level should be obtained before a diagnostic radioiodine dose is administered. Subsequently, the validity of the evaluation can be confirmed by demonstrating that the TSH was indeed sufficiently elevated. Of course, if there is a significant functioning remnant or considerable functioning metastatic tumor, the TSH may not rise vigorously. In this instance, the nuclear medicine physician should proceed with the whole-body scintigraphy despite the relatively low TSH value. The failure of the TSH to rise is likely secondary to thyroid hormone synthesis and secretion by a significant volume of functioning thyroid metastases. Finally, of course, in order for the TSH to rise, pituitary function must be intact. Even if a nuclear medicine service does not routinely use rhTSH to prepare patients for the whole body ^{131}I scintigraphy or radioiodine ablation, it is necessary to use rhTSH for evaluation of patients with pituitary insufficiency. Hence, the nuclear medicine practitioner must be prepared to use rhTSH to prepare patients for evaluation and continue to be familiar with the thyroid hormone withdrawal protocol in the event rhTSH is unavailable or a decision has been made not to use it.[71]

As an alternative approach, patients taking T_4 or T_4 and T_3 can be changed to T_3 (Cytomel) alone for several weeks. Because T_3 has a short biological half-life, it is given in divided doses: 25 μg two or three times a day. The patient remains euthyroid during this period, gradually depleting the serum bound T_4. After several weeks, the T_3 is withdrawn and the patient becomes hypothyroid more rapidly than if he or she had simply had T_4 withdrawn. The advantage of this strategy is that the patient experiences a shorter period of hypothyroidism with its attendant weight gain, fatigue, constipation, and cosmetic changes.

The ^{131}I dose recommended for whole-body imaging has ranged in the past from 1 to 10 mCi. The recently published *Procedure Guideline for Extended Scintigraphy for Differentiated Thyroid Cancer*, developed by the Society of Nuclear Medicine, recommends a 5.0 mCi dose of ^{131}I.[6] The issue of imaging dose has become more complex because there has been increasing concern about **thyroid stunning.** Stunning refers to the potential decrease of tissue uptake as a consequence of the biological impact of the scanning dose. This has led to the suggestion that the scanning dose be no greater then 2.0 mCi of ^{131}I or preferably 2 to 5 mCi of ^{123}I, because the radiobiological effect is principally secondary to the beta particle component of ^{131}I decay. The sensitivity for detection of tumor foci depends upon the dose administered, the tissue or tumor iodine uptake (and turnover), the size of the remnant or tumor, the target-to-background contrast, and, of course, instrumentation. Tumor foci are identifiable on gamma camera imaging even when less than 10 μCi of ^{131}I has accumulated in the focus. This represents 1% of a 1.0 mCi dose. Accordingly, larger diagnostic doses permit identification of smaller foci within the 0.1% range. There is no doubt that therapeutic doses of ^{131}I are indeed handled differently from the preceding scanning dose (2 to 5 mCi of ^{131}I). There is evidence that the decrease in uptake of the therapy dose is a consequence of the therapeutic dose itself rather than the prior administration of a scanning dose of ^{131}I.[79] Despite observations of stunning, ablation success rates are similar in patients who have received a 2 to 5 mCi ^{131}I dose before the ablative dose versus patients who have not received a scanning dose suggesting than stunning is a manifestation of radiation sensitivity and has no effect on outcome. Nevertheless, it has become common practice for scanning to be performed with ^{123}I before therapy with ^{131}I.

Iodine-123 is relatively expensive compared to ^{131}I and less conveniently available. Because of its short half-life, it cannot be stored and it must be ordered in advance based upon a schedule administration. In recent years, these factors have become less of an issue as ^{123}I production has increased and cost has decreased. If ^{123}I is to be used for whole-body scintigraphy, a 2.0 to 5.0 mCi dose is suggested.

The availability of rhTSH has provided another reason to use ^{123}I in screening patients for residual tissue or unexpected tumor. Since it has been demonstrated that remnant ablation can be achieved with rhTSH preparation, the additional cost of a second round of rhTSH injections becomes an issue. A strategy has been developed in which several mCi (at least 2 mCi) of ^{123}I is administered at the time of the second intramuscular injection of rhTSH. Iodine-123 imaging takes place 24 hours later and, provided that there are no surprises, the patient receives the prescribed ablative (therapeutic) dose of ^{131}I after review of the images. This approach allows imaging before therapy and addresses concerns about stunning and insurance carriers' reluctance to reimburse for repeated use of rhTSH.

When ^{131}I is used as the scanning tracer, neck and whole-body images are obtained at 24-hour intervals (Figures 15-10 to 15-12) (Box 15-3). When replacement thyroid hormone is withdrawn, 48- or 72-hour images had been found to be optimal because imaging at these intervals allows sufficient time for reduction of background activity through renal excretion in the hypothyroid patient.[6] Use of rhTSH in patients maintained on thyroid hormone replacement has changed this dynamic. The patient prepared with rhTSH is euthyroid with better cardiac and renal function than a hypothyroid patient and hence there is improved excretion of free iodine from the interstitial fluid space. This results in good contrast images at 24 hours. Because radioiodine is secreted into the saliva and gastric fluids, activity in the gastrointestinal tract can be seen for several days, particularly in the hypothyroid patient who frequently will be constipated.

Even with diagnostic doses involving several mCi of ^{131}I, the count rate in the images is poor. Accordingly, 10-minute image acquisition for static fields is recommended. Radioactive markers may be placed to identify anatomical landmarks, such as the top of the skull, axillae, umbilicus, iliac crests, and knees. If the sternal notch is to be marked, a repeat image without the marker should be obtained so that a thyroid remnant or local tumor focus is not obscured. For whole body scanning, the slowest scan speed possible is recommended.

Radionuclide Therapy. Localization of iodine by thyroid tissue provides the basis for ^{131}I treatment of hyperthyroidism and thyroid cancer. The beta particle emission produces a profound radiobiological effect. With a sufficient dose of ^{131}I, hyperthyroid tissue can be reduced in function and mass, normal thyroid tissue can be ablated, and malignant tumor tissue can be destroyed or at least reduced in mass.

^{131}I Treatment of Hyperthyroidism. Iodine-131 has been used to treat hyperthyroidism regardless of whether the hyperthyroidism is secondary to a diffuse toxic goiter (Graves disease), toxic multinodular goiter, or toxic nodule (adenoma). In the past, ^{131}I was used to perform radiation thyroidectomies to produce hypothyroidism in clinically euthyroid patients with severe coronary artery disease to reduce the metabolic needs of the myocardium. This is no longer an indication for ^{131}I therapy, but

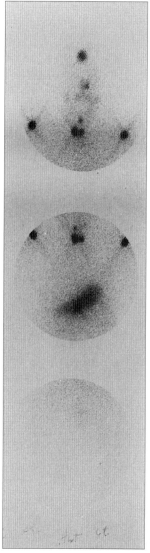

FIGURE 15-10 Whole-body imaging in thyroid carcinoma; 1 to 10 mCi ^{131}I was used as the "diagnostic" tracer with high-energy collimation. This figure illustrates anterior images using gamma camera technique at 24 hours after tracer administration. Markers are placed at the top of the head and shoulders. Background activity is seen throughout the soft tissue, with secretion in the nasal and oral cavities, the parotid and submaxillary glands, and the salivary glands. Residual thyroid tissue is seen in the bed of both the right and left thyroid lobes. A small midline focus cephalad to the thyroid remnants is also seen, representing metastasis to a paratracheal lymph node. Prominent activity is seen in the stomach. No activity is seen in the bladder, although bladder activity is quite common, particularly at 24 hours after tracer administration. Posterior images are also obtained to evaluate possible osseous metastases.

^{131}I is used to avoid surgical resection in euthyroid patients with diffuse or multinodular goiter.

Treatment of hyperthyroidism with ^{131}I is simple, safe, effective, has minimal morbidity, and is relatively inexpensive. Alternatives to ^{131}I therapy include antithyroid drugs or surgery. Before ^{131}I therapy is begun, the benefits and disadvantages of each therapeutic option should be discussed with the patient. In the United States, radioiodine therapy is the most frequently chosen treatment for

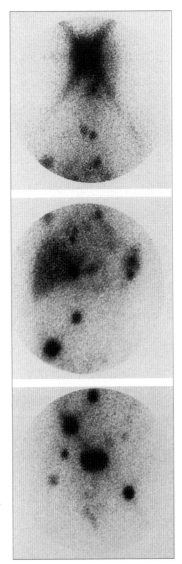

FIGURE 15-11 Whole-body imaging in thyroid carcinoma. Gamma camera images at 72 hours after ^{131}I therapy (134 mCi); 30 sec/frame. Metastases are seen in the brain (with a star artifact caused by septal penetration, readily observed because of the large amount of activity concentrated in a brain metastasis). Additional metastases are seen in the cervical, mediastinal, hepatic, and femoral lymph nodes. Diffuse activity is seen in the liver parenchyma, representing hepatic excretion of radiolabeled thyroid hormone synthesized in the functioning metastases.

BOX 15-3	Whole Body ^{131}I Imaging

1. Confirm whether patient is prepared by thyroid hormone withdrawal or rhTSH (Thyrogen) injections. Obtain blood for thyroglobulin and TSH per departmental protocol.
2. Administer 2-5 mCi of ^{131}I or ^{123}I orally per physician order.
3. Using appropriate collimator (high energy for ^{131}I; low or medium energy for ^{123}I) with patient supine, obtain whole-body images at 24 hours. Scan speed 4 to 5 cm/min or 10 to 15 min per static view.
4. Have images reviewed by nuclear physician before patient departure to ascertain if delayed imaging (48 hours or later) or special acquisitions (SPECT or SPECT/CT) are required.

adults with Graves disease. Surgery is rarely used. Antithyroid drugs require 6 to 12 months of treatment and have a significant failure rate (i.e., recurrence of hyperthyroidism when the antithyroid medication is discontinued). In addition, both surgery and antithyroid drugs have rare but well-defined complications, whereas there is no demonstrable consequence to ^{131}I therapy other than hypothyroidism. Iodine-131 has also been used to good effect in children and adolescents, but unfounded anxiety concerning long-term effects of radiation frequently leads to the choice of antithyroid drugs initially to control the disease in children. This often results in goiter, followed by surgery or ^{131}I therapy after all.

Hypothyroidism occurs frequently as a sequelae of hyperthyroidism regardless of the treatment used (radioiodine, surgery, or drugs).[9,10] Because hypothyroidism is readily treatable with thyroid hormone replacement, there is less reluctance in recent years to treat vigorously with ^{131}I.

The nuclear medicine physician must select a dose of ^{131}I that is appropriate for the clinical indication for therapy. Toxic multinodular goiter (TMNG) is more resistant to ^{131}I than is Graves disease, and a solitary toxic nodule is even more resistant. In addition, certain other clinical conditions are thought to be associated with relative resistance to ^{131}I such as previous treatment with antithyroid medication and ^{131}I.

The three basic approaches to selecting the dose of radioactive iodine (^{131}I) to be administered as therapy for hyperthyroidism are as follows:

1. A relatively fixed dose can be administered in which patients receive 5 to 10 mCi of ^{131}I; the dose chosen depends on a number of factors such as the practitioner's inclination, gland size, diagnosis of Graves disease versus TMNG versus toxic adenoma, and the severity of the hyperthyroidism.
2. A dose based on μCi delivered per gram of thyroid tissue, in which the estimated weight of the thyroid gland is taken into account. Based on clinical judgment, an amount of activity per gram is selected, typically 100 μCi/g. Factors such as the patient's age, whether nodules are present, and the severity of the hyperthyroidism are considered and provide a basis to increase the amount of radioactivity per gram of tissue. The thyroid mass is estimated from palpation and size on the scan. The amount of ^{131}I to be administered is calculated based on the 24-hour uptake:

$$\text{Amount (dose) to be administered } (\mu Ci) = \frac{\mu Ci/g \times \text{Thyroid mass}(g) \times 100}{24 - \text{hour uptake}(\%)}$$

Example: If it is decided that the appropriate thyroid "dose" is 100 μCi/g and the thyroid is estimated to be 40 g, the total amount of thyroid activity is determined to be 40 × 100 mCi = 4.0 mCi. If the 24-hour

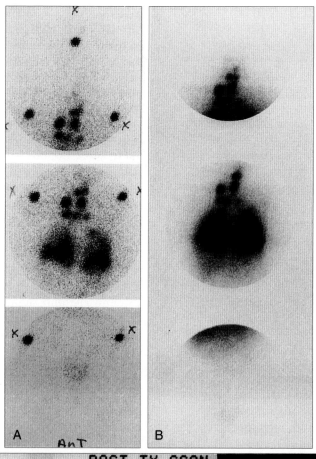

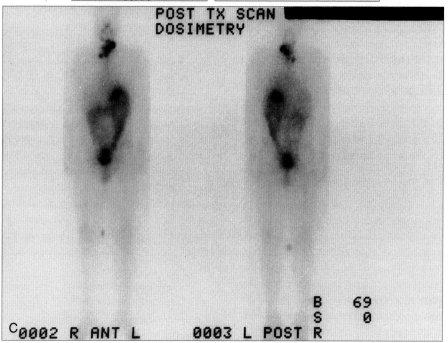

FIGURE 15-12 Whole-body imaging in thyroid carcinoma. Gamma camera technique **(A)** 48 hours after administration of 10 mCi ¹³¹I and **(B)** 72 hours after administration of 200 mCi ¹³¹I (therapeutic dose). In **A,** markers are seen on the top of the skull, at the shoulders, and at the iliac crests. Focal metastases are seen at multiple sites in the neck and superior mediastinum and diffusely throughout the lungs. **C,** Scanning in a different patient at 72 hours after administration of 200 mCi ¹³¹I (therapeutic dose). Prominent activity is seen in the left thyroid lobe remnant, a cervical lymph node lateral to the left lobe, and two small foci in the superior mediastinum. Excreted activity is seen in the stomach, bowel, and bladder. A standard source has been placed between the knees.

TABLE 15-5	Recommended Radiation Absorbed Dose for Treating Thyroid Disease
Condition	Recommended Radiation Absorbed Dose (cGy)
Graves disease	7000
Graves disease with previous failed therapy	10,000 to 12,000
Toxic multinodular goiter	10,000 to 12,000
Toxic nodule	15,000
Ablation of remnant	30,000
Maximum blood dose (thyroid cancer Rx)	200

uptake is 50%, a dose of 8.0 mCi must be administered to result in 4.0 mCi in the gland. If the uptake is 67%, 6.0 mCi would be sufficient to deliver the 4.0 mCi to the thyroid.

The term $\mu Ci/g$ allows the nuclear medicine physician to adjust the retained dose based on experience, the desire for disease control versus ablation, and the clinician's recent experience involving patient response to a particular microcurie per gram dose. Although not a sophisticated formulation, this method integrates patient-specific factors into the selection of the therapeutic dose.

3. A dose based on selecting a radiation absorbed dose (units: rad or cGy) to the thyroid. This approach is slightly more sophisticated in that it accounts for the turnover of ^{131}I by the thyroid. The nuclear physician selects a radiation absorbed dose (in cGy) based on the underlying disease (i.e., 7000 cGy [rad] for uncomplicated Graves disease; 10,000 to 12,000 cGy for toxic multinodular goiter; and 15,000 to 20,000 cGy for toxic adenoma) (Table 15-5). The desired thyroidal radiation absorbed dose is adjusted upward for factors such as age, disease severity, and a history of prior therapy. The dose to be administered is calculated to deliver the selected radiation absorbed dose. The calculation can be performed using either the original Quimby-Marinelli-Hine formula or the medical internal radiation dose (MIRD) formulation. The Quimby-Marinelli-Hine formula has been simplified by Becker and colleagues for the geometry of the thyroid and combining constants.[9,10] The dose to be administered (in mCi) is calculated as follows:

$$\text{Dose to be administered (mCi)} = \frac{\text{cGy (rad) desired} \times \text{thyroid weight (g)} \times 6.67}{t_{1/2eff} \text{ (days)} \times 24 \text{ hr uptake (\%)}}$$

in which $t_{1/2eff}$ is the effective half-life; 6.67 is a constant that corrects for the units and the geometry factors for a thyroid remnant irradiating itself. It is specifically applicable to the ablation of a surgical remnant because it assumes approximately a 10-g spheroid, but the formula provides a convenient method to calculate the ballpark radiation absorbed dose for ^{131}I therapy of small masses and even the entire thyroid. The MIRD uses more elegant corrections for thyroid size and can differ from the Quimby-Marinelli-Hine formulation by about 10%.

It is relatively easy to determine the thyroid gland mass by palpation, by estimate from scans, or by specific calculation based on measurement of areas of functioning tissue. A formula correlating mass and area has been reported: mass (in grams) = $0.86 \times$ area (cm^2). Various methods to estimate weight give different results, and consistency is more important than accuracy. It is important that the nuclear medicine practitioner use a consistent method, because precision (reproducibility) is desired.

All patients must have a 24-hour radioactive iodine uptake and thyroid scan before undergoing radioiodine therapy. The only additional element necessary for the calculation is determining the $t_{1/2eff}$, which is accomplished by determining the thyroid iodine turnover by counting the activity in the thyroid a second and third time after the 24-hour uptake, that is, 24, 48, and 72 or 96 hours. The effective half-life is determined from a semilogarithmic plot of the counts (uncorrected for decay) versus time or with a calculator or computer programmed for this calculation. If a decay corrected uptake is determined, the $t_{1/2bio}$ is obtained from which $t_{1/2eff}$ can be calculated using the following formula:

$$t_{1/2eff} = \left(t_{1/2bio}\right)\left(t_{1/2phys}\right) / \left(t_{1/2bio}\right) + \left(t_{1/2phys}\right)$$
$$t_{1/2phys} \text{ is the physical half-life of } ^{131}I = 8.1 \text{ days}$$

The merit of calculating a radiation absorbed dose versus a simplistic, fixed mCi dose is readily illustrated (Figure 15-13).[9,10] A 5-mCi ^{131}I administered dose can result in a thyroid radiation dose of 3000 to 15,000 cGy (rad), a fivefold range depending on the percentage uptake, the effective half-life, and the thyroid gland weight. Furthermore, to deliver 7000 cGy (a frequently recommended radiation absorbed dose for patients with Graves disease), doses from 3 to 27 mCi may be necessary depending on the variables described (i.e., uptake, weight, $t_{1/2eff}$).

Many patients are in a narrow range for effective half-life values, and the individualized calculated dose to be administered is similar to the simpler calculation and sometimes even to the fixed dose. The effective half-life can vary, however, from 1.5 to 6.0 days. Hence, it is recommended that the nuclear medicine practitioner make this measurement to select a patient-specific treatment dose. The minimal additional effort provides an opportunity to treat patients on a more rational basis by calculating the amount of radioactive material necessary to administer a specific radiation absorbed dose. There is no evidence that the additional effort and calculation

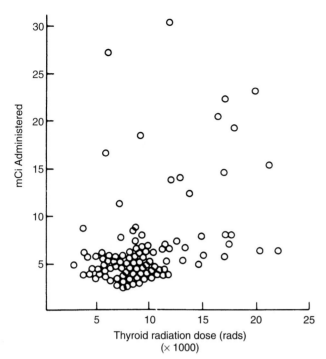

FIGURE 15-13 Relationship of radiation absorbed dose to the thyroid and the amount of ^{131}I administered in 92 hyperthyroid patients.

has a clinical advantage in most patients but it seems appropriate that practitioners who treat patients with ^{131}I have an understanding of the relationship between administered dose and radiation absorbed dose. In addition, this insight serves to clarify the situation encountered in a small (perhaps 5%) subset of hyperthyroid patients who have a rapid biological turnover of ^{131}I, perhaps less than 1 day. These patients would require large doses of ^{131}I to control their hyperthyroidism, and there would be significant whole-body exposure. Rather than administer a dose that will not have a significant impact or deliver a dose perhaps greater than 30 mCi, an understanding of the relationship between turnover rate and the radiation absorbed dose reveals that for a given administered dose of ^{131}I and fractional uptake, the radiation absorbed dose is inversely proportional to the $t_{1/2eff}$. Increasing the biological half-life will increase the effective half-life and in turn increase the radiation absorbed dose to the thyroid and decrease the effective whole-body dose. This can be accomplished by administration of antithyroid drugs for 5 to 7 days and treating the patient while this partial blockade of thyroid turnover is maintained.[10]

[131]I Treatment of Thyroid Carcinoma. In 1946 Seidlin and colleagues[78] reported the complete disappearance of multiple functioning metastases in a patient with thyroid carcinoma treated with [131]I. That report captured the imagination of the public and the press, leading to political support for and subsequent development of a civilian nuclear industry in the United States.

Radioiodine treatment using ^{131}I is involved at several points in the management of patients with thyroid carcinoma, including ablation of the residual thyroid remnant (after variable degrees of surgical thyroidectomy) and treatment of local and distal metastases (see Figures 15-10 to 15-12). Despite 50 years of experience with ^{131}I as a therapeutic agent for thyroid carcinoma, the appropriate dose for therapy in specific clinical settings remains unresolved. For the most part, the therapeutic recommendations are generalizations from observations on a relatively small number of patients: 30 to 75 mCi of ^{131}I to ablate remnants, 75 to 150 mCi to treat local (cervical) metastases, and 150 to 300 mCi to treat distal metastases.[6,32]

Three of the reasons it has been difficult to develop a consensus on a therapeutic dose are the relatively low incidence of thyroid carcinoma, the variety of clinical presentations, and the associated risk and the usually long natural history of the disease. It is suggested that rather than propose a single protocol for all patients, several protocols are described that make use of the several choices and recently available options and that the choice of protocol be made based on patient-specific factors and risk assessment (see Table 15-3).[32]

Thyroid Remnant Ablation. Thyroid ablation is performed in patients with thyroid carcinoma who have had surgical removal of a significant portion of the thyroid gland. Although surgical practice and skill vary, it is well established that many patients have residual thyroid tissue in the region of the thyroid bed (see Figure 15-10). Thyroid ablation refers to elimination of this tissue. It had been the practice to administer 75 to 100 mCi of ^{131}I for this purpose.[32,55,83]

Successful ablation in 87% of patients studied has been reported. In 1983, Snyder and colleagues[82] at the Mayo Clinic reopened the controversy of dose selection by reporting the effectiveness of 30 mCi doses of ^{131}I in remnant ablation. These workers observed complete ablation in 42 of 69 patients (61%) with a single dose of 29 mCi and minimal residual thyroid tissue in another 14. Four more patients responded to a second 29-mCi dose. Some centers routinely administer 75 mCi as an ablative dose. In the past, patients receiving greater than 30 mCi of ^{131}I were classified as radiation sources by the Nuclear Regulatory Commission (NRC). These patients were hospitalized until their body burden (radioactivity) fell to less than 30 mCi. In general, in the United States, this is no longer an issue. Maxon and colleagues at the University of Cincinnati Medical Center have reported the results of quantitative dosimetry of thyroid remnants.[51,56] They report ablation with ^{131}I in 122 of 142 thyroid remnants (86%) in 57 of 70 patients (81%) by delivering 30,000 rad. The range of activity administered was 26 to 246 mCi. Out of 70 patients (37%), 26 received less than 30 mCi of [131]I. This impressive study speaks forcefully for individualized dosimetric determinations in patients undergoing radionuclide thyroid remnant ablation. This method makes it possible to identify patients "likely to respond to outpatient therapy with a higher chance of success" and "those who will require greater administered activities and inpatient treatment."[55,56]

With the relaxation of the requirement to isolate patients receiving more than 30 mCi of ^{131}I, however, this issue has been largely put to rest because the regulatory modification in the United States allows release of patients receiving in excess of 30 mCi of ^{131}I provided that there is no significant increase in the radiation exposure to members of the public. This change eliminates the additional cost and inconvenience of hospital-based radiation isolation. Hence ablation can be performed with 50 to 75 mCi of ^{131}I, a dose that achieves near total ablation in virtually all patients. To this has been added the option of rhTSH stimulation of uptake.[70] It has been demonstrated that preparing patients with rhTSH is as effective in terms of successful ablation as thyroid hormone withdrawal.[70]

Local and Distal Metastases. Cervical lymph nodes and metastases to sites such as mediastinal lymph nodes, pulmonary parenchyma, and bone require larger doses of ^{131}I than ablation of normal thyroid gland remnant, usually 150 to 300 mCi (see Figures 15-10 and 15-11). Leeper and Shimaoka,[52] Beierwaltes and associates,[13] and other researchers have reported satisfactory resolution of lymph node metastases in patients receiving 150 mCi of [131]I. These patients, of course, were followed with radioiodine scans and retreated with similar doses if necessary. Beierwaltes and associates[13] reported 80%, 97%, and 100% ablation of cervical lymph node metastases in patients receiving 150 to 174, 175 to 199, and 200 mCi or more in a series of 35, 37, and 9 patients, respectively, at each level of administered activity. For distal metastases, elimination of the functioning tissue is somewhat less successful but results as good as 75% total ablation of mediastinal nodes were observed in patients receiving less than 200 mCi of [131]I. Patients receiving 175 to 199 mCi had an 89% ablation success rate.

In response to the recent modification of the regulations that no longer require radiation isolation of patients receiving ^{131}I therapy, patients are treated with up to 250 mCi as outpatients provided that they meet the criteria to reasonably ensure that members of the population will not be unnecessarily exposed.

Of course, the uptake in each metastatic lesion varies and it is beyond the control of the treating physician except to ensure that the TSH is elevated. Accordingly, it is not feasible to select a radiation absorbed dose for each tumor site. In some cases, the tumor radiation absorbed dose from 200 or even 250 mCi will be ineffective. It is appropriate to consider whether it is reasonable to administer doses greater than 250 mCi of ^{131}I on appropriate patients, that is, those with metastatic disease. In a small number of patients reported by Beierwaltes and colleagues,[13] patients with lung metastases

had a 67% success rate when greater than 200 mCi was administered (three patients) versus a 20% response rate in patients receiving 175 to 199 mCi (five patients) and a 60% response rate in patients receiving 150 to 174 mCi (five patients). In patients with bone metastases, the response rates were 60% in patients receiving 150 to 174 mCi (five patients), 71% in patients receiving 175 to 199 mCi (seven patients), and 80% in patients receiving greater than 200 mCi of [131]I (five patients). These findings confirm the notion that the administered dose is the one variable in determining the tumor radiation absorbed dose that can be controlled by the nuclear medicine physician. The question arises, therefore, what is the upper limit of ^{131}I therapy dose? What is the maximal tolerated ^{131}I dose? Since the principal toxicity is bone marrow suppression, it would seem appropriate to determine the ^{131}I dose that results in a bone marrow (or blood) radiation absorbed dose associated with hematological toxicity and to set this as the upper limit for ^{131}I therapy in patients with advanced disease. This concept is known as determination of the "maximal tolerated dose (MTD)" based on patient-specific bone marrow dosimetry.

In 1980, Leeper and Shimaoka[52] at the Memorial Sloan-Kettering Cancer Center (MSKCC) in New York determined that hematological toxicity was observed at blood radiation absorbed doses greater than 250 to 300 cGy. Based on this observation, they determined the maximum permissible dose for patients with metastases beyond the cervical lymph nodes based on bone marrow exposure of less than 200 rad per administered dose and limited patients to one therapeutic dose per year. With this strategy, bone marrow depression was avoided despite administration of doses in excess of 300 mCi of [131]I. One patient was reported free of disease or complications 3 years after a 320-mCi administered dose of [131]I. An additional caveat was to limit the pulmonary parenchymal exposure to less than 80 mCi of ^{131}I retained at 24 hours. Experience with this technique at the MSKCC has demonstrated that approximately 80% of patients can tolerate doses in excess of 200 mCi of ^{131}I; in 20% of the patients, impaired renal function or tumor burden and slow ^{131}I turnover limits the dose to less than 200 mCi, but 150 mCi is tolerated by virtually all patients, certainly those with normal renal function.[85]

Maxon and associates[55,56] reported the results of a larger series of thyroid cancer patients who underwent quantitative radiation dosimetry for [131]I. This group had previously reported successful ablation of thyroid remnants at 30,000 rad and treatment of nodal metastases at 8000 rad.[57,58] If the radiation dose to the involved nodes was greater than 8000 rad, 98% of patients responded to treatment, whereas only 20% responded at less than this dose. In the recent series, they observed a success rate of 86% of patients and 90% of involved nodes in situations in which 14,000 rad or more was administered.

In summary, a rational basis exists for the use of quantitative dosimetry for the selection of a therapeutic dose of ^{131}I in the high-risk patient in whom it is desirable to administer ^{131}I doses in excess of 150 mCi. Bone marrow dose is determined as a worst-case calculation, with the assumption that the radiation absorbed dose is equivalent to the blood dose. This is determined by measuring the blood disappearance rate of a tracer dose and assuming a blood volume for the functioning marrow space of 20% of the total blood volume. A maximum "safe" dose is thus determined that will limit the calculated marrow exposure to 200 rad. Tumor dosimetry is problematic and currently is not considered in dose selection. Although it would be of value to know the radiation absorbed dose at various tumor sites, this is not readily accomplished, particularly in a clinical setting. Nevertheless, calculation of the maximum safe dose to be administered provides a basis for administering doses greater than 150 mCi of ^{131}I when this option seems appropriate based upon the presence of metastases (see Tables 15-3 and 15-5).

Another category of patients to consider for therapy are those with elevated serum thyroglobulin levels (>10 ng/ml) but without focal ^{131}I uptake. Two well-documented groups of thyroid carcinoma patients were found to have elevated serum thyroglobulin and negative body ^{131}I scans after total removal of the thyroid gland. Of 83 patients treated at the University of Pisa, Italy, one third had positive scans after a therapeutic dose of 100 mCi of [131]I.[61] Many of the patients had a significant lowering of serum thyroglobulin after radioiodine treatment. At the National Institutes of Health (NIH), 9 of 10 patients with similar diagnostic results (elevated thyroglobulin levels and negative ^{131}I diagnostic scans) had abnormal scans when imaged after a therapeutic dose.[1] Actually, this category of patient would also seem to be appropriate for determination of the maximal tolerated dose based on whole-body (blood) [131]I dosimetry.

With the advent of ^{18}F-FDG imaging, it has been demonstrated that thyroid carcinoma is identified by FDG PET imaging even if ^{131}I imaging is negative. FDG PET identifies disease that may be surgically removable or accessible to focused external beam radiation therapy. The degree of FDG uptake is proportional to the aggressiveness of the tumor.[86,87]

NEUROENDOCRINE SYSTEM

Neuroendocrine system is a term given collectively to cells scattered throughout the body that differentiate from the embryonic neural crest and migrate to various organs, taking on distinct and specialized roles as regulators of diverse processes including secretion of peptide hormones such as insulin, glucagon (by the islets of Langerhans that are embedded in the exocrine pancreas), vasoactive intestinal peptide (VIP), gastrin and **somatostatin** (by the Kolchitsky cells in the gastrointestinal tract), calcitonin (by the parafollicular cells in the thyroid) and vasoactive amines, such as serotonin, dopamine, epinephrine, and norepinephrine (potentially from any of the neuroendocrine cells but the latter particularly from adrenergic tissue). These cells, despite their diverse location and secretory functions, have in common the expression of SSTRs, which regulate the cells themselves. This function, self-regulation (*autocrine*) and local regulation (*paracrine*) are different from the classical *endocrine* system in which biologically active hormones are secreted into the circulation with profound effects on distant organs and tissues. Tumors that evolve from these cells (such as gastrinomas, insulinomas, and **carcinoid tumors**) are known as *neuroendocrine tumors*. These tumors retain the ability to synthesize the peptide and amine hormones of the nonmalignant cells but do so in an uncontrolled manner, often producing symptoms due to systemic effects of uncontrolled production and secretion of hormones and other biologically active substances.

Anatomy and Physiology

The primitive neural crest cells migrate throughout the primitive gut taking on distinct functions at different locations. As the foregut differentiates, the neuroendocrine cells are embedded in the thymus, bronchus, lungs, and stomach; the midgut forms the pancreas, jejunum, ileum, colon, and appendix; and the hindgut forms the colon and rectum. The embedded cells at the various locations have specific functions and elaborate a variety of regulatory hormones. These cells characteristically express SSTRs.

Somatostatin is a 14–amino acid regulatory neuropeptide initially identified as a hypothalamic hormone that inhibits growth hormone release from the anterior pituitary; hence the name "somatostatin." Subsequently, it was observed that somatostatin has effects on diverse organs other than the anterior pituitary and it was concluded that it has a regulatory function via local synthesis and release throughout the gastrointestinal tract, bronchopulmonary system, and some endocrine organs as well. Somatostatin has complex effects also on the immune system, because lymphocytes also express SSTRs. Somatostatin seems to inhibit or at least regulate cell proliferation in general and may be a component of the mechanism that maintains orderly tissue architecture.

There are at least five SSTR subtypes, which are expressed on different tissues. The significance of receptor subtypes is that, whereas somatostatin binds to all receptor subtypes and initiates subsequent biological events, **somatostatin analogs** that are used as drugs react with specific receptor subtypes expressed by some tissues but not by others. Receptors may decrease in affinity or number per cell; indeed, a tumor may dedifferentiate to a point where it no longer expresses SSTR receptors.

This may account for the abrupt deterioration when a tumor dedifferentiates and is no longer receptive to the growth-inhibiting effect of somatostatin (endogenous or pharmacological analogs). Various analogs (octreotide and lanreotide) are used as drugs to inhibit oversecretion of biologically active peptides and amines by neuroendocrine tumors.

Clinical Aspects

Neuroendocrine tumors often present even when quite small because of metabolic syndromes caused by the metabolically active secretions rather than as tumor masses. Conversely, if a neuroendocrine tumor is nonfunctional or secretes active products into the portal venous circulation, the tumors may be quite large or metastatic before presentation. The most common neuroendocrine tumors are carcinoids arising from the Kulchitsky cells, small cells in the bronchial and intestinal mucosa that play a role in mucus secretion, membrane transport, and ciliary and intestinal motility. Sixty percent of carcinoid tumors originate in the gastrointestinal tract; 25% are bronchopulmonary in origin. The tumors retain the capacity to produce any of the active products of neuroendocrine cells but typically bronchopulmonary carcinoids produce adrenocorticotropic hormone (ACTH), islet cell tumors produce peptides (insulin, glucagon, VIP, somatostatin, ACTH), and gastrointestinal tumors produce gastrin or vasoactive amines (serotonin). In addition, there are nonfunctioning bronchial, pancreatic, and gastrointestinal carcinoids. The tumor marker chromogranin A appears in the serum and is a sensitive indicator of neuroendocrine tumor burden even if the neuroendocrine tumor is nonfunctional.

Other neuroendocrine tumors include medullary carcinoma of the thyroid, which arises from the C cells in the thyroid that produce the calcium-regulating polypeptide calcitonin. Calcitonin lowers serum-ionized calcium by inhibiting bone resorption; nevertheless, it is unusual for patients to be symptomatically hypocalcemic despite high levels of calcitonin in patients with advanced disease.

Pheochromocytoma is a tumor that arises from the adrenal medulla. About 10% of pheochromocytomas are malignant and may have metastasized even to remote areas such as the heart or bladder. Ten percent of the pheochromocytomas arise in ectopic locations. Nonfunctioning pheochromocytomas are called paragangliomas and may occur at any location in the autonomic nervous system.

Carcinoid tumors may be discovered as an incidental finding during a surgical procedure or CT. These are usually benign, but histopathological diagnosis of benign versus malignant carcinoid tumors is frequently difficult. Symptoms such as flushing, diarrhea, hives, asthma, and heart valve problems arising from the carcinoid secretory products do not occur unless liver metastases are present, because the portal circulation detoxifies secretions from the primary bowel site. Carcinoid tumors are found in the appendix (38%), the ileum of the small intestine (23%), the rectum (13%), the bronchus (11.5%), at sites throughout the gastrointestinal tract, and rarely in other organs. Nonfunctioning islet cell tumors and medullary carcinoma of the thyroid do not cause metabolic symptoms; therefore, they usually do not become manifest until extensive metastases are present, unless they are identified coincidentally during surgery.

Nuclear Medicine Procedures

The radiolabeled somatostatin analog octreotide is the basis for neuroendocrine tumor imaging. **Octreotide** is an 8–amino acid analog of somatostatin that has a high binding affinity for SSTR subtype 2 and to a lesser extent, subtypes 3 and 5.

Indium-111-DTPA-pentetreotide is a radiolabeled derivative of octreotide that is used to identify tumors that arise from the widely distributed specialized neuroendocrine secretory cells with SSTRs, the so-called *neuroendocrine tumors.*[25,45,46,48,76]

Much of the early clinical evaluation of SSTR scintigraphy (SRS) was performed by Krenning and colleagues,[46,47] who first evaluated a ^{123}I tyrosyl derivative of octreotide. Subsequently, a DTPA derivative of octreotide was prepared. This derivative, DTPA-pentetreotide (OctreoScan, Mallinckrodt, St. Louis), is available in kit form to be labeled with ^{111}In by simple mixing of the two components.

The adult dose of ^{111}In-DTPA-pentetreotide is 6 mCi (222 MBq). Although neuroendocrine tumors are unusual in children and adolescents, the usual approach to pediatric dosage is a fraction of the adult dose based on weight. Indium-111-pentetreotide should be injected slowly intravenously because the pentetreotide (octreotide) component is pharmacologically active. The amount of octreotide injected is only a fraction of the usual pharmacological dose but caution is advised. Instances of a drop in blood pressure in patients with pheochromocytoma, or in the case of insulinoma, a decrease in blood glucose have been observed in patients whose clinical state is dominated by the secretory products of the neuroendocrine tumor.

Sensitivity for identification of tumor sites is dependant upon the absolute amount of radiotracer localized, which is a function of dose administered, tumor size, and receptor expression. Although there is rapid clearance of ^{111}In-pentetreotide from plasma and high-affinity uptake of the tracer, identification of tumor foci increases with time as contrast improves with clearance of tracer from the extracellular space. Hence, although many lesions can be identified at 4 hours, image quality and lesion detection is better at 24 hours because of enhancement

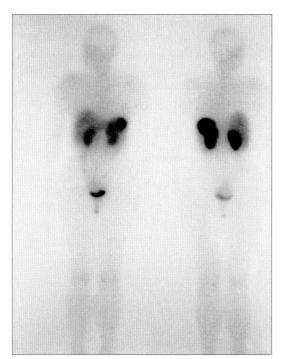

FIGURE 15-14 Anterior and posterior whole-body scan obtained 4 hours after IV injection of 6.0 mCi ^{111}In-pentetreotide. Although patient was referred to locate residual medullary carcinoma of the thyroid, this figure was interpreted as normal. Scan speed is 10 cm/min; at 24 hours, the scan speed is reduced to 8 cm/min. Normal distribution includes mild hepatic uptake and marked spleen and renal uptake. At 4 hours, excretion into the bladder is also seen.

| BOX 15-4 | Somatostatin Receptor Scintigraphy |

1. 5 to 6 mCi ^{111}In-DTPA-pentetreotide IV
2. Individualize protocol per patients needs; physicians request.
3. Usually 4 hours whole body (to mid thigh) images at slow scan speed (6 cm/min desired); alternately, static images, 10 to 15 minutes per image. Medium-energy collimator
4. Repeat step 3 at 24 hours
5. Review planar images with nuclear physician about SPECT or SPECT/CT location. Perform per facility ^{111}In protocol.
6. 48 hours imaging if necessary

hepatic lobe and may both interfere with the identification of metastases in that region and confuse the identification of right adrenal masses and lesions in the head of the pancreas. Tumors in the tail of the pancreas may be obscured by the left kidney. SPECT imaging provides an opportunity to identify lesions that otherwise would be obscured, but there is a limit to the ability of this technique to reconstruct the distribution of activity found in small lesions near the kidneys, which are relatively large and contain a considerable fraction of the administered dose of radioactivity.

Dual energy acquisition is performed with 20% windows centered on the 179- and 267-keV photopeaks of indium-111. High-count static acquisitions of the thorax and abdomen should be obtained in the anterior and posterior projections. Formerly, it was recommended that images be acquired for at least 10 minutes each. Currently, however, the Society of Nuclear Medicine (SNM) guidelines recommend obtaining at least 300,000 counts per image for the head and neck region or up to 15 minutes per view. Because of the nonspecific uptake of the tracer in the liver, spleen, and kidneys, a higher number of counts (500,000) or longer acquisition is recommended for imaging of the torso, specifically the abdomen. Separate acquisition of the chest and abdomen are recommended. When the liver activity is included in the field of view, it accounts for a significant portion of the total counts. There is variable scintigraphic appearance of thyroid gland activity depending on whether the liver is in the field of view. The thyroid is barely visible, whereas in a head-and-neck acquisition, the thyroid is clearly seen (even if normal) since a greater fraction of the total counts are derived from the thyroid gland.[60] It is important to recognize that simply including or excluding another organ in a field of view will influence the intensity of activity in a particular organ of interest. This technical phenomenon should not be interpreted as a clinical finding. This observation is relevant to the accuracy of scintigraphy for the detection of small tumors, particularly in the abdomen, where liver, spleen, and kidney activity may not only directly obscure lesions but also contribute to loss of sensitivity because these organs contribute so many counts to an image taken for a specific number of counts even though the total counts

of the tumor-background contrast. Nevertheless, based on the clinical picture, areas of interest should be imaged at 4 hours for comparison with the 24-hour images to determine if abdominal foci of activity represent tumor deposits or bowel contents. Activity in the bowel is often seen at 24 hours despite bowel preparation because approximately 10% of the ^{111}In-DTPA-pentetreotide is cleared through the hepatobiliary system (Figures 15-14 and 15-15). Accordingly, a gentle laxative should be administered the evening after the injection. Better results are obtained by pretreating the patient with a laxative before injection of the tracer and again the evening after the injection, provided that the patient does not have diarrhea as a prominent symptom of their clinical state.

After IV administration of ^{111}In-DTPA-pentetreotide, whole-body images are obtained at 4 hours (Box 15-4). Activity is normally seen in the liver, spleen, kidneys, and bladder. Approximately 50% is cleared by the kidneys and appears in the urine. On 24-hour images, the bladder is usually clear, and a variable amount of activity is seen in the bowel (see Figures 15-14 and 15-15). Focal accumulation of activity may be seen in the gall bladder. In this regard, SPECT/CT is often necessary to differentiate between hepatic metastases and normal gall bladder accumulation.

Activity in the kidneys remains an obstacle to interpretation because these organs occupy a large portion of the abdomen. The right kidney obscures part of the right

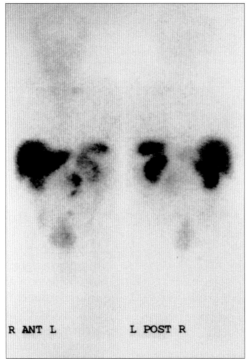

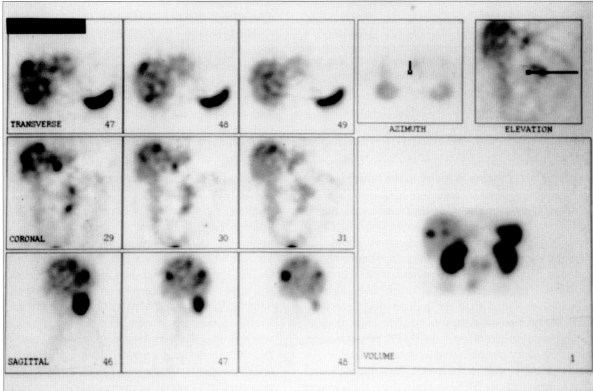

FIGURE 15-15 A, Anterior and posterior scanning gamma camera images obtained at 24 hours after ^{111}In-pentetreotide administration in a patient subsequently confirmed to have metastatic carcinoid tumor. Acquisition was stopped below the pelvis. Uptake in the liver, spleen, and kidneys is seen. Bladder activity is minimal at 24 hours. In addition to the usual organ distribution, two foci are seen in the abdomen slightly to the left of the midline. These represent a primary carcinoid tumor in the wall of the small bowel and a regional nodal metastasis. Neither lesion was identified on abdominal CT or contrast studies. The image is too dark to reveal several metastatic foci in the liver. **B,** Transverse, coronal, and sagittal slices after SPECT acquisition of the same patient. Three distinct foci are seen within the hepatic parenchyma. The bowel and lymph node foci are confirmed.

accumulated may be considerable. It is better technique, therefore, to acquire for a specific time interval or at a slow scan rate for whole-body images than for total counts.

Somatostatin receptor scintigraphy (SRS) has been particularly useful to identify functioning and nonfunctioning islet cell carcinomas. Receptor density and subtype vary with the type of islet cell tumor. Gastrin-secreting tumors (gastrinomas) have virtually 100% detectability, whereas insulin-producing tumors (insulinomas) have 50% detection sensitivity. Of course, identification of the tumor is not tumor-type specific. Indium-111 pentetreotide scintigraphy also detects somatostatin-positive, nonfunctional islet cell tumors. The presence of SSTRs is a more reliable means of differentiating nonfunctioning islet cell tumors from adenocarcinoma of the pancreas than histopathological examination of the tumor. When surgical tissue from patients who have had a prolonged survival after a pathological diagnosis of adenocarcinoma of the pancreas is reevaluated immunohistochemically for SSTRs, the tissue of these prolonged survivors are found to have somatostatin receptors indicating that the initial pathologic diagnosis was incorrect.

In patients with abdominal carcinoid tumors and in patients with gastrinoma, the sensitivity for detection approaches 100%.[31,50] In a study of 80 consecutive patients with Zollinger-Ellison syndrome (recurrent ulcer disease associated with a gastrin-producing tumor), SRS using ^{111}In-octreotide identified liver metastases in 70% of the patients compared to only 45% by MRI, 38% by CT, and 19% by ultrasound.[53,72] Indium-111-DTPA-pentetreotide is also useful for the detection and localization of pheochromocytoma, neuroblastoma, and medullary carcinoma of the thyroid. The frequency of SSTRs on immunopathological examination of medullary carcinoma is approximately 33%, which is less than ideal. In small series, tumors have been identified in 50% to 70% of cases. Results are better in patients presenting early in the course of their disease. This is probably because it is before the tumor has dedifferentiated. More often the initial diagnosis is made after surgical removal of a thyroid nodule that is subsequently reported as a medullary carcinoma. Nuclear imaging is not performed until elevated serum calcitonin levels are observed during follow-up after a total thyroidectomy for medullary thyroid carcinoma. The nuclear medicine facility is asked to identify the source of the recurrent elevation of thyrocalcitonin (the hormonal secretion of the parafollicular C cells). The task is complicated at that time because the tumor may have decreased receptor expression or saturation of the receptors as a result of synthesis of somatostatin by the tumor. In these instances, ^{131}I-MIBG may be of greater value in identifying the site or sites of functioning tissue. As the disease progresses with loss of differentiation, the calcitonin levels may fall; carcinoembryonic antigen (CEA) is expressed and shed into the circulation serving as a tumor marker and indicator of a more differentiated tumor. At this time, it has been noted the ^{18}F-FDG imaging is increasingly positive.[60]

The SNM has published *Procedure Guideline for Somatostatin Receptor Scintigraphy with ^{111}In-Pentetreotide.* The recommended administered ^{111}In-octreotide activity is 222 MBq (6 mCi) in adults and 5 MBq/kg (0.14 mCi/kg) in children. Planar images should be acquired for 10 to 15 minutes per field of view, using either a 256×256 (or even a 512×512) word matrix. Scanning gamma cameras produce good-quality whole-body images but these can be misleading. A negative study does not exclude disease or even provide a complete picture of the extent of disease involvement. Whole-body scintigraphy, though it is convenient to perform and provides aesthetically pleasing studies, contains too little information when performed at a scan speed of 6 to 8 cm/min in order to limit the patient's total time on the imaging table.[5] Whole-body scintigraphy should be performed at a speed of 3 cm/min, or a minimum of 30 minutes for an imaging field from the head to the upper femur, to ensure acquisition of adequate data.

Scintigraphy (either whole body or selected regions of interest) is performed as a rule at 4 and 24 hours after injection. Routine practice currently includes performing SPECT of the appropriate regions of interest, preferably at 24 hours.[5,12,39,40] The SNM guidelines acknowledge inherent differences among various imaging systems but recommends a SPECT protocol including 3-degree angular sampling, with 20 to 30 seconds per stop.

Digital display stations that are increasingly available should be used for image interpretation. Maximum intensity projection (MIP) volume display and SPECT, preferably SPECT/CT, images as well as the possibility for triangulation, are preferable for image interpretation.

SPECT/CT has further improved the sensitivity of detection and overall accuracy of ^{111}In-pentetreotide scintigraphy. In this procedure, CT is performed initially followed by SPECT acquisition on the same imaging table. The CT portion provides an anatomical map that can be viewed in transaxial, coronal, and sagittal slices alongside the corresponding SPECT slice. In addition, a fused image in which the nuclear data is superimposed or overlayed on the CT is displayed. The CT data is also used for attenuation correction of the SPECT images (Figure 15-16).

High-quality SPECT imaging of appropriate areas (thorax or abdomen or both) should be obtained routinely. In patients suspected of having carcinoid or functioning or nonfunctioning islet cell tumors, as well as pheochromocytomas or other chromaffin tissue tumors, complete evaluation includes SPECT or SPECT/CT imaging of the abdomen even if the planar images are negative. Scintigraphy of patients with ectopic ACTH syndrome (frequently the result of a bronchial carcinoid) or medullary carcinoma of the thyroid should include SPECT or preferably SPECT/CT imaging of the thorax.

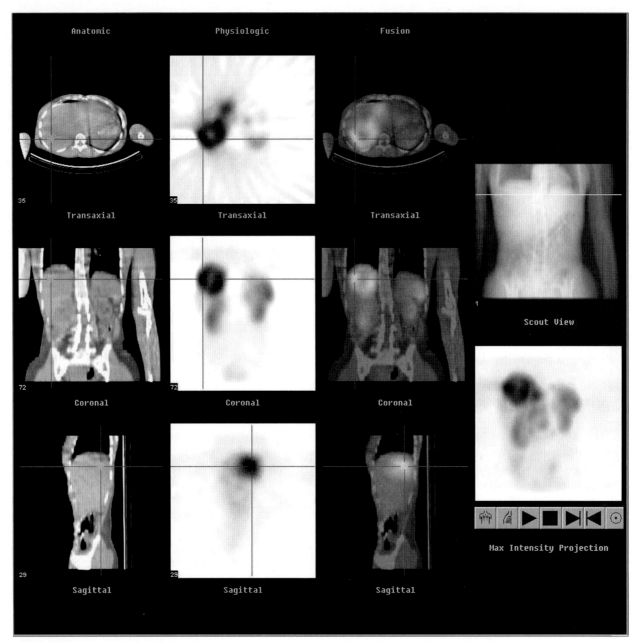

FIGURE 15-16 ^{111}In-DTPA-pentetreotide (OctreoScan) fusion imaging. Selected triangulated slices: *Top* to *bottom:* Transaxial, coronal, and sagittal. *Left* to *right:* CT (anatomy), scintigraphy (physiology), fused anatomy, and physiology. *Extreme right:* Scout CT *(upper)* and volume reconstruction *(lower).*

If plasma markers are present, indicating the presence of tumor, the nuclear medicine technologist should consult with the physician to optimize the protocol for the specific clinical situation.

Many states and regulatory jurisdictions require specific licensing and training of technologists to operate the CT component even though the CT component of the early instruments used is a low-voltage device with few options for the technical acquisition. Recently, other manufacturers have introduced full diagnostic CTs as components of the SPECT/CT imaging devices. Combined with the development and successful marketing of PET/CT, there is pressure to provide training and access

to CT technology for nuclear medicine technologists. Licensed physicians, however, may operate an x-ray (CT) device, which in the case of the initial low-voltage device involves simply pressing "start" after the patient has been properly positioned. One of the drawbacks of the initial version is that the image set available for display, including the MIP or volume display as well as the tomographic slices, is limited to a single bed position; that is, consecutive bed positions can be obtained but they are not "zippered" together. Following the CT acquisition, SPECT is performed in 3- to 6-degree angular steps, 45 to 60 seconds each, with a 128 × 128 matrix. SPECT is reconstructed using the object search engine mapping (OSEM) reconstruction program and images are processed on the accompanying digital processor. A variety of color displays are available. Newer instruments provide images combining at least two bed positions.

Somatostatin receptor SPECT has greater accuracy than planar imaging in patients with neuroendocrine tumors. In a comparison of ^{111}In pentetreotide planar and SPECT SRS with conventional imaging procedures in 149 patients with gastroenteropancreatic (GEP) neuroendocrine tumors, SPECT identified liver metastases in 60 of 65 cases (92% sensitivity) compared to only 38 of 65 (58% sensitivity) for planar imaging and 52 of 65 (80% sensitivity) for conventional imaging including CT and MRI. Indium-111-pentetreotide SPECT was 100% specific (no false-positive images) versus 86% for conventional imaging of the liver. Identification of previously missed metastatic lesions as well as exclusion of equivocal or false-positive findings on conventional imaging by SPECT led to management changes in 28 of 149 patients (19%) compared to 13 of 149 patients (9%) with planar SRS.

In other reports, patients undergoing SRS were imaged with SPECT alone as well as SPECT/CT Simple correlation of SPECT findings with CT findings and images improves accuracy but SPECT/CT (near simultaneous acquisition of both CT [anatomical imaging] and SPECT [functional or molecular imaging]) is more convenient and accurate for direct comparison of anatomy and function particularly in the abdomen where bowel and bladder contents undergo significant changes in volume almost hourly with displacement of other abdominal organs.

Fused or hybrid images combining SPECT and CT have demonstrated abnormal uptake in a normal sized retroperitoneal lymph node. The tracer focus would not have been properly interpreted as a lymph node on SPECT alone nor would it have been identified as abnormal on CT. The fused image accurately demonstrated that the lymph node had a hypermetabolic focus, thus identifying it as a site of metastatic disease. In other patients, a pancreatic tumor that had been previously missed on CT alone was identified. SPECT/CT is more reliable and accurate for the exclusion of extrahepatic, enabling the patient to undergo hepatic chemoembolization. The impact of more accurate and precise localization on selection of therapeutic options cannot be overestimated. SPECT/CT fusion SRS improves image interpretation by providing more precise anatomical localization of lesions detected by SPECT.[27,44,63]

False-positive image interpretation is a result either of misreading normal distribution of activity as lesions (e.g., interpreting gallbladder, bowel, or bladder activity as lesions) or of increased expression of SSTRs on other tissue. False-positive findings are reduced with SPECT/CT. Hybrid imaging improves image interpretation in

general, allowing for precise localization of foci, identifying previously unsuspected metastases in bone and bone marrow versus soft tissue. Of greater clinical significance is the fact that SPECT/CT alters the subsequent management of patients in approximately 15% of patients studied. Results of fused images led to changes in previously planned surgical approaches in some patients and spared two patients from unnecessary surgery based on identification of skeletal metastases.[43,44]

Whenever it is available, SPECT/CT should be used for SRS, because it improves sensitivity and specificity; sensitivity of detection is improved by recognizing that tracer accumulations that may have been interpreted as background noise or bowel contents are in locations that lead to reassessment of their significance; and specificity is improved by confirming that some accumulations cannot possibly be metastases and/or are in fact physiological excretions in the gall bladder, bowel, or urinary collecting system. Hence, there is improvement in the overall accuracy for the detection and staging of neuroendocrine tumors. In addition, it is easier to develop a consensus among scan readers about the significance of a finding, and finally the capacity to demonstrate the anatomical location increases credibility in the result with referring clinicians.

Somatostatin receptor SPECT/CT has been used to demonstrate the complex nature of another disorder of endocrine interest, thyroid associated orbitopathy. Whereas ^{111}In-DTPA-pentetreotide uptake had been demonstrated previously in Graves orbitopathy because activated lymphocytes also express SSTRs, SPECT/CT was able to define the anatomical structures involved.[34]

In summary, SRS is a major element in the clinical management of patients with neuroendocrine tumors. Although at times lesions are readily identifiable on planar imaging, SPECT imaging improves diagnostic performance, which is further enhanced when correlated with CT findings and images. When it is available, SPECT/CT should be used for optimal results in the evaluation of patients with known or suspected neuroendocrine tumors.

Receptor-Targeted Radionuclide Therapy. The same targeting principal that provides the foundation for SRS, the use of a radiolabeled somatostatin analog, can be used to deliver a therapeutic dose of radiation. Clinical trials have demonstrated the utility of tetraazacyclodo-decanetetraacetic acid (DOTA)-labeled somatostatin analogs including octreotide, lanreotide, and octreotate to deliver beta-emitting radionuclides such as yttrium-90 (^{90}Y) and lutetium-177 (^{177}Lu) as therapeutic agents for treatment of disseminated metastatic neuroendocrine tumors expressing SSTR. These radiolabeled peptides have a significant impact in less than one third of the patients and a stabilizing effect for varying intervals in perhaps another 40%. Results are dependant upon patient selection (disease status) and the radiation absorbed dose delivered to the metastases. This work has been performed in Rotterdam, Brussels, Uppsala, Milan, and a few other European centers.[20,24,80,84] In the United States, only a few centers have had access to these compounds during clinical trials. Unfortunately, at the present time, none of these agents are available in the United States. Some investigators have evaluated the potential for the use of ^{111}In-labeled pentetreotide in large doses as a therapeutic agent based upon the radiobiological effect of the Auger electron emitted from the decay of [111]In. The significant amount of gamma emission creates radiation safety difficulties in manufacturing and exposure to medical staff and family members. Although some efficacy has been reported, the results in general have not been as good as those with beta-emitting radionuclides.[23]

PARATHYROID GLANDS

Anatomy and Physiology

The parathyroid glands are located in the neck. They are multifocal (usually four) and found alongside the thyroid gland, lying either adjacent, beneath, or within the substance of the thyroid (see Figure 15-2). The parathyroids migrate from their embryological origins in the branchial clefts into the neck to their usual location alongside the thyroid. Considerable variation may occur, however, in their ultimate location. They can be found within the thyroid gland, elsewhere in the neck, in the mediastinum, within the thymus, among the great vessels (within the carotid sheath above the level of the thyroid to the area around the subclavian and innominate vessels in the thorax).

The parathyroid glands synthesize, store, and secrete parathyroid hormone, a polypeptide hormone that regulates calcium and phosphorus metabolism via action on the bone, kidneys, and gastrointestinal tract. In bone, parathyroid hormone directly stimulates osteoclastic activity, increasing bone resorption and thereby making calcium (and phosphorus) available to the plasma and tissues. In the kidneys, parathyroid hormone increases urinary excretion of phosphorus by inhibiting tubular resorption of phosphate. In the gastrointestinal tract, calcium absorption from the bowel lumen is enhanced by parathyroid hormone.

Synthesis and secretion of parathyroid hormone are regulated by the plasma-ionized calcium level, which is maintained in a physiological range by means of a negative feedback loop: a decline in plasma-ionized calcium stimulates the release of parathyroid hormone, making the calcium ion available.

Clinical Aspects

Failure of the parathyroid tissue to produce parathyroid hormone results in hypoparathyroidism, causing a gradual reduction in serum calcium (hypocalcemia). Clinical manifestations of hypocalcemia are a consequence of delayed repolarization of cell membrane electrical potential, which results in muscle spasm and irritability and cardiac conduction abnormalities.

Excessive secretion of parathyroid hormone (inappropriate secretion despite normal or elevated calcium levels) is known as *hyperparathyroidism*. A principal component of this disorder is elevation of the serum calcium (hypercalcemia). This is associated with increased urinary excretion of calcium, which can cause renal stones and calcification of the kidney (renal calcinosis) and other soft tissues. Because the bones provide a storage source for calcium, orthopedic complications arise from bone mineral loss. There are many causes of hypercalcemia including primary hyperparathyroidism, renal disease, sarcoidosis, and metastatic bone disease. Primary hyperparathyroidism is most frequently associated with a functioning parathyroid adenoma arising from one of the parathyroid glands (80% to 90% of cases). Hyperplasia of the parathyroid glands accounts for the remaining 10% to 20% of cases. The underlying mechanism for diffuse hyperplasia with loss of normal feedback suppression is unknown but probably is a result of receptor autonomy.

In chronic renal disease, the kidneys fail to excrete the phosphate ion adequately and serum phosphate levels rise. Because an upper limit exists for the product of serum calcium and the phosphate ion concentration, calcium is deposited in soft tissues or excreted. Lowering of the serum calcium in this manner stimulates parathyroid hormone secretion and parathyroid gland growth, leading to a clinical condition known as *secondary hyperparathyroidism*. The clinical picture is a mixed one, expressing the underlying chronic renal disease, the secondary hyperparathyroidism (hypocalcemia and increased bone resorption). Therapy should be directed to the underlying renal disease. At times the hyperparathyroidism and related hypercalcemia is so severe that a transplanted kidney would be at risk. Surgical removal of the excess parathyroid tissue is also necessary.[19] Although the excessive parathyroid hormone synthesis and secretion in chronic renal disease begins as a homeostatic response to the hypocalcemia (secondary to the hyperphosphatemia), the hyperactivity may persist after correction of the renal disorder as a consequence of a functioning parathyroid adenoma. This is so-called tertiary hyperparathyroidism.

In the modern era, routine serum calcium determinations result in earlier clinical recognition of hypercalcemia, leading to earlier detection of hyperparathyroidism. This presents an opportunity for nuclear medicine to assist in the localization of the functioning adenoma, because with earlier recognition comes the challenge of locating smaller adenomas.

Nuclear Medicine Procedures

In clinical situations in which hyperparathyroidism is suspected, direct measurement of serum parathyroid hormone by radioimmunoassay provides the basis for the diagnosis. This assay should be conducted before scintigraphy, which is performed to identify the site or sites of parathyroid hormone hypersecretion.

The role of the nuclear medicine imaging is in patients with confirmed hyperparathyroidism in an effort to identify the location of a parathyroid adenoma; not for the differential diagnosis of hypercalcemia. Although experienced surgeons are very successful in finding and removing parathyroid adenoma, performance is improved and anesthesia and operating time are reduced with the use of preoperative imaging for precise localization. In the event the parathyroid tissue is ectopic, the impact of preoperative localization is even greater.[4] Parathyroid adenomas can be found in diverse locations alongside, behind, and within the thyroid and in areas somewhat distant from the thyroid, such as high or low in the neck or mediastinum. Although CT, MRI, and sonography locate parathyroid adenomas, parathyroid scintigraphy is the only technique that confirms the functional nature of the anatomical finding.[54] Parathyroid scintigraphy itself has a high degree of accuracy and is less operator dependant than sonography.[4,36,37,73] The relatively recent introduction of a gamma probe provides assistance in site localization within the operating room as well as serving to confirm completeness of resection.

Technetium-99m-MIBI has emerged as the radiotracer of choice for the localization of parathyroid adenomas.* Two methods are currently available: a dual-tracer method and a so-called dual-phase method (Figure 15-17, Box 15-5). In the dual-tracer technique, ^{99m}Tc-pertechnetate is used to initially identify thyroid tissue. Subsequently, 20 to 25 mCi of ^{99m}Tc-MIBI is administered to identify both thyroid and parathyroid tissue. Both image sets are corrected by background subtraction. The ^{99m}Tc-pertechnetate image is normalized to the ^{99m}Tc-MIBI image by adjusting for the ratio of counts in the thyroid region of interest, and then the normalized ^{99m}Tc-pertechnetate image is subtracted from the secondarily acquired ^{99m}Tc-MIBI thyroid and parathyroid image, effectively leaving the residual image representing parathyroid tissue (Figure 15-18). This process used to involve operator interaction, but contemporary equipment has software that virtually automates the several maneuvers involved in production of the subtracted image.

Thyroid adenoma as well as thyroid carcinoma are frequent false-positive findings because these tumors trap ^{99m}Tc-pertechnetate poorly and therefore will appear cold on ^{99m}Tc-pertechnetate imaging but positive with ^{99m}Tc-MIBI and on the subtraction images. Even with

*References 21, 22, 26, 59, 62, and 82.

Parathyroid scintigraphy

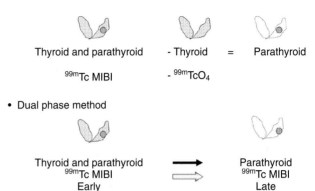

FIGURE 15-17 Schematic of Dual Phase procedure for parathyroid scintigraphy illustrating parathyroid adenoma localization by subtraction (*Dual Tracer*) and delayed imaging (*Dual Phase*) methods.

BOX 15-5 | **Parathyroid Scintigraphy**

1. ^{99m}Tc-pertechnetate/^{99m}Tc-MIBI protocol: Place patient supine; stabilize neck if necessary.
2. Administer 4 to 6 mCi ^{99m}Tc-pertechnetate; use high-resolution collimator.
3. Acquire anterior image for 5 minutes, 20 minutes after injection (use electronic zoom to fill image field with thyroid). Some departments use dynamic acquisition (1-minute frames) to correct for motion.
4. With patient in same position, inject 20 to 25 mCi ^{99m}Tc-MIBI.
5. Acquire anterior image for 10 to 15 minutes, 5 minutes after injection. Use 1-minute frame if preferred.
6. Perform background subtraction for each image set; normalize background subtracted images. Many computer programs perform these maneuvers automatically.
7. Obtain nonzoomed image of anterior thorax to exclude ectopic location.
8. ^{123}I/^{99m}Tc-MIBI protocol:
   a. Administer 200 to 400 µCi of ^{123}I. Patient returns next day.
   b. Acquire ^{123}I anterior cervical image for 10 minutes.
   c. Repeat steps 4 through 7.
   d. Delayed imaging at 90 to 120 minutes after initial ^{99m}Tc-MIBI images.
   e. If SPECT or SPECT/CT desired, obtain at 60 to 90 minutes.

---

this knowledge, thyroid adenoma and carcinoma cannot readily be distinguished from parathyroid adenomas by subtraction imaging. In fact, this situation is the same as the flip-flop phenomenon described for the differential diagnosis of thyroid nodules.

The use of ^{99m}Tc-MIBI has, in general, supplanted the use of ^{201}Tl. Formerly, when ^{201}Tl was used to identify parathyroid adenoma, ^{123}I was used for subtraction of thyroid tissue. Some departments continue to prefer ^{123}I for thyroid localization. Although good quality images are obtained, this protocol involves 2 days of patient

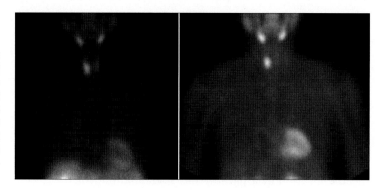

FIGURE 15-18 Anterior neck and upper thorax region images at 10 minutes and 2 hours after administration of 20 mCi ^{99m}Tc-MIBI. In the early images, activity is seen throughout both thyroid lobes. The delayed image shows prominent activity in the lower pole of the right thyroid lobe. This focus of persistent activity is characteristic of a parathyroid adenoma and has a high degree of accuracy in predicting the location of this lesion in an appropriate at-risk population (patients with hyperparathyroidism). False-positive results may be associated with thyroid abnormalities.

visits. ^{123}I (200-300 μCi) are administered on day 1. The patient returns after 24 hours and a thyroid image is acquired. Following this, the patient is injected with the second tracer (currently 20 to 25 mCi ^{99m}Tc-MIBI). Other ^{99m}Tc tracers that were introduced for myocardial perfusion imaging have been used in place of ^{99m}Tc-MIBI in both dual-tracer and dual-phase parathyroid scintigraphy for identification of parathyroid adenomas. These compounds (e.g., ^{99m}Tc-tetrafosmin) have extraction efficiencies and efflux (washout) rates that are slightly different from those of ^{99m}Tc-MIBI. Although satisfactory images have been obtained in many instances, the few comparison studies available suggest that ^{99m}Tc-MIBI is superior to its competitors to localize parathyroid adenomas.[28]

The sensitivity (and specificity) of ^{99m}Tc-MIBI (and ^{99m}Tc tetrafosmin) subtraction scintigraphy is superior to the results obtained with ^{201}Tl subtraction scintigraphy.[2,28] The improvement in overall accuracy is partly the result of the superior imaging characteristics (lower energy) and greater photon flux (larger dose, shorter half-life) of ^{99m}Tc and also the pharmacology or biochemistry of ^{99m}Tc-MIBI and other ^{99m}Tc tumor perfusion agents that bind efficiently to mitochondrial proteins resulting in a greater parathyroid-to-thyroid and parathyroid-to-background ratio than was observed with ^{201}Tl.

In late 1992, Taillefer and colleagues[83] described a so-called double-phase study in which anterior cervical images are obtained at 15 to 20 minutes after injection of 20 to 25 mCi of ^{99m}Tc-MIBI and again at 2 to 3 hours after injection. Ten-minute acquisition was obtained using a parallel-hole, low-energy, high-resolution collimator with a 1.5 zoom factor. The differential washout of the ^{99m}Tc-MIBI (with retention by the parathyroid tissue) resulted in preferential visualization of parathyroid in 19 of 21 instances[83] (see Figure 15-18). It is also convenient with this technique to obtain views of the thorax to detect mediastinal ectopic parathyroid tissue at both the early and late acquisition because the patient is already positioned under a camera with a parallel-hole collimator.

This procedure has been modified since the initial description. ^{99m}Tc-MIBI is injected and the images of the neck are acquired after approximately 30 minutes, the so-called early phase. Repeat imaging of the neck follows at 90 to 120 minutes with comparison of the two image sets. Identification of the parathyroid tissue is based on greater retention of the ^{99m}Tc-MIBI in the metabolically active, mitochondria-dense parathyroid adenoma. However, this mode of identification is not completely parathyroid tissue–specific either, because other focal lesions, specifically thyroid adenomas and carcinomas, preferentially retain ^{99m}Tc-MIBI compared with the surrounding thyroid and other tissue. Nevertheless, in an appropriate clinical setting where the pretest probability of parathyroid adenoma is high because of confirmed elevated parathyroid hormone levels, ^{99m}Tc-MIBI accumulation representing mitochondria-rich tissue is most likely a functioning parathyroid adenoma.

Obviously, the dual-tracer and dual-phase techniques can be combined; that is, the dual radionuclide method can be followed by acquisition of an additional (delayed) ^{99m}Tc-MIBI image. Lesions in this area are quite distinct and can readily be identified because the surrounding tissue is relatively poorly perfused (mediastinum) or less dense (lung). Because the amount of ^{99m}Tc-MIBI activity administered is four to five times that of the ^{99m}Tc-pertechnetate, the ^{99m}Tc-pertechnetate component is trivial and can be ignored when viewing the ^{99m}Tc-MIBI images.

The dual-tracer subtraction parathyroid scintigraphy method is quite dependant on acquisition technique and processing (and requires no patient movement for accuracy). The dual-phase ^{99m}Tc-MIBI method depends upon qualitative interpretation of the degree of contrast, which varies from adenoma to adenoma. Not surprisingly, a wide range of values for sensitivity from 39% to more than 90% have been reported. A cost-effective meta-analysis in the surgical literature concluded that the technique has an overall sensitivity of 91% and a specificity of 99%.[43]

SPECT imaging further improves identification of the surgical location of the hyperfunctioning parathyroid tissue.[16,43] SPECT images of the neck and upper thorax can be obtained about 1 hour after injection, which allows for contrast between activity in the thyroid tissue and a parathyroid adenoma (or even hyperplastic parathyroid tissue) based upon retention of ^{99m}Tc-MIBI by the mitochondria-rich adenoma. This can be followed with the delayed-phase image acquisition.

Initially, the parathyroid ^{99m}Tc-MIBI SPECT images were unimpressive because of the lack of anatomical information and difficulty in assigning a location to the finding (as well as the greater effort involved in acquisition and interpretation). Nevertheless, published reports consistently showed greater sensitivity for ^{99m}Tc-MIBI SPECT than for planar acquisitions alone. The improvement was generally in terms of detection of smaller adenomata, sometimes less than 1 g.

When image fusion SPECT/CT hardware that combined CT images with the SPECT images became available, it became possible to identify the location of the functional activity with a high degree of accuracy. The technique was quite satisfactory and there was an improvement over SPECT alone in terms of identifying the anatomical location of adenoma even when the adenoma is located in a usual location, and more so when an ectopic adenoma is present. Technetium-99m–MIBI SPECT/CT for localization of parathyroid adenomata is highly recommended even though it is essential (in retrospect) in only 10% to 15% of the cases. In one report, there was no difference in the overall high degree of accuracy between SPECT and SPECT/CT ^{99m}Tc-MIBI parathyroid imaging but greater confidence and precision in identification of the site of the hyperfunctioning tissue.[65,66,71] More recently, the author had the opportunity to review SPECT/CT images from an instrument that combined a state-of-the-art, dual-head gamma camera with a full diagnostic CT. The adenoma was located between a thyroid lobe and the trachea, not an unusual location. The detailed anatomical image with the superimposed functional (scintigraphy-derived) information, however, provided a clear road map for surgical intervention that inevitably will pay dividends in terms of reduced morbidity and improve surgical technique.

In essence, parathyroid scintigraphy has undergone a recurring cycle of technological advances that were greeted with enthusiasm by a minority of the nuclear medicine and surgical community but with skepticism and resistance for the most part and then by gradual acceptance.

Despite the progress in refining this noninvasive technique, nuclear medicine physicians and surgeons in some centers have taken advantage of ^{99m}Tc-MIBI localizing preferentially in parathyroid adenoma by combining ^{99m}Tc-MIBI with the use of a gamma probe in the operating room. Used preferably in addition to scintigraphy, intraoperative probe guidance reduces anesthesia and operating time and decreases morbidity following parathyroidectomy.[57,80,88] More than 50% of endocrine surgeons surveyed use ^{99m}Tc-MIBI and the gamma probe to perform minimally invasive parathyroid surgery.[18,35] The probe is used to enhance locating the parathyroid

adenoma and to confirm that all of the hyperfunctioning tissue has been resected.

ADRENAL GLANDS

The adrenal glands consist of an outer adrenal cortex and an interior neurosecretory adrenal medulla. They are located in the retroperitoneum, superior to the kidneys (suprarenal), lying approximately below the eleventh rib. The right adrenal is higher and more posterior than the left (even though the left kidney is frequently higher than the right); the right adrenal is triangular, sitting astride the upper pole of the right kidney. The left adrenal is more crescent shaped and lies anteromedial to the upper pole of the left kidney.

ADRENAL MEDULLA

Anatomy and Physiology

The adrenal medulla is typically located within the adrenal gland surrounded by the adrenal cortex. The medullary tissue is quite small; on sectioning, the area of the adrenal cortex–adrenal medulla is approximately 10:1. The adrenal medulla tissue synthesizes and secretes the catecholamines epinephrine and norepinephrine, hormones that maintain (or increase) smooth muscle tone, heart rate and force of contraction, and other physiological responses associated with stress.

Benign or malignant functioning tumors of this tissue are known as *pheochromocytomas*, which are hyperplastic nodules 1 cm in diameter or larger. Below this size the entity is defined as macronodular hyperplasia. Despite their small size, these tumors may elaborate excessive amounts of epinephrine or norepinephrine, producing a classic picture of undesirable symptoms, particularly hypertension and other consequences of excessive catecholamine product. Pheochromocytomas occur as an apparently spontaneous benign or malignant tumor of the adrenal medulla but may arise from any site of autonomic nervous tissue. They are a frequent component of the hereditary syndrome multiple endocrine neoplasia (MEN) types IIa and IIb. Despite advances in clinical chemistry that make direct assay of catecholamines and even specific assays of plasma and urinary epinephrine and norepinephrine more readily available, the disease is often a clinical enigma, frequently not diagnosed until postmortem examination. Moreover, some tumors elaborate excessive amounts of catecholamines but do not secrete these products into the circulation. Hence, these patients do not present with the typical clinical symptoms associated with pheochromocytoma. These nonsecretory tumors are called paragangliomas. Nevertheless, they may become malignant and then invade surrounding tissue, metastasize throughout the body, or both. The small size of the adrenal medullary tissue and a propensity for ectopic sites make diagnosis even by CT and MRI

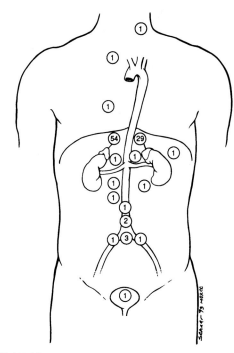

FIGURE 15-19 In a large surgical series, pheochromocytoma was found in the adrenal bed in 83 of 100 patients (three patients had bilateral pheochromocytoma) and in extra-adrenal sites in 17 patients. These sites were distributed principally along the para-aortic tissue as far caudally as the bifurcation and iliac vessels and cephalad above the aortic arch. In one patient a pheochromocytoma was found in the bladder wall.

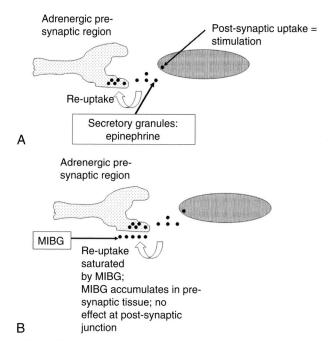

FIGURE 15-20 Metaiodobenzylguanidine (MIBG) uptake mechanism.

unreliable. The aberrant distribution pattern is documented in Figure 15-19, in which 24 of 107 pheochromocytomas were found outside the adrenal glands.[58]

Nuclear Medicine Procedures

The role of nuclear medicine is to identify the location of the catecholamine-synthesizing tumor, either pheochromocytoma or paraganglioma which can occur in one or both adrenals or in an ectopic location related to the distribution of adrenergic tissue. Both benign pheochromocytomas and metastatic sites may be quite small even though there is considerable metabolic activity and life-threatening symptoms associated with the release of excessive amounts of powerful vasoactive amines. Following many years of dedicated research by chemists at the University of Michigan, ^{131}I-MIBG was approved by the U.S. Food and Drug Administration (FDA) over 30 years ago for clinical use as a diagnostic imaging agent. Although cumbersome to work with because of the 364-keV gamma emission and the limited amount of activity used (typically 1 mCi in adults), ^{131}I-MIBG became the imaging agent of choice to identify normal, ectopic, or hyperfunctioning adrenal medullary tissue.[75]

Subsequently, ^{123}I-MIBG was synthesized, but for several years before commercialization and FDA approval, the short half-life of ^{123}I precluded availability of this material except at institutions prepared to

synthesize the radiotracer and perform the required pharmaceutical purity, sterility, and pyrogen testing. Currently, ^{123}I-MIBG is commercially available for routine use in nuclear medicine departments. MIBG labeled with ^{123}I or ^{131}I provides a means to identify the extent of disease in patients with neuroblastoma, a malignant tumor of childhood that can be widely disseminated in the abdomen and bone marrow.

After secretion at the synapse, a portion of the norepinephrine is reabsorbed and stored in granules at the presynaptic site via a presynaptic reuptake mechanism. MIBG has little or no pharmacological effect and does not bind significantly at postsynaptic receptors. As stated, it is incorporated into the presynaptic adrenergic storage granules because of structural similarities to norepinephrine, providing the basis for visualization of adrenergic tissue in general and pheochromocytomas and paragangliomas in particular (Figure 15-20).

At the University of Michigan, analysis of experience with ^{131}I-MIBG in 400 patients with malignant pheochromocytoma demonstrated a sensitivity of 92.4% and a specificity of 100%.[11]

Despite the well-appreciated superiority of ^{123}I as an imaging agent over ^{131}I, many practitioners had initial reluctance to use ^{123}I-MIBG because the short half-life precludes delayed imaging, which was thought to be necessary because the 3- to 5-day interval provided improved target-to-background and hence images of potentially greater diagnostic accuracy. Although ^{123}I-MIBG images were of better quality, studies comparing ^{131}I-MIBG and ^{123}I-MIBG planar scintigraphy showed equivalent performance in terms of detecting pheochromocytoma as well as neuroblastoma, which also localizes MIBG. Nevertheless, the convenience of same-day or 24-hour imaging with ^{123}I-MIBG (as well as the more favorable physical characteristics) was gradually recognized as a practical advantage (Box 15-6). Currently, ^{123}I-MIBG is the preferable imaging agent in doses of 10 mCi (370 MBq) in adults. In addition to improved image quality (despite the lack of evidence of improved sensitivity), ^{123}I-MIBG provides sufficient photon flux for SPECT imaging, which is generally beneficial. SPECT acquisition with ^{123}I-MIBG is made at 3-degree intervals, 128 × 128 matrix, 20 to 30 seconds per stop.

The introduction of SPECT/CT equipment several years ago provided fused images, which improved the ease of interpretation and identification of abnormal accumulations indicative of tumor. In an early report, it was demonstrated that ^{123}I-MIBG SPECT/CT fusion images convincingly excluded a clinically suspected pheochromocytoma in one patient by precisely mapping physiological excretion of MIBG in the ureter.[27] In another series, ^{123}I-MIBG SPECT/CT improved detection of malignant adrenergic tumors and improved specificity over SPECT and CT alone. Fusion images certainly provide a greater degree of confidence for the scan reader as well as the referring physician. Although difficult to quantify, it is believed that SPECT/CT improves

diagnostic information in more than half of the ^{123}I-MIBG performed.[29,41]

Lugol solution or 400 mg of potassium perchlorate should be given to the patient to block thyroid uptake of released iodine at least 1 day before ^{123}I-MIBG or ^{131}I-MIBG administration and continued for 2 and 7 days, respectively. Initial ^{123}I-MIBG images can be obtained at 4 hours and may include SPECT (or SPECT/CT) at that time. The principal diagnostic image set is obtained at 24 hours. Medications that affect the adrenergic system (alpha and beta receptor blockers, decongestants, calcium channel blockers, and tricyclic antidepressants) should be discontinued, but agents that block alpha and beta receptors have no effect on MIBG uptake. As discussed in the section on the thyroid gland, ^{123}I imaging is ideally performed with medium-energy (ME) collimation because septal penetration by high-energy gammas and the scatter from these photons will adversely effect image quality. Nevertheless, it has become common practice to use low-energy, high-resolution collimators.

MIBG should be injected slowly over approximately 5 minutes. Blood pressure and electrocardiogram (ECG) monitoring are optional. A dose of approximately 10 mCi (400 MBq) ^{123}I-MIBG is recommended for diagnostic studies in adults and is adjusted in children based on weight.[64]

Following its initial introduction, radiolabeled MIBG has been used to image the adrenergic cardiac innervation and its impairment in patients with early diabetic neuropathy, or those with arrhythmias.[11,42,77] More recently, MIBG myocardial scintigraphy has been studied in patients with cardiomyopathy and heart failure.[11,30,38,74]

The normal distribution of ^{131}I-MIBG includes the heart (because of the rich neural innervation), liver, spleen, salivary glands, and bladder (the latter two sites because of excretion of free iodine eluted from the tracer). In normal subjects, the adrenal medulla is usually faintly visible. Identification of a pheochromocytoma is usually made based on asymmetrical intense tracer uptake in the adrenal bed or elsewhere in the abdomen or thorax (Figure 15-21). Persistent or increased uptake

---

BOX 15-6	MIBG Imaging (^{123}I-MIBG)

1. Confirm patient has started Lugol solution or saturated solution of potassium iodide (SSKI) drops orally
2. 10 mCi ^{123}I-MIBI IV
3. Individualize protocol per patients needs; physicians request.
4. Medium-energy collimator
5. At 24 hours, acquire whole body (to mid thigh) images at slow scan speed (6 cm/min desired); alternately, static images, 10 to 15 minutes per image. Low- or medium-energy collimator per department protocol.
6. Review planar images with nuclear physician about SPECT or SPECT/CT location. Perform per facility ^{123}I protocol.

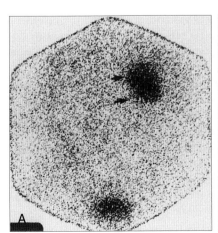 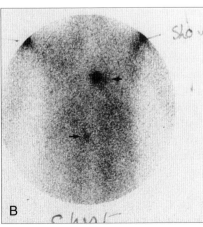

FIGURE 15-21 Imaging at 72 hours after 1 mCi ^{131}I MIBG. **A,** Gamma camera view of the anterior abdomen in a patient with a pheochromocytoma arising from the left adrenal medulla (arrows). **B,** Gamma camera view of the posterior thoracolumbar region in another patient with a recurrent malignant pheochromocytoma. A small residual focus is seen in the left adrenal bed region, and a prominent intense focus is seen in the right thoracic paraspinal region (arrows).

bilaterally suggests bilateral pheochromocytoma, although this diagnosis should not be considered if only faint uptake is seen at 4 hours that does not increase in activity or contrast. In malignant pheochromocytoma, uptake is seen in metastases in the liver, bone, lymph nodes, heart, lungs, mediastinum, and other sites.

Indium-111-DTPA-pentetreotide has also been used to image for the detection pheochromocytomas but this is no longer considered to be the case. ^{123}I-MIBG is currently considered to be the preferred radiotracer for detection of pheochromocytoma and paraganglioma. If ^{111}In-DTPA-pentetreotide scintigraphy is being considered as well as ^{123}I-MIBG scintigraphy, the ^{123}I-MIBG should be used first because of the shorter half-life.

Iodine-131-MIBG therapy is used at a limited number of medical centers as a therapeutic agent to treat malignant pheochromocytoma, paraganglioma, and some cases of neuroblastoma. Its use is limited to investigational protocols requiring a physician-sponsored investigational new drug (IND).

SUMMARY

- The principal endocrine glands are the pituitary (anterior and posterior) gland, thyroid gland, parathyroid glands, the islet cells of the pancreas, adrenal glands (cortex and medulla), and the gonads (ovaries or testes).

- The basis and description of the nuclear medicine procedures approved by regulatory agencies and available clinically for the evaluation of the thyroid gland, the parathyroid glands, the adrenal medulla, and the distributed neuroendocrine system has been reviewed. Nuclear medicine applications in these areas are primarily diagnostic and are based on single photon emitting radiotracers utilizing planar, SPECT, and SPECT/CT scintigraphy.

- There is a great deal of research and development involving new PET tracers, but to date, except for ^{18}F-FDG as an indicator of tumor metabolism, the use of these tracers is investigational.

- Currently, radionuclide therapy is limited to ^{131}I-iodide therapy of the thyroid, specifically hyperthyroidism and thyroid carcinoma.

- Nuclear medicine is a medical discipline and technology that requires specific training and experience for the technologists and physicians involved in the use of these procedures for patient care. The physiological basis for the technology has been discussed in detail, as have the technological aspects of the nuclear medicine procedures currently used to characterize endocrine physiology in health and disease.

- Thyroid hormone synthesis depends on the trapping and organification of iodine ingested in food and water.

- The overall function of the thyroid gland is regulated by the hypothalamus-pituitary axis via TSH, which is produced by the pituitary gland. The hypothalamus communicates with the pituitary gland via TRH (thyrotrophin-releasing hormone).

- A pharmacological block at the organification step of iodine metabolism provides the basis for therapy of hyperthyroidism with antithyroid drugs.

- Diseases of the thyroid can be classified into functional disorders and structural disorders; in many cases both are involved.

- Radioimmunoassay is the most widely used procedure to measure circulating serum T_4, T_3, TSH, TBG, and Tg.

- In vivo testing of thyroid function is based on the degree of iodine uptake.

- Iodine-131 is a mainstay in the therapy of patients with either hyperthyroidism or thyroid carcinoma including ablation of residual normal thyroid tissue or treatment of local or distal metastases.

- Technetium-99m-pertechnetate is trapped but not organified; after trapping, it washes out of the thyroid tissue in a short time.

- Fluorine-18-FDG uptake depends on a tumor's metabolic activity.

- When performing a thyroid uptake test, careful technique is essential so that results accurately reflect patient variables rather than technical variables.

- The principal reason to image a thyroid with palpable findings is to see if the palpable nodule is cold or hot, or similar in function to the rest of the thyroid.

- In thyroid carcinoma, the role of nuclear medicine (aside from identifying suspect nodules as cold) is in the management and treatment of the patient after surgical removal of most or all of the functioning thyroid and readily identifiable cervical lymph node involvement.

- All patients should have a 24-hour radioactive iodine uptake and either a ^{99m}Tc-pertechnetate or ^{123}I-iodide scan before undergoing radioiodine therapy.

- Drug analogs of somatostatin (e.g., octreotide) bind to somatostatin receptors.

- Somatostatin-receptor scintigraphy is a major element in the clinical management of patients with neuroendocrine tumors; when available, SPECT/CT should be used for optimal results.

- Primary hyperparathyroidism is most frequently associated with a functioning parathyroid adenoma arising from one of the parathyroid glands.

- Parathyroid scintigraphy is the only technique that confirms the functional nature of the anatomical findings.

- Pheochromocytomas occur as an apparently spontaneous benign or malignant tumor of the adrenal medulla but may arise from any site of autonomic nervous tissue.

REFERENCES

1. Andros G, Harper PV, Lathrop KA, et al: Pertechnetate-99m localization in man with applications to thyroid scanning and the study of thyroid physiology, *J Clin Endocrinol Metab* 35:250-256, 1972.

2. Apostolopoulos DJ, Houstoulaki E, Grannakenas E, et al: Technetium-99m-tetrafosmin for parathyroid scintigraphy: comparison with thallium-pertechnetate scanning, *J Nucl Med* 39:1433-1441, 1998.

3. Atkins HL, Richards P: Assessment of thyroid function and anatomy with ^{99m}Tc-pertechnetate, *J Nucl Med* 9:7-9, 1968.

4. Attie JN, Kahn A, Rumancik WM, et al: Preoperative localization of parathyroid adenomas, *Am J Surg* 156:323-326, 1988.

5. Balon HR, Goldsmith SJ, Siegel BA, et al. Procedure guideline for somatostatin receptor scintigraphy with ^{111}In-pentetreotide, *J Nucl Med* 42:1134-1138, 2001.

6. Becker DV, Charkes ND, Dworkin H, et al: Procedure guideline for extended scintigraphy for differentiated thyroid cancer: 1.0, *J Nucl Med* 37:1269-1271, 1996.

7. Becker DV, Charkes ND, Dworkin H, et al: Procedure guideline for thyroid scintigraphy: 1.0, *J Nucl Med* 37:1264-1266, 1996.

8. Becker DV, Charkes ND, Dworkin H, et al: Procedure guideline for thyroid uptake measurement: 1.0, *J Nucl Med* 37:1266-1268, 1996.

9. Becker DV, Hurley JR: Current status of radioiodine (^{131}I) treatment of hyperthyroidism. In Freeman L, Weissmann HS, editors: *Nuclear medicine annual 1982*, New York, 1982, Raven Press.

10. Becker DV, Hurley JR: Radioiodine treatment of hyperthyroidism. In Gottschalk A, Hoffer PB, Potchen EJ, editors: *Diagnostic nuclear medicine*, vol 2, Baltimore, 1988, Williams & Wilkins.

11. Beierwaltes WH: Clinical applications of 131-I labeled metaiodobenzylguanidine. In Hoffer PB, editor: *1987 year book of nuclear medicine*, Chicago, 1987, Year Book Medical.

12. Beierwaltes WH: Endocrine imaging: parathyroid, adrenal cortex and medulla, and other endocrine tumors, part II, *J Nucl Med* 32:1627-1639, 1991.

13. Beierwaltes WH, Nishiyama RH, Thompson NW, et al: Survival time and "cure" in papillary and follicular carcinoma with distant metastases: statistics following University of Michigan therapy, *J Nucl Med* 23:561-568, 1982.

14. Berson SA, Yalow RS: Immunoassay of endogenous plasma insulin in man, *J Clin Invest* 35:170-177, 1960.

15. Berson SA, Yalow RS, Glick SA, et al: Immunoassay of protein and peptide hormones, *Metabolism* 13:1135-1140, 1964.

16. Billotey C, Sarfati E, Aurengo A, et al: Advantages of SPECT in technetium-99m-sestamibi parathyroid scintigraphy, *J Nucl Med* 37:1773-1778, 1996.

17. Briganti V, Matteini M, Ferri P, et al: Octreoscan SPET evaluation in the diagnosis of pancreas neuroendocrine tumors, *Cancer Biother Radiopharm* 16:515-524, 2001.

18. Casara D, Rubello D, Cauzzo C, Pelizzo MR: 99mTc-MIBI radio-guided minimally invasive parathyroidectomy: experience with patients with normal thyroids and nodular goiters, *Thyroid* 12:53-61, 2002.

19. Chen H: Surgery for primary hyperparathyroidism: what is the best approach? *Ann Surg* 236:552-553, 2002.

20. Chinol M, Bodei L, Cremonisi M, et al: Receptor-mediated radiotherapy with ^{90}Y-DOTA-DPhe^1-Tyr^3, *Semin Nucl Med* 32:141-147, 2002.

21. Civelek AC, Ozalp E, Donovan P, et al: Prospective evaluation of delayed technetium-99m sestamibi SPECT scintigraphy for preoperative localization of primary hyperparathyroidism, *Surgery* 131:149-157, 2002.

22. Coakley AJ, Kettle AG, Wells CP, et al: ^{99m}Tc sestamibi—a new agent for parathyroid imaging, *Nucl Med Commun* 10:791-794, 1989.

23. de Jong M, Bakker WH, Breeman WAP, et al: Phase I study of peptide receptor therapy with [^{111}In-DTPA^0] octreotide: the Rotterdam experience, *Semin Nucl Med* 32:110-122, 2002.

24. de Jong M, Valkema JF, Kvols LK, et al: Somatostatin receptor–targeted therapy of tumors: preclinical and clinical findings, *Semin Nucl Med* 32:133-140, 2002.

25. de Jong M, Valkema R, Breeman WA, et al: Neuroendocrine neoplasia: scintigraphy and radionuclide therapy. In Khalkhali I, Maublant JC, Goldsmith SJ: *Nuclear Oncology*, Philadelphia, 2001, Lippincott.

26. Denham DW, Norman J: Cost-effectiveness of preoperative sestamibi scan for primary hyperparathyroidism is dependent solely upon the surgeon's choice of operative procedure, *J Am Coll Surg* 186:293-305, 1998.

27. Even-Sapir E, Keidar Z, Sachs J, et al: The new technology of combined transmission and emission tomography in evaluation of endocrine neoplasms, *J Nucl Med* 42:998-1004, 2002.

28. Fjeld JG, Ericksen K, Pfeffer PF, et al: Technetium-99m-tetrafosmin for parathyroid scintigraphy: a comparison with sestamibi, *J Nucl Med* 38:831-834, 1997.

29. Forster GJ, Laumann C, Nickel O, et al: SPET/CT image co-registration in the abdomen with a simple cost-effective tool, *Eur J Nucl Med Mol Imaging* 30:32-39, 2003.

30. Fujimoto S, Inoue A, Hisatake S, et al: Usefulness of (123) I-metaiodobenzylguanidine myocardial scintigraphy for predicting the effectiveness of beta-blockers in patients with dilated cardiomyopathy from the standpoint of long-term prognosis, *Eur J Nucl Med Mol Imaging* 31:1356-1361, 2004.

31. Gibril F, Reynolds JC, Doppman JL, et al: Somatostatin receptor scintigraphy: its sensitivity compared with that of other imaging methods in detecting primary and metastatic gastrinomas, *Ann Intern Med* 125:26-34, 1996.

32. Goldsmith SJ: Thyroid carcinoma: diagnosis, management and therapy. In Khalkhali I, Maublant J, Goldsmith SJ, editors: *Nuclear oncology: diagnosis and therapy*, Philadelphia, 2000, Lippincott Williams & Wilkins.

33. Goldsmith SJ: Thyroid: in vivo tests of function and imaging. In Rothfield B, editor: *Nuclear medicine: endocrinology*, Philadelphia, 1978, JB Lippincott.

34. Goldsmith SJ, Macapinlac HA, O'Brien JP: Somatostatin-receptor imaging in lymphoma, *Semin Nucl Med* 25:262-271, 1995.

35. Goldstein RE, Blevins L, Delbeke D, et al: Effect of minimally invasive radioguided parathyroidectomy on efficacy, length of stay, and costs in the management of primary hyperparathyroidism, *Ann Surg* 231:732-742, 2000.

36. Gotthardt M, Lohmann B, Behr TM, et al: Clinical value of parathyroid scintigraphy with technetium-99m methoxyisobutylisonitrile: discrepancies in clinical data and a systematic metaanalysis of the literature, *World J Surg* 28:100-107, 2004.

37. Haber RS, Kim CK, Inabnet WB: Ultrasonography for preoperative localization of enlarged parathyroid glands in primary hyperparathyroidism: comparison with (99m)technetium sestamibi scintigraphy, *Clin Endocrinol (Oxf)* 57:241-249, 2002.

38. Hanscheid H, Lassmann M, Luster M, et al: Iodine biokinetics and dosimetry in radioiodine therapy of thyroid cancer: procedures and results of a perspective international controlled study of ablation after rh TSH or hormone withdrawal, *J Nucl Med* 47(4):648-654, 2006.

39. Hattori N, Schwaiger M: Metaiodobenzylguanidine scintigraphy of the heart: what have we learnt clinically? *Eur J Nucl Med* 27:1-6, 2000.

40. Ivanovec V, Nauck C, Sandrock D, et al: Somatostatin receptor scintigraphy with ^{111}In-pentetreotide in gastroenteropancreatic endocrine tumors (GEP), *Eur J Nucl Med* 19:736, 1992.

41. Jamar F, Fiasse R, Leners N, et al: Somatostatin receptor imaging with indium-111-pentetreotide in gastroenteropancreatic neuroendocrine tumors: safety, efficacy and impact on patient management, *J Nucl Med* 36:542-549, 1995.

42. Klein M, Kopelewitz B, Krausz Y, et al: Contribution of SPECT/CT to bridging between MIBG scan and diagnostic CT, *J Nucl Med* 45:1138, 2004.

43. Kline RC, Swanson DP, Wieland DM, et al: Myocardial imaging in man with I-123 meta-iodobenzylguanidine, *J Nucl Med* 22:129-132, 1981.

44. Krausz Y, Bettman L, Keidar Z, et al: Contribution of SPECT/CT to preoperative localization of parathyroid adenoma, *J Nucl Med* 44(suppl):144P, 2003 (abstract).

45. Krausz Y, Keidar Z, Kogan I, et al: SPECT/CT hybrid imaging with ^{111}In-pentetreotide in assessment of neuroendocrine tumors, *Clin Endocrinol (Oxf)* 59:565-573, 2003.

46. Krenning EP, Bakker WH, Breeman WA, et al: Localization of endocrine-related tumors with radioiodinated analogue of somatostatin, *Lancet* 1:242-244, 1989.

47. Krenning EP, Bakker WH, Kooij PP, et al: Somatostatin receptor scintigraphy with indium-111-DTPA-D-Phe-1-octreotide in men: metabolism, dosimetry and comparison with iodine-123-Tyr-3-octreotide, *J Nucl Med* 33:652-658, 1992.

48. Krenning EP, Kwekkeboom DJ, Lamberts SWJ: Somatostatin receptor scintigraphy with [111In-DTPA-D-Phe1] and [123I-Tyr3]-octreotide: the Rotterdam experience with more than 1000 patients, *Eur J Nucl Med* 20:716-731, 1993.

49. Krenning EP, Kwekkeboom DJ, Oei HY, et al: Somatostatin-receptor scintigraphy in gastroenteropancreatic tumors: an overview of the European results, *Ann N Y Acad Sci* 733:416-424, 1994.

50. Kusic Z, Becker DV, Saenger EL, et al: Comparison of technetium-99m and iodine-123 imaging of thyroid nodules: correlation with pathologic findings, *J Nucl Med* 31:393-399, 1990.

51. Kvols LK: Metastatic carcinoid tumors and the malignant carcinoid syndrome, *Ann N Y Acad Sci* 733:464-470, 1994.

52. Leeper RD, Shimaoka K: Treatment of metastatic thyroid cancer, *J Clin Endocrinol Metab* 9:383-404, 1980.

53. Lorberboym M, Minski I, Macadziob S, et al: Incremental diagnostic value of preoperative 99mTc-MIBI SPECT in patients with a parathyroid adenoma, *J Nucl Med* 44:904-908, 2003.

54. Lumachi F, Ermani M, Basso S, et al: Localization of parathyroid tumors in the minimally invasive era: which technique should be chosen? Population-based analysis of 253 patients undergoing parathyroidectomy and factors affecting parathyroid gland detection, *Endocr Relat Cancer* 8:63-69, 2001.

55. Maxon HR, Englaro EE, Thomas SR, et al: Radioiodine-131 therapy for well-differentiated thyroid cancer: a quantitative radiation dosimetric approach—outcome and validation in 85 patients, *J Nucl Med* 33:1132-1137, 1992.

56. Maxon HR, Thomas SR, Hertzberg VS, et al: Relation between radiation dose and outcome of radioiodine therapy for thyroid cancer, *N Engl J Med* 309:937-941, 1983.

57. Medrano C, Hazelrigg SR, Landreneau RJ, et al: Thoracoscopic resection of ectopic parathyroid glands, *Ann Thorac Surg* 69:221-223, 2000.

58. Melicow MM: One hundred cases of pheochromocytoma (107 tumors) at the Columbia-Presbyterian Medical Center, *Cancer* 40:1987-2004, 1977.

59. Moka D, Voth E, Dietlein M, et al: Technetium 99m-MIBI-SPECT: a highly sensitive diagnostic tool for localization of parathyroid adenomas, *Surgery* 128:29-35, 2000.

60. Ong SC, Schoder H, Patel SG et al: Diagnostic accuracy of ^{18}F-FDG PET in restaging patients with medullary thyroid carcinoma and elevated calcitonin levels, *J Nucl Med* 48:501-507, 2007.

61. Ozer S, Dobrozemsky G, Kienast O, et al: Value of combined XCT/SPECT technology for avoiding false positive planar 123I-MIBG scintigraphy, *Nuklearmedizin* 43:164-170, 2004.

62. Pacini F, Lippi L, Formica N, et al: Therapeutic doses of iodine-131 reveal undiagnosed metastases in thyroid cancer patients with detectable serum thyroglobin levels, *J Nucl Med* 28:1888-1891, 1987.

63. Perez-Monte JE, Brown ML, Shah AN, et al: Parathyroid adenomas: accurate detection and localization with Tc-99m-sestamibi SPECT, *Radiology* 201:85-91, 1996.

64. Pfannenberg AC, Fachmann SM, Horger M, et al: Benefit of anatomical-functional image fusion in the diagnostic work-up of neuroendocrine neoplasms, *Eur J Nucl Med Mol Imaging* 30:835-843, 2003.

65. Profanter C, Prommegger R, Gabriel M et al: Computed axial tomography-MIBI image fusion for preoperative localization in primary hyperparathyroidism, *Am J Surg* 187:383-387, 2004.

66. Profanter C, Wetscher GJ, Gabriel M, et al: CT-MIBI image fusion: a new preoperative localization technique for primary, recurrent, and persistent hyperparathyroidism, *Surgery* 135:157-162, 2004.

67. Ridgeway EC: Clinician's evaluation of a solitary thyroid nodule, *J Clin Endocrinol Metab* 74:231-235, 1992.

68. Rini JN, Vallabhajosula S, Zanzonico P, et al: Thyroid uptake of liquid versus capsule ^{131}I tracers in hyperthyroid patients treated with liquid ^{131}I, *Thyroid* 9:347-352, 1999.

69. Robbins RJ, Chon JT, Fleisher M, et al: Is the serum thyroglobulin response to recombinant human thyrotropin sufficient, by itself, to monitor for residual thyroid carcinoma? *J Clin Endocrinol Metab* 87:3242-3247, 2002.

70. Robbins RJ, Tuttle RM, Sharaf RN, et al: Preparation by recombinant human thyrotropin or thyroid hormone withdrawal is comparable for the detection of residual differentiated thyroid carcinoma, *J Clin Endocrinol Metab* 86:619-625, 2001.

71. Rubello D, Casara D, Fiore D, et al: An ectopic mediastinal parathyroid adenoma accurately located by a single-day imaging protocol of Tc-99m pertechnetate-MIBI subtraction scintigraphy and MIBI-SPECT-computed tomographic image fusion, *Clin Nucl Med* 27:186-190, 2002.

72. Ruf J, Hanninen EL, Steinmuller T, et al: Preoperative localization of parathyroid glands. Use of MRI, scintigraphy, and image fusion, *Nuklearmedizin* 43:85-90, 2004.

73. Sackett WR, Barraclough B, Reeve TS, et al: Worldwide trends in the surgical treatment of primary hyperparathyroidism in the era of minimally invasive parathyroidectomy, *Arch Surg* 137:1055-1059, 2002.

74. Samnick S, Bader JB, Müller M, et al: Improved labelling of no-carrier-added 123J-MIBG and preliminary clinical evaluation in patients with ventricular arrhythmias, *Nucl Med Commun* 20:537-545, 1999.

75. Sarkar SD, Beierwaltes WH, Ice RD, et al: A new and superior adrenal scanning agent, NP-59, *J Nucl Med* 16:1038-1042, 1975.

76. Schillaci O, Spanu A, Scopinaro F, et al: Somatostatin receptor scintigraphy in liver metastasis detection from gastroentero-pancreatic neuroendocrine tumors, *J Nucl Med* 44:358-368, 2003.

77. Schnell O, Kirsch CM, Stemplinger J, et al: Scintigraphic evidence for cardiac sympathetic dysinnervation in long-term IDDM patients with and without ECG-based autonomic neuropathy, *Diabetologia* 38:1345-1352, 1995.

78. Seidlin SM, Marinelli LD, Oshry E: Radioactive iodine therapy: effect on functioning metastases of adenocarcinoma of the thyroid, *JAMA* 132:838-841, 1946.

79. Sfakianakis GN, Irvin GL III, Foss J, et al: Efficient parathyroidectomy guided by SPECT-MIBI and hormonal measurements, *J Nucl Med* 37:798-804, 1996.

80. Sisson JC, Avram AM, Lawson SA, et al: The so-called stunning of thyroid tissue, *J Nucl Med* 47:1406-1412, 2006.

81. Slooter GD, Mearadji A, Breeman AP, et al: Somatostatin receptor imaging, therapy and new strategies in patients with neuroendocrine tumors, *Brit J Surg* 81:31-40, 2001.

82. Snyder J, Gorman C, Scanlon P: Thyroid remnant ablation: questionable pursuit of an ill-defined goal, *J Nucl Med* 24:659-665, 1983.

83. Taillefer R, Boucher Y, Potvin C, et al: Detection and localization of parathyroid adenomas in patients with hyperparathyroidism using a single radionuclide imaging procedure with technetium-99m sestamibi (double-phase study), *J Nucl Med* 33:1801-1807, 1992.

84. Tuttle RM, Brockhin M, Omry G, et al: Recombinent human TSH-assisted radioactive iodine ablation achieves short-term clinical recurrence rates similar to those of traditional thyroid hormone withdrawal, *J Nucl Med* 49:764-770, 2008.

85. Tuttle RM, Leboeuf R, Robbins CJ, et al: Empiric dosing regimens frequently exceed maximum tolerated activity in elderly patients with thyroid carcinoma, *J Nucl Med* 47:1587-1591, 2006.

86. Wang W, Larson SM, Fazzari M, et al: Prognostic value of [18F] fluorodeoxyglucose positron emission tomographic scanning in patients with thyroid cancer, *J Clin Endocrinol Metab* 85:1107-1113, 2000.

87. Wang W, Macapinlac H, Larson SM, et al: [18F]-2-fluoro-2-deoxy-D-glucose positron emission tomography localizes residual thyroid cancer in patients with negative diagnostic 131I whole body scans and elevated serum thyroglobulin levels, *J Clin Endocrinol Metab* 84:2291-2302, 1999.

Respiratory System

William L. Hubble, Crystal Botkin

OBJECTIVES

After completing this chapter, the reader will be able to:
- Possess a general understanding of normal lung anatomy and physiology.
- Understand how the blood flow within the lung is altered by pathology.
- Understand the mechanism of perfusion imaging.
- Be aware of the special care needed for perfusion imaging of patients with severe pulmonary hypertension.
- Understand the patient preparation requirements for lung imaging.
- Know the importance of the number of particles administered for perfusion imaging.
- Understand the effect of time and decay on particle count.
- Be aware of the effects of gravity on particle distribution in the lung.
- Know the importance of communicating the method of injection to the interpreting physician.
- Be aware of the various techniques for ventilation studies.
- Understand the limitations and advantages of the various ventilation radiopharmaceuticals.
- Possess an understanding of the advantages of the combined diagnostic information of ventilation and perfusion imaging studies.
- Understand how lung imaging studies are used to diagnose disease.
- Possess an understanding of the general applications of lung imaging.
- Be aware of the various references on the subject of lung imaging.
- Identify other methods of detecting and diagnosing pulmonary emboli.

KEY TERMS

aerosol
alveoli
apex
base
chronic obstructive pulmonary
    disease (COPD)
closing capacity
compliance

deep venous thrombosis (DVT)
functional residual capacity
hypoxia
lung quantification
macroaggregated albumin (MAA)
perfusion imaging
pneumonectomy

pulmonary emboli (PE)
residual volume
segment
tidal volume
total lung capacity
venous thromboembolism (VTE)
ventilation imaging

Regional ventilation was first studied by Knipping and colleagues[33] using radioactive xenon in 1955. Much of the current understanding of regional lung function, both in health and in disease, is based on the use of radioactive xenon and other radionuclides by respiratory physiologists working in London and Montreal.[6,58] During this time, considerable advances were also made in understanding the detailed anatomy of the lung[62] and in appreciating the mechanical interrelationships of airways, **alveoli,** and the thoracic cage.[38] Nonrespiratory functions have also been studied, particularly those dealing with lung defense mechanisms[19] and the metabolic activity of the lung.[16]

The development of **macroaggregated albumin (MAA),** at first labeled with iodine-131[56] (^{131}I) and later with technetium-99m (^{99m}Tc), led to the widespread use of perfusion scanning for the diagnosis of pulmonary embolism. The use of radioactive xenon to study regional ventilation has spread from the research laboratory to routine use in the past 30 years. This combined insight into regional ventilation and regional blood flow allows more accurate assessment of disturbances in the lungs' physiology and, at the same time, increases both the diagnostic sensitivity and the specificity of the procedure.[3,37] More than 500,000 patients are diagnosed with **pulmonary emboli (PE)** in the United States annually, resulting in approximately 200,000 deaths.[15,24] The clinical presentation of acute embolism is variable, and it is estimated that more than half of all patients with PE remain undiagnosed. Without treatment, PE is associated with a mortality rate of approximately 30%, primarily the result of recurrent embolism. However, accurate diagnosis with ventilation/perfusion lung scanning, multidetector computed tomography (CT), or

pulmonary angiography followed by effective therapy with anticoagulants results in a significant decrease in mortality to between 2% and 8%.[12,18]

NORMAL ANATOMY AND PHYSIOLOGY

The lungs, shown diagrammatically in Figure 16-1 and schematically in Figure 16-2, lie within the thorax, protected by the rib cage. The ribs anchor the intercostal muscles and the diaphragm. It is the action of these muscles that enlarges the chest during normal breathing. Air enters the lungs, first passing through the nose or mouth and then the pharynx, larynx, and trachea. It is warmed, moistened, and filtered during this time. The trachea divides into right and left mainstem bronchi, and these in turn divide into lobar bronchi (upper, middle, and lower on the right, and upper and lower on the left). The airways continue to divide in a somewhat irregular fashion, sequentially bifurcating about 16 times from the trachea to the terminal bronchioles and a further four to seven times as respiratory bronchioles, alveolar ducts, and alveolar sacs (Figure 16-3). Bronchi have cartilage in their walls, which distinguishes them from bronchioles. Smooth muscle, collagen, and elastic fibers encircle the airways from the trachea to the alveolar ducts. The collagen and elastic fibers continue to the periphery of the lung as a three-dimensional (3D) latticework in the walls of the alveoli. Alveoli first appear in the respiratory bronchioles but are most numerous around the alveolar sacs.

The alveoli are packed together like the cells of a honeycomb (Figure 16-4). Each alveolus offers some support to its neighbors, as well as through the collagen and elastic fibers to the airways. This structural

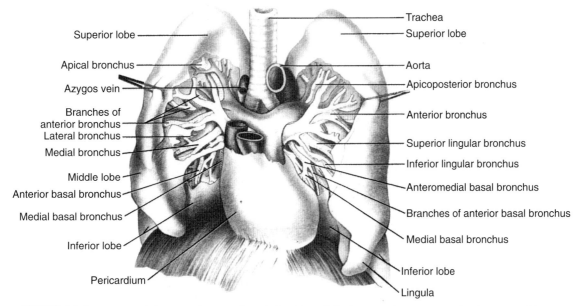

FIGURE 16-1 Anatomical diagram showing the relationships of the heart, pulmonary vessels, airways, and lungs.

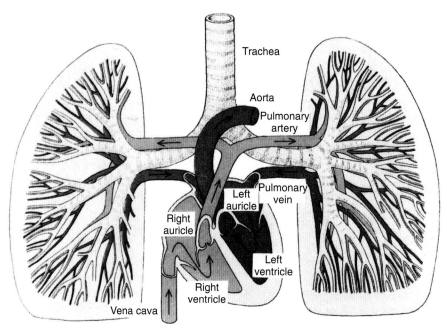

FIGURE 16-2 Schematic diagram of pulmonary circulation and airways.

arrangement and the surfactant that coats the surface of the alveoli are responsible for the elastic properties of the lungs and provide the main force for expiration during normal breathing.

The bronchial epithelium is lined by ciliated cells interspersed with a few goblet cells and the openings of bronchial glands.[9] The alveoli, where oxygen and carbon dioxide are exchanged, are lined by alveolar type I cells. These are very thin and spread over the surface of the alveoli. Pulmonary capillaries lie in contact with these cells (see Figure 16-4). Two other important cell types are found in the alveoli: alveolar type II cells, which make surfactant, and alveolar macrophages, which remove particulate matter that reaches the alveoli.

The pulmonary artery divides to form the right and left pulmonary arteries. These vessels follow the bronchi and bronchioles, dividing with them until they reach the alveoli (see Figure 16-2). Each alveolus, and there are about 250 million to 300 million in an adult, is supplied by a terminal pulmonary arteriole, which has a diameter of about 35 μm and which gives rise to about 1000 capillaries per alveolus. The capillaries are 7 to 10 μm in diameter. The distance between the alveolar surface and the capillaries is only about 0.05 to 0.1 μm. The pulmonary capillaries drain into the pulmonary veins and from there into the left atrium.[62]

The lungs also receive blood from the aorta through the bronchial arteries. These are small but also follow the bronchial tree as far as the respiratory bronchioles. They supply nourishment to the bronchi, surrounding blood vessels, nerves, and lymphatics. Anastomoses are formed between the bronchial and pulmonary circulations at the capillary level around the respiratory

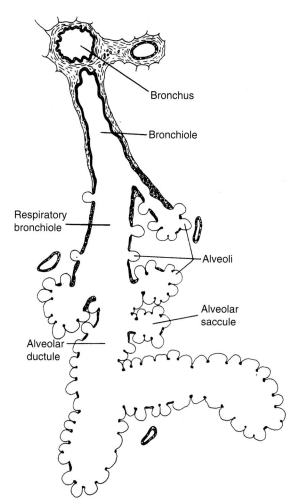

FIGURE 16-3 Schematic cross section of branching of airways from terminal bronchiole to alveolar ductules, saccules, and alveoli.

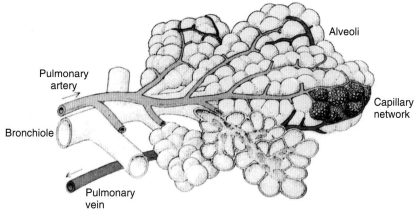

FIGURE 16-4 Schematic drawing of peripheral airways and alveoli and their accompanying blood vessels.

bronchioles. Most of the blood from the bronchial circulation drains into the left atrium through the pulmonary veins.[14]

The lungs are richly supplied with lymphatics. Some course over the pleura and pass into the lungs, whereas others arise in the interstitial spaces of the lungs. Lymphatic vessels travel toward the hilum of the lung, with airways and blood vessels, reaching lymph nodes there and continuing into the mediastinum.

The volume of air breathed out in a normal breath is called the **tidal volume,** and the volume of air in the lungs at the end of a normal breath is called **functional residual capacity. Total lung capacity** is the volume of air in the lungs when as much air has been inhaled as possible, whereas **residual volume** is the volume of air left in the lungs after a complete exhalation. These volumes are measured by standard pulmonary function tests.[66]

During tidal breathing only a small proportion of the total volume of air in the lungs (about 10% to 15%) is exchanged with each breath. A higher percentage is exchanged with deeper breaths or a faster rate of breathing. About one third of each breath is wasted because the air in the bronchial tubes at the end of the breath does not reach the alveoli. This is called *anatomic dead space* because it takes no part in gas exchange.

The structure of the lung is well suited to its chief function of gas exchange—that is, delivering oxygen (O_2) to the bloodstream and removing carbon dioxide (CO_2) so that the body's cellular metabolism can continue. Despite the numerous divisions of the bronchial tree, the resistance to air flow is low. Most of this resistance (80% to 90%) is located in the larger bronchial tubes, where air flow is turbulent. In healthy subjects, only 0.5 to 2.5 cm H_2O pressure is required to generate flows of 1 L/sec at the mouth. Large increases in the resistance of the smaller airways (as occurs in obstructive lung disease) can result in increased airways resistance and make the work of breathing more taxing. The change in volume for a change in pressure is called **compliance,** which is a measurement of the distensibility of the lungs. The compliance of the lungs can be altered by diseases of the lung

parenchyma, such as pulmonary fibrosis. The pressure in the pulmonary artery is considerably lower than that in the systemic circulation, and there is very little resistance to blood flow. The entire cardiac output passes through the pulmonary capillaries, in an almost continuous sheet of fluid over the alveolar walls. These thin walls, which have a total surface area of 70 to 80 m^2, offer an almost negligible barrier to the diffusion of gases from alveoli to blood or vice versa.

As the lung ages, its elastic properties diminish and the smaller bronchial tubes tend to collapse during a full expiration. The volume of air in the lungs when closure begins is the **closing capacity.** Both radioactive xenon and nonradioactive tracer gases (e.g., nitrogen, helium, argon) have been used to measure this volume. Early damage to the small airways from any cause increases this volume, an increase that therefore is a sensitive but nonspecific indication of small-airway disease.[4,10]

In the 1960s it was shown that both ventilation and blood flow are not evenly distributed within the lungs. Posture and the direction of gravity or of acceleration play an important part in healthy lungs.

In the upright position, ventilation of the upper parts of the lung increases about 1½ to 2 times from the upper third of the lung to the lower third.[6,30,65] In the supine position, the distribution is more uniform from the **apex** (top) to the **base** (bottom), but there is then a gradient from the anterior (front) to the posterior (back). If a person lies on one side, more air is exchanged in the lower part of the lungs compared with the upper part. The distribution is modified by exercise, the rate of breathing, and diseases that affect the bronchial tubes or the lung parenchyma.

In the upright position, blood flow is threefold to fivefold higher in the base than in the upper parts of the lung. In fact, the upper one fourth of the lungs gets very little blood flow at rest while a person is sitting upright.[5,65] In the supine position, blood flow is more uniform from apex to base, but then a gradient exists from front to back. Lying on one side causes more blood to flow to the lowermost part of the lung. Apart from the disease states that usually alter blood flow within the lung, exercise results in a more even distribution. Lowering the oxygen tension in the bronchial tubes also alters blood flow by causing local constriction of the pulmonary arterioles and diverting blood flow away from this region.

The distribution of blood flow within the upright lung shows the largest gradient from top to bottom when the measurements are made at total lung capacity. At functional residual capacity, blood flow increases from the apex to about the level of the fourth or fifth rib and then decreases a little toward the base. If the distribution of blood flow is measured at residual volume, it is almost even throughout the lungs.[25]

The ratio in which ventilation and blood flow are mixed is not uniform from top to bottom in the upright position. Ventilation exceeds blood flow by about 2:1 to 3:1 in the upper zones. In the midzones they are more closely matched, whereas in the lower parts of the lung blood flow exceeds ventilation. The closer the matching of ventilation and blood flow, the better the oxygenation of the blood. Whenever ventilation is reduced in comparison to blood flow, the oxygenation of the blood is also reduced. If ventilation exceeds blood flow, the red

cells quickly take up their maximum load of oxygen (4 molecules per hemoglobin molecule, or 1.34 ml of O_2 per gram of hemoglobin), and the excess ventilation is then wasted,[66] for no further exchange can occur.

PATHOPHYSIOLOGY

The distribution of blood flow within the lungs is altered by many disease processes that affect the lungs, the heart, the chest wall, or the diaphragm. The mechanisms underlying these disturbances are outlined schematically in Figure 16-5. Figure 16-5, *A* to *C*, represents disease processes that affect the pulmonary vasculature. The most obvious cause, represented by *A*, is pulmonary embolism, in which the embolus (usually a small blood clot) blocks one of the branches of the pulmonary artery so that no blood can flow past this obstruction. The defect produced on the perfusion scan corresponds to the anatomic **segment** or lobe of the lung involved. Pulmonary emboli usually arise from thrombi originating in the deep venous system of the lower extremities (**deep venous thrombosis [DVT]**); however, they may also originate in the pelvic, renal, or upper-extremity veins and the right

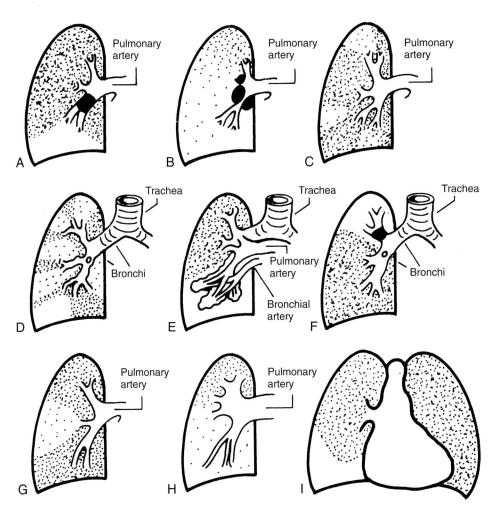

FIGURE 16-5 Schematic representation of major mechanisms of abnormal perfusion scans (**A** to **I**). *Spotted areas,* Blood flow; *clear areas,* regions with absent blood flow.

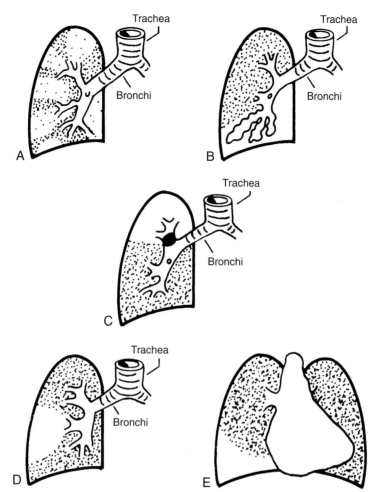

FIGURE 16-6 Schematic representation of major mechanisms of abnormal ventilation studies (**A** to **E**). *Spotted areas,* Ventilation; *clear areas,* regions of abnormal ventilation.

heart. Iliofemoral thrombi appear to be the source of most clinically recognized PE.[31,63] Only about 10% of emboli cause pulmonary infarction, usually in patients with preexisting cardiopulmonary disease. Most PE are multiple, with the lower lobes being involved in the majority of cases.[39,45]

Other causes of defects in blood flow from disease processes that affect the pulmonary vessels are shown in Figure 16-5, *B* and *C*. Figure 16-5, *B*, represents enlarged lymph nodes at the hilum of the lung, as might be seen in advanced lung cancer, causing compression of the pulmonary vessels and hence alterations in blood flow. Figure 16-5, *C*, represents disease processes that involve the smaller pulmonary arterioles, such as a vasculitis or multiple small PE.

Figure 16-5, *D* to *F*, represent diseases in which the initial problem is in the airways (or bronchial tubes), and blood flow is reduced as a result of the diminution in ventilation. Figure 16-5, *D*, is a composite diagram that represents the changes seen in chronic bronchitis, emphysema, and asthma. Figure 16-5, *E*, represents bronchiectasis in which there is dilatation of the peripheral bronchi and surrounding inflammation. The bronchial arteries to the affected region are often greatly enlarged. There is

virtually no blood flow through the pulmonary artery and very little exchange of air in the bronchiectatic segment. Figure 16-5, *F*, represents obstruction of a bronchus by a tumor or foreign body. Blood flow is reduced in part by the effects of local **hypoxia.**

Figure 16-5, *G* to *I*, represent miscellaneous conditions. In *G* the lung parenchyma is filled with inflammatory exudate, as is seen in pneumonia, or with blood, as is seen in a pulmonary infarction. Blood flow is greatly reduced, and there is no ventilation of the affected region. Figure 16-5, *H*, represents the interesting phenomenon of a reversal of the normal gradient of blood flow. This is seen when the pressure in the left atrium is elevated, such as in mitral stenosis or left ventricular failure. Figure 16-5, *I*, represents a condition in which a pleural effusion or a large heart is compressing lung tissue, reducing blood flow in that region.

The mechanisms responsible for the disturbances in ventilation are shown in Figure 16-6. Figure 16-6, *A*, represents diseases that cause obstruction to air flow by narrowing or distorting the airways. Chronic bronchitis, for example, is marked by excess mucus production and some inflammatory swelling of the bronchial walls. Both processes narrow the lumen of the airways, usually in an irregular fashion, producing variable patterns of airway obstruction. In emphysema the main damage is in the alveoli, which are steadily destroyed, resulting in loss of surface area and capillaries. The small airways are not properly supported; they become kinked and distorted and collapse readily on expiration, which leads to inefficient exchange of air. Chronic bronchitis and emphysema are usually found together because both diseases are caused by the same mechanisms and, for the most part, by cigarette smoking.

Bronchial asthma is marked by spasm of the bronchial smooth muscle, which causes narrowing of the airways and increased mucus production and edema of the bronchial mucosa. Severe abnormalities of ventilation and blood flow may be seen.

Figure 16-6, *B*, represents bronchiectasis. Little or no air exchange takes place in the dilated bronchi, which are often the sites of chronic infection. Figure 16-6, *C*, represents narrowing or complete obstruction of a bronchus caused by a tumor or foreign body. The worse the obstruction, the more obvious the abnormality in ventilation. If the obstruction is in a lobar bronchus, the affected lobe of the lung collapses as its lumen closes off. If the obstruction is in a segmental or smaller bronchus, collateral ventilation through the pores of Kohn can prevent complete collapse by allowing air to enter the obstructed segment from a neighboring segment. Figure 16-6, *D*, represents the condition in pneumonia or pulmonary infarction, in which the alveoli are filled with exudate or blood and hence cannot exchange any air.

Figure 16-6, *E*, represents pleural fluid or a large heart, both of which occupy lung volume, thus reducing ventilation.

PERFUSION IMAGING

Perfusion imaging shows the distribution of pulmonary arterial blood flow and is usually demonstrated by intravenous (IV) injection of radioactive particles. The method was shown to be effective by Haynie and colleagues,[23] who injected labeled ceramic microspheres into dogs. The development of MAA, labeled with ^{131}I by Taplin and colleagues[56] and Wagner and colleagues[61] in 1964, led to the first successful lung scans in humans. After IV injection the particles, which range from 10 to 90 μm in diameter,[34] pass through the right atrium and right ventricle, where they are well mixed with blood, and then into the pulmonary artery. They pass into the blood vessels of the lung until they become impacted in the terminal arterioles and capillaries because they are too large to pass through them. The usual diameter of human albumin microspheres corresponds to the size of the smallest pulmonary arteriole. The distribution of particles has been shown experimentally to be closely related to the distribution of pulmonary arterial blood flow.[46] This was accomplished by comparing the relative distribution of particles to the uptake of oxygen by each lung and the distribution of particles to that of labeled red blood cells (RBCs).[58] A normal perfusion scan is shown in Figure 16-7.

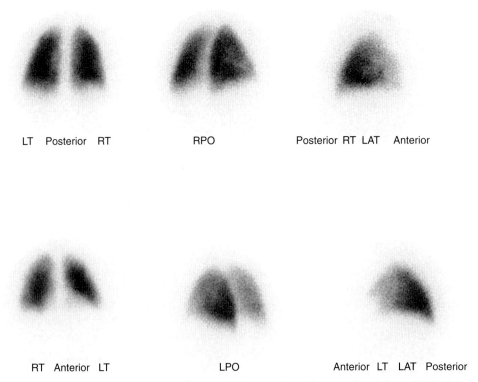

LT   Posterior   RT   RPO   Posterior RT LAT   Anterior

RT   Anterior   LT   LPO   Anterior LT LAT Posterior

FIGURE 16-7 Normal six-view perfusion scan. *Clockwise from top left:* Posterior, right posterior oblique *(RPO)*, right lateral *(RT LAT)*, left lateral *(LT LAT)*, left posterior oblique *(LPO)*, and anterior.

It is important to remember that what is seen on the images reflects the distribution that existed at the time of injection.

Macroaggregated albumin, human albumin microspheres, and other particles break up and pass through the pulmonary capillaries and are removed from the circulation in the liver and spleen. These particles have variable biological half-lives in the lung, which depend not only on the nature of the particles, including particle hardness due to the method of preparation and treatment, but also to some extent on the underlying disease processes. Clearance is delayed in chronic lung disease and heart failure.

With the usual dose of particulate material of the appropriate size, fewer than 1 in 1000 pulmonary arterioles are blocked.[20,55] No abnormalities of pulmonary function can be demonstrated after such an injection.[17,47] Perfusion scanning has a reputation for great safety, but special care should be taken to administer half of the usual dose and therefore a reduced number of particles to patients who are known to have severe pulmonary hypertension, because the available vascular bed is reduced in diameter[13]; who have right-to-left shunts,[43] because the particles can pass through to the systemic circulation and embolize to the brain, kidneys, heart, and other organs; and who have had a **pneumonectomy.**

Radioactive xenon dissolved in saline solution is occasionally used to demonstrate the distribution of blood flow. It is given intravenously, and because the gas is relatively insoluble, it comes out of solution as it reaches the air contained in the alveoli. Its distribution can be measured during breath holding and corresponds to pulmonary capillary blood flow. Regions of the lung that are collapsed or consolidated, as in pneumonia, appear to have no blood flow because the alveoli contain no air.

Preparation

No special patient preparation is required for either ventilation or perfusion lung imaging; however, a few things should be done in advance of the examination. A recent chest radiograph (ideally within 4 hours, but acceptable up to 24 hours) should accompany the patient to the nuclear medicine facility. The radiograph allows the physician to compare the images of the two modalities and therefore be more specific when interpreting the images. A good patient history is important to the diagnosing physician. The most common risk factors for PE identified in the Prospective Investigation of Pulmonary Embolism Diagnosis (PIOPED) study were immobilization, surgery (within last 3 months), stroke, history of **venous thromboembolism (VTE)**, and malignancy.[60] Physicians may also request that a blood gas or D-dimer assay report accompany the patient. Overall, arterial blood gas measurements do not play a major role in excluding or establishing the diagnosis of PE.[39,45,64] The utility of

measuring D-dimer, a degradation product of cross-linked fibrin, has been extensively studied for the diagnosis of both DVT and PE. D-dimers are detectable at levels greater than 500 ng/ml in nearly all patients with PE. However, an elevated D-dimer concentration is insufficient to establish the diagnosis of PE because such values are nonspecific and are commonly present in hospitalized patients, particularly those with malignancy or who have had recent surgery.[20,42,44,64] Specificity may decrease further with increasing patient age. Despite this low specificity, the sensitivity and negative predictive value of the D-dimer assay in most patients with suspected VTE appear to be high, especially in patients with a low pretest probability.[20,42,44] Again, this additional information can provide another clue to the correct diagnosis of the patient. Computed tomography is another modality being used to diagnose PE.[32] In fact, CT angiography (CTA) has replaced ventilation/perfusion VQ scanning as the predominant imaging modality for PE diagnosis in the United States. However, CT angiography has limitations, which include cost, relatively high radiation doses, and inapplicability in patients who have contraindications (e.g., reduced renal function or iodine allergy) to iodinated contrast material.[53,54,59] In recent studies, such as PIOPED II, ventilation/perfusion scintigraphy has been found to be diagnostically definitive in a majority of patients. It is therefore considered an appropriate pulmonary imaging procedure for patients of whom CT is disadvantageous.[53] It is not the technologist's responsibility to set laboratory policy with regard to the type of examination that should be ordered for the diagnosis of PE. However, it generally is the technologist's responsibility to understand the role of complementary diagnostic tests and provide any additional information to the diagnosing physician.

Dosage

In addition to the amount of radioactivity given, the number of particles and the amount of albumin injected are of special importance. Because, as previously discussed, a small percentage of the capillary bed is obstructed during the perfusion imaging, care must be taken to ensure that the patient's respiratory ability is not further impaired by a test intended to help them.[21] In a normal patient, a satisfactory perfusion image can be obtained using 1 to 4 mCi ^{99m}Tc MAA with 200,000 to 700,000 particles.[41,57] An appropriate reduction in the number of particles should be applied for pediatric patients, patients with pulmonary hypertension, patients with right-to-left shunts, and those who have had a pneumonectomy. To help control the number of particles used in perfusion imaging, aggregated albumin kits should be prepared to the same volume every day, and patients should be scheduled as close as possible to the preparation time. Every technologist in the laboratory should know the total number of particles in whichever kit the laboratory uses and the viable time span for the constituted kit.

If too few particles are given, the scans have an obvious blotchy appearance. An even more blotchy appearance is seen if small blood clots or incompletely separated or clumped particles are inadvertently injected.

Method of Injection

The patterns of perfusion are different, depending on whether the particles are injected with the patient in the upright or the supine position. As indicated earlier, gravity plays an important role in the pressure gradient and vascular relationships within the lungs. Patients injected when upright tend to have a larger proportion of the particles distributed toward the bases. Patients injected when supine demonstrate a more homogeneous distribution of particles from the bases to the apices; therefore a supine injection is recommended. However, there are arguments and situations favoring each position for injection. As long as both the technologist and the physician are aware of the difference, either method is satisfactory. The method of injection should be noted somewhere on the film, film jacket, or digital image. An important consideration is that albumin appears to have an affinity for the plastic tubing of IV sets, catheters, and syringes. If these avenues of administration are used, a variable proportion of the dose never reaches the patient. One recommended setup for aggregated albumin injections is a saline syringe, three-way stopcock, and dose syringe (Figure 16-8). This arrangement also eliminates the drawing of blood back into the dose and prevents the possible formation of small thrombi as a result of the mixing of whole blood and MAA.

Agitation of the syringe before the injection will reduce the risk of agglutination of the particles. Having the patient take a few deep breaths during the injection may promote homogeneous distribution of the particles.[41]

Positioning

Although SPECT acquisition can be used, the standard planar perfusion imaging includes the six basic views: posterior, anterior, right and left laterals, and right and left posterior obliques.[11,40,49] A common procedure is performing the posterior view first, for 500,000 counts (with a range of 500,000 to 1,000,000), and then each of the other views for the same time that it takes to do the posterior view. The lateral views can then be compared more easily. Because of shine-through, about one third of the counts from the contralateral lung are included during lateral imaging; therefore imaging for a set time rather than for a set number of counts will maintain relative count density between images.

Unlike many radiographic procedures, the radionuclide images provide the physician with very few landmarks that indicate rotation or distance from the collimator face.[51] Therefore it is essential that the technologist properly position the patient when performing the study. Please review the description of the procedure for perfusion imaging found in Box 16-1.

VENTILATION IMAGING

Table 16-1 shows some of the radiopharmaceuticals used to study regional ventilation. Xenon-127, krypton-81m generator, and ^{99m}Tc-technegas have all been used

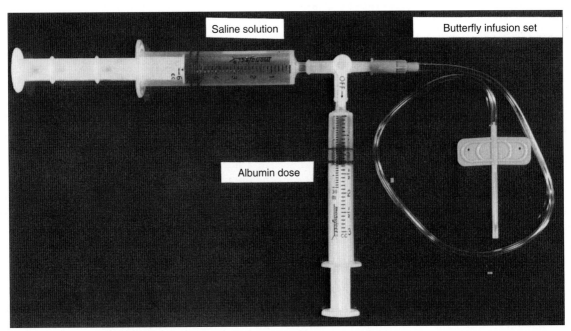

FIGURE 16-8 Arrangement of recommended injection set for albumin particles.

BOX 16-1 | 99mTc-MAA Perfusion Imaging

1. Explain the exam to the patient and position patient supine (if possible) for injection.
2. Select and prepare site for injection of 1-4 mCi of 99mTc-MAA. The number of particles should be 200,000-700,000.
3. Administer 99mTc-MAA through IV injection. To minimize blood mixing with the 99mTc-MAA one may use a 3-way stop cock with saline attached for easy flushing.
4. Remove needle from patient and place bandage on injection site.
5. Properly position patient to obtain the posterior view for 500,000-1,000,000 counts. Note the time that it takes.
6. Obtain the remainder of the standard six views: anterior, right lateral, left lateral, right posterior oblique, and left posterior oblique, for the same time it took to do the posterior view. Anterior oblique views are optional.
7. SPECT images can also be obtained if necessary.
8. Process and film the images appropriately for physician review.

TABLE 16-1 | Radiopharmaceuticals Used for Ventilation Lung Imaging

	Agent	
	99mTc-DTPA Aerosol	133Xe
Physical half-life	6.0 hours	5.3 days
Principal gamma energy	140 keV	80 keV
Radiation absorbed dose per mCi in lungs	112.5 mrad*	12 mrad†

*Actual dose delivered to lung is approximately one fifth because lung deposition is on the order of 200 µCi.

†Radiation absorbed dose has been estimated with a rebreathing time of 3 minutes.

for **ventilation imaging** and are still used outside the United States. Xenon-133 (133Xe) has been used for quasistatic measurement of regional ventilation and blood flow, for dynamic measurement of regional ventilation, for measurement of regional lung volumes, for measurement of closing volume, and for studying factors that influence the distribution of a single breath. Clinical studies of regional ventilation are usually done with 133Xe.

Techniques for ventilation studies are not standardized, but three aspects of ventilation are often examined: (1) the distribution of a single breath, (2) the distribution of lung volume, and (3) the distribution of the efficiency of ventilation from the clearance of radioactive xenon. Single-breath studies show the distribution of an inhaled bolus of radioactive xenon and air, to total lung capacity—a somewhat unphysiological situation (Figure 16-9, A). If the tracer gas is rebreathed to equilibrium (i.e., until the concentration of xenon in the lungs and in the rebreathing system is constant), the distribution of xenon within the lungs corresponds to lung volume (see

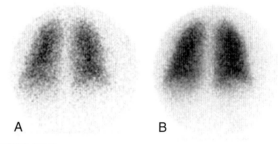

FIGURE 16-9 **A,** Normal distribution of a single breath of 133Xe in the posterior projection. **B,** Wash-in equilibrium image of the same patient.

Figure 16-9, *B*). Measurements made during a wash-in of xenon to equilibrium reflect the efficiency of ventilation; the faster a region reaches equilibrium, the better its ventilation and vice versa. When air is breathed after a wash-in, the subsequent washout provides excellent evidence of the regional variations in ventilation (Figure 16-10). The best-ventilated regions clear fastest, and the poorly ventilated ones stand out by contrast as regions in which the clearance of radioactivity is delayed.[1]

Xenon-133 Ventilation Imaging

Currently the most readily available nuclide for performing ventilation studies is xenon-133 (133Xe). Although it is not an ideal nuclide for this study because of its low energy, beta emission, and solubility in fat and blood, its price and ready availability have forced it into prominence. The energy, 80 keV, is not optimal for the Anger camera because so much scattered activity is included in the window.

The perfusion study could be done first so that if a ventilation study is necessary, the patient can be positioned for it on the basis of the perfusion scan. Some institutions do the perfusion image first, using only 1 mCi of 99mTc-labeled particles, and then proceed with a ventilation study using 5 to 20 mCi of 133Xe or more.[41] However, because the energy of 133Xe is lower than that of 99mTc and the Compton scatter from the 99mTc would interfere with the images, and because of the importance of the washout phase, it is technically advantageous to perform the ventilation study before the perfusion examination. This is the most frequently employed technique.

A number of commercial gas delivery and rebreathing units are available for ventilation studies, but one can be built with a little imagination and some engineering skill[50] (Figure 16-11). Figure 16-12 shows one commercially available ventilation unit with the front panel open. The illustration shows the infusion pump used to introduce xenon into the system, as well as the chambers associated with carbon dioxide and moisture absorption. Carbon dioxide is absorbed in the closed system by soda lime crystals, while moisture is removed by calcium sulfate or cobalt chloride crystals. The crystals from

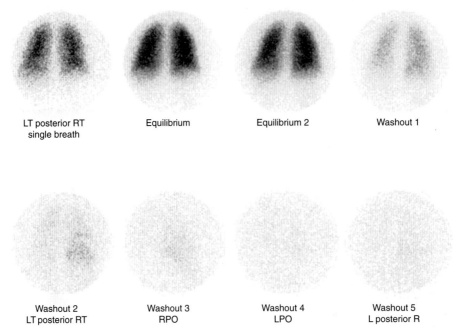

LT posterior RT single breath	Equilibrium	Equilibrium 2	Washout 1

Washout 2 LT posterior RT	Washout 3 RPO	Washout 4 LPO	Washout 5 L posterior R

FIGURE 16-10 Posterior projection of xenon ventilation study. *Top row, left to right:* Single-breath posterior view, first and second equilibrium images, and first image of washout phase. *Bottom row, left to right:* Second washout image, right posterior oblique *(RPO)* washout, left posterior oblique *(LPO)* washout, final washout image.

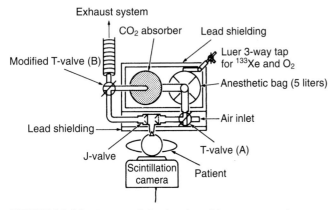

FIGURE 16-11 Diagram of simple rebreathing apparatus that can be constructed from commercially available parts.

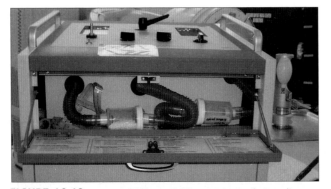

FIGURE 16-12 Commercially available xenon ventilation dispensing system. The infusion pump is shown at far right. Open front panel shows carbon dioxide and moisture absorbing chambers.

both of these chambers must be changed at regular intervals.

One consideration with xenon ventilation studies is the safe disposal of the xenon after the study is finished. Many laboratories, if suitably located, simply vent the diluted xenon (half-life of 5.27 days) into the atmosphere. The Nuclear Regulatory Commission Derived Air Concentration is 5×10^{-7} µCi/ml for ^{133}Xe for an unrestricted area. It is unlikely that released xenon gas would pose a risk to any member of the public in such dilute concentrations. A negative-pressure room is required for xenon ventilation studies to maintain ALARA for staff members and patients in the event of a leak during the study. Commercial ventilation units employ xenon traps that use activated charcoal to prevent the release of radioactive xenon during the washout phase of a study.[36] These charcoal filters must be changed regularly.

Several methods can be used to do a ventilation study. Patients may be imaged supine or upright. Patients who are cooperative and able may be more comfortable in an upright position for the ventilation portion of the study. Figure 16-13 demonstrates upright patient positioning during a ventilation study using a commercially available ventilation unit. Some laboratories use the single-breath technique, in which the patient inhales a bolus of 5 to 20 mCi of ^{133}Xe and holds their breath for 10 to 20 seconds while a static image is taken. Serial washout images are then made at 30- to 60-second intervals as the xenon clears from the lungs. This method works well but requires a good deal of patient cooperation in taking a deep breath and then holding it for 10 to 20 seconds.

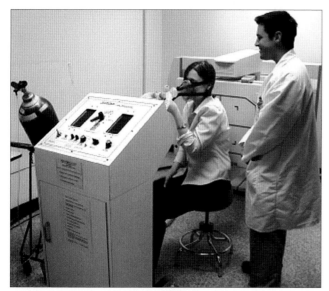

FIGURE 16-13 Technologists simulate xenon ventilation exam performed in the upright position. The patient is in the right posterior oblique position for the demonstrated view.

The more straightforward wash-in–washout method is preferred and can be used even on comatose patients. In this method, 5 to 20 mCi of ^{133}Xe diluted in 2 L of oxygen are rebreathed from a simple rebreathing apparatus for approximately 3 minutes while a static wash-in image is taken. Air is then breathed, and serial images are taken at 30- to 60-second intervals as the xenon clears from the lungs. With the variety of mouthpieces, respiratory masks, and harnesses available, a technologist can perform a ventilation study without assistance from the patient. This type of examination has been successfully completed on many patients, and if the patient is breathing, a ventilation study can be performed. Such studies can also be performed on patients who require mechanical ventilation.

The ventilation study may be done in any position. The routine technique is to use the posterior view in the upright position because this provides the best view of the greatest area of lung. The patient should be seated comfortably with their back to the scintillation camera and should be encouraged to keep as still as possible during the study. The first few breaths of xenon, which are seen on the monitor, can be used to adjust the position of the camera before the wash-in images are started. Please review the description of the procedure for xenon ventilation imaging found in Box 16-2.

Aerosol Ventilation Imaging

Aerosols are deposited in the bronchial tree in relation to particle size, air flow rates, and turbulence. The delivery tubing effectively filters out larger particles, 10 to 15 μm in diameter. Smaller ones are deposited in the larger airways during both inspiration and expiration.

Particles less than 2 μm can reach the alveoli and be deposited there, whereas even smaller particles, less than 0.1 μm, probably escape in the expired air. Radioactive aerosols have been used for more than three decades to study the patency of the airways. It is important that aerosol particle size be well controlled for reproducible studies. Many radiopharmaceuticals have been used, specifically ^{99m}Tc-diethylenetriamine pentaacetic acid (^{99m}Tc-DTPA), ^{99m}TcO$_4^-$, ^{99m}Tc–sulfur colloid, ^{99m}Tc-HAS, and ^{113m}In-Cl$_2$.

The aerosol is generated from an ultrasonic nebulizer or a positive-pressure nebulizer. It is inhaled through a mouthpiece or a face mask. If older systems are used, exhaled material must be collected, and the procedure is best done near a fume hood with an extraction fan. This is not necessary, however, with the newer systems that incorporate a bacterial filter at the outlet. The oxygen flow rate should be set at 10 L/min to be inhaled with 5 ml of fluid containing up to 35 mCi of the nuclear pharmaceutical. Only 2% to 5% actually reaches the lungs.[34] During inhalation, it is preferable to have the patient in an upright position. Images can be acquired using the six standard views (Figure 16-14). Normal aerosol scans look much like perfusion scans except that the trachea and mainstem bronchi usually can be seen. The esophagus and stomach may also be seen because of swallowed material.

With obstructive disease of the airways, central deposition in the larger bronchial tubes, with little or no peripheral filling, may occur, a pattern seen in severe bronchial asthma and emphysema. Less central but definitely patchy peripheral filling tends to be seen in chronic bronchitis, cystic fibrosis, and mild bronchial asthma. Delayed views, 4 to 6 hours after the initial images, can help resolve some central deposition. This is cleared by mucociliary transport in otherwise normal individuals, resulting in normal delayed images. Aerosol scans are

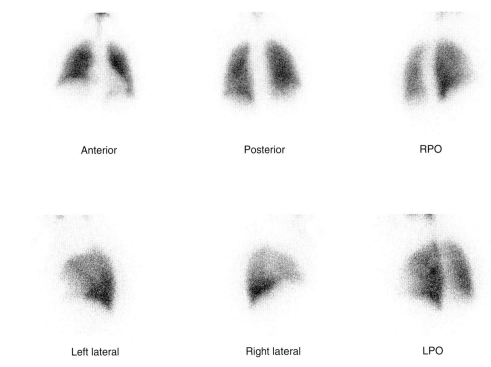

Anterior   Posterior   RPO

Left lateral   Right lateral   LPO

FIGURE 16-14 ^{99m}Tc-DTPA aerosol ventilation images. *Clockwise from top left:* Anterior, posterior, right posterior oblique *(RPO)*, left posterior oblique *(LPO)*, right lateral, and left lateral views.

almost as sensitive as xenon studies for detecting early disease of small airways. Sequential images for several hours after aerosol inhalation have been used to measure mucociliary clearance rates in smokers, nonsmokers, and children with cystic fibrosis.[48]

The development of small, disposable nebulizers has renewed interest in the use of aerosols for lung imaging.[22] These light, portable units have been greatly improved over the cumbersome systems designed during the development of this technique. Bedside procedures are possible with a cooperative patient. Even with these improvements, however, the aerosol technique remains one of the more difficult nuclear medicine procedures. It requires detailed attention to variables such as tubing length and diameter, air flow, and pressure. Please review the description of the procedure for aerosol ventilation imaging found in Box 16-3.

VENTILATION-PERFUSION STUDIES

By combining studies of ventilation and perfusion, it can be determined whether defects in blood flow are associated with defects in ventilation. The pulmonary diseases commonly seen in clinical nuclear medicine tend to fall into two categories: (1) those with abnormal regional pulmonary blood flow but normal (or near normal) regional ventilation (pulmonary embolism is by far the most important of these, but early heart failure, interstitial lung diseases, some lung cancers, and other abnormalities of the pulmonary vasculature may also show

BOX 16-3	Aerosol Ventilation Imaging

1. Ventilation study using aerosol should be completed before the perfusion study.
2. Explain the exam to the patient and position upright.
3. Add up to 35-40 mCi of ^{99m}Tc-DTPA to the nebulizer.
4. Administer to the patient using a mask or mouthpiece with nose clips for 3-5 minutes.
5. Nebulizer should contain 5 ml of fluid and set at 10 L/min oxygen flow rate.
6. After the administration of aerosol is complete, properly position patient to obtain the posterior view for 200,000-300,000 counts. Note the time that it takes.
7. Obtain the remainder of the standard six views: Anterior, right lateral, left lateral, right posterior oblique, and left posterior oblique, for the same time it took to do the posterior view. Anterior oblique images are optional.
8. Process and film images appropriately for physician review.

this pattern); and (2) those with abnormal ventilation and abnormal blood flow. The most common conditions are chronic bronchitis, emphysema, and asthma; however, cystic fibrosis and bronchiectasis cause similar patterns. Cancers of the bronchus, other bronchial tumors, or foreign bodies obstructing a bronchus can all produce localized abnormalities of ventilation and blood flow. In general, the disturbance of ventilation is more pronounced than that of blood flow and is detected as a regional delay in the clearance of xenon. When this delay

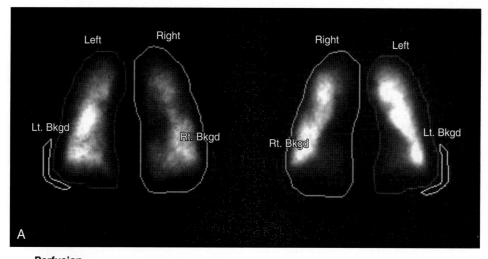

Perfusion

	Posterior	
	Left	Right
Total counts	285K	257K
% Ratios	52.58	47.42

	Anterior	
	Left	Right
Total counts	275K	249K
% Ratios	52.48	47.52

	Geometric mean	
	Left	Right
Total counts	270K	248K
% Ratios	52.12	47.88

FIGURE 16-15 A, Lung images with ROIs drawn. **B,** Full lung quantification analysis of perfusion images.

is significant, a corresponding defect is usually visible on the wash-in image as an area of diminished activity, where this part of the lung has not reached equilibrium with the tracer gas.

Pneumonias, pulmonary infarctions, and severe pulmonary edema are all associated with defects in the equilibrium images, which correspond to the infiltrates seen on the chest radiograph. No retention of radioactive xenon is seen during the washout because no radioactive xenon can enter the fluid-filled alveoli.

Normal perfusion scans show an even gradation of activity, with more activity visible in the lower lobes than in the upper lobes, if the injection is given with the patient in the upright posture. The outline of the lungs and mediastinum corresponds closely to that seen on the chest radiograph. A normal wash-in image shows an even distribution of activity throughout the lungs, and a normal washout is usually complete within 3 to 4 minutes of breathing air. Occasionally the bases clear slightly faster than the upper zones.

Computer Processing of Ventilation-Perfusion Images

The ready access to digital computer processing of image data has led to several methods of processing the

information from ventilation-perfusion imaging. The partitioning of ventilation, lung volume, and blood flow between the lungs can be obtained with considerable ease; however, measurements of regional ventilation and regional ventilation-perfusion ratios are less readily obtained. In most instances the numeric values obtained do not correspond to how much air is exchanged or to the physiological ventilation-perfusion ratios.[51]

Lung Quantification

Patients who are facing lung reduction surgery because of lung cancer, emphysema, or both; or who have a reduction in lung function due to cystic fibrosis, lung transplant, or congenital heart disease may benefit from a quantification lung study. The **lung quantification** information is easily obtained using the ventilation and perfusion images obtained during a VQ study.

Regions of interest (ROI) can be drawn using the appropriate computer software that accompanies the imaging systems. These ROIs can be placed around the left and right lung (Figure 16-15), and each lung can be further divided into lobes and segments. A geometric mean and percentages are calculated by the computer software for each region. These data are used to determine the feasibility of the lung reduction surgery and the extent of function in each region. The quantification is more commonly done using the perfusion images, but can also be done using the ventilation images. Please review the description of the procedure for lung quantification found in Box 16-4.

Pulmonary Embolism

In PE the defects in blood flow correspond to anatomical subdivisions of the lung, such as segments or lobes, in 75% of patients. The remaining 25% have ill-defined nonsegmental defects (Figure 16-16). If the patient had previously healthy lungs, ventilation is usually well maintained to the affected parts of the lung because their bronchial tubes are patent. Only a small proportion

(10% to 15%) of patients with emboli develop pulmonary infarction, with its associated infiltrates, as seen on the chest radiograph.

Interpretation is more difficult and less reliable when the patient already has **chronic obstructive pulmonary disease (COPD)**, such as chronic bronchitis, emphysema, or asthma.[2] Retrospective studies from the 1970s suggested that the true positive rate, or sensitivity, and the true negative rate, or specificity, of ventilation-perfusion scanning were more than 90%.[3,37] Subsequent studies have not shown this to be true.[2,7,8]

Two prospective studies of the accuracy of ventilation-perfusion scanning in comparison to pulmonary angiography showed PE to be present in about 90% of patients with high-probability lung scan interpretations.[26,60] However, for other interpretations, such as intermediate, indeterminate, or low probability, the proportion of patients with angiographically proven PE ranged from 14% to 40%. When the perfusion scan was completely normal, PE were rarely found.[26,29]

For patients with ventilation-perfusion scans that are neither high probability nor normal, further diagnostic studies are indicated. Noninvasive tests for proximal vein thrombosis, such as B-mode ultrasound or impedance plethysmography, should be considered, or even the more invasive venography if these noninvasive tests are

BOX 16-4	Lung Quantification

1. Complete the ventilation/perfusion images as directed.
2. Using the appropriate computer software, draw regions of interest (ROI) around each lung and/or around regions corresponding to the lobes or segments of the lung that are being evaluated.
3. A geometric mean and percentages are calculated for each lung and region.

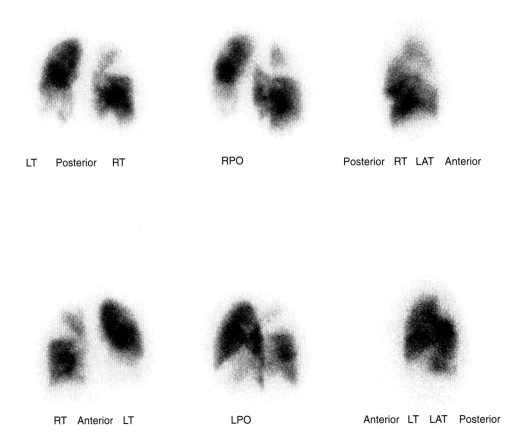

LT   Posterior   RT   RPO   Posterior   RT LAT   Anterior

RT   Anterior   LT   LPO   Anterior   LT LAT   Posterior

FIGURE 16-16 Markedly abnormal perfusion scan of the lungs demonstrating multiple segmental defects. *Clockwise from top left:* Posterior, right posterior oblique *(RPO)*, right lateral *(RT LAT)*, left lateral *(LT LAT)*, left posterior oblique *(LPO)*, and anterior views.

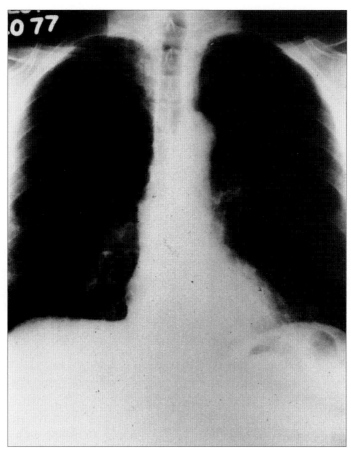

FIGURE 16-17 Chest radiograph of a 64-year-old man with severe emphysema. He has large lungs and bullous areas in the upper lobes.

not available.[28,35] Finding evidence of venous thrombosis would lead to treatment for VTE.[28] If the diagnosis is still in doubt, pulmonary angiography, if available, may be needed to resolve the problem.[7,8,27] Most PE are eventually lysed by the body's own fibrinolytic systems; therefore defects in blood flow tend to disappear with time. Most improvement is seen in the first few days. Further improvement occurs more slowly over the next 3 to 4 weeks and can continue for several months.[52] Anticoagulant treatment is important; it prevents the formation of new blood clots and the extension of those already present in the lungs.

Chronic Obstructive Pulmonary Disease

Radioactive ventilation studies provide one of the most sensitive ways of detecting damage to the small airways.[56] Patients with chronic bronchitis and emphysema show an endless variety of defects in blood flow and ventilation. Eighty percent of the time the defects in blood flow cannot be strictly related to anatomic subdivisions of the lung. In general, both lungs tend to be affected to a similar although rarely identical degree. In some patients most of the damage is in the lower zones; in others, the damage is in the upper zones; and in yet others, the damage is scattered throughout both lungs. It is by no means rare for one lung to be distinctly more severely affected than the other (Figures 16-17 and 16-18).

In chronic bronchitis, ventilation tends to be more severely affected than blood flow, and some changes in the pattern of ventilation and blood flow can be seen with exacerbations of this disease. In emphysema the defects in ventilation and blood flow correspond more closely and tend to be more stable from year to year.

Patients with bronchial asthma also show considerable changes in both ventilation and blood flow, with ventilation being more severely affected. If just a perfusion scan is done, often the defects are recognizably segmental, or even lobar, leading to a false diagnosis of pulmonary embolism.

In cystic fibrosis, the upper lobes usually are the more severely affected, and fissure signs are often seen on the lateral views. This sign is attributable to a defect in blood flow along the greater fissure. It is also seen in other obstructive airway diseases, as well as in pulmonary edema with pleural fluid and occasionally in pulmonary embolism. The segments or lobes of lung involved with bronchiectasis are clearly outlined by lack of ventilation and absent pulmonary arterial blood flow.

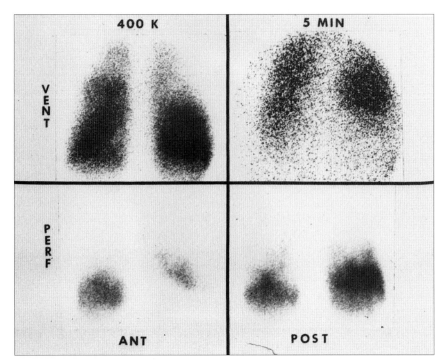

FIGURE 16-18 Selected ventilation (VENT) and perfusion (PERF) images of the patient in Figure 16-17. Perfusion images show decreased perfusion in the upper half of both lung fields. Diminished filling of both upper lung fields is seen on equilibrium (wash-in) images (upper left) and delayed clearance from both lungs during washout (upper right). ANT, Anterior; POST, posterior.

Lung Cancer

In various types of primary lung cancer, ventilation-perfusion studies can be used to determine individual lung function when a pneumonectomy is planned. The relative distribution of blood flow calculated from a posterior upright (or supine) perfusion scan enables postoperative lung function to be predicted with considerable accuracy. A successful resection of the tumor tissue is less likely if the affected lung receives less than about 25% to 30% of the total pulmonary blood flow. Occasionally the site of a tumor can be identified by ventilation-perfusion scanning when it cannot be found by more conventional means. After radiation treatment for lung cancer, ventilation usually improves, but blood flow is restored in a much smaller proportion of such patients.

The most important indication for ventilation-perfusion scanning is in the differential diagnosis of pulmonary embolism. Lesser indications are for the follow-up of this condition and for the assessment of regional and individual lung function in the preoperative assessment of patients with lung cancer or other conditions in which lung tissue may be resected. Ventilation-perfusion scans can sometimes be helpful in the management of patients with COPD. They may also play some part in the follow-up of patients who have had surgical correction of certain congenital heart defects.

SUMMARY

- Alveoli are packed together like cells in a honeycomb.
- Surfactant coats the surface of alveoli.
- Alveoli are where the exchange of oxygen and carbon dioxide takes place.
- Adults have about 250 million to 300 million alveoli.
- Capillaries are 7 to 10 μm in diameter.
- Tidal volume is the volume of air breathed out in a normal breath.
- Functional residual capacity is the volume of air in the lungs at the end of a normal breath.
- Total lung capacity is the volume of air in the lungs when as much air has been inhaled as possible.
- Residual volume is the volume of air left in the lungs after a complete exhalation.
- Compliance is the change in volume for a change in pressure.
- Closing capacity is the volume of air in the lungs when closure begins.
- In the upright position, ventilation of the upper parts of the lung increases by about 1½ to 2 times from apex to base and blood flow increases 3 to 5 times.
- In the supine position, blood flow is more uniform from apex to base, but there is a gradient from anterior to posterior.
- Distribution of blood flow within the upright lung shows the largest gradient from apex to base when measurements are made at total lung capacity.
- Ventilation exceeds blood flow by about 2:1 to 3:1 in the upper zones of the lungs.
- If there is a blood clot, the defect produced on the perfusion scan corresponds to the anatomic segment or lobe of the lung involved.

- PE usually arise from DVT.
- Most PE are multiple with the lower lobes being involved in the majority of the cases.
- MAA particles measure 10 to 90 μm in diameter.
- The usual dose of particulate material blocks less than 1 in 1000 pulmonary arterioles.
- Half the number of particles is given to patients with severe pulmonary hypertension, patients with right-to-left shunts, and patients who have had a pneumonectomy.
- Injection of MAA should be given while the patient is in the supine position to give a more homogeneous distribution of the particles from apex to base.
- Patients injected with MAA while upright show a larger proportion of particles distributed in the bases.
- Because the energy of ^{133}Xe is less than that of ^{99m}Tc, the ventilation study should be performed first.
- In aerosol imaging the trachea, the mainstem bronchi, and sometimes the esophagus and stomach appear.
- PE are demonstrated in images by an abnormal regional blood flow but normal or near normal regional ventilation.
- Obstructive airway diseases are demonstrated in images by abnormal blood flow and corresponding abnormal ventilation.
- Patients with primary lung cancer should have a lung function study performed before a pneumonectomy or lobotomy.
- Functional information can be obtained by performing a lung quantification analysis on perfusion and/or ventilation images.

REFERENCES

1. Alderson PO, Biello DR, Khan AR, et al: Comparison of ^{133}Xe single-breath and washout imaging in the scintigraphic diagnosis of pulmonary embolism, *Radiology* 137:481-486, 1980.
2. Alderson PO, Biello DR, Sachariah KG, et al: Scintigraphic detection of pulmonary embolism in patients with obstructive pulmonary disease, *Radiology* 138:661-666, 1981.
3. Alderson PO, Rujanavech N, Secker-Walker RH, et al: The role of ^{133}Xe ventilation studies in the scintigraphic detection of pulmonary embolism, *Radiology* 120:633, 1976.
4. Anthonisen NR, Danson J, Roberson PC, et al: Airway closure as a function of age, *Respir Physiol* 8:58, 1969.
5. Anthonisen NR, Milic-Emili J: Distribution of pulmonary perfusion in erect man, *J Appl Physiol* 21:760, 1966.
6. Ball WC Jr, Stewart PB, Newham IGS, et al: Regional pulmonary studies with xenon 133, *J Clin Invest* 41:519, 1962.
7. Biello DR, Mattar AG, McKnight RC, et al: Ventilation-perfusion studies in suspected pulmonary embolism, *AJR Am J Roentgenol* 138:661-666, 1981.
8. Biello DR, Mattar AG, Osei-Wusu A, et al: Interpretation of indeterminate lung scintigrams, *Radiology* 133:189-194, 1979.
9. Breeze RG, Wheeldon EB: The cells of the pulmonary airways, *Am Rev Respir Dis* 116:705, 1977.
10. Buist AS, Van Fleet DL, Ross BB: A comparison of conventional spirometric tests and the test of closing volume in an emphysema screening center, *Am Rev Respir Dis* 107:735, 1973.
11. Burdine JA, Murphy PH: Clinical efficacy of a large-field-of-view scintillation camera, *J Nucl Med* 16:1158, 1975.
12. Carson JL, Kelley MA, Duff A, et al: The clinical course of pulmonary embolism: one year follow-up of PIOPED patients, *N Engl J Med* 326:1240, 1992.
13. Child JS, Wolfe JD, Tashkin D, et al: Fatal lung scan in a case of pulmonary hypertension due to obliterative pulmonary vascular disease, *Chest* 67:308, 1975.
14. Daly I de B, Hebb C: *Pulmonary and bronchial vascular systems*, Baltimore, 1966, Williams & Wilkins.
15. Dismuke SE, Wagner EH: Pulmonary embolism as a cause of death. The changing mortality in hospitalized patients, *JAMA* 255:2039, 1986.
16. Fishman AP, Pietra G: Handling of bioactive materials by the lung, *N Engl J Med* 291(18):953-959, 1974.
17. Gold WM, McCormack KR: Pulmonary function response to radioisotope scanning of the lungs, *JAMA* 197:146, 1966.
18. Goldhaber, SZ. Pulmonary embolism, *N Engl J Med* 339:93, 1998.
19. Green GM: The J. Burns Amberson Lecture: in defense of the lung, *Am Rev Respir Dis* 102:691, 1970.
20. Guidelines on diagnosis and management of acute pulmonary embolism. Task Force on Pulmonary Embolism, European Society of Cardiology, *Eur Heart J* 21:1301, 2000.
21. Harding LK, Horsfield K, Singhal SS, et al: The proportion of lung vessels blocked by albumin microspheres, *J Nucl Med* 14:579, 1973.
22. Hayes M, Taplin GV, Chopra SK, et al: Improved radioaerosol administration system for routine inhalation lung imaging, *Radiology* 131:256-258, 1979.
23. Haynie TP, Calhoon JH, Nasjleti CE, et al: Visualization of pulmonary artery occlusion by photoscanning, *JAMA* 185:306, 1963.
24. Horlander KT, Mannino DM, Leeper KV: Pulmonary embolism mortality in the United States, 1979-1998: an analysis using multiple-cause mortality data, *Arch Intern Med* 163:1711, 2003.
25. Hughes JMB, Glazier JB, Maloney JE, et al: Effect of lung volume on the distribution of pulmonary blood flow in man, *Respir Physiol* 4:78, 1968.
26. Hull RD, Hirsch J, Carter CJ, et al: Diagnostic value of ventilation-perfusion lung scanning in patients with suspected pulmonary embolism, *Chest* 88:819-828, 1985.
27. Hull RD, Hirsch J, Carter CJ, et al: Pulmonary angiography, ventilation lung scanning, and venography for clinically suspected pulmonary embolism with abnormal perfusion lung scan, *Ann Intern Med* 98:891-899, 1983.
28. Hull RD, Raskob GE, Coates G, et al: A new noninvasive management strategy for patients with suspected pulmonary embolism, *Arch Intern Med* 149:2549-2555, 1989.
29. Hull RD, Raskob GE, Coates G, et al: Clinical validity of a normal perfusion lung scan in patients with suspected pulmonary embolism, *Chest* 97:23-26, 1990.
30. Kaneko K, Milic-Emili J, Dolovich MB, et al: Regional distribution of ventilation and perfusion as a function of body position, *J Appl Physiol* 21:767, 1966.
31. Kistner RL, Ball JJ, Nordyke RA, et al: Incidence of pulmonary embolism in the course of thrombophlebitis of the lower extremities, *Am J Surg* 124:169, 1972.
32. Kleine JA, Johns KL, et al: New diagnostic tests for pulmonary embolism, *Ann Emerg Med* 35:2, 2000.
33. Knipping HW, Bolt W, Vanrath H, et al: Eine neue Methode zur Prüfung der Herz- und Lungenfunktion, *Deutsch Med Wochenschr* 80:1146, 1955.
34. Kowalski RJ, Falen SW: *Radiopharmaceuticals in nuclear pharmacy and nuclear medicine*, Washington, D.C., 2004, APhA.

35. Lensing AWA, Prandoni P, Brandjes D, et al: Detection of deep-vein thrombosis by real-time b-mode ultrasonography, *N Engl J Med* 320:342-345, 1989.
36. Luizzi A, Keaney J, Freedman G: Use of activated charcoal for the collection and containment of Xe-133 exhaled during pulmonary studies, *J Nucl Med* 13:673, 1972.
37. McNeil BJ: A diagnostic strategy using ventilation-perfusion studies in patients suspect for pulmonary embolism, *J Nucl Med* 17:613, 1976.
38. Mead J, Takishima T, Leith D: Stress distribution in lungs: a model of pulmonary elasticity, *J Appl Physiol* 28:596, 1970.
39. Moser, KM: Venous thromboembolism, *Am Rev Respir Dis* 141:235, 1990.
40. Nielsen PE, Kirchner PT, Gerber FH: Oblique views in lung perfusion scanning: clinical utility and limitations, *J Nucl Med* 18:967, 1977.
41. Parker JA, Coleman RE, Hilson AJW, et al: *Procedure guideline for lung scintigraphy*, Reston, Va, 2004, Society of Nuclear Medicine.
42. Rathbun SW, Whitsett TL, Vesely SK, et al: Clinical utility of D-Dimer in patients with suspected pulmonary embolism and nondiagnostic lung scans or negative CT findings, *Chest* 125:851, 2004.
43. Rhodes BA, Stem HS, Buchanan JA, et al: Lung scanning with Tc-99m microspheres, *Radiology* 99:613, 1971.
44. Righini M, Goehring C, Bounameaux H, et al: Effects of age on the performance of common diagnostic tests for pulmonary emboli, *Am J Med* 109:357, 2000.
45. Rodger MA, Carrier M, Jones GN, et al: Diagnostic value of arterial blood gas measurement in suspected pulmonary embolism, *Am J Respir Crit Care Med* 162:2105, 2000.
46. Rogers RM, Kuhl DE, Hyde RW, et al: Measurement of the vital capacity and perfusion of each lung by fluoroscopy and macroaggregated albumin lung scanning, *Ann Intern Med* 67:947, 1967.
47. Rootwelt K, Vale JR: Pulmonary gas exchange after intravenous injection of ^{99m}Tc sulphur colloid albumin macroaggregates for lung perfusion scintigraphy, *Scand J Clin Lab Invest* 30:17, 1972.
48. Sanchis J, Dolovich M, Rossman C, et al: Pulmonary mucociliary clearance in cystic fibrosis, *N Engl J Med* 288:651, 1973.
49. Sasahara AA, Belko JS, Simpson RC: Multiple view lung scanning, *J Nucl Med* 9:187, 1968.
50. Secker-Walker RH, Barbier J, Weiner SN, et al: A simple ^{133}Xe delivery system for studies of regional ventilation, *J Nucl Med* 15:288, 1974.
51. Secker-Walker RH, Evens RG: The clinical application of computers in ventilation-perfusion studies, *Progr Nucl Med* 3:166, 1973.
52. Secker-Walker RH, Jackson JA, Goodwin J: Resolution of pulmonary embolism, *Br Med J* 4:135, 1970.
53. Sostman DH, Stein PD, Gottschalk A, et al: Acute pulmonary embolism: sensitivity and specificity of ventilation-perfusion scintigraphy in PIOPED II study, *Radiology* 246:3, 2008.
54. Sostman DH, Miniati M, Gottschalk A, et al: Sensitivity and specificity of perfusion scintigraphy combined with chest radiography for acute pulmonary embolism in PIOPED II, *J Nucl Med Technol* 49:11, 2008.
55. Taplin GV, Johnson DE, Dore EK, et al: Lung photoscans with macroaggregates of human serum radioalbumin: experimental basis and initial clinical trials, *Health Phys* 10:1219, 1964.
56. Taplin GV, Tashkin DP, Chopra SK, et al: Early detection of chronic obstructive pulmonary disease using radionuclide lung imaging procedures, *Chest* 71:567, 1977.
57. Taylor A, Schuster DM, Alazraki N: *A clinician's guide to nuclear medicine*, ed 2, Reston, Va., 2006, Society of Nuclear Medicine.
58. Tow DE, Wagner HN, Lopez-Majano V, et al: Validity of measuring regional pulmonary arterial blood flow with macroaggregates of human serum albumin, *Am J Roentgenol Radium Ther Nucl Med* 96:664, 1966.
59. Trowbridge RL, Araoz PA, Gotway MB, et al: The effect of helical computed tomography on diagnostic and treatment strategies in patients with suspected pulmonary embolism, *Am J Med* 40:751, 2004.
60. Value of the ventilation/perfusion scan in acute pulmonary embolism. Results of the prospective investigation of pulmonary embolism diagnosis (PIOPED). The PIOPED Investigators, *JAMA* 263:2753-2759, 1990.
61. Wagner HM, Sabiston DC, McAfee JG, et al: Diagnosis of massive pulmonary embolism in man by radioisotope scanning, *N Engl J Med* 271:377, 1964.
62. Weibel ER: *Morphometry of the human lungs*, New York, 1963, Academic Press.
63. Weinman EE, Salzman EW: Deep vein thrombosis, *N Engl J Med* 331:1630, 1994.
64. Wells PS, Anderson DR, Rodger M, et al.: Excluding pulmonary embolism at the bedside without diagnostic imaging: management of patients with suspected pulmonary embolism presenting to the emergency department by using a simple clinical model and D-dimer, *Ann Intern Med* 135:98-107, 2001.
65. West JB: Pulmonary function studies with radioactive gases, *Ann Rev Med* 18:459, 1967.
66. West JB: Respiratory physiology: the essentials, Baltimore, 1975, Williams & Wilkins.

Cardiovascular System

Neeta Pandit-Taskar, Ravinder K. Grewal, H. William Strauss

OUTLINE

OBJECTIVES

After completing this chapter, the reader will be able to:
- Diagram the structures of the heart.
- Describe the mechanical and electrical activity of the heart.
- List the acquired abnormalities of the cardiovascular system that can be evaluated with radionuclide techniques.
- State the preparation, dosage, and injection technique for radionuclide evaluation of ventricular function.

- Explain how an ejection fraction is calculated.
- Describe an exercise and a pharmacological stress test and explain when each is used.
- Discuss radiopharmaceuticals used for myocardial perfusion imaging.
- Describe the imaging techniques for SPECT and PET myocardial perfusion imaging.
- Discuss the advantage of PET radionuclides for cardiac imaging.

KEY TERMS

angina
cardiac cycle
cardiac output
cardiomyopathy
cinematic display
congestive heart failure (CHF)
coronary artery disease (CAD)
dipyridamole

end-diastolic volume
horizontal long axis
hypertension
ischemia
multiple gated acquisition (MUGA)
myocardial infarction
myocardial ischemia
redistribution

regadenoson
short axis
stenosis
stroke volume
vasodilator
vertical long axis

Radionuclide studies of the cardiovascular system are primarily used to detect and determine the severity of acquired heart diseases, particularly coronary artery disease (CAD), cardiotoxicity of antineoplastic drugs, and determine the severity of congestive heart failure. Assessments of patients with congenital heart disease and valvular heart disease are generally made by a combination of echocardiography and magnetic resonance imaging (MRI). This chapter focuses on the current clinical applications of nuclear techniques; the reader is referred to other sources for procedures of historical importance.

Nuclear medicine laboratories use both single-photon and positron-emitting radiopharmaceuticals to evaluate myocardial perfusion and ventricular function. Single-photon tracers are imaged with multiple-detector gamma cameras and hybrid gamma cameras equipped with an associated CT (SPECT-CT) for attenuation correction and anatomic localization. Positron-emitting agents are imaged with a positron emission tomograph coupled to a CT (PET-CT) instruments. PET instruments have higher spatial resolution (4-5 mm) than single-photon systems (6-8 mm) and can be used to acquire data on myocardial perfusion, ventricular function, and viability, in similar fashion to single photon devices. In contrast to single-photon imaging, PET has the added capability of absolute quantitation (e.g., expressing myocardial perfusion as ml/min/g of myocardium). This chapter describes various practical aspects of both single-photon and PET imaging of the heart.

CLINICAL PROBLEM

Approximately 81 million people in the United States have one or more forms of acquired disease of the heart or blood vessels. Elevated blood pressure (**hypertension**) is present in 74.5 million adults; coronary artery disease (CAD, partial or total blockage of one or more of the coronary arteries) in 17.6 million (10.2 million have **angina**, or chest pain of cardiac origin); **congestive heart failure (CHF)**, the inability of the heart to pump sufficient blood to meet the demands of the body in approximately 5.8 million; and stroke in 6.4 million. Coronary artery disease (CAD) caused about 425,000 deaths in the United States in 2006, making CAD the number one killer in the United States. About 935,000 people will suffer a new or recurrent heart attack each year. In addition to CAD, heart failure is becoming increasingly prevalent as the population ages. In patients older than 40 years, CHF occurs in about 0.3% of the population, but in patients older than 80 years, more than 13% of the population have CHF. A major reason for the increased prevalence of CHF with age is that heart failure is often the final phase of other forms of heart disease, such as hypertension, CAD, valvular heart disease, or cardiomyopathy.[1] **Cardiomyopathy,** is a disorder of the heart muscle, which limits the ability of the heart to function as a pump. There are two major forms of cardiomyopathy. The first is associated with an abnormal increase in the thickness of the myocardium (hypertrophic cardiomyopathy), due to either a congenital abnormality, or more often, due to prolonged hypertension. The thick heart muscle is stiff, reducing the ability of the cardiac chambers to fill with blood during diastole. The second type of cardiomyopathy is caused by a reduced ability the myocardium to contract effectively, despite an adequate blood supply, limiting the ability of the heart to pump blood to the lungs and body. This usually results in dilatation of the cardiac chambers, with thinning of the muscle (dilated cardiomyopathy).

Coronary artery disease leads to **myocardial ischemia** and **myocardial infarction.** Myocardial ischemia is a reversible condition caused by a temporary reduction in the delivery of oxygen to the myocardium, usually as a result of narrowing of one or more of the coronary arteries. Myocardial infarction is associated with death of heart muscle, caused by a more prolonged, severe reduction of blood flow, usually as a result of occluded arteries. Early identification of myocardial infarction allows restoration of blood flow within a few hours of onset, resulting in preservation of myocardium and improved function.

Although myocardial infarction can occur with no warning and can cause sudden death, the underlying disease of the coronary arteries evolves over decades. The arterial lesions begin around puberty, progressing from lipid deposits in the wall of the vessel, called *fatty streaks*, to raised lesions that intrude on the arterial lumen. This progression occurs over 30 to 50 years (Figure 17-1). The rate of progression is accelerated in patients with hypercholesterolemia, diabetes, elevated homocysteine levels, and diets rich in saturated and trans fats. Atheromatous narrowings that occupy more than 50% of the lumen diameter restrict the maximum amount of blood that can flow through a vessel, but may not be associated with symptoms. Narrowings of at least 70% of the lumen are often symptomatic, causing dyspnea on exertion, angina when the demand for blood flow (oxygen) through the coronary arteries exceeds the supply of oxygen and nutrients that can be supplied by the narrowed artery, or both. This condition of myocardial ischemia is associated with decreased contraction in the affected area. Prolonged **ischemia** leads to damage of the myocardium, and may result in myocardial infarction. These changes can be readily detected by radionuclide imaging studies.

ANATOMY

The adult heart (Figure 17-2) weighs about 300 g and holds approximately 500 ml of blood. The heart is actually two pumps (the right heart and left heart) operating in parallel to eject the same amount of blood with each beat. The right heart accepts blood from the body and

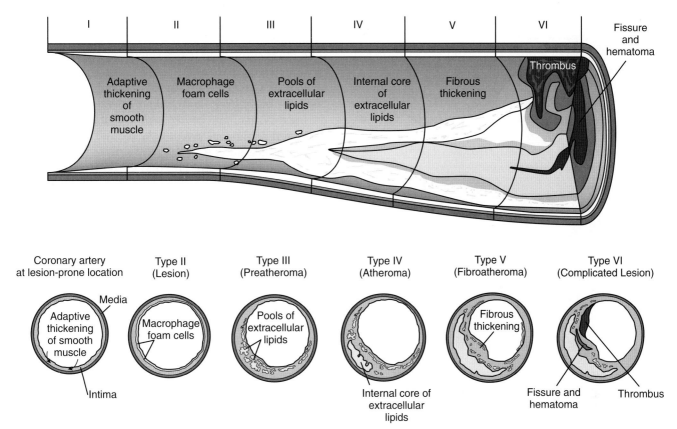

FIGURE 17-1 Advanced types of atherosclerotic lesions and histological classification. The top row shows a vessel in longitudinal section; the bottom row shows sections through the vessel in cross section. The Roman numerals represent the stages of atheroma, using the American Heart Association classification. There are no major vessel narrowings until lesions are type IV.

pumps this blood to the lungs, where it is oxygenated. The left heart accepts the oxygenated blood returning from the lungs and pumps it to the body. The right heart and left heart each have two chambers, a thin-walled atrium, which holds about 100 ml, and a more muscular ventricle, with a capacity of about 150 ml. Atria serve as temporary reservoirs for blood returned to the heart, and the ventricles do the major work of pumping the blood away from the heart. The right atrium accepts deoxygenated blood returning from the body through the superior and inferior vena cava. The right atrium pumps the blood into the right ventricle, which in turn pumps the blood to the lungs, where it is oxygenated before returning to the left atrium. The left atrium pumps the oxygenated blood to the left ventricle, which pumps the oxygenated blood to the body.

The right and left atria are separated by a thin, muscular wall, the interatrial septum; the right and left ventricles are separated by the thicker, muscular interventricular septum. Valves separate the atria from the ventricles and the ventricles from the arteries. The valves prevent blood from flowing backward. The tricuspid valve (named for its three leaflets, or cusps) separates the right atrium from the right ventricle, and the mitral valve (with two cusps) separates the left atrium from the left ventricle. The pulmonic valve separates the right ventricle from the pulmonary artery, and the aortic valve separates the left ventricle from the aorta. The pulmonic and aortic valves each have three cusps.

The heart muscle (myocardium) receives its blood supply through arteries that specifically supply its needs. Oxygen and nutrients are delivered to the myocardium by the left and right coronary arteries (Figure 17-3). The left main coronary artery divides into two main branches. The left anterior descending artery supplies oxygen and nutrition to the interventricular septum and the anterior wall of the left ventricle; the left circumflex artery supplies the left atrium and the posterior and lateral walls of the left ventricle. The right coronary artery supplies the inferior wall of the left ventricle, the free wall of the right ventricle, and the right atrium. Blood drains from the myocardium to the coronary veins, which run alongside the coronary arteries and terminate in the coronary sinus of the right atrium, where the deoxygenated blood from the myocardium mixes with deoxygenated blood carried by the vena cava.

PHYSIOLOGY

Circulation

Deoxygenated venous blood, carrying carbon dioxide and waste products, returns from the body to the heart via the superior and inferior venae cavae (Figure 17-4).

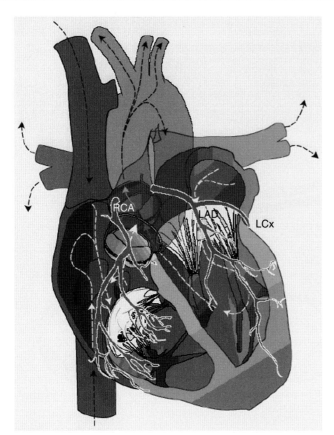

FIGURE 17-2 Gross anatomy of the heart. Cutaway drawing of the heart, showing the four chambers, atria, ventricles, tricuspid and mitral valves, pulmonic and aortic valves, and the right and left coronary arteries. The *dotted lines* and *arrows* depict the flow of blood in each chamber.

Blood flows through the large veins at 40 cm/sec on its way to emptying into the right atrium at a pressure of less than 5 mm Hg. Blood traverses the tricuspid valve to enter the right ventricle, which pumps it through the pulmonic valve into the pulmonary artery and lungs for oxygenation. The right ventricle pumps blood into the lungs at a pressure of 25 mm Hg. In the enormous capillary bed of the lungs, the velocity of blood slows to 1 mm/sec in the capillaries of the alveoli, where carbon dioxide is eliminated and oxygen is taken up.

The oxygenated blood returns to the left atrium via the pulmonary veins at a pressure of less than 5 mm Hg. The blood then flows through the mitral valve to the left ventricle, which expels blood through the aortic valve, at a velocity of about 15 m/sec, into the aorta at a systolic pressure of about 120 mm Hg.

Mechanical Activity of the Heart

Each **cardiac cycle** (i.e., one beat) consists of systole—the period of ventricular contraction—and diastole—the period of ventricular relaxation (Figure 17-5). The two sides of the heart contract in unison. During most of

diastole, both the atria and the ventricles are relaxed. Atrial pressures are slightly higher than ventricular pressure, the tricuspid and mitral valves are open, and blood passes from the atria into the ventricles. Eighty to ninety percent of ventricular filling takes place in this passive fashion. The aortic and pulmonic valves are closed during this time, preventing backflow of blood from the aorta and pulmonary arteries. At the end of diastole the atria contract, adding 10% to 20% more volume to the ventricles. The quantity of blood in the ventricles at the end of diastole is called the **end-diastolic volume** (about 150 ml in the left ventricle of an average 70-kg adult, and about 170 ml in the right ventricle).

During systole, the myofibrils of the ventricular myocardium shorten and ventricular pressure rises, causing the tricuspid and mitral valves to close. This is followed by the interval of isovolumetric (i.e., no change in volume) contraction, when the continued shortening of the myofibrils causes ventricular pressure to exceed the pressure in the pulmonary artery and aorta. The pulmonic and aortic valves open, and ventricular ejection begins. During the interval of ventricular ejection, blood is also returned to the atria. As a result, both right and left atrial volumes and pressures rise during the interval of ventricular ejection. At the conclusion of ventricular ejection, the myofibrils rapidly relax, ventricular pressure falls, the aortic and pulmonic valves close, the tricuspid and mitral valves open, and the ventricles start to refill. Filling occurs rapidly during early diastole and slows as atrial pressure and volume decrease. This filling pattern ensures the heart's ability to function effectively during times of increased heart rate (as with exercise and emotional stress), when the length of diastole is shortened. The amount of blood ejected from the left ventricle over a 1-min interval is the cardiac output (usually expressed in liters per minute). A normal 70-kg adult has a cardiac output of approximately 5 to 6 L/min at rest. The amount of blood ejected in a single beat is the stroke volume (usually expressed in milliliters). The normal adult stroke volume is approximately 80 to 100 ml. The cardiac output is distributed to the organs in proportion to their oxygen requirements, which change from rest to exertion (Table 17-1).

Electrical Activity of the Heart

Heart muscle has an intrinsic rate of contraction. The sinoatrial node, a small mass of specialized cells embedded in the wall of the right atrium near the entrance of the superior vena cava, has the fastest inherent rate and supersedes other similar sites in the heart (Figure 17-6). Consequently, the sinoatrial node usually serves as the impulse generator for the remainder of the heart. The wave of electrical depolarization spreads to the surrounding atrial muscle cells and stimulates mechanical contraction. There are no specialized conduction fibers within the atria, and the impulse spreads from cell to cell

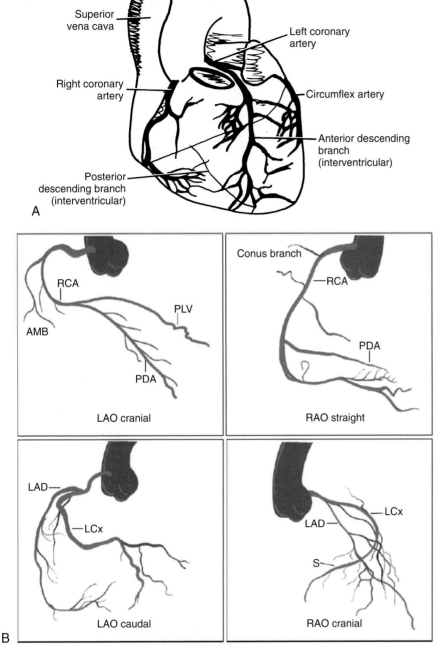

A, Anterior view of the heart, showing the coronary arteries. Aorta; Superior vena cava; Left coronary artery; Right coronary artery; Circumflex artery; Anterior descending branch (interventricular); Posterior descending branch (interventricular).

B, LAO cranial: RCA, AMB, PLV, PDA. RAO straight: Conus branch, RCA, PDA. LAO caudal: LAD, LCx. RAO cranial: LAD, LCx, S.

FIGURE 17-3 A, Anterior view of the heart, showing the coronary arteries. **B,** Typical coronary angiographic views: *LAO cranial; RAO straight; LAO caudal; RAO cranial. AMB,* Acute marginal branch; *LAD,* left anterior descending; *LAO,* left anterior oblique; *LCx,* left circumflex; *PDA,* posterior descending artery; *PLV,* posterior left ventricular artery; *RAO,* right anterior oblique; *RCA,* right coronary artery; *S,* septal.

to cover the entire atria within 0.08 sec. Mechanical contraction requires approximately 0.1 sec, much longer than the spread of the electrical signal.

There is a delay in the transmission of the electrical signal from the atria to the ventricles, to allow the atria to complete their mechanical contraction before the ventricles start to contract. As the signal enters the atrioventricular (AV) node there is a delay of more than 0.1 second before the electrical impulse enters the specialized conduction system in the interventricular septum.

Propagation of the electrical signal from the AV node to the ventricular myocardium is followed by the onset of mechanical systole. Mechanical systole requires approximately 0.3 second.

The electrocardiogram (ECG) reflects the electrical activities of the heart (Figure 17-7). It typically consists of a P wave, QRS complex, and T wave. The P wave is the electrical signal that starts atrial contraction, the QRS complex serves the same function in the ventricles, and the T wave identifies an electrical reset of the

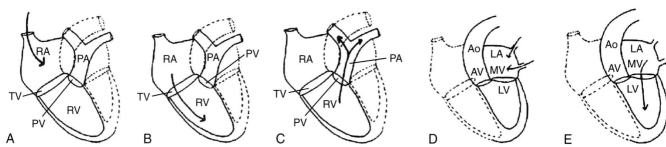

FIGURE 17-4 Poorly oxygenated blood returning to the heart from the organs enters the right atrium *(RA)* and is stored there until the RA contracts. When the RA contracts, the tricuspid valve *(TV)* opens, allowing blood to enter the right ventricle *(RV)*. When the RV contracts, the pulmonic valve *(PV)* opens, and blood is propelled into the pulmonary artery *(PA)*. The PA carries the blood to the lungs, where it picks up oxygen. Well-oxygenated blood returning to the heart from the lungs enters the left atrium *(LA)* and is stored there until the LA contracts. When the LA contracts, the mitral valve *(MV)* opens, allowing the blood to enter the left ventricle *(LV)*, from which it is pumped into the aorta during systole and distributed to various organs and tissues.

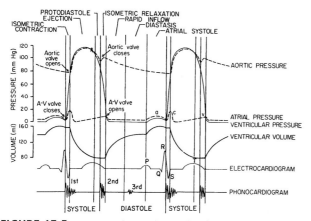

FIGURE 17-5 Events in the cardiac cycle, showing the simultaneous relationship of the electrocardiogram and phonocardiogram to the measured pressures in the left atrium, the left ventricle, and the aorta and the volume of the ventricles. *A-V,* Atrial-ventricular.

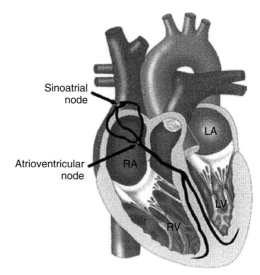

FIGURE 17-6 Conduction system of the heart. *LA,* Left atrium; *LV,* left ventricle; *RA,* right atrium; *RV,* right ventricle.

TABLE 17-1	Cardiac Output at Rest and Exercise	
	Fraction of Cardiac Output	
Organ	**Rest (5 L/min)**	**Exercise (15 L/min)**
Brain	15%	4%
Heart	4%	5%
Kidneys	20%	5%
Liver	10%	1%
Gastrointestinal tract	15%	1%
Skeletal muscle	20%	70%
Skin	6%	10%
Other	10%	4%

Compiled from McCardle WD, et al: *Exercise, physiology, energy, nutrition and human performance*, Philadelphia, 1981, Lea & Febiger.

ventricles for the next cardiac cycle. During much of diastole the heart is electrically silent.

Irregularities or abnormalities of conduction are quite common and can have substantial effects on ventricular function and radionuclide studies. Some of the more common conduction abnormalities are listed in Box 17-1.

RADIONUCLIDE IMAGING CONSIDERATIONS

Tracers Used for Cardiac Imaging

Radiopharmaceuticals determine which functional aspect of the heart is depicted in the image. The four major categories of radiopharmaceuticals used in clinical cardiac imaging include (1) perfusion tracers, which measure the regional (and with PET tracers, absolute) distribution of blood flow to the heart muscle; information from gated perfusion images can also be used to measure global and regional ventricular function; (2) blood-pool tracers, used for more detailed measurements of atrial and ventricular function; (3) analogs of epinephrine to measure sympathetic innervation; and (4) glucose

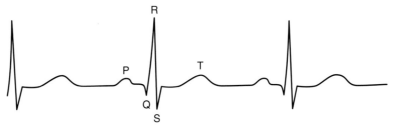

FIGURE 17-7 A normal electrocardiogram (ECG) tracing showing the P, Q, R, S, and T waves.

BOX 17-1	**Common Conduction Abnormalities**

- **Premature systoles** may originate in the atria (PACs) or ventricles (PVCs) or may be coupled. If the extrasystoles occur every other beat, the rhythm is called *bigeminy.*
- **Ventricular tachycardia** originates in a focus in the ventricle. This type of arrhythmia is potentially life-threatening and should be treated immediately. Ventricular tachycardia can proceed to ventricular fibrillation, which if left untreated results in death.
- **Atrial fibrillation** is defined as a totally disorganized firing at multiple sites in the atria that causes a rapid, irregular ventricular rate.
- **Bundle branch block** (either left or right) is an abnormal conduction pattern associated with slower depolarization of the conducting pathway through one ventricle compared to the other (e.g., LBBB results in a delay of conduction to depolarize the left ventricle)

LBBB, Left bundle branch block; *PACs,* premature atrial contractions; *PVCs,* premature ventricular contractions.
From Zipes DP: *Heart disease: a textbook of cardiovascular medicine,* Philadelphia, 1984, Saunders.

BOX 17-2	**Radiopharmaceuticals for Clinical Cardiac Imaging**

Myocardial perfusion
  Single photon agents
    Thallium-201
    Technetium-99m tracers
      Sestamibi
      Tetrofosmin
  Positron emitting tracers
    Rubidium-82
    Nitrogen-13–ammonia
    Oxygen-15–labeled water
Ventricular function
  Technetium-99m–labeled red blood cells
Measurement of myocardial metabolism
  Fluorine-18–fluorodeoxyglucose
  Iodine-123–betamethyliodophenylpentadecanoic acid
Measurement of sympathetic innervation
  Iodine-123–metaiodobenzylguanidine

and fatty acid analogs to measure metabolism (Box 17-2).

Planar and SPECT Data Acquisition

The majority of cardiac studies are performed with single-photon radiopharmaceuticals and imaged with single photon emission computed tomography (SPECT). Planar imaging is rarely used, except in morbidly obese patients, where the quality of SPECT images is reduced.

SPECT cardiac images are recorded as a series of individual projections, usually in steps of 3 degrees in an arc spanning at least 180 degrees, beginning at 45 degrees right anterior oblique (RAO) and moving to 45 degrees left posterior oblique (LPO). Images are recorded with multidetector scintillation cameras with extrinsic resolution better than 5 mm full width at half maximum (FWHM). The projection images are each recorded in 64 × 64 or preferably a 128 × 128 matrix (see Chapter 9). The individual projections are reconstructed using iterative algorithms into a series of transverse slices through the imaged volume. The transverse slices are reoriented along the long axis of the left ventricle, to produce three standard cardiac views: **vertical long axis** (corresponding to coronal images, presented from the septum to lateral wall), **horizontal long axis** (corresponding to transverse sections, presented from the inferior to the anterior surface), and **short axis** (corresponding to sagittal views, presented from the apex to the base). These reoriented images depict the myocardium or blood pool in a standard presentation, which simplifies interpretation (Figure 17-8). (See Chapter 9 for details of SPECT acquisition and processing.)

Transverse section images should provide six to eight slices through the heart (typical reconstructions are 1 to 2 pixels thick with no spaces between the slices). Before reconstruction, the projection images should be reviewed as a **cinematic display** to detect patient motion, major changes in cardiac position during acquisition, and technical problems, such as missed or duplicated angles. Single episodes of motion of less than 2 pixels can usually be tolerated. Although motion-correction software is available in many of the reconstruction software programs, the corrections are often incomplete and may result in artifacts in the reconstructed data. Multiple episodes of motion, movement greater than 2 pixels, or loss of more than one set of projection data creates significant artifacts that can lead to erroneous

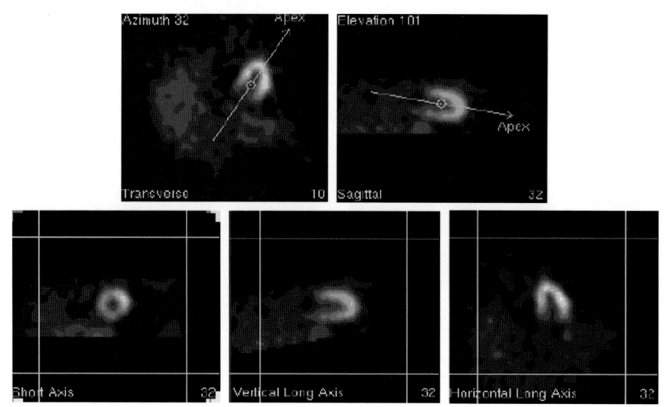

FIGURE 17-8 Reorientation of transverse slices into standard orientation. The long axis of the left ventricle is identified on the transverse and sagittal images *(top row)*. The standard short-axis, vertical long-axis, and horizontal long-axis images are then generated by the computer.

interpretation. In these circumstances, the acquisition should be repeated.

The most common multidetector cameras have two detectors, which can assume positions ranging from 90 to 180 degrees apart. A dual-detector system with the detectors oriented 90 degrees to each other is preferable for recording cardiac SPECT because the detectors are closest to the heart for each image. This maximizes collimator resolution and eliminates the highly attenuated photons arising from the back of the patient and the attenuation artifacts that may be caused by the spine that would be recorded if a full 360-degree acquisition were used.

New collimator and detector designs for dedicated cardiac cameras permit continuous acquisition of data from the entire myocardium simultaneously, eliminating the need to move the detector during acquisition. Since the entire heart is viewed by the detectors simultaneously, image acquisition time can be shortened without decreasing image quality. An alternative use of this increased sensitivity is reduction of the administered dose (and the radiation burden to the patient) while the imaging time is maintained.

The use of CT for attenuation correction reduces artefacts from the diaphragm and breast in myocardial perfusion images. Before applying the CT attenuation correction to the emission SPECT data, it is important to check the two data sets for misregistration. The CT attenuation data and emission scan data should be reconstructed in the transaxial, sagittal, and coronal planes and the images superimposed, to be certain that all slices of the emission data fit in the cardiac silhouette. If the CT was acquired during a breath hold, it is likely that the diaphragm will be in a different position than if the CT was recorded during free breathing. If necessary, the images can be realigned, before the attenuation correction is applied to the emission data.

To maximize spatial resolution, high-resolution or ultra–high-resolution collimation should be used and the detectors should be as close as possible to the surface of the patient when recording each image. Mechanically, it is easiest to rotate the detector through a circle when recording data for 15 to 60 sec at each step. Inadequate sampling (step angles greater than 6 degrees or gaps between steps) can result in an artifact that resembles the spokes of a wheel (i.e., star artifact). To avoid this, angular sampling of about 3 degrees is recommended. An alternative is sampling during continuous motion of the detector. Unfortunately, this approach leads to blurring of the individual projections, making it less desirable for routine use.

A circular orbit maximizes the distance between the collimator and the body surface in the anterior and posterior positions, resulting in a spatial resolution of approximately 12 to 19 mm in the reconstructed data. Moving the detector through an ellipse as it traverses the chest keeps the detectors closer to the heart, resulting in some improvement in resolution. However, setting up a noncircular acquisition is more complex, and even though the detector is closer to the body surface, the heart is not in the center of the body. Because the gain in resolution is small, especially for large patients, a circular orbit generally is used.

During the 20- to 30-minute SPECT data acquisition, the patient lies supine with the left arm above the head (a fairly uncomfortable position). SPECT images may also be recorded with the patient prone, to minimize attenuation from the diaphragm. Prone patients also elevate the left arm to minimize attenuation. Although prone image acquisition may provide better images of the inferior wall, the improvement comes at a cost of marked patient discomfort.

Myocardial perfusion data is usually recorded with synchronization to the patient's cardiac cycle (ECG gating). Gated myocardial perfusion acquisitions can be processed to show regional wall motion and ejection fraction, in addition to the myocardial perfusion data. The information about regional function increases the diagnostic value of the procedure. Because the photon flux available from technetium-99m (^{99m}Tc)–labeled perfusion agents (typically administered in 10- to 30-mCi doses of ^{99m}Tc-sestamibi or ^{99m}Tc-tetrofosmin) provides higher count density gated myocardial perfusion SPECT studies than those obtainable with thallium-201 (^{201}Tl; 4 mCi), ^{99m}Tc agents are preferred for these studies. However clinically useful gated acquisitions can be recorded with ^{201}Tl.

Attenuation Correction. The soft tissue of the chest musculature, breast, and diaphragm attenuate the emission signal and may resemble perfusion defects. Generally attenuation is more pronounced for the lower energy photons of thallium and less significant for technetium. However, this is not always true. Technetium has only 20% less attenuation than thallium, and because of higher photon flux, the artifacts may actually be more pronounced.

Attenuation can be corrected by measuring the attenuation coefficients using a radionuclide transmission source or x-ray CT. The information is incorporated into the reconstructed emission data to compensate for the attenuation. An x-ray source is preferred to a radioactive source because the higher photon flux from the x-ray tube make the x-ray determined attenuation map much more precise than that available from a radioactive source. Typically, the attenuation correction CT is recorded immediately before the emission SPECT images.

While attenuation correction is an important tool to distinguish artifacts, attenuation correction itself can cause artifacts. To minimize these problems, it is important to review both corrected and noncorrected images and correlate the data with the raw cine images and

gating. In addition the alignment of the emission and transmission data should be reviewed on the transaxial, sagittal, and coronal planes to assure that the myocardium fits within the cardiac silhouette.

MYOCARDIAL PERFUSION IMAGING

As the heart does more work (either by increasing heart rate, pumping at a higher pressure, or both), the amount of oxygen delivered to the myocardium must increase. Normal coronary arteries are 3 mm in diameter at the origin of the vessel. The three coronary arteries (see Figures 17-2 and 17-3) supply about 0.6 to 1 ml/min/g of blood to the left ventricular muscle under basal conditions. When the myocardial oxygen demand increases, the coronary arteries dilate and coronary blood flow increases by threefold to fivefold. If a coronary artery is narrowed by more than 50%, blood flow cannot increase sufficiently to meet the maximum demand for oxygen. When myocardial oxygen demand exceeds the oxygen supply, myocardial ischemia results. The inadequately perfused zone of myocardium stops contracting within a few seconds (if the mismatch is severe, or contraction is reduced if the mismatch is less severe), causing a regional wall motion abnormality on images recorded during ischemia. If the area supplied by the stenosed coronary artery is extensive, overall function of the ventricle may be impaired, reducing the ejection fraction.

Myocardial perfusion imaging is performed to detect myocardial ischemia and to determine its location and extent. Two sets of perfusion images are recorded: one following injection at rest and the second during peak stress. The rest injection defines the distribution of myocardial perfusion when there is basal coronary blood flow. Regions of decreased perfusion identified at rest are usually caused by regions of myocardial scar, typically due to prior myocardial infarction. The peak stress injection defines the distribution of myocardial perfusion when there is maximal coronary blood flow. A region of decreased perfusion seen on the stress injected images that was not present at rest signifies an area of myocardial ischemia. An unchanged region of diminished perfusion seen at rest and stress signifies myocardial scar. Perfusion imaging with injection of a radiotracer during stress detects a relative decrease in blood flow in the ischemic regions.

Following injection of the technetium-labeled agents the myocardial distribution remains stable for about an hour. This allows imaging at some time after tracer administration. On the other hand, following myocardial uptake of thallium-201, the tracer does not remain fixed in the myocardium. Over the course of about 4 hours, the myocardial concentration of thallium will decrease by 30% to 50%, with more rapid clearance from areas of normal perfusion than from regions of diminished perfusion. This nonuniform clearance causes thallium to "redistribute," making it very difficult to detect areas of ischemia on images that are recorded hours after tracer administration. For diagnostic purposes thallium images must be recorded within ~20 minutes of tracer administration to depict the distribution of myocardial perfusion at the time of injection.

For the stress portion of myocardial perfusion imaging, large muscle dynamic exercise is the preferred approach (Box 17-3). In patients who cannot exercise, pharmacological stress may be used. Exercise stress is typically performed using a treadmill. The patient's heart rate, ECG, blood pressure, and symptoms are continuously monitored during the stress procedure. The perfusion tracer is administered at the peak of exercise, and the patient is urged to continue exercising for 1 to 2 additional minutes to permit the tracer to clear from the blood. The indications to stop the exercise procedure are listed in Box 17-5.

A uniform pattern of myocardial perfusion at rest and stress makes it very unlikely that the patient has a significant risk of sudden death or myocardial infarction within the next 2 years. An abnormal scan with injection at stress and a normal scan with injection at rest suggests myocardial ischemia. Depending on the site and extent of the abnormality, the risk of a significant cardiac event (myocardial infarction, angina, or sudden death) in the next 2 years varies from 1% to 2% for a small area of ischemia involving the inferior or lateral wall up to about 15% for a large lesion involving the anterior wall. Myocardial scar is less likely to cause an acute event.

Single-Photon Agents Used for Perfusion Imaging

See Box 17-2 for a list of agents used for perfusion imaging. Thallium-201 is produced by proton bombardment of thallium-203 (^{203}Tl) in a cyclotron. An intermediate product, lead-201 (^{201}Pb), is produced, which decays to ^{201}Tl. Thallium-201 has physical half-life of 74 hours. It decays by electron capture with the production of mercury x-rays of about 80 keV (90% abundant) and

gamma photons of 135 and 167 keV (2% and 8% abundance, respectively). The final decay product is stable mercury-201 (^{201}Hg). Images are usually recorded with multiple windows surrounding the mercury x-ray and each of the gamma rays. Thallium is minimally excreted through the bowel and kidneys (only 10% is lost from the body over 10 days), resulting in a long biological half-life. After intravenous (IV) injection, about 3.5% of the injected dose localizes in the myocardium.*

Kidneys concentrate about 10% of the injected dose, which has an effective half-life of approximately 57 hours, resulting in a radiation burden of about 1.7 rad/mCi to the kidney. The long effective half-life limits the dose that can be injected to about 4 mCi.

Two technetium-labeled tracers, sestamibi (methoxyisobutyl isonitrile [MIBI]) and tetrofosmin, are in wide clinical use (Table 17-2). Sestamibi and tetrofosmin have lower myocardial extraction (about 60% for MIBI and 50% for tetrofosmin versus 88% for thallium); therefore a smaller fraction of the injected dose per millicurie of injected activity localizes in the myocardium. These agents have slightly slower blood clearance than thallium, making it particularly important to continue the stress for about 2 minutes after injection instead of the 1 minute usually used for thallium. Tetrofosmin and MIBI have more favorable dosimetry (20 mCi of ^{99m}Tc-sestamibi delivers 3.6 rad to the large bowel, and 20 mCi of ^{99m}Tc-tetrofosmin delivers 1.5 rad to the large bowel). The higher administered dose results in a much greater photon flux from the myocardium and allows recording of high-quality gated data after injection at rest and injection at stress. Because technetium agents have minimal **redistribution**, separate injections are required to depict perfusion at rest and stress. ^{99m}Tc-Sestamibi and ^{99m}Tc-tetrofosmin have biological half-lives of longer than 5 hours in the myocardium, allowing images to be recorded up to 90 minutes after injection. When possible, earlier images are preferred, and most laboratories image these agents 15 to 45 minutes after injection.

Imaging Protocols Using Single-Photon Radiopharmaceuticals. Table 17-3 shows the commonly used protocols. When thallium alone is used, stress injection is given first and redistribution imaging at 3 to 4 hours later. Also, 24-hour imaging may be done for additional information about ischemic viable myocardium.

Imaging with technetium-labeled tracers can be done with either a 1- or 2-day protocol. In the 2-day protocol, the rest and stress examinations are done on separate days, each with a dose of 20 to 30 mCi (typically 30 mCi). For the 1-day study, patients can have either the rest or stress study performed first, typically with a dose of 10 mCi, followed about 4 to 6 hours later (to

---

*The myocardium receives 4% of cardiac output. Thallium has a myocardium extraction of 88%, resulting in the myocardium uptake of about 3.5% of the administered dose.

TABLE 17-2	Technetium-Labeled Perfusion Tracers			
Agent	Myocardial Concentration	Myocardial $t_{1/2}$	Comments	
Sestamibi	2.4%	6 hours	Slight redistribution (not nearly as much as with thallium, but images should be recorded within 45 minutes of injection to maximize detection of ischemic lesions); myocardial images can be recorded with gating, allowing an estimate of left ventricular ejection fraction and regional myocardial thickening.	
Tetrofosmin	2.0%	8 hours	Slight redistribution; images should be recorded within 45 minutes of injection to maximize sensitivity for detection of ischemia; myocardial images can be recorded with gating to estimate ventricular function and regional thickening.	

TABLE 17-3	Imaging Protocols
Protocol	Comments
Technetium Agents: ^{99m}Tc-sestamibi or ^{99m}Tc-tetrofosmin	
Two-day stress-rest: Inject 20 to 30 mCi at peak exercise. Begin imaging at 15 to 30 minutes after injection during exercise. On day 2, give same dose at rest. Begin imaging at 45 to 60 minutes after injection at rest.	Observing a waiting period after injection allows adequate hepatobiliary clearance. For sestamibi, the recommended wait after injection is at least 15 to 20 minutes for exercise stress, 45 minutes for pharmacological stress, and 45 to 60 minutes for rest. For tetrofosmin, the recommended wait after injection is at least 10 to 15 minutes after exercise stress, 45 minutes after pharmacological stress, and 30 to 45 minutes after rest.
One-day rest-stress: This is a same-day imaging protocol using a low-dose (8 to 10 mCi) resting study followed by a high-dose (20 to 30 mCi) stress study. This protocol is preferred over the stress-rest technique (see next entry).	
One-day stress-rest: Give stress injection of 10 to 15 mCi, followed by an interval of 2 to 4 hours; then give rest injection of 20 to 30 mCi.	
Thallium-201 (^{201}Tl)	
Stress and delay (standard): Inject 2.5 to 4.0 mCi at peak stress. Record images within 20 minutes of injection. Wait 2 to 4 hours (3 hours is preferred) and record "redistribution" images. After recording the stress images, an additional 1.5 mCi of ^{201}Tl may be injected, before recording the rest images at 3 to 4 hours.	
Rest redistribution: Inject 3 mCi at rest and obtain initial image. Delayed image is acquired at 3 hours. Further imaging may be done at 24 hours without reinjection.	
Dual Isotope	
^{201}Tl rest and ^{99m}Tc-sestamibi/tetrofosmin stress studies are performed the same day. Inject 3 mCi of thallium and image. Later inject 20 to 30 mCi of technetium agent at stress. Image at appropriate times.	Cross talk occurs between the energies of thallium and technetium; however, when imaging is done in this sequence, the energy spill is minimal compared with imaging thallium after technetium.

permit both physical decay and biological loss of radio-pharmaceutical from the myocardium) by the other examination, with a dose of 30 mCi. Typically, the rest study is performed with the low dose first, followed by the stress study several hours later.

A dual isotope technique, using thallium for the rest imaging and a technetium agent (sestamibi or tetrofosmin) for the stress-imaging is an alternative approach for a one day imaging protocol. There is a minimal amount of activity in the technetium window from the rest-injected thallium (caused by a 12% incidence of gamma photons from ^{201}Tl). The advantage of this approach is that activity in the bowel is minimized, and the stress test can be performed immediately after the rest thallium images are obtained, eliminating the waiting time between the rest and stress studies when a technetium-labeled tracer is used for both the rest and stress images.

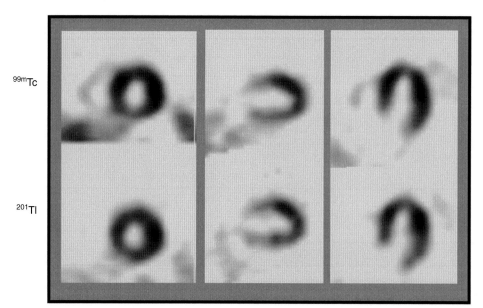

FIGURE 17-9 Effect of photon energy on images. Thallium images *(bottom row)* demonstrate slightly less activity in the inferobasal, antero-basal, and posterobasal segments compared with technetium images *(upper row)* because of attenuation caused by the overlying right ventricle in the vertical long-axis view and the attenuation effect in the horizontal long-axis view.

BOX 17-4	Indications for Pharmacological Stress

1. Patients with functional impairment due to injury, arthritis, orthopedic problems, peripheral neuropathy, myopathies, or peripheral vascular disease in which a maximal heart rate is not easily achieved with routine exercise stress testing, usually because of an early onset of fatigue due to musculoskeletal, neurological, or vascular problems rather than cardiac ischemia
2. Elderly patients with decreased functional capacity and possible CAD
3. Patients with chronic debilitation and possible CAD
4. Other cases, including patients taking β-blockers or other negative chronotropic agents that would inhibit the ability to achieve an adequate heart response to exercise
5. Atrial fibrillation

CAD, Coronary artery disease.

BOX 17-5	Indications to Stop Exercise

1. Marked arrhythmia induced by exercise (e.g., ventricular tachycardia, PVCs in pairs or triplets, and atrial fibrillation)
2. Decrease in BP > 20 mm Hg below the starting BP or heart rate as exercise progresses
3. Extreme elevation in blood pressure (systolic pressure >250 mm Hg or diastolic pressure >120 mm Hg)
4. Severe chest pain, marked dyspnea, and dizziness
5. Achievement of greater than 85% (preferably 100%) of predicted heart rate for age, computed as 220 − age (yr)
6. Severe ST depression (>3 mm) or >1 mm ST elevation in leads without pathological Q waves
7. Onset of advanced atrioventricular block
8. Onset of bundle branch block
9. Failure of monitoring system
10. Severe fatigue, leg pain, or breathlessness

BP, Blood pressure; *PVC,* premature ventricular contraction; *ST,* changes on electrocardiogram.

For the detection of ischemia, thallium and technetium agents perform equally well. When there is a question of myocardial viability, thallium is preferred. Although gated SPECT studies can be recorded with thallium, the higher photon flux of the technetium agents provides better quality data (Figure 17-9). The sensitivity of myocardial perfusion imaging for the detection of CAD is greater than 85% and the specificity is 80% to 90%.

Before the stress procedure, a history and cardiac directed physical examination should be completed to evaluate the patient's overall status and determine whether the patient is likely to perform sufficient exercise to achieve the target heart rate. If it appears the patient is too frail or has a medical problem that would preclude exercise, pharmacological stress should be used (Boxes 17-4 and 17-5). A complete medication history is obtained to determine if any medication would alter the sensitivity of the stress procedure. If the test is being done to determine if medical therapy reduces the incidence of ischemia, it is helpful to perform the procedure while the patient is taking the medication. If the test is done to make the diagnosis of coronary disease, β-blocking medication and calcium channel–blocking medication should be stopped for at least 24 hours before the stress (Table 17-4).

TABLE 17-4	Drugs That Can Affect Exercise Test Response and Interpretation
Drug	**Discontinuation Before Exercise Test**
Antiarrhythmics	48 hours
Antihypertensives	4 days
β-adrenergic blockers	48 hours
Calcium channel blockers	48 hours
Digitalis/digoxin	1 to 2 weeks
Diuretics	4 days
Long-acting nitrates	At least 12 hours
Sedatives and tranquilizers	1 day
Sublingual nitroglycerin	2 hours

TABLE 17-5	Bruce Protocol			
Stage	**Duration (min)**	**Total Time**	**Speed (mph)**	**Grade (%)**
1	3	—	1.7	0
2	3	6	1.7	5
3	3	9	1.7	10
4	3	12	2.5	12
5	3	15	3.4	14
6	3	18	4.2	16
7	3	21	5.0	18

BOX 17-6	Contraindications for Stress Test

1. Uncontrolled unstable angina; however, patients with suspected unstable angina at presentation who are otherwise stable and pain free can undergo stress testing
2. Patient with decompensated or inadequately controlled congestive heart failure
3. Uncontrolled hypertension (BP > 200/115 mm Hg)
4. Acute myocardial infarction within last 2 to 3 days
5. Severe pulmonary hypertension

BP, Blood pressure.

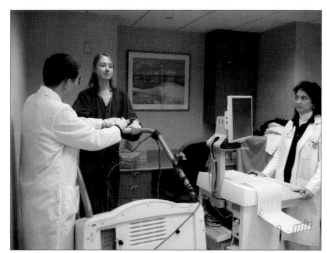

FIGURE 17-10 Patient on treadmill with supervising physician and technologist observing electrocardiogram and monitoring vital signs.

Exercise Stress. Treadmill exercise (Figure 17-10) is usually done using the standard Bruce protocol (Table 17-5). The protocol can be altered if indicated. A modified Bruce protocol starts at a lower work level, and is usually used for less physically fit individuals. Stages 1 and 2 of the modified Bruce protocol are at a functional class 3 workload (2.9 and 3.7 metabolic equivalents [METS]) and the third stage corresponds to the first stage of the standard Bruce protocol. Thus the person who does 9 minutes in the modified protocol does the same workload as 3 minutes on the Bruce protocol; 12 minutes on the modified is the same as 6 minutes on the Bruce. The modified Bruce protocol is used for exercise testing patients who are frail or expected to have poor exercise tolerance for other reasons, or for those within 1 week of myocardial infarction. The longer exercise duration makes the patient more susceptible to fatigue before achieving the required heart rate. Both Bruce and modified Bruce protocols give satisfactory results. For an exercise test to be "adequate," the patient should achieve at least 85% of maximum heart rate (220 − patient's age in years), in the absence of other indications to stop the stress procedure. During the stress test, patients must be continuously observed, a 12-lead ECG must be recorded each minute, and blood pressure must recorded at least every 3 minutes. Indications to stop the stress test are summarized in Box 17-5. Contraindications to performing a stress test are summarized in Box 17-6.

To maximize the likelihood of detection of CAD with stress perfusion imaging, the radiopharmaceutical should be administered at the peak of exercise and the exercise should continue for an additional 1 to 2 minutes to permit the tracer to clear from the blood and localize in the myocardium in proportion to perfusion at the peak of exercise. If exercise is terminated prematurely, particularly in patients with small zones of minimal ischemia, part of the tracer dose is delivered at a time when the tissue has decreased flow and part of the dose is delivered when perfusion is normal. This phenomenon reduces contrast between the normal and ischemic tissue, making detection of the lesion difficult.

An IV line is placed before the stress procedure to facilitate injection at the peak of stress. Because glucose alters the clearance rate of ^{201}Tl from the myocardium, the IV line should be kept open with saline. Injection of the radiopharmaceutical should be followed by a flush of 10 ml of saline to minimize the time that the radiopharmaceutical is in contact with the veins of the arm. After injection, exercise should continue for 1 to 2 minutes. If the patient has difficulty maintaining peak exercise levels, the workload can be reduced to maintain the increased heart rate and blood pressure during the brief interval of tracer clearance.

ECG and blood pressure monitoring continue for at least 5 minutes or until the heart rate has decreased to within about 20% of baseline. If transient ECG changes, symptoms of ischemia, markedly increased blood pressure, or arrhythmias occur, monitoring should continue until the findings have resolved, or treatment is initiated. Imaging should commence within 10 minutes of injection with thallium and within 15 to 45 minutes for ^{99m}Tc-sestamibi and ^{99m}Tc-tetrofosmin. Imaging within a short time of the conclusion of stress increases the likelihood of detection of transiently increased lung uptake, transient enlargement of the left ventricular cavity and a fall in the ejection fraction. When the patient is stable and breathing normally, SPECT images are recorded with ECG gating.

If thallium is the only tracer used for recording myocardial perfusion images, the stress examination is performed first and followed by immediate imaging. Because thallium redistributes, delayed images are obtained 3 to 4 hours later. The patient should be instructed not to eat any food containing carbohydrates, because ingestion of glucose accelerates the rate of ^{201}Tl clearance from both normal and ischemic myocardium, minimizing the differential clearance necessary to detect ischemia. Occasionally, to improve count statistics, an additional 1-mCi dose of thallium is administered at rest before the delayed images are recorded.

Pharmacological Stress. Some patients cannot exercise because of peripheral vascular disease, neurological problems, or musculoskeletal abnormalities. In these patients, instead of large muscle dynamic exercise myocardial blood flow can be increased using drugs to cause vasodilation of the coronary arteries or to increase heart rate and blood pressure (and secondarily increase coronary blood flow; see Box 17-4 for indications). The **vasodilator** method is used more often. Dipyridamole, adenosine, or regadenoson can be used; adenosine or regadenoson are preferred because of their short biological half-life, compared to dipyridamole. These agents are agonists of the adenosine receptors. **Regadenoson** is a newer synthetic selective A2 adenosine receptor agonist, which is associated with bronchoconstriction. Adenosine and dipyridamole both increase tissue levels of adenosine. Both adenosine and dipyridamole may cause bronchoconstriction, and are contraindicated in patients who are actively wheezing or have a history of significant bronchospastic disease. These agents cause a generalized vasodilation, and are not specific for the heart.

Dipyridamole reduces the metabolism of endogenously produced adenosine by inhibiting *adenosine deaminase and by reducing the uptake of adenosine into red blood cells,* which results in increased tissue concentrations of adenosine. Adenosine that is infused, on the other hand, increases the tissue concentration of adenosine directly. Regadenoson selectively occupies the adenosine A2 receptor sites, resulting in coronary, abdominal, and peripheral vasodilation. Dipyridamole lasts for hours after administration, adenosine has a biological half-life of only 10 seconds, and regadenoson has a biologic half-life of approximately 30 minutes.

When the drugs are infused, coronary arteries dilate to increase myocardial blood flow to the myocardium. If tracer is administered at the time of the maximum effect of the drug, all areas of the myocardium supplied by normal vessels show homogeneous increased uptake. If a vessel is markedly narrowed, or fails to vasodilate appropriately (caused by endothelial dysfunction, a phenomenon that occurs in areas with underlying inflamed atheroma) flow distal to the narrowing does not increase to the same degree as that in myocardial territories supplied by normal coronary arteries, and areas of low uptake can be seen (Figure 17-11). Although this phenomenon does not usually cause ischemia, as in exercise tests, the underlying basis for detection of abnormalities (the **stenosis** of a coronary artery) remains the same.*

The effects of dipyridamole, adenosine and regadenoson can be reversed by administration of aminophylline. Because the vasodilator properties of adenosine, regadenoson, and dipyridamole may result in decreased blood pressure, patients should be either lying supine or performing low-level exercise at the time of drug administration. Typically hypotension is mild, causing a reduction in blood pressure of 10 to 15 mm Hg. In some patients, however, the reduction in blood pressure can be significant, requiring immediate supportive treatment. In the unlikely event that a patient develops serious complications, such as third-degree heart block or severe hypotension, aminophylline should be available for immediate intravenous administration. Because adenosine is very short lived, stopping the infusion usually will decrease the symptoms within about 1 minute. As with exercise tests, serious side effects such as arrhythmias, severe hypotension, cerebral ischemia, stroke, and death have been reported with pharmacological stress tests. Therefore, the examination should be performed only in facilities equipped to handle medical emergencies.

In addition to the cardiovascular effects, the vasodilator agents may also cause a transient headache, a sense of gastrointestinal fullness, a feeling of breathlessness, and a choking sensation. If symptoms occur, they rapidly dissipate when adenosine is the stress agent. However, with dipyridamole or regadenoson, it may be necessary to administer aminophylline.

---

*Vasodilation can cause ischemia if the territory is perfused primarily by collateral vessels that are relatively narrow and require normal blood pressure to maintain adequate flow. When blood pressure decreases, as often occurs during infusion of adenosine or dipyridamole, flow through collaterals may also decrease, resulting in myocardial ischemia.

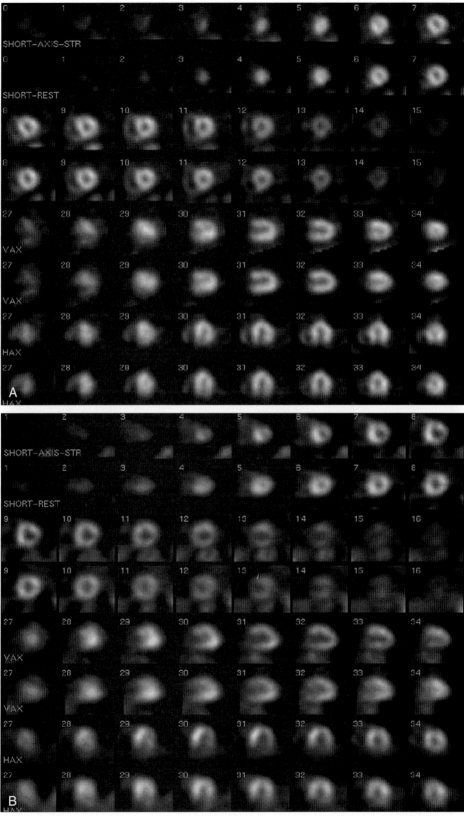

FIGURE 17-11 A, Normal gated rest and stress SPECT myocardial perfusion images. Stress images *(top row of each pair)* following injection of 99mTc-tetrofosmin and rest images *(bottom row of each pair)* following injection of 201Tl. **B,** Gated stress and rest SPECT myocardial perfusion images. Stress images *(top row of each pair)* following injection of 99mTc-tetrofosmin, and rest images *(bottom row of each pair)* following injection of 201Tl. This is a 73-year-old woman with quadruple coronary artery bypass grafting, hypertension, and hypercholesterolemia for preoperative evaluation before colon surgery. The scan shows stress-induced ischemia of anterolateral, inferolateral, and mid-distal anterior walls.

Patients should prepare for the test by fasting for at least 4 hours, abstaining from food or beverages containing caffeine (e.g., coffee, tea, most soft drinks) for at least 24 hours, and discontinuing all xanthine-containing medications 36 hours before the study. Caffeine and xanthine-containing medications reduce the effectiveness of the vasodilator, especially dipyridamole, and may produce a negative test result in patients with coronary stenoses.

The test is performed after administration of 0.56 mg/kg dipyridamole over 4 minutes or 0.140 mg/kg/min of adenosine for 4 minutes while serial blood pressure and ECG recordings are made. Dipyridamole and adenosine are injected intravenously using an infusion pump at a rate determined by the patient's weight, whereas regadenoson is administered over 10 to 20 seconds as a "flat dose." The perfusion tracer is administered approximately 3 to 4 minutes after the conclusion of the dipyridamole infusion, during the third minute of adenosine infusion, or 20 to 30 seconds following administration of regadenoson.

Administration of adenosine, regadenoson, or dipyridamole may be accompanied by a pounding headache, a sensation of heaviness in the chest, nausea, a feeling of abdominal fullness, and a feeling of breathlessness. These symptoms can be minimized with low-level exercise, either by walking on the treadmill at about 1 mile/hr or using arm weights of 2 to 5 pounds during the infusion. Adenosine or regadenoson infusion are often combined with a low-level exercise to minimize the side effects and improve the image quality.

An alternative to vasodilator pharmacological stress uses dobutamine, a sympathomimetic drug that increases the heart rate and blood pressure. This agent increases myocardial work and hence the need for increased flow in the coronary arteries. In contrast to other drugs in this category, dobutamine has a low incidence of cardiac arrhythmia. The drug has a half-life of about 1 to 2 minutes, which limits the duration of effect. As with the vasodilator agents, the heart rate, ECG, and blood pressure should be monitored continuously during administration of the drug. Because the drug causes increased oxygen consumption, it can cause ischemia, similar to exercise.

Dobutamine is infused at a graduated rate, starting at 5 μg/kg/min. After 3 minutes, the dose is increased to 10 μg/kg/min. Three minutes later, if the heart rate response is still insufficient, it is helpful to elevate the legs on a pillow (to increase venous return), and increase the infusion rate to 20 μg/kg/min. The dose is increased every 3 minutes by 10 μg/kg/min to a maximum of 40 μg/kg/min. If the heart rate has not achieved 85% of maximum and the blood pressure is still in an acceptable range, atropine is administered in divided doses up to a total of 1 mg to produce a tachycardia. Once the patient's heart rate has achieved 85% of predicted maximum, the tracer is injected and the infusion continued for at least

1 minute. It typically requires 8 to 12 minutes for the patient's heart rate to return to baseline following cessation of dobutamine infusion.

Although pharmacological testing is useful in patients who cannot exercise, the vasodilator agents cause a marked increase in blood flow to the liver, which can make it difficult to see lesions of the inferior wall. Neither the vasodilators nor dobutamine provide the breadth of information about cardiac performance that is available with an exercise study. Exercise testing offers information about the overall status of the patient's cardiovascular fitness, the duration and severity of exercise that causes symptoms, and the timing of symptoms versus objective indicators of ischemia (ST segment changes on ECG or perfusion scan abnormalities). This information frequently plays a key role in planning of therapy.

Nitrates. Nitroglycerin is often used to relieve myocardial ischemia. The drug works by causing both venodilation and arterial dilation. As a result of the venodilation, the amount of blood returning to the heart is reduced, decreasing myocardial oxygen requirements. The arterial dilation results in increased blood flow to the myocardium. In patients with severe CAD, lesions narrowing the lumen 95% to 99%, may limit blood flow even at rest. Administration of nitroglycerin before injection at rest in patients with severe coronary disease enhances the detection of viable but ischemic myocardial tissue. Typically, nitroglycerin is administered as a single, 0.4-mg sublingual tablet, or as a sublingual spray about 2 minutes before the rest tracer injection. The patient should be seated for the procedure, and the pulse and blood pressure should be recorded at baseline and at the time of tracer administration.

SPECT Imaging

SPECT data are collected using a 180-degree orbit, with the left arm extended above the head to be out of the field of view. Right arm can be at the side. Data acquisition for the 180-degree orbit typically begins at 45 degrees RAO and ends at 45 degrees LPO. Image acquisition time is about 30 minutes using a dual detector camera with the detectors at 90 degrees following injection of 30 mCi (the dose typically used at stress) and a 3-degree step angle. A typical SPECT protocol requires 64 stops for 180-degree acquisition.

Two types of artifacts occur fairly frequently on SPECT images: attenuation (caused by breast or stomach tissue) and motion (caused by slight patient movement or differences in the phase of respiration as a projection is being recorded). Both of these artifacts tend to cause areas of decreased counts in the reconstructed data that can be mistaken for zones of decreased perfusion. These artifacts can be readily appreciated if the projection data are reviewed in a cinematic display. When attenuation is seen, its impact on the data can be anticipated, and the images can be interpreted correctly. An alternative

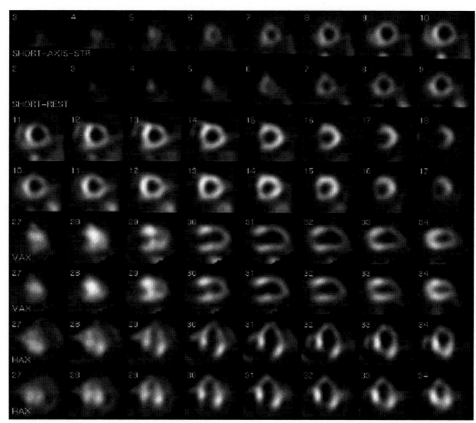

FIGURE 17-12 Gated stress and rest SPECT myocardial perfusion images. Stress images *(top row of each pair)* following injection of ^{99m}Tc tetrofosmin, and rest images *(bottom row of each pair)* following injection of ^{201}Tl. This is a 62-year-old woman with shortness of breath, recent electrocardiogram changes, hypertension, sarcoidosis, peripheral neuropathy, alcohol abuse, and squamous cell carcinoma of the oral cavity referred for preoperative evaluation. The myocardial perfusion scan demonstrates predominantly fixed defect in the distal septum, apical, mid-distal anterior, lateral, and inferior walls.

approach corrects for attenuation using a transmission scan, such as CT. Gross patient motion, or changes in the level of the diaphragms, are difficult to correct. If multiple motion episodes are seen or if a discrete movement changes the data by more than 2 pixels, the reconstructed data probably will have focal artifacts. If artifacts are seen, another acquisition should be recorded rather than attempting to motion correct the data.

After high-level exercise (>10 METS), SPECT imaging should not commence until respiration has returned to normal. This will eliminate an artifact caused by a change in the extent of diaphragmatic excursion during SPECT acquisition. This phenomenon of *upward creep* typically results in an artifactual lesion in the inferior or inferoseptal regions of the left ventricle.

Gated Perfusion Imaging

Gated perfusion SPECT is typically recorded using 8 frames per cardiac cycle. When 64 angles are recorded with 8 frames/cycle at each location, a total of 512 images are obtained. Although end-systole is not correctly identified under this circumstance, the apparent loss of ejection fraction is typically on the order of 5%

and is most apparent in patients with high ejection fractions at rest. This type of study has sufficient precision to differentiate patients with normal ejection fractions from those with depressed function.

Data Analysis. Myocardial perfusion images are initially interpreted subjectively to detect zones of diminished tracer localization in the left and right ventricular myocardium (Figure 17-12). The images are also evaluated using quantitative techniques to determine the relative activity in each segment of myocardium. On the tomographic images the quantitative data compares the relative distribution in each segment to a database of normal subjects. Regions with diminished activity are highlighted. Qualitative interpretation reviews the images for the factors listed in Box 17-7. SPECT images are usually quantified by stacking the reconstructed/reoriented short-axis slices onto a bull's-eye display, where the apex is at the center and the basal slice is at the periphery (Figure 17-13).

Gated Image Display. After reconstructing the data, the gated slices usually are displayed as multiple cine loops for visual assessment of wall motion. Thereafter the endocardial borders of the midventricular horizontal and vertical long-axis slices are defined, and the ejection

LAO, Left anterior oblique; *LV,* left ventricular; *RV,* right ventricular.

fraction and ventricular volumes are calculated. These data can be appended to the evaluation of myocardial perfusion and are particularly useful for determining regional function in areas of diminished perfusion. Because the gated study is performed at rest, after the ischemic episode is over, zones of ischemia may have normal function (i.e., appear as areas of decreased intensity with normal thickening). Areas of scar, on the other hand, should have decreased perfusion and diminished function.

POSITRON EMISSION TOMOGRAPHY OF THE HEART

Stress and rest myocardial perfusion studies can be performed using positron emitters and a PET-CT camera.

Myocardial Perfusion Tracers

Positron-emitting radiopharmaceuticals for assessment of myocardial perfusion include generator produced rubidium-82 [^{82}Rb] chloride, nitrogen-13 [^{13}N] ammonia, and oxygen-15 [^{15}O] labeled water (see Box 17-2). A new fluorine-18 labeled perfusion tracer, flurpiridaz, is in clinical trials.

Rubidium-82 chloride has a physical half-life of 75 seconds. The tracer is eluted from a strontium-82 (^{82}Sr) generator, directly into the patient. Strontium-82 has a half-life of about 25 days. Rubidium-82 behaves

physiologically like ^{201}Tl and is initially concentrated in the myocardium in proportion to regional myocardial perfusion, with an extraction fraction of 70%. Retention of ^{82}Rb chloride depends at least partly on sodium-potassium adenosine triphosphatase (Na$^+$/K$^+$-ATPase) transport. The short physical half-life of this tracer permits recording rest and stress images within about 15 minutes of each other. A tracer dose of 30 to 50 mCi (1110 to 1850 MBq) is used for measuring perfusion at rest and stress. The total volume of rubidium eluate infused is 20 to 50 ml, at a rate of ~1 ml/sec. The short half-life requires imaging within a few seconds of tracer administration, which limits the options for the stress procedures to pharmacological agents.

Usually a vasodilator stress is employed. Dipyridamole or regadenoson are the preferred stress agents. Adenosine can be employed, but the requirement for continuous infusion of adenosine at the time the generator is eluted into the patient requires venous access with an 18-gauge venous catheter. Dipyridamole or regadenoson, on the other hand, are administered before infusion of the generator eluate, allowing venous access with a 20- or 22-gauge venous catheter. Box 17-8 is a more detailed protocol for recording ^{82}Rb images.

Figures 17-14 and 17-15 are examples of a normal rubidium-82 rest and stress myocardial perfusion scan and an abnormal scan indicating ischemia.

Flow reserve, the relative increase in myocardial perfusion from rest to stress, is a sensitive and specific indicator of the health of the coronary arteries. In patients with hyperlipidemia and diabetes and current smokers, perfusion reserve is diminished. Adding flow reserve data to information on the regional distribution of myocardial perfusion enhances the sensitivity of myocardial perfusion imaging. Flow reserve can be readily calculated from dynamic acquisitions at rest and stress using commercially available software.

PET and SPECT have similar sensitivities for detecting myocardial ischemia (80% to 95%), but the specificity of PET is about 10% to 15% higher than that of SPECT.

Myocardial Viability

Viability is typically assessed in a patient with a history of coronary disease and multiple infarcts, with a reduced ejection fraction and heart failure. In these patients, rest injected perfusion images are compared to the regional distribution of fluorodeoxyglucose (FDG) in the myocardium (after glucose loading) to detect regions of relatively increased utilization of glucose in regions of decreased perfusion. Areas of decreased perfusion but relatively increased FDG identifies ischemic but viable tissue. Patients with this outcome are successfully treated with revascularization. A nonradionuclide approach to this problem utilizes delayed enhancement on contrast myocardial MRI. Regions of myocardial scar enhance. If there is delayed enhancement on an MRI in a

SPECT myocardial perfusion

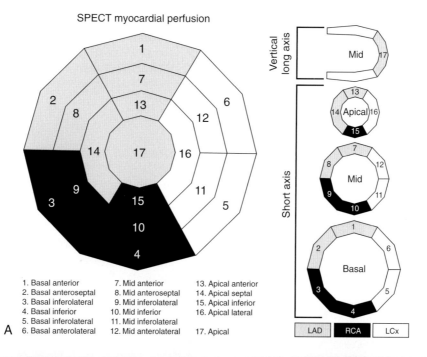

1. Basal anterior
2. Basal anteroseptal
3. Basal inferolateral
4. Basal inferior
5. Basal inferolateral
6. Basal anterolateral

7. Mid anterior
8. Mid anteroseptal
9. Mid inferolateral
10. Mid inferior
11. Mid inferolateral
12. Mid anterolateral

13. Apical anterior
14. Apical septal
15. Apical inferior
16. Apical lateral
17. Apical

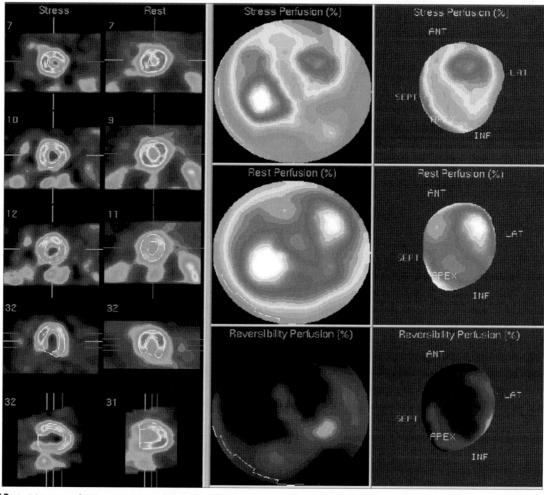

FIGURE 17-13 A, Diagram of 17-segment model. *Left,* Bull's-eye format of concentric short-axis views; *right,* the location of the segments in the short and vertical long axes. The gray segments are in the left anterior descending *(LAD)* territory, the black segments are right coronary artery *(RCA)* territory, and the blank segments are left circumflex *(LCx)*. **B,** The AutoQuant display of the Bull's-eye (ADAC) showing the ischemic lesion in the LAD and LCx territories *(middle column)* and selected short-axis and vertical long-axis views *(stress left and rest right),* and the bullet depiction *(right column)*. Several manufacturers offer variations of this display.

BOX 17-8 | **Detailed Protocol for Recording ^{82}Rb Images**

Indications
1. Detect stress induced myocardial ischemia.
2. Evaluate myocardial perfusion in patients BMI greater than 28.
3. Evaluate patients with suspected multivessel or small vessel coronary artery disease, since the images can be quantified to measure myocardial flow reserve.
   Dose: 30 to 50 mCi in 50 ml saline

EKG Gating
All patients are monitored with continuous EKG for arrhythmia and/or ischemia, and serial blood pressures during the stress procedure. Defibrillator and cardiac crash cart should be available in the stress area. AHA, ACC, SNM and ASNC guidelines are followed for the stress procedures.

Patient Preparation
1. Patient should be NPO for at least 4 hours. We ask patients to not routinely withhold medications unless instructed by the patient's physician.
2. A brief cardiovascular history and physical examination performed. The lungs are auscultated to detect obstructive lung disease.
3. The risks and benefits of the procedure are reviewed with the patient, and informed written consent for stress is obtained.
4. The patient is placed on the imaging table, and a topogram (scout view) is acquired to determine the scanning area of the patient. The topogram is acquired with 30 mAs, 120 to 130 kVp, with a setting to include the entire scanning area. A commercially-available program is used to acquire prospectively gated CT images for the Coronary Calcium Score. 120 kVp and 250 mAs are typical parameters for a small person, and 400 mAs is typical for a large person. Following the calcium score acquisition, the table is repositioned, and a low dose attenuation correction scan area is acquired at 30 mAs.

5. With the patient at rest, rubidium infusion (generally 50 ml saline containing 30 to 50 mCi of rubidium over 30 seconds) is started, and LM acquisition with gating is started. Data are acquired in dynamic mode with LM option "on." The EKG triggers are also saved on the PET console simultaneously for retrospective LM cardiac gating of the rest images. LM acquisition is continued for 7 minutes.
6. The rest emission and CT images are reviewed to determine if the emission cardiac silhouette is located within the cardiac region on the CT. If there is misregistration, the scans are realigned prior to reviewing the attenuation-corrected emission data. If the data cannot be aligned, the CT attenuation-correction data are reacquired.
7. Following rest, image acquisition vasodilator stress is performed.

Dipyridamole Stress
Dipyridamole is infused at a rate of 0.14 mg/kg/min for 4 minutes (a total of 0.56 mg/kg). About 5 minutes after completion of dipyridamole infusion, the patient is repositioned in the scanner for the stress acquisition. LM acquisition and rubidium infusion are started simultaneously and for 6 to 7 minutes. **Regadenoson** may be used in place of dipyridamole. A flat dose of 0.4 mg is administered over approximately 20 seconds. About 20 to 30 seconds after injection of regadenoson, the rubidium infusion is started, and LM data are acquired over 6 to 7 minutes.

If flow reserve will be calculated, it is important to record the blood pressure multiple times (at least every minute), starting about 30 seconds after regadenoson administration. Most patients develop an increase in heart rate of 10 to 30 bpm, and they sustain a transient decrease in blood pressure of 10 to 30 mm Hg systolic. The flow reserve data should be normalized for changes in rate pressure product to the rest value.

ACC, American College of Cardiology; *AHA*, American Hospital Association; *ASNC*, American Society of Nuclear Cardiology; *BMI*, body mass index; *CT*, computed tomography; *EKG*, electrocardiogram; *LM*, list mode; *NPO*, nothing by mouth (nil per os); *PET*, positron emission tomography; *SNM*, Society of Nuclear Medicine.

---

myocardial region with decreased perfusion, that tissue will not benefit from revascularization.

Myocardial Metabolism

A fundamental characteristic of the myocardium is its continuous requirement for oxygen and metabolic substrates to meet its energy needs.

Metabolic Tracers. Fluorine-18–fluorodeoxyglucose (^{18}F-FDG), carbon-11 (^{11}C)-palmitate, and ^{11}C-acetate are typical PET radiopharmaceuticals used for metabolic cardiac studies. Fluorodeoxyglucose mirrors glucose utilization (Figure 17-16); myocardial uptake and clearance of palmitate reflects the myocardial utilization of fatty acid; and acetate labeled with ^{11}C is a promising tracer of overall oxidative metabolism. These metabolic tracers are often employed for research studies.

PET-CT, SPECT-CT, and CT Angiography. Nuclear medicine images are fused with CT for anatomical localization and for attenuation correction. Although "fusion"

software has been available for many years, transmission and emission data were often obtained under circumstances of breath holding for the CT and free breathing for the emission scan. This disparity results in misregistration of the images. The registration problem can be overcome by blurring the CT, decreasing the mA on the x-ray tube, and acquiring the CT data over 30 to 120 seconds. This "blurred" CT data is used for attenuation correction on the emission scan.

Prospectively gated low dose CT can be used to determine the extent of coronary artery calcification. The calcium score has prognostic value to the myocardial perfusion data. In the evolution of atheroma, vascular calcification reflects an end-stage of the process, often seen in more advanced lesions (see Figure 17-1). Vascular calcium provides definitive evidence that the vessel contains atheroma. Several scoring systems are available to quantify coronary calcium. One of the most common is the Agatston score, which combines both the extent and density of coronary calcium. The Agatston score increases

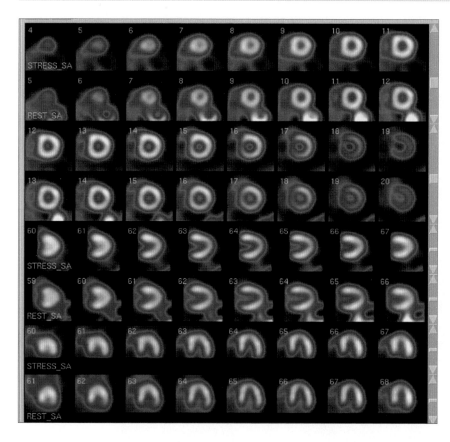

FIGURE 17-14 Normal myocardial perfusion with PET. A 47-year-old man with no risk factors was examined with a history of atypical chest pain. A rest/stress dipyridamole [82]Rb PET study was done. The stress and rest images are shown in the short, vertical, and long axes. Uniform tracer distribution is seen in all segments, with no perfusion defects.

with age: normal patients who are younger than 60 years have coronary scores of less than 100, whereas those over age 65 may have normal scores up to 400. High scores in young subjects are associated with increased risk of coronary events. Coronary calcium indicates the presence of atheroma in a specific vascular territory, which is particularly useful as an addition to myocardial perfusion studies: in patients with a high calcium score and a normal myocardial perfusion scan there is a higher incidence of cardiac events then in patients without elevated calcium scores, similar to the findings in patients with an abnormal stress electrocardiogram and a normal scan.

If a 64-slice (or higher) CT scanner is available, a CT coronary angiogram can be recorded following injection of intravenous contrast. CT angiography can be particularly useful in patients with abnormal perfusion scans to determine if lesions involve the proximal portion of the vessel. The CT is acquired during diastole to minimize the radiation exposure. The data are reconstructed with special software to depict the coronary arteriogram. CT coronary angiograms have a sensitivity greater than 95% for the detection of lesions with greater than 50% narrowing found on selective coronary angiograms. The presence of flow-limiting disease ($\geq$75% stenosis) in proximal vessels, especially the left main coronary artery and the proximal left anterior descending, suggests the need for revascularization. Natural history studies of the prognostic value of coronary angiograms demonstrate that as the number of atheromas in each vessel and the

number of diseased vessels increase, there is an increased risk of coronary events.

RADIONUCLIDE EVALUATION OF VENTRICULAR FUNCTION

The heart's ability to function as a pump can be measured by recording data with gating during myocardial perfusion imaging or by imaging a radiopharmaceutical that is retained in the blood pool. In perfusion imaging, the tracer allows visualization of wall motion, change in cavity size, and thickening of the myocardium from diastole to systole. An alternative approach labels the blood in the cardiac chambers. Blood-pool imaging allows assessment of both global and regional right and left ventricular function (Figure 17-17).

There are two approaches to evaluating ventricular function with tracers in the blood pool: first pass and equilibrium. The equilibrium technique is preferred, since higher count density images are recorded, allowing a more detailed assessment of regional wall motion.

Equilibrium Gated Blood-Pool Studies

An equilibrium gated blood-pool study (GBP) is a preferred method over first-pass method for assessment of the left ventricular function because of the simplicity of technique and processing of data. Table 17-6 shows the labeling techniques used for red blood cells (RBCs). The in vivo method is simple and does not require the

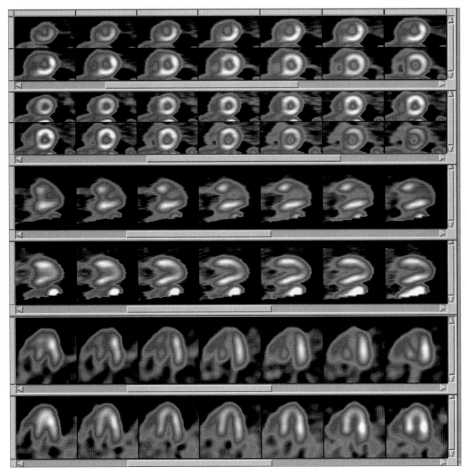

FIGURE 17-15 A 68-year-old asymptomatic obese man with a history of smoking, hypertension, and hyperlipidemia and a family history of heart disease had a rest/stress dipyridamole ⁸²Rb PET study. The images show severe apical, anterior, and septal defects during stress and a normal perfusion pattern at rest, indicating severe ischemia and high-grade occlusion of the left anterior descending (LAD) coronary artery. Angiography showed a 95% proximal LAD lesion, which was treated with stent placement.

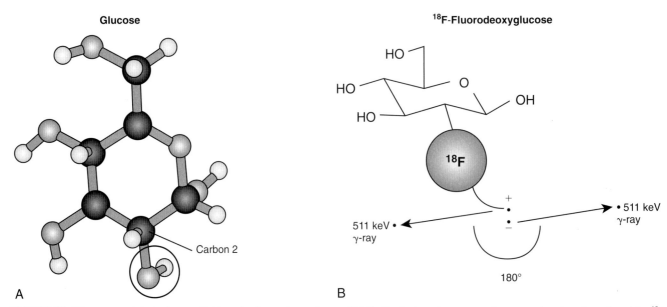

FIGURE 17-16 A, A model of glucose. **B,** To make fluorodeoxyglucose (FDG), the hydroxyl group on the second carbon is replaced by ¹⁸F.

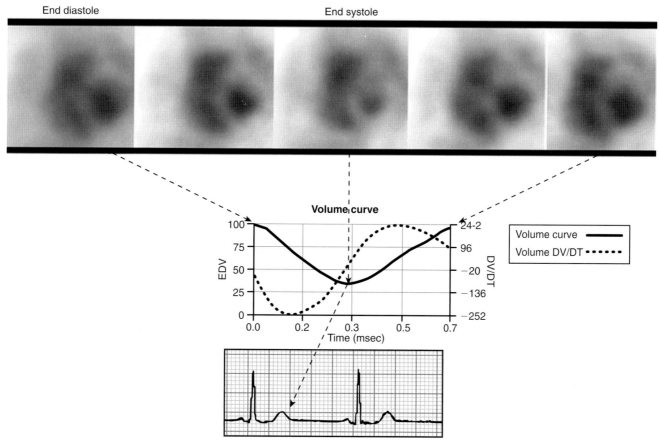

FIGURE 17-17 Selected frames from a planar left anterior oblique radionuclide ventriculogram, shown in relation to the left ventricular volume curve (obtained from region-of-interest analysis of the left ventricle) and the electrocardiogram. *DV/DT,* Rate of emptying/filling of the left ventricle; *EDV,* end diastolic volume.

handling of blood outside the body; however, the average labeling efficiency is lower, and the noncardiac blood-pool counts are higher than that with the in vitro or modified in vivo methods. Radiolabeled autologous RBCs are the preferred tracer for determining cardiac function with GBP imaging (see Table 17-6).

Because multiple points in the cardiac cycle are recorded, the technique is often called *multiple gated acquisition (MUGA)*. After the tracer has equilibrated in the blood pool (about 5 to 10 minutes after administration of the labeled red cells), data are recorded in synchrony with the patient's cardiac cycle. The R wave of the patient's electrocardiogram is used as a physiological marker for the beginning of systole. The heart rate is expressed in milliseconds per cycle. The length of the cardiac cycle is usually divided into 16 frames (but may also be divided into 32 or 64 frames for determination of filling rates). The computer is programmed to record data from the first portion of the cardiac cycle into the first frame, the second portion of the cycle into the second frame, and so on until the last frame is reached or the next R wave is sensed, which resets the recording to the first frame to repeat the process. Data from about 500 to 1000 cycles are added to obtain an "average" cardiac cycle.

Equilibrium GBP imaging can be done as a planar or SPECT acquisition.

- The planar images are usually recorded in three views: (1) the anterior view (to examine right atrial size and motion and right ventricular size and motion); (2) the 45-degree LAO (optimized to separate the right and left ventricles and to determine the timing and motion of the anterior wall, posterior wall, and motion and thickening of the septum of the left ventricle); and (3) either the left lateral or LPO view (to view the inferior and posterior surfaces of the left ventricle and the size and motion of the left atrium). In planar imaging, the left atrium overlaps the left ventricle posteriorly in the LAO view and the right ventricle obscures the inferior wall of the left ventricle in the RAO or anterior view. Because the left atrium and left ventricle beat out of phase with each other (i.e., the atrium fills while the ventricle empties and vice versa), including the left atrium in the left ventricular region of interest reduces the calculated left ventricular ejection fraction (LVEF) (see Figure 17-17).
- Gated blood-pool SPECT images are acquired in similar fashion to myocardial perfusion studies, with

TABLE 17-6	Techniques Used for Labeling RBCs to Be Used as Radiolabeled Autologous Red Blood Cells	
Technique		**Comments**
Red Blood Cell Labeling Techniques		
In vivo labeling: Give stannous pyrophosphate intravenously (3 to 4.5 mg of stannous ion, usually as stannous phosphate). Wait 15 to 30 minutes. Use separate IV access to inject 20 mCi of ^{99m}Tc-pertechnetate.		Overall poor labeling is seen in patient with a hematocrit <30%. Plasma characteristics may be altered with lower temperature, very sick patients. Stannous citrate/stannous diphosphonate, stannous pyrophosphate/stannous glucoheptonate produce good labeling results. Separate IV access prevents adherence of tracer to catheter. Labeling efficiency is 60% to 90%. Heart to background ratio is 2:1. Radiation dose to bladder is 2.2 rad.
In vitro labeling: Draw 12 ml of blood into syringe with heparin/ACD plus stannous ion. Incubate 10 to 20 minutes at room temperature. Centrifuge and remove supernatant plasma. Add 20 mCi of pertechnetate to RBCs. Incubate 10 minutes and centrifuge again. Remove supernatant and inject RBCs.		Labeling efficiency is 95%. Ultratag,* a kit available for tagging RBCs, is simple and easier to use.
Modified in vivo labeling: Inject stannous pyrophosphate intravenously. Wait 15 to 30 minutes. Withdraw 1 to 5 ml of blood into a heparin syringe with 20 mCi of pertechnetate. Mix. Incubate syringe 10 minutes at room temperature. Reinject whole blood.		Labeling efficiency is 90% to 95%.
Labeled Albumin		
A commercial kit is available in Europe but not in the United States. The albumin is reconstituted and labeled with pertechnetate.		Albumin is available immediately and requires minimal handling or exposure to blood. The kit can be used for multiple doses. Disadvantages include diffusion out of the vasculature and high background and liver activity.

*Mallinckrodt, St. Louis, Mo.
ACD, Acid-citrate-dextrose; *RBCs,* red blood cells.

two detectors at 90 degrees recording information from the 45-degree RAO to the 45-degree LPO positions. High-resolution, low-energy collimators should be used (Figure 17-18). The acquisition matrix is 128 × 128. Zoom may be applied to a factor of 1.2 to 1.5, depending on the size of the detectors; 64 views are acquired at 30 sec/frame. Typical counts acquired may be in the range of 30 million to 40 million. The data are reconstructed in similar fashion to perfusion images, with reorientation of the blood-pool data to produce a standard cardiac orientation. The reconstructed and reoriented tomographic display permits more accurate assessment of right and left atrial and ventricular function and chamber size.

Patient Preparation. Electrocardiogram electrodes should be placed (Figure 17-19) and a baseline recording obtained. Usually four electrodes are placed to record one of the standard limb leads of the ECG. The ECG waveform should be reviewed to determine that gating is adequate. Also, it should be determined if the initial portion of the QRS complex is positive (Figure 17-20) because there can be slight temporal offset in the data when the initial waveform is negative as some triggers seek positive wave. Consequently, it is best to

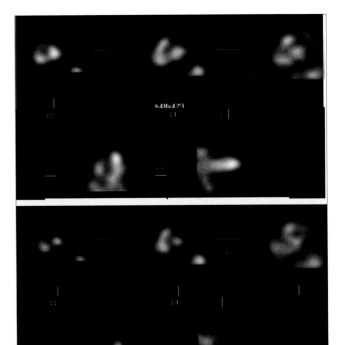

FIGURE 17-18 Selected slices from gated blood-pool SPECT in the short axis *(top row)* vertical and horizontal long axes *(second row)* at end-diastole *(top)* and end-systole *(bottom)*.

standardize on one polarity. If the initial waveform is negative, the electrodes should be moved, or the leads reversed, to provide a positive complex. The ECG waveform should also be reviewed to determine that gating is adequate (Figure 17-20) and that the double gating (due to a tall peaked P wave or T wave) does not occur. If the patient has a low-voltage QRS complex, the electrodes should be relocated until a single gating signal occurs with each beat.

Usually a single, well-defined QRS complex is observed with each cardiac cycle, which triggers the gate only once; however, the gate may trigger twice on a single beat in patients with pacemakers or tall, peaked T waves or less frequently in patients with tall P waves. If more than one complex per cycle is seen, the electrodes should be moved until the waveform of one complex is

maximized and the other minimized. If the patient has a markedly irregular heart rate (greater than 10% variation in the R-R interval in more than 10% of the beats), as occurs in atrial fibrillation or with multiple premature contractions, the rates of filling and emptying of the heart change substantially from beat to beat. As a result, gating becomes difficult and wall motion and ejection fraction (EF) cannot be optimally assessed.

Data Analysis. The planar LAO or best septal view is analyzed to calculate the ejection fraction from the total counts in the left ventricle at end-systole and end-diastole (after background correction) (Figure 17-21). Regions of interest can be drawn over the left ventricle automatically (using either a second derivative or threshold algorithm) or manually. Identification of the ventricular border often is facilitated by smoothing the data spatially by applying a resolution recovery (Wiener) filter before analysis. Temporal smoothing should be used only when the heart rate is regular. If the R-R interval has significant variation, temporal smoothing causes errors. The latter frames of the acquisition, which contain fewer counts, are averaged with the initial frames, thereby lowering the counts in the early frames. If these data are used to calculate the ejection fraction, the end-diastolic counts in

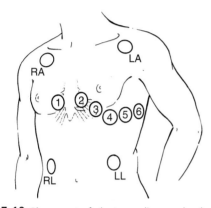

FIGURE 17-19 Placement of electrocardiogram leads. *Limb leads:* Both supraclavicular and abdominal regions (adjacent to the pelvic crest) bilaterally. *Chest leads:* These leads are placed in the following sequence and positions: V_1, second intercostal space to the immediate right of the sternum; V_2, second intercostal space to the immediate left of the sternum; V_4, left midclavicular line in the fifth intercostal space; V_3, halfway between V_2 and V_4; V_6, left midaxillary line in the fifth intercostal space; V_5, midway between V_4 and V_6. *LA,* Left anterior; *LL,* left lateral; *RA,* right anterior; *RL,* right lateral.

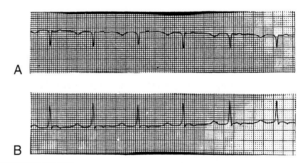

FIGURE 17-20 A, Negative QRS complex. **B,** Positive QRS complex.

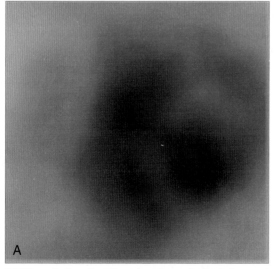
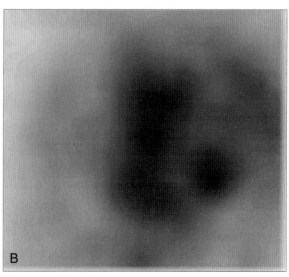

FIGURE 17-21 End diastolic **(A)** and end systolic **(B)** left anterior oblique radionuclide ventriculographic images showing optimal septal visualization.

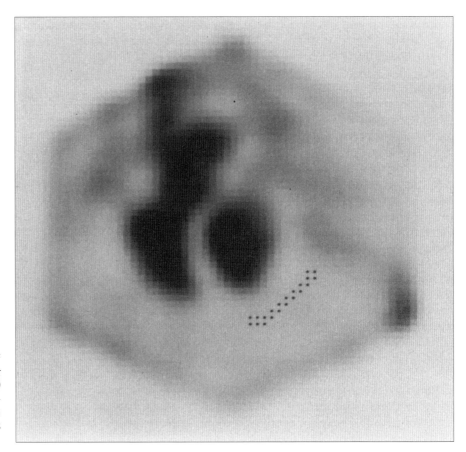

FIGURE 17-22 Background region of interest (ROI) selection *(light dots adjacent to posteroinferior margin of left ventricle)* from end-diastolic image of equilibrium-gated study. Multiple gated acquisition (MUGA) amplitude and phase analysis image.

the left ventricle are lower than they should be, resulting in a calculated ejection fraction that is too low.

A background region is selected, located between the 3 o'clock and 6 o'clock positions from the left ventricle away from pulmonary artery, left atrium, and spleen (Figure 17-22). The background subtraction step is crucial to the subsequent calculation of the EF. Subtraction of too much background results in a falsely elevated EF, and subtraction of too little produces a falsely depressed EF.

The total background-corrected counts in the left ventricle on each frame are then normalized to the counts in the end-diastolic frame, and the time-activity curve from the left ventricular region of interest is displayed. The EF is calculated from the time-activity curve. Normal values for the LVEF range from 50% to 75%. Normal LVEF in women is generally about 5% higher than men, because female hearts are slightly smaller. In addition to the EF, the time of filling and emptying and the ejection and filling rates of the ventricles can be readily computed from these curves. An alternative approach to calculate the EF uses a single region of interest, based on the end-diastolic frame, to measure the time-activity curve. The LVEF can also be calculated from the gated SPECT data, by counting the pixels in the left ventricular region of interest at diastole and systole. The equation for calculation of the left ventricular ejection fraction expressed as a percentage is as follows:

$$EF = (\text{end diastolic counts} - \text{end systolic counts})/\text{end diastolic counts}$$

Regional motion of the left and right ventricles can be readily appreciated from visual assessment of the cinematic display. One approach applies a qualitative assessment to specific segments in the left ventricle (Figure 17-23). Each segment is evaluated as normal, hypokinetic, akinetic, or dyskinetic. An alternative approach to depicting regional function is the stroke-volume image, obtained by subtracting the end-systolic image from the end-diastolic image. Similarly, a "dyskinesis" image can be recorded by subtracting the end-diastolic image from the end-systolic image. Phase and amplitude images can also be generated. Phase analysis assumes that the heart contracts in a specific pattern that resembles the waveform of a cosine function. Each pixel in the image can be evaluated for the timing (phase) of these changes in activity and for its amount of change (amplitude) between the maximum and minimum count values in the pixel. This information can be calculated and presented as a functional image, in which specific colors or brightness represent information about amplitude or phase.

Chemotherapy Cardiotoxicity. A major application of rest GBP images is the evaluation of left ventricular function in patients receiving potentially cardiotoxic chemotherapy (Table 17-7). Patients frequently are evaluated before administration of these agents and at the

Equilibrium radionuclide angiography

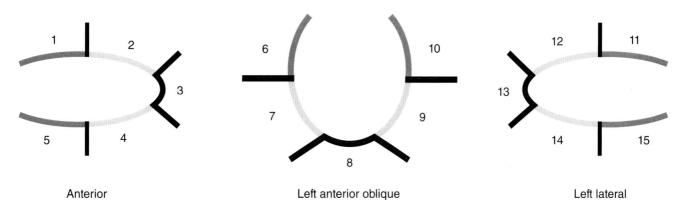

Anterior   Left anterior oblique   Left lateral

FIGURE 17-23 Diagram of left ventricular segments on equilibrium radionuclide angiography. Each segment is scored for normal wall motion, hypokinesis, akinesis, or dyskinesis.

TABLE 17-7	Cardiotoxic Chemotherapeutic Drugs
Agent	**Cardiac Toxicity**
Anthracycline agents (e.g., doxorubicin)	Cardiomyopathy
Cyclophosphamide	Cardiomyopathy and myocardial necrosis
Cisplatin	Cardiomyopathy
Fluorouracil (rare)	Ischemia and angina
Trastuzumab (Herceptin)	Cardiomyopathy
Aldesleukin (Proleukin)	Pericarditis, myocarditis; rarely cardiomyopathy and endocarditis
Arsenic	Prolonged QT intervals
Capacitabine (Xeloda)	Cardiomyopathy, dysrhythmias
Fludarabine	Angina and heart failure
Pacitaxol	Hypertension, bradycardia, congestive failure
Pegaspargase	Cardiomyopathy
Pentostatin	Electrocardiographic abnormalities, chest pain, and hypertension
Procarbazine	Tachycardia, hypertension

conclusion of a course of therapy. Patients with a drop in the LVEF of 5% or greater from a prior determination or whose LVEF is below 50% are likely to be experiencing significant cardiotoxicity from the therapy. Patients with antecedent heart disease are at particular risk.

Gated Blood-Pool Stress

Measurement of cardiac function at rest is valuable for evaluating cardiac function in patients with a history of myocardial infarction, valvular disease, shortness of breath, and suspected heart failure. Measurement of cardiac functional reserve by recording information while the subject is performing exercise adds both

prognostic and diagnostic information. Most blood-pool exercise studies are performed using bicycle ergometer exercise. The initial workload is 20 to 25 watts, with increments every 3 minutes. Planar LAO view images are obtained during the last 2 minutes of each stage. The LVEF should increase by at least 5% from rest to exercise in normal subjects.

Patient Preparation. Patient preparation and performance of stress blood-pool imaging is similar to that for myocardial perfusion imaging. When patients cannot exercise, a pharmacological stress test using dobutamine can be performed.

IMAGING CARDIAC NEUROTRANSMISSION

Imaging of the regional myocardial distribution of adrenergic and cholinergic innervation has been used to assess certain cardiomyopathies and to assess the regional changes of myocardial innervation in ischemic heart disease.

Neurotransmission Assessment

Generally, radiolabeled tracers using physiological neurotransmitters or their structural analogs are used. Each differs in its binding characteristics and selectivity of binding (Box 17-9).

Iodine-123–metaiodobenzylguanidine

Iodine-123–metaiodobenzylguanidine (^{123}I-MIBG) was the first radiopharmaceutical used for the assessment of adrenergic innervation and is the most commonly used tracer for assessing neuronal status of the heart. Iodine-123–MIBG is a guanethidine derivative that is known to be a potent neuron-blocking agent acting selectively on sympathetic nerve endings. MIBG has a molecular

---

BOX 17-9 | **Radiopharmaceuticals for Cardiac Neurotransmission Assessment**

Presynaptic:
    Norepinephrine synthesis
        ^{18}F-fluorodopamine
    Presynaptic reuptake and storage
        ^{11}C-hydroxyephedrine
        ^{11}C-epinephrine
        ^{11}C-ephedrine
        ^{123}I-MIBG
Postsynaptic:
    β-adrenoceptor expression and density
        ^{11}C-CGP
        ^{11}C-carazolol

---

structure similar to noradrenaline and therefore increased affinity for neuronal uptake. It also utilizes the same uptake and storage mechanism as noradrenaline. Iodine-123–MIBG shows increased uptake in the heart because of its dense sympathetic innervation. Myocardial MIBG uptake and retention is reduced in patients with congestive heart failure.

Imaging. Before administration of MIBG, the thyroid is blocked with either 500 mg potassium perchlorate orally or 10 drops of saturated solution of potassium iodide (SSKI) in water. Thirty minutes later, about 370 MBq of ^{123}I-MIBG is administered intravenously. Planar and SPECT images of the heart are acquired at 20 minutes and 4 hours after tracer administration using the 159-keV ^{123}I photopeak and a 20% window. A heart-to-mediastinum ratio (HMR) is obtained by drawing regions of interest (ROIs) over the mediastinum and the myocardium in the anterior view. A heart-to-mediastinum ratio less than 1.4 is considered abnormal.

A visual assessment is made using a point scale for detecting reduction in MIBG concentration in given myocardial segments. A semiquantitative measurement of myocardial MIBG uptake is preferred. ROIs are drawn over the left ventricular myocardium and the noncardiac portion of the mediastinum and an HMR is calculated. SPECT imaging is preferred because lung and LV myocardial activity can be separated. In conditions such as heart failure or following myocardial infarction, myocardial MIBG uptake is markedly decreased and the image quality may not be optimal for proper analysis and interpretation.

Other Compounds. Fluorine-18–fluorodopamine, ^{11}C-hydroxyephedrine, and ^{11}C-CGP-12177 (4-[3-*t*-butylamino-2-hydroxypropoxy]-benzimidazol-one), are also undergoing evaluation as markers of myocardial adrenergic receptor activity.

SUMMARY

- Radionuclide studies of the cardiovascular system are primarily used to detect and characterize acquired heart diseases, such as coronary artery disease, cardiotoxicity of antineoplastic drugs, and congestive heart failure.

- Atheromatous narrowings that occupy at least 50% of the lumen diameter restrict the maximum amount of blood that can flow through a vessel but may not be associated with symptoms. Narrowings of at least 70% of the lumen are often symptomatic.

- Cardiac output for a normal 70-kg adult is approximately 5 to 6 L/min at rest, and the stroke volume is approximately 80 to 100 ml.

- The sinoatrial node usually serves as the impulse generator for the remainder of the heart.

- The five major categories of radiopharmaceuticals used in clinical cardiac imaging are (1) perfusion tracers, (2) blood-pool tracers, (3) glucose and fatty acid analogs to measure metabolism, (4) analogs of epinephrine to measure sympathetic innervation, and (5) tracers that localize in areas of acute myocardial necrosis.

- The three standard views are vertical long axis (corresponding to coronal images), horizontal long axis (corresponding to transverse images), and short axis (corresponding to sagittal images).

- Multiple episodes of motion, movement greater than 2 pixels or loss of more than one set of projection data creates significant artifacts that can lead to erroneous interpretation, and acquisition should be repeated.

- Gated acquisitions show regional wall motion and ejection fraction in addition to the myocardial perfusion data.

- The soft tissue of the chest musculature, breast, and diaphragm are known to cause attenuation of the signal and to lead to artifacts that resemble perfusion defects.

- Perfusion imaging is performed to detect myocardial ischemia and to determine its location and extent.

- Redistribution makes thallium very useful for identifying ischemic myocardium.

- Technetium agents do not redistribute; therefore separate injections are required to depict perfusion at rest and with stress.

- For detection of ischemia, thallium and technetium agents perform equally well. When there is a question of severe myocardial ischemia and the issue is myocardial viability, thallium is preferred.

- Treadmill exercise is usually done using the standard Bruce protocol. The modified Bruce protocol is used for patients who are frail or expected to have poor exercise tolerance, or for those within 1 week of myocardial infarction.

- Pharmacological stress is used for patients who cannot exercise.

- Active asthma is a contraindication for use of dipyridamole or adenosine.

- Dobutamine is a sympathomimetic drug that increases heart rate and blood pressure.
- Neither the vasodilators nor dobutamine provide the breadth of information about cardiac performance that is available with an exercise study.
- Two types of artifacts in SPECT imaging that occur fairly frequently are attenuation and motion. Both tend to cause decreased counts in the reconstructed data that can be mistaken for zones of decreased perfusion.
- SPECT images are usually quantified by stacking the reconstructed/reoriented short-axis slices onto a bull's-eye display where the images are arranged concentrically from the apex of the ventricle (center) to the base (periphery).
- Positron-emitting radionuclides and PET-CT are very useful for defining regional myocardial perfusion, the coronary artery calcium score, perfusion reserve, and if necessary, CT coronary angiography
- Gated blood-pool studies are preferred over the first-pass method for assessment of the left ventricular function because of simplicity of technique and processing of data.
- Stress tests can cause ischemia, arrhythmias, hypotension, infarction, and death; therefore they should be performed only by qualified personnel who are familiar with the procedure and who know CPR.
- Iodine-123–MIBG is the most commonly used tracer for assessing neuronal status of the heart.

REFERENCE

1. Lloyd-Jones D, et al: Heart disease and stroke statistics: 2010 update. A report from the American Heart Association, (circulation) 121(7):e46-e215, 2010.

SUGGESTED READING

Alessi AM, et al: *Nuclear cardiology technology study guide*, Reston, 2010, SNM.
Zaret BL, Beller GA: *Clinical nuclear cardiology, state of the art and future directions*, St Louis, 2010, Mosby.

Gastrointestinal System

Jean-Luc C. Urbain, Leon S. Malmud

OBJECTIVES

After completing this chapter, the reader will be able to:
- Diagram and describe the organs and structures of the gastrointestinal system.
- Describe the physiology of the gastrointestinal system, including the esophagus, stomach, liver, hepatobiliary collecting system and gallbladder, small intestine, and large intestine.
- Describe the technique for parotid glands imaging.
- Describe various techniques for evaluating esophageal transit using computerized regions-of-interest studies.
- Discuss gastroesophageal reflux procedures and imaging techniques for esophageal reflux, pulmonary aspiration, and calculation of a gastroesophageal reflux index.
- Explain the clinical aspects of performing radionuclide gastric emptying studies.

- Diagram the hepatobiliary system (e.g., common duct, cystic duct, gallbladder, and bile duct).
- Describe the procedure for liver and spleen scintigraphy using colloidal materials.
- Describe imaging procedures using labeled red blood cells to detect hepatic hemangioma.
- Discuss imaging procedures for the hepatobiliary system and identification of cholecystitis.
- Explain procedures that can be used for the determination of enterogastric reflux.
- Differentiate the advantages of 99mTc–sulfur colloid imaging from 99mTc–labeled red blood cell imaging for the identification of gastrointestinal bleeding.
- Describe the principles of performing breath-test studies with 14C-labeled compounds.

KEY TERMS

cholecystokinin (CCK)
cholescintigraphy
enterogastric reflux
enterogastric reflux index (EGRI)
esophageal transit time

gallbladder ejection fraction (GBEF)
gastric half emptying time
gastroesophageal reflux
lag phase
Meckel diverticulum

peristalsis
sialography
whole-gut transit
xerostomia

The gastrointestinal (GI) system consists of the GI tract, or alimentary canal, and several accessory organs. The alimentary canal is a continuous tube running through the ventral body cavity; it originates at the mouth and is followed by the pharynx, esophagus, stomach, small intestine, and large intestine (Figure 18-1).

The purpose of the alimentary canal is to provide a route of intake for nourishment, to digest and absorb nutrients, and to eliminate waste products. For the purpose of this chapter, the accessory organs involved are the salivary glands, pancreas, liver, and gallbladder. Although not a part of the GI system, the spleen is mentioned, but only its morphology is considered.

A variety of radionuclide techniques are available for evaluation of the GI tract, including techniques for imaging specific organs and those that characterize function. In this chapter, methodologies are described in detail for procedures used to study the movement of luminal contents in the GI tract. These techniques take advantage of the unique features offered by the use of radiotracers in the study of physiological processes; that is, they permit quantitative measurement of GI function but do not disturb the process under study. These methodologies include evaluation of the swallowing function and esophageal transit, detection and quantitation of **gastroesophageal reflux,** measurement of gastric emptying, and qualitative and quantitative evaluation of gallbladder function and **enterogastric reflux.** Other techniques include detection of pulmonary aspiration and Carbon-14 (^{14}C) breath testing. Techniques that long have enjoyed clinical acceptance, such as colloid liver and spleen scanning, GI bleeding studies, and salivary gland imaging, are also reviewed in detail.

SALIVARY GLANDS

The salivary glands consist of three paired exocrine glands that produce saliva. Saliva, a fluid that initiates the chemical breakdown of food, is continuously secreted into the mouth. The primary set of salivary glands is the parotid glands, which are located in the cheeks, below and in front of the ears (see Figure 18-1). The parotid glands empty into the oral cavity through Stensen ducts. The second pair of salivary glands is the submandibular glands, which are located beneath the tongue in the posterior aspect of the floor of the mouth; these empty directly into the oral cavity. The third pair of sublingual

glands is also located beneath the tongue and is anterior to the submandibular glands.

Salivary gland imaging, also known as nuclear **sialography,**[39] is used primarily to determine the function and confirm the location of the salivary glands including ectopic glands. Rarely is it now used to evaluate Warthin tumors.

The salivary glands indiscriminately trap a number of ions, among them the iodides and the technetium-99m (^{99m}Tc)-pertechnetate ion. Also, these ions are actively excreted by the glands into the saliva. Hence, the production and excretion of saliva can be evaluated using ^{99m}Tc-pertechnetate.

The main clinical indication for salivary gland imaging is the evaluation of the symptoms of dryness of the mouth, or **xerostomia.** Xerostomia is a difficult clinical symptom to assess, because it may have a significant psychosomatic contribution in its origin. However, the possibility must be considered that the xerostomia is caused by blockage of one or several of the salivary gland ducts by a benign or neoplastic mass. Xerostomia is also an important feature and often a presenting complaint in several systemic disease complexes, notably the collagen-vascular diseases, particularly Sjögren syndrome.[39] Xerostomia can also be associated with thyroiditis and should be taken into account in the interpretation of salivary gland images. Xerostomia occurs in sarcoidosis, after radiation therapy to the head and neck, during states of dehydration, and as a result of administration of certain drugs and pharmacological agents.

Imaging Procedure

No patient preparation is necessary. Rinsing of the mouth before the examination may reduce pertechnetate excretion into the oral cavity. The patient is seated comfortably facing the scintillation camera. The camera is peaked for ^{99m}Tc with a 20% energy window and fitted with a low-energy, parallel-hole collimator. To prevent superimposition of the thyroid gland on the salivary glands, the patient's head should be tilted backward with the neck extended as far as possible, allowing the chin to make contact with the camera face.

Technetium-99m-pertechnetate (1 to 5 mCi) is administered intravenously after the patient has been properly positioned. Dynamic sequential anterior images of the

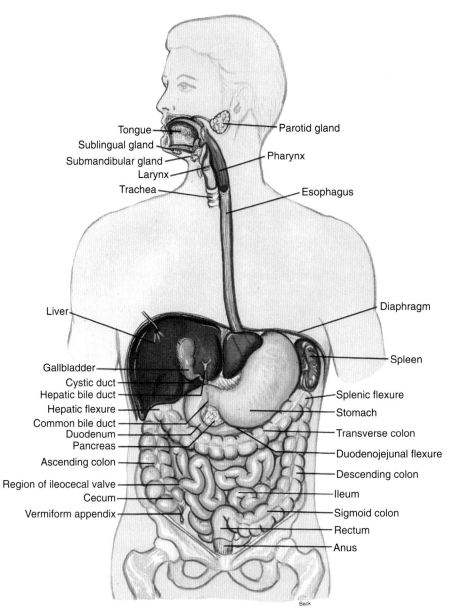

FIGURE 18-1 Location of gastrointestinal system organs.

face and neck are obtained at 1- to 2-second intervals for 15 to 20 seconds (Figure 18-2). The review of the images by cine display enables visual evaluation of the secretory process. Quantitative evaluation of secretion is achieved by drawing regions of interest around each gland and generating time-activity curves. These should demonstrate simultaneous and symmetrical uptake of the radiotracer in the parotid, submandibular, and sublingual glands. Thereafter the study often is useful for obtaining anterior and lateral views of the head and neck (Figure 18-3) to confirm the normal presence of radiotracer in the saliva in the oral cavity.

It may be useful at this point to test the salivary gland response to gustatory stimulation.[5] A 1:1 dilution of commercial lemon juice (pH approximately 2.6) may be used; alternatively, fresh-squeezed lemon juice diluted equally with tap water may be substituted. The patient is instructed to take a mouthful of the lemon juice solution, swish it throughout the mouth for approximately 5 seconds, and then expectorate fully into a disposable beaker. The patient may then be repositioned in front of the camera and imaged dynamically for an additional 20 minutes. In normal individuals, a rapid, symmetrical, and profound diminution in radiotracer localization in the salivary glands usually is seen (Figure 18-4) and can be easily assessed by time-activity curves generated over each gland.

Prior administration of perchlorate should be avoided, because it would partly block salivary gland uptake of the radiotracer.

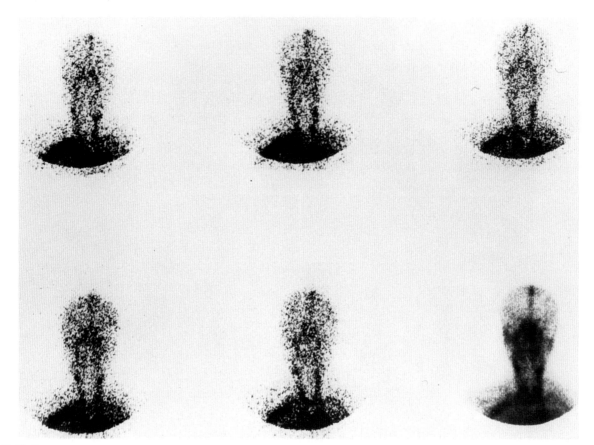

FIGURE 18-2 Rapid sequential images of the head and neck in the anterior projection at 2-second intervals. There is symmetrical perfusion with simultaneous and rapid localization in the salivary glands.

Clinical Aspects

Normally, simultaneous, rapid, and symmetrical uptake and localization of the radiotracer occurs in all three pairs of salivary glands (see Figure 18-2), with homogeneous distribution and parallel excretion of the pertechnetate (see Figure 18-3). It originally was hoped that this examination could be used to discern a wide variety of mass lesions in the salivary glands, but this has not been the case. Only two types of neoplasm have a consistent appearance on nuclear sialography: (1) Warthin tumors, which appear as focal areas of increased uptake (Figure 18-5), and (2) metastatic lesions, which are characteristically cold focal areas. Benign mixed tumors of the salivary glands may appear as focal areas of increased or decreased uptake. Focal cold areas are seen with other types of malignancy, cysts, some mixed tumors, enlarged lymph nodes, and inflammatory diseases. Decreased or absent uptake in a single gland or set of glands may be seen in congenital aplasia or obstructive sialolithiasis and after sialectomy, trauma, or radiotherapy. In Sjögren syndrome and other types of vascular and connective tissue diseases, either asymmetrical arrival of the radiotracer in the salivary glands is seen or radiotracer uptake in the salivary glands is delayed and decreased compared with radiotracer uptake in the thyroid. On delayed images, bilaterally decreased excretion can be seen in these diseases, and a response after administration of a gustatory stimulant may be absent or blunted.[5] Bilaterally decreased uptake and excretion in the salivary glands can also be seen in acute suppurative parotitis and multicentric sialoangiectasis and in some aged individuals.

Poor response to gustatory stimulation is seen in the systemic connective tissue diseases, acute parotitis (mumps), and after radiotherapy of the head and neck. If a single salivary gland or group of salivary glands fails to excrete, this is suggestive of stenosis or blockage of the salivary duct.[30]

Despite lack of anatomical detail, salivary gland imaging plays a useful clinical role in the evaluation of certain morphological and functional diseases.

OROPHARYNX

The oropharynx lies posterior to the mouth. It is a complex organ composed of numerous small muscles, cartilage, and tendons. The oropharynx functions in both a respiratory and digestive capacity and its components function in a very finely coordinated manner to accept food from the mouth and propel it from the esophagus while suspending respiration. Although radiographic studies of swallowing have been in use for some

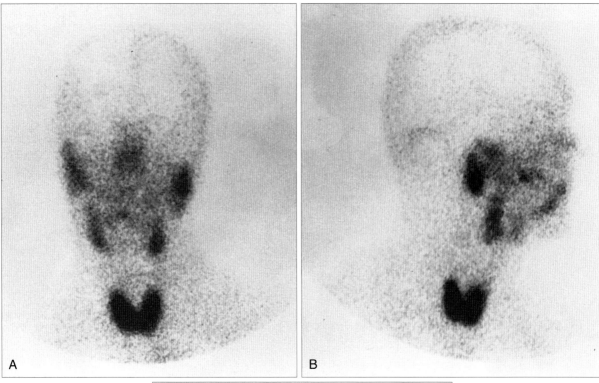

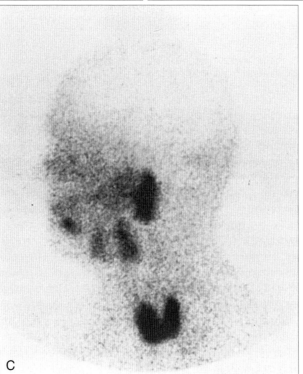

FIGURE 18-3 A, Anterior view of the head 15 minutes after injection. Normal salivary glands display homogenous distribution of ^{99m}Tc-pertechnetate. Localization is symmetrical in the parotid, submandibular, and sublingual glands. Uptake is also seen in the thyroid gland. **B,** Right lateral view of the head and neck. **C,** Left lateral view of the head and neck. The parotid and submandibular glands are seen particularly well in these lateral views.

time, they are accompanied by a relatively high radiation burden and do not readily provide quantitative information of the swallowing function. Radionuclide studies generally are very sensitive and are able to provide physiological and quantitative information. The radionuclide

oropharyngeal study was developed as a method of measuring clearance of liquids from the oropharynx and to detect and possibly assess aspiration of food in patients with oropharyngeal dysfunction. This technique is usually combined with esophageal transit and

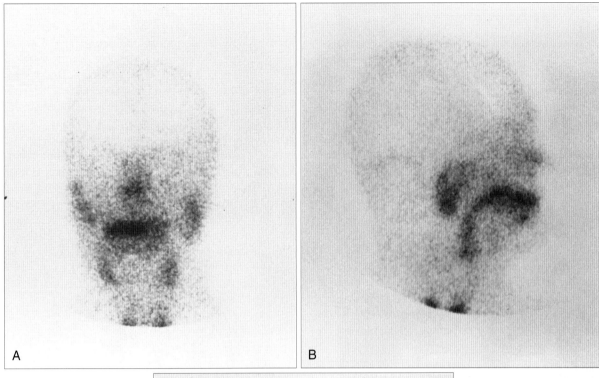

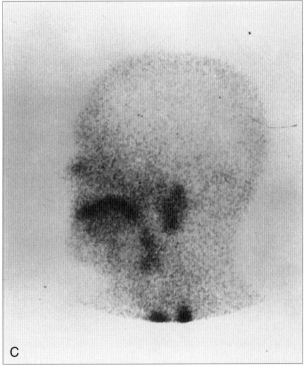

FIGURE 18-4 Anterior **(A)**, right lateral **(B)**, and left lateral **(C)** views of the head 20 minutes after oral administration of dilute lemon juice. Rapid, symmetrical, and profound diminution of radiotracer localization in the salivary glands has occurred. Compared with Figure 18-3, most of the activity is now in the oral cavity.

gastroesophageal reflux studies. Recently it has been used in patients with laryngopharyngeal reflux.[19]

Imaging Procedure

Cold tap water (10 ml) is mixed with 1 mCi of ^{99m}Tc–sulfur colloid by shaking for 30 seconds immediately

before this study. A liquid sample of approximately 10 ml is used, because this volume is easily swallowed as a bolus.

A large–field-of-view scintillation camera fitted with a high-sensitivity collimator is used. Images should be acquired on a computer. The patient is seated erect in front of the camera in the anterior position with the neck

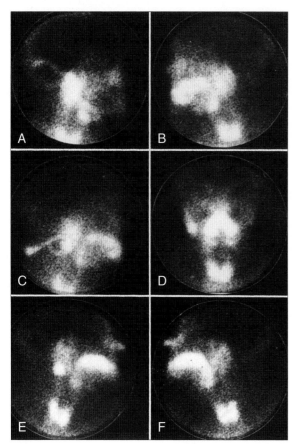

FIGURE 18-5 Warthin tumor of the right parotid gland. Immediate right (**A**) and left lateral (**B**) views. **C**, Delayed right lateral view with radioactive string marker around palpable nodule. One-hour delayed views taken in the anterior (**D**), right (**E**), and left lateral (**F**) positions.

rotated to the left. The right cheek is positioned at the surface of the collimator, as is the chest, such that a right lateral view of the mouth and oropharynx and an anterior view of the chest are obtained.

The patient is instructed to sip the fluid through a straw and to hold the entire amount of the material in the mouth. On command, the patient is instructed to swallow all the material at once. It may be useful to review the procedure with the patient using sips of plain water before administration of the test dose. After swallowing the radiopharmaceutical, the patient is instructed to dry swallow every 15 seconds on command. The patient should breathe quietly through the nose during the remainder of the study.

Images are acquired dynamically for 5 minutes in the computer for subsequent analysis. The initial 30 seconds of the examination are acquired at 0.1 sec/frame, and the following 270 seconds are acquired at 1 sec/frame (Figure 18-6).

Images for the first 30 seconds are added by the computer to yield a composite image for anatomical definition of the oropharynx. From this summed image a manually outlined region of interest is drawn and stored in the computer. The region of interest is used to generate a time-activity curve from the raw data. The time-activity curve, representing the oropharyngeal count rate, can be fitted to a biexponential clearance model, which consists of fast- and slow-clearing components (Figure 18-7), each associated with an amplitude and half-life.

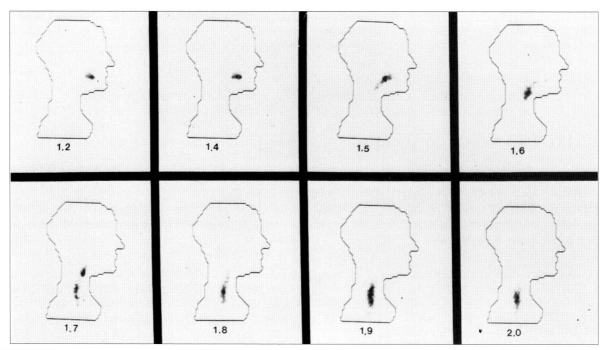

FIGURE 18-6 Normal oropharyngeal 0.1-second images obtained with the patient positioned with the right side of the face at the surface of the collimator.

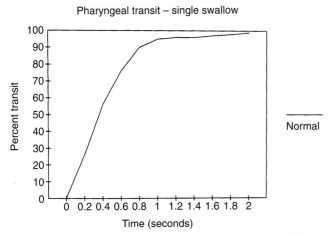

Pharyngeal transit – single swallow

FIGURE 18-7 Normal time-activity curve representing oropharyngeal function. Function is biexponential with fast- and slow-clearing components.

Clinical Aspects

This radionuclide imaging procedure is useful for documenting the swallowing function and pharyngeal transit time in patients with neurological or connective tissue disorders in whom no demonstrable abnormality can be seen either by direct inspection or by other methods, such as the barium swallow. A prolonged high-amplitude slow component appears to be characteristic of an abnormal swallowing function.

ESOPHAGUS

The esophagus is a muscular tube that is approximately 20 cm long and extends from the pharynx at the level of the sixth cervical vertebra to the stomach at the level of the tenth thoracic vertebra. Its function is to transport a swallowed food bolus from the pharynx to the stomach, which is accomplished by coordinated contractions of its muscular layers, termed **peristalsis.** The esophagus is located posterior to the trachea in the thorax and in its resting state remains collapsed (see Figure 18-1).

Histologically, the proximal third consists primarily of striated muscle; the distal third is exclusively composes of smooth muscle; and the middle portion is a transitional mixture of the two. Anatomically, three specialized areas can be identified: the upper esophogeal sphincter, the body, and the lower esophogeal or gastroesophogeal sphincter. Proper relaxation of the lower esophageal sphincter is necessary to allow the passage of the food bolus into the stomach. Incoordinate lower esophageal sphincter function has been implicated in a number of disorders that affect esophageal transit, as well as in gastroesophageal reflux.

Esophageal Transit

The act of swallowing triggers the coordinated motor pattern of the esophagus. First, a pharyngeal contraction transfers the bolus through a relaxed upper esophageal sphincter into the esophagus. The sphincter then contracts and a peristaltic wave carries the food bolus from the upper esophagus into the stomach through a relaxed lower esophageal sphincter. This peristaltic process is called *primary peristalsis*. Secondary peristaltic waves also occur in the esophageal body in response to residual food or refluxed gastric content. Tertiary nonperistaltic contractions are seen occasionally as a normal phenomenon in the young and more commonly in the elderly; these contractions are induced by intrinsic intramural reflex mechanisms. Radionuclide esophageal transit studies[15] are useful as a noninvasive screening test and for the quantitative assessment of suspected esophageal motor disorders. They may also be employed to evaluate the efficacy of surgical or mechanical interventions on lower esophageal stricture.

Difficulty or discomfort associated with swallowing can be associated with anatomical lesions of the esophagus or an esophageal motor disorder. Severely painful swallowing can be associated with mucosal destruction of the esophagus from infection, reflux esophagitis, ulcerations, or tumor. Esophageal studies are also useful for evaluating patients with suspected regurgitation or aspiration pneumonias. Motility disorders of the esophagus may be the result of innate muscular or innervation disorders or can occur secondary to a systemic disease, such as a connective tissue disease. Amotility, which is seen in achalasia and scleroderma, may be a factor. Hypomotility, or decreased pressure of swallowing, can be seen in older individuals, and hypermotility can be seen in diffuse esophageal spasm.

Imaging Procedure. The patient should fast for at least 2 hours before the examination. The radiopharmaceutical is prepared by mixing 300 µCi of ^{99m}Tc–sulfur colloid in 15 ml of tap water.

The patient is placed supine under the camera for an anterior view of the thorax. The camera is fitted with a high-sensitivity or low-energy, all-purpose collimator and interfaced to a computer. The patient is positioned with the stomach at the bottom of the field of view. The radiopharmaceutical is administered orally through a straw, and the patient is instructed to take the entire volume into the mouth but not to swallow until instructed to do so. The computer is started, and the patient is instructed to swallow the contents of the mouth as a single compact bolus. The patient is instructed to dry swallow every 15 seconds for the next 10 minutes. Images are acquired every 0.25 seconds for the first 2 minutes and at 15-second intervals for the remaining 8 minutes (Figure 18-8). At the conclusion of the study, the data are retrieved from the computer for analysis.

A few methods of data analysis can be used to evaluate and measure esophageal transit. A global measure of esophageal emptying can be made by recording the counts present in the total esophagus after multiple swallows using a computer-generated rectangular region of

FIGURE 18-8 Normal esophageal images. Images of the esophagus are acquired in the anterior projection at the initial swallow and then every 15 seconds with each dry swallow for the next 10 minutes. Individual images are shown for the first, fourth, eighth, sixteenth, thirty-second, and fortieth swallows. Images are acquired online, stored on a digital computer, and later retrieved for analysis. NOTE: In normal subjects, no activity is seen in the esophagus after the initial swallow.

Multiple swallow technique—normal subject

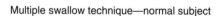

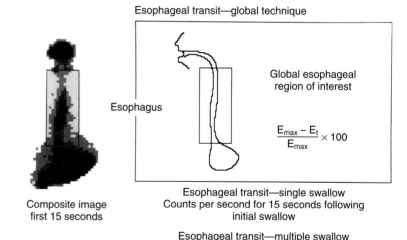

Composite image
first 15 seconds

Esophagus

Global esophageal
region of interest

$$\frac{E_{max} - E_t}{E_{max}} \times 100$$

Esophageal transit—single swallow
Counts per second for 15 seconds following
initial swallow

Esophageal transit—multiple swallow
Counts per 15 second interval following each
swallow for ten minutes

FIGURE 18-9 The esophageal region of interest when esophageal transit is measured as a global function.

interest over the entire esophagus (Figure 18-9). The count rate in the esophageal region of interest is used to determine the rate of esophageal transit according to the following formula[15]:

$$C_t = \frac{(E_{max} - E_t)}{E_{max}} \times 100$$

where C_t represents the esophageal transit at time t; E_{max} is the maximum count rate in gaesophagus; and E_t is the esophageal count rate at time t.

The second method analyzes regional esophageal transit by dividing the esophagus into proximal, middle, and distal regions of interest. Three equal-size, rectangular regions of interest are drawn on the esophagus and a fourth region encompasses the fundus of the stomach (Figure 18-10). In this segmental approach, four parameters are derived from the time-activity curves: (1) the **esophageal transit time**, defined as the time interval between the peak activity of the proximal esophageal curve and the peak activity of the distal esophageal curve; (2) the segmental emptying time, defined as the

Data processing

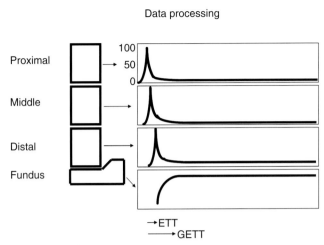

FIGURE 18-10 Schematic representation of a normal esophageal transit study. The esophageal transit time *(ETT)*, the segmental emptying time, the global esophageal emptying time, and the esophagogastric transit time *(GETT)* can be derived from the time-activity curves.

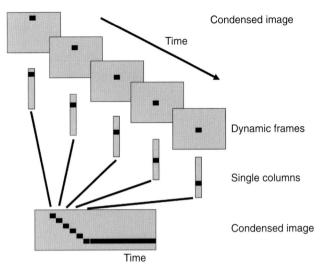

FIGURE 18-11 Condensed images of the esophagus. In its simple form, the activity of all rows of each dynamic frame are summed into a single column. Columns are then added together so that the vertical axis demonstrates the spatial distribution of the radioactivity in the esophagus, and the horizontal, long axis represents time. In the gated format, dynamic images from different swallows are gated to generate single, condensed columns. A composite image is generated from the temporal sum of the condensed columns.

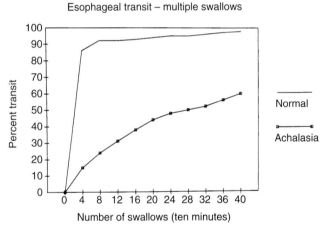

FIGURE 18-12 Time-activity curves of percentage transit versus the number of swallows for 10 minutes. Both a normal individual (patient in Figure 18-8) and a patient with achalasia (patient in Figure 18-13) are illustrated.

time required for more than an arbitrary percentage of the maximal radioactivity (usually 90%) in each region of interest to be eliminated; (3) the global esophageal emptying time, represented by the time from entry of the bolus in the proximal esophagus to the clearance of more than 90% from the entire esophagus; and (4) the **esophagogastric transit time,** defined as the time interval between peak activity of the proximal esophageal curve and maximal gastric activity.[44]

The concept of the condensed image refers to the summing of all computer frames during the transit of the bolus that produces a "topographical picture" or "condensed picture" of the esophagus.[25,43, 46] The condensed image consists of the summation of the activity in the pixel rows into a single column for each frame of the swallowing test data series. The vertical axis shows the spatial distribution of the radioactivity from the mouth to the stomach and the horizontal axis shows time (Figure 18-11). This method of display depicts a complete dynamic sequence in one single image, facilitates qualitative assessment of radionuclide esophageal transit, and improves diagnostic ability.[24] To integrate the dynamic sequences after each bolus swallow into one single, condensed image, a "pseudo gating" technique of condensed esophageal images can also be performed.[45] This method has the advantage of displaying into one single image the average esophageal transit of multiple boluses and dry-swallow sequences and appears to be very sensitive. The built-in disadvantage of this approach is that it sums dynamic sequences, which may not be "gatable" because of the occurrence of the dry swallows at different time intervals and the resultant large intraindividual swallowing variability.

Clinical Aspects. Esophageal activity decreases rapidly, usually within 5 to 10 seconds after the first swallow, and the activity is no longer visible (see Figure 18-8),

although count rates of approximately 10% of peak activity may be found until the eighth swallow (2 minutes) (Figure 18-12). As the initial bolus passes through the esophagus, a smooth progression of sequential peaks of activity in the proximal, middle, and distal esophagus are demonstrated (see Figure 18-10). By the fortieth swallow (10 minutes), less than 5% of peak activity remains in the whole esophageal region of interest (see Figure 18-12). Using these methods, it is possible to differentiate patients with achalasia (see Figures 18-12 and 18-13) from those with scleroderma, because in scleroderma most of the bolus activity is able to enter the stomach, whereas in achalasia a more marked delay

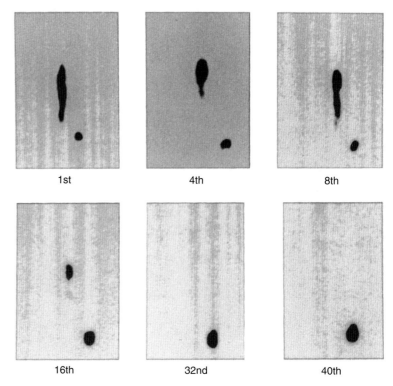

1st   4th   8th

16th   32nd   40th

Multiple swallow technique in a patient with achalasia

FIGURE 18-13 Anterior views of the esophagus in a patient with achalasia. Note poor passage of liquid bolus in the esophagus (retention) despite repeated dry swallows. Percentage transit is illustrated in Figure 18-12.

in esophageal emptying is seen. With diffuse esophageal spasm, the radionuclide study shows incoordinate activity, which is different from patients with nonspecific abnormalities.

The radionuclide method has demonstrated 100% sensitivity for detecting achalasia, diffuse esophageal spasm, and scleroderma. Radionuclide esophageal transit studies can also be useful in the evaluation of esophageal strictures and esophageal diverticula and after radiotherapy for carcinoma of the esophagus.

A routine esophageal transit study may be combined with delayed images of the thorax in the anterior and posterior projections for the detection of aspirated radionuclide. Delayed images of the thorax can be particularly useful in an adult patient with nonspecific pulmonary symptoms in whom the diagnosis of pulmonary aspiration is often difficult to confirm. Overnight pulmonary aspiration of a radionuclide from the stomach, when demonstrable, is seen as a highly specific though insensitive method for detecting this disorder (Figure 18-14). Unfortunately, because aspiration is intermittent and dependent upon a number of factors, such as position, gravity, pH, fat content, and gastric content, the result of a pulmonary aspiration scan can be negative even in patients with clear symptoms.

Gastroesophageal Reflux

Gastroesophageal reflux refers to the symptom complex of heartburn, regurgitation, and chest pain. Esophageal

reflux occurs when either gastric or duodenal contents enter the esophagus. Some of the anatomical abnormalities that can result in incompetence of the lower esophageal sphincter and symptomatic gastroesophageal reflux include enlargement of the diaphragmatic hiatus, disruption of the phrenoesophageal ligament, loss of the acute cardioesophageal angle of Hiss, loss of the gastric mucosal rosette, and a change in the distal paraesophageal pressure from an intraabdominal to an intrathoracic level. In short, lower esophageal sphincter incompetence must be present for acid reflux to occur.

There is now a vast battery of tests to demonstrate and evaluate gastroesophageal reflux, including esophagography, endoscopy with or without biopsy, Bernstein test, esophageal manometry, 24-hour pH monitoring, and esophageal scintigraphy. Of these studies, gastroesophageal scintigraphy is possibly the most useful in the detection and the quantitative assessment of reflux and its therapy.[14,31] The clinical significance of minimal degrees of esophageal reflux is questionable at best. It has been suggested that diminished muscle tone in the lower esophagus, rather than hiatal hernia, is the cause of most reflux.[37] Simple, inexpensive regimens, such as the use of antacids and changes in the diet to include more protein, may resolve symptoms in most patients (only 5% of whom may eventually require surgery). Small degrees of reflux are hardly grounds for surgery, and a trial of therapy (known to be innocuous) can satisfy both patient and referring physician much more than the results of complicated diagnostic tests.[8]

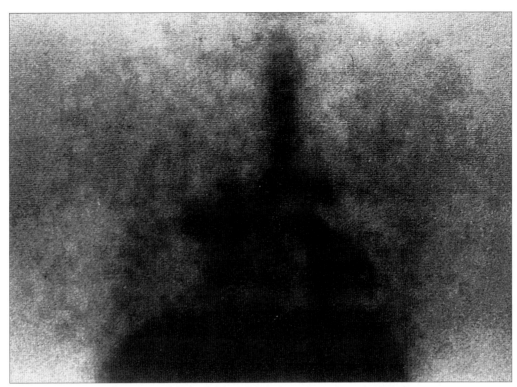

FIGURE 18-14 Pulmonary aspiration. Anterior view of the thorax obtained 24 hours after instillation of ^{99m}Tc–sulfur colloid into the stomach via nasogastric tube. Activity is seen in the trachea, bronchi, and peripheral lung fields, indicating overnight aspiration of gastric contents.

Many esophageal disorders disrupt neural and muscular mechanisms that control the activity of the lower esophageal sphincter. Fat, alcohol, chocolate, and cigarette smoking are some of the factors that commonly cause depression of the lower esophageal sphincter pressure, and these have also been associated with symptomatic gastroesophageal reflux. Consequences of recurring gastroesophageal reflux are esophagitis, unrelenting heartburn, and eventual dysphagia. Often these symptoms are associated with abnormalities in esophageal clearance, and it may be beneficial routinely to perform esophageal and gastroesophageal scintigraphic studies as a single examination.

Imaging Procedure. The patient must fast at least 8 hours before the examination; then, the esophageal transit study should be performed first. This allows the technologist to note all the obvious abnormalities that can impair esophageal clearance. After these data for the esophagus have been stored for later processing, the gastroesophageal reflux study may be performed.

The patient is given an oral solution containing 300 μCi of ^{99m}Tc–sulfur colloid mixed with 150 ml of orange juice and 150 ml of 0.1 N hydrochloric acid. The entire 300 ml of solution should be administered, because this volume of liquid in the stomach opposes induced abdominal pressure. The patient then is fitted with an abdominal binder similar to a large blood pressure cuff. The patient is positioned supine under the camera, and the abdominal binder is readjusted so that the inflatable bladder within it is centered over the stomach and below the costal margin. In female patients, care should be taken not to pinch the breasts. The binder should be positioned carefully so that its pressure on the abdomen forces the stomach superiorly. Compression of the lower ribs should be avoided because this forces the stomach inferiorly, away from the diaphragm.

Four factors are required to induce reflux successfully in a patient who is prone to gastroesophageal reflux: (1) oral administration of an acidified solution; (2) successive, increased pressure applied to the abdomen; (3) maintenance of a supine position; and (4) at least a 300-ml volume in the stomach to oppose the applied pressure.

No longer than 10 minutes after oral administration of the ^{99m}Tc–sulfur colloid solution, the patient is centered under the camera so that the stomach is positioned at the bottom of the field. The entire stomach must be included on all images. As pressure is increased with the abdominal binder, the stomach image is seen to rise, but immediate repositioning is not necessary unless the esophageal region is excluded from the field of view. If activity is seen in the esophagus during positioning, either a delay in esophageal clearance or a spontaneous reflux has occurred. An additional 30 ml of tap water should clear this activity.

Use of a parallel-hole collimator on a large–field-of-view camera is best, although a diverging collimator with a small–field-of-view camera may be used. Images are

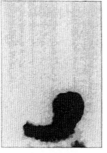
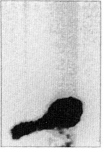
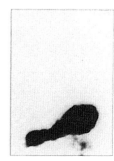

| 10 mm Hg | 15 mm Hg | 20 mm Hg |

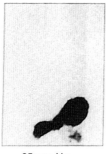
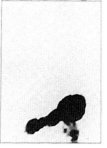
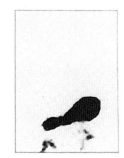

| 25 mm Hg | 30 mm Hg | 35 mm Hg |

FIGURE 18-15 Serial scans of a gastroesophageal reflux study in a normal individual. The resting pressure across the lower esophageal sphincter is 10 mm Hg, and with each successive inflation of the abdominal binder, a corresponding pressure increase of 5 mm Hg is seen across the lower esophageal sphincter. Throughout the study no gastroesophageal reflux is visualized.

acquired for 30 seconds at the following pressure points, which are obtained by inflating the abdominal binder: 0, 20, 40, 60, 80, and 100 mm Hg. A postdeflation image also is obtained. Increments of 20 mm Hg on the abdominal binder are successively applied while the sphygmomanometer attached to the binder is monitored (increments of 20 mm Hg applied externally have been shown to increase the pressure across the lower esophageal sphincter in increments of 5 mm Hg) (Figure 18-15). Images should be acquired as quickly as possible so that patient discomfort is not prolonged. It is important not to deflate the binder between successive stages of pressure. Most patients can tolerate pressure of 100 mm Hg, but it should be kept in mind that some patients cannot withstand this level because of debilitating surgery or their present symptoms.

It is best that a display monitor with a high persistence be used as a visual aid during the performance of the examination. Reflux can be visualized during the course of the test (Figure 18-16). Computer images might warrant adjustment of contrast in cases of subtle reflux. Subtly visualized activity in the esophagus has been shown to correspond to 3% to 4% of the 300 μCi ^{99m}Tc dose and can be used to confirm reflux. (In patients in whom the esophageal transit study is done before the gastroesophageal reflux study, a greater amount of activity will be noted in the stomach at the beginning of the examination.)

Patients with a known esophageal motor disorder or with a large hiatal hernia should have an endogastric

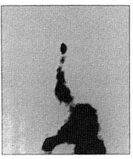

Patient with reflux

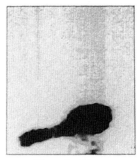

Normal subject

FIGURE 18-16 Anterior images of the thorax obtained in a patient with reflux and in a normal subject, respectively. An oscilloscope with a high persistence should be used as a visual aid during the performance of this examination, because reflux can be readily visualized on the oscilloscope face.

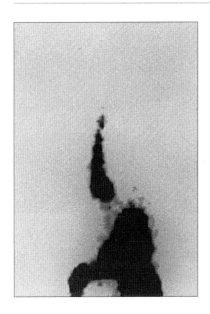
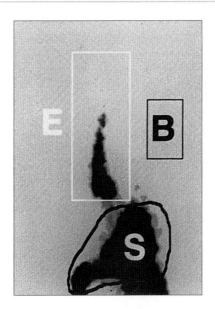

FIGURE 18-17 Anterior view of the thorax is recalled from the computer for analysis. Regions of interest are drawn for the esophagus *(top left)*, the stomach *(S)*, and the background *(B)*. Counts in each region of interest are recorded for each pressure level and then used to calculate the gastroesophageal reflux indices.

tube placed before performance of the reflux study. In this way the radiopharmaceutical solution can be delivered into the stomach through the tube, bypassing the esophagus. The tube can be flushed with 10 to 15 ml of tap water and removed before the imaging study is begun. This technique prevents retention of activity in the esophagus, which can be related to the motor disorder or hiatal hernia.

Computer analysis of this study is accomplished by recalling the separate images and drawing regions of interest for the stomach and esophagus (Figure 18-17). The counts in the stomach region of interest and in the esophageal region of interest are noted and used to calculate a gastroesophageal reflux index for each level of abdominal pressure using the following formula:

$$GERI = \left(\frac{E_p}{G_{max}} \right) \times 100$$

where GERI is the gastroesophageal reflux index in percent, E_p is the esophageal counts at a specific pressure point p, and G_{max} is the maximum gastric count obtained for one image in this study.

Clinical Aspects. A normal gastroesophageal reflux study has a reflux index of less than 4%; this is the level at which gastroesophageal reflux cannot be visualized (see Figure 18-16). An index greater than 4% is considered to be abnormal and usually can be visualized in the images (Figure 18-18). This quantitative feature is unique to the scintigraphic study and permits the evaluation of patients before and after medical or surgical therapy for gastroesophageal reflux.

Delayed images of the thorax can be obtained up to 24 hours to detect reflux leading to pulmonary aspiration (see Figure 18-14). This is particularly useful in children and infants, in whom the radionuclide solution can be delivered through intubation or by placing the radiopharmaceutical in a bottle with the infant's formula or juice. Radionuclide studies are superior to barium studies for diagnosing reflux in children, not only because of the lower radiation burden, but also because reflux occurs intermittently and fluoroscopy cannot be performed continuously because of its associated high radiation exposure.

STOMACH

The stomach is a J-shaped muscular pouch, located in the upper abdomen (Figure 18-19). It has three major roles: (1) it provides a reservoir for food; (2) it breaks down solid food into small particles that, when combined with its secretion of gastric juice, form a semiliquid mixture called *chyme;* and (3) it controls the rate of emptying of gastric content into the duodenum.

Anatomically, the stomach is divided in three regions: (1) the fundus (proximal portion to the gastroesophageal junction), (2) the corpus (between the gastroesophageal junction and the incisura angularis), and (3) the antrum (between the incisura angularis and the duodenum) (see Figure 18-19).

Physiologically, the human stomach consists of two integrated but electromechanically distinct parts: (1) the proximal stomach, which encompasses the fundus and the orad corpus; and (2) the distal stomach, which includes the mid and caudad corpus and the proximal, middle, and distal antrum. The proximal portion of the stomach is a reservoir for solid and liquid food. It controls emptying by generating a pressure gradient between the stomach and the duodenum. The distal stomach is the prime propeller, grinder, and sieve of solid food and is characterized by phasic peristaltic waves that spread out circumferentially from the corpus to the pylorus at a rate of three contractions per minute.

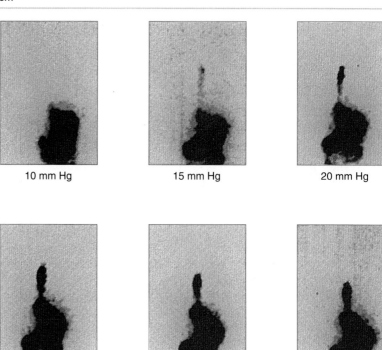

10 mm Hg   15 mm Hg   20 mm Hg

25 mm Hg   30 mm Hg   35 mm Hg

FIGURE 18-18 Anterior views of the thorax illustrating an abnormal examination result. With progressive inflation of the abdominal binder, causing incremental pressure increases of 5 mm Hg across the lower esophageal sphincter, an increase in the amount of induced gastroesophageal reflux is seen.

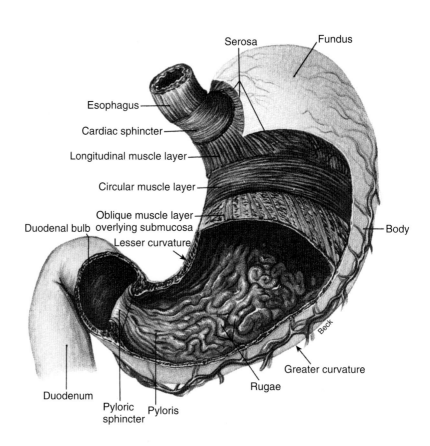

FIGURE 18-19 Stomach regions and structure.

Gastric emptying is a complex process affected by the physical and chemical composition of the ingested meal, the intrinsic and extrinsic nervous innervation of the stomach, and circulating neuroendocrine transmitters. The rate of gastric emptying is determined by many factors including the volume, physical state, caloric content, caloric density, concentration of nutrients, meal distribution, salinity, acidity, and viscosity of the test meal used.

The main determinant of the rate of liquid gastric emptying is volume. Saline, neutral, isosmolar, and calorically inert solutions (such as water) empty in a single exponential manner. Gastric emptying of liquids is precisely controlled by osmolytes, acid, fatty acids (particularly medium-chains), and carbohydrate and protein receptors along the small bowel. These receptors limit the rate at which food enters the duodenum either by release of intestinal hormones or by triggering neural receptors and autonomic reflexes.

The gastric emptying curve for solid food is sigmoidal and characterized by (1) an initial **lag phase** during which no or little solid is evacuated, (2) a prolonged phase with a constant emptying rate, and (3) a late, much slower phase, when the stomach is nearly empty. Gastric emptying is very sensitive to intestinal feedback inhibition during the lag phase and rather insensitive to solid nutrients entering the bowel during the prolonged linear period. The physical characteristics of solid foods determine their lag phase duration and emptying rate. Preground food is evacuated quickly, without any lag phase, and small particles empty faster than larger ones[51]. High-calorie meals increase the lag phase and decrease the emptying rate of solids.[49] An increase of solid emptying due to increased volume is overridden by intestinal inhibition as additional calories enter the small intestine. High nutritive density (number of calories per volume unit) decreases the volume emptied. Isocaloric concentrations of fat, carbohydrate, and protein produce an equal slowing of gastric emptying.

With a combined solid-liquid test meal, liquids empty much more rapidly than solids, but at a slower rate than if given alone. The rapid passage of water from the stomach while solid is retained has been popularly designated as *solid-liquid discrimination*.[34]

The symptoms of gastric stasis include nausea, vomiting, postprandial bloating, epigastric pain, and early satiation. Early or late postprandial anxiety, weakness, dizziness, tachycardia, sweating, and flushing can occur with rapid emptying and constitute the so-called *dumping syndrome*. *Dyspepsia* refers to the whole constellation of gastric symptoms such as abdominal pain or discomfort, early satiety, fullness, distension, bloating, nausea, vomiting, belching, and epigastric or retrosternal burning. It is very common in the normal adult population, with 38% of patients reporting a history of dyspeptic symptoms in the last 6 months. Dyspepsia also accounts for 3% to 4% of visits to general practitioners. The pathophysiology of dyspepsia remains unclear and complex. Objective detailed evaluation does not necessarily establish a dominant etiological factor. Based on the presence or the absence of underlying structural and/or biochemical abnormalities, dyspepsia has been categorized as either organic or functional.

Whereas a large variety of methods including intubative techniques, barium x-rays, ultrasound, computed tomography (CT), magnetic resonance imaging (MRI), epigastric impedance, breath tests, and scintigraphy have all been used to assess gastric emptying, the major

advantages of scintigraphy include (1) the digital acquisition and quantification of the data, (2) the use of a physiological test meal, (3) the potential for simultaneous measurement of both solid and liquid emptying, (4) the noninvasiveness of the test, (5) the low radiation burden permitting repetitive testing, and (6) the ability to analyze fundal, antral, and overall gastric motility.

Numerous methods[11,12,32] have been proposed for a simultaneous radionuclide study of the liquid and solid components of a meal using different radionuclide labels for the solid and liquid portions of the test meal and dual isotope counting. Because the rate of gastric emptying varies with meal size, each laboratory must standardize meal size and composition according to the amount of carbohydrate, fat, protein, nondigestible solids, and caloric content. A wide variety of meals including meat, potatoes, porridge, pancakes, cornflakes, chicken liver, eggs, French toast, and chemical resins have been used.[9,21,35,52] Indium-111 (^{111}In) and ^{99m}Tc are the radionuclides most often used, because they are well suited for imaging with the scintillation camera. Adequate images and good counting statistics can be achieved with small doses, and the radiation burden to the patient is kept to a minimum.[42]

The simplest approach to measurement of gastric emptying with the scintillation camera involves giving a dual solid/liquid labeled test meal and serially imaging and plotting anterior count rates from the stomach with the patient either upright or supine (Figures 18-20 to 18-22). Corrections for attenuation, physical decay, and downscatter from ^{111}In in the ^{99m}Tc window may be necessary to measure accurately the amount of activity remaining in the stomach during the study.[11] This is particularly true because the examination may continue over several hours. Therefore each laboratory must perform its own phantom studies to determine the appropriate correction factors.

Conventional gastric emptying is a simple procedure that measures the transit of a standardized radiolabeled test meal through the stomach; it requires static imaging at defined time intervals, minimal processing, and analysis. Conventional gastric emptying provides little information on gastric physiology and pathophysiology. Over the past 15 years, mathematical modeling of the gastric emptying curves, compartmental analysis of the stomach, and more recently dynamic antral scintigraphy (DAS) have provided new tools to evaluate the pathophysiology of gastric motor disorders.

Imaging Procedure

Gastric emptying is performed after a 12-hour overnight fast and discontinuation of any medication likely to interfere with gastric motility. Patients should refrain from smoking since it may delay gastric evacuation. Diabetic patients should be studied early in the morning, after receiving two thirds of their usual insulin dose.

Dual phase radionuclide gastric emptying study

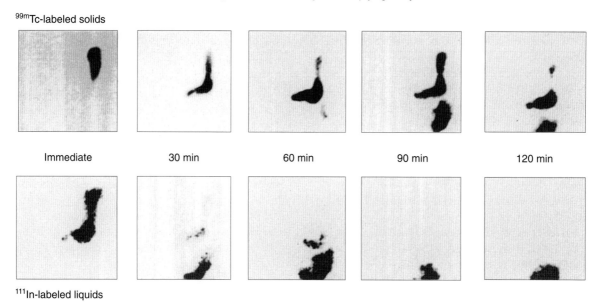

FIGURE 18-20 Dual isotope gastric scintigraphy. Anterior images of the abdomen obtained in a normal subject after oral administration of a scrambled egg sandwich prepared with ^{99m}Tc–sulfur colloid and the liquid portion consisting of ^{111}In-DTPA in water. Images were obtained for 1 minute at regular intervals at both ^{99m}Tc and ^{111}In window settings. Note the emptying of both liquids and solids from the stomach.

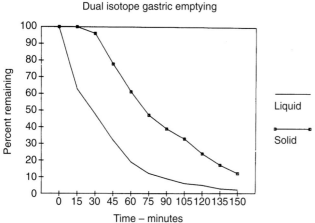

FIGURE 18-21 Normal dual isotope gastric emptying. Time-activity curves for both liquids and solids are graphed as percentage remaining as a function of time. Note emptying of both liquids and solids. These data are from the same individual used for Figure 18-20.

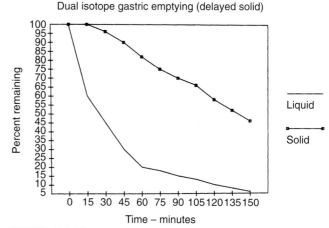

FIGURE 18-22 Abnormal dual isotope gastric emptying curves, generated for the patient in Figure 18-24. When compared with the normal curve study, liquids empty normally, whereas solids are delayed.

There is currently no consensus on the optimal test meal to study gastric emptying. However, radiolabeled eggs, which are readily available, easy to prepare, and stably labeled are used in most nuclear medicine laboratories. The eggs are mixed with 20 to 40 MBq (0.5 to 1.0 mCi) ^{99m}Tc–sulfur colloid, cooked until firm in a Teflon-coated pan, and given to the patient as an egg sandwich. To evaluate liquid emptying, 3 MBq (75 µCi) of ^{111}In-DTPA is administered orally with water. Ingestion of the test meal should be completed within 10 minutes.

Imaging is preferably performed with the subject sitting or standing. A ^{57}Co marker placed on the xiphoid process or iliac crest facilitates repositioning of the patient and automated processing. Immediately after the completion of the meal, the patient is positioned in front of the camera fitted with a medium-energy, parallel-hole collimator. An initial 1-minute image of the stomach is acquired in the 140-keV ± 20% technetium window. The patient then ingests the water and a second 1-minute image is taken in the technetium window to calculate the downscatter percentage of indium into the technetium window.

Simultaneous anterior and posterior static images (dual-head system), or an anterior, immediately followed by a posterior, view (single-head system) of the stomach are taken in a 64 × 64 or 128 × 128 matrix in the technetium and indium windows at regular time intervals up to 50% emptying. Depth attenuation must be corrected for by calculation of the geometric mean (i.e., the square root of the anterior activity multiplied by the posterior activity) of gastric counts. Counts are then corrected for

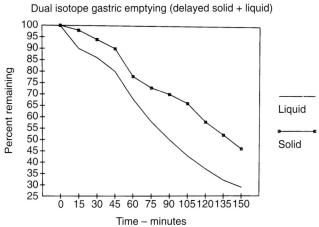

FIGURE 18-23 Abnormal dual isotope gastric emptying curves (same patient as Figure 18-25). Retention of both liquids and solids is seen during the course of the examination. Compare with normal subject in Figure 18-21.

decay and downscatter, and normalized to 100% based on total gastric counts obtained immediately following ingestion of the meal (time [t] = 0). Solid and liquid data are then plotted as percentage retention of food in the stomach over time (Figures 18-23 to 18-25). The procedure steps are found in Box 18-1.

Measurement of the **gastric half emptying time** ($t_{1/2}$), or time required by the stomach to empty 50% of the ingested meal, is the simplest way to assess gastric transit. It is routinely and commonly used for clinical evaluation. Modeling of gastric emptying curves can be used to quantitate the emptying of the test meal component(s). Liquid emptying curves are usually adequately described by the single exponential function $y = e^{-kt}$ In this equation, $y(t)$ is the fractional meal retention at time t, and k the emptying rate (in minutes) − 1; $t_{1/2}$ is equal to ln 2/k.

Gastric emptying of solids is sigmoid in shape and characterized by an initial shoulder with little emptying (lag phase, or t_{lag}), followed by a prolonged linear phase and finally a much slower phase. The lag phase corresponds qualitatively and quantitatively to the redistribution of solid food particles from the fundus to the distal stomach and more specifically to the time to peak activity in the distal stomach.[51] The modified power exponential function (Figure 18-26) adequately fits biphasic solid emptying data: $y(t) = (1 - [1 - e^{-kt}]^{\beta})$ where $y(t)$ is the fractional meal retention at time t, k is the gastric emptying rate (in minutes^{-1}), and β is the extrapolated y-intercept from the terminal portion of the curve. The

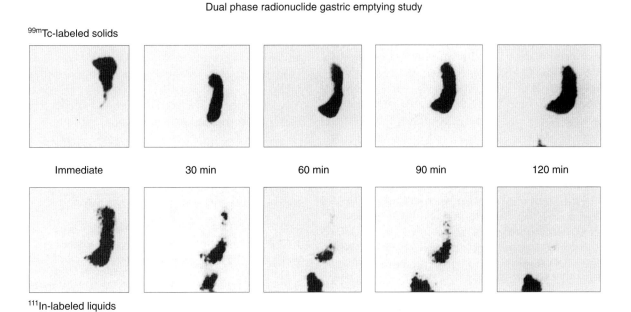

FIGURE 18-24 Abnormal dual isotope gastric scintigraphy. Anterior images of the abdomen were obtained in this patient with delayed emptying of solids and normal emptying of liquids. Compare images with normal individual in Figure 18-20.

Dual phase radionuclide gastric emptying study

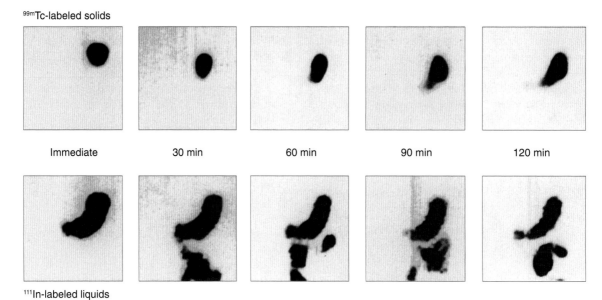

^{99m}Tc-labeled solids

| Immediate | 30 min | 60 min | 90 min | 120 min |

^{111}In-labeled liquids

Abnormal patient—delayed emptying of solids
and delayed emptying of liquids

FIGURE 18-25 Abnormal dual isotope gastric scintigraphy. Anterior images of abdomen obtained at 30-minute intervals reveal delayed emptying of both liquids and solids. Compare with normal individual in Figure 18-20.

| BOX 18-1 | Gastric Emptying Procedure |

1. Have the patient fast for 12 hr.
2. Prepare the test meal as per laboratory protocol.
3. Ask the patient to eat the test meal within 10 min.
4. Enter the imaging acquisition parameters into the computer to acquire anterior and posterior views of the stomach and abdomen into a 128 × 128 matrix.
5. Acquire images at time zero (immediately after meal ingestion) and at regular time intervals until 50% emptying. An alternative is to follow the Society of Nuclear Medicine guidelines with static images at 0, 1, 2, and 4 hr as described by Abell and colleagues.[1] The percent retention at each time is then reported and compared to normal values.
6. Using ROIs, determine the stomach counts in the stomach on each image.
7. Correct ROI counts for isotope decay (^{99m}Tc).
8. Perform geometric mean calculation to compensate for movement of gastric radioactivity.
9. Calculate half-emptying time or percent retention in the stomach at each time point.
10. Compute these data points in the appropriate software program to generate a gastric emptying curve with the % of meal remaining in the stomach (y-axis) over time (x-axis)
11. Fit the gastric emptying curve with the appropriate fitting function to determine the lag phase (solid meal) and the half emptying time ($t_{1/2}$; solid and liquid meals).

ROI, Region of interest.

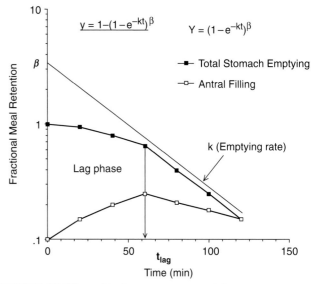

$$y = 1-(1-e^{-kt})^{\beta}$$

$$Y = (1-e^{-kt})^{\beta}$$

■ Total Stomach Emptying
□ Antral Filling

k (Emptying rate)

Lag phase

Fractional Meal Retention

t_{lag}

Time (min)

FIGURE 18-26 Modified power exponential function representation. This fitting function allows for the calculation of the lag phase (t_{lag}), emptying rate (k) and half emptying time for solid emptying. β is the extrapolated y-intercept from the terminal portion of the curve. The lag phase is numerically equal to ln β/k and corresponds to the inflection point of the total gastric emptying curve and to the peak antral filling.

parameters k and β are determined by a nonlinear least-squares algorithm using the measured fractional retention $y(t)$ and time t as input. Four parameters can be derived from the gastric emptying curve: (1) the β value (the initial shoulder); (2) t_{lag}, in minutes; (3) the emptying rate, in percent of emptying per minute; and (4) the half emptying time $(t_{1/2})$, in minutes.

Recently a consensus document has been published relating to the performance of gastric emptying studies and the analysis of data. This document, published in the *Journal of Nuclear Medicine Technology*[1] recommends the meal composition and meal size, imaging techniques, and data analysis and interpretation procedures that should be followed to produce normal data that can be compared to accepted expert values. This standardized protocol recommends a meal of the equivalent of two large eggs, two slices of toast with jam and water. Imaging is performed at 0, 1, 2 and 4 hrs and the percent meal retention in the stomach is reported for geometric mean, decay corrected data. Any variations in meal content, meal size, imaging times, region of interest (ROI) definition, data analysis techniques, and so on, will all change the resultant data and percent retention at various imaging times or half-emptying time values.

Clinical Aspects

Diabetes Mellitus. Rapid gastric emptying can be observed in the early stages of diabetic autonomic neuropathy. Delay in solid gastric emptying is very common in symptomatic and asymptomatic longstanding diabetes. This delay is essentially due to a prolonged lag phase while the emptying rate is preserved. Advanced gastroparesis is characterized by a markedly prolonged gastric emptying, with a linear solid emptying curve. A prolonged lag period with a normal $t_{1/2}$ has also been recently described in patients with longstanding disease.[50] Liquid emptying is only abnormal when solid food emptying is severely impaired.

Idiopathic Dyspepsia. In functional dyspepsia associated with gastroparesis, there is a prolonged lag phase and slow emptying rate that reflects the retention of food in the distal stomach.

Gastric Surgery. In patients with partial gastrectomy, such as the Roux-en-Y anastomosis, there is an initial precipitous emptying followed by a slow evacuation phase, resulting in a delay in both solid and liquid emptying. There is no lag phase, and both liquids and solids empty in a similar fashion.[48]

Compartmental Analysis of the Stomach

Scintigraphy, like electrophysiological and manometric studies, allows for the characterization of the respective role of the proximal and distal stomach in the gastric emptying process. To that effect, distinct regions of interest are drawn over the proximal and distal stomach.

Food retention in each compartment is normalized to the total maximum gastric activity at time zero and displayed on time-activity curves. In normal subjects, total and proximal liquid gastric curves are almost identical because there is no retention of liquid in the distal stomach. In contrast, solids are retained in the stomach by the pylorus, and the distal stomach emptying curve for solids takes an asymmetrical bell-shaped pattern. In diabetic gastroparesis, there is a significant retention of food in the proximal stomach, which might correspond to a decrease in fundic motor activity.[50] In contrast, patients with functional dyspepsia with or without gastroparesis display a normal proximal stomach emptying, which corroborates the normal electromechanical findings.[47]

SMALL BOWEL AND COLON

The small intestine is a lengthy, hollow tube extending from the pyloric sphincter of the stomach to the ileocecal valve at the large intestine. The small intestine is divided into the duodenum, the jejunum, and the ileum (see Figure 18-1). It is responsible for digestion and absorption of all nutrients in the body. The inner lining of the small intestine contains glands that secrete intestinal digestive enzymes. The lining is also especially adapted for absorption of all needed nutrients; microvilli cover the entire 20-foot length of the small intestine.

The large intestine, or colon, extends from the ileocecal valve to the anus. The large intestine is divided into the cecum, ascending colon, transverse colon, descending colon, sigmoid colon, and rectum (see Figure 18-1). Very little absorption of nutrients occurs in the large intestine, with the notable exception of some vitamins. The major function of the large intestine is reabsorption of water; this results in the formation of fecal material, which is expelled through the anus.

Colon Transit

Studies of colonic transit are difficult to perform because the colon is relatively difficult to access noninvasively and the techniques used are time-consuming. Methods using oral tracers are dependent upon gastric emptying and small bowel transit. Radiopaque markers used for serial radiographic imaging of the abdomen are at best semiquantitative and nonphysiological.

Imaging Procedure. Patients are asked to discontinue any medications likely to affect colon transit for at least 3 days before the test. No dietary change is needed. The study should not be performed within the 4 weeks following a colonoscopy. Because of the physical half-life of ^{111}In, oral administration of ^{111}In-DTPA is the most commonly used radionuclide to assess colon transit. It can be administered in encapsulated nondigestible capsules, plastic particles, or methylacrylate-coated resin particles that dissolve in the ileocecal region. However, the easiest method consists of the oral administration of 4 MBq (100 μCi) of ^{111}In-DTPA in water.

Imaging is typically performed at 6, 24, 48, 72, and 96 hours following the oral administration of ^{111}In-DTPA. Anterior and posterior images of the abdomen are obtained for 10 minutes, using a large–field-of-view camera with medium-energy collimator. Different methods exist to analyze colon transit images. The simplest method consists of determining the percentage of retention in each colonic segment (cecum, ascending, transverse, descending colon, and rectosigmoid colon) over time and calculating the time required to clear 50% of the initial radioactivity. Quantitation of residual activity in the different colonic regions at 4 and 24 hours provides accurate colon transit information. Colon transit time can also been assessed by the condensed images technique.

The geometric-mean-center (GMC) technique is now widely used to determine the segmental emptying of the anatomical regions of the colon.[29] To calculate the GMC, the colon is divided into numbered anatomical regions: cecum and ascending colon (region 1), hepatic flexure (region 2), transverse colon (region 3), splenic flexure (region 4), descending colon (region 5), rectosigmoid region (6), and excreted stool (region 7). The geometric center is the weighted average of the proportion of total colon counts in each region (Figure 18-27). Therefore a low geometric center (1 to 2) indicates that the majority

of the radiolabel is closer to the cecum. A higher value (5 to 7) indicates that most of the activity has progressed to the left side of the colon or has been eliminated as stool.

Clinical Aspects. In normal subjects the ascending colon empties in a linear manner after an initial lag phase suggesting its storage role. Periods of no emptying alternating with periods of emptying can be observed. A linear progression through the colon is also demonstrated when using the GMC analysis. Solid or liquid tracers produce similar patterns of colon transit. Significant interstudy variability in transit can be observed. Colon transit is slower and more variable in females than in males, but there is no effect of aging. In patients with idiopathic constipation, the GMC analysis makes it possible to differentiate colonic inertia from pelvic obstruction of defecation. Colonic inertia is a pancolonic disorder characterized by a very slow transit throughout the entire length of the colon, in patients with significant stasis of radioactivity in the esophagus. In contrast, obstructed defecation is associated with an abnormal retention in the rectosigmoid.

The most common clinical application of colon transit scintigraphy is the evaluation of patients with idiopathic constipation and the effect of the prokinetic drugs such as cisapride or naloxone.

Whole-Gut Transit

Several methods have been proposed to investigate **whole-gut transit,** the entire GI tract (gastric emptying, small bowel, and colonic transit), in a single test. At Temple University Hospital, ^{111}In-DTPA in water is given with a solid meal. The egg sandwich (discussed under Imaging Procedure) is labeled with ^{99m}Tc to simultaneously study gastric emptying of solids. In normal subjects, water empties from the stomach rapidly (90% within 2 hours) and a geometric mean of abdominal counts is obtained at 2 to 3 hours to determine 100% of the administered ^{111}In-DTPA activity. This determination enables us to generate terminal ileum filling rates as well as the input bolus into the colon to measure the GMC. Whole-gut transit techniques may be of limited value in patients with severe gastroparesis, particularly when liquid emptying is markedly delayed, leading to delays in the more distal gut.

INTESTINAL TRACT

Gastrointestinal Bleeding

During the past 20 years, the management of patients with acute gastrointestinal bleeding has changed dramatically. The widespread availability of upper and lower GI endoscopy and the progress in interventional radiology and embolization techniques have given nuclear medicine a new role in the diagnostic and

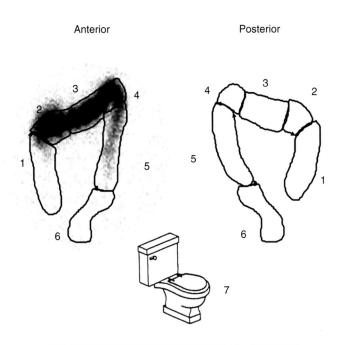

Anterior   Posterior

Geometric Center = Σ ROI ι $_{(1-7)}$ / Total Counts × ι $_{(1-7)}$ = 3.1

FIGURE 18-27 Calculation of the geometric center of a colonic transit study. On this image the geometric center was calculated at 3.1. *1,* Cecum and ascending colon; *2,* hepatic flexure; *3,* transverse colon; *4,* splenic flexure; *5,* descending colon; *6,* recto-sigmoid colon; *7,* stools; *ROI,* region of interest.

therapeutic algorithms of GI bleeding. Acute bleeding scans are performed in patients with active lower GI bleeding to evaluate the presence of the bleed and, more importantly, to localize the site of bleeding before selective catheterization and embolization or surgery.[28]

Technetium-99m heat-treated red blood cells (RBCs) and ^{99m}Tc–sulfur colloid techniques have for the most part been replaced by non–heat-treated ^{99m}Tc-labeled RBC procedures for performing GI bleeding studies. Both in vivo and in vitro RBC-labeling methods are now available. In vivo labeling using the injection of stannous ion followed 20 to 30 minutes later by ^{99m}Tc-pertechnetate is convenient and easy to perform. However, labeling efficiency is variable and inconsistent, varying from 60% to 90%. When present in significant amount, free pertechnetate is secreted by the gastric mucosa and the kidneys. This may interfere significantly with the ability to detect a bleed in the stomach, proximal small bowel, and/or colon. The in vivo/vitro technique consists of the intravenous (IV) administration of the stannous ion, the ^{99m}Tc-pertechnetate labeling of a blood sample collected in a syringe containing an anticoagulant and ^{99m}Tc-pertechnetate, and the reinjection of the labeled sample. The labeling efficiency approaches 95%. The absence of blood manipulation and risk of contamination is a significant advantage of these two techniques. In the in vitro technique, a sample of blood is withdrawn from the patient and an anticoagulant and stannous solution are added. Sodium hypochlorite and acid-citrate-dextrose (ACD) solution are then added to oxidize the extracellular stannous ion. Technetium-99m-pertechnetate is added to the blood sample and diffuses into the RBCs, where it is reduced and trapped. Labeling efficiency is high and image quality appears superior.[33]

Technetium-99m–sulfur colloid has the advantage of minimizing background activity and promoting the highest contrast ratios. However, its rapid clearance requires that the patient be actively bleeding at the time of injection (or within minutes after injection). Non–heat-treated ^{99m}Tc-labeled RBCs, with their prolonged retention in the intravascular pool, are preferred by investigators who maintain that GI bleeding is most often intermittent and slow. In addition, they allow repetitive imaging for up to 36 hours after injection with a far lower radiation dose to the liver and spleen and have the ability to detect GI bleeding better in the upper abdominal region.

Imaging Procedure

^{99m}**Tc–Sulfur Colloid Technique.** The patient is placed supine under a large–field-of-view scintillation camera equipped with a low-energy, parallel-hole collimator so that the view includes the inferior margin of the liver to the symphysis pubis. Freshly made ^{99m}Tc–sulfur colloid (7 to 10 mCi) is injected as an IV bolus, and an anterior flow study of the abdomen is obtained at 1 to 2 sec/frame

for 2 to 3 minutes. Thereafter 500,000- to 750,000-count anterior images of the abdomen are obtained every 1 to 2 minutes for 20 to 30 minutes at intensity settings such that the bone marrow can be visualized. If an area of bleeding is identified, more detailed views of that area can be obtained with oblique, lateral, or posterior views. If no bleeding site is identified at the end of 30 minutes, a 1 million–count image of the upper abdomen is obtained with oblique views to better delineate the hepatic and splenic flexures. If these views are negative, repeat lower abdominal views can be obtained in 15 to 20 minutes to check for activity that may have been obscured in the areas of the hepatic and splenic flexures by liver and spleen activity. Any bowel movements by the patient during the course of the study should be scanned in the bedpan to ensure that a very low rectal source of bleeding has not been obscured by genital activity. If the scan result is negative, repeat injections of the tracer may be necessary if clinical evidence exists of renewed active bleeding.

The flow study clearly delineates the aorta and other vascular structures, including the liver, spleen, kidneys, and small and large bowel. As the ^{99m}Tc–sulfur colloid clears the intravascular space, it accumulates in the liver and spleen and bone marrow and fades from the vascular structures. The genital areas have a significant accumulation of the ^{99m}Tc–sulfur colloid, and a lateral view may be helpful to avoid confusion with a possible source of lower rectal bleeding. If a fresh preparation of ^{99m}Tc–sulfur colloid is used, renal and bladder activity will be minimized, because the amount of free ^{99m}Tc will be less than 2%.

Care should be taken in positioning the patient so that only small margins of the liver and spleen are seen in the images. This brings out any activity in the abdominal cavity.

^{99m}**Tc-Labeled Red Blood Cells Procedure.** After the IV administration of the ^{99m}Tc-labeled RBCs, sequential sets of 15-minute continuous dynamic study with 15-second framing for a total of 60 images is acquired in a 128 × 128 byte matrix. Every 15 minutes, the acquisition is saved at completion. The study is stopped when the bleeding site is identified. If the patient is not bleeding during the initial hour following the administration of the labeled red cells, the study is terminated. Patients can be brought back to the department within the next 24 hours for additional imaging if an acute onset of recurrent bleeding occurs. Procedure steps are listed in Box 18-2.

Clinical Aspects. Using ^{99m}Tc–sulfur colloid, areas of active bleeding may be seen on the flow study, but they are more commonly identified after the first 5 minutes. They usually appear as focal areas of increased activity that can become more intense with time as background activity decreases. Because blood is both a stimulant and an irritant in the bowel, the activity can pass more quickly through the colon. Retrograde motion that can occur may make localization of the site of bleeding difficult. Both arterial and venous bleeding can be identified from both small and large bowel sources. False-positive results can occur if there is asymmetrical bone marrow accumulation of the tracer, as can be seen with replacement of marrow by tumor, after radiation therapy, or as a result of some other pathological process, such as Paget disease. In such cases, the area of involvement has decreased uptake, and the more normal-appearing area on the other side of the abdomen may possibly be misinterpreted as an area of bleeding. False-positive study results can also occur in renal transplants, which accumulate ^{99m}Tc–sulfur colloid during rejection.

BOX 18-2 | **Gastrointestinal Bleeding Procedure**

1. Prepare the ^{99m}Tc–sulfur colloid injection or label the patient's red blood cells (RBCs) per laboratory protocol.
2. Place the patient supine under the camera to include the inferior margin of the liver at the top of the field of view.
3. For studies with ^{99m}Tc–sulfur colloid, the acquisition should include a flow phase with 1-2 sec/frame for about 2 min followed by 500,000-750,000 counts images every 1-2 min for 20-30 min (128 × 128 or 256 × 256 matrix).
4. Inject the ^{99m}Tc–sulfur colloid and start acquisition.
5. Additional views might be needed if a site of bleeding is identified.
6. For ^{99m}Tc–labeled RBC studies, place the patient to visualize the entire abdomen and acquire 4 sequential sets of 15 min continuous dynamic imaging at a rate of 15 sec/frame in a 128 × 128 matrix.
7. When using ^{99m}Tc–labeled RBCs, consider delay imaging up to 24 hr delayed images if no bleeding is seen on the early images.

Using the non–heat-treated ^{99m}Tc-labeled RBC method, the flow study outlines the great vessels of the abdomen and the general position of the kidneys, spleen, small and large bowel, and genital organs (particularly in women, when the uterus may be highly vascularized). Occasionally, if marked bleeding is occurring, it can be seen on the flow study. Additionally, vascular tumors can be seen as abnormal tracer collections on the arterial phase that disappear during the venous phase. An abnormal scan demonstrates a focus of tracer activity, which usually becomes more intense with time and is not related to normal abdominal structures (Figure 18-28). Generally speaking, the tagged RBC method can identify colonic bleeding more easily than small-bowel bleeding sites. If early views are negative and only delayed views show activity in the cecum, it may be difficult to pinpoint the site of bleeding, because bleeding may have occurred in the upper small bowel, right side of the colon, or transverse colon and merely collected in the cecum. This is especially true if suboptimum RBC labeling has occurred and gastric activity is noted on the initial views. False-positive results may occur if anatomical variants of vascular structures are present in the abdomen.

With labeled RBCs, bleeding rate detection varies from 0.05 to 0.1 ml/min depending on the efficiency of the labeling procedure and other technical and processing factors. The cine display of the continuous dynamic set of images allows in most cases for the visualization and the precise localization of the bleeding site by tracking down the progression of blood within the bowel. If active bleeding is not identified during the first hour, delayed views at 2-, 4-, and 6-hour intervals can be obtained as clinically suggested by changes in vital signs or evidence of recurrent bright red blood per rectum.

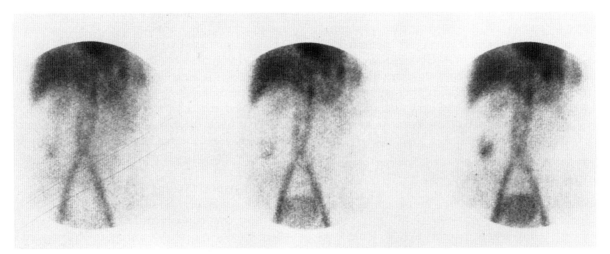

FIGURE 18-28 ^{99m}Tc–labeled red blood cell study. Anterior views of the abdomen were obtained to visualize an intermittent bleeding site. In this patient, images were obtained at approximately 5-minute intervals. Progressive accumulation of the tagged red blood cells is seen in the right lower quadrant of the abdomen, with apparent tracking of these cells in the ascending colon toward the hepatic flexure. Note the structures normally visualized with this method: the liver, spleen, abdominal vessels, kidneys, bladder, and stomach.

Delayed views for up to 36 hours after injection can be obtained with good results.

If the patient is bleeding profusely, a quick transfer is organized, either to interventional radiology for selective catheterization and embolization or to the operating room for surgery.

Meckel Diverticulum

Meckel diverticulum, a congenital defect in which a small sac forms in the ileum, is a common cause of GI tract bleeding in children. Meckel diverticulum imaging is most frequently performed on children. The acute remnant is a small invagination of the intestine that can contain gastric mucosa. Bleeding is the presenting symptom in almost three fourths of patients, but other symptoms may include inflammation, obstruction, intussusception, or perforation of the bowel. Most Meckel diverticula are located in the ileum, usually within 1 m of the ileocecal valve. Most patients with GI bleeding are found to have gastric parietal cells in the Meckel diverticulum. These cells cause peptic ulceration of the bowel by acid secretion.

Technetium-99m-pertechnetate concentrates in gastric mucosa and can be used to detect and localize a symptomatic Meckel diverticulum (Figure 18-29). Since this disease most often occurs in children, the details of this procedure may be found in Chapter 22.

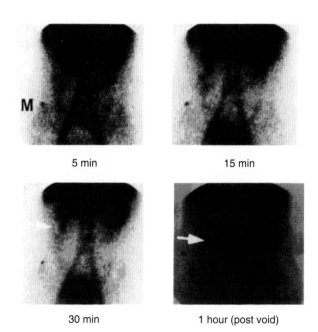

5 min   15 min

30 min   1 hour (post void)

Anterior views of abdomen following premedication with
H-2 blocker and pentagastrin, and 25 mCi ^{99m}Tc pertechnetate IV

FIGURE 18-29 Meckel diverticulum in the right side of the abdomen. The patient received H_2 blockers for 2 days before the study, and 20 minutes before the examination pentagastrin was given. Progressive accumulation of the radiotracer is seen in the diverticulum *(arrow)*. M, Marker at right iliac crest.

Barrett Esophagus

The presence of ectopic gastric mucosa in the distal esophagus is called *Barrett esophagus.* Scintigraphic detection of this ectopic gastric mucosa in the distal esophagus was proposed because the parietal cells contained in gastric mucosa are known to concentrate ^{99m}Tc-pertechnetate. However, scintigraphy can only support the diagnosis of Barrett esophagus; mucosal biopsy still is necessary to confirm it. With the widespread use of fiber-optic endoscopy, use of this examination has declined. However, it may still serve as an aid in locating a more specific region for biopsy.

Imaging Procedure. The patient should fast for 2 hours before the examination. Technetium-99m-pertechnetate (5 mCi) is given intravenously. Dental sponges are placed in the oral cavity to prevent the patient from swallowing pertechnetate excreted in the saliva and to avoid confusion of the origin of esophageal activity. The patient then is placed in a sitting position with the anterior chest against a large–field-of-view camera with a parallel-hole collimator. Images are acquired at 5-minute intervals for 30 minutes.

Prior administration of atropine or atropine-like compounds or administration of potassium perchlorate is to be avoided. These agents are known to reduce uptake of pertechnetate ions by gastric mucosa.

Clinical Aspects. Normally, activity is visualized only in the stomach and salivary glands. Pertechnetate activity above the level of the diaphragm suggests the presence of ectopic gastric mucosa in the distal esophagus. Barrett esophagus is associated with dyspepsia, esophagitis, and upper GI bleeding. Gastric mucosal imaging has also been used for preoperative diagnosis of pulmonary and mediastinal enterogenous cysts containing gastric mucosa.

LIVER AND SPLEEN

The liver is a solid, lobulated organ located in the right upper quadrant of the abdomen beneath the right side of the diaphragm (Figure 18-30). In an adult male, the liver weighs about 1800 g and is divided into two principal lobes, the right lobe and the left lobe, which are separated by the falciform ligament. The inferior quadrate and posterior caudate lobes are associated with the right lobe. The configuration of the normal liver varies widely; however, the right lobe generally is larger than the left.

The liver is composed of two major cell populations, the reticuloendothelial cells (Kupffer cells) and hepatocytes. The hepatocytes perform a variety of functions, among them the conversion of bilirubin to bile. The hepatocytes secrete bile into small canaliculi that empty into the intrahepatic ducts, which merge to become the common hepatic duct. The common hepatic duct joins the cystic duct of the gallbladder to form the common

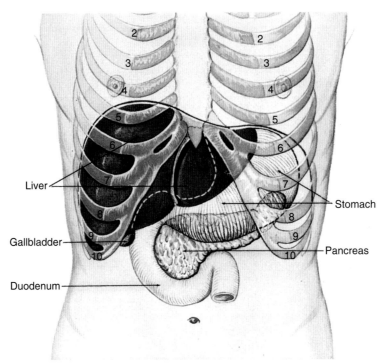

FIGURE 18-30 Liver in its normal position relative to the rib cage, diaphragm, stomach, and pancreas.

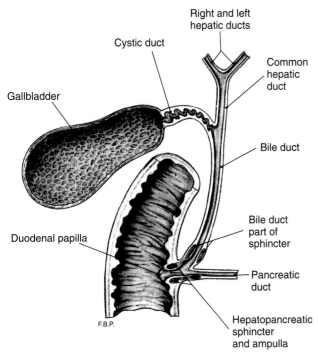

FIGURE 18-31 Schematic representation of extrahepatic biliary apparatus.

bile duct, which drains into the duodenum via the ampulla of Vater (Figure 18-31).

The liver possesses a dual blood supply: arterial oxygenated blood is received from the hepatic artery, which is a branch of the abdominal aorta, and venous blood draining from the intestines is carried through the hepatic portal vein into the liver. The hepatic portal system carries nutrients absorbed from the intestines into the liver for processing by hepatocytes.

The spleen is an oval mass of lymphatic tissue located in the left upper quadrant of the abdomen. It is situated between the fundus of the stomach and the left half of the diaphragm. The spleen is part of the reticuloendothelial system but not part of the gastrointestinal system.

Liver and Spleen Scintigraphy

Before the advent of fast (spiral) and multidetector CT,[2] liver and spleen scintigraphy had been the only noninvasive imaging modality available for the evaluation of functional liver diseases that involve the Kupffer cells, such as cirrhosis, hepatitis, and metabolic disorders. Liver and spleen scintigraphy remains of use for the evaluation of hepatomegaly, chronic liver diseases, focal nodular hyperplasia, liver enzyme abnormalities of uncertain cause, functional asplenia, ectopic spleen, and accessory splenic tissue after splenectomy.

The large–field-of-view scintillation camera allows simultaneous imaging of the liver and spleen in most patients. Approximately 1 million counts should be obtained in the anterior image of the liver and spleen and other projection views should be acquired for this same time.

Technetium-99m–sulfur colloid and ^99mTc–albumin colloid are the radiopharmaceuticals most commonly used for imaging the liver and spleen. However, this study can be combined with other imaging agents to raise the specificity of detection of certain lesions.

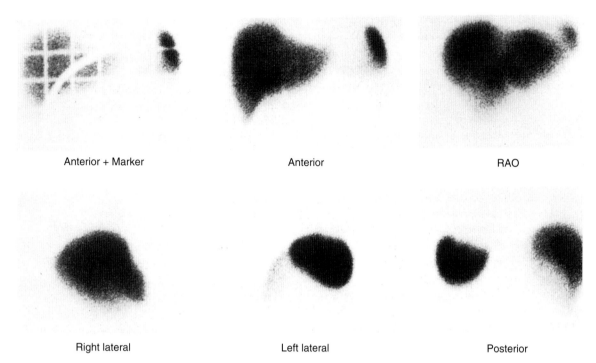

Anterior + Marker   Anterior   RAO

Right lateral   Left lateral   Posterior

FIGURE 18-32 Normal ^{99m}Tc–sulfur colloid liver and spleen scan demonstrating the size and costal margin marker image and the anterior, right anterior oblique *(RAO)*, right lateral, left lateral, and posterior projections. The size of the lead grid is 5 cm between bars. Note the normal distribution of ^{99m}Tc– sulfur colloid to the liver (85%) and spleen (10%); the remaining 5% is extracted by the bone marrow and is not normally visualized.

Hepatobiliary agents, ^{99m}Tc-labeled RBCs, and gallium-67 (^{67}Ga)-citrate imaging[26,27] all can be helpful for imaging certain lesions.

Rapid serial perfusion imaging[53] has been found increasingly useful and is performed routinely in some institutions. The flow images can identify the vascular nature of certain defects seen on the standard static image. All reported studies conclude that liver and spleen scintigraphy is a good screening test with high sensitivity but relatively poor specificity.[7]

Imaging Procedure. No patient preparation is needed; however, liver and spleen scintigraphy should be performed before administration of any iodinated or barium-containing contrast agents. Such agents, if retained in the body (particularly barium in the colon), can result in artifactual defects in the liver or spleen.

The radiopharmaceutical is given as an IV bolus; the usual adult dose is 5 to 10 mCi for sulfur colloid and 1 to 8 mCi for albumin colloid. For the perfusion study, the patient should be positioned supine under a large–field-of-view scintillation camera fitted with a low-energy, parallel-hole collimator. The patient should be positioned with the upper abdomen included in the field of view. The computer should be set to acquire a dynamic sequence of 2- to 3-second intervals. The radiopharmaceutical should be administered in the right antecubital vein, and the image acquisition should then be started. Blood-flow imaging should continue for at least 1 minute, possibly longer, and then an immediate

postinjection static image, or blood pool image, should be obtained.

After a wait of approximately 15 minutes, planar static imaging may begin. A waiting period is necessary for the colloid particles to be completely localized in the liver and spleen. Images should be obtained for 1 million counts total. Usually, images are obtained for the same time as the anterior image in the right anterior oblique (RAO), left anterior oblique (LAO), right lateral, left posterior oblique (LPO), and posterior projections (Figure 18-32). One image should be obtained using a standard-size reference marker. This is usually done in the anterior view with the marker placed along the costal margin. Inspiration and expiration breath-holding views of the liver can be obtained for approximately 20 seconds. These images frequently can aid in the identification of defects caused by compression of the liver by the ribs.[20,26,36] If a defect moves with the liver, the source most likely is intrinsic disease.

Additional views can be obtained, depending on the clinical problem, or decubitus views may add valuable information.[13] The study may be combined with other imaging agents (e.g., hepatobiliary agents, ^{99m}Tc-labeled RBCs, ^{67}Ga-citrate[26,27]) or may follow oral administration of small amounts of ^{99m}Tc–sulfur colloid mixed with water to outline the stomach.

Images of the upper abdomen by single photon emission computed tomography (SPECT) are now also routinely obtained after the planar projections based on 360

| BOX 18-3 | Liver-Spleen Scintigraphic Procedure |

1. Prepare ^{99m}Tc–sulfur colloid (^{99m}Tc-SC) as per radiopharmacy procedure.
2. Position the patient underneath the camera to include the upper abdomen in the field of view.
3. Enter the acquisition parameters on the camera's computer including a flow phase with 2-sec images in a 128 × 128 matrix for 60 sec.
4. Inject the patient and start the computer acquisition at the time of ^{99m}Tc-SC injection.
5. At 15 min postinjection images in the anterior, posterior, RAO, LAO and LPO projections for 1 million counts per image.
6. Inject the ^{99m}Tc-SC and start the imaging session. SPECT images should also be acquired based on a 360 degrees of rotation in a 128 × 128 matrix with 120 projections of 20 sec each.
7. Reconstruct the images to generate transaxial, sagittal, and coronal views.

LAO, Left anterior oblique; *LPO,* left posterior oblique; *RAO,* right anterior oblique.

degrees of rotation in a 128 × 128 matrix, 120 projections of 20 seconds each acquisition protocol. Transverse, sagittal, and coronal images and in some instances three-dimensional (3D) viewing are then reconstructed using specific filter selections available on the computer platform used. Procedure steps for liver spleen imaging are listed in Box 18-3.

Clinical Aspects. Review of the early perfusion images usually reveals the normal dual blood supply of the liver. Absence of blood flow in these systems may be assessed during the angiographic phase, and the presence of collateral flow may be apparent. Occasionally, perfusion images help in the identification of the vascular nature of a focal defect seen on the static imaging, but this has not been shown to be of value in differentiating benign from malignant lesions. The perfusion study[53] can aid the identification of extrahepatic disease, such as pericardial or pleural effusion. It may also reveal separation of lung and liver by a subdiaphragmatic mass.[40]

A characteristic pattern seen on the perfusion images in inferior vena caval obstruction (Budd-Chiari syndrome) is the concentration of ^{99m}Tc–sulfur colloid in the quadrate lobe of the liver, the result of collateral circulation. Following injection, 80% to 90% of the sulfur colloid is taken up by the Kupffer cells of the liver and 5% to 10% is taken up by the spleen. A small portion is also absorbed by the bone marrow. The sulfur colloid clears rapidly from the bloodstream ($t_{1/2}$ = 2 minutes). In normal patients, imaging may begin 5 to 10 minutes after injection. If the patient has known compromised hepatic function, portal hypertension, or both, optimal concentration of the sulfur colloid will take longer and imaging should not begin before 20 to 30 minutes postinjection. Planar static images are reviewed for the size and shape[15] of the liver and spleen, the relative concentration and distribution of the radiopharmaceutical in these organs, and any defects or displacements. A size marker (see Figure 18-32, *upper left*) is useful for estimating the liver's size.[10] Normally the longitudinal axis of the right lobe of the liver is about 15 cm, measured from the dome of the right lobe. The size and shape[15] of the liver are particularly important when following the course of diseases by serial studies. The size of the spleen can also be estimated from the images. The maximum length of the spleen in one of the routine views is approximately the same as that of the liver, about 14 cm, measured diagonally.

Normally the stomach lies between the spleen and the left lobe of the liver. This may be outlined by giving the patient a small oral dose of ^{99m}Tc–sulfur colloid or ^{99m}Tc–albumin colloid mixed in water. Artifacts from other organs and anatomical structures are commonly seen on the liver and spleen images. In females, the breasts may cause a variety of attenuation artifacts that can mimic an intrahepatic lesion. Usually the crescent pattern of the breast artifact is easily recognizable. Retained barium in the colon, particularly in the hepatic or splenic flexure, can produce image artifacts as well. Generally, artifacts created by overlying structures can be elucidated by obtaining supine and upright views. These demonstrate movement of the "defects." If tomographic imaging is available, the defects are seen to lie outside the liver or spleen parenchyma.

In addition to spiral CT, liver scintigraphy remains a readily available method for detecting the presence of focal disease. Detection of pathology is based on size. Currently, with the use SPECT imaging, defects as small as 5 mm can be detected. Planar imaging can routinely detect lesions as small as 20 mm.[38] The closer the lesion is to the surface of the liver, the more easily it will be detected, because there is less attenuation from surrounding structures.

If there is increased sulfur colloid uptake in the spleen and bone marrow with associated decreased uptake in the liver, this is a sign of diffuse liver disease and/or portal hypertension. This phenomena is called *colloid shift.* In renal transplant patients, increased activity within the transplant kidney is a sign of rejection. Increased activity within the lungs may occur in patients with cirrhosis, pulmonary infections, neoplasms, or possibly related to excess aluminum in the technetium preparation. With liver scintigraphy, hepatic diseases usually cause defects in uptake of the radiopharmaceutical. However, focal hot spots within the liver may occur with cirrhosis and collateralization of veins, Budd-Chiari syndrome, and focal nodular hyperplasia. Overall, hepatic abnormalities are usually divided into focal or diffuse disease.

Focal Lesions. Focal lesions present as photopenic regions within the liver. Unfortunately, unless pertinent history is provided, specific diagnoses are difficult to make without the use of other imaging modalities such as CT, MRI, or ultrasonography. However, the ability to detect lesions on ^{99m}Tc–sulfur colloid scans is comparable to ultrasonography and only slightly less sensitive than CT. Currently the sensitivity of detecting a lesion with planar scintigraphy is 86% and the specificity is 83%. Slight improvement of detectability can occur with the use of SPECT.[1a] A single defect or multiple focal defects on a liver scintigram in a patient with cirrhosis suggests hepatoma. If suspicious of a hepatoma, a ^{67}Ga-citrate scan could also be performed because these lesions are gallium avid.[23] Other conditions associated with the development of a hepatoma are glycogen storage diseases, hemochromatosis, schistosomiasis, thorotrast exposure, and alpha toxins. Other entities associated with focal photopenic regions on liver scintigraphy include liver cysts, hematomas, adenomas (usually occurring in young females using oral contraceptives), and hepatic injuries including infarcts, which are usually seen as peripheral defects within the liver.

Focal nodular hyperplasia (FNH) and liver hemangiomas are special cases of focal liver disease. FNH is a benign entity of the liver that is usually asymptomatic, occurring most often in young females. The tumor is composed of bile ducts, hepatocytes, and Kupffer cells. Because of the presence of Kupffer cells, these lesions usually take up ^{99m}Tc–sulfur colloid normally; therefore if a CT or an MRI shows a liver tumor with a normal appearing liver scan, FNH should be considered as the primary diagnosis. Unfortunately there are exceptions to this rule; sometimes FNH will actually appear hot or even cold on a liver scan. If a hemangioma is suspected, an additional ^{99m}Tc blood pool scan should be performed (see following section).

Diffuse Lesions. Cirrhosis and hepatitis are perhaps the most common diffuse liver diseases detected with liver scintigraphy. The appearance of hepatitis is similar to the early stages of cirrhosis. The liver will be enlarged and have a mottled appearance. As cirrhosis progresses, fibrosis develops and causes the liver to shrink. Usually the right lobe decreases in size the most, leaving the appearance of a large left and caudate lobe. Over time, portal hypertension and ascites may develop causing a "colloid shift" with splenomegaly and a photopenic halo around the liver, respectively. As liver function wanes, very little ^{99m}Tc–sulfur colloid will get taken up by the liver. Therefore much activity will be seen in odd places such as the heart, because the radiopharmaceutical remains in the blood pool and in the reticuloendothelial system of the bones and lungs. Liver scintigraphy, of course, is correlative with cross-sectional imaging or ultrasonography. Metastatic disease is another common entity that may present with diffuse defects on a liver scan. It is virtually impossible to correlate imaging findings with histology; however, some tumors cause characteristic liver metastasis that may help narrow the spectrum. For example, colon and renal cell carcinomas cause "cannonball" defects. Other tumors such as breast and lung are much less specific in appearance. Liver scintigraphy is better suited for monitoring effectiveness of treatment at reducing metastatic lesion. Of importance, though, is that certain chemotherapeutic agents such as methotrexate and nitrosoureas may actually cause changes in the appearance of the liver that may mimic the presence or progression of diffuse disease.

Hepatomegaly with little or no compromise in liver function can be caused by a large number of diseases. Some of these diseases include diabetes mellitus, metastases, leukemia, lymphoma, passive congestion, and hepatitis. The liver may also appear large if there is fatty infiltration or may actually be a normal variant if the patient is large.

Despite the advent of CT[2,3] and MRI scans, liver and spleen scintigraphy remains in use in the evaluation of congenital hepatic abnormalities, nutritional and metabolic diseases, infectious diseases, primary and secondary malignant neoplasms,[17] benign hepatic cell adenomas and FNH, hepatic and splenic trauma, functional asplenia, splenomegaly, and splenic variations.

Liver Hemangioma Detection Using ^{99m}Tc-Labeled Red Blood Cells

Hemangiomas are probably the most common benign tumor of the liver. Because of their prevalence, they often are discovered during CT or ultrasound examination of the abdomen. Yet, the specific criteria for diagnosis of a hemangioma by CT or ultrasound might not always be present in an individual lesion. The radionuclide technique described here, if performed properly, is virtually 100% accurate in the diagnosis of a hemangioma. Accurate diagnosis is essential, because inadvertent biopsy of a hemangioma can lead to significant hemorrhage.

Imaging Procedure. No special patient preparation is necessary, although as with any radionuclide liver imaging procedure, there should be no retained radiographic contrast agents in the abdomen.

Before the imaging procedure is begun, the position of the lesion in question in the liver should be ascertained by referring to the initial CT or ultrasound examination. If the lesion is located anteriorly in the right or left lobe of the liver, the patient is positioned supine for an anterior radionuclide angiogram. If the lesion is located posteriorly in the right lobe, a posterior flow study is performed. If multiple lesions are suspected, the largest lesion should be chosen as the reference. Any non–heat-treated method for labeling the patient's RBCs can be used, and several of these techniques are outlined in the section on detection of GI bleeding. Once the patient has been positioned for the radionuclide angiogram, the bolus of 15 to 25 mCi of ^{99m}Tc-labeled RBCs can be given and rapid sequence imaging at 1 to 3 sec/frame can be done to record blood flow through the liver. Next, blood pool images should be obtained, usually in the anterior, right lateral, and posterior projections at minimum. Steep or shallow oblique views are obtained

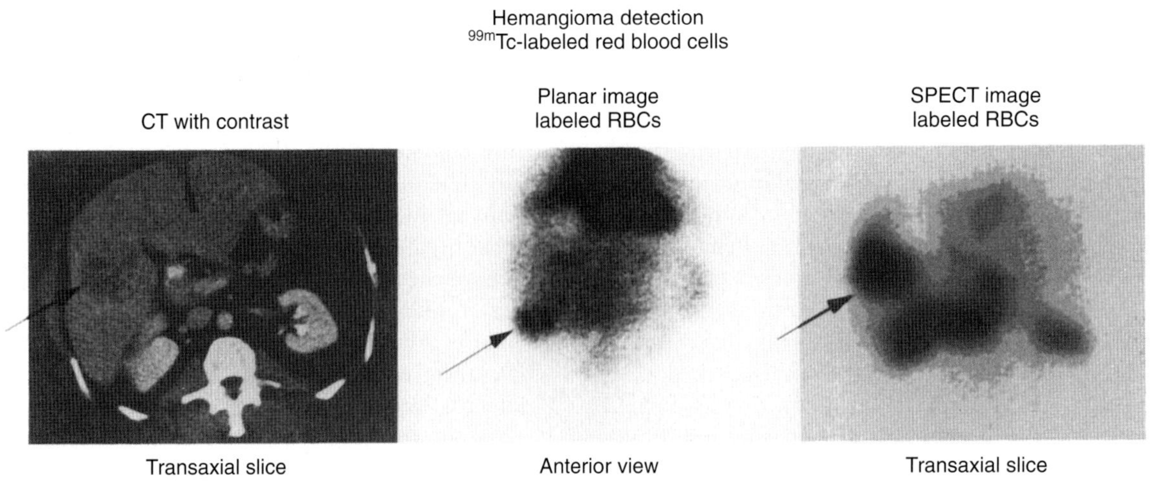

Hemangioma detection
^{99m}Tc-labeled red blood cells

CT with contrast

Planar image
labeled RBCs

SPECT image
labeled RBCs

Transaxial slice

Anterior view

Transaxial slice

FIGURE 18-33 Example of the use of ^{99m}Tc-labeled red blood cells *(RBCs)* to detect hepatic hemangioma. The initial image is a transaxial CT slice revealing a space-occupying lesion in the right lobe of the liver *(arrow)*. Planar and SPECT images obtained at least 2 hours after in vivo labeling of the patient's RBCs show accumulation of the radiolabeled cells in the lesion *(arrows)*, indicating a hemangioma.

as necessary, depending on the position of the lesion. These images should be recorded at high-count rates, usually for 500,000 to 1 million counts. At 2 hours after the dose, delayed imaging can begin. This can consist of planar images, which should be obtained in the same projections and for the same time intervals as the initial blood pool images, SPECT imaging of the liver, or a combination of planar and SPECT imaging. Generally, single large lesions can be adequately visualized using the planar technique alone; small lesions (less than 2 cm) and multiple lesions require SPECT imaging.[6]

Clinical Aspects. Using the previously described method, the characteristic features of a hemangioma are (1) little or no blood flow to the lesion on the early angiographic images, although late angiographic images might show early uptake; (2) early accretion of the tagged cells, usually from the periphery of the lesion inward on the blood pool images; and (3) accretion of the tagged cells equal to but usually greater than the surrounding liver parenchyma on the delayed planar or SPECT images. Other types of lesions, such as hepatic carcinoma and metastatic disease, can show increased blood flow and early accretion of the radiolabeled cells, but they do not retain the cells for long. Only hemangiomas retain RBCs until the 2-hour interval. Adequate time must be allowed for the hemangioma to accumulate a sufficient quantity of the radiolabeled cells to be identified (Figure 18-33).

GALLBLADDER

The gallbladder is a hollow, pear-shaped organ about 7 to 10 cm long (see Figure 18-31). It is located against

---

BOX 18-4 | **Hepatobiliary Imaging: Clinical Indications**

1. Acute (or chronic) cholecystitis
2. Calculation of gallbladder ejection fraction
3. Evaluation of enterogastric reflux (bile reflux)
4. Evaluation of the biliary system after surgery
5. Jaundice (obstructive versus nonobstructive)
6. Pediatrics (biliary atresia versus neonatal hepatitis; presence of choledochal cyst)
7. Evaluation of cold defects seen on radiocolloid liver images
8. Biliary leak

---

the visceral surface of the liver, where it occupies a small indentation, the gallbladder fossa. The gallbladder concentrates and stores bile, which it receives from the common hepatic duct through the cystic duct. After ingestion of a fatty meal, the gallbladder is stimulated to contract, and it discharges the stored bile into the duodenum. Bile is useful in digestion in the breakdown and emulsification of fats.

Hepatobiliary Imaging

Radiopharmaceutical agents that localize in the hepatobiliary system can be extremely valuable in several clinical situations.[16,17,54] The most common clinical indications are listed in Box 18-4. The most commonly used radiopharmaceuticals are derivatives of ^{99m}Tc-iminodiacetic acid (^{99m}Tc-IDA)[54] such as ^{99m}Tc-hepatoiminodiacetic acid (^{99m}Tc-HIDA), ^{99m}Tc–diisopropyl iminodiacetic acid (^{99m}Tc-DISIDA), and ^{99m}Tc-mebrofenin. These agents are

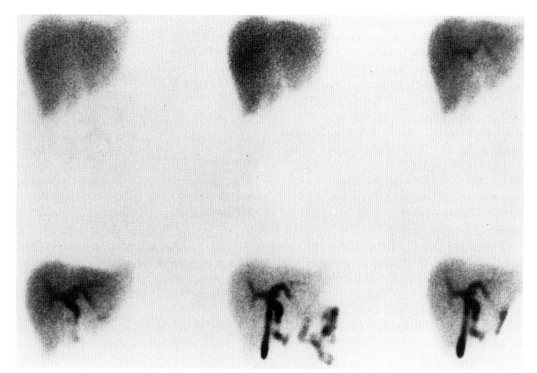

FIGURE 18-34 Normal hepatobiliary scan. Anterior images of the abdomen reframed at approximately 10-minute intervals after intravenous administration of 5 mCi ^{99m}Tc-IDA. Rapid uptake of the radiotracer by the liver is seen, with excretion into the biliary ducts, gallbladder, and small bowel.

superior to older iodine-131 (^{131}I) rose engal, because ^{99m}Tc-IDA derivatives provide a relatively low radiation dose to the patient,[55] have a 6-hour half-life, and provide very high-count images.

Cholescintigraphy is a valuable method for investigating patients with upper abdominal pain. Because acute cholecystitis generally is caused by cystic duct obstruction, visualization of the gallbladder with the radionuclide tracers virtually excludes the diagnosis of acute cholecystitis. Conversely, lack of gallbladder visualization with these agents carries a high probability of acute cholecystitis. In this way, obstructive causes of clinical jaundice may be differentiated from hepatocellular causes. In the neonate, suspected biliary atresia can be evaluated with these agents. Technetium-99m–IDA derivatives are selectively removed from the blood circulation by hepatocytes; therefore these agents are specific for liver tissue. This high specificity allows cold defects demonstrated on colloidal liver and spleen scans to be identified as anatomical variants of the biliary anatomy. However, if the defect is not adequately explained by hepatobiliary imaging, other causes, such as benign or malignant mass lesions, must be considered.

The clinical indications for biliary tract imaging are summarized in Box 18-4.

Imaging Procedure. Patients need to be fasting for 2 to 5 hours before the test to enable visualization of the gallbladder. Prolonged fasting (longer than 12 hours) and parenteral alimentation may also cause the gallbladder not to fill in despite a patent cystic duct because of increased intraluminal pressure and viscous, concentrated bile. Pain medications that contain opium or morphine derivatives or their synthetic counterparts should be discontinued 2 to 6 hours before the study, because these medications can prevent transit of the radiotracer through the biliary system.

The usual adult dose is 1 to 5 mCi of the ^{99m}Tc-IDA given intravenously. Imaging may begin immediately, with the patient supine under a large–field-of-view scintillation camera with a low-energy, all-purpose, parallel-hole collimator. The patient is positioned so that the liver appears in the upper left corner of the field of view. An angiographic phase consisting of 60 images of 1 second each in a 128×128 byte mode matrix is first obtained and followed by a function study consisting of 59 continuous dynamic images of 1 minute each in a 128×128 word mode matrix (Figure 18-34). Supplemental views in the anterior oblique or right lateral projection may be useful for separating the gallbladder and common bile duct from the duodenum and underlying structures such as the kidneys.

If the gallbladder or biliary ducts fail to visualize by 1 hour, imaging can be continued for up to 4 hours or longer, because delayed visualization of the gallbladder and biliary tree could indicate chronic cholecystitis. Complementarily and/or alternatively, a morphine challenge test can be performed. Morphine sulfate contracts the sphincter of Oddi and generates an increase in pressure in the common bile duct and cystic duct. If these ducts are not patent, the radiopharmaceutical refluxes back in the gallbladder. Typically 0.02 mg/kg of morphine sulfate and a second lower (3 mCi) dose of tracer is administered intravenously if there is not enough activity left in the liver. The serial dynamic acquisition is then continued for another 30 minutes.

To assess the **gallbladder ejection fraction (GBEF)** and/or the sphincter of Oddi response to **cholecystokinin (CCK),** the C-terminal octapeptide portion of CCK, sincalide (Kinevac), is given intravenously at a concentration of 0.02 mg/kg in normal saline over a period of 3 to 30 minutes. The administration of fatty foods may also enhance gallbladder emptying.

The GBEF is calculated from dynamically acquired image data by placing a region of interest over the region of the gallbladder (taking into account patient motion) and a background region of interest over the adjacent liver. The liver region of interest should be selected to exclude ductal activity. GBEF is calculated from the gallbladder time-activity curve by

$$GBEF(\%) = \frac{(\text{net GB cts}_{max}) - (\text{net GB cts}_{min})}{(\text{net GB cts}_{max})} \times 100.$$

The GBEF is generally considered normal if it >33% within 3 minutes and >50% within 10 minutes of the completion of CCK or fatty meal administration.[18]

The count rate of the liver changes constantly during the study because of the metabolism and excretion of the radiotracer into the bile ducts. Cameras with good resolution can delineate the path of the biliary ducts and the gallbladder. Supplemental pinhole views may be useful for further evaluation. Procedure steps are listed in Box 18-5.

Clinical Aspects. In the normal individual, the radiopharmaceutical begins to concentrate in the liver during the first few minutes after injection. By 15 to 30 minutes after injection, most of the radiopharmaceutical has been removed from the bloodstream and is concentrated in the liver. This is followed by concentration of the tracer in the biliary ducts and gallbladder (Figure 18-35). The gallbladder is typically well visualized by 45 to 60 minutes, and radioactivity is identified in the gastrointestinal tract (duodenum and proximal jejunal loops) by 30 minutes after injection (Figure 18-36).

In acute cholecystitis, the liver, common bile duct, and GI tract are visualized within 60 minutes after injection. A rim of activity caused by inflammation can be seen around the gallbladder on the angiographic phase. However, the gallbladder is not visualized at 60 minutes and if further imaging is obtained, it will still fail to visualize up to 4 hours after injection. The lack of visualization of the gallbladder is the result of functional or anatomical obstruction of the cystic duct of the gallbladder, which is the basis for acute cholecystitis. In chronic cholecystitis, the liver, common bile duct, and GI tract

---

BOX 18-5   Hepatobiliary Scintigraphic Procedure

Baseline Study
1. The patient should be fasting for 2-5 hr.
2. Prepare the radiopharmaceutical as per laboratory procedure.
3. Place the patient supine under the camera to capture the liver and as much of the rest of the abdomen as possible.
4. Set up the acquisition parameters with a 60-sec angiographic phase made of 60 images of 1 sec each and a function study with 59 images of 1 min each, next using a 128 × 128 matrix.
5. Inject the radiopharmaceutical and start the acquisition. Acquire delayed additional planar and tomographic views if required.

Gallbladder Function Assessment
1. If activity is present in the intestines and assessment of the gallbladder function is needed, inject CCK at 0.02 μg/kg over a period of 3 to 30 min while taking dynamic set of 30 images of 1 min each.
2. Process the data to determine the gallbladder ejection fraction.

Cystic Duct Obstruction Assessment
1. If the gallbladder is not visualized and a cystic duct obstruction is suspected (most of the time due to acute cholecystitis), 0.02 mg/kg of morphine sulfate and eventually a second dose of tracer can be administered.
2. An additional set of dynamic images is acquired for the next 30 to 60 min.

---

may visualize by 60 minutes; there will usually be delayed visualization of the gallbladder after 60 minutes, usually 2 to 4 hours after injection.

The use of pharmacokinetic agents, such as CCK analogs[18] and morphine sulfate, has been advocated by some practitioners to separate patients with acute cholecystitis from those with chronic cholecystitis without the need for imaging to 4 hours. In general, if administration of either of these agents during a study in which the gallbladder does not visualize by 60 minutes causes gallbladder visualization to occur, cystic duct obstruction is not present.

Occasionally the liver, common bile duct, and gallbladder visualize within 60 minutes after injection but no radiotracer is seen in the GI tract. In these instances it might be necessary to obtain delayed views of the abdomen up to 24 hours after injection. Absence of excretion of the radiotracer into the GI tract is evidence of common bile duct obstruction, either functional or anatomical.

In the evaluation of cold defects seen on a ^{99m}Tc–sulfur colloid liver and spleen scan, use of a biliary agent can answer the question of whether the cold defect seen on the sulfur colloid liver image is the result of normal anatomical structures of the biliary system. This is particularly useful when the defect is in the region of the porta hepatis or when it must be determined whether an apparent lesion is caused by an intrahepatic gallbladder.

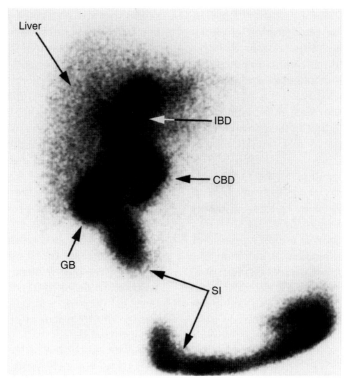

FIGURE 18-35 Normal hepatobiliary scan. This is a single anterior image of the abdomen obtained at 60 minutes after intravenous administration of a ^{99m}Tc-IDA compound. The scan shows normal visualization of the gallbladder *(GB)*, intrahepatic biliary duct *(IBD)*, common bile duct *(CBD)*, and small intestine *(SI)*.

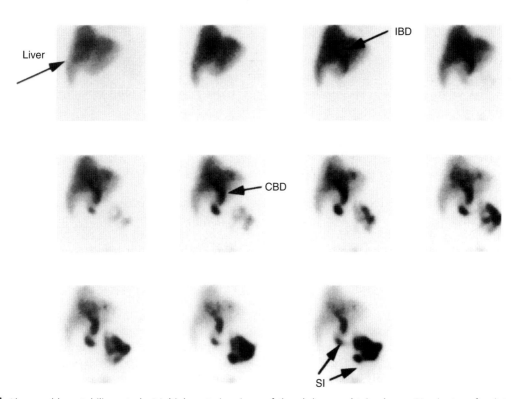

FIGURE 18-36 Abnormal hepatobiliary study. Multiple anterior views of the abdomen obtained over 60 minutes after intravenous administration of a ^{99m}Tc-IDA compound. Normal excretion of the radiotracer through the intrahepatic biliary ducts *(IBD)*, common bile duct *(CBD)*, and small intestine *(SI)* is seen. However, no radiotracer localization is seen in the expected area of the gallbladder. Compare with Figure 18-34.

In pediatric and congenital abnormalities, ^{99m}Tc-IDA agents are extremely helpful in the detection of choledochal cysts, biliary atresia, and other congenital abnormalities. The radiation dose to the child is minimal, the study can be performed without sedation or restraints, and there is no danger of morbidity.

A common problem in performing this examination is the presence of profound jaundice in the patient. When the serum bilirubin approaches 15 to 20 mg/dl, extraction of the ^{99m}Tc-IDA compounds by the hepatocytes is severely reduced. Spurious excretion of the radiotracer through the urinary system may occur, causing circulating background activity to be high. In these instances delayed images may be useful up to 24 hours.

Hepatobiliary imaging is not a useful method for detecting gallstones in the gallbladder or common bile duct. Oral cholecystography, ultrasonic examination, and CT are the methods of choice for detecting gallstones, although the presence of gallstones alone is not a true indicator either of acute or chronic cholecystitis.

Enterogastric Reflux (Bile Reflux) Imaging

Functional scintigraphy can help detect and quantitate enterogastric reflux with the use of hepatobiliary (^{99m}Tc-IDA) agents.[46] Enterogastric scintigraphy has been used to confirm the reflux of bile into the stomach in patients with symptoms of bile reflux gastritis.

Both alkaline gastritis and bile reflux gastritis have been used to describe patients with symptoms of nausea, bile vomiting, abdominal fullness, heartburn, gastric pain, weight loss, and anemia. In severe cases the patient may vomit bile-stained fluid that does not contain food. These patients also have high concentrations of bile acid in fasting gastric aspirates, gastritis or esophagitis, and no peptic ulcerations.

The enterogastric reflux (bile reflux) study is particularly useful in individuals who have undergone gastric surgery in which the pyloric sphincter mechanism was rendered incompetent, removed, or bypassed. Although gastric endoscopy may confirm the presence of bile in the stomach in these individuals, the scintigraphic study has the advantage of being noninvasive and can also quantitate the amount of refluxed bile.

Imaging Procedure. The patient fasts overnight, and any medication that might affect GI motility is stopped. Although patients can be imaged supine, sitting, or standing, supine imaging is preferred because there is less chance of patient movement, repositioning is easier, and overlap of the stomach and small bowel is minimal.

For identifying the stomach, a dual radiopharmaceutical imaging technique with a radiolabeled test meal is helpful. A 2- to 5-mCi dose of ^{99m}Tc-IDA is prepared for IV injection, and a fatty meal is prepared by mixing 100 to 250 mCi of ^{111}In-DTPA with a commercial fatty meal preparation of 250 ml. Any fatty meal preparation may be used, although it is most convenient to use one of the several bottled or canned preparations available on the market (e.g., Meritene).

After IV injection of the ^{99m}Tc-IDA, the patient is immediately positioned under a large–field-of-view camera with a low-energy, all-purpose collimator. The patient is positioned so that the liver appears in the left upper quadrant of the image. Dynamic images are recorded for 45 minutes until peak filling of the gallbladder is seen on the persistence scope. At this point the patient is instructed to drink the fatty meal labeled with the ^{111}In-DTPA. At this time the liver and biliary tree are identified by imaging the technetium window, and the stomach is identified by imaging the indium window (Figure 18-37). Images are obtained at 15-minute intervals for 2 hours at both the technetium and the indium window settings for 1 minute each. Between imaging intervals, the patient is permitted to assume the upright position, to sit, or to stand. At each imaging interval, the liver, gallbladder, and biliary tree are identified by the pattern of ^{99m}Tc activity seen before the meal was given (Figure 18-38).

At the conclusion of the study, regions of interest are created for the stomach and for the hepatobiliary area, which includes the liver, bile ducts, and gallbladder (Figure 18-39). The counts for both the ^{111}In and the ^{99m}Tc images are recorded in both regions of interest for time zero (ingestion of the fatty meal) and for each subsequent 15-minute interval (Figure 18-40) and graphed. Corrections must be made for the ^{111}In downscatter into the ^{99m}Tc window, and the technetium counts must be decay corrected.

Enterogastric reflux index (EGRI) is defined as the increase in ^{99m}Tc activity in the stomach area of interest divided by the decrease in ^{99m}Tc activity in the hepatobiliary tree, using the following formula:

$$EGRI_t = \frac{(S_t - S_o)}{(HB_o - HB_t)} \times 100$$

where $EGRI_t$ is the enterogastric reflux index at time t, S_o represents the ^{99m}Tc activity in the stomach at time zero (immediately after ingesting the fatty meal), HB_o represents the activity in the hepatobiliary area of interest immediately following the fatty meal, and S_t and HB_t indicate the activity in the stomach and hepatobiliary area at subsequent time intervals.

Clinical Aspects. In the normal individual without previous gastric surgery, very little, if any, of the ^{99m}Tc counts can be expected in the stomach, usually less than 15% at 15 to 30 minutes. In patients who have undergone previous peptic ulcer surgery in which a portion of the stomach was removed and the pyloric sphincter mechanism was removed, rendered incompetent, or bypassed, enterogastric reflux usually is observed, even in asymptomatic patients. In studies with asymptomatic postsurgical patients, an enterogastric reflux index of approximately 25% at 15 to 30 minutes may be expected.

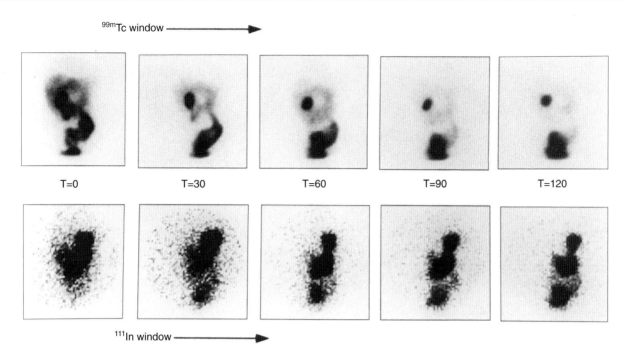

FIGURE 18-37 Enterogastric (bile) reflux study. Anterior images of the abdomen were obtained after intravenous administration of one of the ^{99m}Tc-IDA compounds and after oral ingestion of a fatty meal containing ^{111}In-DTPA. Images are shown for the ^{99m}Tc window and the ^{111}In window. The presence of ^{99m}Tc tracer in the stomach is evidence of enterogastric reflux at each time *(T)* in minutes.

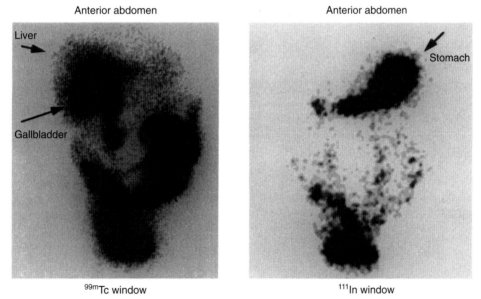

FIGURE 18-38 Enterogastric reflux study. Anterior images of abdomen were obtained after intravenous administration of one of the ^{99m}Tc-IDA compounds and oral ingestion of a fatty meal labeled with ^{111}In-DTPA. The liver, gallbladder, and stomach are seen.

In postsurgical patients with symptoms of nausea, bile vomiting, and abdominal burning, the enterogastric reflux index can be greater than 80% at 15 to 30 minutes. This study is useful in postsurgical patients in whom the degree of enterogastric reflux can be used to determine the response to therapy. A trial of medical therapy can be instituted and followed by repeat examination to determine if the degree of enterogastric reflux has diminished.

Several variations in the performance of this particular examination have been proposed, in particular the use of CCK analogs to replace the fatty meal. Also, several sources of error are inherent in the scintigraphic determination of enterogastric reflux. Each laboratory

Anterior abdomen

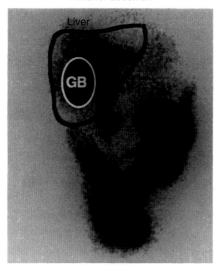

⁹⁹ᵐTc window

Anterior abdomen

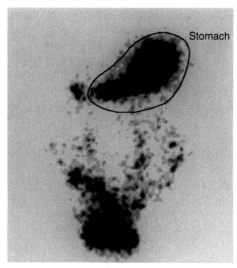

¹¹¹In window

FIGURE 18-39 Calculation of the enterogastric reflux index. Anterior images of the abdomen are recalled from the computer, and regions of interest are created for the stomach, liver, and gallbladder *(GB)*. The hepatobiliary area includes the liver, bile ducts, and gallbladder. Both the ¹¹¹In and the ⁹⁹ᵐTc counts are recorded in both regions of interest at each 15-minute interval.

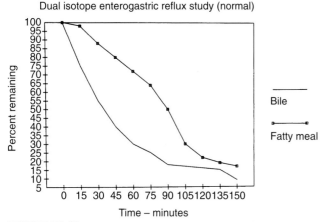

Dual isotope enterogastric reflux study (normal)

Bile

Fatty meal

FIGURE 18-40 Normal dual isotope enterogastric reflux study. The percentage normalized remaining ¹¹¹In counts and ⁹⁹ᵐTc counts are graphed as a function of time. Smooth emptying of the fatty meal from the stomach area is seen, with a nearly parallel decrease in the labeled bile.

must establish methods for background activity correction, tissue attenuation, scatter correction, and interference correction resulting from liver and small bowel overlap. Normal values must be established for each laboratory. Simple visual interpretation of the images can be used to determine if reflux is present (see Figure 18-37).

BREATH TESTING WITH ¹⁴C-LABELED COMPOUNDS

Breath testing is now primarily used to assess the presence or absence of a specific type of bacteria

(*Helicobacter pylori*) in the stomach. These bacteria are responsible for, and are present in, the majority of gastric ulcers. The bacteria can be eradicated with proper antibiotic therapy. Breath testing can also be used to diagnose bacterial overgrowth and carbohydrate malabsorption and to evaluate the liver function.

Gas produced in the stomach, bowel lumen, or both by various acid/base or metabolic reactions, diffuses to some degree into the body circulation and is excreted by respiration into the breath. Of the five principal colonic gases (carbon dioxide, hydrogen, methane, nitrogen, and oxygen), carbon dioxide and hydrogen are the two most important for breath analysis.

The isotopic carbon dioxide breath tests[41] use ¹⁴C-labeled substrates, which are given orally. Labeled carbon dioxide is then excreted in the breath as a result of carbon dioxide (CO_2) production from absorption and breakdown of ¹⁴C-labeled material.

¹⁴C-labeled carbon dioxide can be measured directly by passing the expired breath through plastic filament detectors or by liquid scintillation counting of specimens in which ¹⁴C–carbon dioxide breath is trapped as labeled carbonic acid by a known amount of alkali such as hyamine hydroxide.

¹⁴C-Urea Breath Test

The *H. pylori* breath test is used to detect stomach infection by the bacterium *H. pylori* and determine the efficacy of the antibiotic therapy that is given to infected patients. *H. pylori* produces a significant amount of the enzyme urease, which is not present in normal human tissue.

When ^{14}C-labeled urea is administered orally to the patient and urease activity is present in the stomach, ^{14}C urea is split into ammonia and $^{14}CO_2$, which is absorbed into the blood and exhaled though the lungs. The ^{14}C activity is trapped in an alkaline solution and measured.

Details about the procedure and protocol to perform this test are specific to each laboratory and are based on information about the radiopharmaceuticals, reagents, and the apparatus; recommendations provided by the suppliers; and the type of scintillation counter used. The overall procedure can be summarized as follows. Patients are fasted for at least 6 hours and given a solution or capsule containing 1 mg of urea labeled with 1 mCi of ^{14}C-urea with 20 ml of lukewarm water. Twenty minutes after ingestion, the patient is asked to take a deep breath and hold it for about 10 seconds and then exhale it through a straw into an alkaline solution to trap the CO_2. A scintillation solution is then added to the sample, and the activity in the sample and a blank and a standard is then counted in a liquid scintillation counter. The activity in the sample is background-corrected and expressed in *dpm* after correcting for the efficiency of the scintillation counter according to the following formula:

$$dpm = \frac{(Sample\ cpm - Blank\ cpm)}{Counter\ efficiency}$$

Based on reference dpm values recommended by the manufacturer and/or established within the laboratory, the study is generally interpreted as negative for *H. pylori* when the number of dpm is less than the background activity, and positive when the activity is at least 4 times the background level. It is deemed indeterminate if activity is between the background level and the cutoff value for positivity.[3]

Liver Function Analysis

Measurement of ^{14}C-labeled carbon dioxide after either oral or IV administration of ^{14}C-labeled aminopyrine provides an estimate of hepatic mixed oxidase function.[4,22] The radiolabeled aminopyrine breath test has the clinically useful potential for differentiating patients with the cholestatic form of chronic active hepatitis from those with primary biliary cirrhosis. Correct categorization of such patients is not easily accomplished by other means, and simple blood tests do not measure actual liver function; therefore the aminopyrine test has important therapeutic implications.

Fat Absorption Test

One of the earliest reported uses of the labeled carbon dioxide breath test was breath analysis after oral administration of fat labeled with isotopic carbon.[41] Despite earlier encouraging reports, simple carbon dioxide testing never adequately distinguished those with moderate fat malabsorption from normal subjects. The steps between ingestion of labeled fat and excretion of labeled carbon dioxide are much more complicated than those encountered with other labeled carbon dioxide breath tests.

SUMMARY

- Many procedures of the gastrointestinal system measure physiological process and may be time-consuming in order to observe the transit of radiotracer through a segment of the alimentary system.
- Salivary imaging is performed with ^{99m}Tc-pertechnetate in both dynamic and static modes. Stimulation of the salivary glands is done using lemon juice and tap water followed by dynamic imaging.
- Esophageal transit studies may be performed with ^{99m}Tc–sulfur colloid in 15 ml of tap water with dynamic imaging and computer analysis to measure the esophageal transit time of the total esophagus or its regions.
- Esophageal reflux is measured using ^{99m}Tc–sulfur colloid. The procedure may include the application of an abdominal binder that is raised to various pressures, and imaging is used to identify and quantitate gastroesophageal reflux as $GERI = E_p / G_{gm} \times 100$.
- Gastric emptying is measured using a meal of standard volume and caloric content that contains a non-absorbed radionuclide to measure liquids, solids, or both. The simplest technique involves continuous or periodic imaging to measure the amount of activity remaining in the stomach during the study, which is most commonly plotted as a time-activity curve and the time to half-emptying is determined. The normal rate of emptying is dependent upon the volume and caloric density of the meal.
- Colonic transit time is measured using ^{111}In-DTPA in water and imaging periodically for 96 hours to determine the time to clear 50% of the decay-corrected radioactivity.
- Gastrointestinal bleeding studies are performed with either ^{99m}Tc–sulfur colloid for rapid bleeding or ^{99m}Tc-labeled RBCs for intermittent or slow bleeding. Imaging is performed dynamically.
- Imaging of the liver and spleen may be performed following the administration of ^{99m}Tc–sulfur colloid and imaging dynamically from the anterior projection followed at 15 to 20 minutes with static images from the anterior, posterior, lateral, and oblique projections.
- Hemangiomas of the liver may be imaged using ^{99m}Tc-labeled RBCs. Both planar and SPECT images are commonly used, and imaging is commonly performed following a 2-hour delay from the time of injection.

- Hepatobiliary imaging is performed dynamically using ^{99m}Tc-HIDA, ^{99m}Tc-DISIDA, or ^{99m}Tc-mebrofenin. Patients are imaged only in a fasting state and when no opium- or morphine-derivative medications have been administered. Dynamic anterior images are obtained during the uptake phase. Pharmacological intervention may be done using morphine sulfate to contract the sphincter of Oddi or CCK; or fatty foods may be administered to enhance gallbladder emptying.

- The gallbladder ejection fraction may be calculated during the interventional washout phase of imaging, and the gallbladder ejection fraction is calculated by:

$$GBEF(\%) = \frac{(net\ GB\ cts_{max}) - (net\ GB\ cts_{min})}{(net\ GB\ cts_{max})} \times 100$$

REFERENCES

1. Abell TL, Camilleri M, Donohoe K, et al: Consensus recommendations for gastric emptying scintigraphy: a joint report of the American neurogastroenterology and motility society and the society of nuclear medicine, *J Nucl Med Technol* 36:44-54, 2008.

1a. Adam A, Allison DJ, Bydder G, et al: The liver. In Granger RG, Allison DJ, editors: *Diagnostic radiology*, London, 1992, Churchill Livingstone.

2. Alfidi RJ, Haaga J, Meaney TF, et al: Computed tomography of the thorax and abdomen: a preliminary report, *Radiology* 117:257, 1975.

3. Alfidi RJ, Laval-Jeanet M: AG 60.99: A promising contrast agent for computed tomography of the liver and spleen, *Radiology* 121:491, 1976.

4. Balon H, Gold CA, Dworkin HJ, et al: Procedure guideline for carbon-14-urea, *J Nucl Med* 39:2012, 1998.

5. Blue PW, Jacison JH: Stimulated salivary clearance of technetium-99m pertechnetate, *J Nucl Med* 26:308, 1985.

6. Brodsky RI, Friedman AC, Maurer AH, et al: Hepatic cavernous hemangioma: diagnosis with ^{99m}Tc-labeled red cells and single-photon emission computed tomography, *AJR Am J Roentgenol* 148:125-129, 1987.

7. Bryan PJ, Dunn WM, Grossman ZD: Correlation of computerized tomography, gray scale ultrasonography and radionuclide imaging of the liver in detecting space-occupying processes, *Radiology* 124:387, 1977.

8. Castell DO: The lower esophageal sphincter: physiologic and clinical aspects, *Ann Intern Med* 83:390, 1975.

9. Chaudhuri TK, Heading RC, Greenwald A, et al: Measurement of gastric emptying (GET) of solid meal using ^{99m}Tc DTPA, *J Nucl Med* 15:483, 1974.

10. Christian PE, Coleman RE, Harris CC: An accessory for estimating organ size from gamma camera images, *J Nucl Med Technol* 8:211, 1980.

11. Christian PE, Datz FL, Sorenson JA, et al: Technical factors in gastric emptying studies, *J Nucl Med* 24:264, 1983.

12. Cooperman AM, Cook SA: Gastric emptying: physiology and measurements, *Surg Clin North Am* 56:1277, 1976.

13. Crandell DC, Boyd M, Wennemark JR, et al: Liver-spleen scanning: the left lateral decubitus position is best for lateral views, *J Nucl Med* 13:720, 1972.

14. Datz FL: The role of radionuclide studies in esophageal disease, *J Nucl Med* 25:1040, 1984.

15. DeNardo GL, Stadalnik RC, DeNardo SJ, et al: Hepatic scintiangiographic patterns, *Radiology* 111:135, 1974.

16. Fonseca C, Greenberg D, Rosenthall L, et al: Assessment of the utility of gallbladder imaging with ^{99m}Tc-IDA, *Clin Nucl Med* 3:437, 1978.

17. Fonseca C, Rosenthall L, Greenberg D, et al: Differential diagnosis of jaundice by ^{99m}Tc-IDA hepatobiliary imaging, *Clin Nucl Med* 4:135, 1979.

18. Freeman LM, Sugarman LA, Weissman HS: Role of cholecystokinetic agents in ^{99m}Tc IDA cholescintigraphy, *Semin Nucl Med* 11:186, 1981.

19. Galli J, Volante M, Parrilla C, et al: Oropharyngoesophageal scintigraphy in the diagnostic algorithm of laryngopharyngeal reflux disease: a useful exam? *Otolaryngol Head Neck Surg* 132:717, 2005.

20. Garcia AC, Yeh SDJ, Benua RS: Accumulation of bone-seeking radionuclides in liver metastasis from colon carcinoma, *Clin Nucl Med* 2:265, 1977.

21. Heading RC, Tothill P, Laidlaw AJ, et al: An evaluation of indium DTPA chelate in the measurement of gastric emptying by scintiscanning, *Gut* 12:611, 1975.

22. Hepner GW, Vesell ES: Quantitative assessment of hepatic function by breath analysis after oral administration of (^{14}C) aminopyrine, *Ann Intern Med* 83:632, 1975.

23. Hiraki Y, Nakajo M, Uchiyama N: A case of multiple primary cancers, hepatoma, and seminoma, detected by ^{67}Ga citrate and ^{99m}Tc-Hida scintigraphy. *Jpn J Nucl Med* 28:1497, 1991.

24. Klein HA: Applications of condensed dynamic images, *Clin Nucl Med* 11:178, 1986.

25. Klein HA, Wald A: Computer analysis of radionuclide esophageal transit studies, *J Nucl Med* 25:957, 1984.

26. Kumar B, Coleman RE, Alderson PO: Gallium citrate Ga-67 imaging in patients with suspected inflammatory processes, *Arch Surg* 110:1237, 1975.

27. Lomas F, Dibos PE, Wagner HN Jr: Increased specificity of liver scanning with the use of 67 gallium citrate, *N Engl J Med* 286:1323, 1972.

28. Lull RJ, Morris GL: Scintigraphic detection of gastrointestinal hemorrhage: current status, *J Nucl Med Technol* 14:79, 1986.

29. Madsen JL, Fuglsang S, Graff J: Reference values for the geometric centre analysis of colonic transit measurements with 111indium-labelled diethylenetriamine penta-acetic acid. *Clin Physiol Funct Imaging* 23:204, 2003.

30. Makdissi J, Escudier MP, Brown JE, et al: Glandular function after intraoral removal of salivary calculi from the hilum of the submandibular gland, *Br J Oral Maxillofac Surg* 42:538, 2004.

31. Malmud LS, Fisher RS: Quantitation of gastroesophageal reflux before and after therapy using the gastroesophageal scintiscan, *South Med J* 71(suppl 1):10, 1978.

32. Malmud LS, Fisher RS, Knight LC, et al: Scintigraphic evaluation of gastric emptying, *Semin Nucl Med* 12:116, 1982.

33. Maurer AH, Urbain JL, Krevsky B, et al: Effects of in vitro versus in vivo red cell labeling on image quality in gastrointestinal bleeding studies, *J Nucl Med Technol* 26:87, 1998.

34. Meyer JH: Motility of the stomach and gastroduodenal junction. In Johnson LR, editor: *Physiology of the gastrointestinal tract*, New York, 1987, Raven Press.

35. Meyer JH, MacGregor IL, Gueller R, et al: ^{99m}Tc-tagged chicken liver as a marker of solid food in the human stomach, *Am J Dig Dis* 21:296, 1976.

36. Oppenheimer BE, Hoffer PB, Gottschalk A: The use of inspiration-expiration scintiphotographs to determine the intrinsic or extrinsic nature of liver defects, *J Nucl Med* 13(7):554, 1972.

37. Pope CE II: Pathophysiology and diagnosis of reflux esophagitis, *Gastroenterology* 70:445, 1976.

38. Salvatori M: Imaging of hepatic focal lesions by nuclear medicine, *J Surg Oncol Suppl* 3:189, 1993.

39. Schmitt G, Lehmann G, Strotges W, et al: The diagnostic value of sialography and scintigraphy in salivary gland diseases, *Br J Radiol* 49:326, 1976.

40. Selby JB: Radiological examination of subphrenic disease process, *CRC Crit Rev Diagn Imaging* 9:229, 1977.

41. Shreeve WW: Labeled carbon breath analysis. In Rocha AFG, Harbert JC, editors: *Textbook of nuclear medicine: basic science*, Philadelphia, 1978, Lea & Febiger.

42. Siegel JA, Wu RK, Knight LC, et al: Radiation dose estimates for oral agents used in upper gastrointestinal disease, *J Nucl Med* 24:835, 1983.

43. Svedberg JB: The bolus transport diagram: a functional display method applied to oesophageal studies, *Clin Phys Physiol Meas* 3:267, 1982.

44. Taillefer R, Beauchamp G: Radionuclide esophagogram, *Clin Nucl Med* 9:465, 1984.

45. Tatsch K, Schroettle W, Kirsch CM: Multiple swallow test for the test for the quantitative and qualitative evaluation of esophageal motility disorders, *J Nucl Med* 32:1365-1370, 1991.

46. Tolin RD, Malmud LS, Stelzer F, et al: Enterogastric reflux in normal subjects and patients with Bilroth II gastroenterostomy, *Gastroenterology* 77:1027, 1979.

47. Urbain JL, Vekemans MC, Parkman H, et al: Dynamic antral scintigraphy to characterize gastic antral motility in functional dyspepsia, *J Nucl Med* 36(9):1579-1586, 1995.

48. Urbain JL, Penninckx F, Siegal JA, et al: Effect of proximal vagotomy and Roux-en-Y diversion on gastric emptying kinetics in asymptomatic patients, *Clin Nucl Med* 15:688, 1990.

49. Urbain JL, Siegal JA, Mortelmans L, et al: Effect of solid-meal caloric content on gastric emptying kinetics of solids and liquids, *Nuklearmedizin* 28:120, 1989.

50. Urbain JL, Vekemans MC, Bouilon R, et al: Characterization of gastric antral motility disturbances in diabetes using the scintigraphic technique, *J Nucl Med* 34:576, 1993.

51. Urbain JL, Siegal JA, Charkes ND, et al: The two-component stomach: effects of meal particle size on fundal and antral emptying, *Eur J Nucl Med* 15:254, 1989.

52. van Dam APM: The gamma camera in clinical evaluation of gastric emptying, *Radiology* 110:155, 1974.

53. Waxman AD, Apaw R, Siemsen JK: Rapid sequential liver imaging, *J Nucl Med* 13:522, 1972.

54. Wistow BW, Subramanian G, Van Heertum RL, et al: An evaluation of ^{99m}Tc-labeled hepatobiliary agents, *J Nucl Med* 18:455, 1977.

55. Wu RK, Siegel JA, Rattner Z, et al: Tc-99m HIDA dosimetry in patients with various hepatic disorders, *J Nucl Med* 25:905, 1984.

SUGGESTED READING

Klein HA: Esophageal transit scintigraphy, *Semin Nucl Med* 25:306, 1995.

Krevsky B, Malmud LS, D'Ercole F, et al: Colonic transit scintigraphy: a physiologic approach to the quantitative measurements of colonic transit in humans, *Gastroenterology* 91:1102, 1986.

Krevsky B, Maurer AH, Fisher RS: Patterns of colonic transit in chronic idiopathic constipation, *Am J Gastroenterol* 84:127, 1989.

Kumar R, Tripathi M, Chandrashekar N, et al: Diagnosis of ectopic gastric mucosa using 99Tcm-pertechnetate: spectrum of scintigraphic findings, *Br J Radiol* 78:714, 2005.

Lin EC, Kuni CC: Radionuclide imaging of hepatic and biliary disease, *Semin Liver Dis* 21:179, 2001.

Lin HC, Prather C, Fisher RS, et al: Task Force Committee on Gastrointestinal Transit Measurement of gastrointestinal transit, *Dig Dis Sci* 50:989, 2005.

Mariani G, Boni G, Barreca M, et al: Radionuclide gastroesophageal motor studies, *J Nucl Med* 45:1004, 2004.

Maurer AH, editor: Gastrointestinal nuclear imaging. I. Functional studies, *Semin Nucl Med* 25:4, 1995.

Maurer AH, editor: Gastrointestinal nuclear imaging. II. Other studies, *Semin Nucl Med* 26:1, 1996.

Smart RC, McLean RG, Gaston-Parry D, et al: Comparison of oral iodine-131 cellulose and indium-111-DTPA as tracers for colon transit scintigraphy: analysis by colon activity profiles, *J Nucl Med* 32:1668, 1991.

Urbain JL, Charkes ND: Gastrointestinal nuclear imaging. Recent advances in gastric emptying scintigraphy, *Semin Nucl Med* 25 4:318, 1995.

Zuckier LS: Acute gastrointestinal bleeding, *Semin Nucl Med* 33:297, 2003.

Genitourinary System

Henry D. Royal, Akash Sharma

OBJECTIVES

After completing this chapter, the reader will be able to:
- Describe the anatomy and physiology of the genitourinary system.
- List the radiopharmaceuticals used for renal studies and discuss their characteristics.
- Describe the differences in excretion of renal radiopharmaceuticals.
- List common renal nuclear medicine studies and their indications.
- Describe the performance of functional renal study.

- Discuss the procedure for diuretic renal scintigraphy.
- Describe the procedure for performing renal scintigraphy with angiotensin converting enzyme (ACE) inhibition.
- Describe the performance of scintigraphy for morphological renal imaging.
- Discuss the anatomy, physiology, and indications for testicular scintigraphy.
- Define ERPF and GFR and describe methods to obtain these measurements.

KEY TERMS

acute tubular necrosis (ATN)
angiotensin-converting enzyme
  (ACE)
effective renal plasma flow (ERPF)
filtration fraction
foreshortening

functional agents
glomerular filtration rate (GFR)
glomeruli
horseshoe kidney
hydronephrosis
ileal loop

morphological agents
nephron
relative renal function
renal artery stenosis (RAS)
torsion
vesicoureteral reflux (VUR)

ANATOMY

The top of each kidney usually is located at the level of the lowest ribs in the back (Figure 19-1), spanning the distance from about the twelfth thoracic vertebra to the third lumbar vertebra. In the adult, each kidney measures about 11 to 12 cm long, 5 to 7.5 cm wide, and 2 to 3 cm thick.[17] Because it is displaced by the liver, the right kidney usually is slightly lower than the left kidney.

Determining the size of the kidney by planar scintigraphy is less accurate than determining the size of the kidney by ultrasound. With planar scintigraphy, the kidney may appear smaller than its actual size if the long axis is not parallel to the surface of the crystal of the gamma camera. This artifact is called **foreshortening** (Figure 19-2). Single photon emission computed tomography (SPECT) imaging using a morphological renal imaging agent such as 2,3-dimercaptosuccinic acid

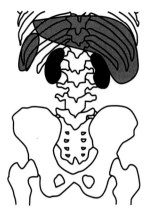

FIGURE 19-1 Location of the kidneys on the posterior view. The right kidney is normally slightly lower than the left kidney, because it is displaced by the liver. The background activity for the right kidney is usually higher than that for the left because of activity that accumulates in the liver. Blood flow to the spleen can be misinterpreted as blood flow to the left kidney, especially when the blood flow to the left kidney is reduced.

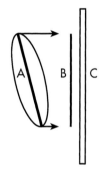

FIGURE 19-2 Foreshortening. The true length of the long axis of the kidney (A) will be underestimated (B) if the long axis of the kidney is not parallel to the plane of the gamma camera crystal (C).

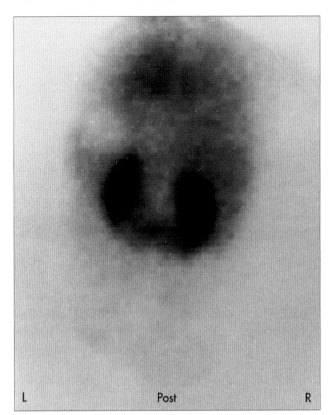

L   Post   R

FIGURE 19-3 Horseshoe kidney. Posterior image of the kidneys of a 10-month-old girl acquired 0 to 2 minutes after injection of ^{99m}Tc-MAG3. Ultrasound examination had shown bilateral hydronephrosis. Hydronephrosis is frequently seen with horseshoe kidneys because the connecting band of tissue compresses the ureters. The decreased activity noted superior and lateral to the left kidney is caused by a full stomach. This decrease in activity is often seen in infants after feeding.

(DMSA) is a more accurate technique for measuring renal size.[23]

Normally the kidneys are about an equal depth from the skin of the back, but in some patients the depths of the kidneys may be unequal. When the kidneys are at unequal depths, measurement of the relative activity in each kidney is inaccurate because of greater attenuation of the radiation from the deeper kidney. Consequently, the relative function of the deeper kidney is underestimated. One way to tell whether asymmetrical activity in the kidneys is related to a difference in kidney depth is to obtain an anterior view of the kidneys. If relatively more activity is seen on the anterior view in the kidney that has decreased activity in the posterior view, a difference in kidney depth is at least partly responsible for this difference in activity.

When a kidney study is obtained with a mobile camera in the intensive care unit, imaging must be performed by placing the patient in a lateral decubitus or prone position. Either of these positions may exaggerate the asymmetrical depth of the kidneys, because one kidney may fall forward more than the other. It is sometimes tempting to perform a mobile study in the anterior view; however, anterior images of normally positioned kidneys are rarely satisfactory.

Sometimes the bottoms of the two kidneys are joined; this congenital abnormality is called a **horseshoe kidney** (Figure 19-3). Because the spine attenuates the activity coming from the thin band of tissue connecting the lower poles of the kidneys, this congenital abnormality may be missed because usually only posterior views are obtained. A clue to the presence of a horseshoe kidney is the orientation of the kidneys: the lower ends of horseshoe kidneys appear closer together than in normal kidneys whereas the upper ends are further apart than normal. An anterior view often clearly shows the band of functioning tissue that connects the lower poles of the kidneys.

Another disease that can grossly distort the anatomy of the kidney is polycystic kidney disease. Patients with this inherited disease have multiple large cysts in the kidneys and often in the liver as well (the latter more common in autosomal dominant form) (Figure 19-4). These cysts increase in size as the patient ages, often resulting in renal failure.

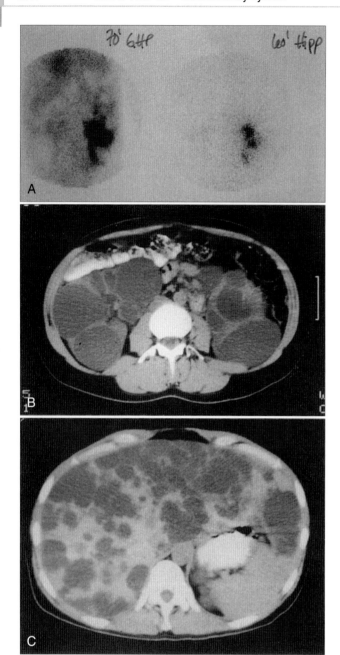

FIGURE 19-4 Polycystic kidneys. **A,** Posterior images of the kidneys obtained 70 minutes after injection of ^{99m}Tc-glucoheptonate *(left)* and 60 minutes after injection of ^{131}I-hippuran *(right)*. Both images are very abnormal (this patient had polycystic kidney disease and renal failure). The function of the left kidney is considerably worse than that of the right kidney. The areas of decreased activity seen on the glucoheptonate images are caused by the renal cysts. Despite the poor renal function, most of the hippuran is in the collecting system at 60 minutes. The glucoheptonate is cleared from the rest of the body more slowly than hippuran and is retained in the renal parenchyma. **B,** CT scan of the kidneys shows nearly complete replacement of the renal tissue by cysts. **C,** CT scan of the liver shows extensive cystic disease of the liver. Patients with polycystic kidney disease often have cysts in the liver.

Occasionally a kidney may be in an unusual location, such as in the pelvis, particularly if the patient is sitting or standing. When the patient is imaged in the supine position, the kidney may return to a more normal position. A mobile kidney in an abnormal position is called *ptotic*. Transplanted kidneys are most often placed in the anterior pelvis. Before beginning a kidney study, the technologist should inquire whether it is likely that the patient's kidneys are in an unusual location so as to make certain that the camera is optimally positioned.

Another important clinical determination, in some cases, is what proportion of renal function can be ascribed to a transplanted kidney and what proportion to the patient's native kidneys. This question is best answered by obtaining simultaneously an anterior view of the transplanted kidney and a posterior view of the native kidneys, using a large–field-of-view, dual-headed camera.

The urine produced by the kidneys is excreted into the renal pelvis and then transported to the bladder through the ureters (Figure 19-5). Dilation of the renal pelvis and ureters is called **hydronephrosis**. This dilation may be due to an acute obstruction somewhere in the collecting system or may be the result of a prior insult to the same.

The bladder is a hollow, distensible, muscular baglike organ that stores urine until it is eliminated through the urethra. Sometimes a patient's bladder is removed to treat bladder cancer. A new "bladder" (neobladder) can be fashioned from the patient's gastrointestinal tract, and is most commonly made from a portion of the small bowel (ileum), thus called an **ileal loop** (Figure 19-6). Less commonly, a small portion of the colon can be used to construct a neobladder. When imaging, it is important to note if the patient has had a recent radiographic procedure that included administering contrast agents in the rectum, because barium in the rectum can cause an attenuation artifact that overlies the bladder (Figure 19-7).

The scrotum is a skin pouch suspended from the lower pelvis that contains the testes, epididymis, and vas deferens (ductus deferens). The testes produce spermatozoa and the hormone testosterone. The epididymis is a tortuous tubular structure in which spermatozoa mature and are stored before they are transported. The vas deferens is contiguous to the epididymis and is the excretory duct of the testes.

The blood flow to and from the kidney usually is through a single artery and vein that subsequently divide into interlobar arteries (Figure 19-8). A common variation of normal anatomy of the renal artery is to have two main renal arteries to a kidney, usually one to the upper pole of the kidney and one to the lower pole. When this occurs, there can be differential function of the upper and lower poles of the kidney if one of these arteries becomes narrowed or obstructed. These main arteries subdivide until they form the afferent arteriole to a web of capillaries called **glomeruli** (Figure 19-9).

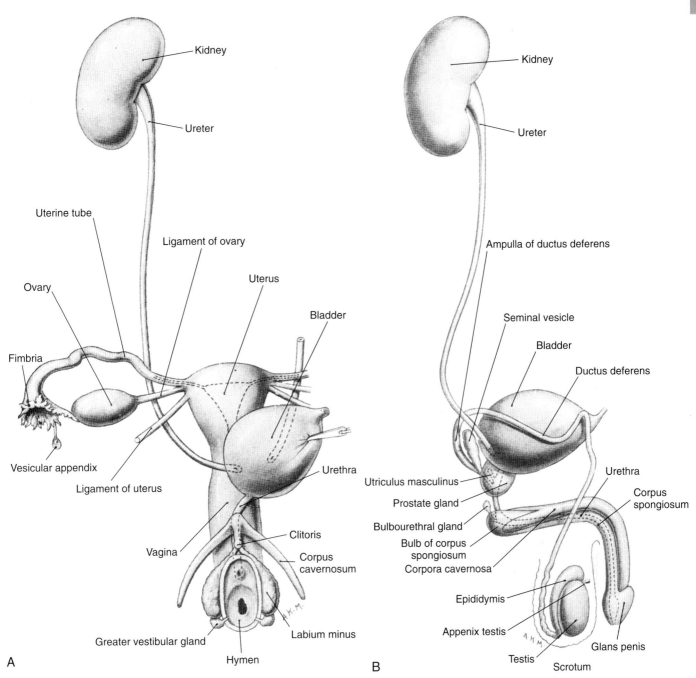

FIGURE 19-5 Schematic representation of urogenital organs in the female **(A)** and the male **(B)**.

The blood leaves the glomerulus through the efferent arteriole, which courses deep into the medulla (the central portion of the kidney closest to the collecting system), forming the peritubular capillaries and the vasa recta.

PHYSIOLOGY

The kidney has several major functions, including excretion of waste products, resorption of important body constituents, maintenance of acid-base balance, and maintenance of fluid balance. To accomplish these functions, the kidney requires a large blood flow. Approximately 20% to 25% of the cardiac output goes to normally functioning kidneys. Because the resting cardiac output is 5 L/min, total renal blood flow is about 1.2 L/min (Box 19-1). Because plasma constitutes about 50% of the total blood volume, the **effective renal plasma flow (ERPF)** is about 600 ml/min. When the plasma and red blood cells pass by the glomerulus, approximately 20%

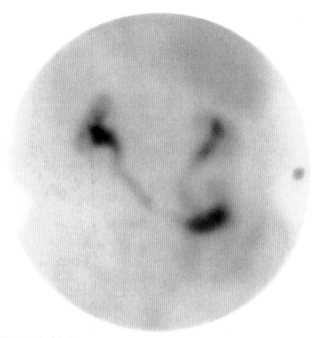

FIGURE 19-6 Ileal bladder. This patient's bladder has been removed. Excreted activity collects in an artificial bladder that has been created using a section of ilium. The ileal bladder usually drains into a collecting bag.

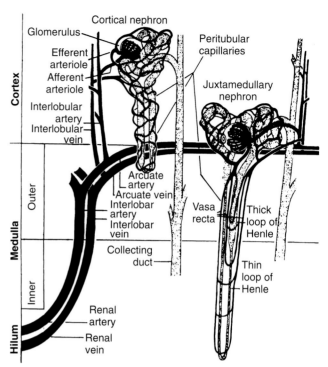

FIGURE 19-8 Schematic representation of a nephron, circulation, and respective locations in the kidney.

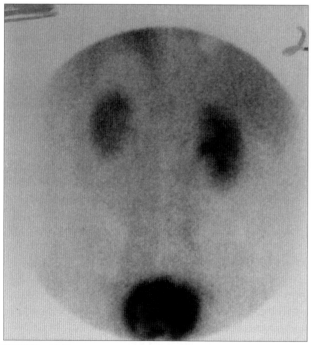

FIGURE 19-7 Barium in the rectum. The serpiginous area of apparent decreased activity overlying the bladder is caused by barium in the rectum.

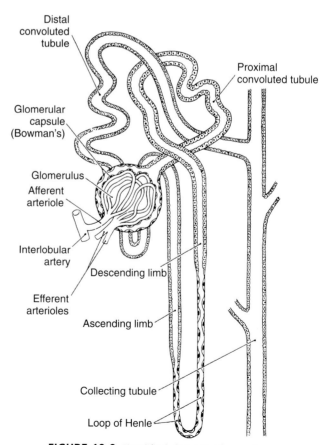

FIGURE 19-9 Simplified diagram of a nephron.

BOX 19-1	Normal Physiology Flow Rates
Cardiac output	5 L/min
Renal blood flow	1.2 L/min
Effective renal plasma flow	600 ml/min
Glomerular filtration rate	120 ml/min
Filtration fraction	20%

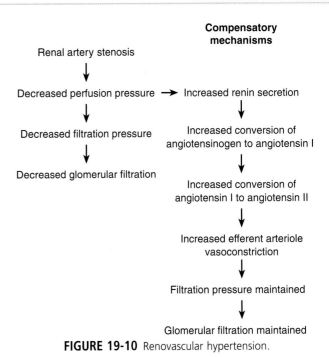

FIGURE 19-10 Renovascular hypertension.

of the plasma passes through the glomerulus into the renal tubules, resulting in a **glomerular filtration rate (GFR)** of 120 ml/min. Most of the filtrate is reabsorbed. The proportion of plasma that reaches the kidney and is filtered by the glomerulus is called the **filtration fraction.** Normally, the filtration fraction is about 20% (GFR/ERPF).

Only 1000 to 1500 ml of urine is produced each day. More than 170 L of urine would be produced per day if none of the plasma that was filtered through the glomerulus was reabsorbed by the tubular cells. On average the body contains only about 42 L of water; therefore tubular cell dysfunction that prevents resorption of the filtrate would rapidly result in death from dehydration. Fortunately, when tubular dysfunction occurs, a number of reflex mechanisms cause a dramatic decrease in renal blood flow and glomerular filtration. Although these compensatory mechanisms have significant long-term adverse effects, rapid death from acute dehydration is prevented.

The basic functional unit of the kidney is called a **nephron** (see Figure 19-8). A normally functioning kidney has millions of nephrons. The nephron consists of an afferent arteriole that delivers blood to a web of capillaries (vascular tuft) in the glomerulus. The blood leaves the glomerulus through the efferent arteriole. Between the afferent and efferent arterioles is an important hormone-producing mass of cells called the *juxtaglomerular apparatus*. The hormone (renin) produced by these cells has important effects on blood pressure.

The porous surface of the glomerulus permits filtration of water and solutes into Bowman's capsule (see Figure 19-9). The major factor that determines whether a substance is filtered is its molecular size. Substances with a molecular size of less than 150,000 dalton are freely filterable if they are not protein bound. Filtration is a passive process, and the rate is primarily determined by the perfusion pressure. The large volume of filtrate (125 ml/min) is transported to the proximal and distal renal tubules. More than 99% of the filtrate is selectively reabsorbed by the tubular cells. The nephron is oriented with the glomerulus in the cortex (outermost layer) of the kidney, whereas the tubules are primarily in the medulla.

The kidney produces a number of important hormones. The physiology of the renin-angiotensin system is important for understanding renovascular

hypertension. When **renal artery stenosis (RAS)** is present, the perfusion pressure decreases (Figure 19-10). This results in a decrease in pressure in the afferent renal arteriole and thus a decrease in filtration pressure and the GFR. Fortunately the kidney has an important reflex mechanism to maintain the glomerular filtration pressure even with RAS. The decrease in perfusion pressure in the afferent renal arteriole is a potent stimulus for the release of renin from the juxtaglomerular apparatus. Renin converts angiotensinogen to angiotensin I, which subsequently is converted to angiotensin II by the **angiotensin-converting enzyme (ACE)**. Angiotensin II causes vasoconstriction of the efferent glomerular arteriole, thus helping to preserve filtration pressure and the GFR. In addition, angiotensin II increases the secretion of aldosterone by the adrenal glands, which in turn causes increased sodium resorption by the tubular cells. The increased salt retention increases the systemic blood pressure, and the increased blood pressure helps preserve the perfusion/filtration pressure of the kidney.

Patients with hypertension are often given an ACE inhibitor for treatment of their hypertension. The ACE inhibitor blocks the conversion of angiotensin I to angiotensin II and therefore blocks one of the mechanisms that contributes to hypertension. Usually the overall effect is beneficial. However, RAS is a significant contributor to hypertension (renovascular hypertension) in about 5% of patients; In these patients, the loss of the efferent glomerular arteriolar vasoconstriction caused by the ACE inhibitor results in a decreased filtration pressure and a subsequent decrease in GFR. This can result in renal failure in some patients. Using nuclear medicine techniques, these physiological changes can be observed and used to diagnose renovascular hypertension in patients. ACE inhibitor decreases the vascular resistance of the abnormal kidney; therefore the blood flow to the kidney is usually maintained or may increase despite the decrease in GFR. For this reason, when an ACE inhibitor is given, the initial uptake of a blood flow agent such as technetium-99m (^{99m}Tc)–mercaptoacetyltriglycine (MAG3) may be preserved even though the initial uptake of a GFR agent such as ^{99m}Tc–diethylenetriamine pentaacetic acid (DTPA) may be markedly decreased. For both agents there is prolonged retention of the radiopharmaceutical in the cortex of the kidney due to the decrease in GFR.

RADIOPHARMACEUTICALS

Conceptually, it is best to divide renal radiopharmaceuticals into two categories: **functional agents** and **morphological agents** (Table 19-1).[13,43,44] Functional radiopharmaceuticals are rapidly taken up and excreted by the kidneys by a single, simple physiological mechanism such as ERPF or GFR. Morphological tracers are also rapidly taken up by the kidney but by more complicated mechanisms that usually involve a complex interaction of ERPF, GFR, tubular secretion, and tubular resorption. The hallmark of a morphological tracer is that some of the tracer is retained in the renal parenchyma for a prolonged period. Prolonged retention of the tracer in the kidney makes relatively high-resolution imaging of the renal parenchyma possible, even several hours after injection of the tracer.

Functional agents (see Table 19-1) include iodine-labeled hippuran, ^{99m}Tc-MAG3,[41] and ^{99m}Tc-DTPA. Iodine-labeled hippuran is no longer available because the radiation dose and imaging properties of iodine-131 (^{131}I)–labeled hippuran are undesirable. Iodine-123 (^{123}I)-labeled hippuran is not commercially available in the United States and would be expensive because of the short half-life (13 hours).

Hippuran is the classic agent that has been used to measure ERPF. The ideal characteristics of an agent to measure ERPF or the GFR are listed in Box 19-2. Hippuran fulfills these requirements because first-pass extraction of this agent is high as it passes through the kidney. A high first-pass extraction means that almost all of the agent delivered to the kidney remains in the kidney. For hippuran the ratio of activity in the renal vein to the activity in the renal artery is about 0.15, because about 85% of the activity is retained in the kidney. The most accurate blood flow agent is microspheres, because they have the highest first-pass extraction (about 100%). Hippuran has such high first-pass extraction because it is

TABLE 19-1	Renal Radiopharmaceuticals
Functional Radiopharmaceuticals	**Comments**
^{131}I-hippuran	Effective renal plasma flow agent; para-aminohippuric acid analog
	High first-pass extraction
	Freely filtered; near-total tubular secretion; no tubular resorption
	High target to background even with poor renal function
	^{131}I has poor imaging characteristics and gives a relatively high radiation dose to patient
	^{123}I-labeled hippuran has much better imaging characteristics and gives a relatively low radiation dose to patient; however, it is expensive and not readily available because of its short half-life (13 hours)
^{99m}Tc-DTPA (diethylenetriamine pentaacetic acid)	Glomerular filtration agent; inulin analog
	Freely filtered; no tubular secretion; no tubular resorption
	Readily available
	Very good imaging characteristics; low radiation dose to patient
^{99m}Tc-MAG3 (mercaptoacetyltriglycerine)	Effective renal plasma flow agent; biokinetics are different from those of hippuran
	High first-pass extraction
	Freely filtered; near-total tubular secretion; no tubular resorption
	High target to background even with poor renal function
	Very good imaging characteristics; low radiation dose to patient
	Recently introduced; likely to replace all other renal radiopharmaceuticals for most applications
Morphological Radiopharmaceuticals	
^{99m}Tc-DMSA (dimercaptosuccinic acid)	Hepatobiliary excretion with poor renal function can interfere with delayed imaging of renal parenchyma
	Physiological mechanisms for uptake; excretion and retention are complex
	66% of dose is excreted; 34% is retained by renal cortex at 6 hours after injection
^{99m}Tc-glucoheptonate	Physiological mechanisms for uptake; excretion and retention are complex
	More than 90% of dose is excreted; 6% to 10% is retained by renal cortex

efficiently secreted by the renal tubule cells and is not reabsorbed from the tubular lumen.

Technetium-99m–MAG3 has replaced hippuran as a functional agent.[44] Like hippuran, MAG3 has a high first-pass extraction fraction. Unlike hippuran, MAG3 is taken up by red blood cells (RBCs); therefore it clears the plasma even more rapidly than hippuran.[45] Technetium-99m–MAG3 is preferred over hippuran because of its superior imaging characteristics.

Technetium-99m–DTPA is cleared from the plasma almost exclusively by glomerular filtration by the kidney. Several other radiopharmaceuticals (e.g., iodine-125 [^{125}I] iothalamate) also have the necessary characteristics for measuring the GFR[25,29] using multiple blood samples to measure a plasma clearance curve, but imaging is possible only with ^{99m}Tc-DTPA.

Technetium-99m–DMSA and ^{99m}Tc-glucoheptonate are considered morphological imaging agents (see Table 19-1), because accumulation in the kidney is the result of a complex interaction of blood flow, GFR, tubular secretion, and tubular resorption. ^{99m}Tc-glucoheptonate can also be used as a functional agent due to adequate early accumulation in the renal parenchyma.[40] Approximately 30% of DMSA is retained in the renal parenchyma, compared with 5% to 10% of glucoheptonate.

The choice of radiopharmaceutical to use for renal imaging depends on the clinical question that is being asked. A technetium-labeled agent is required to obtain a flow study (Figure 19-11). For evaluation of the renal collecting system for obstruction, an agent that is rapidly excreted into the collecting system is best. For optimum visualization of the renal cortex to detect evidence of renal scarring, an agent that is retained in the renal parenchyma is preferred.

Before the introduction of ^{99m}Tc-MAG3 in 1989, different radiopharmaceuticals and different combinations thereof were chosen for different indications. Since the introduction of MAG3, a functional radiopharmaceutical, most institutions have used it for most indications. With MAG3 it is even possible to evaluate the morphology of the renal parenchyma, because very good images of the kidney can be obtained within the first few minutes after injection of the tracer (Figure 19-12).

BOX 19-2	Ideal Characteristics of ERPF/GFR Agents

- ERPF agent is completely removed from plasma during its passage through the kidney (high first-pass extraction).
- GFR agent is freely filterable by the glomerulus.
  - Agent is not protein bound.
  - Agent is not metabolized.
  - No significant excretion by other organs occurs.

ERPF, Effective renal plasma flow; *GFR,* glomerular filtration rate.

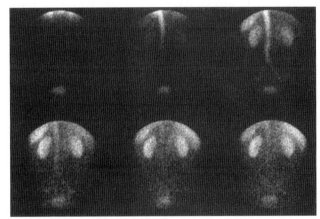

FIGURE 19-11 Radionuclide flow study of the kidneys. A flow study of the kidneys is obtained as the tracer is being injected. These images have been added on the computer so that each image contains 10 seconds of data. Activity initially is seen in the descending aorta, then in the kidneys and the spleen. Note that the activity in the liver does not appear until well after the activity in the spleen, because most of the hepatic blood flow is from the portal circulation.

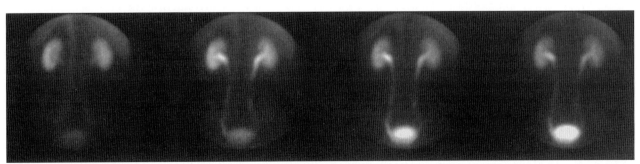

FIGURE 19-12 Evaluation of the renal parenchyma with ^{99m}Tc-MAG3. Relatively high-quality images of the renal parenchyma can be obtained using MAG3. Images from the dynamic study have been added so that each image contains 5 minutes of data. Evaluation of the renal parenchyma is not compromised by collecting-system activity on the earliest images.

BOX 19-3	Major Indications for Radionuclide Renal Scintigraphy

Relative renal function
Renal transplant evaluation
Acute renal failure
Obstructive uropathy
Renovascular hypertension
Infection and inflammation
Vesicoureteral reflux

RADIONUCLIDE PROCEDURES

Practical Considerations

To maximize the clinically relevant information obtained from radionuclide renal imaging, the reasons for doing the study must be determined before it is started. Major indications for radionuclide imaging are listed in Box 19-3. Pertinent clinical information includes the number, location, and size of the kidneys; the results of other imaging tests; the patient's creatinine level and current medications; and any specific instructions regarding the physiological conditions under which the test is to be performed.

Common physiological variables include the state of hydration and the position of the patient. Normally patients are hydrated by having them drink two or three 8-ounce glasses of water. Renal imaging usually is performed with the patient supine, except for diuretic renal imaging, which is best performed with the patient upright when possible. Less common but potentially important physiological variables include whether various draining tubes (e.g., Foley catheter, nephrostomy tubes, wound drains) should be clamped.[5,6]

In general, no patient preparation is necessary, although ideally the patient should be well hydrated. A number of drugs can significantly affect the function of the kidney or directly interfere with the uptake of the radiopharmaceuticals.[34] If a renal arteriogram using intravenous iodinated contrast has been performed within a few days before the radionuclide renal study, an inaccurate impression of renal function (absolute and relative) may be obtained because of transient contrast-induced **acute tubular necrosis (ATN)**. Drugs that block tubular secretion (e.g., probenecid) may interfere with the uptake of certain tracers despite otherwise normal renal function.

Technologists should reassure patients about the safety of the examination. These agents are extremely safe because such small amounts are injected. Patients often express concern about having a radioactive material injected into their bodies. The radiation dose is similar to that from a CT scan.[42] The overall risk of a radionuclide examination is much less than the risk from a CT scan because of the extreme rarity of hypersensitivity reactions with radiopharmaceuticals in comparison to intravenous contrast agent that is commonly administered with a CT scan.

Common Procedures

Functional Renal Imaging. Functional renal imaging using ^{99m}Tc-MAG3 or ^{99m}Tc-DTPA is the most common radionuclide renal imaging study performed at most medical centers. Common indications for this study include (1) measurement of **relative renal function,** (2) evaluation of a renal transplant, and (3) evaluation of acute renal failure.[16,31,46]

In general, ^{99m}Tc-MAG3 is the preferred radiopharmaceutical over ^{99m}Tc-DTPA. Because ^{99m}Tc-MAG3 is primarily excreted via tubular secretion and because it has a very high first-pass extraction, it is possible to see perfusion and function even in a failing kidney that would not be as easily seen if a predominantly GFR-based agent such as ^{99m}Tc-DTPA was used. Since elevated serum creatinine would affect both native kidneys equally, assessment such as relative function or response to a diuretic is possible even in dysfunctional kidneys. There is some evidence that ^{99m}Tc-DTPA imaging may be more sensitive in detecting very early perfusion decrease in a transplanted kidney.[1] Still, there is no significant difference in the clinical implication of renal function in most situations, even in a transplanted kidney, to warrant preferential ^{99m}Tc-DTPA use.

For most common indications, a visual assessment of the renal perfusion and function is performed, followed by quantitative analysis of relative renal function. As with any other procedure, patient identification, appropriate requisition and indication should be verified. If the need for assessing renal response to diuretic administration exists, this can be done immediately following the functional assessment.[33] The procedures for Standard Functional Assessment and Diuretic Scintigraphy can be found in Boxes 19-4 and 19-5 respectively.

As described Box 19-4, a typical protocol for functional renal imaging consists of a rapid sequence of blood flow images (e.g., one 128×128 image every 2 to 3 seconds for the first minute), followed by a sequence of functional images obtained at a slower rate (e.g., one 256×256 image every 20 to 30 seconds for the next 19 minutes). Functional renal imaging can be used to determine both absolute and relative renal function. Most medical centers do not measure absolute renal function (ERPF or the GFR) because the most accurate methods are time-consuming and cumbersome, requiring several timed blood samples.[32] Measurements of absolute renal function based on imaging alone are done infrequently because these are not as reliable and in most clinical settings serum creatinine is a satisfactory indicator of absolute renal function.

Much more useful is the ability of radionuclide renal imaging to provide an index of relative individual kidney function. A major factor in the decision to treat or remove a diseased kidney is the degree to which the diseased kidney contributes to total renal function. Usually little effort is expended to repair a kidney that contributes less than 10% of total renal function.

BOX 19-4 | Standard Functional Assessment

1. Patient preparation: Patients are hydrated orally (2 to 3 8 oz cups of water) or via intravenous fluids and are encouraged to void before beginning the imaging procedure.
   a. After ensuring a functioning venous access for the radiopharmaceutical injection, the patient is positioned supine on the table for the initial part of the exam. Position so kidneys are near the top of the field of view.
2. Instrumentation: Usual camera setup is a large–field-of-view single head camera with a low energy all-purpose (LEAP) collimator. In pediatric patient, a diverging collimator may be optimal.
3. Procedure: With the correct acquisition protocol initiated, the radiopharmaceutical is injected as a bolus and radionuclide angiogram acquired. It is important to ensure the appropriate position of the kidneys (near the top of the field) early in order to adjust the camera, if needed. Thereafter, motion should be kept to a minimum, because the first 3 minutes of acquisition will be summed into the relative function analysis.
   a. Imaging protocol: The first minute of imaging, 30 frames at 2 seconds/frame, is immediately followed by 20 minutes of imaging, 20 seconds/frame, usually displayed as 2 minute compressed images.
   b. At the end of the acquisition, the patient is asked to void, and an upright postvoid image is obtained.
   c. If a urinary (Foley) catheter is in place, it is useful to acquire an image of the catheter drainage bag.
   d. The initial set of images—flow, function, and postvoid upright—are usually reviewed by the nuclear medicine physician to assess for completion and to determine whether additional imaging with diuretic administration is required.
4. Quantitative analysis of relative renal function is performed using a standard application. (If the patient is to undergo diuretic scintigraphy, this analysis can be deferred until completion of the additional imaging to ensure timely acquisition of data).

BOX 19-5 | Diuretic Renal Scintigraphy

1. Patient positioning: This portion of the study is acquired with the patient ideally in an upright position. Ensure that the patient can maintain an upright position with their back against the camera without movement for the duration of the study (20 minutes). If this is not possible, patient may be kept supine for this phase as well.
   a. Ensure that the camera is in proper dynamic acquisition mode.
   b. Ensure that a urinary catheter, if present, is not clamped.
2. Administration: Diuretic administration is done by the approved staff member (physician, nurse, or technologist) and should be done as a slow injection over 2 to 3 minutes.
3. Procedure: As with the prior phase, a 20-minute acquisition, 20 seconds/frame usually compressed into 2-minute static images, is performed.
   a. A radioactive marker flashed at the edge of the field of view at the midpoint of diuretic administration is a useful integral quality control for visually assessing response to diuretic administration.
   b. Again, the patient is asked to void (unless a catheter is in place) and a postvoid image is obtained.
4. Quantitative analysis for the diuretic phase is performed using standardized programs, with results including $t_{1/2}$ of radiopharmaceutical clearance in response to the diuretic administration.

Functional renal imaging also has been used to predict postoperative renal function after removal of a kidney for a renal malignancy. In this setting, postoperative renal function may be underestimated because of compensatory mechanisms.[21,26]

Relative renal function is calculated using an early image of the kidneys (1 to 3 minutes or 2 to 3 minutes after injection). The relative renal function is calculated by dividing the background-corrected kidney counts by the sum of the background-corrected counts from both kidneys. An early image is used because the radiopharmaceutical is primarily in the parenchyma (functioning tissue) of the kidney at this time. In later images the radiopharmaceutical may be retained in the collecting system. Collecting system activity does not correspond to relative renal function. To measure relative renal function, regions of interest are drawn around the entire kidney. Partial kidney regions of interest (in an attempt to avoid collecting system activity) would be unsatisfactory.

The time-activity curve (renogram) from a normal MAG3 study shows prompt uptake of the tracer, with the activity in the kidney peaking at 3 to 5 minutes after injection and decreasing to less than 50% of peak value by 20 minutes. Abnormal curves can result because of abnormal renal function, retention of activity in the collecting system, or patient movement (Figure 19-13, *A*). The cause of an abnormal curve usually can be easily determined from visual inspection of the images, with careful attention paid to the fate of activity seen in the peripheral parenchyma (cortex) of the kidney. A carefully drawn, crescent-shaped region of interest that excludes the collecting system may be helpful if significant retention of activity is seen in the renal pelvis.

Several caveats attend the determination of relative renal function. First, calculation of the relative renal function requires estimates of the number of counts in each kidney and the number of counts in a background region of interest (see Figure 19-13, *B*).[19] Normally, this calculation is quite robust; however, as renal function deteriorates, the number of counts in the background region of interest increases and becomes much more important in the calculation. Under these circumstances (low kidney counts and high background counts), the choice of the background region of interest can significantly change the measured contribution of the diseased

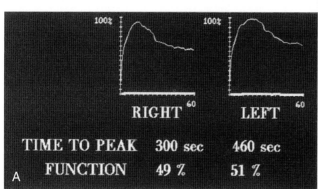
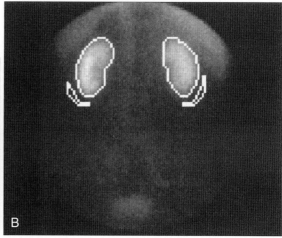

FIGURE 19-13 A, Renogram. The background-corrected activity versus the time curve from the kidney regions of interest is called the *renogram.* The renograms from the right and left kidneys are shown. The renogram represents only the function of the kidney when there is no significant retained activity in the collecting system. Retained activity in a dilated collecting system can give the false impression of decreased renal function. To avoid this error, both the images and the curves must be examined. **B,** Relative renal function. The percentage of renal function contributed by each kidney is calculated by drawing a region of interest around each kidney. In addition, a background region of interest is drawn for each kidney. The contribution of each kidney to total renal function is calculated by dividing the background-corrected counts for each kidney at 1 to 3 (or 2 to 3) minutes after injection by the background-corrected counts at 1 to 3 (or 2 to 3) minutes from both kidneys. The results usually are expressed as a percentage.

kidney; therefore a subjective estimate of the relative function may be just as accurate. Unfortunately, no universally accepted standards have been adopted for defining regions of interests.

A second source of error for the measurement of relative renal function is attenuation. Some of the radiation coming from the kidneys is absorbed by the soft tissue between the kidney and the gamma camera. If there is a significant difference in the depths of the kidneys, the contribution of the deeper kidney will be underestimated.

Finally, under some conditions (e.g., acute urinary obstruction, especially in young children) the loss of renal function may be reversible.

Functional renal imaging in the routine postoperative management of renal transplant patients has become uncommon.[11,12] Routine postoperative radionuclide imaging is not performed at most medical centers because unexpected surgical complications from renal transplantation are rare. In selected patients, radionuclide imaging can be useful for identifying urine leaks, obstruction of the urinary collecting system, and renal infarctions (Figures 19-14 to 19-16). Differentiation of acute tubular necrosis, rejection, and cyclosporine toxicity with radionuclide imaging is imperfect.[12]

Treatable causes of acute renal failure include dehydration (hypovolemia), infection, urinary collecting-system obstruction, and acute vascular obstruction. Radionuclide renal imaging is most helpful in excluding acute vascular obstruction as the cause of acute renal failure. Acute vascular obstruction is an uncommon cause of acute renal failure. One clinical setting in which vascular obstruction is likely to be considered is the

aftermath of abdominal aortic aneurysm repair. Decreased renal function after aortic stent placement or surgery is most likely caused by the transient ischemia of the kidneys that commonly occurs during repair of the aorta; however, an alternative cause is vascular obstruction, especially if the renal arteries had to be reimplanted at the time of surgical repair. If the kidney failure is the result of transient ischemia, renal function probably will improve; if it is the result of vascular obstruction, the loss of renal function is likely to be permanent.

Another potential use for radionuclide renal imaging in patients with acute renal failure is to determine their prognosis. Patients with little or no detectable renal activity on radionuclide renal imaging with hippuran (and presumably with ^{99m}Tc-MAG3) are unlikely to recover significant renal function.[41] Determination of the likelihood of recovery of renal function is helpful in deciding whether an arteriovenous shunt should be placed for future hemodialysis.

Diuretic Renal Imaging. The standard method used to differentiate a dilated renal collecting system from an obstructed renal collecting system is called the *Whitaker test.*[49] This invasive test requires placement of an infusion catheter (nephrostomy tube) through the skin (percutaneously) overlying the kidney into the collecting system proximal to the suspected point of obstruction. Saline is infused at high, nonphysiological flow rates (about 10 ml/min) while the pressure in the proximal collecting system is monitored. If no significant increase in pressure is seen, no urodynamically significant obstruction is present. Because it is invasive, the Whitaker test cannot be used routinely to follow patients for urinary

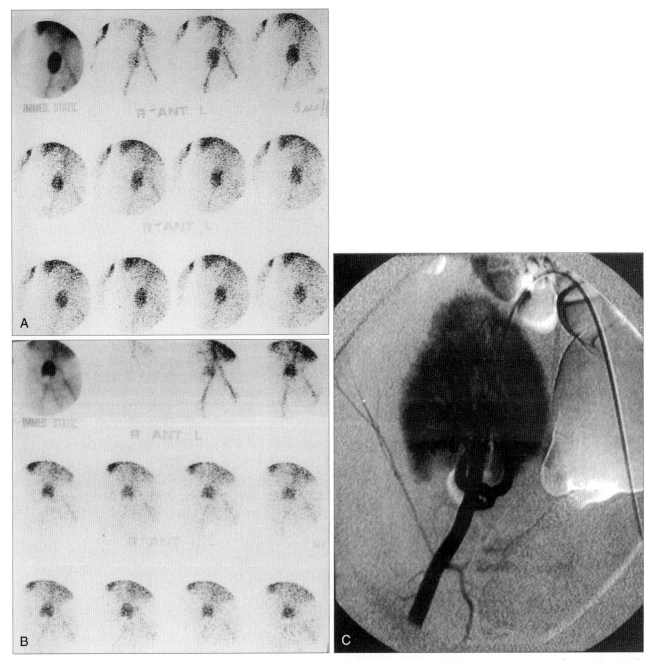

FIGURE 19-14 Infarction of the lower pole of a transplanted kidney. **A,** Flow study and immediate static image 1 day after renal transplant. The donor kidney was supplied by two renal arteries. **B,** Flow study and immediate static image 7 days after renal transplant when the patient was having pain and swelling of the transplanted kidney. **C,** Arteriogram of the transplanted kidney confirming the occlusion of the artery to the lower pole of the transplanted kidney.

tract obstruction. In addition, some question the significance of increased pressure at high, nonphysiological flow rates.

Diuretic renal imaging is particularly useful for differentiating a dilated renal collecting system from an obstructed renal collecting system (Figure 19-17, *A*).[22] Many dilated but unobstructed collecting systems empty spontaneously during routine radionuclide renal imaging. If collecting-system activity persists on a sitting post void image of the kidneys obtained 20 minutes after injection of the radiopharmaceutical, intravenous (IV) injection of furosemide (Lasix) (e.g., 0.5 mg/kg) is very useful. After injection of the furosemide, an additional 20 to 30 minutes of functional images are obtained. If a urodynamically significant outflow obstruction is present, the affected kidney is unable to increase its urine flow rate significantly in response to the furosemide injection. Because the urine flow rate does not increase, washout of the activity from the collecting system is prolonged (clearance half-time [$t_{1/2}$] of longer than 20 minutes). A

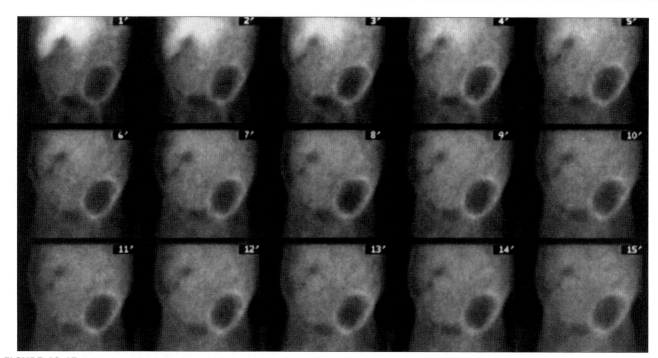

FIGURE 19-15 Infarction of a transplanted kidney. A 20-minute dynamic study (1 minute per image) after injection of ^{99m}Tc-MAG3 reveals decreased activity and no function of the renal transplant. The ring of increased activity is caused by an inflammation surrounding the infarcted kidney.

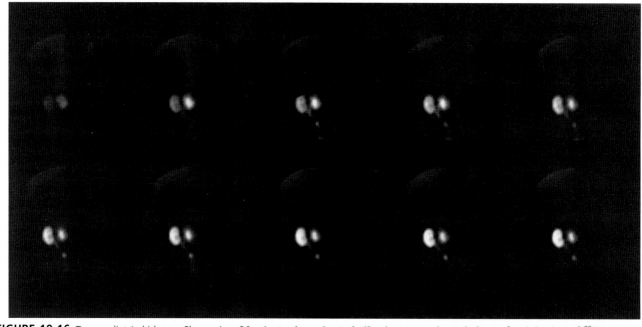

FIGURE 19-16 Two pediatric kidneys. Shown is a 20-minute dynamic study (2 minutes per image) done after injection of ^{99m}Tc-MAG3 in an adult patient who received both kidneys from a child donor. The kidney at the iliac bifurcation is functioning normally; the other kidney has prolonged retention of activity consistent with acute tubular necrosis (ATN), probably caused by a longer ischemic time.

dilated but unobstructed kidney can increase its urine flow rate in response to furosemide; therefore, the washout of activity from the collecting system is in the normal range ($t_{1/2}$ of less than 10 minutes) (Figure 19-17, B). When the $t_{1/2}$ for washout is 10 to 20 minutes, the results are equivocal. Some nuclear medicine departments inject furosemide 15 minutes before or at the time of the radiopharmaceutical injection.[10,24]

Compared with the Whitaker test, diuretic renal imaging has a high sensitivity for the detection of urodynamically significant ureteral narrowings. False-positive results and equivocal interpretation may arise

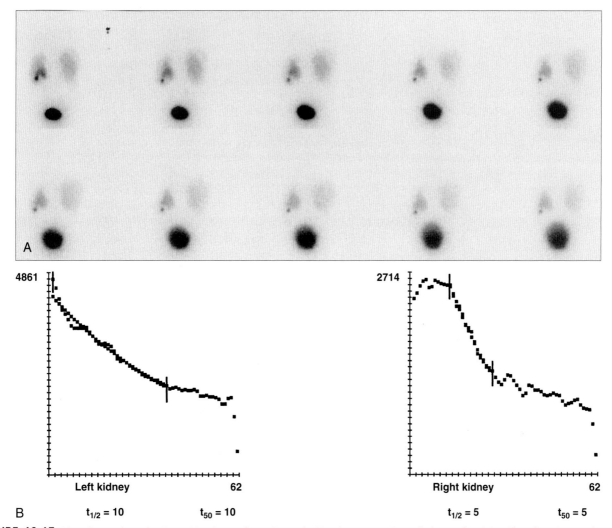

FIGURE 19-17 Diuretic renal study. **A,** A 20-minute dynamic study (2 minutes per image) done after injection of Lasix reveals normal washout of the radiopharmaceutical from the dilated but unobstructed left renal collecting system. **B,** Renogram reveals that both kidneys have a normal response to Lasix ($t_{1/2} \leq 10$ minutes).

when (1) a diseased kidney is not responsive to furosemide injection (such as with immature renal function in neonates, severe dehydration, and poor baseline renal function); (2) the collecting system is grossly dilated; and (3) **vesicoureteral reflux (VUR)** or a fully distended bladder (e.g., neurogenic bladder) is present.[27]

Renal Scintigraphy Augmented by ACE Inhibitor. The relationship between RAS and renovascular hypertension is complex.[8,39,47] Patients with hypertension may be classified into three groups: (1) those with hypertension and no significant RAS, (2) those with hypertension in whom RAS is a major contributor to the hypertension, and (3) those with hypertension in whom RAS is an insignificant contributor to the hypertension. Renal imaging with and without an ACE inhibitor is intended to identify patients in whom RAS is a major contributor to the hypertension (group 2). These patients have renovascular hypertension, and the hypertension is likely to be more easily controlled if the RAS is repaired.[2]

The physiology of renovascular hypertension has been reviewed. If an ACE inhibitor is given, less efferent arteriolar constriction occurs, the glomerular filtration pressure decreases, and the GFR declines. The ACE-dependent change in renal function can be detected using radionuclide imaging with and without an ACE inhibitor (Figure 19-18).

A number of different parameters can be used to document the change in renal function, including a decrease in renal uptake, prolongation of renal parenchymal transit, a decrease in the relative function of the affected kidney, and an increase in the time to peak activity.[18,38] Different investigators have used different parameters and combinations of parameters to detect renovascular disease.[14,43] Studies have documented the accuracy of this test in the prediction of normalization of blood pressure after revascularization.[9,36]

Morphological Renal Imaging. Morphological renal imaging after injection of ^{99m}Tc-glucoheptonate or

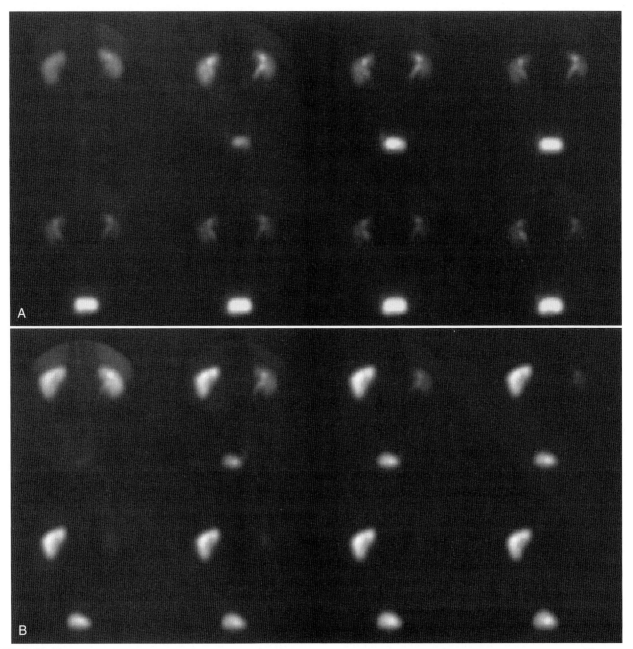

FIGURE 19-18 Renovascular hypertension. **A,** Baseline renal imaging (2.5 min/image) shows prompt symmetrical uptake of ^{99m}Tc-MAG3. A small amount of retained activity is seen in the renal collecting system bilaterally. Little retained activity is seen in the renal parenchyma. **B,** Renal imaging (2.5 min/image) after administration of an angiotensin-converting enzyme (ACE) inhibitor shows prompt uptake of activity in both kidneys. There is marked prolonged retention of activity in the left kidney. The patient had left renal artery stenosis.

^{99m}Tc-DMSA can be used to document global and regional changes in renal function. In patients with acute pyelonephritis, areas of decreased function may improve with appropriate treatment. In children with VUR and a history of urinary tract infections, the decision to repair the ureters may be influenced by the presence or absence of persistent renal cortical defects as demonstrated by radionuclide imaging.[30,33,35,37] SPECT imaging also may be useful.[7,28]

Morphological renal imaging may also be used to detect the presence or absence of small renal infarctions.

These infarctions may occur in patients at increased risk of systemic emboli, such as patients with atrial fibrillation or a left ventricular aneurysm. Infarctions that can occur as the result of a complicated renal procedure, such as percutaneous angioplasty of a stenotic renal artery or repair of an abdominal aortic aneurysm, also can be detected with renal imaging.

Vesicoureteral Reflux Study. A conventional contrast-voiding cystourethrogram is the initial investigation of choice in selected children with urinary tract infections. The anatomical information provided by this study is far

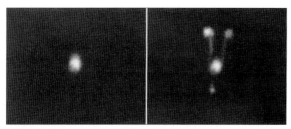

FIGURE 19-19 Vesicoureteral reflux (VUR) study. Two images from the first 2 minutes of a VUR are shown. Activity initially is seen only in the bladder *(left)*. There is prompt, severe reflux of activity to the level of both renal collecting systems *(right)*.

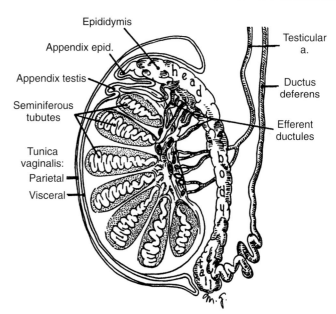

FIGURE 19-20 Testicular anatomy.

superior to the functional information provided by the radionuclide VUR study. Because of its lower radiation dose, a VUR study is preferred for follow-up when the primary concern is the severity and presence (or absence) of reflux rather than anatomy.[1a,48] Radionuclide cystography can be performed by catheterizing the patient and directly instilling the radionuclide into the bladder (Figure 19-19) or by injecting the patient with the tracer and allowing the bladder to fill with the tracer as it is excreted from the kidneys. Direct catheterization has a higher sensitivity and specificity than the indirect method and is the preferred method for radionuclide cystography. The clinical importance of reflux in children is its association with chronic pyelonephritic scarring and subsequent increased risk of hypertension in later years.

TESTICULAR IMAGING

Anatomy and Physiology

The testicles develop in the abdomen and descend to their normal position in the scrotum at about the time of birth. During their descent, the testicles are draped with a fold of parietal peritoneum called the *tunica vaginalis* (Figure 19-20). Normally the tunica vaginalis covers only the anterolateral surface of the testicle. The blood supply enters the posterior aspect of the testicle and prevents it from rotating in the scrotum. In a common variant of this normal anatomy, the tunica vaginalis more fully envelops the testicle. The blood supply that normally would enter posteriorly enters superiorly and no longer tethers the testicle, preventing it from rotating. This common variant, called the *bell clapper deformity*, is always present in cases of acute testicular **torsion.** Because the bell clapper deformity is usually bilateral, corrective surgery on the unaffected testicle is indicated when testicular torsion has been diagnosed.

Torsion, which most commonly occurs in males between 10 and 19 years of age, usually is marked by a sudden onset of testicular pain. Because the torsed testicle remains viable only for several hours, it is imperative that the diagnosis be suspected and the patient undergo surgery quickly. Some testicles are no longer

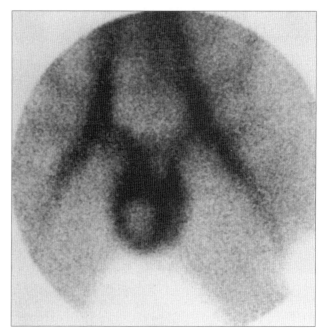

FIGURE 19-21 Delayed torsion. Testicular scintigraphy reveals a central area of decreased activity with a surrounding area of increased activity. The increased activity is caused by inflammation that occurs after the testicle becomes nonviable.

salvageable after 4 hours of torsion. None are salvageable after 12 to 24 hours of torsion. When testicular torsion lasts longer than 24 hours (delayed torsion), the testicle becomes necrotic and an inflammatory reaction occurs (Figure 19-21). Occasionally, testicular torsion can be intermittent, and the patient can have recurrent episodes of pain. Because acute testicular torsion is a surgical emergency, surgery should not be delayed. Patients suspected of having acute torsion should be sent directly to the operating room. Testicular scintigraphy should be reserved for patients who are unlikely to have acute testicular torsion.

Other diseases that can cause testicular pain include epididymo-orchitis, tumor, torsion of the appendix testis, trauma, and abscess. These causes of testicular pain usually can be differentiated from acute torsion by the patient's history and a physical examination.

Testicular Scintigraphy

Use of testicular scintigraphy to diagnose testicular torsion has largely been replaced by Doppler ultrasound examination of the testicles. In addition to morphological information, Doppler ultrasound is able to measure blood flow to the testicles.

Testicular scintigraphy consists of a flow study and immediate static images.[20] Technetium-99m-pertechnetate is the most commonly used radiopharmaceutical. The penis of the supine patient should be taped over the pubis. A tape sling should be used to support the testicles between the thighs. Cephalic angulation of the camera can help separate the activity from the thighs and pelvis from the activity from the testicles. Lead shielding can be used on the immediate static images but may make interpretation of the flow study more confusing. When lead shielding is used on the immediate static images, it must be carefully placed to shield both testicles symmetrically.

The blood flow study is primarily used to detect asymmetric blood flow. It usually is impossible to distinguish low testicular blood flow from normal testicular blood flow. The main purpose of the flow study is to detect areas of increased blood flow that would be seen with diseases such as epididymo-orchitis, delayed torsion, tumor, trauma, and abscess. Acute torsion probably will produce normal-appearing blood flow images. In acute torsion, the immediate static images reveal a central area of decreased activity with normal surrounding activity. A central area of decreased activity can also be seen with a hydrocele (fluid in the space formed by the tunica vaginalis). Hydroceles usually are painless and can be identified by transillumination on physical examination. Abscesses, necrotic tumors, hematomas, and delayed torsion usually have a central area of decreased activity surrounded by an area of increased activity caused by the surrounding inflammatory reaction.

MEASUREMENT OF EFFECTIVE RENAL PLASMA FLOW AND THE GLOMERULAR FILTRATION RATE

Effective renal plasma flow and the GFR can be quantified by measuring the plasma clearance of the selected radiopharmaceutical (see Table 19-1).[3,4,32] Plasma clearance of substances can be measured using two fundamentally different approaches. The first approach is called the *UV/P* (UV divided by P) method (Table 19-2).

TABLE 19-2	UV/P Method
U (urine concentration)	= 4000 cpm/ml
V (timed urine collection)	= 60 ml urine produced/20 min
P (plasma concentration)	= 100 cpm/ml

$$GFR = \frac{UV}{P} = \frac{60\,ml \times 4000\,cpm \times 1\,ml}{20\,min \times 1\,ml \times 100\,cpm}$$

$$= \frac{240,000\,ml}{2000\,min} = 120\,ml/min$$

This method requires (1) measurement of the plasma concentration of the substance (P [mg/ml]), (2) the rate of urine production (V [ml/min]), and (3) the concentration of the substance in the urine (U [mg/ml]). The units of clearance are milliliters per minute. Conceptually, clearance is how much plasma is completely cleared of the substance (ml) per unit time (minute).

The UV/P method has two major limitations. First, it works best with a steady plasma concentration of the substance of interest. In practice this requires that the patient be given a constant infusion of the substance over a few hours. Second, although the plasma and urine concentrations of the substance are readily measured, accurate measurement of urine production requires timed, complete urine collections. Hydration (to increase urine production) and bladder catheterization are needed to increase the reliability of the method.

A second way to determine how well the kidneys clear a substance from the plasma is to measure the plasma disappearance curve. This method produces reliable results only when the kidneys are the only significant pathway for excretion. This important requirement is adequately met by only a few radiopharmaceuticals. Typically, the plasma clearance curve is modeled as two compartments (Figure 19-22). The first compartment is the intravascular compartment (plasma), and the second compartment is the extravascular compartment. Initially, the concentration of the tracer in the plasma is very high. The initial rapid clearance of the tracer from the plasma (often called the *fast component*) is primarily the result of diffusion into the extravascular compartment. During this time a small amount of tracer is also cleared from the intravascular space by kidney excretion. Once the tracer reaches equilibrium in the two compartments, any decrease in activity in the intravascular compartment is the result of kidney excretion alone. Mathematically, the clearance curve that results from this model consists of the sum of two monoexponential equations. The plasma clearance curve method does not require the urine collections that are needed for the UV/P method. However, the plasma clearance curve method also is laborious because at least eight blood samples collected over a 4-hour period are needed to estimate accurately the biexponential clearance of the tracer. Methods using only one or two blood samples have been described.[15]

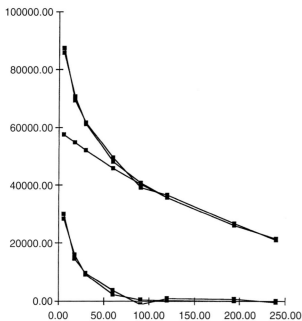

FIGURE 19-22 Glomerular filtration rate (GFR) plasma clearance curve and plasma clearance curve after intravenous injection of ^{99m}Tc-DTPA. The x-axis is minutes and the y-axis is counts per milliliter. The GFR is calculated by fitting a monoexponential to the slow component (the last four points) of the plasma clearance curve. The fitted curve is subtracted from the original data. A monoexponential curve is then fitted to the first four points of the resulting curve (the curve on the bottom of the graph). The GFR can be calculated based on the results of the two fitted monoexponential equations.

SUMMARY

- The kidneys are located in the back, spanning the distance from the twelfth thoracic vertebra to the third lumbar vertebra, with the right kidney usually slightly lower than the left.
- With planar scintigraphy the kidney may appear smaller than its actual size if the long axis is not parallel to the surface of the crystal of the gamma camera; this is called *foreshortening*.
- SPECT imaging using a morphological renal imaging agent is a more accurate technique for measuring renal size.
- Normal ERPF is about 600 ml/min and normal GFR is about 120 ml/min.
- The basic functional unit of the kidney is the nephron.
- The major factor that determines whether a substance is filtered is its molecular size.
- Filtration is a passive process and the rate is primarily determined by the perfusion pressure.
- When RAS is present, there is a decrease in perfusion pressure resulting in a decrease in filtration pressure and GFR.
- RAS is a significant contributor to renal hypertension. Patients with renal hypertension are often on an ACE inhibitor medication.

- Renal imaging with and without an ACE inhibitor is intended to identify patients in whom RAS is a major contributor to hypertension.
- Functional radiopharmaceuticals are taken up by the kidneys by a single, simple physiological mechanism such as ERPF or GFR and have a high first-pass extraction.
- Functional renal imaging is used to measure relative renal function, evaluate a renal transplant, and evaluate acute renal failure.
- Morphological radiopharmaceuticals are taken up by the kidneys by a complicated mechanism and have prolonged retention allowing evaluation of the morphology of the parenchyma. They can be used to document global and regional changes in renal function.
- If a renal arteriogram has been performed within a few days before a radionuclide renal study, inaccurate information of renal function may be obtained.
- Diuretic renal imaging is particularly useful for differentiating a dilated renal collecting system from an obstructed renal collecting system.
- A vesicoureteral reflux (VUR) study is the preferred follow-up study when the primary concern is the severity and presence (or absence) of reflux rather than anatomy. VUR can be performed by a direct or indirect method.
- Testicular scintigraphy to diagnose testicular torsion has largely been replaced by Doppler ultrasound.
- ERPF and GFR can be quantified by measuring the plasma clearance of the selected radiopharmaceutical.

REFERENCES

1. Aktaş A, et al: Comparison of Tc-99m DTPA and Tc-99m MAG3 perfusion time-activity curves in patients with renal allograft dysfunction, *Transplant Proc* 38:449-453, 2006.
1a. Ascenti G, et al: Vesicoureteral reflux: comparison between urosonography and radionuclide cystography, *Pediatr Nephrol* 18:768-771, 2003.
2. Black HR: Captopril renal scintigraphy: a way to distinguish functional from anatomic renal artery stenosis, *J Nucl Med* 33:2045-2046, 1992.
3. Blake GM, et al: Reference ranges for 51Cr-EDTA measurements of glomerular filtration rate in children, *Nucl Med Commun* 26:983-987, 2005.
4. Chiou YY, Wang ST, Tang MJ, et al: Renal fibrosis: prediction from acute pyelonephritis focus volume measured at ^{99m}Tc dimercaptosuccinic acid SPECT, *Radiology* 221:366-370, 2001.
5. Conway JC: The principles and technical aspects of diuresis renography, *J Nucl Med Technol* 4:208-214, 1989.
6. Conway JJ, Maizels M: The "well tempered" diuretic renogram: a standard method to examine the asymptomatic neonate with hydronephrosis or hydroureteronephrosis: a report from combined meetings of the Society for Fetal Urology and members of the Pediatric Nuclear Medicine Council, the Society of Nuclear Medicine, *J Nucl Med* 33:2047-2051, 1992.

7. Craig JC, et al: Reliability of DMSA for the diagnosis of renal parenchymal abnormality in children, *Eur J Nucl Med* 27:1610-1616, 2000.

8. Davidson RA, Wilcox CS: New tests for diagnosis of renovascular disease, *JAMA* 268:3353-3358, 1992.

9. Dondi M, et al: Prognostic value of captopril renal scintigraphy in renovascular hypertension, *J Nucl Med* 33:2040-2044, 1992.

10. Donoso G, et al: 99mTc-MAG3 Diuretic renography in children; a comparison between F0 and F20, *Nucl Med Commun* 24:1189-1193, 2003.

11. Dubovsky EV, et al: Report of the Radionuclides in Nephrourology Committee for evaluation of transplanted kidney (review of techniques), *Semin Nucl Med* 29:175-188, 1999.

12. Dubovsky EV, Russell CD: Radionuclide evaluation of renal transplants, *Semin Nucl Med* 3:181-198, 1988.

13. Eshima D, Fritzberg AR: Radiopharmaceuticals for renal imaging. In Henkin RE et al, editors: *Nuclear medicine*, St Louis, 1996, Mosby.

14. Fine EJ: Interventions in renal scintirenography, *Semin Nucl Med* 29:128-145, 1999.

15. Fleming JS, Persaud L, Zivanovic MA: A general equation for estimating glomerular filtration rate from a single plasma sample, *Nucl Med Commun* 26:743-748, 2005.

16. Fommei E, Volterrani D: Renal nuclear medicine, *Semin Nucl Med* 25:183-194, 1995.

17. Gates GF: Glomerular filtration. In Henkin RE, et al, editors: *Nuclear medicine*, St Louis, 1996, Mosby.

18. Geyskes GG, et al: Renovascular hypertension identified by captopril-induced changes in the renogram, *Hypertension* 1:36-42, 1987.

19. Harris CC, et al: Effect of region assignment on relative renal blood flow estimates using radionuclides, *Radiology* 151:791-792, 1984.

20. Holder LE, et al: Testicular radionuclide angiography and static imaging: anatomy, scintigraphic interpretation, and clinical indications, *Radiology* 125:739-752, 1977.

21. Johansson M, Moonen M: Prediction of postoperative glomerular filtration rate after nephrectomy for renal malignancy, *Clin Physiol* 21:688-692, 2001.

22. Konda R, et al: Ultrasound grade of hydronephrosis and severity of renal cortical damage on 99m-technetium dimercaptosuccinic acid renal scan in infants with unilateral hydronephrosis during follow-up and after pyeloplasty, *J Urol* 167:2159-2163, 2002.

23. Lin E, et al: Reproducibility of renal length measurements with ^{99m}Tc-DMSA SPECT, *J Nucl Med* 41(10):1632-1635, 2000.

24. Liu Y, et al: The F+O protocol for diuretic renography results in fewer interrupted studies due to voiding the F-15 Protocol, *J Nucl Med* 46:1317-1320, 2005.

25. Majd M, Rushton HG: Renal cortical scintigraphy in the diagnosis of acute pyelonephritis, *Semin Nucl Med* 22:298-311, 1992.

26. Marks LS, Maxwell MH: Renal vein renin: value and limitation in the prediction of operative results, *Urol Clin North Am* 2:311-317, 1975.

27. Niemczyk P, et al: Use of diuretic renogram in evaluation of patients before and after endopyelotomy, *Urology* 53:271-275, 1999.

28. Peng NJ, et al: ^{99m}Tc dimercaptosuccinic acid renal scintigraphy for detection of renal cortical defects in acute pyelonephritis: posterior 180-degree SPECT versus planar image and 360-degree SPECT, *Nucl Med Commun* 22:417-422, 2001.

29. Perrone RD, et al: Utility of radioisotopic filtration markers in chronic renal insufficiency: simultaneous comparison of ^{125}I iothalamate, ^{169}Yb-DTPA, ^{99m}Tc-DTPA, and inulin, *Am J Kid Dis* 16:224-235, 1990.

30. Piepsz A, et al: Consensus on renal cortical scintigraphy in children with urinary tract infection, Scientific Committee of Radionuclides in Nephrourology, *Semin Nucl Med* 29:160-174, 1999.

31. Piepsz A, Ham HR: Pediatric applications of renal nuclear medicine, *Semin Nucl Med* 36:16-35, 2006.

32. Piepsz A, Ham R, DeSadeleer C: Guidelines for the measurement of glomerular filtration rate using plasma sampling, *Nucl Med Commun* 26:175-176, 2005.

33. Pohl HG, et al: Early diuresis renogram findings predict success following pyeloplasty, *J Urol* 165:2311-2315, 2001.

34. Prescott MC, Johnson WG: Influence of drugs on the renogram. In O'Reilly PH, Shields RA, Testa HJ, editors: *Nuclear medicine in urology and nephrology*, Boston, 1989, Butterworth.

35. Rossleigh MA: Renal cortical scintigraphy and diuresis renography in infants and children, *J Nucl Med* 42:91-95, 2001.

36. Roubidoux MA, et al: Renal vein renins: inability to predict response to revascularization in patients with hypertension, *Radiology* 178:819-822, 1991.

37. Rushton HG, et al: Renal scarring following reflux and nonreflux pyelonephritis in children: evaluation with 99mtechnetium-dimercaptosuccinic acid scintigraphy, *J Urol* 147:1327-1332, 1992.

38. Setaro JF, et al: Simplified captopril renography in diagnosis and treatment of renal artery stenosis, *Hypertension* 18:289-298, 1991.

39. Sfakianakis GN, et al: Single-dose captopril scintigraphy in the diagnosis of renovascular hypertension, *J Nucl Med* 28:1383-1392, 1987.

40. Shapiro E, et al: Optimal use of 99mtechnetium-glucoheptonate scintigraphy in the detection of pyelonephritic scarring in children: a preliminary report, *J Urol* 40:1175-1177, 1988.

41. Sherman RA, Sherman B: Clinical significance of nonvisualization with I-131 hippuran renal scan. In Hollenberg NK, Lange S, editors: *Radionuclides in nephrology*, Stuttgart, Germany, 1980, Thieme.

42. Snyder WS, et al: *Absorbed dose per unit cumulated activity for selected radionuclides and organs*, MIRD Pamphlet No 11, New York, 1975, Society of Nuclear Medicine.

43. Taylor A: Radionuclide renography: a personal approach, *Semin Nucl Med* 29:102-127, 1999.

44. Taylor A, et al: Clinical comparison of I-131 orthoiodohippurate and the kit formulation of Tc-99m mercaptoacetyltriglycine, *Radiology* 170:721-725, 1989.

45. Taylor A Jr, et al: Comparison of iodine-131OIH and technetium-99m MAG3 renal imaging in volunteers, *J Nucl Med* 27:795-803, 1986.

46. Taylor A Jr, Nally JV: Clinical applications of renal scintigraphy, *AJR Am J Roentgenol* 164:31-41, 1995.

47. Van Bockel JH, et al: Renovascular hypertension: collective review, *Surg Gynecol Obstet* 169:471-478, 1989.

48. Vlajkovic M, et al: Radionuclide voiding patterns in children with vesicoureteral reflux, *Eur J Nucl Med Mol Imaging* 30:531-537, 2003.

49. Whitaker RH: Methods of assessing obstruction in dilated ureters, *Br J Urol* 45:15-22, 1973.

Skeletal System

Kristen M. Waterstram-Rich, Gary Dillehay

OBJECTIVES

After completing this chapter, the reader will be able to:
- Explain the composition of bone and list the general types of bones.
- Name the major bones and joints of the skeleton.
- Explain the accumulation mechanism of bone-imaging agents.
- Discuss the advantages of whole-body imaging techniques versus spot imaging.
- Describe adequate acquisition parameters for static bone imaging using spot-film and whole-body imaging devices.
- Explain the advantages of performing SPECT bone scans.
- Describe imaging techniques and acquisition parameters for obtaining flow studies and blood pool imaging.
- Explain the advantages of performing delayed imaging in the diagnosis of osteomyelitis.
- Discuss the use of gallium and white cell imaging techniques in correlation with bone scans.
- Describe the principles of bone therapy and discuss the characteristics of radioactive strontium.
- Identify the appropriate radiopharmaceutical dose and administration technique for strontium bone therapy.

KEY TERMS

analog
avascular necrosis (AVN)
blood pool image
epiphysis

equal-time imaging
heterionic exchange
hydroxyapatite
photopenic

spot views
superimposition

The skeleton performs several functions for the body, including support, protection, movement, and blood formation. Bone consists of living cells and a predominant amount of nonliving intercellular substance that is calcified. It is a metabolically active tissue with large amounts of nutrients being exchanged in the blood supplying the bone. Thus the skeleton and body fluids are in equilibrium. Tracer techniques have been used for many years to study the exchange between bone and blood,[5] and radionuclides have played an important role in the understanding of normal bone metabolism, in addition to the metabolic effects of pathological involvement of bone.

Radionuclide imaging of the skeleton is frequently used in the evaluation of abnormalities involving bones and joints.[6] Several studies have demonstrated that different information can be obtained from radionuclide bone imaging compared with radiography and blood chemistry analysis.[18,22,28,37,40] Radionuclide joint imaging for the evaluation of many diseases involving the joints has been used for a shorter period than has bone imaging.*

To fully understand the technical and clinical aspects of radionuclide imaging of the skeletal system, a thorough knowledge of the anatomy and physiology of bones and joints is necessary. The first part of this chapter reviews skeletal anatomy and physiology. The remainder of the chapter discusses radionuclide imaging of the bones and joints, including the technical aspects and applications of the imaging procedure. Radionuclide bone therapy and information on the three radionuclides—[89]Sr-chloride, [153]Sm-lexidronam and ^{32}P-sodium phosphate—currently approved by the U.S. Food and Drug Administration (FDA) for palliative therapy can be found in Chapter 22.

COMPOSITION OF BONE

Bone, as well as other connective tissue in the body, is maintained by living cells in addition to having amorphous ground substance and fibers. The main difference between bone and other connective tissue is that it is calcified; thus it is harder. Bone matrix, the other major constituent of bone, consists of collagen, amorphous ground substance, and mineral.

The periosteum is fibrous connective tissue containing blood vessels that cover the bone. The cells involved in the formation and growth of bone include osteoprogenitor, osteoblasts, osteoclasts, and osteocytes.[12] Osteoblasts are associated with bone growth and osteoclasts are associated with absorption and removal of bone. Bone is under a constant cycle of absorption and growth.

There are two types of bone tissue, compact and spongy. Compact bone is dense, hard tissue that normally composes the shafts of long bones and the outer layer of other bones. This type of bone is made up of cylindrical units called osteons or haversian systems. Each unit has mature bone cells (osteocytes) forming concentric circles around blood vessels.[12] Spongy bone is lined with endosteum. This helps reduce the weight of the bones and it provides a space for red bone marrow which produces red blood cells.

The composition by weight of normal adult cortical bone is approximately 5% to 10% water, 25% to 30% organic matter (collagen, ground substance, and cellular elements), and 65% to 70% inorganic matter (bone mineral). Collagen is the main protein constituent and accounts for 90% to 95% of the organic matter of bone.

Collagen is present in the form of fibrils bunched together into bundles of fibers. The ground substance is the interfibrillar cement substance in which the fibrils are embedded. The bone salt mineral (inorganic matter) has the crystalline form of an apatite and is composed of the following ions: calcium, phosphate, hydroxyl, carbonate, and citrate, with lesser amounts of sodium, magnesium, potassium, chloride, and fluoride. Approximately 27% of the weight of cortical bone is calcium. The main anion constituent of bone is phosphorus (as phosphate), which contributes approximately 12% of the weight of cortical bone. The bone mineral consists of individual crystals so small that the electron microscope is needed for visualization of the crystals. The crystalline structure is **hydroxyapatite,** with the empirical formula of $Ca_{10}(PO_4)_6(OH)_2$.

GROSS STRUCTURE OF BONE

Bones have obvious differences in size and shape but also certain features in common. They have a cortex (compact bone) surrounding various amounts of cancellous (spongy or trabecular) bone, which contains blood-forming (myeloid) elements or fatty marrow (Figures 20-1 and 20-2). In the adult, most of the myeloid marrow is in the bones of the trunk, with some in the calvarium and upper ends of the humeri and femora. Another similarity in bones is that they are covered by periosteum, except in areas of articulation or where tendons and ligaments connect them. The differences in bones include general architecture and gross structure, which can be divided into in the following groups: tubular, short, flat, and irregular.

Tubular Bones

The long tubular bones include the humerus, radius, ulna, femur, tibia, and fibula. The short tubular bones include the metacarpals, metatarsals, and phalanges. Often the tubular bones are all classified as long bones. The tubular bones have a shaft (diaphysis) consisting of a cortex of compact bone surrounding the medullary cavity, which contains bone marrow (see Figure 20-1). In the adult this is mainly yellow, or fatty, marrow except for the proximal humerus and femur, where it is red (blood-forming) marrow (see Figure 20-2). The cortex is thickest at the midshaft and tapers toward the ends of the shaft. The end of a bone that previously in childhood had an **epiphysis** is known as an *epiphyseal bone end*. The juncture of the cancellous bone of the epiphyseal bone end and the spongy bone of the diaphysis is called the *metaphysis*.

Short Bones

The short bones include the wrist (carpals), ankle (tarsals), sesamoids (small bones forming in a tendon or

---

*References 15, 31, 38, 39, 52.

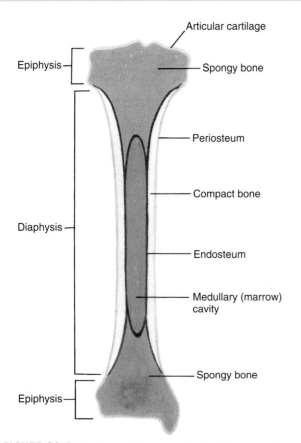

FIGURE 20-1 Structure of long bone in longitudinal section.

joint capsule), and other anomalous or extra bones. These bones are generally cubic and have spongy osseous tissue covered by a shell of compact bone.

Flat Bones

The flat bones include the ribs, sternum, and scapulae and several of the skull bones. These bones are thin and have little spongy bone between two layers of compact bone. The flat bones of the skull consist of an inner and outer table (layers of cortical bone) separated by a thin layer of spongy bone (diploe). The spongy layer of the ribs and sternum contains considerable red marrow.

Irregular Bones

The irregular bones include the bones of the spine and pelvis and some of the skull. Part of an irregular bone may fit into one of the other categories, but the entire bone does not fit into any of the previous categories. The largest part of these bones often consists of large amounts of spongy osseous tissue with a very thin surrounding cortex, whereas another part of the same bone may have no spongy tissue and may be composed of two layers of compact bone (Figure 20-3).

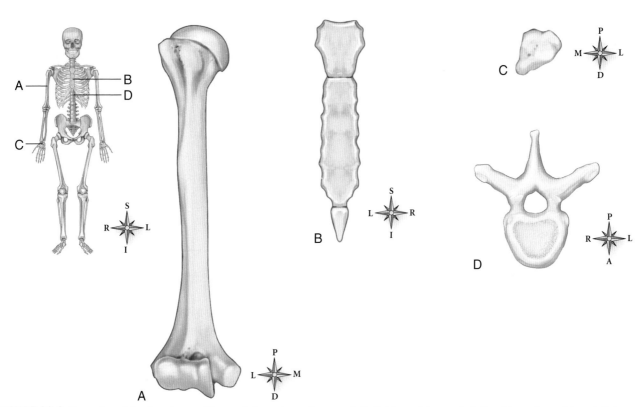

FIGURE 20-2 Examples of the four types of bone. **A,** Long bone (humerus). **B,** Flat bone (sternum). **C,** Short bone (carpal bone). **D,** Irregular bone (vertebra).

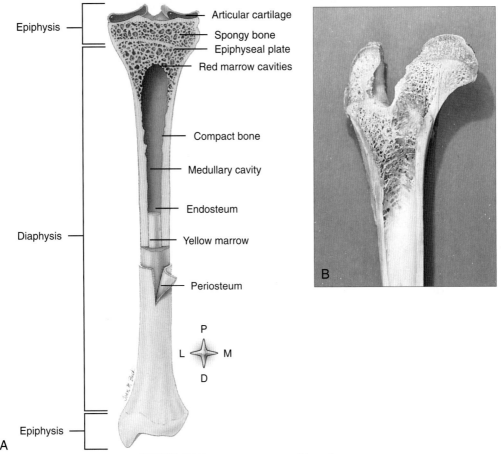

FIGURE 20-3 Cutaway section of long bone.

SKELETON

The human skeletal system (Figures 20-4 and 20-5 usually contains 206 bones; it provides a supporting framework for the body and forms protective chambers, such as the skull and thorax. The skeleton is divided into two main parts, the axial skeleton and the appendicular skeleton (Table 20-1). The axial skeleton is composed of the bones of the skull, thorax, and vertebral column, which form the axis of the body. The appendicular skeleton is composed of the bones of the shoulder, upper extremities, hips, and lower extremities. A detailed structure of the vertebrae is shown in Figure 20-6.

JOINTS

Joints (articulations) are spaces where bones come into contact and are bridged in some manner. The articulations have variable amounts of movement and have been classified into two main types according to the amount of movement: rigid (synarthroses) or freely movable (diarthroses).

With a synarthrosis there is absence of a joint space, with little or no movement allowed. In the formation of a synarthrosis, the tissue connecting the bones is replaced

TABLE 20-1	Skeletal System
Skeletal Parts	**Number of Bones**
Axial Skeleton	
Skull and hyoid	29
Vertebrae	26
Ribs and sternum	25
Subtotal	**80**
Appendicular Skeleton	
Upper limbs	64
Lower limbs	62
Subtotal	**126**
Total	**206**

by the ends of the bone growing together. The sutures of the skull are examples of synarthroses, with only a thin, fibrous membrane separating the ends of the bones (Figure 20-7, A). In some synarthroses, cartilage grows between the articular surfaces of the bones and may allow some motion. Examples of the cartilaginous synarthroses are the symphysis pubis and the joints between the vertebral bodies (see Figure 20-7, B and C).

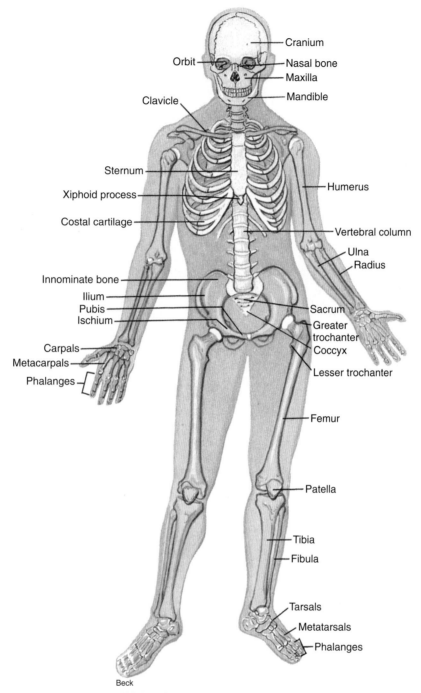

Cranium
Orbit
Nasal bone
Maxilla
Mandible
Clavicle
Sternum
Xiphoid process
Costal cartilage
Humerus
Vertebral column
Ulna
Radius
Innominate bone
Ilium
Pubis
Ischium
Sacrum
Greater trochanter
Coccyx
Carpals
Metacarpals
Phalanges
Lesser trochanter
Femur
Patella
Tibia
Fibula
Tarsals
Metatarsals
Phalanges

Beck

FIGURE 20-4 Skeleton, anterior view.

A diarthrosis permits freedom of movement and is the most common type of joint in the body. A diarthrosis has a well-defined articular cavity that contains fluid (synovia) and is lined by a synovial membrane (see Figure 20-6, *D* and *E*). Intraarticular structures such as ligaments and menisci may be present. A thin layer of hyaline cartilage, known as *articular cartilage,* cushions the ends of each bone in the joint. The synovial joint develops from undifferentiated mesenchyme between the bone rudiments. Part of the undifferentiated mesenchyme differentiates into synovial mesenchyme and subsequently into synovial membranes, menisci, and ligaments. The outer portion of the undifferentiated mesenchyme condenses and forms the joint capsule, which attaches to the bone ends of the joints beyond their articular cartilages.

RADIONUCLIDE IMAGING

Of the many different imaging procedures performed in clinical nuclear medicine, radionuclide bone and joint studies especially require the technologist to be thoroughly knowledgeable of anatomy and imaging techniques so that excellent images of the radiopharmaceutical

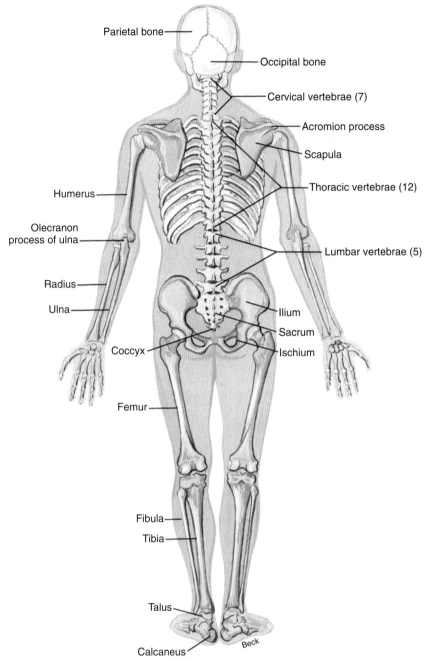

Parietal bone

Occipital bone

Cervical vertebrae (7)

Acromion process

Scapula

Thoracic vertebrae (12)

Humerus

Olecranon process of ulna

Lumbar vertebrae (5)

Radius

Ulna

Ilium

Sacrum

Coccyx

Ischium

Femur

Fibula

Tibia

Talus

Beck

Calcaneus

FIGURE 20-5 Skeleton, posterior view.

distribution can be obtained. Because early disease involvement of bone initially may be subtle, improper positioning of the patient for imaging, improper exposure of the film, or improper manipulation of the computer images may lead to an inaccurate interpretation. Furthermore, because these studies frequently are used to follow therapy, the technique must be reproducible to allow careful comparison with a previous study. Several different types of radionuclide studies can be performed in the evaluation of bone and joint disorders. The most commonly performed procedure is radionuclide bone imaging with a technetium-99m (^{99m}Tc) phosphate compound. Joint imaging is used in the

evaluation of suspected inflammatory processes involving bones and joints.

Past and Present Radiopharmaceuticals

The earliest applications of radionuclides to study the bone were performed with phosphorus-32 (^{32}P) and calcium-45 (^{45}Ca) for observation of bone structure and function.[2,38] These radionuclides are pure beta particle emitters and accumulate in regions of increased bone mineral deposition, but their lack of gamma radiation limits external measurement. Clinical application became

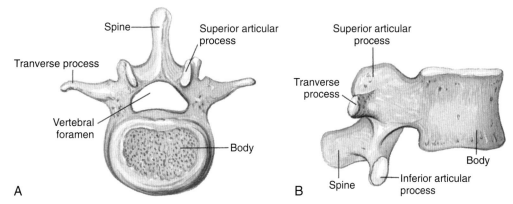

FIGURE 20-6 Third lumbar vertebra from above (**A**) and the side (**B**).

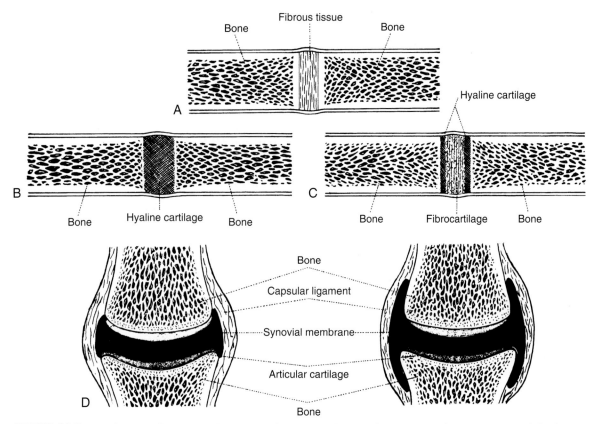

FIGURE 20-7 Classification of joints. **A,** Fibrous synarthrosis. **B** and **C,** Cartilaginous synarthroses. **D,** Synovial diarthrosis.

possible in the 1960s with the introduction of the rectilinear scanner only and the use of strontium-85 (^{85}Sr), a calcium **analog** that produced gamma rays that could be detected externally.[4,10,11] ^{85}Sr has a half-life of 65 days and emits gamma rays at 513 keV. The long effective half-life of this radionuclide limited the amount of activity injected to 100 mCi. With this small amount of activity, scanning time was extensive and the information density of the image was extremely low. Although the accumulation of strontium in bone is rapid, blood and gastrointestinal clearances are slow; therefore a 2- to 7-day interval between the times of injection and scan was needed. In addition, because of the high radiation

dose involved, its use was limited to patients with documented malignancy.

Another isotope of strontium used for bone scanning was strontium-87m (^{87m}Sr), which has a half-life of 2.9 hours and has a gamma ray energy of 388 keV.[46] Its short half-life allowed the administered dose to be increased to a range of 1 to 4 mCi and scans to be performed 2 to 3 hours after injection. Strontium-87m is a generator-produced isotope from a parent product of yttrium-87 (^{87}Y), which has a half-life of 80 hours. Unfortunately, ^{87m}Sr was rather expensive.

In the late 1960s and early 1970s, wider application of bone imaging occurred with the introduction of fluorine-18 (^{18}F), a hydroxyl analog. ^{18}F was the first bone-seeking radiopharmaceutical that gave an acceptable radiation dose to the patient and provided a higher quality scan than the strontium isotopes.[8] The rapid blood clearance of ^{18}F is advantageous for the performance of bone scans because the blood and tissue activity levels are low compared with that of bone at the time of imaging and therefore give a high ratio of bone to soft tissue. The disadvantage of using ^{18}F is its half-life of 1.87 hours, which makes it expensive to manufacture and deliver to a large number of hospitals at any great distance from a production facility. The annihilation radiation (511 keV) from its positron emission requires special consideration and instrumentation for imaging.

Although the development of ^{99m}Tc-labeled phosphate complexes for bone imaging was introduced by Subramanian in 1971,[47,48] ^{99m}Tc in the form of pertechnetate does not localize to any useful extent in bone. Technetium-99m has excellent physical properties for nuclear medicine imaging because of its ideal characteristics for use with the Anger scintillation camera, and its short half-life allows several millicuries of activity to be injected, which allows images with high information density to be obtained.

Because of its ideal characteristics for imaging, ^{99m}Tc became the radionuclide of choice, and the phosphate compound that produced the best image needed to be determined. Figure 20-8 shows the structure of four phosphate compounds that have been used in routine clinical bone imaging. To evaluate these various phosphate compounds, their distribution in the body relative to the rate and amount of accumulation in various organ systems and bone was determined.

Polyphosphate was the first commercially available ^{99m}Tc-labeled compound for bone imaging. The structural formula of polyphosphate includes a group of phosphates with a chain length of approximately 40 to 55. Extremely long phosphate chains can result in the formation of a radiocolloid in the bloodstream, causing hepatic localization of the pharmaceutical. Further development of this agent moved from longer phosphate chains toward shorter, more stable phosphate complexes. Among these were pyrophosphate and ethylenehydroxydiphosphonate (EHDP).

Pyrophosphate is a naturally occurring compound in the body, and its P—O—P bond is subject to breakdown by phosphatase enzymes. The carbon–carbon bond of EHDP is believed to offer greater stability than pyrophosphate. Both pyrophosphate and EHDP have a faster blood and tissue clearance than does polyphosphate.

Methylene diphosphonate (MDP) and hydroxymethylene diphosphonate (HMDP) are similar to pyrophosphate and EHDP but have faster blood clearance.[34] The blood clearance of MDP and HMDP in the initial 3 to 4 hours after administration is very similar to that of fluorine. MDP and HMDP labeled with ^{99m}Tc provide a better image of the bones, because the lower blood and tissue concentrations give a higher ratio of bone to tissue. MDP and HMDP give comparable quality bone images.

Mechanism of Accumulation

The accumulation of radionuclides in bone is related both to vascularity and to the rate of bone production (osteoblastic activity).[19, 47] Osteoclastic activity is not involved in the accumulation of radionuclides and therefore does not appear in the image. Increased blood supply to an area of bone results in a **blood pool image** (obtained immediately after radiopharmaceutical administration) with increased activity.

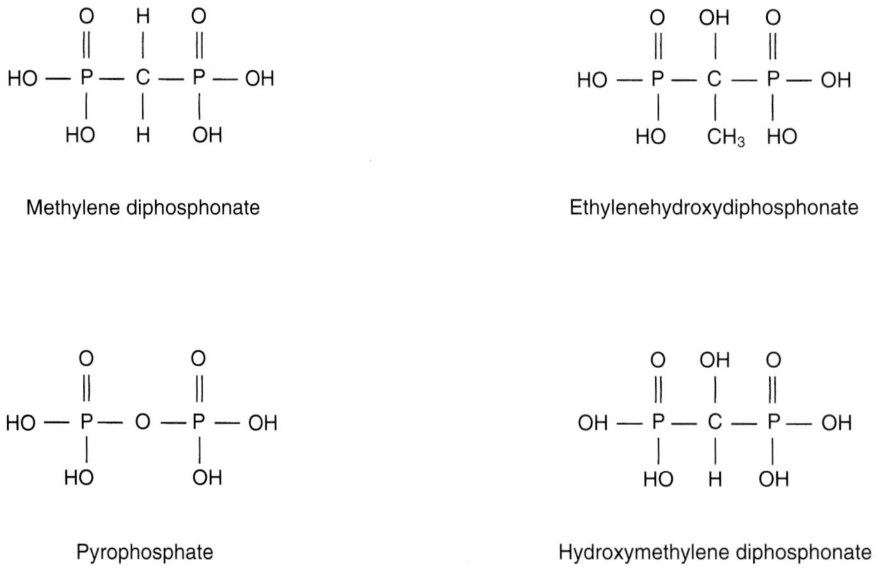

Methylene diphosphonate

Ethylenehydroxydiphosphonate

Pyrophosphate

Hydroxymethylene diphosphonate

FIGURE 20-8 Structural formulas of various phosphate pharmaceuticals in acid form.

Localization of various bone-imaging agents is related to their exchange with ions in the bone, and although these mechanisms are not completely understood, the principle of bone imaging is fairly basic. The principle of bone imaging relies on the exchange of an ion native to bone for a labeled, bone-seeking ion, a process called **heterionic exchange.**[9, 27] Calcium phosphate is the main inorganic constituent of bone; however, calcium is also found in the form of carbonate and fluoride. Calcium is located in microcrystals of hydroxyapatite.[39] Analog elements of calcium, such as strontium, are believed to exchange with the calcium. Fluorine-18 exchanges with the hydroxyl (OH) ion in the hydroxyapatite. The accumulation of labeled phosphate compounds probably is related to the exchange of the phosphorus groups onto the calcium of hydroxyapatite.

Calcium analogs or phosphate compounds have a low concentration in blood and tissue; however, radiopharmaceuticals used for bone imaging can localize in soft-tissue areas, demonstrating not only calcification but also infarction, inflammation, trauma, and tumor. The portion of any radiopharmaceutical that does not accumulate in bone or tissue or that stays in circulation is eliminated from the body by various routes, depending on the radiopharmaceutical. Strontium-85 has some concentration in the gastrointestinal tract for several days. ^{18}F- and ^{99m}Tc-labeled phosphate compounds demonstrate activity in the kidneys and bladder, because these agents are excreted through the urinary tract.

Technical Considerations

The physical characteristics of the radionuclides that have been used for bone imaging present several important factors in radiopharmaceutical selection. These factors relate primarily to the amount of activity that may be administered to the patient, the gamma ray energy, and the amount of accumulation of radiopharmaceutical in the bone.

Before the introduction of ^{18}F and ^{99m}Tc phosphate compounds, bone imaging was a time-consuming procedure associated with a high radiation dose to the patient and poor information content in the images. The subsequent development of better radiopharmaceuticals and improved instrumentation produced images of higher quality with better information about bone physiology. In conjunction with the improved information in the images, the need for carefully controlling the technical aspects of the procedure became apparent.

Selection of the best radionuclide for bone imaging is a simple choice based on the physical characteristics. The strontium and fluorine isotopes have high-energy gamma rays and require the use of coarse-resolution collimators with thick lead septa. The high-energy gamma rays have a low attenuation coefficient, resulting in a poor detection efficiency in the thin, sodium iodide crystal of the Anger scintillation camera. Also, these radionuclides must be administered in amounts of activity smaller than those of ^{99m}Tc, yielding lower information-density images. ^{99m}Tc –labeled compounds allow larger quantities of activity to be administered with a resultant lower radiation dose than do the other radionuclides. The monoenergetic gamma ray emission of 140 keV and the absence of particulate radiation make ^{99m}Tc well suited for use with the scintillation camera. ^{99m}Tc is also readily available to all laboratories at a very low cost, unlike other radionuclides for bone imaging.

Patient Preparation

Preparation of the patient for bone imaging is minimal when any of the ^{99m}Tc-labeled agents are used, but several factors must be taken into consideration. The patient needs to have a complete understanding of the procedure, especially the reason for the delay between radiopharmaceutical administration and imaging. A delay of approximately 3 hours is generally an adequate time to achieve good bone accumulation and a low soft-tissue level of the radiopharmaceutical. Radiopharmaceuticals with fast blood and tissue clearance, such as MDP and HMDP, allow imaging as early as 2 hours after administration. Unless contraindicated, patients should be hydrated to aid clearance of the radiopharmaceutical from the body. Administration of four to six glasses of liquid during the delay period is adequate, and the patient should be encouraged to void frequently to reduce the radiation dose to the bladder. Patients must also void immediately before imaging begins so that the image of the pelvis is not obscured by a large amount of radioactivity in the bladder. Because of the high concentration of radioactivity in the urine, care must be taken by both the patient and technologist to avoid contamination of the patient, the patient's clothing, or the bed sheets, which can lead to a false-positive result on the study. Box 20-1 shows the skeletal imaging protocol.

INSTRUMENTATION

Several types of instruments have been used for bone imaging. Wider application of this procedure has been responsible for the design of new instruments and accessories.

The Anger scintillation camera is currently the most versatile and most commonly used imaging device for ^{99m}Tc-labeled compounds. Because the skeleton is one of the most extensive organ systems in the body, application of the mobile camera with an approximately 10-inch standard field of view requires 25 to 30 separate views for complete imaging. Performing bone imaging by this technique requires a large amount of the technologist's time and effort in positioning the patient for all these views. High-resolution or medium-resolution (140 keV) collimators are well suited for bone imaging with a standard-field camera (high-sensitivity collimators

---

BOX 20-1   Skeletal (Bone) Imaging Protocol

Instrumentation: Gamma camera: Large field of view, preferably with two heads.
Collimator: Low energy, high resolution, parallel hole.
Energy window: 20% window centered at 140 keV
Radiopharmaceutical: ^{99m}Tc-MDP; ^{99m}Tc-HMDP
Activity: 25 mCi (925 MBq)
Imaging field: Entire body

1. Provide patient with information regarding scan, including reasoning for and length of delay between injection and imaging and information regarding injection technique if dynamic imaging is required (see Box 20-4).
2. Position patient for imaging during injection, if a dynamic study is required.
3. Inject patient intravenously with radiopharmaceutical.
    a. Avoid injecting in an area of interest.
    b. Take images during injection if a dynamic study is required.
4. Instruct patient to return 2 to 3 hours later to be scanned and to drink 4 to 6 glasses of water and void frequently during the interim and immediately prior to the scan.
5. Position patient supine (if possible) for the scan.
6. Acquire whole-body (WB) images
    a. The scan speed should be set using count rate or ID or by selecting the total time for the WB scan based on manufacturer protocols.
    b. The same scan speed should be used for both the anterior and the posterior images.
    c. Acquire spot views of areas of interest as indicated.
    d. If a WB scan images can not be acquired, spot views of the entire body should be taken using equal-time technique.*

---

*Counts over the sternum are taken; between 400,000 and 600,000 counts are accumulated for a standard-field camera and between 500,000 and 1 million for a large-crystal camera. All subsequent images are taken for the same interval that had been recorded for the first image. Alternatively, if available, the ID feature available on the scintillation camera can be used.

should not be used). A 140-keV diverging collimator can maintain good resolution and allows a reduction of the total number of images taken because of the larger effective field of view but results in slight spatial distortion and loss of resolution at the image edges. Use of a large-crystal (≥15-inch) scintillation camera (square, rectangular, or circular) with a parallel-hole collimator allows inclusion of a larger area of the body in each view.

SPOT VIEWS

When performing a bone scan, individual images of certain areas can be obtained with the scintillation camera after the initial image of the total skeleton on another type of instrument has been performed. Because the bone area and activity in the field of the camera can be highly variable for different portions of the body, some images may require a long imaging time to achieve high information density (ID). Commonly, multiple individual images (or **spot views**) are taken for an equal amount of time, which is termed **equal-time imaging.**

This equal-time technique allows comparison of the film density in one image with that in another image, because the exposure is made for equal amounts of time. This method is effective as long as adequate statistics are achieved. First, one area of the body (e.g., the anterior or posterior view of the chest) is imaged for a preset number of counts and the time recorded. Between 400,000 and 600,000 counts are accumulated for a standard-field camera and between 500,000 and 1 million for a large-crystal camera. All subsequent images are taken for the same interval that had been recorded for the first image. An alternative method of performing equal-time imaging is to use the ID feature available on some scintillation cameras. An area of normal bone in the sternum or spine is selected with the ID marker, and an exposure is made until the ID in this region reaches a range of 2500 to 4000 counts. The time for this exposure is then used to obtain the other images.

The spot films provide detailed images of areas that are not well visualized on the whole-body imaging instruments or supply additional views that aid the determination of the presence (or absence) of abnormality. For example, a detailed view of the pelvis can be degraded by whole-body imaging devices because of activity accumulated in the bladder before the imaging device reaches the pelvis. Images of the pelvis should be obtained immediately after the patient has voided, which can be before or after the whole-body image. In addition, images of the scapula with the arms moved forward or up can be used to differentiate activity in the scapula and underlying ribs.[17,19]

WHOLE-BODY IMAGING

The production of an image of the total body area (Figure 20-9) onto one film is accomplished by an accessory that moves either the camera detector or the patient through the camera field of view. As the body moves past the detector, the area seen by the camera is minified and advances across the film at a speed proportional to that of the patient.

When a scintillation camera is used with a whole-body imaging accessory, a portion of the crystal may be masked either electronically or by collimation into a rectangular field of view. It is essential that this region of the detector be proportional in its speed over the patient compared with the motion of the minified image area that moves across the cathode ray tube (CRT).

The technique for establishing imaging parameters is determined by monitoring the count rate or ID or by selecting the total time for the whole-body scan. A region for measuring the count rate usually is selected anteriorly over the chest or posteriorly over the spine. The same scan speed should be used for both the anterior and the posterior images. The scan speed is determined by one of several techniques. Most camera manufacturers supply a table, chart, or nomogram for determining the proper

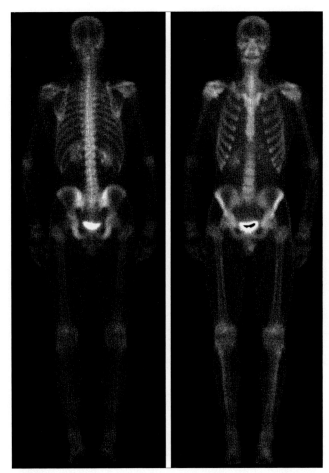

FIGURE 20-9 Normal whole-body bone scan, anterior and posterior.

BOX 20-2   **SPECT Imaging**

Image parameters:
1. Degrees of rotation: 360 degrees
2. Image matrix: 64 × 64
3. Time per image: 20 seconds

Data processing:
1. Reconstruct transverse, sagittal, and coronal images
2. Filter selection based on computer software

SPECT IMAGING

Single photon emission computed tomography (SPECT) is of interest for bone imaging because of the improved image contrast for lesions; the removal of **superimposition** of bony structures, which results in better localization of abnormal accumulation; and the additional three-dimensional information about the disease; and it occasionally shows lesions not seen on planar images. However, SPECT studies of poor quality or those performed improperly are inferior to quality planar images. The importance of quality control in SPECT is stressed in Chapter 9. Box 20-2 shows the SPECT imaging protocol.

Bone studies using SPECT have mainly involved patients with suspected disease of the hips, lumbar spine, knees, temporomandibular joints, and facial bones. Bone SPECT has been demonstrated to be the most sensitive noninvasive test for evaluation of the extent of arthritis in patients with chronic knee pain who have been examined by conventional radiography, bone scanning, and subsequent arthroscopy. SPECT offers advantages over planar imaging in the evaluation of patients with suspected **avascular necrosis (AVN)** of the hip. A **photopenic** area (area devoid of activity) is frequently seen on SPECT imaging that is not seen on planar imaging. SPECT has also been shown to be more sensitive than planar imaging in the evaluation of patients with evidence of spondylolysis or spondylolisthesis. It is also better than planar imaging in identifying the site of abnormality in symptomatic patients with defects in the pars interarticularis, and SPECT is superior to planar imaging in the evaluation of patients with temporomandibular joint dysfunction who undergo preoperative evaluation.

Bone SPECT imaging of the axial skeleton should be performed with high-resolution collimators. When imaging the lumbar spine, the patient's legs should be slightly elevated to make the spine straight. As with usual SPECT imaging, the detector-to-patient distance should be minimized. High-quality images can be obtained only with an adequate imaging time (i.e., 30 to 45 minutes). Imaging with a single-head camera is most commonly performed using a 64 × 64 image matrix; some cameras have high enough resolution to warrant the use of a 128 × 128 matrix. Studies should be acquired using a large

scan speed, based on the desired ID in the image and the count rate from the patient. Some systems may have a microcomputer for automatically calculating the scan speed, determined from monitoring the count rate from the patient. All these methods are basically the same, but some additional variations from the manufacturer's method may give improved image quality. Digital cameras record the whole-body scan in a high-resolution matrix for photographing after data acquisition.

It is recommended that the whole-body image include more than 2.5 million counts. The best positioning of the patient is to have the detector under the table and have the patient lie prone and supine to produce the anterior and posterior images, respectively. Using this technique, the detector can be nearer the patient during imaging.

Whole-body imaging with the scintillation camera provides a good relationship of overall radiopharmaceutical distribution with only a small loss in resolution generated from the motion synchronization of the table and the CRT recording. Less manipulation of the patient is necessary, and little effort is required of the technologist during the imaging procedure.

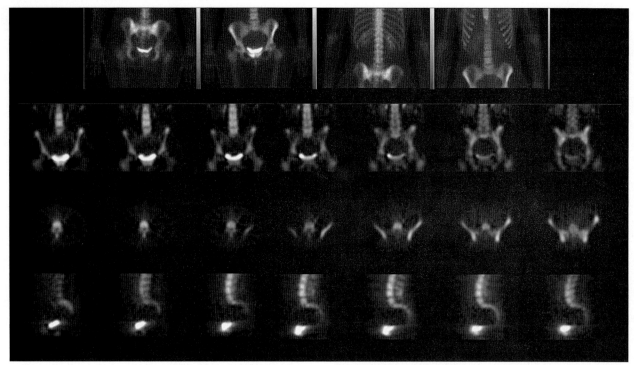

FIGURE 20-10 Planar and SPECT bone images compared.

number of views (120 to 128) in 360 degrees to obtain good angular sampling. SPECT studies acquired with these parameters have very high counts and very high resolution and therefore should be reconstructed with high-resolution prefiltering and reconstruction filters. Reconstructed images should be reviewed by the technologist for proper orientation and should be free of artifacts. Reconstructed transverse, coronal, and sagittal slices should be oriented to the patient's anatomy for interpretation and comparison with planar images. Figure 20-10 shows a SPECT study of the lumbar spine compared with planar images.

CLINICAL ASPECTS

The skeleton is a complex organ system subjected to many different types of adversities. Bone disease can be generally classified into two broad categories—congenital and acquired. In the congenital bone diseases, radionuclide imaging has essentially no role, because most of these diseases have a characteristic radiographic appearance. However, radionuclide bone imaging is important in the evaluation of several acquired bone diseases. These can be classified as traumatic, neoplastic, inflammatory, metabolic, degenerative, vascular, and other bone diseases that do not fit into these listed categories.

Localization of the bone-seeking radiopharmaceuticals depends mainly on two factors—bone blood flow and bone production; however, the relative importance of each of these parameters is not well defined. Increased radiopharmaceutical deposition accompanying increased

BOX 20-3	Indications for Bone Imaging

1. Staging of malignant disease (screening of high-risk patients and localization of biopsy sites)
2. Evaluation of primary bone neoplasms
3. Diagnosis of early skeletal inflammatory disease
4. Evaluation of skeletal pain of undetermined etiology
5. Evaluation of elevated alkaline phosphatase of undetermined etiology
6. Determination of bone viability
7. Evaluation of painful total joint prostheses

bone production is well exemplified by the epiphyseal growth plate in bone imaging in children (Figure 20-11). Occasionally an abnormality is detected as a focal area of decreased radiopharmaceutical accumulation (photopenic area) (Figure 20-12). This decreased accumulation can be related to impaired blood flow or to complete destruction or replacement of bone by a tumor, an inflammatory mass, or radiation.

Indications for bone imaging are listed in Box 20-3. The most frequent reason for ordering a bone scan is to stage malignant disease by determining whether spread to bone has occurred. The other indications are used less frequently but are important reasons for bone imaging.

When performing a bone scan, anterior and posterior images of the whole body generally are obtained (see Figure 20-9). The anterior skull, facial bones, mandible,

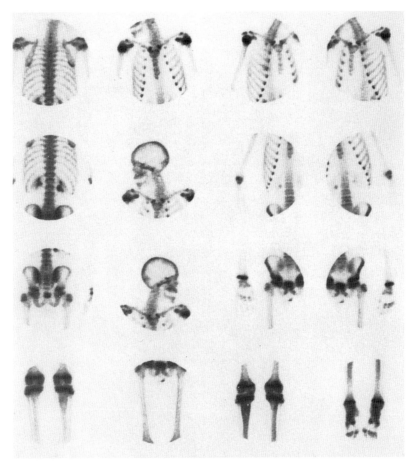

FIGURE 20-11 Multiple gamma camera images from a large-crystal camera of a 15-year-old boy with an aneurysmal bone cyst of the right tibia. The epiphyseal activity in multiple areas is apparent.

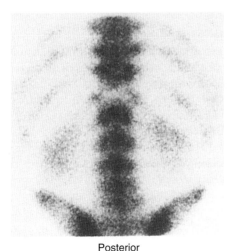

Posterior

FIGURE 20-12 Absent accumulation of radiopharmaceutical in vertebral body.

clavicle, sternum, anterior ribs, anterior iliac spine, and pubic rami are best visualized on the anterior images. The posterior skull, spine, posterior ribs, scapulae, sacroiliac joints, and ischia are best visualized on the posterior images. The shoulders, hips, and extremities are commonly seen well on both views, primarily depending on patient positioning.[10] The activity in the skeleton is usually symmetrical from side to side; however, some asymmetry may be seen in the skull, shoulders, sternoclavicular joints, and anterior ends of the ribs without a pathological condition present.[3] Since ^{99m}Tc-MDP or ^{99m}Tc-HMDP are excreted via the urinary system, visualization of the kidneys is common. This activity is variable but is usually less than the surrounding bone activity. Kidney disease associated with pronounced asymmetry of renal activity, a focal area of absent activity (cyst or tumor), or ureteric visualization, suggesting ureteric obstruction,[7,35] may be visualized. In addition, accumulation of the bone-imaging radiopharmaceutical can occur in the normal female breast and with various diseases of the breast[3] (Figure 20-13).

Metastatic Disease

Metastases to bone are common in several primary malignancies, including lung, breast, and prostate carcinomas. In most institutions, radionuclide bone imaging has replaced the radiographic skeletal survey for evaluation of skeletal metastatic disease because metastases to

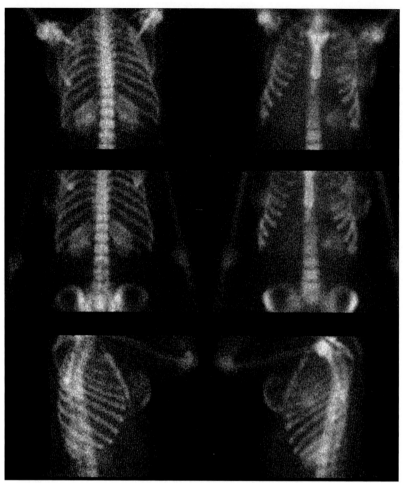

FIGURE 20-13 Chest images in a bone scan of a female patient demonstrating bilateral accumulation of the radiopharmaceutical in normal breasts.

the spine are difficult to detect radiographically. Loss of approximately 50% of the mineral content of the bone must occur before lytic lesions are detected radiographically.[15] Whereas 10% to 40% of adult patients with metastatic bone disease and an abnormal bone scan may have normal radiographs, fewer than 5% of bone scans are negative when the radiograph demonstrates metastatic disease.[29,45] In the pediatric population, one study has demonstrated 68% of metastases were identified by radionuclide imaging alone.[23] False-negative scans have been related to several factors. If the skeleton is diffusely involved with metastatic disease, the focal nature of the lesions might not be apparent.[16] A diffusely abnormal scan may be difficult to differentiate from a normal scan, but with quality images irregularities of radiopharmaceutical deposition can generally be noted (Figure 20-14). Metastatic lesions that have no associated osteoblastic activity may not be detected by bone scan or may be detected as a photon-deficient area.[24] An example of a disease in which the lesions might not produce an abnormality on the bone scan is multiple myeloma, which has a high false-negative rate. In general, after the bone

images are performed, radiographs of the abnormal areas are often recommended for a more definitive diagnosis and to exclude other etiologies of an abnormal scan in the patient with suspected metastatic disease.

The usual pattern of skeletal metastatic disease is multiple focal lesions throughout the skeleton, with the greatest involvement generally in the axial skeleton[26,28] (Figure 20-15). The area of abnormal radiopharmaceutical deposition represents the edge of the metastatic deposit where osteoblastic repair is attempted. There are some primary cancers that metastasize to tissue rather than bone but accumulate bone-seeking radiopharmaceuticals. These tumors generally tend to be calcified and can be seen on radiographs, but the bone scan is abnormal before the radiographs[42] (Figure 20-16). In addition, a few bone-producing metastatic lesions do occur such as those attributable to osteogenic sarcoma (Figure 20-17). Metastatic accumulation of the agent in soft-tissue metastases may prove helpful in detecting extraskeletal involvement and can be detected by scan before the appearance of radiographic abnormalities.[42]

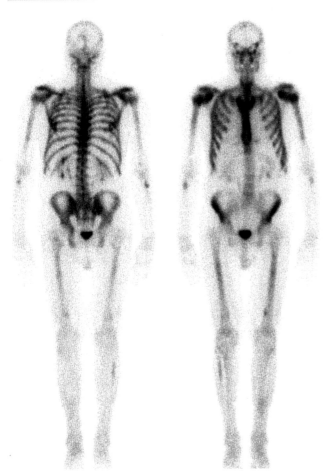

FIGURE 20-14 Bone scan of a patient demonstrating diffusely increased activity with an irregular distribution. This is a superscan of widespread metastatic disease.

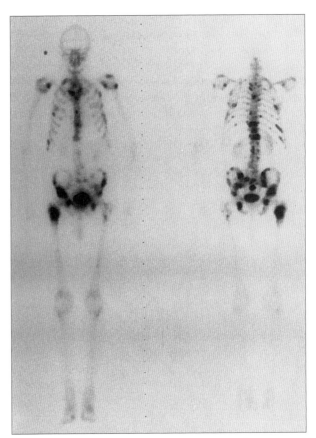

FIGURE 20-15 Multiple focal lesions in the bone of a patient with prostate carcinoma.

Bone imaging has demonstrated importance for the staging of malignant disease in breast, lung, and prostatic carcinomas,[28,37,41] because these are common malignancies with a high incidence of bony metastatic disease. However, because other malignancies spread to the bone, most patients with malignancies have a bone scan as part of their evaluation.

Primary Bone Neoplasms

Bone scanning is also used for the evaluation of primary bone neoplasms. Usually the patient has already had radiographs of the primary tumor, and the bone scan offers no additional information about that area. The extent of the abnormality on the bone scan is generally not much different from that of the radiographically apparent lesion. The value of bone scanning in patients with primary bone malignancy lies in the detection of the disease elsewhere.[25] As many as 30% of patients with Ewing sarcoma may have lesions in other bones, a finding that significantly alters the therapy of the disease.[6,23,50]

Inflammatory Diseases

Radionuclide bone imaging also is used in the evaluation of several nonmalignant processes. It has been demonstrated to be useful in the evaluation of patients with suspected osteomyelitis and diskitis.[20,31,43,51] The bone scan may be positive within 24 hours after the onset of symptoms, whereas the radiographic changes are not apparent for 10 to 14 days.

Early images are important in the evaluation of inflammatory processes; therefore a three- or four-phase bone scan should be performed. The first phase, or dynamic phase, is performed by acquiring a rapid flow sequence of images every 2 to 4 seconds for 40 to 60 seconds over the area of interest during radiopharmaceutical injection. The second phase, or blood pool phase, is accomplished by immediately obtaining static images for 300,000 to 500,000 counts without moving the patient Additional projection images are taken as necessary. Both osteomyelitis and cellulitis cause early increased activity as a result of an increased vascular response to the affected area. The third phase, or osseus or delayed phase, is routine scanning at 2 to 3 hours after injection. This scan typically includes static images as well as a whole-body scan. If necessary, a fourth phase,

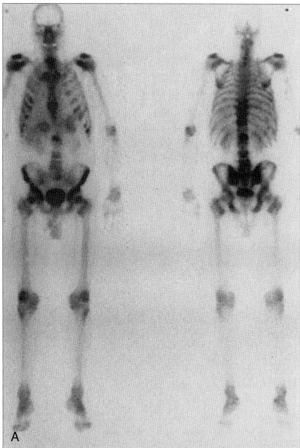

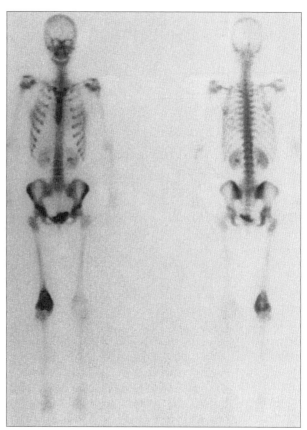

FIGURE 20-17 Osteogenic sarcoma of distal femur in a 16-year-old girl shows tumor restricted to femur without evidence of metastatic disease.

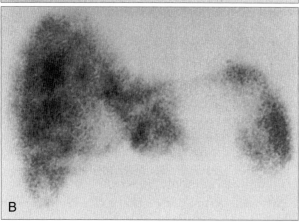

FIGURE 20-16 Metastatic colon cancer. **A,** Anterior whole-body scan reveals a doughnut-shaped area of abnormal accumulation in the right upper quadrant. **B,** ^{99m}Tc–sulfur colloid liver-spleen scan reveals areas of diminished colloid localization. This abnormality is a metastatic lesion from a primary colon cancer.

BOX 20-4	Three Phase Bone Scan

1. Position patient and field of view as determined by the area of interest; include both sides of the body.
2. Administer the radiopharmaceutical as a bolus injection.
3. Acquire serial images for 5 seconds each for 60 seconds starting at the time of injection.
4. Acquire blood pool image for approximately 1 minute.
5. Have patient return for delayed images, and take images as required for a bone scan (see Box 20-1).

or delayed/delayed phase is performed to evaluate persistent increased activity at 5 hours to 24 hours postinjection. The third- and fourth-phase spot images should be taken for 100,000 to 250,000 counts to allow comparison of these delayed images with respect to changes in activity in the affected area (Figure 20-18). Box 20-4 shows the Three Phase Bone scan protocol.

With cellulitis, increased blood pool activity may be seen diffusely throughout the area of involvement, as well as some diffusely increased activity on the regular bone images obtained 2 to 3 hours after injection. Osteomyelitis, however, demonstrates focally increased activity in the involved bone on both the blood pool and routine images (see Figure 20-18). Since bone imaging came to be used for detecting osteomyelitis, it has been found that several patients do not subsequently develop the typical radiographic changes, because the early diagnosis and treatment prevents the development of radiographic abnormalities.

Diskitis, an inflammatory process of the disk space, usually occurs secondary to a bacterial infection.

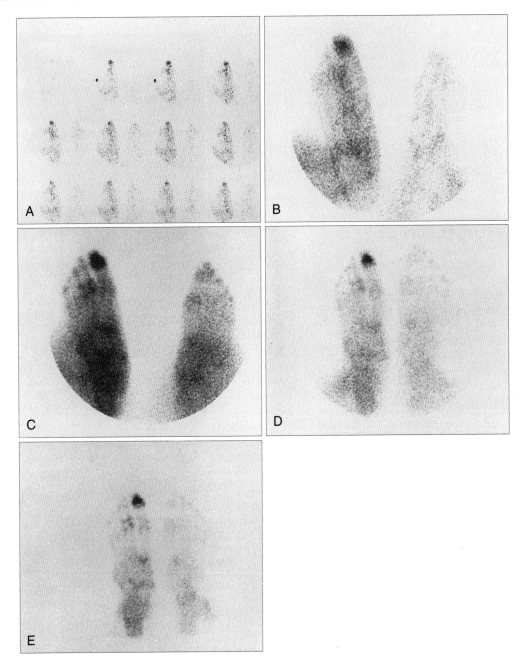

FIGURE 20-18 **A,** Plantar view flow images at 4 sec/frame show increased perfusion to the first right distal phalanx. **B,** Blood pool images also demonstrate abnormal accumulation. Images at 2 hours **(C)**, 5 hours **(D)**, and 24 hours **(E)** show persistent radiopharmaceutical collection consistent with osteomyelitis.

The bone scan can reveal increased activity in the vertebral bodies on each side of the disk space (Figure 20-19).

Trauma

The bone scan has been used to evaluate patients who have experienced trauma[40] when fractures are suspected and the radiographs are normal (Figure 20-20). Immediately after a fracture, for the first day or two, there may be decreased activity visualized at the site. After the third day, there is generally diffusely increased activity in the area of fracture, which becomes focally increased by the tenth day. Depending on the angulation of the fracture and stress, for example, the activity decreases with time but may remain abnormal for years if the fracture is complicated and bone remodeling continues.

OTHER USES FOR BONE IMAGING

Radionuclide bone imaging is also used with several other conditions. Paget disease is associated with greatly

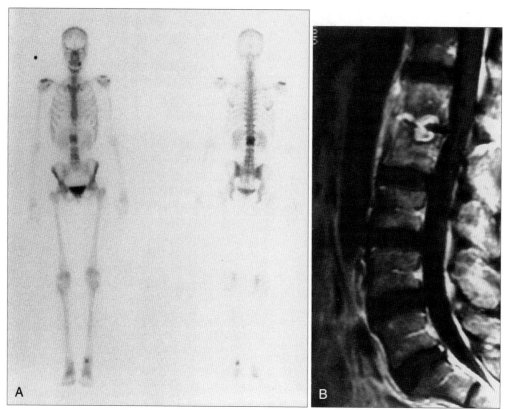

FIGURE 20-19 A, Whole-body bone scan reveals diffusely increased radiopharmaceutical accumulated in T10 and L2 vertebral bodies. **B,** T$_2$-weighted MRI image reveals abnormal signal intensity in disk space between L1 and L2 with the abnormal signal extending into the vertebral bodies. This patient had diskitis.

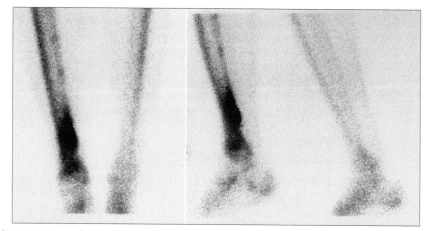

FIGURE 20-20 Delayed static images of the lower extremities of a 20-year-old male athlete with pain in the tibia (plain radiographs were normal). The bone scan shows marked abnormal accumulation in the distal tibia (anterior and lateral) with the abnormality extending through the cortex, characteristic of a stress fracture.

abnormal radiopharmaceutical accumulation, typically involving the greater part of a bone[1,44] (Figure 20-21). The bone scan has been used to evaluate therapy for this disease.[1] Another use for bone scanning is in the evaluation of the cause of pain after a total joint replacement. Determination of pain in this situation is frequently difficult, and radionuclide imaging has been demonstrated to be a sensitive method of detecting a complication, such as loosening or infection of the prosthetic implant[21]

(Figures 20-22 and 20-23). Radionuclide imaging is also very sensitive for the detection of osteoid osteomas, a cause of skeletal pain that may go undetected for years.[33]

Avascular necrosis of the hip is difficult to diagnose by clinical examination and radiographs of the hips. Radionuclide imaging frequently is used in the evaluation of these patients. Early in the course of the disease, decreased activity in the blood flow and blood pool

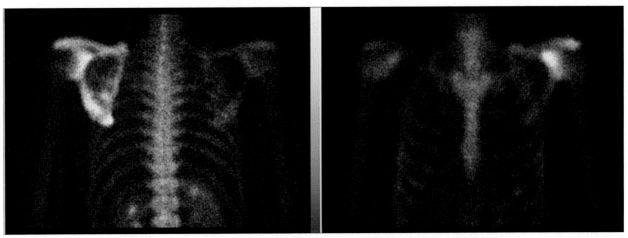

FIGURE 20-21 Paget disease. Whole-body images demonstrate abnormal uptake.

PET Imaging

The use of ^{18}F as a bone imaging agent has reemerged with positron emission tomography (PET) imaging. PET bone imaging alone or PET images fused with another modality such as CT or MRI have proven its value in the areas of oncology, general orthopedics, and sports medicine. ^{18}F-FDG (fluoro-D-glucose) PET scans promise improved imaging quality for both benign and malignant bone disease, with significantly improved sensitivity and specificity over conventional planar and SPECT bone scans.[8] An advantage to imaging with PET/CT or fusing PET images with CT or MRI images is the result of an image that displays anatomy and physiology. Because of the rapid blood clearance of ^{18}F, dynamic imaging times are shorter; and because of the short half-life, the time delay between injection and scan is shorter than with ^{99m}Tc imaging agents. ^{18}F bone scans can be used for the same indications as are bone scans performed with the ^{99m}Tc imaging agents. The increased sensitivity and specificity of PET bone scans, approaching 100%, may provide a more thorough and conclusive evaluation of bone disease.[8]

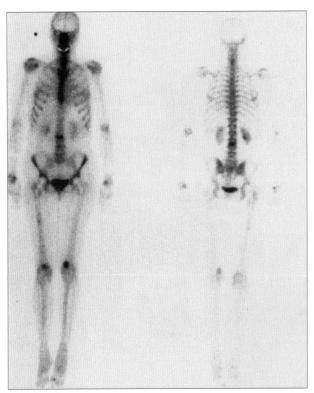

FIGURE 20-22 Loosened total hip prosthesis. Patient with bilateral hip prostheses has focal abnormal accumulation in the right femoral lesser and greater trochanters and the tip of the prosthesis, typical of loosening.

images, in addition to decreased accumulation of the bone-scanning radiopharmaceutical on delayed images, can be seen. In AVN, magnetic resonance imaging (MRI) may also detect abnormalities before radiographic changes (Figure 20-24).

Intraoperative bone imaging may be used to localize lesions for surgical resection. The specimen may also be imaged to document that the lesion has been removed.[30,52]

Joint Imaging

Radionuclide imaging of the joints can be used for the evaluation of inflammatory joint disease.* This imaging is performed with either ^{99m}Tc-pertechnetate or ^{99m}Tc-phosphate compounds. When using ^{99m}Tc-pertechnetate, images are obtained immediately after injection of the radiopharmaceutical, and abnormal accumulation is noted in areas of increased blood flow, such as are found in synovitis. Technetium-99m phosphate compounds localize in areas of joint inflammation that show an increased turnover rate and vascularity of the adjacent bone, as well as increased vascularity of the synovium

---

*References 5, 13, 29, 34-37, 48, 49.

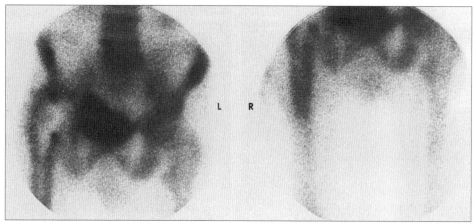

FIGURE 20-23 Infected total hip prosthesis. Diffusely abnormal accumulation around the entire prosthesis in right hip is characteristic of an infected implant.

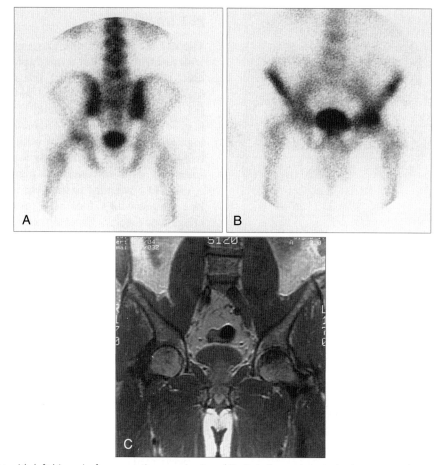

FIGURE 20-24 Patient with left hip pain from aseptic necrosis. **A** and **B,** Anterior and posterior bone scan demonstrates increased uptake in left femoral head with slightly increased uptake in right femoral head. **C,** Coronal MRI demonstrates decreased signal in 30% to 40% of left femoral head and 10% to 15% of right femoral head.

(Figure 20-25). Either of these radiopharmaceuticals can be used to detect early joint inflammation, often before radiographic abnormalities occur. Compared with a physical examination, radiographs, and arthrography, joint imaging with the ^{99m}Tc phosphate complex is the most sensitive indicator of early degenerative disease of the knee.[49]

In addition, several studies have demonstrated the utility of ^{99m}Tc-phosphate imaging in the early detection of sacroiliac inflammatory disease[14] (Figure 20-26).

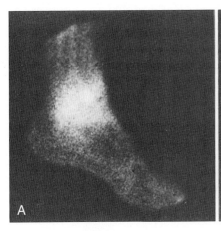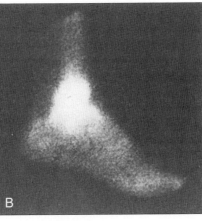

FIGURE 20-25 Septic arthritis of tibiotalar joint. **A,** Blood pool image obtained after administration of ^{99m}Tc methylenediphosphonate (^{99m}Tc-MDP) demonstrates abnormal accumulation in ankle joint area. **B,** Routine image obtained 2½ hours later demonstrates focal accumulation in distal tibia and talus. Joint fluid was aspirated, and the aspirate grew pathogenic organisms. Radiographs revealed no joint abnormality.

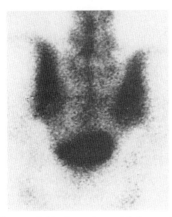

FIGURE 20-26 Sacroileitis. Posterior pelvic image in a patient with low back pain. Quantification revealed ratio of activity in sacroiliac area to midsacrum to be greater than 2 (normal is less than 1.5).

Detection of the inflammatory process before radiographic changes have occurred has been demonstrated. The technique uses a computer to quantify areas of bone activity and compares the activity in the sacroiliac joint region with an area of equal size in the midsacrum. Radiosynoviorthesis, the radionuclide procedure that provides an alternative treatment for inflammatory joint disease associated with rheumatoid arthritis, osteoarthritis, and hemophiliac arthropathy is described in Chapter 22.

Radionuclide Therapy of Painful Bone Metastases

Some neoplasms, such as those of the breast, lung, prostate, kidney, and thyroid, frequently spread to bone and cause pain.[33] The method of treatment for painful bone metastases is a dilemma for the oncologist. Narcotic medication is widely used in the treatment of bone pain, but lethargy and constipation are major side effects of these drugs that limit their usefulness. Biphosphonates originally were used to treat the hypercalcemia resulting from bone metastases, and they are now used alone or

in combination with cytotoxic agents in the palliation of painful bone metastases.[33] Details of radionuclide therapy for the treatment of bone pain as an effective palliative treatment for patients with osteoblastic bone metastasis and bone pain is also located in Chapter 22.

Gallium-67 and Indium-111 White Blood Cell Imaging in Bone and Joint Disease

Several studies have recently demonstrated the value of gallium-67 (^{67}Ga)-citrate scanning in patients with inflammatory bone and joint disease.[25,31-33] Some patients with osteomyelitis or septic arthritis may have normal ^{99m}Tc-phosphate complex images but abnormal ^{67}Ga images.

Indium-111 (^{111}In)-labeled white blood cells have also been used in the evaluation of patients with suspected bone and joint infections.[13] The results of using ^{111}In–white blood cells have varied, which is most likely related to the patient populations studied. One study had only a 50% sensitivity in detecting skeletal infection (Figure 20-27), but the patient population included many individuals with chronic infection. Another study reported a 98% sensitivity in patients with suspected bone and joint infection, and it has been reported that patients with diabetes mellitus and skin ulcers of the feet have demonstrated a high frequency of osteomyelitis and a high accuracy of ^{111}In–white blood cell imaging in this patient population. Although ^{111}In–white blood cell imaging can be comparable to ^{67}Ga-citrate imaging in detecting inflammatory bone and joint disease, ^{67}Ga-citrate imaging does not require the handling of blood products and is the preferred procedure at some institutions.

In addition to detecting inflammatory bone and joint, ^{67}Ga-citrate imaging is used to stage certain malignancies, such as Hodgkin lymphoma and malignant melanoma. The study typically is used to detect the soft tissue involvement of these malignancies, but skeletal involvement can be detected (Figure 20-28). Detailed information on the radiopharmaceuticals for inflammatory

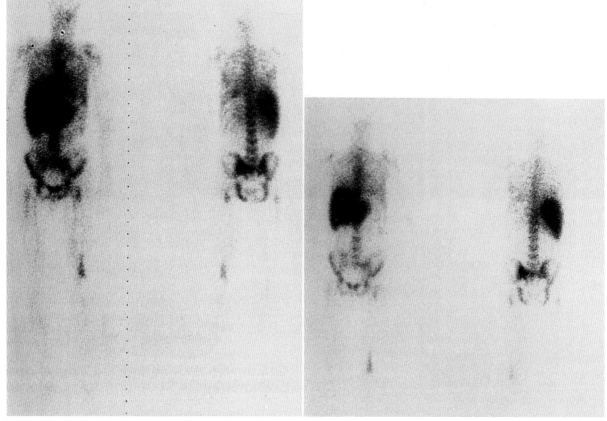

FIGURE 20-27 Osteomyelitis. Whole-body images obtained 4 hours (*left*) and 18 hours (*right*) after administration of ^{111}In-leukocytes following a splenectomy. Abnormal accumulation is seen in the left sacroiliac joint, left ischium, left proximal femur, and left distal femur in this patient with multifocal osteomyelitis.

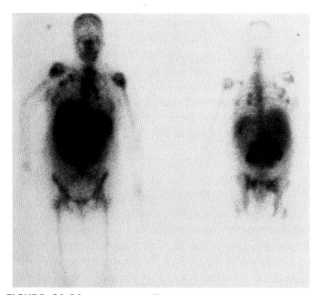

FIGURE 20-28 Whole-body ^{67}Ga-citrate imaging demonstrates markedly abnormal accumulation in abdominal lymphoadenopathy and in multiple ribs in this patient with Hodgkin lymphoma.

imaging (^{67}Ga-citrate and ^{111}In-oxine–labeled white blood cells) as well as imaging protocols can be found in Chapter 22.

SUMMARY

- Composition of bone by weight in the normal adult is approximately 5% to 10% water, 25% to 30% organic matter, and 65% to 70% inorganic matter (bone mineral).
- Bone salt mineral has the crystalline form of an apatite composed of the following ions: calcium, phosphate, hydroxyl, carbonate, and citrate, with lesser amounts of sodium, magnesium, potassium, chloride, and fluoride. The main ion of bone is phosphorus as phosphate. The crystalline structure is called *hydroxyapatite*.
- Because early disease involvement of bone may be subtle, improper positioning of the patient for imaging, improper exposure of the film, or improper manipulation of computer images may lead to an inaccurate diagnosis.

- Because bone studies are used to follow therapy, the imaging technique must be reproducible to allow careful comparison with a previous study.
- The accumulation of radionuclides in bone is related to both vascularity and to the rate of bone production.
- Localization of various bone-imaging agents is related to their exchange with ions in the hydroxyapatite crystal of the bone. Examples of these changes include strontium exchanges with calcium, ^{18}F exchanges with the hydroxyl ion, and the phosphate compounds' exchanges with the phosphorous groups.
- The patient should have a complete understanding of the procedure, especially the reason for the 2- to 3-hour delay between administration of the radiopharmaceutical and the imaging.
- Equal-time technique allows comparison of the film density in one image with that in another.
- SPECT is of interest for bone imaging because of the improved image contrast for lesions, the removal of superimposition of bony structures, and the ability to obtain three-dimensional information about the extent of the disease.
- The value of bone scanning in patients with primary bone malignancy lies in the detection of metastases.
- Early images are important in the evaluation of inflammatory processes.

REFERENCES

1. Altman RD, Johnston CC, Khairi MRA, et al: Influence of disodium etidronate on clinical and laboratory manifestations of Paget's disease of bone (osteitis deformans), *N Engl J Med* 28:1379, 1973.
2. Anderson J, Emergy EW, McAlister JM, et al: The metabolism of a therapeutic dose of calcium-45 in a case of multiple myeloma, *Clin Sci Mol Med* 15:567, 1956.
3. Bassett LW, Gold RH, Webber MM: Radionuclide bone imaging, *Radiol Clin North Am* 19:675, 1981.
4. Bayer GCH, Wendeberg B: External counting of Ca-47 and Sr-85 in studies of localized skeletal lesions in man, *J Bone Joint Surg Br* 41B:558, 1959.
5. Belchier J: An account of the bones of the animals being changed to a red color by aliment only. In Bauer GCH, editor: Tracer techniques for the study of bone metabolism in man, *Adv Biol Med Phys* 10:228, 1965.
6. Bhansali SK, Desai PB: Ewing's sarcoma: observations in 107 cases, *J Bone Joint Surg* 45A:541, 1963.
7. Biello D, Coleman RE, Stanley RJ: Correlation of renal images on bone scan and intravenous pyelogram, *Am J Roentgenol Radium Ther Nucl Med* 127:633, 1976.
8. Bridges RL, Wiley CR, Christian JC, et al: An introduction to Na^{18}F bone scintigraphy: basic principles, advanced imaging concepts, and case examples, *J Nucl Med Technol* 35:64-76, 2007.
9. Charkes ND, Philips CM: A new model of ^{18}F-fluoride kinetics in humans. In *Medical radionuclide imaging*, vol 2, Vienna, 1977, International Atomic Energy Agency.
10. Charkes ND, Sklaroff DM: Early diagnosis of metastatic bone cancer by photoscanning with strontium-85, *J Nucl Med* 5:168, 1964.
11. Charkes ND, Valentine G, Cravitz B: Interpretation of the normal ^{99m}Tc polyphosphate rectilinear bone scan, *Radiology* 107:563, 1973.
12. Colbert B, Ankney J, Lee KT: *Anatomy & physiology for health professionals: an interactive journey*, Upper Saddle River, N.J., 2007, Prentice Hall.
13. Coleman RE, Welch DM, Baker WJ, et al: Clinical experience using indium-111–labeled leukocytes. In Thakur ML, Gottschalk A, editors: *Indium-111–labeled neutrophils, platelets, and lymphocytes*, New York, 1980, Trivirium.
14. Davis P, Thomson ABR, Lentle BC: Quantitative sacroiliac scintigraphy in patients with Crohn's disease, *Arthritis Rheum* 21:234, 1978.
15. Edelstyn GA, Gillespie PJ, Grebbel FS: The radiological demonstration of osseous metastases: experimental observations, *Clin Radiol* 18:158, 1967.
16. Frankel RS, Johnson KW, Mabry JJ, et al: "Normal" bone radionuclide image with diffuse skeletal lymphoma, *Radiology* 111:365, 1974.
17. Freeman L, Fink-Bennett D: The "hug" view: an image that results in optimal visualization of the upper posterior thorax, *Clin Nucl Med* 24:63, 1999.
18. Galasko CSB: The detection of skeletal metastases for mammary cancer by gamma camera scintigraphy, *Br J Surg* 56:757, 1969.
19. Galasko CSB: The mechanisms of uptake of bone-seeking isotopes by skeletal metastases. In *Medical radionuclide imaging*, vol 2, Vienna, 1977, International Atomic Energy Agency.
20. Gelfand MJ, Silberstein EB: Radionuclide imaging: use in diagnosis of osteomyelitis in children, *JAMA* 237:245, 1977.
21. Gelman MI, Coleman RE, Stevens PM, et al: Radiography, radionuclide imaging, and arthrography in the evaluation of total hip and knee replacement, *Radiology* 128:467, 1978.
22. Gerber FH, Goodreau JJ, Kirchner PT, et al: Efficacy of preoperative and post-operative bone scanning in the management of breast carcinoma, *N Engl J Med* 297:300, 1977.
23. Gilday DL, Ash JM, Reilly BJ: Radionuclide skeletal survey for pediatric neoplasms, *Radiology* 123:399, 1977.
24. Goergen TG, Alazraki NP, Halpern SE, et al: "Cold" bone lesions: a newly recognized phenomenon of bone imaging, *J Nucl Med* 12:1120, 1974.
25. Handmaker H, Giammona ST: The "hot joint": increased diagnostic accuracy using combined ^{99m}Tc phosphate and ^{67}Ca citrate imaging in pediatrics, *J Nucl Med* 17:554, 1976.
26. Hart G, Hoerr SO, Hughes CP: Detection of bone metastases from breast cancer: an accurate, four film roentgenographic survey, *Cleve Clin Q* 38:1, 1971.
27. Jones AG, Francis MD, Davis MA: Bone scanning: radionuclide reaction mechanisms, *Semin Nucl Med* 6:1, 1976.
28. Krishnamurthy GT, Tubis M, Hiss J, et al: Distribution pattern of metastatic bone disease: a need for total body skeletal imaging, *JAMA* 237:2054, 1977.
29. Legge DA, Tauxe WN, Pugh DG, et al: Radioisotope scanning of metastatic lesions of bone, *Mayo Clin Proc* 45:755, 1970.
30. Leitha T, Staudenherz A, Korpan M, et al: Pattern recognition in five-phase bone scintigraphy: diagnostic patterns of reflex sympathetic dystrophy in adults, *Eur J Nucl Med* 23:256-262, 1996.
31. Lisbona R, Rosenthall L: Observations on the sequential use of ^{99m}Tc-phosphate complex and ^{67}Ga imaging in osteomyelitis, cellulitis, and septic arthritis, *Radiology* 123:123, 1977.
32. Lisbona R, Rosenthall L: Radionuclide imaging of septic joints and their differentiation from periarticular osteomyelitis and cellulitis in pediatrics, *Clin Nucl Med* 2:337, 1977.
33. Lisbona R, Rosenthall L: Role of radionuclide imaging in osteoid osteoma, *Am J Roentgenol Radium Ther Nucl Med* 132:77, 1979.

34. Littlefield JL, Rudd TG: Tc-99m hydroxymethylene diphosphonate and Tc-99m methylene diphosphonate: biologic and clinical comparison: concise communication, *J Nucl Med* 24:463, 1983.

35. Maher FT: Evaluation of renal urinary tract abnormalities noted on scintiscans, *Mayo Clin Proc* 50:370, 1975.

36. Maisano R, Pergolizzi S, Cascini S: Novel therapeutic approaches to cancer patients with bone metastases, *Crit Rev Oncol Hematol* 40:239, 2001.

37. Merrick MV: Review article: bone scanning, *Br J Radiol* 48:327, 1975.

38. Pecher C: Biological investigations with radioactive calcium and strontium, *Proc Soc Exp Biol Med* 46:86, 1941.

39. Rasmussen H: Parathyroid hormone, calcitonin, and calciferols. In Williams RH, editor: *Textbook of endocrinology*, ed 5, Philadelphia, 1974, WB Saunders.

40. Rosenthall L, Hill RO, Chuang S: Observation on the use of ^{99m}Tc-phosphate imaging in peripheral bone trauma, *Radiology* 119:637, 1976.

41. Schaffer DL, Pendergrass HP: Comparison of enzyme, clinical, radiographic, and radionuclide methods of detecting bone metastases from carcinoma of the prostate, *Radiology* 121:431, 1976.

42. Schall GL, Zeiger L, Primack A, et al: Uptake of ^{85}Sr by an osteosarcoma metastatic to lung, *J Nucl Med* 12:131, 1971.

43. Shirazi PH, Rayudu GVS, Fordham EW: ^{18}F bone scanning: review of indications and results in 1500 cases, *Radiology* 112:361, 1974.

44. Shirazi PH, Rayudu GVS, Ryan WG, et al: Paget's disease of bone: bone scanning experience with 80 cases, *J Nucl Med* 14:450, 1973.

45. Sklaroff DM, Charkes DN: Diagnosis of bone metastasis by photoscanning with strontium 85, *JAMA* 188:1, 1964.

46. Spencer R, Herbert R, Rish MW, et al: Bone scanning with ^{85}Sr and ^{18}F: physical and radiopharmaceutical considerations and clinical experience in 50 cases, *Br J Radiol* 40:641, 1976.

47. Subramanian G, McAfee JG, Blair RJ, et al: Radiopharmaceuticals for bone and bone-marrow imaging. In *Medical radionuclide imaging*, vol 2, Vienna, 1977, International Atomic Energy Agency.

48. Sy WM, Bay R, Camera A: Hand images: normal and abnormal, *J Nucl Med* 18:419, 1977.

49. Thomas RJ, Resnick D, Alazraki NP, et al: Compartmental evaluation of osteoarthritis of the knee: comparative study of available diagnostic modalities, *Radiology* 116:585, 1975.

50. Wang CC, Schulz MD: Ewing's sarcoma: a study of 50 cases treated at the Massachusetts General Hospital, 1930-1952 inclusive, *N Engl J Med* 284:571, 1953.

51. Waxman AD, Bryan D, Siemsen JK: Bone scanning in the drug abuse patient: early detection of hematogenous osteomyelitis, *J Nucl Med* 14:647, 1973.

52. Wioland M, Serfent-Alaoui A: Didactic review of 175 radionuclide-guided excisions of osteoid osteomas, *Eur J Nucl Med* 23:1003-1011, 1996.

SUGGESTED READING

Probst-Proctor SL, Dillingham MF, McDougall IR, et al: The white blood cell scan in orthopedics, *Clin Orthop Relat Res* 168:157, 1982.

Subramanian G, McAfee JF: A new complex of ^{99m}Tc for skeletal imaging, *Radiology* 99:192, 1971.

Hematopoietic System

Kristen M. Waterstram-Rich, Helen H. Drew

OBJECTIVES

After completing this chapter, the reader will be able to:
- List the normal components of blood in the plasma compartment and cellular compartments.
- Define a hematocrit value, how it is derived, and how to interpret it.
- Describe the function, life span, and survival problems of a red blood cell.
- Describe how to label platelets with ^{111}In-oxine.
- State the isotope dilution principle.
- Explain the ascorbic acid technique for labeling red blood cells with ^{51}Cr.
- Describe the correct procedure and calculation for performing a total red cell volume measurement,

including sample collection, processing, and counting.
- Describe the correct procedure and calculation for performing a total plasma volume measurement, including sample collection, processing, and counting.
- Describe the limitations imposed when attempting to compare measured red blood cell and plasma volumes to normal volumes.
- Describe the technique used to perform a red blood cell survival and calculate the results.
- Describe the technique used to perform a splenic sequestration.

KEY TERMS

acid-citrate-dextrose (ACD)
anemia
anticoagulant
buffy coat

cohort (pulse) labeling
hematocrit (Hct)
hemolysis
plasma

plasmacrit
random labeling
sequestration
serum

BLOOD

Circulating blood is complex mixture of various kinds of cells or formed elements. The average blood volume of a normal adult is 5000 ml to 3000 ml of plasma and 2000 ml of red blood cells. Of the total 40 liters of fluid in the body, 25 liters comprise the intracellular fluid found in the 75 trillion cells of the body.[4]

Blood has three categories of functions: transportation, regulation, and protection. Blood transports oxygen, hormones, and nutrients to cells throughout the body. It also transports carbon dioxide and wastes from metabolic processes to the lungs or kidneys for excretion from the body. Another function of blood is regulation. Blood plays a major role in homeostasis by regulating pH and electrolytes within parameters of normal levels to maintain tissue fluids at normal levels, thereby ensuring efficient and proper cell function. It also plays a role in regulating or maintaining body temperature by absorbing heat generated by skeletal muscles, spreading it throughout the body and radiating excess heat out of the body through the skin.[2] In addition, blood adjusts fluid levels as needed by various parts of the body to maintain a proper fluid balance. Lastly, the blood has the function of protection. It serves to protect the body from infection and invasion of pathogens or toxins by white blood cells (WBCs) and antibodies, and it clots to prevent loss of blood.

BLOOD COMPONENTS

Circulating blood is an extraordinarily complex mixture consisting of a solid portion that contains cells (also referred to as formed elements) and a liquid portion called **plasma** (Figure 21-1). When blood is separated by a centrifuge, the blood will divide into two major components, plasma and formed elements.[2] The cellular compartment which consists of formed elements will sink to the bottom of the tube. The formed elements that make up approximately 45% of the blood volume include red blood cells (RBCs), or erythrocytes; WBCs,

or leukocytes; and platelets, or thrombocytes. The upper portion of the sample or the liquid clear straw-colored portion is called plasma, which comprises approximately 55% of the total blood volume and contains about 100 different substances dissolved within.[2] Plasma is about 90% water and contains a variety of substances, including nutrients, salts, a small amount of oxygen, hormones and other cell activity–regulating substances. [2] Proteins found in plasma include albumin, globulin, and fibrinogen. Albumin aids in keeping the correct amount of water in the blood; fibrinogen is a substance needed for clotting; and globulins are used to form antibodies.[2] The amount of plasma can vary based on the hydration of the individual. Therefore a decrease in water intake or an increase in water excretion will decrease the level of plasma in the blood.

If blood is collected without an **anticoagulant,** a clot is formed consisting of the cellular elements and the proteins consumed in the coagulation process. The fluid from which the clot is separated is called **serum.** Serum is plasma without the clotting factors (Figure 21-2). Many of the anticoagulants routinely used by hematologists are not applicable to nuclear hematological studies because they prevent clotting by chelating calcium (a requirement for normal clotting) and other heavy ions

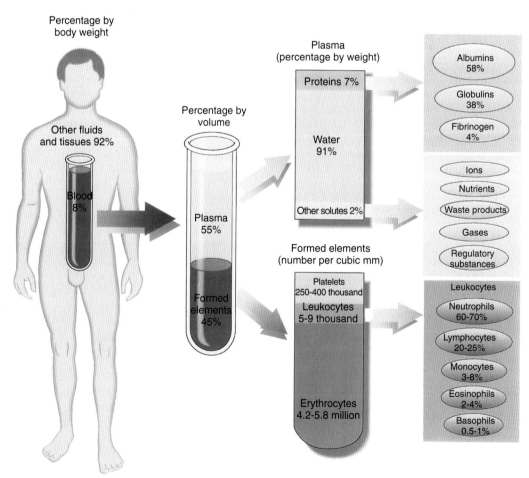

FIGURE 21-1 Normal blood sample.

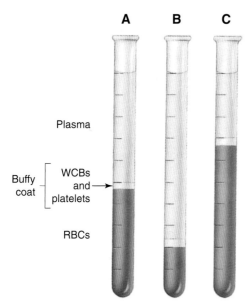

A **B** **C**

Plasma

Buffy coat { WCBs and platelets →

RBCs

FIGURE 21-2 Cellular elements have been separated from plasma by centrifugation. **A,** A normal percent of red blood cells. **B,** Anemia (a low percent of red blood cells). **C,** polycythemia (a high percent of red blood cells).

such as tracer iron, which are used in some nuclear medicine studies.

Although the total blood volume is dependent on the size and gender of the individual and normally ranges from 4 to 6 liters, the relative percentage of the basic cellular types present in circulating blood under normal conditions fall within a certain range and are listed in Figure 21-1 and described in Table 21-1. RBCs are the most abundant elements in the cellular compartment of the blood. They contain a red iron-containing pigment called hemoglobin, which is responsible for the transport of oxygen from the lungs to the rest of the body. Mature circulating RBCs are critical to the survival and proper function of each cell in all tissues of the body. They are shaped like biconcave disks, which allow them to change shape as they travel through different size vessels throughout the body. They are produced from stem cells in the bone marrow through a process called hematopoiesis and have a life span of approximately 120 days. The type of hematopoiesis for RBC production is called erythropoiesis and it is regulated by the hormone erythropoietin, which is released from the kidney. The location of RBC production changes during the course of one's life. In infants, RBCs are produced in the red marrow of all bones, but as an adult, production primarily occurs in the red marrow of the skull, ribs, sternum, vertebrae, and pelvic bones.[11] Under normal circumstances the bone marrow replaces 1% of the total circulating mass of RBCs daily. The bone marrow also stores a reserve of mature RBCs that can be quickly released into the circulation when needed. In situations of continuing stress, normal marrow can gradually increase its daily rate of production manyfold (up to eight times normal in the case of RBCs). At the end of their life spans

or if damaged, most RBCs are removed from circulation by phagocytic cells in the liver and spleen called macrophages. In the process of phagocytosis, principle components of the cell are made available for reuse. The hemoglobin is broken into components for either reuse or excretion; for example, iron is recovered and either stored or recirculated for reuse by the bone marrow, and the heme portion is degraded and excreted as bile pigments by the liver.[11]

Other blood cells include WBCs and thrombocytes, both of which are produced in the marrow by hematopoiesis. There are different types of WBCs or leukocytes and just as with RBCs, the production and circulating number cells is regulated. WBCs can be categorized as granular or agranular, and examples of types of WBCs are found in Table 21-1. WBCs serve as the body's protection against the invasion of microorganisms, often through phagocytosis of microorganisms. Thrombocytes are often referred to as platelets. Their function is to form clots to prevent blood loss.

The percentages and numbers of the different types of blood cells vary from one another. The blood test used to measure the percentage of RBCs in whole blood is called the **hematocrit (Hct)**. The name of the test is often synonymous with what it represents. An Hct is often ordered as part of routine blood work; when there are signs of anemia, leukemia, dietary deficiency; or when the patient has any medical condition. To obtain an Hct, a blood sample is taken usually from the patient's antecubital vein or a vein on back of the hand. The well-mixed sample of anticoagulated blood is placed in a suitable tube and centrifuged for an appropriate period of time to allow for the separation of the cellular elements from the plasma. When Hcts are performed on normal blood, the RBCs compose most of the volume of packed cells (see Figure 21-1) because of their number and size. The grayish-colored layer just above the red cells, known as the **buffy coat,** is the WBC population in that sample of blood. Just above the buffy coat is an even more minute layer of creamy-colored cells, representing the platelets.

The Hct value represents the ratio of the cellular compartment volume to the total volume of a given sample of blood; therefore, alterations in the plasma compartment (or plasma volume) can result in a misleading hematocrit. If a patient has a low plasma volume the Hct will be falsely elevated, or if the patient has an increased plasma volume the Hct will be falsely low.[15] Dehydration is an example of a physical condition that can cause an Hct to be falsely elevated. Careful examination of the Hct tube is necessary to verify that the packed cells consist of a normal RBC population and not an excess of WBCs or platelets. The existence of an excess of WBCs or platelets in the packed cells will give false and misleading results. The use of a handheld magnifying glass or the magnifier supplied with the reading equipment aids in a more accurate reading if

TABLE 21-1	Classes of Blood Cells		
Cell type	Description	Function	Life Span
Erythrocyte	7 μm in diameter; concave disk shape; entire cell stains pale pink; no nucleus	Transportation of respiratory gases (O_2 and CO_2)	105 to 120 days
Neutrophil	12 to 15 μm in diameter; spherical shape; multilobed nucleus; small, pink-purple–staining cytoplasmic granules	Cellular defense—phagocytosis of small pathogenic microorganisms	Hours to 3 days
Basophil	11 to 14 μm in diameter; spherical shape; generally two-lobed nucleus; large, purple-staining cytoplasmic granules	Secretes heparin (anticoagulant) and histamine (important in inflammatory response)	Hours to 3 days
Eosinophil	10 to 12 μm in diameter; spherical shape; generally two-lobed nucleus; large, orange-red–staining cytoplasmic granules	Cellular defense—phagocytosis of large pathogenic microorganisms such as protozoa and parasitic worms; releases antiinflammatory substances in allergic reactions	10 to 12 days
Lymphocyte	6 to 9 μm in diameter; spherical shape; round (single lobe) nucleus; small lymphocytes have scant cytoplasm	Humoral defense—secretes antibodies; involved in immune system response and regulation	Days to years
Monocyte	12 to 17 μm in diameter; spherical shape; nucleus generally kidney bean– or horseshoe-shaped with convoluted surface; ample cytoplasm often "steel blue" in color	Capable of migrating out of the blood to enter tissue spaces as a macrophage—an aggressive phagocytic cell capable of ingesting bacteria, cellular debris, and cancerous cells	Months
Platelet	2 to 5 μm in diameter; irregularly shaped fragments; cytoplasm contains very small, pink-staining granules	Releases clot-activating substances and helps in formation of actual blood clot by forming platelet "plugs"	7 to 10 days

From Thibodeau G, Patton K: *Anatomy and physiology*, ed 6, St Louis, 2007, Mosby.

microhematocrit tubes are used. Because of the smaller number of WBCs and platelets (and, in the case of platelets, minute size) compared to RBCs, the Hct value cannot be relied on to measure the quantity of WBCs and platelets, and only an estimated plasmacrit can be calculated. Typically WBCs and platelets are counted in a medical laboratory.

Anemia is a blood condition in which here is a less than normal number of RBCs or there is abnormal or deficient production.[2] Anemia can be a result of bone marrow dysfunction, low levels of iron or vitamins, or the improper formation of RBCs.[2] The basic causes of anemia are summarized as follows:

- Excessive rate of removal of RBCs from the circulation
  - Blood loss (chronic or acute)
  - **Hemolysis**

- Deficient production of RBCs
  - Lack of proper building blocks (e.g., iron, vitamin B_{12}, folic acid); iron deficiency anemia is a common, simple, and rapidly curable condition
  - Suppression of marrow activity by a wide variety of acute and chronic diseases
  - Primary disorders of the bone marrow

Acute, self-limited, or rapidly cured disorders, such as the common cold or acute pneumonia, cause temporary, essentially complete cessation of marrow RBC production. Such a short-term illness does not result in a recognizable degree of anemia. However, in patients with certain disease states, such as a compensated hemolytic anemia (a condition where RBCs have a significantly shortened life span, but a normal Hct value is maintained by very active marrow that increases the rate of erythrocyte production) a severe degree of anemia may very rapidly develop because of marrow suppression from such otherwise mild illnesses. A wide variety of chronic diseases (e.g., rheumatoid arthritis, malignant disorders) may cause chronic suppression of marrow activity and consequent anemia.

ISOTOPIC LABELING OF CELLULAR ELEMENTS

Valuable information can be obtained from the isotopic labeling of cellular elements followed by the appropriate procedure to obtain information. Isotopic labels of the cellular elements of the blood are of two general types: (1) cohort, or pulse, labels; and (2) random labels. It is important to recognize the fundamental difference in the information to be gained with each of them.

Cohort (Pulse) Labels

Cohort (pulse) labeling is available only to the marrow precursors of a given cell type for a specific and limited length of time; therefore cells that are already circulating will not be cohort labeled. Incorporation of this type of label in the marrow erythroid precursors results in the appearance in the circulation of mature labeled RBCs of the same age. An ideal cohort label with the appropriate gamma-emitting nuclide would permit study of the rate of production of RBCs, their kinetics, longevity, manner of death, and ultimate disposal in the body. However, none of the currently available radioisotopes for cohort labeling of RBCs satisfies all these requirements, and as result are not used in routine clinical studies.

Random Labels

Random labeling of cells refers to the in vitro tagging of circulating cells of the peripheral blood with a radioisotope. This process labels all cells in the sample, thereby labeling blood cells of random age. These labels are applicable to the study of mean cell survival or other direct measurements of the circulating cells of the blood. It is important to emphasize that isotopic labeling of circulating blood cells provides reasonably precise data only if separation, labeling, and reinfusion of these cells are performed so as to minimize damage to the cells.

PLATELET KINETICS

The only isotopic labels available for platelets are of the random type. Chromium-51 (^{51}Cr)-chromate has been extensively used as a random platelet label, but the physical characteristics of the radionuclide result in limitations of its use. Only 9% of the emissions of ^{51}Cr are useful gamma photons. The 27.8-day half-life of ^{51}Cr is long for studies of human platelets, which have a mean survival of approximately 10 days. In addition, since there is low platelet labeling efficiency of ^{51}Cr-chromate, large amounts of blood (up to 500 ml) must be drawn to maximize the final platelet-bound ^{51}Cr activity. Even with optimum harvesting and labeling procedures, the amount of ^{51}Cr infused to platelets is limited to approximately 10 to 30 mCi. As a consequence of these factors, external quantitative organ localization or imaging studies cannot be performed with ^{51}Cr despite its 320-keV gamma energy.

Indium-111 (^{111}In)-oxine as a random cellular label allows for precise platelet kinetic and organ distribution studies.[14] The ^{111}In-oxine complex easily penetrates the cell membrane because of its lipophilic nature, and the ^{111}In label has been shown to possess great stability. The viability of the cells reportedly is not affected by the ^{111}In-oxine labeling procedure if care is taken to avoid cell damage during separation and washing procedures and if labeling is carried out in the presence of plasma.

Because all cellular elements of the blood (RBCs, WBCs, and platelets) will concentrate ^{111}In-oxine, platelets must first be separated by differential centrifugation before the ^{111}In labeling complex is introduced. After incubation of the platelets with ^{111}In-oxine, the unbound ^{111}In radioactivity must be removed. For this purpose, the cells are washed with plasma, centrifuged, and resuspended in fresh plasma.[13-16] The 2.8-day half-life of ^{111}In, its gamma photon energies of 173 and 247 keV, and their relatively high yields (84% and 94%, respectively) allow quantitative external imaging of platelet distribution and deposition in addition to precise determination of platelet survival.

Indium-111–labeled platelets are used for the study of platelet kinetics and for in vivo quantification of sites of platelet distribution and deposition. They have also been used in the investigation of thrombotic and vascular disorders and in monitoring the therapeutic effectiveness of platelet-active drugs in these conditions.

ERYTHROKINETICS

Measurement of Circulating Red Blood Cell Volume

The determinations of the RBC and plasma volumes are based on the simple radioisotope dilution technique.[1] The larger the volume into which the label is mixed, the lower the counts in the sample withdrawn; conversely the smaller the volume, the higher the counts in the sample. This dilution technique is true only when a closed system is used and no radiopharmaceutical is allowed to leak out of the system being measured. Also, the volume of the unknown must not change significantly during the measurement.

To measure circulating RBC volume, a sample of whole blood is collected with the use of an appropriate anticoagulant in the correct ratio to the volume of whole blood. If **acid-citrate-dextrose (ACD)**-NIH solution A or Strumia ACD solution is used, the ratio is 1:5. Because of the wide variance in the composition of the many citric acid, sodium citrate, sodium biphosphate, and citrate phosphate dextrose (CPD) solutions, when using these anticoagulants, the manufacturer's recommendation should be consulted regarding the proper ratio of whole blood to the solution being used. Heparin and ethylenediaminetetraacetic acid (EDTA) are unsatisfactory for use in this procedure. Several satisfactory methods are available both for preparing the ^{51}Cr-labeled RBCs and for performing the necessary measurements.

Chromium-51 is not an ideal label for RBC volume measurements. With gamma rays as only 9% of its emissions, its relatively long half-life (27.8 days), and a relatively slow rate of removal from circulating RBCs (1% per day), serial RBC volume measurements require undesirable increases in the amount of ^{51}Cr injected for each subsequent study. For these reasons, labeling RBCs with technetium-99m (^{99m}Tc) and trace amounts of stannous ions is a useful alternative method of measuring RBC volume.[3,5,8] Because ^{99m}Tc is essentially monoenergetic and has a short half-life, it can be used in amounts that greatly reduce the radiation dose to patients who undergo serial RBC volume measurements. But, because of the more rapid loss of the ^{99m}Tc label, ^{51}Cr-labeled RBCs should be used when sampling times for a single study must extend beyond 60 minutes after injection.

^{51}Cr–Ascorbic Acid Method for Labeling Red Blood Cells

The procedure used when labeling RBCs with ^{51}Cr–ascorbic acid is summarized in Table 21-2. During this method, about 80% to 95% of the chromate ion is promptly transported across the RBC membrane and binds to the beta chain of the hemoglobin molecule. During labeling within the RBCs, the hexavalent chromate ion is reduced to a trivalent chromic ion.

TABLE 21-2	Procedure for Labeling Red Blood Cells with ^{51}Cr–Ascorbic Acid	
Step	**Action**	**Comment**
1	Withdraw 10 ml of venous blood from the patient into a 20-ml syringe containing 2 ml of citric acid, sodium citrate, and ACD—Strumia's formula.	
2	Transfer prepared blood into a 20-ml vacutainer.	
3	Add 30 μCi of ^{51}Cr in the form of chromate ion to vacutainer.	^{51}Cr is transported across erythrocyte membrane.
4	Incubate blood sample for 10 to 15 minutes.	
5	Add ascorbic acid (50 mg).	Reduces the free chromate to chromic ion, which immediately stops the tagging procedure; within the erythrocyte the chromate ion is converted to chromic.
6	Withdraw exactly 5 ml of blood into syringe and save the remainder of the blood to use as the standard.	
7	Inject patient intravenously with the 5 ml of blood.	
8	Wait about 10 minutes and withdraw sample from a vein other than the one used for injection.	Ensures complete patient circulation; disease states can affect the timing.
9	Perform hematocrit determinations.	

ACD, Acid-citrate-dextrose.

Chromium-51 should not be added to the ACD solution before the patient's blood is added to the vial. Dextrose contained in the ACD solution acts as a reducing agent. Ascorbic acid is added after incubation to reduce the free chromate to chromic ion, which immediately stops the tagging procedure, because the chromic ion is unable to penetrate the RBC membrane.

As noted in the procedure found in Table 21-2, the labeled blood is drawn into a syringe and injected into the patient intravenously. The remainder is kept to make a standard. After adequate time to ensure complete mixing of the labeled RBCs in the circulation, a sample is drawn from a vein other than that used for the injection. In normal subjects, 10 minutes is sufficient to ensure complete mixing; however, disease states can affect the mixing time. Splenomegaly and severe polycythemia may result in greatly delayed mixing time, whereas other disease states may cause a less pronounced delay. Because of this, serial samples should be taken until no significant difference in counts is seen.

Hematocrit value determinations are performed on the well-mixed standard and blood samples. Four counting tubes are prepared to contain 1-ml volumes of the following:

Whole blood from the standard = Std WB
Plasma from the standard = Std Plas
Whole blood from the sample = Samp WB
Plasma from the sample = Samp Plas

The standards and samples are counted in a well counter with the spectrometer centered on the 320-keV photopeak of ^{51}Cr. Samples should be counted for sufficient time to ensure a counting accuracy of 1% error or less. Usually there are so few counts in the postinjection plasma sample that a shorter counting time is acceptable for this tube.

$$\text{RBC Volume (ml)} = [cpm\,\text{Std WB} - (cpm\,\text{Std Plas} \times \text{Std Plct})] \times$$
$$\frac{\text{Volume injected} \times \textit{Samp Hct}}{[cpm\,\textit{Samp WB} - (cpm\,\textit{Samp Plas} \times \textit{Samp Plct})]}$$

where *Plct* is the decimal **plasmacrit** (1.00 − decimal Hct) and *Samp Hct* is the decimal Hct of sample (a 42% Hct = 0.42 decimal Hct.).

Falsely high results are found if:

- Faulty intravenous injection technique is used and the entire dose is not injected into a vein.
- RBCs are damaged.
- Excessive binding of the ^{51}Cr by WBCs or platelets occurs.

Falsely low values are caused by:

- Failure to obtain a preinjection blood sample in a patient who has had previous administration of radioactive tracers
- Contamination of equipment with radioactivity

It should be noted that for measurement of the circulating RBC mass, 10 μCi of ^{51}Cr is an adequate amount of activity and provides enough counts so that statistically significant sample counting can be performed in a reasonable time. The specific activity of the ^{51}Cr chromate must be such that less than 2 mg of chromium ion is present per milliliter of packed RBCs. This becomes particularly critical when this technique is used for RBC survival studies that require larger doses of ^{51}Cr.

Plasma Volume

Iodinated human serum albumin is the conventional agent used for estimation of plasma volume. Albumin does not remain in the intravascular space but diffuses rapidly into extravascular compartments. Because this vascular space is now an open system, use of the closed-system isotope dilution principle for calculations causes errors in the plasma volume measurement. An extrapolation procedure can be used to calculate the volume if the injected tracer leaves the open system at a rate that is slow compared with the rate of mixing uniformly within that system, and samples are taken only after mixing has been completed.[17]

Iodine-125 (^{125}I)-labeled human serum albumin is provided by radiopharmaceutical manufacturers in a concentration of 10 mCi per 1.5 ml. Not more than 2% of the radioactivity can be in the free form because the free form is removed from the intravascular space more rapidly than the labeled albumin, which would result in an overestimation of plasma volume. Technetium-99m–labeled albumin can also be used but must be 98% bound on injection.

When performing plasma volume measurements, the patient should not have had a transfusion or phlebotomy in the 4 weeks before the procedure. In addition, if the patient has undergone any previous studies involving radionuclides, a 4-ml sample of blood should be drawn and counted to determine if the blood counts are above background. Usually both plasma and RBC volume measurements are done. When this is the situation, the plasma volume determination should be done first unless the measurements are being performed simultaneously.[15] The procedure for plasma volume measurements can be found in Box 21-1. It should be noted that the patient should be supine for at least 10 to 15 minutes before the study is started; this is done because in the standing position, plasma volume decreases from an increase in venous pressure in the legs, which causes water to move from the intravascular to the extravascular space.[17] Also, it is recommended that thyroid blockage of radioiodine be performed at least 30 minutes before injection of the radiotracer by means of oral administration of 5 drops (150 mg) of a supersaturated solution of sodium iodide (SSKI).

Blood Volume Measurements

Under normal conditions, blood volumes are regulated and kept constant by various mechanisms. A decrease in blood volume, which results in a decrease in cardiac output and arterial pressure, causes an increase in fluid retention by the kidneys to return the volume to normal limits. The converse is true with an increase in blood volume.

In normal subjects, with a precisely measured RBC or plasma volume and venous Hct value, the volume of the other compartment can be calculated and the total blood volume estimated. This is true only for normal subjects, because in normal subjects a fixed relationship exists between the whole body Hct (Hct$_b$) and the venous Hct

---

BOX 21-1   Plasma Volume Measurement (^{125}I–Human Serum Albumin)

1. Patient preparation: Thyroid blockage of radioiodine should be performed 30 minutes prior to beginning the study (for example, 5 drops, 150 mg, of a supersaturated solution of sodium iodide [SSKI]).
2. Patient position: Supine (or at rest) for at least 10 to 15 minutes before the study is started
3. Procedure:
   - Administer by intravenous injection of 10 µCi of ^{125}I RISA with care being taken that it all enters the vein.
   - Collect three timed heparinized blood samples at 10, 20, and 30 minutes post injection at a site different from the injection site.
   - From each of the patient's timed samples, duplicate whole blood specimens are obtained and counted as a duplicate blood sample in a well counter. Duplicate microhematocrits on the samples are also measured.[7]
4. Samples are centrifuged, and 1 ml aliquots of plasma are counted.
5. The radioactivity in each of these samples is measured and plotted against time on semilogarithmic paper:

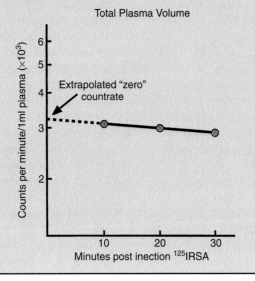

Total Plasma Volume

6. The best straight line is drawn through these points, and only the earlier points are used if the later points deviate from the initial linear slope. The zero-time activity is estimated by extrapolation and used to calculate the plasma volume.
7. A standard solution (Std) is prepared by diluting a known volume of ^{125}I RISA with water to a known and exact volume (for example, 1000 ml) utilizing an identical injection/flushing technique to that used for patient injection.[7]
   - The dilution factor (DF) is calculated: DF = volume or RISA/total volume of standard.[7]
8. Calculation:

$$\text{Plasma volume (ml)} = \frac{\text{Volume injected} \times \text{cpm in 1 ml Std} \times \text{dilution factor}}{\text{cpm of plasma sample obtained by extrapolation}}$$

If whole blood is counted instead of plasma the calculation is as follows:[7]

$$\text{Plasma volume (ml)} = \frac{\text{Volume injected} \times \text{cpm in 1 ml Std} \times (1\text{-Hct})}{\text{cpm/ml whole blood @ T} = 0}$$

Volume injected = ml RISA injected

Although in healthy subjects the difference between the 0-minute and the 10-minute counts may be negligible, the extrapolated 0-minute value yields the most accurate final plasma volume result, because in states of rapid protein, disappearance from the intravascular space, significantly lower counts will be obtained in serial samples. Use of these lower counts would result in false overestimation of the plasma volume.[7]

(Hct_v); the ratio of Hct_b to Hct_v on the average is 0.90. It is believed that two factors are responsible for the difference observed between the Hct_b and the Hct_v: (1) the Hct value of blood in small capillaries is lower than that found in larger vessels, and (2) the iodinated albumin used to measure the plasma space is immediately distributed into a space larger than that of the vascular space in which the RBCs are distributed. In patients with moderate or gross splenomegaly, the ratio of Hct_b to Hct_v may be substantially and unpredictably increased to greater than 1; in patients with severe polycythemia, abnormalities may be present in the plasma volume as well as the RBC volume. In clinical circumstances, therefore total blood volume can be reliably estimated only by measuring RBC volume and plasma volume simultaneously.

A limitation in the interpretation of these studies is that normal values for blood volume in any given individual cannot be simply predicted from such parameters as height and weight despite the many elaborate formulas that have been proposed. Factors such as obesity, recent weight loss, or prolonged bed rest may make it impossible to estimate the RBC and plasma volume from height and weight measurements, because RBC volume is related to lean body mass. The measured values of patients who are exceptionally obese or who have had a recent significant weight loss should be compared with values based on ideal or recent body weight.

In interpreting studies in adults, the simplest method of calculating the values in milliliters per kilogram is probably at least as reliable as using any of the various formulas or nomograms. The normal values published

TABLE 21-3	Normal Blood Volume Compartment Values (ml/kg)	
	Males	**Females**
Total blood volume	55 to 80	50 to 75
Red blood cell volume*	25 to 35	20 to 30
Plasma volume†	30 to 45	30 to 45

*95% confidence limits.
†Because of the many variables that may influence plasma volume in normal subjects, it is not possible to place confidence limits on these values.

by the International Panel on Standardization in Haematology are shown in Table 21-3. The wide range in plasma volume observed in normal subjects is indicative of the lack of preciseness with this test. The undesirable rapid diffusion of the radiolabeled albumin from the vascular space is but one factor making this procedure less than precise, even in normal subjects. Body position, recent exercise, and a number of other factors cause rapid, significant changes in plasma volume. Therefore, although the circulating RBC volume can be measured and reported precisely, the plasma volume should always be reported as an estimate.

Blood volume measurements have proved to be of considerable value in several specific circumstances. Use of ^{51}Cr-labeled RBCs to measure the RBC volume allows a precise determination of whether true polycythemia is present or the patient has an elevated Hct because of a reduced plasma volume. Patients who have a persistent elevation of the Hct, but in whom the RBC volume is normal when measured by the ^{51}Cr technique, are usually normal subjects whose RBC volume is near the upper limits of normal and whose plasma volume is near the lower limits of normal. Undergoing this procedure to determine blood volume, which proves that the RBC volume is normal, spares these patients an elaborate, expensive, and prolonged series of other diagnostic procedures.

Patients with polycythemia vera and myelofibrosis may have pronounced expansion of the plasma volume, which is apparent only if this parameter is directly measured. Because of the combined abnormality of plasma volume and RBCs, serial measurements of both the ^{99m}Tc-RBC and plasma volume may become essential to the management of patients with polycythemia vera. Paradoxically, in an acutely hemorrhaging patient or a patient suffering from recent severe trauma, the Hct may remain normal or disproportionately high for some time. In these circumstances direct measurement with ^{51}Cr-labeled RBCs reveals the true RBC volume. The procedure for RBC volume measurement can be found in Box 21-2. As with plasma volume measurements, the patient should not have had a transfusion or phlebotomy in the 4 weeks before the procedure. In addition, if the patient has undergone any previous studies involving

radionuclides, a 4-ml sample of blood should be drawn and counted to determine if the blood counts are above background. Usually both plasma and RBC volume measurements are done. When this is the situation, the plasma volume determination should be done first unless the measurements are being performed simultaneously.[15]

Erythrocyte Survival and Splenic Sequestration Studies

It is sometimes necessary to study the half-life of RBCs. In patients with suspected hemolytic anemia, a RBC survival study may be performed. To determine if the spleen is the cause of a patient's increased destruction of RBCs, survival and splenic sequestration studies are performed.

For these procedures, red blood cells are labeled using the same technique as that for RBC volume determination except that the dose of ^{51}Cr is adjusted to 1.5 mCi per kilogram of body weight. After labeling, the cells are reinjected, and the first 6-ml sample is obtained 24 hours later and placed in a tube containing an anticoagulant (preferably solid EDTA or concentrated heparin). Samples are then obtained every other day for the next 3 weeks. Before samples are pipetted and Hct values are determined, a tiny amount of saponin powder is added to each tube, and the tubes are gently inverted 12 to 15 times to ensure mixing and complete lysis of the RBCs. Care is taken not to allow the sample to touch the cap of the counting tube. Each day of collection, 5 ml of whole blood is pipetted from the tubes and Hct determinations are made on each sample.

On the last day of the study, all the samples are counted on the gamma spectrometer with settings of 280 to 360 keV for ^{51}Cr. The samples are counted for approximately 10 minutes to give a sample error of ≤1%.

For calculation of the half-time ($t_{1/2}$) of disappearance of the labeled RBCs, the net counts per minute of each sample are plotted on semilogarithmic paper as a function of time (Figure 21-3). The best straight line is drawn through all the points. The $t_{1/2}$ is obtained as follows:

1. The line to time zero is extrapolated; this is the y-intercept.
2. The y-intercept value is divided by 2. At this value on the y-axis, a straight line is drawn parallel to the x-axis until it intersects the best straight line drawn through the observed data points.
3. A perpendicular line is dropped to the x-axis; this is the labeled RBC half-time disappearance rate or survival time as measured by the ^{51}Cr technique, not corrected for elution of the isotope.

The mean half-life of normal ^{51}Cr-labeled RBCs is 25 to 35 days. Normal RBCs are removed from the

---

BOX 21-2 | **Red Cell Volume Measurement (^{51}Cr–Red Blood Cells)[9]**

1. Patient preparation: The study is often performed with plasma volume measurements.
2. Patient position: Supine
3. Radiopharmaceutical, dose, and administration: radiopharmaceutical: ^{51}Cr labeled RBCs; dose: 10-30 μCi; IV administration
4. Procedure: Specimen acquisition
   a. Perform a venipuncture with a 19-gauge infusions set; secure it to the patients arm
   b. Using a 50-ml syringe containing 5 ml of ACD solution, withdraw 40 ml of blood for a total of 45 ml.
   c. Inject 0.5 ml of heparin solution into the infusion set.
   d. Label the patient's blood samples.
   e. Place a 21-gauge infusion set in the patient's opposite arm and inject 0.5 ml of heparin solution.
   f. Inject 20 mL of labeled patient's blood through the 21 gauge infusion set into the patient.
   g. After 20 minutes (for adequate mixing), using the 19-gauge infusion set withdraw 20 ml of blood into a heparinized syringe (do not use the 21-gauge set through which the radiopharmaceutical was administered) and remove both infusion sets.
5. Data processing
   a. Determine the microhematocrit of the whole blood standard and 20 minute blood specimen, each in duplicate.
   b. Label the necessary 5 vials for counting.
   c. Pipette 1 ml of standard whole blood (from the ACD tagging vial) into the dilution flask and add 99 ml of water; mix for uniformity.
   d. Centrifuge the remaining whole blood standard and pipette 1 ml of plasma into a second dilution flask; add 99 ml of water; mix for uniformity.
   e. Pipette 5 ml of the diluted whole blood standard and 5 ml of diluted plasma into counting vials.
   f. Pepette 5 mL of the 20 minute blood specimen into a counting vial.
   g. Centrifuge the 20-minute blood specimen and pipette 5 ml of plasma into a counting vial.
   h. Count all vials for 10,000 counts and reduce the results to cpm/ml.
6. Calculations:
   a. Calculate average microhematocrits and microplasmacrits, all in decimal form.
   b. Calculate net counts per minute per ml for all samples.
   c. Calculate total RBC counts injected (cpm):
   Dilution factor = 100; volume injected = 20 (or actual volume if different) (std WB dil – [std Pl dil × std WB Plct]) × vol inj × dil fact = RBC cts injected
   d. Calculate the cpm per ml in the sample RBC:

$$\frac{20 \text{ min WB(cpm/ml)} - [20 \text{ min Pl(cpm/mL)} \times 20 \text{ Plct}]}{20 \text{ min Hct}} =$$
   sam.RBC (cpm/ml)

   e. Calculate RCV (ml)

$$\frac{\text{RBC counts injected(cpm)}}{\text{Sample RBCs(cpm/ml)}} = \text{RCV (ml)}$$

dil fac, dilution factor; *Hct,* hematocrit; *Pl,* plasma; *std WB dil,* standard whole blood dilute; *std Pl dil,* standard plasma dilute; *std WB Plct,* standard whole blood plasmacrit; *vol inj,* volume injected; *WB,* whole blood.

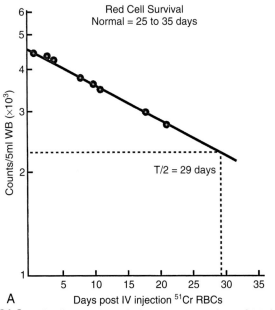

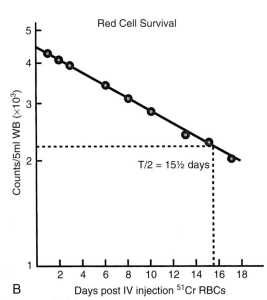

A

B

FIGURE 21-3 Red cell survival graph showing a normal $t_{1/2}$ of 29 days **(A)**, compared with an abnormal $t_{1/2}$ **(B)**, which indicates a hemolytic process resulting in shortened survival of ^{51}Cr-labeled erythrocytes. *IV,* Intravenous.

circulation as they reach their age limit at a rate of approximately 1% per day; the true mean life span of the normal RBC therefore is 50 to 60 days. However, this approximately 1% per day removal of senescent RBCs from the circulation coupled with the approximately 1% per day elution of the ^{51}Cr label from the RBCs gives a mean half-life of 25 to 35 days when measured with this technique. Tables are available for correcting for this elution, but they were derived from studies in normal subjects, and their relevance in disease states in which the elution rate is known to vary is uncertain. However, the more severe the hemolytic process or bleeding, and thus the more rapid the rate of removal of the ^{51}Cr-labeled RBCs, the less significant this ^{51}Cr elution becomes.

Determination of the mean RBC life span from a label randomly applied to cells of all ages is meaningful only in a patient who is in a steady state rate of production and destruction of RBCs. If either of these rates changes, the mean age of the circulating RBCs is changed and the ^{51}Cr results will be affected, even though the actual longevity of the individual RBC has not changed. A constant Hct value before and during the period of study is one index of a steady state. Obviously, inaccurate results are obtained in a patient who is being or has recently been transfused.

The study of splenic **sequestration** (removal or destruction) of RBCs should be a routine part of any ^{51}Cr-RBC survival study. Organ counting is begun 24 hours after labeled cells are reinjected and is continued approximately every other day for the next 3 weeks. The counting probe should be equipped with a flat-field collimator designed to exclude radiation from areas other than the organs of interest but that still permits sampling of a large enough organ volume to give adequate count rates. The spectrometer is adjusted to count gamma rays from 280 to 360 keV. The patient is positioned on the examining table as follows:

- *Precordium:* The patient is placed supine, and the detector is centered over the left third intercostal interspace at the sternal border.
- *Liver:* The patient is placed supine, and the detector is placed over the ninth and tenth ribs on the right, in the midclavicular line. In elderly subjects and patients with chronic obstructive pulmonary disease, the exact location of the liver should be checked by percussion.
- *Spleen:* The patient is placed prone, and the detector is placed two thirds of the distance from the spinous process to the lateral edge of the body at the level of the ninth and tenth ribs.

The skin is marked with indelible ink, which in turn is covered by transparent nonallergenic tape to indicate the position of the external detector from one day to the next. Each area must be counted with the same geometry each time by having the detector touch the patient's

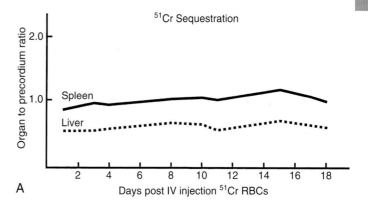

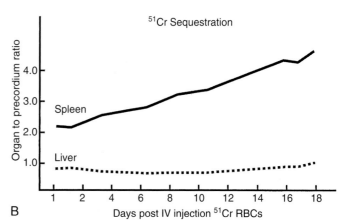

FIGURE 21-4 Organ localization of ^{51}Cr-labeled erythrocytes. Normal liver-to-precordium and spleen-to-precordium ratios **(A)** compared with increasing spleen-to-precordium ratios **(B)**, showing active splenic sequestration. *IV,* Intravenous; *RBCs,* red blood cells.

skin. The areas are counted to give a sample error of 5% or less.

The results are expressed as ratios of count rates: the count rate over the spleen to the count rate over the precordium, and the count rate over the liver over to the count rate over the precordium. These ratios are graphed as a function of time on linear graph paper (Figure 21-4). In normal subjects, the spleen-to-liver ratio is less than or may approximate 1:1. In patients with active splenic sequestration of cells, this ratio often rises to 2:1 or even to 4:1. The spleen-to-precordium ratio is judged to be clearly abnormal if the ratio is greater than 2:1. An initial and persistent elevation of the spleen-to-precordium ratio is attributable to an increased splenic blood pool. A progressive gradual increase indicates active sequestration of the labeled cells.

Sources of Error

Sources of error study of splenic sequestration include the following:

- Inaccurate probe positioning, which causes false results

- Blood loss from the gastrointestinal tract or surgical sites, which results in a shortened half-life
- Blood transfusions during the procedure, which also cause an apparent shortening of the half-life because of the increased volume of the unlabeled cells from the transfusion

MEASUREMENT OF ABSORPTION AND SERUM LEVELS OF ESSENTIAL NUTRIENTS

Vitamin B$_{12}$ (Cyanocobalamin) Absorption

Vitamin B$_{12}$, also known as cobalamin, is an essential water-soluble vitamin. The organ systems most profoundly affected by vitamin B$_{12}$ deficiency are the bone marrow, GI and neurologic systems.[4] Nuclear medicine has furnished important tools for the diagnosis of vitamin B$_{12}$ deficiency. The consequences of untreated vitamin B$_{12}$ deficiency include anemia, thrombocytopenia, leukopenia, crippling spinal cord degeneration, and death. The importance of measuring vitamin B$_{12}$ (or **cyanocobalamin,** a form of vitamin B$_{12}$) absorption in patients with unexplained anemia deserves emphasis, because the principle that anemia is not a disease per se but only a symptom of some underlying disorder is not always reflected in practice. The onset of clinical symptoms from vitamin B$_{12}$ deficiency can be insidious, and the initial complaints of patients can be vague; in the early stages the classic RBC changes are not present.[8]

Box 21-3 summarizes the causes of vitamin B$_{12}$ deficiency. Box 21-4 summarizes factors important in vitamin B$_{12}$ nutrition and absorption in humans. Absorption of this vitamin through the terminal ileum depends on secretion of intrinsic factor, a protein secreted by the parietal cells of the stomach. Intrinsic factor itself is not absorbed at the sites in the terminal ileum, but it is required in an active transport mechanism. Ionic calcium and a pH of ileal contents greater than 6 are also required. Once absorption takes place, a normal transport protein, transcobalamin II, must be present in the bloodstream to convey the B$_{12}$ to areas of the body for utilization or storage. Isolated "pure" dietary deficiency (apart from severe prolonged protein deprivation) is very rare. Therefore, the overwhelming number of cases of vitamin B$_{12}$ deficiency are caused by some underlying disorder attributable to malabsorption. The most common cause of vitamin B$_{12}$ malabsorption is a deficiency in intrinsic factor.

The availability of radioactive vitamin B$_{12}$ for specific testing of a patient's ability to absorb physiological amounts of this essential nutrient has been of great clinical value. Vitamin B$_{12}$ is a complex corrinoid compound (Figure 21-5), of which the central ligand is cobalt. Several radioisotopes of cobalt are available for labeling the vitamin. The earliest radioisotope of cobalt to be used was cobalt-60 (^{60}Co), but cobalt-57 (^{57}Co) and

---

BOX 21-3	Causes of Vitamin B$_{12}$ Deficiency

I. Inadequate intake
II. Malabsorption
  A. Caused by gastric abnormalities
    1. Absence of intrinsic factor
      a. Congenital
      b. Addisonian pernicious anemia
      c. Total gastrectomy
      d. Subtotal gastrectomy
    2. Excessive excretion of hydrochloric acid (Zollinger-Ellison syndrome)
  B. Caused by intestinal malabsorption
    1. Destruction, removal, or functional incompetence of ileal mucosal absorptive sites
    2. Competition with host for available dietary vitamin B$_{12}$
      a. *Diphyllobothrium latum* (fish tapeworm)
      b. Small bowel lesions associated with stagnation and bacterial overgrowth (e.g., jejunal diverticula, strictures, blind loops)
    3. Drug therapy*
      a. Para-aminosalicylic acid (PAS)
      b. Neomycin
      c. Colchicine
      d. Calcium-chelating agents
  C. Caused by genetic abnormality in the transport protein transcobalamin II

*Although any of these agents may cause abnormalities in vitamin B$_{12}$ absorption, only patients undergoing long-term PAS therapy have been reported to develop clinical evidence of vitamin B$_{12}$ deficiency.

BOX 21-4	Absorption of Dietary Vitamin B$_{12}$ in Humans*

1. Vitamin B$_{12}$ is available for human nutrition only from animal food sources.
2. Vitamin B$_{12}$ is bound to the intrinsic factor by the gastric mucosa.
3. Normal ileal mucosal absorptive sites depend on the presence both of ionic Ca^{2}+ and of ileal contents with a pH higher than 6.
4. Normal transport protein (transcobalamin II) conveys vitamin B$_{12}$ from ileal absorptive sites to areas of active utilization and storage.

*The same factors apply to absorption of tracer amounts of the radioactive vitamin B$_{12}$ used in absorption studies.

---

cobalt-58 (^{58}Co) are now preferred for routine clinical studies because of their shorter half-lives and smaller radiation doses (Table 21-4).

The Schilling test of urinary excretion is generally accepted as the standard method of measuring absorption of radioactive vitamin B$_{12}$. This test requires (1) oral administration of a tracer dose of vitamin B$_{12}$ in the range of 0.25 to 2 mg, an amount similar to one that might be present in a normal meal; amounts above this level may be absorbed by mechanisms not dependent on intrinsic factor; and (2) an injection of a flushing dose of 1 mg of nonradioactive vitamin B$_{12}$, which causes transient saturation of normal binding sites in the plasma.

Patients should have nothing to eat after midnight on the day before the test and should remain fasting for 2 hours after the oral dose of ^{57}Co vitamin B$_{12}$; however, they may drink water before and after the test. The patient's physician should be instructed not to give enemas or laxatives or to schedule the patient for a barium enema or intravenous pyelogram for the duration of this study. In addition, certain medications interfere with the results of the test, (e.g., vitamin B$_{12}$ injections, colchicine corticosteroids, and adrenocorticotropic hormone [ACTH]). If large (1 mg or greater) daily doses of vitamin B$_{12}$ are administered, it is theoretically possible to block all the absorptive sites (in the terminal ileum) due to hepatobiliary recirculation. If the patient

has normal renal function, however, all excess vitamin B$_{12}$ is promptly excreted in the urine, and the test needs to be delayed only 24 to 48 hours after discontinuation of the vitamin B$_{12}$ injections.

Schilling Technique

The Schilling technique is as follows:

- Twenty-four–hour urine collection is obtained for background if the patient has previously been given radioactive materials.
- 0.5 µCi of ^{57}Co vitamin B$_{12}$ is administered orally.
- Two hours later a 1-mg flushing dose of stable vitamin B$_{12}$ is given by intramuscular injection.
- Patient obtains two 24-hour urine collections, one for each 24-hour period. The patient is instructed to collect all urine during this period and avoid losing any urine during defecation.

The total volume of each 24-hour collection is measured. The urine samples and a standard are counted in a well counter with the spectrometer set to count gamma rays from 105 to 145 keV.

$$\% \text{ of } ^{57}\text{Co Vitamin B}_{12} \text{ in 24-hour urine} = \frac{\text{cpm in urine} \times \dfrac{\text{Urine volume}}{\text{Sample volume}} \times 100}{\text{cpm in Std} \times \text{Dilution factor}}$$

A result of less than 9% of the administered dose in the first 24-hour urine collection is indicative of malabsorption of vitamin B$_{12}$.

Pitfalls associated with the test include the dependence on a complete 24-hour urine collection. The loss of one urine specimen may cause falsely low results. The 24-hour test also requires that urinary function be intact. Erroneously low values result from abnormal urinary retention, as in men with benign prostatic hypertrophy or in patients with renal disease. In such patients, the

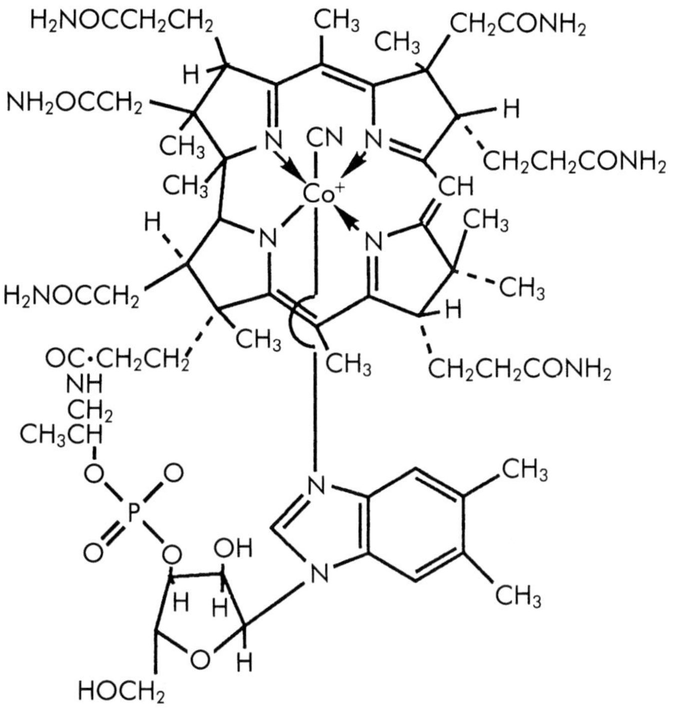

FIGURE 21-5 Structure of cyanocobalamin, the most widely administered form of vitamin B$_{12}$.

		Effective half-life		**Principal photon**	**Relative dose**
Isotope	Physical half-life	in liver*	Radiation	energies (meV)	to liver
^{57}Co	270 days	161 days	Electron capture	0.122 (87%)	1†
^{58}Co	72 days	60 days	Electron capture, β⁺, γ	0.810 (99%)	2
				0.511 (30%)	
^{60}Co	52 years	331 days	β⁻, γ	1.17 (100%)	29
				1.33 (100%)	

TABLE 21-4 Characteristics of Selected Radioisotopes of Cobalt

*Assuming a biological half-life of 400 days after administration as radioactive cobalt-labeled vitamin B$_{12}$.
†Approximately 0.051 rad per 0.5 µCi of ^{57}Co-labeled vitamin when parenteral dose of 1 mg of vitamin B$_{12}$ is given, resulting in renal excretion of approximately 30% of the absorbed dose of radioactive vitamin B$_{12}$.
Complied from McIntyre PA: *Textbook of nuclear medicine: clinical applications,* Philadelphia, 1979, Lea & Febiger; adapted from Heinrich HC, editor; *Vitamin B-12 and intrinsic factor. II. Europäisches Symposium über Vitamin B-12 und Intrinsic Factor,* Hamburg, Germany, 1961, Stuttgart, Germany, 1961, Ferdinand Encke Verlag.

amount excreted in the first 24 hours is reduced, but significant radioactivity continues to be excreted for the next 24 to 48 hours; total excretion eventually is within normal limits. This is the rationale for having the patient collect two separate 24-hour urine specimens and making calculations with each specimen separately after the single flushing dose.

If less than 6% of the dose is excreted in 24 hours, a stage II Schilling test should be performed. A period of 3 to 7 days must elapse after the first Schilling test before the stage II test can be performed. In the stage II test, 10 mg of intrinsic factor is given along with the [57]Co-labeled vitamin B_{12}. If the patient's urinary excretion value is normal after the administration of intrinsic factor, an intrinsic factor deficiency is indicated.

Several factors can contribute to a false-negative result on the stage II Schilling test. When radioactive vitamin B_{12} and intrinsic factor are given in separate capsules, incomplete binding of the two in the stomach may result. To prevent this, before administration, the radioactive vitamin B_{12} and intrinsic factor should be mixed together in water.[10] Another factor that can contribute to a false-negative result is if hog intrinsic factor is used. In this situation, a negative result does not completely rule out intrinsic factor–dependent malabsorption, because some patients who have previously been exposed to hog intrinsic factor (as present in many multivitamin preparations) may have antibodies against it. Finally, vitamin B_{12} deficiency can produce small bowel megaloblastosis with atrophy, which can cause ileal malabsorption. In these situations, vitamin B_{12} therapy may be necessary to allow the ileum to heal before a stage II study is performed.[6]

If it is determined that the stage II study result is truly abnormal, other causes of malabsorption must be investigated and treated if possible, followed by another stage I Schilling test.

Dual-Isotope Method for Measuring Vitamin B_{12} Absorption

The conventional Schilling test for vitamin B_{12} absorption is done in two stages, requiring at least 1 week for a final result if stage I is abnormal. To obtain faster results, a dual-isotope method is available in which vitamin B_{12} labeled with two different isotopes of cobalt is administered. One form, [57]Co vitamin B_{12}, is bound to intrinsic factor by prior incubation with normal human gastric juice; the other form contains non–protein-bound [58]Co vitamin B_{12}.

The two capsules are ingested orally by a fasting patient, after which a flushing injection of 1 mg of non-radioactive vitamin B_{12} is given. Two 24-hour urine samples are collected. Differential isotope counting is performed to determine the percentage of administered dose of each isotope that has been excreted in the urine. A patient with normal vitamin B_{12} absorption excretes

equal amounts of the two isotopes, whereas a patient lacking intrinsic factor excretes greater amounts of intrinsic factor–bound [57]Co vitamin B_{12}.[12] In patients with bacterial overgrowth or bowel lesions resulting in vitamin B_{12} malabsorption, both isotopes are excreted in abnormally low amounts.

The dual-isotope Schilling test has advantages over the conventional method. One advantage is time. Results can be obtained in 2 days compared with 1 week, which leads to earlier diagnosis and treatment and saves money. Another advantage is that the use of [57]Co vitamin B_{12} bound to human gastric juice eliminates the use of hog intrinsic factor preparations, against which some patients may have developed antibodies.

False-negative results may occur if small bowel changes caused by vitamin B_{12} deficiency are not considered. These changes can result in the absorption of the [57]Co vitamin B_{12} bound to gastric juice being falsely low, along with a low [58]Co vitamin B_{12} absorption.

At the time of this writing, the cobalt radionuclides necessary for this procedure are difficult to obtain and as a result the Schillings Test is not used, however, the test is still in use in other parts of the world.

SUMMARY

- When blood is collected with an anticoagulant, it divides into a cellular component and fluid component called *plasma.*
- When blood is collected without an anticoagulant, it divides into a clot and a fluid component called *serum.*
- Hematocrit is the ratio of the cellular compartment volume to the total volume of a given blood sample, and it can be affected by alterations in the plasma compartment.
- Anemia can result from either an excessive rate of removal of RBCs from the circulation or a deficient production of RBCs.
- Random labeling of cells refers to the in vitro tagging of circulating cells of the peripheral blood with a radioisotope.
- The determination of the RBC volume and plasma volume is based on the simple radioisotope dilution technique.
- The study of splenic sequestration should be a routine part of any ^{51}Cr-RBC survival study.
- Reproducibility in counting is essential in a splenic sequestration study.

REFERENCES

1. Belcher EH, Berlin NI, Eernisse JG, et al: Standard techniques for the measurement of red cell and plasma volume, *Br J Haematol* 25:801-814, 1973.
2. Colbert B, Ankney J, Lee K: *Anatomy and physiology for health professions: an interactive journey,* Upper Saddle River, N.J., 2006, Prentice Hall.

3. Ducassou D, Arnaud D, Bardy A, et al: A new stannous agent list for labeling red blood cells with ^{99m}Tc and its clinical application, *Br J Radiol* 49:344-347, 1979.
4. Early PJ, Sodee DB: *Principles and Practice of Nuclear Medicine*, St Louis, 1995, Mosby-Year Book Inc.
5. Eckelman W, Richards P, Hausen W, et al: Technetium-labeled red blood cells, *J Nucl Med* 12:22-24, 1971.
6. Haurani FI, Sherwood N, Goldstein F: Intestinal malabsorption of vitamin B_{12} in pernicious anemia, *Metabolism* 13:1342-1348, 1964.
7. Henkin R, et al: *Nuclear Medicine Volume 1*, St Louis, 1996, Mosby.
8. Jones J, Mollison PL: A simple and efficient method of labeling red cells with ^{99m}Tc for determination of red cell volume, *Br J Haematol* 38:141, 1978.
9. Klingensmith WC III: *Nuclear Medicine Procedure Manuel*, Eaglewood, C.O., 2003, Wick Publishing, Inc.
10. Kubasik NP, Volosin MT, Sine HE: Comparison of commercial kits for radioimmunoassay. III. Radioassay of serum folate, *Clin Chem* 21:1922-1926, 1975.
11. Mader S: *Human Biology*, ed 7, New York, 2002, McGraw-Hill.
12. McDonald JW, Barr RM, Barton WB: Spurious Schilling test results obtained with intrinsic factor enclosed in capsules, *Ann Intern Med* 83:827-829, 1975.
13. Nickoloff EL, Drew H, Hagan J: *In vitro techniques: radionuclides in haematology*, London, 1986, Churchill Livingstone.
14. Scheffel U, Tsan MF, McIntyre PA: Labeling of human platelets with (^{111}In)-8-hydroxyquinoline, *J Nucl Med* 20:524-531, 1979.
15. Scheffel U, Tsan MF, Mitchell TG et al: Human platelets labeled with In-111-8-hydroxyquinoline: kinetics, distribution, and estimates of radiation dose, *J Nucl Med* 23:149-156, 1982.
16. Tsan MF, Hill-Zobel RL: Should platelets be radio-labeled in plasma medicine? *Am J Hematol* 25:355-359, 1987.
17. Wright RR, Tono M, Pollycove M: Blood volume, *Semin Nucl Med* 5:63-77, 1975.

Inflammatory/Tumor/Oncology Imaging and Therapy

Kathy S. Thomas, Frances L. Neagley

OUTLINE

OBJECTIVES

After completing this chapter, the reader will be able to:
- Explain the role nuclear medicine plays in the diagnosis and treatment of infections and tumors.
- Discuss the evolution of infection imaging from ^{67}Ga to ^{111}In to ^{99m}Tc.
- Describe the imaging procedures for parathyroid, prostate, colorectal, neuroendocrine, adrenal, breast, and lung tumors.
- Describe radioimmunotherapy in lymphomas and radionuclide therapies for metastatic bone pain and other maladies.

KEY TERMS

antibodies
antibody fragment (Fab)
cancer
Hodgkin lymphoma (HD)

murine
murine monoclonal antibody (mab)
neuroblastoma
non-Hodgkin lymphoma (NHL)

pheochromocytoma
radioimmunotherapy
radiosynoviorthesis (RSV)
somatostatin

Inflammatory and tumor imaging requires a multidisciplinary approach to accurately diagnose, stage, and follow-up malignancy or infectious processes. Computed tomography (CT), magnetic resonance imaging (MRI), and ultrasound offer anatomic and limited physiological assessment of the body. Nuclear medicine maps metabolism and physiology and, when combined with other diagnostic imaging procedures, provides the clinician with the most accurate diagnostic information possible.

Fever of unknown origin, abscess, osteomyelitis, and other inflammatory processes can be difficult to locate or accurately assess. Computed tomography, MRI, and ultrasound offer an anatomic assessment of known areas of infection; however, radionuclides, labeled white cells, and **murine** (from mice) antibodies map the physiology of the infection, thus assisting the clinician in identifying unknown areas of infection.

If left undetected, **cancer,** a broad term used to describe genetic changes that result in the uncontrolled growth and spread of abnormal cells in the body, may become life-threatening and result in death. Cancer is not selective. It attacks all areas of the body and is rarely limited by age, race, or gender. Early diagnosis, accurate staging, effective treatment protocols, and consistent follow-up to detect recurrent disease provide the best possible long-term outcome.[42]

Nuclear medicine plays an important role in the diagnosis and treatment of a selected number of life-threatening cancers. Although positron emission tomography (PET) has taken a leading role in oncology, radionuclides, radiolabeled **antibodies,** and peptides continue to play an important supporting role in the patient's clinical assessment and treatment.

Regardless of the clinician's objective for identifying infection or tumor, optimal diagnostic data can be acquired only by careful patient assessment before imaging. Assessment should include a detailed review of the patient's current clinical and medication history, recent blood chemistry, therapeutic treatments (surgery, radiation therapy, chemotherapy, etc.), and diagnostic imaging procedures with special emphasis for procedures using murine antibodies.

INFLAMMATORY IMAGING

Infections, abscesses, and other inflammatory process are a major concern to the clinician and to the patient. Inflammatory processes have an increased number of neutrophilic granulocytes present as the body attempts to combat the infection. Clinical indications for inflammatory imaging include[47]:

- Fever of unknown origin (FUO)
- Retroperitoneal fibrosis
- Suspected osteomyelitis or diskitis (see Chapter 20)
- Pulmonary and mediastinal inflammation/infection
- Lymphocytic or granulomatous inflammatory processes (e.g., sarcoidosis/tuberculosis)
- Drug-induced pulmonary toxicity
- Acute or chronic inflammation/infection

^{67}Ga-Citrate

There are several radiopharmaceuticals used to image infectious conditions. Gallium-67 (^{67}Ga) citrate, an iron analogue, is absorbed by lysosomes and endoplasmic

---

BOX 22-1	**Inflammatory Imaging ^{67}Gallium**

1. Complete a comprehensive patient assessment, including review of clinical history, current medications, laboratory tests, and recent imaging procedures.
2. Explain imaging procedure, including multiple imaging days, time requirements for each imaging set, and physical requirements (supine position, arm position, etc.) during the imaging procedure.
3. Inject the patient with the appropriate activity and discharge to home with written instructions for imaging days and times, bowel prep (if indicated), and contact information should the patient have additional questions.
4. For the initial imaging sequence, perform a whole body (WB) scan with additional static images or SPECT or SPECT/CT of the area of interest using a medium- or high-energy collimator.
   a. Count rate for the WB images should be in the range of 1 to 2 million counts.
   b. Static images should be acquired for 800,000 to 1 million counts.
   c. SPECT images are acquired at 64 × 64 or 128 × 128 matrix; 360-degree rotation with 3- to 6-degree sampling for 40 to 50 seconds/stop.
   d. Obtain CT images as per manufacturer's protocol.
5. Repeat imaging sequence as directed by the interpreting physician for all subsequent imaging sets.
6. Process the images as per institution's protocol for filtration and display.

---

reticulum of the white blood cells and is attracted by inflammatory leucocytes and low molecular weight molecules of bacteria.[52] From abscesses to osteomyelitis to fevers of unknown origin, ^{67}Ga continues to have a role in diagnosing infections (Box 22-1).

Gallium has 14 known isotopes, ranging in number from 63 to 78. Only ^{67}Ga, ^{68}Ga, and ^{72}Ga have appropriate half-life, emission, and production processes to be useful for clinical nuclear medicine. Gallium-67 was first used in 1965 at the Oak Ridge Institute of Nuclear Studies for bone imaging.[3] Edwards and Hayes[17] began research with ^{67}Ga as a tumor localizer in 1969. Bell and colleagues[6] began reporting on ^{67}Ga in inflammatory processes in 1971.

Gallium-67 is cyclotron produced by proton bombardment of a zinc oxide target: ^{67}Zn (p,n) ^{67}Ga. It has a half-life of 78 hours (3.25 days) and decays by electron capture. It has four principal gamma-ray energies (Table 22-1).[26] The radiation absorbed dose for 5 mCi of ^{67}Ga-citrate is shown in Table 22-2.[5]

Imaging with ^{67}Ga can begin any time from 6 hours to 1 week following injection. The gallium concentration in tissue remains while the target-to-background ratio increases as the blood clearance progresses over time. The actual imaging time is usually determined by weighing the urgency of the patient's condition and the increased scanning time required for significantly delayed images.[45,46]

TABLE 22-1 ⁶⁷Ga Radionuclide Characteristics

Nuclide	Production	Half-Life	Principal Radiations meV	%
⁶⁷Ga	⁶⁷Zn(p,n)⁶⁷Ga	78 hours	0.093	40
	⁶⁸Zn(p,2n)⁶⁷Ga			
			0.184	24
			0.296	22
			0.388	7

From The Bureau of Radiological Health: *Radiological health handbook*, Washington, DC, 1970, U.S. Department of Health, Education, and Welfare.

TABLE 22-2 Radiation Dosimetry for ⁶⁷Ga Citrate

Organ	⁶⁷Ga-Citrate (rad/5 mCi)
Whole body	1.3
Skeleton	2.2
Liver	2.3
Bone marrow	2.9
Spleen	2.65
Kidney	2.05 (calyx)
Ovary	1.4
Testes	1.2
Stomach	1.1
Small intestine	1.8
Upper colon	4.5

From Medical Internal Radiation Dose (MIRD): Dose estimate report no 2, *J Nucl Med* 14:755, 1973.

Initially, rectilinear scanners were used for gallium imaging. The evolution of scintillation cameras with their larger fields of view and multiple pulse height analyzers has significantly improved the resolution and efficacy of gallium imaging. Single photon emission computed tomography (SPECT) or SPECT/CT has further enhanced the potential of gallium studies.

The patient receives 5 to 10 mCi (185 to 370 MBq) of ⁶⁷Ga, and imaging begins after an appropriate delay. Anterior and posterior whole-body images in the 2 million–count range are recommended, along with 1 million count static images and/or SPECT or SPECT/CT imaging as desired (Figure 22-1).

Although medium-energy collimators (rated at a minimum of 300 keV) can be used, high-energy collimators are recommended because of the physical characteristics of the photon emissions. Optimally, the 93-keV and 185-keV or the 93-keV, 185-keV, and 300-keV photopeaks are used. Regardless of whether two or three photopeaks are used, a high-energy collimator is necessary to collimate the higher energies and reduce septal penetration. A symmetrical energy window of 15% to 20% centered over each photopeak is customary.

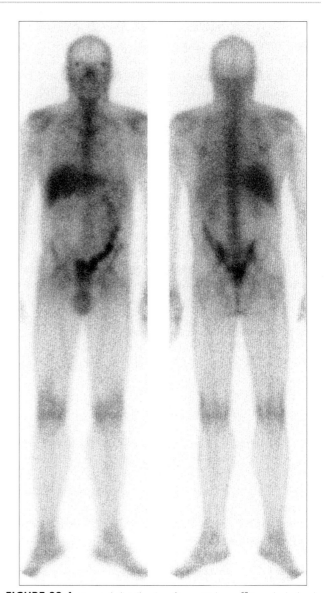

FIGURE 22-1 Normal distribution for a 48-hour ⁶⁷Ga whole-body scan.

Whereas careful attention to imaging is required, careful interpretation is equally important. Excretion of the radionuclide into the bowel can be problematic. In the past, a bowel preparation was recommended. The current belief is that the bowel preparation, which can irritate the colon and increase uptake, is unnecessary, and delayed reimaging is preferable.

¹¹¹In-Oxine–Labeled White Blood Cells

In the early 1970s, Indium-111 (¹¹¹In)-chloride was used to image tumors and abscesses. It had an advantage over ⁶⁷Ga because it did not concentrate in the gastrointestinal (GI) tract, but it was nonetheless inferior. Later in the decade Thakur and associates[70] developed ¹¹¹In-oxine–labeled white blood cells (WBCs) and demonstrated it to be superior to ¹¹¹In-chloride and ⁶⁷Ga. Indium-111 has

TABLE 22-3	¹¹¹In Radionuclide Characteristics		
		Principal Radiations	
Nuclide	**Half-Life**	**keV**	**%**
¹¹¹In	67.4 hours	171	90.0
		247	94.2

TABLE 22-4	Radiation Dosimetry for ¹¹¹In-Labeled White Blood Cells
Organ	**¹¹¹In-Labeled White Blood Cells (rad/mCi)**
Whole body	0.50 to 0.53
Liver	1 to 5
Spleen	18 to 20.4

From Freeman LM, Weissman HS, editors: *Nuclear medicine annual*, New York, 1982, Raven Press; Segal AW: Radiation dosimetry for ¹¹¹In-labeled white blood cells, *Lancet* 2:1056-1058, 1976.

BOX 22-2	Inflammatory Imaging: White Blood Cells

1. Complete a comprehensive patient assessment including review of clinical history, current medications, laboratory tests, and recent imaging procedures.
2. Explain imaging procedure, including blood labeling technique, time requirements for imaging, and physical requirements (supine position, arm position, etc.) during the imaging procedure.
3. Blood labeling may be performed by a local radiopharmacy or in-house.
4. Withdraw a minimum of 50 ml of blood using a large bore needle (18 to 20 gauge).
5. Label blood sample and complete appropriate paperwork before sending to radiopharmacy or labeling in-house.
6. If labeling product in-house, follow the approved protocol for labeling ¹¹¹In-oxine or ⁹⁹ᵐTc-HMPAO.
7. Correctly identify the patient before reinjecting the labeled blood product using a large bore needle (18 to 20 gauge, if possible).
8. At the appropriate time interval, ask the patient to void and remove any articles of clothing or metal objects that may cause attenuation artifacts on the images.
9. Perform an initial whole-body and/or static image protocol followed by a SPECT or SPECT/CT of the selected area. *Note:* Imaging parameters depend on radiopharmaceutical used for labeling.
10. Perform the delayed imaging protocol as per the interpreting physician's request. *Note:* The delayed protocol may include additional static and SPECT or SPECT/CT images, as requested.
11. Process the SPECT or SPECT/CT images as per institution protocol.

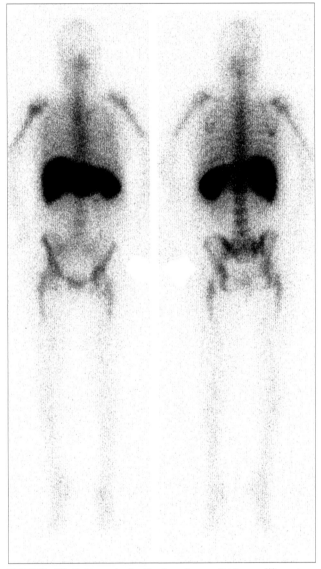

FIGURE 22-2 Normal distribution for a 24-hour ¹¹¹In-oxine–labeled white blood cell whole-body scan.

a physical half-life of 67.4 hours (2.8 days) and it decays by electron capture, producing two gamma photons (Table 22-3 and Box 22-2).[46]

The radiation absorbed dose per millicurie (dependent on the number of red cells present) is shown in Table 22-4.[19]

Imaging can be performed from 3 to 24 hours following an injection of 500 to 600 µCi (18.5 to 22.2 MBq) ¹¹¹In-WBCs. Early imaging will demonstrate some retention of the labeled WBCs in the lungs, which will clear after several hours[46] (Figure 22-2).

Anterior and posterior whole-body images and selected static images are acquired after an appropriate time interval with medium-energy collimators and a symmetrical 20% window centered on each gamma photopeak.

The drawback for ¹¹¹In-WBCs is that it requires a large volume of blood (50 ml) to be withdrawn from the patient and a 2- to 3-hour labeling procedure. The

TABLE 22-5	Radiation Dosimetry for ^{99m}Tc Leukocytes		
Radiopharmaceutical	Administered Activity MBq (mCi)	Organ Receiving the Largest Radiation Dose mGy/MBq (rad/mCi)	Effective Dose mSv/MBq (rem/mCi)
Radiation Dosimetry: Adults			
^{99m}Tc-exametazime (HMPAO) leukocytes	185 to 370 IV (5 to 10)	0.15 Spleen (0.56)	0.017 (0.063)
Radiation Dosimetry: Children (5 Years Old)			
^{99m}Tc-exametazime (HMPAO) leukocytes	3.7 IV (0.1 to 0.2)	0.48 Spleen (1.8)	0.054 (0.020)

From Palestro CJ, Brown ML, Forestrom LA, et al: *Society of nuclear medicine procedure guideline for 99mTc-exametazime (HMPAO)-labeled leukocyte scintigraphy for suspected infection/inflammation,* version 3.0, June 2, 2004 (publication available online): http://interactive.snm.org/docs/HMPAO_v3.pdf. Accessed August 16, 2010.
IV, Intravenous.

reward is that the ^{111}In study has a specificity of 97%, whereas the ^{67}Ga study has a specificity of 64%.[22] Unfortunately, the ^{111}In-WBCs study has significantly lower counting statistics compared to ^{67}Ga and does not lend itself to delayed imaging much beyond 24 hours.

The longer half-life and high-energy photons of ^{67}Ga and the labeling procedure and poor counting statistics of ^{111}In have always detracted from their usefulness. In recent years, there has been increasing interest in the development of ^{99m}Tc agents for infection imaging.

^{99m}Tc Exametazime (Ceretec)

Technetium-99m (^{99m}Tc)-exametazime (Ceretec), initially known as hexamethylpropylene amine oxine (HMPAO), was originally developed for regional cerebral blood flow scintigraphy. The compound received approval by the U.S. Food and Drug Administration (FDA) in 1988.

In 1990, ^{99m}Tc-exametazime–labeled leukocytes began to be used for suspected sites of acute inflammation/infection in patients with fevers, abdominal pain, or positive blood cultures. As with ^{111}In-WBC labeling, ^{99m}Tc-exametazime requires the withdrawal of 40 to 50 ml of the patient's blood. The adult administered dose is 7 to 25 mCi (259 to 925 MBq).

The estimated absorbed radiation dose for a 10-mCi injection of ^{99m}Tc-leukocytes is shown in Table 22-5.[28]

Anterior and posterior whole-body images are acquired after a delay of 4 to 24 hours. A high-resolution, low-energy collimator is recommended; however, the low count rate on delayed images may benefit from the use of a low-energy, all-purpose collimator. Additional static images and SPECT or SPECT/CT imaging can be helpful.[47]

^{99m}Tc-Fanolesomab (NeutroSpec)

In July 2004 the FDA approved ^{99m}Tc-fanolesomab (NeutroSpec) for imaging patients (age 5 years or older) with equivocal signs and symptoms of appendicitis. Technetium-99m-fanolesomab is an anti-CD15 monoclonal antibody that selectively binds to neutrophils in vivo. The average adult dose is 10 to 20 mCi (370 to 740 MBq). Imaging is performed 2 to 4 hours following injection. One million–count images of the abdomen with a high-resolution collimator is the sole requirement (Figure 22-3); however, SPECT or SPECT/CT may further enhance the diagnostic quality of the images.

In late December, 2005, NeutroSpec was voluntarily removed from the market as the result of several adverse events associated with the off-label use of the monoclonal antibody; however, follow-up clinical trials were performed and submitted to the FDA for re-approval of the product. The outcome of that submission is pending at the time of this writing.

TUMOR IMAGING

For many years, ^{67}Ga was nuclear medicine's cornerstone in tumor imaging. It was used to diagnose lung tumors, mediastinal involvement, and the presence or extent of lymphoma and other tumors. It was also used to evaluate response to therapy. All of these roles have, for the most part, been replaced by other radiopharmaceuticals or diagnostic imaging modalities.[5]

The use of receptor-specific radiolabeled monoclonal antibodies and their fragments has gained wide acceptance in the detection and treatment of selected tumors including colorectal, lung, prostate, **non-Hodgkin lymphoma (NHL)**, and others.[25] Antibodies are immunoglobulins produced by B lymphocytes or plasma cells in response to an antigen (foreign substance). The successful targeting of a radiolabeled antibody relies, in part, on its affinity to the antigens expressed by the cells. Today, commercially available radiolabeled antibodies successfully localize disease with sensitivities and specificities equal to, or at times exceeding, those of standard diagnostic imaging procedures.

Parathyroid

Primary hyperparathyroidism is a relatively common disease. The Endocrine and Metabolic Diseases Information Service of the National Institutes of Health (NIH) estimated that 100,000 people will be diagnosed in 2009. The number of women diagnosed each year outnumbers men two to one and the risk increases with age. Approximately 2 in 1000 women over the age of 60 will be diagnosed with hyperparathyroidism each year.[27] The suspicion of a parathyroid adenoma is usually based on findings of persistently elevated serum calcium and parathyroid hormone (PTH) levels. Because these glands are not palpable and not easily imaged by other modalities, radionuclide imaging plays an important role in their diagnosis and surgical intervention.

Initially, parathyroid imaging was performed with a dual-phase, dual-isotope study utilizing thallium-201 (^{201}Tl)–thallous chloride and ^{99m}Tc-pertechnetate. In 1992, Taillefer and colleagues[68] reported on their dual-phase study with ^{99m}Tc-sestamibi, and this technique has become the standard imaging protocol. (Technetium-99m-sestamibi is [99m]Tc-[MIBI]$_6$ where MIBI is 2-methoxy isobutyl isonitril and marketed as Cardiolite.)

The average adult dose of ^{99m}Tc-sestamibi is 20 mCi (740 MBq). The estimated radiation absorbed dosimetry is illustrated in Table 22-6.

Whereas a flow study can be acquired immediately after injection, the first (or thyroid) phase of imaging should begin 15 to 20 minutes postinjection. The second (or parathyroid) phase is performed 2 hours postinjection.

There is some controversy over whether to use pinhole or parallel-hole collimators; nonetheless, high-resolution images of the neck and mediastinum are acquired at early and late time intervals. SPECT and SPECT/CT imaging may improve sensitivity and anatomic location of suspected abnormalities.

The net retention of the ^{99m}Tc-sestamibi in the thyroid gland decreases more rapidly than in the parathyroid adenoma over time. A positive study for the presence of a parathyroid adenoma is defined as a focal area of increased uptake in the thyroid bed and surrounding areas that demonstrates a progressive intensity over time or a fixed uptake that persists as the normal thyroid activity decreases (Figure 22-4).

Prostate Cancer

Prostate cancer is the second leading cause of cancer death in men. The American Cancer Society estimates

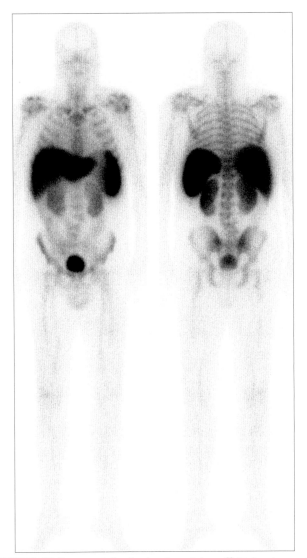

FIGURE 22-3 Normal distribution for a 3-hour ^{99m}Tc-fanolesomab whole-body scan.

TABLE 22-6	Radiation Dosimetry for ^{99m}Tc-Sestamibi		
Radiopharmaceutical	Administered Activity MBq (mCi)	Organ Receiving the Largest Radiation Dose mGy/MBq (rad/mCi)	Effective Dose mSv/MBq (rem/mCi)
[99m]Tc-sestamibi	185 to 925 IV (5 to 25)	0.039 Gallbladder 0.014	0.0085 (0.031)

From Palestro CJ, Brown ML, Forestrom LA, et al: *Society of nuclear medicine procedure guideline for 99mTc-exametazime (HMPAO)-labeled leukocyte scintigraphy for suspected infection/inflammation,* version 3.0, June 2, 2004 (publication available online): http://interactive.snm.org/docs/HMPAO_v3.pdf. Accessed August 16, 2010.

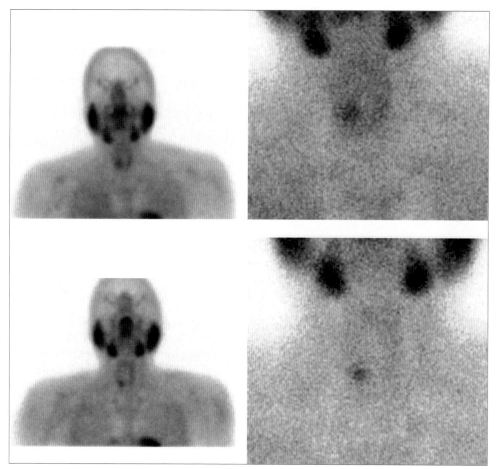

FIGURE 22-4 Abnormal parathyroid scan demonstrating a focal area of activity on the delayed images overlying the right lobe of the thyroid gland consistent with a parathyroid adenoma.

that one in six men will be diagnosed with prostate cancer in 2009 and 1 in 34 will die of the disease. Early detection, enhanced treatment options, and improved accuracy in diagnosis and follow-up have slowed the mortality rate of this disease.[9] Indium-111–capromab pendetide (ProstaScint) is a monoclonal antibody used in the diagnostic assessment and clinical management of prostate cancer.

Indium-111–capromab pendetide is an IgG1 **murine monoclonal antibody (mab)** directed toward prostate-specific membrane antigen (PSMA), a glycoprotein expressed by prostate epithelium. It is nonreactive with serum markers for prostate cancer including prostate-specific antigens (PSA).[25,74]

Clinical indications for imaging include newly diagnosed patients with biopsy-proven prostate cancer being considered for definitive therapy (surgery or radiation) that may be at risk for lymph node metastasis or for posttreatment patients with a rising PSA and negative or equivocal metastatic workup including CT, MRI, and bone scan.[16,25,29]

The procedure is performed over 96 to 120 hours. Day one begins with an injection of 5 mCi (185 MBq)

[111]In–capromab pendetide infused over 3 to 5 minutes. The effective dose equivalent for a 5-mCi (185 MBq) dose is 50 mSv; the critical organ is the liver.

Although reported hypersensitivity to the monoclonal antibody is small, adverse reactions including hypotension, hypertension, flulike symptoms, and changes in blood chemistries have been reported. A slow infusion may help to minimize possible adverse events.

Patient preparation should include a laxative 24 hours before imaging and an enema on the morning of the procedure. Additionally, an indwelling urinary catheter inserted before imaging will minimize urine activity in the pelvic region. Bladder irrigation may also improve visualization of the pelvic region including the prostate fossa.

To improve the accuracy of interpretation, blood pool activity should be mapped or an anatomical localization of the area of interest should be created using a SPECT/CT protocol. Blood pool activity can be imaged 30 minutes to 4 hours following the ^{111}In–capromab pendetide injection or using a dual-isotope technique on the day of imaging. A dual-isotope technique with 20 mCi (740 MBq) ^{99m}Tc-labeled red blood cells (RBCs) and

[111]In–capromab pendetide ensures accurate registration of image sets and improved lesion detection with subtraction analysis.

For optimal targeting and minimal blood pool activity, imaging should be performed at 96 to 120 hours postinjection. Imaging is performed with a medium-energy collimator and a symmetrical 15% to 20% energy window centered over the 140-keV photopeak for ^{99m}Tc and the 171- and 245-keV photopeaks for [111]In. Whole-body or 800,000 to 1 million planar anterior/posterior images from the top of the head to midcalf are acquired followed by SPECT or SPECT/CT imaging of the abdomen and pelvis. Recommended SPECT acquisition parameters for a multidetector camera system include a 128 × 128 matrix, 360-degree rotation, 3-degree sampling, and a 50- to 60-second acquisition time/stop. Image reconstruction should be approximately 1-cm slice thickness with appropriate filtering to adequately reconstruct the low-count images.[70] The CT protocol should be per manufacturer's recommendations for kVp, mA, slice thickness, and so on, to optimize final image quality.

Normal distribution of the radionuclide (Figure 22-5) is liver, spleen, bone marrow, and genitalia.

Colorectal Cancer

Colorectal cancer is the third leading cause of cancer death in both men and women and when the statistics for the male and female population are combined, colorectal cancer becomes the second leading cause of cancer death in the United States. Although colorectal cancer has demonstrated a decline over the past 20 years, the American Cancer Society estimates that approximately 146,970 new cases of colorectal cancer will be diagnosed in 2009 and an estimated 49,920 will die of the disease in the same year. The continued decline in diagnosed cases is due in part to increased awareness, improved nutritional habits, appropriate screening, and early removal of polyps. The continued decline in mortality is due to early detection and improved treatment options.[9] Technetium-99m-arcitumomab (CEA-Scan) is used in the diagnostic evaluation of recurrent or metastatic colorectal cancer.

Technetium-99m-arcitumomab is **antibody fragment (Fab)** generated from IMMU-4, a murine IgG1 monoclonal antibody. IMMU-4 reacts with carcinoembryonic antigen (CEA), a tumor-associated antigen expressed on a variety of carcinomas including those found in the gastrointestinal tract.[10,25]

Clinical indications for CEA-Scan are detection of the presence, location, and extent of recurrent or metastatic colorectal carcinoma involving the liver, extrahepatic abdomen, and pelvis in patients with histologically confirmed diagnosis of colorectal carcinoma. Additionally, CEA-Scan may be useful in evaluating patients with no evidence of disease by standard diagnostic screening but

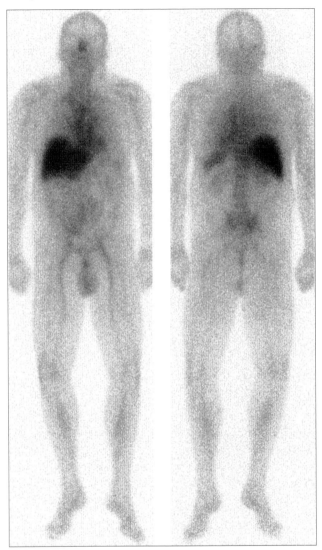

FIGURE 22-5 Normal distribution for a 96-hour ^{111}In–capromab pendetide (ProstaScint) whole-body scan.

with a rising serum CEA or documented recurrent disease.[10]

Patient preparation should include adequate hydration before injection. Imaging is performed with a low-energy, high-resolution collimator or a low-energy, all-purpose collimator and a symmetrical 15% to 20% energy window centered on the 140-keV peak of [99m]Tc. Anterior/posterior 800,000 to 1 million planar or whole-body images of the chest, abdomen, and pelvis are acquired 2 to 5 hours following an injection of 20 to 30 mCi (740 to 1110 MBq) of ^{99m}Tc-arcitumomab, followed by SPECT or SPECT/CT imaging of the chest, abdomen, and pelvis. The effective dose equivalent for a 20- to 30-mCi (740 to 1110 MBq) dose is 13.1 µSv/MBq; the critical organ is the kidney.

Recommended SPECT parameters for a multidetector camera system are 64 × 64 or 128 × 128 matrix, 360-degree rotation, 3- to 6-degree sampling, and 30- to 45-second acquisition time/stop. For optimal results, the

SPECT/CT protocol should be per manufacturer's recommendations including mA, keV and slice thickness. To minimize blood pool activity, the optimal imaging time is 4 to 5 hours postinjection. Insertion of a urinary catheter may be indicated for patients unable to empty their bladder. Additionally, to minimize contamination artifacts, it is recommended that colostomy bags be changed before imaging.[65,75]

Normal distribution of ^{99m}Tc-arcitumomab includes blood pool (heart, lungs, major blood vessels), liver, spleen, kidneys, intestine, and bladder.[10]

Neuroendocrine Tumors

Somatostatin is a naturally occurring neuropeptide that possesses a wide range of pharmacological properties including inhibition of growth hormone release and suppression of insulin and glucagon secretion. Somatostatin receptors are found in endocrine cells throughout the body and in numerous endocrine tumors. Indium-111-pentetreotide (OctreoScan) is used to visualize primary neuroendocrine tumors and neuroendocrine metastasis.[11,20,62]

Indium-111-pentetreotide is a radiolabeled analog of somatostatin. It is a conjugate of octreotide, a somatostatin analog that binds to somatostatin receptors found in neuroendocrine and some nonneuorendocrine tumors with somatostatin receptors. Numerous tumors carrying somatostatin receptors may be imaged including adrenal medullary tumors, gastroenteropancreatic tumors, carcinoid tumors, pituitary adenomas, paragangliomas, small cell lung carcinoma, and medullary thyroid carcinomas.[4,36,44]

Patient preparation should include adequate hydration before injection and for 24 hours following injection. A mild laxative is recommended the evening before injection and the evening following injection. Additionally, for insulinoma patients, an intravenous (IV) solution containing glucose should be administered before and during ^{111}In-pentetreotide administration to avoid severe hypoglycemia. The recommended activity for ^{111}In-pentetreotide is 6 mCi (222 MBq) for an adult and 0.14 mCi/kg (5 MBq/kg) for children. The effective dose equivalent for a 6-mCi (222 MBq) dose is 26.06 mSv/222 MBq; critical organs are spleen, kidney, and urinary bladder wall.

Because ^{111}In-pentetreotide is eliminated primarily by the genitourinary system, patients should void before whole-body imaging and again before the acquisition of planar and SPECT images of the pelvis. Images are acquired at 4, 24, and 48 hours. Imaging is performed with a medium-energy collimator and a symmetrical 15% to 20% energy window centered over the 171- and 245-keV photopeaks for [111]In. Whole-body or 800,000 to 1 million planar anterior/posterior images are acquired at 4 hours and anterior/posterior whole-body and/or planar images in addition to SPECT or SPECT/CT

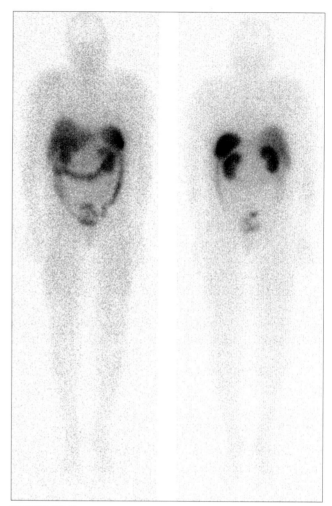

FIGURE 22-6 Normal distribution for a 24-hour ^{111}In-pentetreotide (OctreoScan) whole-body scan.

images of the relevant clinical site are acquired at 24 and 48 hours. Delayed SPECT or SPECT/CT images may be compared with earlier images to differentiate bowel activity from underlying disease. Recommended SPECT acquisition parameters for a multidetector camera system are 128 × 128 matrix, 360-degree rotation, 3-degree sampling, and a 30- to 45-second acquisition time/stop.[4] Recommended SPECT/CT acquisition parameters are per manufacturer's recommendation for an optimal diagnostic or attenuation correction image.

The normal distribution for ^{111}In-pentetreotide includes pituitary, thyroid, liver, spleen, kidneys, bowel, gallbladder, ureters, bladder, and stimulated adrenal glands (Figure 22-6).[44]

Pheochromocytoma and Neuroblastoma

Pheochromocytomas are catecholamine-secreting tumors from the pheochromocytes of the adrenal medulla. Although the incidence rate of pheochromocytomas is unknown, approximately 0.01% to 0.5% of hypertensive patients are estimated to have the unusual tumor

TABLE 22-7	Physical Properties Data for ^{131}I and ^{123}I			
Radionuclide (Half-Life)	Decay Constant	Mode of Decay	Principal Emissions (keV)	Mean Number of Emissions per Disintegration
^{123}I (13.2 hours)	0.0533 hr^{-1}	Electron capture	Gamma (159)	0.83
^{131}I (8.08 days)	0.00358 hr^{-1}	Beta	Beta (191.6)	0.90
			Gamma (364.5)	0.81

From Palestro CJ, Brown ML, Forestrom LA, et al: *Society of nuclear medicine procedure guideline for 99mTc-exametazime (HMPAO)-labeled leukocyte scintigraphy for suspected infection/inflammation,* version 3.0, June 2, 2004 (publication available online): http://interactive.snm.org/docs/HMPAO_v3.pdf. Accessed August 16, 2010.

that in many cases is not diagnosed during the patient's lifetime. Hypertension is the primary clinical symptom of pheochromocytoma. Approximately 90% of the lesions are benign and have been found anywhere from the base of the skull to the pelvic floor.

Neuroblastomas are malignant tumors of the sympathetic nervous system and are found most often in infants and children (<10 years). Most neuroblastomas (approximately two thirds) originate in the adrenal glands or sympathetic nervous system ganglia of the abdomen. The remaining one third are found in the chest, neck, pelvis, or spinal cord. Neuroblastomas are the most common cancer in infants and the fourth most common cancer in children, with an estimated 650 new cases diagnosed each year.[9,67]

Iobenguane or meta-iodobenzylguanidine (MIBG) is an analog of norepinephrine and is taken up by the adrenergic nervous system of tissues that are derived from the neural crest. Iodine-131 (^{131}I)- or iodine-123 (^{123}I)-labeled iobenguane sulfate (AdreView)[1] has been shown to be effective in the localization of primary or metastatic pheochromocytomas and neuroblastomas.[39,40] The physical properties of ^{123}I and ^{131}I are described in Table 22-7.

Patients should be screened for medications that are contraindicated for MIBG imaging, including cocaine, calcium channel blockers, adrenergic blockers, some foods, selected cold preparations and decongestants, antipsychotics, catecholamine agonists, and reserpine. Additionally, patient preparation should include a thyroid blocking agent 24 hours before injection and continued for 5 to 6 days following injection to block thyroid uptake of free iodine.[73]

In adults, the recommended patient dose is 0.5 to 1.0 mCi ^{131}I-MIBG or 10 mCi ^{123}I–iobenguane sulfate. In children, the imaging dose is physician directed with a minimum recommended activity for ^{131}I-MIBG of 0.135 mCi.[56] The effective dose equivalent for ^{123}I-MIBG based on age and weight ranges from 13.7-162 μSv/MBq.[1] The effective dose equivalent for ^{131}I MIBG is 0.20 mSv/MBq; critical organs are the bladder wall and liver.

Imaging is performed with a high-energy collimator and a symmetrical 15% to 20% energy window centered over the 364-keV photopeak for ^{131}I or a low-energy, high-resolution or general-purpose collimator and a symmetrical 15% to 20% energy window centered over the 159-keV photopeak for ^{123}I. Anterior/posterior planar images of the head, chest, abdomen, and pelvis are acquired on days 1 and 3 for ^{131}I-MIBG and at 6 and 24 hours for ^{123}I-MIBG. SPECT or SPECT/CT images are recommended at 24 hours for ^{123}I-MIBG (Figure 22-7). Recommended SPECT acquisition parameters for a multidetector camera system consist of a 64 × 64 matrix, 360-degree rotation, 3- to 6-degree sampling, and 30- to 45-seconds/stop.[21,41,51] Recommended CT acquisition parameters are per manufacturer's guidelines for diagnostic or attenuation correction images.

The normal distribution of MIBG includes the salivary glands, nasopharynx, heart, liver, spleen, and urinary bladder. Bowel activity is observed in 20% of patient studies (Figure 22-8).

Breast Cancer

Breast cancer is the second leading cause of cancer death in women. Approximately 209,060 new breast cancers will be diagnosed in 2010 and an estimated 40,230 will die of the disease in the same year. The American Cancer Society predicts that women living in the United States have a 12% risk factor, or a 1 in 8 lifetime risk of developing breast cancer.[9]

Mammography remains the most widely used imaging method for breast cancer screening with a sensitivity of approximately 85%; however, in dense breasts, the sensitivity of mammography decreases to 68%. Breast biopsies to examine abnormalities found on mammography identify malignancies in 15% to 30% of the cases sampled. Technetium-99m-sestamibi (Miraluma) provides the clinician with an additional diagnostic tool to assess breast abnormalities in dense breast tissue or in patients with equivocal mammography findings.[8,31-33,72]

Technetium-99m-sestamibi is a cationic ^{99m}Tc complex that accumulates in viable myocardial tissue. The mechanism of localization in malignant, inflamed, benign, or fibrous tissue has not been established; however, the increased blood flow and metabolic rate of the neoplastic cells are most likely the primary contributing factors.[32]

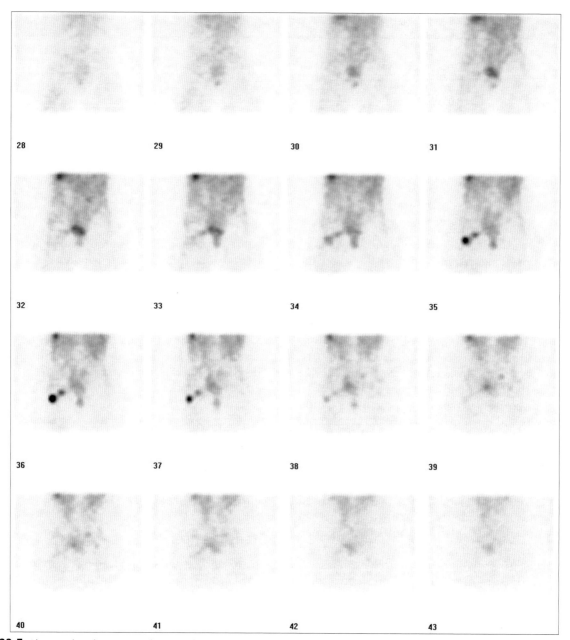

FIGURE 22-7 Abnormal 24-hour coronal SPECT abdomen/pelvis demonstrating increased ^{123}I-MIBG activity in the right femoral head, neck, and right femoral trochanteric region, as well as the left posterior medial iliac bone, suggestive of bone metastasis.

No special preparation is required for the examination; however, breast scintigraphy should be delayed 2 weeks following a fine needle aspiration and 4 to 6 weeks following a core biopsy. Imaging begins 10 minutes following the administration of 20 to 30 mCi (740 to 1110 MBq) of ^{99m}Tc-sestamibi. The effective dose equivalent for a 20- to 30-mCi dose is 0.0085 mSv/MBq; the critical organ is the gallbladder.

The radionuclide should be administered in the contralateral arm followed by a 10 ml 0.9% saline flush. If bilateral disease is suspected, the injection should be administered in a foot vein. Planar anterior and lateral images of each breast are acquired for 10 minutes each using a high-resolution collimator and a symmetrical 10% energy window centered over the 140-keV photopeak. The anterior chest image may be performed with the patient in the upright or supine position with the arms extended above the head. The image should include both breasts and both axilla in the field of view. Prone lateral images are acquired with the patient's arms extended to expose the axilla and a breast-positioning device that allows the imaged breast to hang freely. The contralateral breast should be compressed against the table to minimize cross talk in the image. The field of view should include the breast, axilla, and anterior wall of the chest and should exclude any internal organ activity. For optimal resolution, the detector should be positioned as closely to the patient's side as possible.

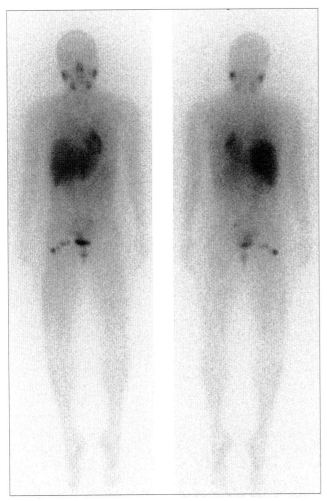

FIGURE 22-8 A 24-hour ^{123}I-MIBG whole-body scan demonstrating normal distribution of the radionuclide, as well as increased activity in the right femoral head, neck, and trochanteric region.

Additional oblique images and images with markers to identify palpable lesions may help in the final interpretation of the study; however, the markers should not be placed until after the patient is placed in the prone position. SPECT imaging, imaging with multidetector systems to allow simultaneous acquisition of prone lateral images, and imaging with high-resolution breast-specific gamma camera (HRBGC) systems are being used in a number of clinical settings; however, no consensus within the imaging community has been reached regarding the added utility of these imaging techniques.[8,13,32]

The normal distribution of ^{99m}Tc-sestamibi is the salivary and thyroid glands, myocardium, gallbladder, liver, intestines, muscle, kidneys, and bladder.[32]

Lung Cancer

Lung cancer is the primary cause of cancer-related deaths in both men and women in the United States. Approximately 225,520 new cases of lung cancer will be diagnosed in 2010 with an estimated 157,300 dying of the disease in the same year. The incidence of lung cancer

and mortality has steadily declined over the past decade as the result of decreased smoking rates, early detection when surgical intervention offers the best option for survival, and improved chemotherapeutic protocols.[9] Technetium-99m-depreotide injection (NeoTect) offers the clinician an additional diagnostic tool to assess pulmonary lesions found on CT, chest x-ray, or both.

Technetium-99m-depreotide is a 10–amino acid synthetic peptide that contains a somatostatin receptor (SSTR) binding domain that has demonstrated a high affinity for SSTR-expressing tumors. Somatostatin receptors are expressed on normal tissues and overexpressed on many malignant tumors as well as some inflammatory processes. The overexpression of SSRT has been clinically demonstrated on most neuroendocrine tumors including small cell lung carcinoma.

Technetium-99m-depreotide is indicated for the identification of SSTR-bearing pulmonary masses in patients with pulmonary lesions on CT and/or chest radiograph who have known malignancy or who are highly suspect for malignancy.[43]

Patient preparation includes hydration before and following injection and instructions to void frequently for the first few hours following injection.

SPECT or SPECT/CT images of the entire lung fields are acquired 2 to 4 hours following the intravenous administration of 15 to 20 mCi (555 to 740 MBq) of ^{99m}Tc-depreotide. Technetium-99m-depreotide should not be administered with total parenteral solutions or through intravenous lines that have administered total parenteral solutions.[65] The patient's arms should be extended above the head and immobilized to ensure minimal motion during imaging. Images are acquired with a low-energy, high-resolution collimator or a low-energy, general-purpose collimator and a symmetrical 15% to 20% energy window centered over the 140-keV photopeak. SPECT acquisition parameters for a multidetector camera system consist of a 128 × 128 matrix, 360-degree rotation, 3-degree sampling, and a 30- to 40-minute acquisition time/stop. Optional 800,000 to 1 million anterior/posterior planar images may be acquired, as needed.[43] For optimal results, the CT acquisition parameters should be per manufacturer's recommendations.

Normal distribution of the radionuclide includes the kidneys, liver, spleen, and bone marrow.

LYMPHOSCINTIGRAPHY

Elective lymph node dissection (ELND) or axillary lymph node dissection (ALND) does not improve the prognosis for patients diagnosed with melanoma, squamous cell carcinoma of the head and neck, vulvar and penile malignancies, or breast cancer; however, histological sampling and examination of lymph tissue for tumor cell migration is considered to be the gold standard for staging a patient with a confirmed diagnosis of one of these malignancies.[2,15,38] Post-operative complications and morbidity associated with the removal of 10 to 30 lymph nodes for ELND or ALND includes seroma, infection, pain, paresthesias, and severe lymphoedema. Lymphoscintigraphy is an imaging technique that, when combined with an interoperative gamma probe and/or blue dye technique during the surgical procedure, offers an alternative to ELND or ALND. The first, or sentinel, lymph nodes that receive lymphatic drainage from the tumor site represent the primary site for metastasis. The ability of the surgeon to accurately identify and remove only the sentinel lymph nodes for physical and histological examination can reduce post-operative complications as well as improve the accuracy of sampling errors associated with blind dissection of the entire lymphatic bed. ELND and ALND continues to be performed when sentinel lymph nodes are not found or when physical examination at the time of surgery is suggestive for disease.[15,18,38] Lymphoscintigraphy is most often performed for patients diagnosed with melanoma and breast cancer and will be discussed here.

Melanoma

Staging of melanoma tumors is based on the thickness of the tumor, the level of the skin invasion, and lymphatic involvement of lymph nodes draining from the tumor site. ELND has been described as a controversial staging technique for those patients with early or intermediate-stage melanoma without clinical evidence of metastasis because of the unpredictability of lymphatic drainage and the associated cost and morbidity of the procedure. Lymphoscintigraphy, when combined with an interoperative gamma probe and/or blue dye technique, pinpoints sentinel lymph nodes as well as provides the surgeon with a visual representation of the lymphatic pathway during surgery.[2,18,50]

No specific patient preparation is required for the imaging procedure; however, in most cases, patients scheduled for same day surgery will follow the instructions provided by the surgical department.

The U.S. Food and Drug Administration (FDA) has not approved a radiopharmaceutical for lymphoscintigraphy studies performed in the United States; however, Tc-99m sulfur colloid is most often used for this procedure. Although unfiltered sulfur colloid has been used, smaller particle size has been shown to more readily visualize the lymphatic channel; thus sulfur colloid filtered through a 0.22-mm filter is most often used. Outside of the United States, other commercially available radiopharmaceuticals used for lymphoscintigraphy include Tc-99m antimony trisulfide colloid (particle size 0.015-0.3 μm), Tc-99m rhenium colloid (50-100 μm), and Tc-99m human serum albumin nanocolloid (particle size 0.05-0.8 μm).[2,50]

Depending on the location of the lesion or biopsy site, one to eight (1-8) intradermal peritumoral injections are administered as closely as possible to the lesion or biopsy scar. Each injection should contain at least 3.7 MBq (100 μCi) in a volume of approximately 0.1 ml. The appropriate number and location of injections is determined by the site and size of disease as well as the possibility of the injection masking a sentinel node that may be in close proximity to the primary lesion (for example, head and neck lesions where inferior injections may obscure the sentinel lymph node).[2,50]

The Society of Nuclear Medicine's Procedure Guidelines for this procedure specify a high resolution or general purpose collimator with a symmetrical 10% to 20% energy window centered over the 140 keV photopeak to perform planar dynamic or sequential static imaging immediately post injection and continuing for 30 to 60 minutes. Dynamic images are acquired at 30 seconds per frame for 2 to 30 minutes. Static sequential images are acquired every 5 minutes for 60 minutes or until the sentinel lymph node is identified. The site of the lesion will define the required patient position. When the lesion is located in the trunk region, bilateral anterior/posterior axillary and inguinal regions must be imaged with additional oblique and/or lateral images acquired, as necessary, to separate overlapping injection sites from sentinel lymph nodes. Head and neck lesions also require anterior/posterior as well as oblique and/or lateral images to accurately separate overlapping activity. If the lesion is located on an extremity, images should include the knee or elbow. SPECT or SPECT/CT images have also been successfully used when the tumor is located in areas of the body where lymphatic drainage is unpredictable.[18] Transmission images using a Co-57 flood source placed with the patient between the camera and the source helps to define the patient's body contour to facilitate a more accurate interpretation of the acquired images. An alternative to transmission imaging is the use a radioactive source to trace the patient's outline during the static image, which will define the patient's body contour and help to clarify the anatomical location of the injection site and sentinel lymph nodes.[2]

Skin marking is performed using either the gamma probe or a radioactive source marker to locate the sentinel lymph node. In most cases, the skin is marked in two planes (for example, anterior and lateral) or as the patient might be positioned during the surgical procedure. Skin markings should be confirmed with static planar images to support accurate placement for the interpreting physician and surgeon.

The normal distribution of the radiopharmaceutical will include the injection site, lymphatic channel and the sentinel and secondary lymph nodes.[2]

Breast

Staging of breast cancer relies on the TNM system which includes the size of the tumor (T), the nodal status (N), and distant metastasis (M). Nodal status is reported to be the most important factor used to define the patient's 5 to 10 year survival rate.[15]

Based on overwhelming data for success rate, sensitivity and accuracy, sentinel lymph node biopsy has successfully replaced ALND in most clinical sites. Clinical studies over the past decade have demonstrated that histological examination of the sentinel lymph node is superior when compared to the histological examination of lymph nodes from ALND in patients with small invasive breast cancer and clinically negative lymph nodes.[37]

Patient preparation is not required for the imaging procedure; however, the patient must follow the preoperative instructions provided by the surgical department.[37,38]

A universally accepted technique for breast lymphoscintigraphy has yet to be determined. There continues to be significant diversity in radiopharmaceutical attributes, volume, and injection techniques.[37] Additionally, the usefulness of patient images versus identification of the radioactive sentinel node using the blue dye technique and/or an interoperative gamma probe continues to be controversial.

Because the FDA has not approved a radiopharmaceutical for lymphoscintigraphy, sulfur colloid remains the only commercially available radionuclide in the United States that meets the particle size criteria for the procedure. Consensus on the use of filtered versus unfiltered sulfur colloid has yet to be resolved. Outside of the United States, Tc-99m sulfur colloid (filtered and unfiltered), Tc-99m human serum albumin nanocolloid, and Tc-99m antimony sulfur colloid are routinely used.

Injection techniques are also site dependent. Lymphatic drainage from a breast cancer is variable; however, drainage from the mammary gland as well as overlying skin is described as a single biological unit.[38] Successful injection techniques described in the literature include intratumoral, interdermal, subdermal, periareolar, subtumoral, subareolar, peritumoral, and intraparenchymal. Intratumoral and subtumoral are seldom used in today's practice; however areolar/periareolar injections are gaining in popularity over peritumoral injections.[15,34]

There is significant diversity of practice for the number of injections, as well as volume and depth of injection. For every article that cites improved success with high volume injections, there are an equal number describing the benefits of low volume injections. The same is true for depth of injection, location of injection, and the number of injections. Total volume of activity ranges from 2 ml to 8 ml. The total number of injections ranges from 1 to 4. The total injected activity ranges from approximately 7 to 185 MBq (190 µCi-5 mCi). Breast massage for 2 to 5 minutes post injection can improve overall circulation and transit time.[34,35,38,77]

Although 2-day imaging protocols have been reported, most clinical sites use a same-day protocol as the surgical procedure. Images post injection are most often acquired using a high resolution collimator and a 15% to 20%

symmetrical window centered over the 140 keV gamma peak. Static sequential images begin immediately post injection and are acquired at 5 to 10 minute intervals until the sentinel lymph node is identified. Patient images are most often acquired in the anterior and/or oblique position to separate the injection sites from the sentinel lymph node. SPECT or SPECT/CT may be useful techniques to separate overlying activity.[18] The use of transmission scanning or body contour marking can assist the interpreting physician and surgeon with location of the sentinel lymph node. Based on the surgeon's preference, skin marking may be performed or optional. If skin markings are made, they should be verified with static planar images.

The normal distribution of the radiopharmaceutical includes the injection site, lymphatic channel and the sentinel and secondary lymph nodes.[2]

THERAPY

Radioimmunotherapy

Radioimmunotherapy combines the killing efficiency of radiation with a monoclonal antibody engineered to target specific proteins expressed by a tumor cell. The monoclonal antibody is designed to activate the patient's own macrophages and monocytes (killer cells) to attack and destroy cancer cells that it binds. Adding a beta-emitting radionuclide to the monoclonal antibody enhances the killing power by delivering radiation to the bound cells as well as to surrounding cells, including large, bulky tumors that may be poorly vascularized.[25,30]

Two radioimmunotherapy regimens have been approved by the FDA that target antibodies to the CD20 antigen expressed in 90% of all B-cell NHLs.

Lymphoma is the fifth most common cancer in the United States.[9] It is a hematological malignancy that is further categorized as HD or NHL. Non-Hodgkin lymphoma is seven times more prevalent than HD and although it is found in all age groups, the patient population at highest risk is those over the age of 60 years. Despite improved treatment options, patients diagnosed with low-grade NHL continually relapse following treatment and ultimately fail to respond to therapy; therefore time off therapy becomes a quality of life indicator for this patient population.

Patient Assessment/Contraindications for Treatment. Not all patients with B-cell NHL will qualify for a radionuclide therapeutic regimen. To ensure optimal outcome, cautious patient assessment should confirm the following[7,23,78]:

- Appropriate diagnosis (i.e., B-cell NHL) and clinical indication as dictated by the therapeutic regimen
- Bone marrow involvement ≤25%, as confirmed by a recent (within 6 weeks) bone marrow biopsy

- Adequate marrow reserves: platelet count ≥100,000 cells/μl; absolute neutrophil count (ANC) ≥1500 cells/mm^3
- Previous external beam therapy less than 25% of active marrow
- No previous myeloablative therapies with bone marrow or stem cell replacement
- No known allergies to murine proteins or components of the therapeutic regimens
- Negative serum pregnancy test; not breast-feeding
- Normal renal function (serum creatinine less than 1.5 times the upper limit of normal—tositumomab [Bexxar])
- Dosimetric whole-body scans performed 1 week before the therapeutic dose demonstrates expected biodistribution and residence time

Standard Patient Preparation

- Patient may eat and take prescribed medication, as necessary before treatment.
- Administration of acetaminophen, 650 mg, and diphenhydramine, 50 mg, to reduce infusion-related adverse events (flulike symptoms) administered 30 to 60 minutes before infusion of the unlabeled tositumomab or rituximab antibody.
- Establish venous access and verify venous patency before and during administration of unlabeled and labeled monoclonal antibodies.

^{131}I-Tositumomab (Bexxar)

Iodine-131 (^{131}I)-tositumomab is a murine IgG2a lambda monoclonal antibody directed against the CD20 antigen found on the surface of normal and malignant B lymphocytes (Box 22-3).[6] Iodine-131 has a physical half-life of 193 hours (8.04 days). It decays by emission of beta particles and gamma radiation. The principal beta emission has a maximum energy of 0.606 MeV with an average penetrating range of 0.8 mm in soft tissue. The principal gamma emission is 364.5 keV.

The therapeutic dose in mCi is calculated based on the activity hours to deliver the prescribed dose (65 cGy for patients with mild thrombocytopenia [platelet counts of 100,000 to 149,000] or 75 cGy for patients with platelet counts greater than 150,000) and the total body residence time as follows:

$$^{131}\text{I idoine activity (mCi)} = \frac{\text{Activity hours (mCi hr)}}{\text{Residence time (hr)}} \times \frac{\text{Desired total body dose}}{75\,\text{cGy}}$$

The activity hours are based on patient gender and weight obtained from a provided look-up table. The total body residence time is determined from a "best fit" line from whole-body scan data performed following the administration of the dosimetric dose of 5 mCi ^{131}I-tositumomab on day 0, day 2 or 3, and day 6 or 7.

BOX 22-3 ^{131}I-Tositumomab (Bexxar)

1. Complete a comprehensive patient assessment, including review of clinical history, current medications, laboratory tests, and recent imaging procedures including those using murine proteins.
2. Confirm that a signed consent form has been obtained for the therapeutic procedure.
3. Review the diagnostic and therapeutic infusion technique including location, time frame for injection, involved personnel, pre-dose medication, etc.
4. Reinforce the importance of thyroid blocking medication throughout the diagnostic and therapeutic protocol.
5. Explain the imaging procedure, including multiple imaging days, time requirements for each imaging set, and physical requirements (supine position, arm position, bladder full/empty, etc.).
6. Working with the Radiation Safety Officer (RSO) or other appropriate hospital personnel, verify the home environment and review the patient's understanding of the required safety precautions following the therapeutic procedure.
7. All instructions and information pertaining to the therapeutic protocol should be discussed verbally with the patient and at least one family member or friend, then provided in writing for later review. Written instructions should always include the physician's emergency contact information.
8. Following the diagnostic infusion of the cold antibody and ^{131}I-tositumomab, perform a WB scan of the (1) patient, (2) standard, and (3) background immediately following infusion; then repeat at day 2 or 3 and day 6 or 7. Maintain consistent acquisition parameters including camera, collimator, speed, matrix, camera height, etc.
9. Process image data per protocol and calculate the therapeutic dose or forward the completed data to appropriate hospital personnel.
10. The therapeutic infusion of the cold antibody and ^{131}I-tositumomab may be performed by the nuclear medicine physician, radiation oncologist, hospital physician, or technologist as per state regulatory guidelines and/or the institution's radioactive materials license.

Consistent imaging parameters are required for data accuracy including the same camera, energy window, field of view, collimators, scanning distance in cm (anterior/posterior head-to-toe images), collimator distance from the patient (auto contour *off*), and scanning speed for each imaging session.[55] The median radiation dose to total body is approximately 0.24 mGy/MBq (range 0.2 to 0.3 MGy/MBq), and the critical organs are identified as urinary bladder wall and bone surface.

Patient Preparation

- Thyroid blocking agent (saturated solution of potassium iodide [SSKI], Lugol solution, or potassium iodide tablets) administered 1 day before the dosimetric dose and continued for 2 weeks following the therapeutic dose.

- Administer 450 mg tositumomab in 50 ml over 60 minutes followed by a 0.9% NaCl flush.
- Administer the patient-specific therapeutic dose of ^{131}I-tositumomab in 30 ml over 20 minutes followed by a 0.9% NaCl flush.

Patient Discharge/Radiation Safety Considerations.

In most states, patient release for high-dose ^{131}I therapy is based on 10 CFR 35.75,[72a] which specifies that patients can be discharged providing that a total effective dose equivalent (TEDE) to another individual does not exceed 500 mrem (5 mSv). To determine patient releasability, a thorough evaluation should include the following:

- *Patient-specific conditions:* ability to understand and follow clearly defined safety instructions; ability to perform self care with minimal assistance from others; ability to delay return to work for a prescribed period of time; and no history of recent urinary incontinence
- *Home environment:* must include separate bed and bathroom and adequate space to maintain appropriate distance from children and adults
- *Public exposure:* ability to avoid public transport and long trips for a prescribed period of time

Safety instructions must be followed for a period of 1 to 2 weeks and include sleeping in a separate bed (>6 feet apart), avoiding sexual contact, using a separate bathroom, sitting when urinating, using separate eating utensils, washing laundry separately, avoiding use of disposable items, maintaining a distance of >6 feet from children and pregnant women, avoiding long trips with others (>4 hours), avoiding public transportation, not returning to work, and limiting time spent in public. If the patient cannot or is unwilling to follow the required safety instructions, hospitalization may be required.[54,59]

^{90}Y–Ibritumomab Tiuxetan (Zevalin)

^{90}Y–ibritumomab tiuxetan is a murine IgG$_1$ kappa monoclonal antibody directed against the CD20 antigen found on the surface of normal and malignant B cells.[78] Yttrium-90 has a physical half-life of 64.1 hours (2.67 days). It decays by emission of beta particles. The principal beta emission has a maximum energy of 2.28 MeV with an average penetrating range of 5 mm in soft tissue.

The therapeutic dose is calculated from the patient's weight and platelet count: 0.3 mCi/kg for platelet counts between 100,000 and 149,000, and 0.4 mCi/kg for platelet counts greater than 150,000. Regardless of the patient's weight, the maximum therapeutic dose should not exceed 32 mCi (1184 MBq). The median radiation dose to total body is approximately 60 cGy (range: 23 to 79 cGy) and the critical organ is identified as the liver (532 cGy [range: 234 to 1856 cGy]).

Patient Preparation

- Administer 250 mg/m^2 rituximab (Rituxan) (infusion time approximately 2 to 6 hours).
- Administer the therapeutic dose of ^{90}Y–ibritumomab tiuxetan (in 4 to 8 ml) over 10 minutes followed by a 0.9% NaCl flush. (NOTE: Therapeutic dose must be administered within 4 hours of the cold antibody.)[65]

Patient Discharge/Radiation Safety Considerations.

Yttrium-90 is a pure beta emitter and requires minimal precautions as follows[51]:

- For 3 days following administration:
  - Wash hands carefully
  - Avoid transfer of bodily fluids (e.g., saliva, blood, stool)
  - Clean up spilled urine and dispose of blood-contaminated material so that others will not inadvertently handle it
- For 1 week following administration:
  - Use a condom for sexual relations
- For 1 year following treatment:
  - Use effective contraceptive methods

Radionuclide Therapy for Bone Pain

Radionuclide therapy for the treatment of bone pain is an effective palliative treatment for patients with osteoblastic bone metastasis and bone pain (Box 22-4). Pain relief and improved quality of life is attributed to cell death of tumor cells in bone allowing the patient to

---

BOX 22-4 ^{89}Sr-Chloride (Metastron)

1. Complete a comprehensive patient assessment, including review of clinical history, current medications, laboratory tests, recent bone scan, and review of therapeutic procedures including chemotherapy or radiation therapy.
2. Confirm that a signed consent form has been obtained for the therapeutic procedure.
3. Review the therapeutic procedure, including IV access and infusion of the therapeutic dose; answer any last minute questions, as necessary.
4. Working with the RSO or other appropriate hospital personnel, verify the home environment and review the patient's understanding of the required safety precautions following the therapeutic procedure.
5. All instructions and information pertaining to the therapeutic protocol should be discussed verbally with the patient and at least one family member or friend, then provided in writing for later review. Written instructions should always include the physician's emergency contact information.
6. The therapeutic infusion of ^{89}Sr-chloride may be performed by the nuclear medicine physician, radiation oncologist, hospital physician, or technologist as per state regulatory guidelines and/or the institution's radioactive materials license.

TABLE 22-8	Approved Radionuclides for the Treatment of Bone Pain					
Radionuclide	Commercial Name	$t_{1/2}$	Max Energy (MeV)	Mean Energy (MeV)	Average Penetration (mm)	Gamma Energy (MeV)
[89]Sr-chloride	Metastron	50.5 days	1.46	0.58	2.44	—
[153]Sm-lexidronam	Quadramet	46.7 hours	0.81	0.23	0.60	0.103
[32]P–sodium phosphate	—	14.2 days	1.72	0.70	3.00	—

From Silberstein EB, Buscombe, JR, McEwan A, et al: *Society of nuclear medicine procedure guidelines for palliative treatment of painful bone metastases,* version 3.0, January 2003 (publication available online): http://interactive.snm.org/docs/pg_ch25_0403.pdf. Accessed August 16, 2010.
$t_{1/2}$, Half-life.

resume many daily activities. Although numerous radionuclides have been successfully used in the treatment of bone pain, only three are currently approved by the FDA: ^{89}Sr-chloride, [153]Sm-lexidronam, and ^{32}P–sodium phosphate (Table 22-8).

These radionuclides are rapidly cleared from the blood and localize in bone. They actively target osteoblastic lesions and remain within boney metastases up to five times longer than normal bone. This extended biological half-life enhances the therapeutic effectiveness of the treatment. Pain relief is reported as early as 5 days and as late as 4 weeks with an overall average of 7 to 14 days posttherapy; however, in some cases increased bone pain, also known as bone flare, may be reported within the first 2 to 3 days following treatment. Bone flare should be anticipated and treated as necessary.[12,25,48,58]

[89]Sr-Chloride (Metastron). Strontium-89-chloride is a calcium analog that clears rapidly from the blood and localizes in bone. It actively targets osteoblastic bone lesions. The biological half-life of ^{89}Sr-chloride in bone metastasis is five times longer than normal bone (i.e., 50.5 days versus 14 days, respectively). Therapeutic doses are calculated at 40 to 60 µCi/kg (1.5 to 2.2 MBq/kg) and are administered intravenously.[16] As anticipated, the bone surface and red bone marrow are cited as the critical organs for this radionuclide. Radiation dosimetry for the bone surface is estimated to be 17.0 mGy/MBq (63.0 rad/mCi).

[153]Sm-Lexidronam (Quadramet). Samarium-153-lexidronam (Quadramet) is a phosphate compound that concentrates in bone mineral. The therapeutic dose is calculated as 1 mCi/kg (37 MBq/kg) administered intravenously. Although [153]Sm-lexidronam is not indicated for diagnostic bone imaging, the 103-keV photopeak allows for excellent visualization of bone and metastases 24 to 72 hours following treatment.[55] The bone surface and red bone marrow are cited as the critical organs for this radionuclide. Radiation dosimetry for the bone surface is estimated to be 6.8 mGy/MBq (25.0 rad/mCi).

[32]P–Sodium Phosphate. Phosphorous-32–sodium phosphate is distributed in bone in the same manner as stable phosphate. It accumulates primarily in the hydroxyapatite crystal of bone as well as nonosseous tissue. The intravenous therapeutic dose is calculated as 5 to 10 mCi (185 to 370 MBq); the oral therapeutic dose is calculated as 10 to 12 mCi (370 to 444 MBq).[61] The bone surface and red bone marrow are cited as the critical organs for this radionuclide. Radiation dosimetry for the bone surface is estimated to be 10.0 mGy/MBq (37.0 rad/mCi).

Patient Assessment—Pretreatment
- Recent bone scan (within 4 to 8 weeks) demonstrating increased osteoblastic activity
- Adequate blood counts: platelets ≥60 to 100,000/µl; leukocytes ≥2400 to 3000/µl; granulocytes ≥2000/µl
- Negative serum pregnancy test; not breast-feeding
- No chemotherapy or radiation therapy scheduled for 6 to 12 weeks following treatment unless part of a clinical trial for combined therapy
- Signed informed consent

Patient Preparation
- Patient may eat and take prescribed medication, as necessary.
- Hospitalization is not required.
- Catheterize incontinent patients for 3 to 5 days posttherapy.
- Establish patent IV access.
- Administer radionuclide over 2 to 4 minutes; flush with 20 to 30 ml 0.9% normal saline.

Patient Discharge/Radiation Safety Considerations. Minimal radiation safety considerations are required for pure beta emitters (^{32}P–sodium chloride and ^{89}Sr-chloride) or a beta/low-energy gamma emitters ([153]Sm-lexidronam). Refer to the ^{90}Y radioimmunotherapy protocol for discharge instructions.

Additional [32]P Therapeutic Protocols

Phosphorus-32 has been used to successfully treat patients with hematological blood disorders, malignant effusions, and inflammatory joint disease for many decades.

Polycythemia Vera. Polycythemia vera (PV), an increase in total RBC volume or an increased concentration of RBC to decreased plasma volume, is a life-threatening hematological blood disorder. Phosphorus-32 sodium phosphate has been successfully used to treat PV since 1939 and is considered to be the treatment of choice in the elderly patient population with uncomplicated PV.[25,65]

Phosphorus-32 sodium phosphate is a clear aqueous solution that is absorbed by rapidly proliferating tissue. Contraindications for the treatment protocol include leukocyte counts below 5000/mm^3 or a platelet count below 150,000/mm^3. Therapeutic doses are calculated based on specific clinical factors (weight and blood counts) as well as extent of disease. Intravenous doses range from 1 to 20 mCi (37 to 740 MBq) with an average dose range of 1 to 8 mCi (37 to 296 MBq). Repeat doses are adjusted, as necessary for individual patient needs.[61] Dosimetry for treatment of PV is the same as for the treatment of bone metastases. The bone surface and red bone marrow are cited as the critical organs with dosimetry for the bone surface estimated to be 10.0 mGy/MBq (37.0 rad/mCi).

Malignant Effusion. Although chemotherapeutic protocols are most often the treatment of choice for malignant effusion in the thoracic and peritoneal cavities, ^{32}P–chromic phosphate continues to provide an alternative treatment option for a select patient population including those with stage II epithelial ovarian cancer.[49,63,66,69]

Phosphorus-32–chromic phosphate suspension is a blue-green colloidal suspension for intracavitary administration only. If the colloidal suspension is administered intravenously, it will be cleared by the Kupffer cells in the liver resulting in severe localized radiation damage to the liver.[63,64] Contraindications for ^{32}P–chromic phosphate therapy include the presence of ulcerative tumors or where loculation would limit the uniform distribution of the colloidal suspension, which may cause tissue necrosis and suboptimal therapy results. For abdominal protocols, loculation of the abdominal cavity is assessed pretreatment with 5 mCi ^{99m}Tc–sulfur colloid mixed in 1000 ml normal saline followed by patient rolling from side to side for 60 to 90 minutes. For pleural effusions, a thoracentesis is performed to drain the effusion followed by the instillation of 5 mCi (185 MBq) ^{99m}Tc–sulfur colloid and patient rolling before imaging. Imaging of the abdominal or thoracic cavity will identify overall distribution of the colloid and provide a mechanism to quantify percent loculation, if present.

The suggested dose range for intraperitoneal treatment is 10 to 20 mCi (370 to 740 MBq). The suggested dose range for intrapleural treatment is 6 to 12 mCi (222 to 444 MBq). The estimated dose rate must be calculated on an individual basis and is based on the depth in tissue, activity administered, and uniformity of distribution.

Radiosynoviorthesis. Radiosynoviorthesis (RSV) is the destruction of synovitis in individual joints by an intraarticular injection of radiocolloid such as ^{32}P. The procedure provides an alternative treatment for inflammatory joint disease associated with rheumatoid arthritis, osteoarthritis, and hemophiliac arthropathy that has not responded to or failed other pharmacological therapies including intraarticular steroid injections. As an alternative to surgery, RSV has comparable results to the more invasive and expensive surgical procedure, may be repeated, and has an improved quality of life outcome because the patient remains ambulatory following each procedure.

Radiosynoviorthesis has also been shown to be effective in reducing effusions following surgical implantation of prosthesis.[53]

Ideal radiocolloids for RSV must be appropriately sized (2 to 10 μm) to be engulfed or ingested by phagocytes and not leak from the joint and to remain tightly bound to the particle throughout the radionuclide's half-life, and should be able to distribute uniformly throughout the intraarticular space without causing an inflammatory response. Yttrium-90–citrate silicate, ^{186}Re–colloid sulfide, and ^{169}Er-citrate are routinely used for RSV in European countries. Additional radiocolloids including ^{198}Au-colloid, ^{32}P–chromic phosphate, and ^{165}Dy–ferric hydroxide macroaggregate are used in the United States; however, because of the disadvantages associated with lymphatic transport, they are no longer included in European guidelines.[24,57]

Contraindications for treatment include ruptured Baker cyst (knee), local skin infection, and significant bleeding into the joint. Additional patient assessment should include evaluation for significant cartilage loss or joint instability associated with bone destruction.[24,53]

The suggested therapeutic dose is based on the size of the joint and the radionuclide selected and ranges from less than 1 mCi (10 to 20 MBq) for proximal interphalangeal joints to 5 to 6 mCi (185 to 222 MBq) for knee joints.[53] The estimated dose rate must be calculated on an individual basis and is based on the depth in tissue, activity administered, and uniformity of distribution.

^{90}Y Microspheres for Selective Internal Radiation Therapy

Primary and metastatic liver cancer accounts for the largest cancer-related adult mortality in the world.[9] The liver is the most common site of metastases for cancer of the abdominal organs and approximately one third of all cancers ultimately spread to the liver. Because most patients present with nonresectable disease, alternative treatment protocols have been developed including hepatic arterial embolization with and without chemotherapy, external radiation, and systemic chemotherapy. Unfortunately no single treatment protocol has demonstrated improved patient survival.

Selective internal radiation therapy (SIRT) offers an additional therapeutic option to treat metastatic liver cancer. SIRT relies on two key factors: the increased vascularity of tumor nodules in the liver and the predominant blood supply of the liver nodules by the hepatic artery. Yttrium-90–embedded microspheres administered through the hepatic artery offer targeted therapy to tumor nodules while sparing normal surrounding liver tissue. Yttrium-90 particles (TheraSphere yttrium-90 glass microspheres or SIR-Spheres yttrium-90 resin microspheres) are sized to allow delivery to tumor nodules via the hepatic artery while limiting the spheres passing from tumor vasculature into venous circulation.[60,71]

TheraSphere is indicated for radiation treatment or as a neoadjuvant to surgery or transplantation in patients with unresectable hepatocellular carcinoma (HCC) who can have placement of appropriately positioned hepatic arterial catheters.[14,71] SIR-Spheres is indicated for the treatment of unresectable metastatic liver tumors from primary colorectal cancer with or without adjuvant intrahepatic arterial chemotherapy (IHAC) of floxuridine (FUDR).[60] Contraindications include patients with previous external beam radiation to the liver; ascites or clinical liver failure; markedly abnormal liver function tests; lung shunting exceeding 20%; abnormal vascular anatomy that would result in significant reflux of hepatic arterial blood to the stomach, pancreas or bowel; disseminated extrahepatic malignant disease; treatment with capecitabine within 2 months or scheduling for capecitabine following treatment; or portal vein thrombosis.[58,71]

Therapeutic activity ranges from 50 to 150 Gy (5000 to 15,000 rad) and is based on tumor size, liver size, and lung shunting. The liver and tumor size are calculated from a recent abdominal CT scan. Following the administration of 5 mCi (185 MBq) ^{99m}Tc–macroaggregated albumin (MAA) administered during the diagnostic hepatic angiogram, lung shunting is quantified with planar images of the chest and abdomen. The therapeutic dose is administered in multiple small incremental infusions during the therapeutic hepatic angiogram. Vascular status is mapped with contrast between each infusion. Administration of the microspheres continues until the full dose is administered or until stasis is reached. Adverse events include fever, transient decrease of hemoglobin, mild to moderate abnormal liver function tests, abdominal pain, nausea, vomiting, and diarrhea. Radiation safety precautions for the pure beta emitter are institution-specific. Universal precautions should be practiced by hospital personnel if the patient is admitted for overnight observation following the therapeutic procedure.[76]

SUMMARY

- The use of radionuclides continues to be an important clinical tool in the diagnosis, treatment, and follow-up of inflammatory and oncological processes.
- The efficacy of patient assessment and treatment relies on a thorough understanding of the disease state and its pathophysiological processes.
- The efficacy of imaging and therapy relies on an understanding of these processes and careful adherence to approved clinical guidelines.

REFERENCES

1. *AdreView (iobenguane sulphate) prescribing information*, Chalfont St. Giles, U.K., 2008, GE Healthcare.
2. Alazraki N, Glass EC, Castronovo F, et al: *Society of nuclear medicine procedure guideline for lymphoscintigraphy and the use of intraoperative gamma probe for sentinel lymph node localization in melanoma of intermediate thickness*, version 1.0, June 15, 2002 (publication available online): http://interactive.snm.org/docs/pg_ch24_0403.pdf. Accessed August 16, 2010.
3. Andrews GA, Knisley RM, Wagner HN: *Radioactive pharmaceuticals*, AEC Symposium Series 6, Washington, DC, 1966, Division of Technical Information, U.S. Atomic Energy Commission.
4. Balon HR, Goldsmith SJ, Siegel BA, et al: *Procedure guideline for somatostatin receptor scintigraphy with ^{111}In-pentreotide*, version 1.0, February 2001 (publication available online): http://interactive.snm.org/docs/pg_ch27_0403.pdf. Accessed August 16, 2010.
5. Bartold SP, Donohoe KJ, Haynie TP, et al: *Society of nuclear medicine procedure guideline for gallium scintigraphy in the evaluation of malignant disease*, version 3.0, June 2001 (publication available online): http://interactive.snm.org/docs/pg_ch23_0403.pdf. Accessed August 16, 2010.
6. Bell EG, O'Mara RE, Henry CA, et al: Non-neoplastic localization of ^{67}Ga citrate, *J Nucl Med* 12:338, 1971 (abstract).
7. *Bexxar (tositumomab and iodine I-131 tositumomab) prescribing information*, Seattle, 2005, Corixa.
8. Brem RF, Schoonjans JM, Kieper DA, et al: High resolution scintimammography: a pilot study, *J Nucl Med* 43:909-915, 2002.
9. *Cancer facts and figures, 2010* (publication available online): http://www.cancer.org/acs/groups/content/@nho/documents/document/acspc-024113.pdf. Accessed August 16, 2010.
10. *CEA-Scan (arcitumomab) prescribing information*, Morris Plain, NJ, 1999, Immunomedicas.
11. Christian PE, Bernier DR, Langan JK, editors: *Nuclear medicine and PET: technology and techniques*, ed 5, St Louis, 2004, Mosby.
12. Clark MT, Galie E: Radionuclide therapy of osseous metastatic disease, *J Nucl Med Technol* 21:3-6, 2001.
13. Coover LR, Caravaglia G, Kuhn P: Scintimammography with dedicated breast camera detects and localizes occult carcinoma, *J Nucl Med* 45:553-558, 2004.
14. Dancey JE, Shepherd FA, Paul K, et al: Treatment of nonresectable hepatocellular carcinoma with intrahepatic ^{90}Y-microspheres, *J Nucl Med* 41:1673-1681, 2000.
15. Davey S, White SJ, Curie GM, et al: Injection techniques for breast lymphoscintigraphy: a review, *The Internet Journal of Oncology*, 2009
16. Dickinson CZ, Hendrix NS: Strontium-89 therapy in painful bony metastases, *J Nucl Med Technol* 21:133-137, 1993.
17. Edwards CL, Hayes RL: Tumor scanning with ^{67}Ga citrate, *J Nucl Med* 10:103-108, 1969.
18. Even-Sapir E, Hedva L, Lievshitz G, et al: Lymphoscintigraphy for sentinel node mapping using a hybrid SPECT/CT system, *J Nucl Med* 44:1413-1420, 2003.
19. Freeman LM, Weissman HS, editors: *Nuclear medicine annual*, New York, 1982, Raven Press.
20. Gabriel M, Decristoforo C, Donnemiller E, et al: An intrapatient comparison of ^{99m}Tc EDDA/HYNIC-TOC with ^{111}In DTPA octreotide for the diagnosis of somatostatin receptor-expressing tumors, *J Nucl Med* 44:708-716, 2003.
21. Gelfand MJ, Elgazzar AH, Kriss VM, et al: Iodine-123-MIBG SPECT versus planar imaging in children with recurrent crest tumors, *J Nucl Med* 35:1753-1757, 1994.

22. Goodwin DA, Doherty RW, McDougall IR: Clinical use of indium-111-labeled white cells: an analysis of 312 cases. In *Neutrophils, platelets and lymphocytes*, New York, 1982, Trivirum.

23. Gregory SA: Selecting patients for treatment with ^{90}Y-ibritumomab tiuxetan (Zevalin), *Seminars in Oncology* 30:17-22, 2003.

24. Harbert JC, Eckelman WC, Neumann RD, editors: *Nuclear medicine diagnosis and therapy*, New York, 1996, Thieme Medical Publishing.

25. Haynie T, editor: *Nuclear medicine self-study program IV—nuclear medicine oncology*, Reston, Va, 2004, Society of Nuclear Medicine.

26. Hurralde MP, editor: *CRC dictionary and handbook of nuclear medicine and clinical imaging*, Boca Raton, Fla, 1990, CRC Press.

27. *Hyperparathyroidism* (website): www.endocrine.niddk.nih. gov/pubs/hyper/hyper.htm. Accessed July 28, 2010.

28. International Commission on Radiologic Protection: *Radiation dose to patients from radiopharmaceuticals*, IRCP 53, New York, 1988 ICRP.

29. Jani AB, Blend MJ, Hamilton R, et al: Influence of radioimmunoscintigraphy on post-prostatectomy radiotherapy treatment decision making, *J Nucl Med* 45:571-578, 2004.

30. Juweid ME: Radioimmnotherapy of B-Cell non-Hodgkin's lymphoma: from clinical trials to clinical practice, *J Nucl Med* 43:1507-1592, 2002.

31. Khalkhali I, Baum JK, Villanueva-Meyer J, et al: 99mTc-sestamibi breast imaging for the examination of patients with dense and fatty breasts: multi-center study, *Radiology* 222:149-155, 2002.

32. Khalkhali I, Caravaglia G, Abdel-Nabi HH, et al: *Society of nuclear medicine procedure guidelines for breast scintigraphy*, version 2.0, June 2004 (publication available online): http://interactive.snm.org/docs/BreastScintigraphyGuideline_V1.0.pdf. Accessed August 16, 2010.

33. Khalkhali I, Villanueva-Meyer J, Edell SL, et al: Diagnostic accuracy of ^{99m}Tc-sestimibi breast imaging: multi-center trial results, *J Nucl Med* 40:1973-1979, 2000.

34. Kim SH, Shim J, Kim CK, et al: Reverse echelon node and a lymphatic ectasia in the same patient during breast lymphoscintigraphy: the importance of injection and imaging technique, *Br J Radiology* 77: 1053-1056, 2004.

35. Krynyckyi BR, Kim CK, Mosci K, et al: Areolar-cutaneous "junction" injections to augment sentinel node count activity, *Clinical Nuc Med* 28:97-107, 2003.

36. Lebtahi R, Le Cloirec J, Houzard C, et al: Detection of neuroendocrine tumors: ^{99m}Tc-P829 scintigraphy compared with ^{111}In pentetreotide scintigraphy, *J Nucl Med* 43:889-895, 2002.

37. Liberman L, Lymphoscintigraphy for lymphatic mapping in breast cancer, *Radiology*, 228: 313:315, 2003.

38. Mariani G, Moresco L, Viale G, et al, Radioguided sentinel lymph node biopsy in breast cancer surgery, *J Nucl Med* 42:1198-1215, 2001.

39. Maris J: MIBG/I-131 therapy yields high response, low toxicity in children with relapsed neuroblastoma. May 17, 2005, SNM Hot Topics (serial online): http://interactive.snm.org/index.cfm?PageID=3971. Accessed August 16, 2010.

40. Maurea S, Klain M, Mainolfi C, et al: The diagnostic role of radionuclide imaging in evaluation of patients with non-hypersecreting adrenal masses, *J Nucl Med* 42:884-892, 2001.

41. Mozley PD, Kim CK, Mohsin J, et al: The efficacy of iodine-123 MIBG as a screening test for pheochromocytoma, *J Nucl Med* 35:1138-1144, 1994.

42. Murphy GP, Lawrence W Jr, Lenhard RE: *Clinical oncology*, ed 2, Atlanta, 1995, The American Cancer Society.

43. *NeoTect technical user's guide*, Wayne, N.J., 2002, Berlex Laboratories.

44. *OctreoScan (Indium In-111 Pentetreotide) prescribing information*, St Louis, 1994, Mallinckrodt Nuclear.

45. Palestro, CJ, Brown ML, Forestrom LA, et al: *Society of nuclear medicine procedure guideline for gallium scintigraphy in inflammation*, version 3.0, June 2, 2004 (publication available online): http://interactive.snm.org/docs/Gallium_Scintigraphy_in_Inflammation_v3.pdf. Accessed August 16, 2010.

46. Palestro CJ, Brown ML, Forestrom LA, et al: *Society of nuclear medicine procedure guideline for ^{111}In-leukocyte scintigraphy for suspected infection/inflammation*, version 3.0, June 2, 2004 (publication available online): http://interactive. snm.org/docs/Leukocyte_v3.pdf. Accessed August 16, 2010.

47. Palestro CJ, Brown ML, Forestrom LA, et al: *Society of nuclear medicine procedure guideline for 99mTc-exametazime (HMPAO)-labeled leukocyte scintigraphy for suspected infection/inflammation*, version 3.0, June 2, 2004 (publication available online): http://interactive.snm.org/docs/HMPAO_v3.pdf. Accessed August 16, 2010.

48. Pandit-Taskar N, Batraki M, Divgi CR: Radiopharmaceutical therapy for palliation of bone pain from osseous metastases, *J Nucl Med* 45:1358-1365, 2004.

49. Pattillo RA, Collier BD, Abdel-Dayem H, et al: Phosphorus-32 chromic phosphate for ovarian cancer: I. Fractionated low dose intraperitoneal treatments in conjunction with platinum analog chemotherapy, *J Nucl Med* 36:29-36, 1995.

50. Rossi CR, De Salvo GL, Trifiro G, et al: The impact of lymphoscintigraphy technique on the outcome of sentinel node biopsy in 1313 patients with cutaneous melanoma: an Italian multicentric study (SOLISM-IMI), *J Nuc Med* 47:234-241, 2006.

51. Rufini V, Fisher GA, Shulkin BL, et al: Iodine-123 MIBG imaging of neuroblastoma: utility of SPECT and delayed imaging, *J Nucl Med* 37:1464-1468, 1996.

52. Shackett P: *Nuclear medicine technology: procedures and quick reference*, ed 2, Philadelphia, 2009, Lippincott Williams & Wilkins.

53. Schneider P, Farahati J, Reiners C: Radiosynovectomy in rheumatology, orthopedics and hemophilia, *J Nucl Med* 46:48S-54S, 2005.

54. Seldin DW: Techniques for using Bexxar for the treatment of non-Hodgkin's lymphoma, *J Nucl Med Technol* 30:109-114, 2002.

55. Serafini A: Samarian Sm-153 lexidronam for the palliation of bone pain associated with metastases, *Cancer* 88:2934-2939, 2005.

56. Shulkin BL, Shapiro B: Current concepts on the diagnostic use of MIBG in children, *J Nucl Med* 39:679-688, 1998.

57. Siegel HJ, Luck JV, Siegel ME: Advances in radionuclide therapeutics in orthopaedics, *J Am Acad Orthop Surg* 12:55-64, 2004.

58. Silberstein EB, Buscombe, JR, McEwan A, et al: *Society of nuclear medicine procedure guidelines for palliative treatment of painful bone metastases*, version 3.0, January 2003 (publication available online): http://interactive.snm.org/docs/pg_ch25_0403.pdf. Accessed August 16, 2010.

59. Silverman D, Delpassand ES, Torabi F, et al: Radiolabeled antibody therapy in non-Hodgkin's lymphoma: radiation protection, isotope comparisons and quality of life issues, *Cancer Treat Rev* 30:165-172, 2004.

60. *SIR-Spheres (Yttrium-90 Resin Microspheres) prescribing information*, Lake Forest, Ill., 2004, Sirtex Medical.

61. *Sodium Phosphate (P-32 Solution) prescribing information*, St Louis, 2000, Mallinckrodt.

62. *Somatostatin receptor imaging for neuroendocrine tumors*, St Louis, 1994, Mallinckrodt Medical (product monograph).

63. Soper JT, Berchuck A, Dodge R, et al: Adjuvant therapy with intraperitoneal chromic phosphate (^{32}P) in women with early ovarian carcinoma after comprehensive surgical staging, *Obstet Gynecol* 79:993-997, 1992.

64. Sprengelmeyer JT, McDermott RL: Phosphorus-32 colloidal chromic phosphate: treatment of choice of malignant pericardial effusion, *J Nucl Med* 31:2034-2036, 1999.

65. Stevens AM, Wells PC, *editors: Review of nuclear medicine technology: preparation for certification examinations*, ed 3, Reston, Va, 2004, Society of Nuclear Medicine.

66. Sullivan DL, Harris CC, Currie JL, et al: Observation on intraperitoneal distribution of chromic phosphate (^{32}P) suspension for intraperitoneal therapy, *Radiology* 146:539-541, 1983.

67. Taasan V, Shapiro B, Hoefnagel CA: *Clinical use of I-131 MIBG scintigraphy in localization of pheochromocytoma and neuroblastoma*, Bedford, Mass, 1994, CIS-US.

68. Taillefer R, Boucher Y, Potvin C, et al: Detection and localization of parathyroid adenomas in patients with hyperparathyroidism using a single radionuclide imaging procedure with 99mTc-Sestimibi (double phase study), *J Nucl Med* 33:1801-1807, 1992.

69. Taylor A, Baily NA, Halpern SE, et al: Loculation as a contraindication to intracavitary ^{32}P chromic phosphate therapy, *J Nucl Med* 16:318-319, 1975.

70. Thakur ML, Coleman RE, Welch MS: Indium-111 labeled leukocytes for the localization of abscess: preparation, analysis, tissue distribution and comparison with gallium-67 citrate in dogs, *J Lab Clin Med* 89:217-218, 1977.

71. *TherasSphere (Yttrium-90 Glass Microspheres) prescribing information*, Ottawa, 2005, MDS Nordion.

72. Tiling R, Stephan K, Sommer H, et al: Tissue specific effects on uptake of ^{99m}Tc-sestamibi by breast lesions: a targeted analysis of false scintigraphic diagnoses, *J Nucl Med* 44:1822-1828, 2004.

72a. U.S. Nuclear Regulatory Commission: Title 10, *Code of Federal Regulations*, Part 35: Human uses of byproduct material, Washington, DC, 2009, U.S. Nuclear Regulatory Commission.

73. William S: Adrenal imaging meta-iodobenzylguandine MIBG (publication available online): http://www.auntminnie.com/index.asp?sec=ref&sub=ncm&pag=get&itemid=54419#MIBG. Accessed on August 16, 2010.

74. William S: Prostascint (111In-Capromab Pendetide) (CYT-356) (publication available online): http://www.auntminnie.com/index.asp?Sec=ref&sub=ncm&pag=dis&ItemId=55327. Accessed on August 16, 2010.

75. Willkom P, Bender H, Bangard M, et al: FDG PET and immunoscintigraphy with ^{99m}Tc-labeled antibody fragments for the detection of recurrence of colorectal carcinoma, *J Nucl Med* 41:1657-1663, 2000.

76. Wong CO, Salem R, Qing F, et al: Metabolic response after intraarterial ^{90}Y glass microspheres treatment for colorectal liver metastases: comparison of quantitative and visual analysis by 18F-FDG PET, *J Nucl Med* 45:1892-1897, 2004.

77. Yeung HW, Cody HS, Turlakow A, et al: Lymphoscintigraphy and sentinel node localization in breast cancer patients: a comparison between 1-day and 2-day protocols, *J Nuc Med* 42:420-423, 2001.

78. *Zevalin (ibritumomab tiuxetan) prescribing information*, San Diego, 2004, Biogen Idec.

Pediatric Imaging

*Helen R. Nadel, Jan Leggett, Derek McGuire,
Susan C. Weiss, James J. Conway*

OUTLINE

OBJECTIVES

After completing this chapter, the reader will be able to:
- Discuss the considerations involved in dealing with pediatric patients and parents.
- List and discuss methods of immobilizing pediatric patients.
- Describe techniques for interacting with pediatric patients and their parents.
- List the materials needed to perform injections in pediatric patients, and list possible injection sites.
- Discuss techniques for determining the administered dose of radiopharmaceuticals for pediatric patients.
- Describe imaging considerations for bone scintigraphy in pediatric patients.

- Discuss renal scintigraphy, renography, cystography, and diuresis studies.
- Describe imaging procedures for the pediatric gastrointestinal system, including hepatobiliary conditions, Meckel diverticulum, gastroesophageal reflux, and gastric emptying.
- Describe imaging procedures for pediatric cardiovascular nuclear medicine.
- Discuss the concept of Image Gently.
- Describe imaging procedures and special considerations for PET-CT imaging in pediatrics.

KEY TERMS

child abuse
Ewing sarcoma
gastroesophageal reflux (GER)

Legg-Calvé-Perthes
neonatal hydronephrosis
neuroblastoma

pediatric immobilization
techniques

---

*Klaus Hahn and Sibylle Fischer contributed to the "Pet Imaging" section.

All examinations performed in adults can be performed in children and even young infants; however, the disease processes of the pediatric age group and the technical requirements of imaging of children differ significantly from those encountered in adults. The pediatric age group includes children from newborn to adulthood. It is because of their size and different stages of development throughout this age span that modifications to techniques are required for their successful accomplishment. Hence pediatric nuclear imaging requires an understanding of the disease processes that affect these children in order to correctly modify technical aspects of their examinations to provide for their needs. This chapter will discuss some of the instrumentation, distraction techniques, immobilization, safety measures, and procedure modifications needed to be used to obtain high-quality diagnostic studies in children, as well as specific pediatric considerations for hybrid imaging to include positron emission tomography and computed tomography (PET-CT) and single photon emission computed tomography and computed tomography (SPECT-CT). Clinical applications of the more common pediatric examinations will then be discussed.

TECHNICAL CONSIDERATIONS

Instrumentation

As with all of medical imaging, resolution is an important technical consideration to achieve diagnostic quality of the images. All pediatric imaging should be performed with an imaging instrument that has the highest state-of-the-art resolution. Another consideration is the positioning of the patient. The area of interest should be centered in the field of view and whenever possible, only the area of interest should be included in the field of view. This will reduce unnecessary activity from areas of noninterest. Another consideration when imaging children is the use of magnification. Since children differ in size from adults, magnification is often necessary to ensure that the area of interest is properly centered and appropriate detail is achieved. When using magnification, maximum camera zoom should be applied to obtain the images. In addition, small parts imaging can be enhanced with the use of pinhole collimators. The pinhole collimator provides excellent resolution for imaging and is particularly useful for example in imaging the hips during bone imaging for **Legg-Calvé-Perthes** disease. Still another technical consideration in pediatric imaging is the use of single photon emission computed tomography (SPECT) imaging. SPECT should be used liberally in pediatric imaging to increase the diagnostic value of the procedure. Examples of when SPECT is most useful include imaging small parts such as the hands and feet, performing a Meckel diverticulum scintigram, performing a biliary scintigram, and evaluating the spine. To aid in the positioning and immobilization of smaller children for an imaging procedure, some gamma camera manufacturers offer pediatric pallets and head holders.

SPECT techniques require stringent quality control that is very time-consuming. In addition to the routine daily quality control procedures for the gamma camera, pediatric SPECT scintigraphy requires generation of flood correction matrices and center of rotation (COR) measurements for every possible combination of collimator and magnification factor that might be used. Because of the age range of patients imaged, this may require a 2-week cycle of nightly quality control acquisitions. When a single-head SPECT instrument is used, data acquisition requires 45 to 60 minutes to obtain adequate statistics. Younger patients might require sedation or immobilization for SPECT, SPECT-CT, or PET-CT examinations,[43,77] sometimes even when they are cooperative.

SPECT-CT. SPECT-CT is used mainly for bone imaging and metaiodobenzylguanidine (MIBG) scintigraphy. To ensure the best possible image fusion, the patient should not be moved between the SPECT and CT acquisitions. Because of the inability for the patient to move between studies, when it is anticipated that CT might be added to the examination, extra caution should be taken to ensure that there are no artifacts such as metal in the anticipated field of view at the start of the SPECT acquisition. Positioning of feet for SPECT in particular needs to be the same as that used for routine CT evaluation of the feet.

Hybrid imaging with PET-CT or SPECT-CT should be performed with attention to the radiation exposure from the CT study depending upon the quality of CT study that is needed; a low-dose CT is used for attenuation correction only and a higher quality CT is used for correlating anatomy.[1] Written protocols should be in place and the nuclear medicine physician should be consulted on a case by case or diagnosis driven protocol regarding the CT exposure. Weight-based protocols for low-dose CT with lower kVp and mAs for attenuation correction scans and for diagnostic and contrast CT imaging. A single postcontrast diagnostic evaluation with lower kVp and mAs can be performed as the CT portion of the PET-CT study, and that can be used for attenuation correction.[1,29,59]

Patient Safety and Care

Safety is paramount in pediatric imaging. At no time should a child be left alone in an imaging room or on an imaging table, whether or not a procedure is in progress. To ensure that a child is not left alone, it is often necessary to have two individuals, at least one of whom is a technologist, to perform studies in children. In addition to ensuring that a child is not left alone, having two individuals working to accomplish the study can also help to ensure cooperation of the child and efficiency of the procedure. Immobilization techniques may also be necessary to restrain children who are unable to remain still during the procedure.

Other aspects of safety are associated with the standards of care in their respective hospitals and include fire safety and adverse event reporting. Additional technologist responsibilities required to ensure a safe environment may include certification in cardiopulmonary resuscitation (CPR) that covers pediatric resuscitation techniques, and working with various intravenous (IV) infusion equipment and monitoring devices, such as pulse oximeters.

There is always an interest and concern regarding exposure to ionizing radiation during diagnostic procedures. The Society for Pediatric Radiology has taken the lead in creating a program targeting appropriate imaging techniques using the principle of "as low as reasonably achievable" (ALARA) principle to promote dose reduction in pediatric imaging. The Alliance for Radiation Safety in Pediatric Imaging has created the Image Gently campaign and has a website to provide resources for health professionals and parents.[7,35,36]

Immobilization Techniques

As with all patients, it is necessary for children to be informed about the study they are about to have and what will be expected of them, and it is important for this explanation to be tailored for the child's age and level of comprehension. However, there are situations when the child is either unable or unwilling to remain still for the time required to complete the examination. In these situations, immobilization is required. **Pediatric immobilization techniques** include the use of Velcro straps, masking tape, sandbags, and swaddling techniques (using blankets or a papoose type of apparatus), Immobilization, particularly with infants, can also be accomplished by the technologist or the parent simply by holding the child in place with gentle pressure on the body area being imaged.

In addition, distraction techniques, such as reading books; blowing bubbles; watching television or movies; and listening to music are examples of methods that may be employed to entertain the child in an effort to keep them still and cooperative during the examination. In addition, encouraging parents to bring along the child's favorite toy, blanket, or special object that may provide comfort to the child is a good practice. Sleep deprivation or delaying the patient's normal nap time before the scheduled study might induce sleep. Many younger children are accustomed to having a story read to them just before bedtime, and simulation of that situation might induce calm or even sleep.

Problems Associated with Immobilization Techniques. Each of the immobilization techniques just mentioned has its advantages and disadvantages and should be used judiciously. Wrapping or swaddling effectively immobilizes the child, but monitoring of the respiratory rate, skin tone, pulse, and blood pressure is inhibited by this technique. Overheating can occur as well. If an emergency arises with the patient's condition, the time needed to unwrap the child can be detrimental and frustrating.

Sandbags are also used to stabilize the patient's arms or legs in an appropriate position. A sheet or towel placed over the area of interest and sandbag placed alongside or atop the sheet can effectively immobilize the patient when using a posterior imaging position with the camera beneath the imaging table. However, in the neonate or infant, sandbags may be too heavy or may cause ischemia, particularly if used for prolonged imaging times. Sandbags also attenuate photons and can create artifacts in the image. They are primarily used as safety devices positioned alongside the body to prevent the child from rolling off the table.

Surgical adhesive tape can be used to help immobilize, but tape should never be applied directly to the skin. Many children are allergic to adhesive tape, and it can stick to the skin or hair and cause pain on removal. Adhesive tape is more practical as a safety device and should be used like a seat belt. Allergy to rubber tourniquets is also a problem and every patient should be queried about rubber allergy. It is not uncommon in children that undergo frequent exams. Velcro strap devices attached to the imaging table may be preferable to adhesive tape.

Sedation Techniques. Sedation, to include conscious and general anesthesia, is an effective means of achieving immobilization.[72] However, sedation should be used judiciously and with the appropriate monitoring protocol so that complications are minimized and the patient can adequately recover from the effects of the sedation before discharge.[2] Situations in which the use of sedation is considered need to be assessed individually. Rarely, with idiosyncratic reactions to the sedation, it may be necessary to keep the child in the hospital overnight to ensure complete recovery. Sedation is most often used for patients 1 to 5 years old, especially for bone imaging, SPECT, PET, and hybrid imaging. Patients of any age who have neurodevelopmental handicaps or behavior problems may need sedation. Special consideration must be given to sedating a child with a brain injury, respiratory distress, cyanosis, or a history of an adverse reaction to sedation. The technologist and physician must be aware of all medications the child is receiving and the time of the last administered dose.

The American Academy of Pediatrics has published guidelines for the sedation and recovery of children.[11] These guidelines emphasize the use of approximate administered doses to reach various levels of consciousness and appropriate monitoring of vital signs using modern devices such as electronic oxygen saturation monitors. Children with severe systemic disease should be cared for by an anesthesiologist if sedation is required. All personnel monitoring sedated children must be certified in pediatric CPR, and all information regarding the pharmaceutical, dose administered, monitoring, and recovery must be permanently documented as part of the patient's record. State or local laws may also regulate sedation, such as who can administer it, but in all cases a physician must be readily available on-site. If anesthesia is considered, appropriate information should be given to the parents at the time the appointment is scheduled. Finally, the parent must be cautioned that delayed reactions can occur and they must be given written instructions and emergency phone numbers to call if any are observed. It is highly preferable that an institutional policy (and procedure) for the use of sedation, which follows established guidelines, be in place before any sedatives are used. The policy should also include quality improvement processes and oversight.[52]

Examples of pharmaceuticals used for sedation of a healthy child include chloral hydrate and midazolam. Chloral hydrate can be administered orally or rectally and is generally effective within 20 to 30 minutes. Midazolam can be administered as a nasal spray[48] to achieve patient cooperation, particularly for studies of the bladder. Lesser doses of all sedatives are recommended for children who are debilitated or who have respiratory or neurological deficits.

The effectiveness of chloral hydrate and other sedation pharmaceuticals is variable. Some children may require a longer time to go to sleep and others may never fall asleep completely but are quieted enough to enable the technologist to perform the imaging procedure. An occasional child might exhibit an adverse or opposite effect to the sedation, that is, become more combative and uncontrollable. This is more likely if the child is allowed to become extremely agitated before sedation. Frequently, a history of sedative use indicates whether a given pharmaceutical is appropriate to use for sedation. If chloral hydrate is not indicated or if there are other medical reasons, an anesthesiologist should be consulted. Very rarely, the child may need to be admitted to the hospital and be given a general anesthetic so that the procedure can be performed. In all situations, appropriate emergency equipment is necessary to respond to possible allergic reactions or other emergencies. The equipment should be kept close by, and all technologists must be aware of the location of these supplies and how to activate an emergency response team.

Patient–Parent Interaction

A major consideration in pediatric imaging is the psychological interaction between the child and the parent or family unit.[81] A pediatric study usually necessitates dealing with a family unit, that is, the parent, the child, and at times other members of the family as well. Frequently, either the parent or the child indicates apprehension about the procedure. The examination should be explained to the child as well as the parent. One explanation is given in terms that the parent will understand and another at the level of the child's understanding. The nuclear medicine technologist must assess the situation and determine which of the explanations should be given first. If the patient is younger than 3 years, it is of little value to discuss the study with the child. If the patient is an older child, the parent's explanation becomes secondary.

If the patient is of childbearing age, the importance of inadvertent radiation exposure of a fetus must be considered. The technologist should directly address the issue of possible pregnancy (a girl's sexual activity may begin as early as 10 years of age). It is appropriate to determine the date of the patient's last menstrual cycle and to inquire if the patient is sexually active. The adolescent may deny sexual activity in the presence of the parent or others; therefore the technologist should question the patient privately.[13] There may be occasions or policies that require females of a certain age to have a blood pregnancy test before having an imaging procedure or therapy performed. The information should be noted in the patient's nuclear medicine record.

Assessment of the patient–parent relationship and interaction is important for successful performance of a nuclear medicine examination of a pediatric patient. The parent may convey apprehension or other emotions to the child in many ways, both verbally and nonverbally. This communication has a direct effect on the child's behavior. The parenting philosophy may have a direct effect on the child's behavior as well. For example, if the parent is permissive, the child might refuse to cooperate, and the parent might not intervene or even perceive a need to intervene to correct the child's behavior. Other parents exhibit strict, authoritarian parenting techniques, and the child might be passive.

It might be appropriate for the technologist or the nuclear medicine physician to privately discuss with the parent the effect of the parent's behavior on the child and the technologist's ability to perform a successful examination. Generally, it is preferable to allow the parent to accompany the child into the imaging room to observe the entire procedure.[10] It is usually more comforting to the child to have the parent in attendance. However, if a child is uncooperative and the technologist cannot gain the child's cooperation with the assistance of the parent, it may be necessary to ask the parent to leave the room until the child agrees to cooperate. The technologist must be firm and authoritative in the approach to the child to maintain control of the situation. Patient cooperation should be praised, both to the child and to the parent. Allowing the child to participate in the study, for example, by letting the child control the remote stop-start switch on the gamma camera, enhances further cooperation.

Cooperation is often accomplished by dealing truthfully with the child. For example, if an injection is necessary, it is preferable to tell the child that there will be some discomfort. To do otherwise ensures loss of trust and cooperation. The technologist must also listen to the child's complaints and respond to them appropriately (Table 23-1). The technologist should never allow the child to become abusive, either physically or verbally, and the child should be rewarded for good behavior and cooperation. Presenting small toys or other items as gifts to the patient upon completion of the study is a good method of reinforcing the child's perception of the experience as being nontraumatic. In many institutions, technologists provide children with a choice of rewards from a "goodie box" before discharging them from the department.

Dose Administration: Injection Technique

For successful intravenous administration of a radiopharmaceutical to the pediatric patient, the injection should be performed by individuals whose attributes include a delicate manual dexterity, calmness under stressful conditions, and an empathetic nature. Nuclear medicine technologists might be the most capable for this task, because they receive formal training in phlebotomy and, unless otherwise prohibited by state regulation, are readily available to perform most radiopharmaceutical administrations.

It is commonly believed that an IV injection in an infant or child is more difficult. However, when proper technique is used, the procedure is successful in the vast majority of cases. The following technique has been used with a very high success rate.[18] The technique requires an appropriate explanation to the child, ready availability of the required materials, and preferably two individuals, one to insert the needle and the other to assist in immobilizing the patient. The child should be told that the injection will cause a small sensation of pain and that it is appropriate to cry when it hurts. In fact, many times when the child is told to scream "ouch" when it hurts, the child concentrates so heavily on the expectation of pain, that the injection is completed without the child realizing the needle has been inserted.

A tray should be prepared that includes all the necessary items for administration of the radiopharmaceutical. Included on the tray should be winged infusion sets of a variety of sizes, usually 21-, 23-, and 25-gauge needles, and a three-way disposable stopcock with the radionuclide syringe attached to one port and a syringe of normal saline (minimum 10 ml) attached to the side port (Figure 23-1). Alcohol wipes, dry 2 × 2 sterile sponges, a pediatric-size tourniquet, disposable sterile gloves, hypoallergenic tape for fixation of the needle, and various sizes of support boards are also needed. The tray is lined with plastic-backed disposable paper to prevent

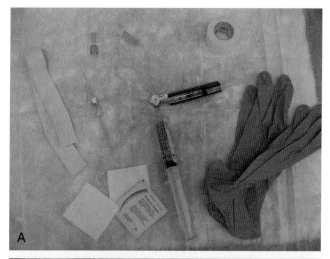

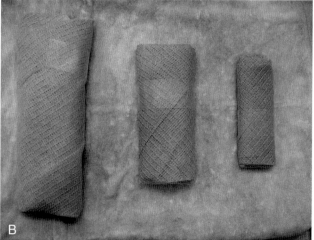

FIGURE 23-1 Injection tray used to transport all required materials from the preparation area to the injection room. **A,** Note that some materials are duplicated in case more than one attempt must be made to insert the intravenous line. **B,** IV arm boards of various sizes are used to restrict movement of an extremity.

contamination in case the radionuclide spills. The syringe containing the radiopharmaceutical should be enclosed in a lead syringe shield.

The injection should be performed using aseptic technique and universal precautions. The selection of an injection site is of utmost importance. All the preferred injection sites should be examined before an attempt is made to insert the needle. Several sites are objectionable and should be used only under unusual circumstances. The antecubital veins are often deeply situated and are not visible or palpable in young children. They are often used for blood sampling and, as a consequence, have often been traumatized before the child reaches the nuclear medicine department. It is possible to infiltrate the entire radiopharmaceutical dose into the antecubital space without observing any indication of extravasation. Scalp veins are not only aesthetically objectionable and more frightening to the child, but often trauma to the scalp and extravasation produce significant injection

TABLE 23-1	Child Growth and Development and Strategies for Working with Children in Health Care Settings			
Normal Development	**Child's Understanding**	**Related Responses**	**Interventions**	
Infants (0-18 months)				
Closely attached to parent Explores self and environment Calls for attention Experiences separation anxiety; "makes strange" with strangers	May sense anxiety transmitted by parent	Distress/protest, crying Developmental regression Clinging Rejection of new relationships/strangers Rejection of activities/objects Withdrawal	Maximize parental information and involvement Encourage touch, swaddling, and/or comfort positioning before, during, or after procedures Provide multisensory stimulation (visual, auditory, tactile, kinesthetic, vestibular) Promote sucking reflex where possible Incorporate familiar toys/play	
Toddlers (18 months-3 years)				
Achieves developmental milestones: language, walking, feeding, toileting Able to recall images Interacts socially (e.g., makes eye contact, shows off) Asks for information Begins use of symbolization; will engage in dramatic play Highly egocentric view of the world	Interpret experience in egocentric perspective (i.e. she caused pain, illness, hospitalization) May sense anxiety transmitted by parent	Protest (verbal and physical) Temper tantrums Developmental regression Sleep disturbances Separation anxiety Withdrawal	Maximize parental information and involvement Talk to the child as well as the parent Whenever possible, allow the child to hold or see a familiar object/toy Minimize use of excessive restraint	
Preschool (3-6 years)				
Transitions between dependence upon perception and logical thinking Learns by watching and listening; interested in purpose and function of objects Extremely sensitive and concerned with body integrity	May view hospitalization as punishment; fear of abandonment May watch other patients and believe they will receive the same treatment May sense anxiety transmitted by parent	Developmental regression Anger directed at primary caregiver Acting out Protest, aggression, physically defense Dependency Withdrawal	Maximize parental involvement and information Involve the child as much as possible (i.e., give them a specific "job" to master) Offer choices when available Build rapport using clues about the child (e.g., referencing his toy, T-shirt, etc.)	
School-Aged (6-12 years)				
Begins to think logically and can comprehend a series of actions Understands basic descriptions of internal functions Understands analogies Becomes aware of personal strengths and limitations Increases in independence and competitiveness	Expects things to make sense Senses physical limitations of hospital, frustration with rules Disruption of normal routine with family, friends, at school Fear of loss of control, loss of mastery, bodily mutilation, bodily injury, illness, disability, and death	Confusion (i.e., needles used to stop pain) Developmental regression Withdrawal Depression Displaced anger and hostility	Maximize parental information and involvement Give choices whenever possible Explain procedures simply, fully, and honestly; clarify misconceptions Encourage opportunities for peer support	
Adolescents (12-18 years)				
Develops capacity for abstract thinking Increases in independence; spends more time with friends Increases in need for privacy Concerns about body image and sexuality Goal- and future-oriented	Experience loss of independence, increased dependency on staff and caregiver(s) Discomfort/anxiety with exposing her body to unfamiliar people Understand implications of illness and hospitalization on future plans/peer group status Fear of bodily injury and pain, loss of identity	Anxiety (especially re: body image); embarrassment (re: altered physical appearance) Developmental regression (deference to caregivers, staff) Noncompliance Withdrawal Feelings of loss and sadness associated with unfulfilled goals	Explain procedures fully and honestly Provide privacy; ask permission to touch Encourage self-expression/advocacy Respect independence and decision-making capacity Encourage opportunities for peer support Respect the adolescent's choice/need re: degree of caregiver involvement in care	

Courtesy of Deidre Tamlin, Catia Stuart, and Catherine Leung, Child Life Specialists, BC Children's Hospital.
From Rollins J, Bolig R, Mahan C: *Meeting children's psychosocial needs across the health-care continuum,* Austin, Tex., 2005, PRO-ED.

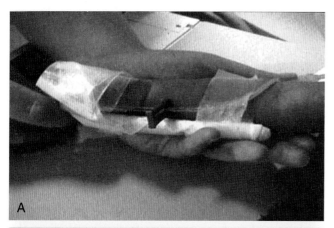

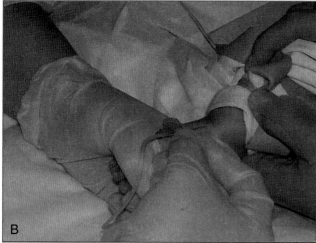

FIGURE 23-2 **A,** Immobilization of the hand for injection. **B,** Foot injection technique.

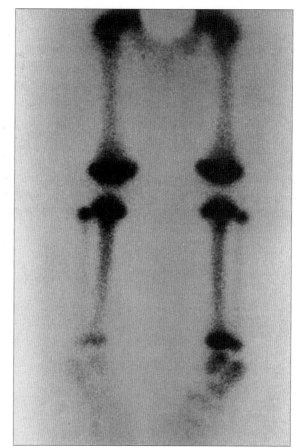

FIGURE 23-3 Increased localization of radiopharmaceutical in the left lower extremity caused by tourniquet effect of the restraint during injection of radionuclide in to the foot.

artifacts on subsequent images. Femoral and jugular vein injections should not be routinely used and should only be attempted by a professional trained in these techniques. Serious complications such as hip joint infection and femoral artery thrombosis have been reported from attempting to use the femoral veins.[53] And the use of jugular veins is difficult because of the manipulations necessary to produce venous dilation, such as extending the head and neck and forcibly restraining the child's head to one side. This technique is also aesthetically objectionable to the parents and a very frightening experience for the child.

Preferred sites include the veins on the dorsum of the hand and the foot. The veins in these sites usually are not already traumatized, because they are rarely used for blood sampling, are usually visible because of their superficial location, and are usually oriented linearly. In addition, during a dynamic study the hands and feet are usually more accessible if the child is beneath the camera, and they are easily immobilized for the injection.[15]

Immobilization of the hand or the foot can easily be accomplished by holding the wrist or the foot between the index and middle finger and holding the patient's fingers or toes down with the thumb (Figure 23-2). Extension of the joint at the elbow and flexion at the

wrist further immobilizes the hand veins and reduces the patient's ability to withdraw the extremity. Extension of the knee and ankle joints helps immobilize the veins on the dorsum of the foot. In older children it is helpful to have a second person gently restrain the arm or leg. If this is done, the technologist must remember to loosen all restraints for a short interval before injecting the radiopharmaceutical so as not to produce a tourniquet effect artifact[83] (Figure 23-3).

The size of the needle should match the size of the vein. The needle is connected to the three-way stopcock with the valve on the stopcock positioned such that the saline syringe portal is open to the needle. Saline is flushed through the needle before use. The venipuncture should be performed with the bevel of the needle in the down position. In this manner the needle bevel enters parallel to the vein and not at an angle. It is preferable to direct the needle between the confluence of branching vessels into a single vein. As soon as the needle has entered the vein, blood immediately refluxes into the infusion tubing at the needle hub. Application of suction by drawing back on the saline syringe is unnecessary in children because blood in the needle hub does not appear unless the needle is intravenously located, and it can safely be concluded that the vein has been entered. In adults the larger diameter veins may not exhibit suffi-cient pressure beyond the tourniquet to reflux blood into the needle hub.

When blood is seen in the tubing, no further manipu-lation of the needle should be attempted, such as thread-ing the needle into the vein, because further manipulation frequently results in perforation of the opposite venous wall or dislodgment from the vein. At this point, the needle should be secured in place with appropriate tape or transparent film dressing. The tourniquet should be immediately released and a test injection of saline made to confirm the intravenous placement. Any immediate swelling around the site of the needle tip indicates an extravascular location and necessitates removal of the needle and use of another site. If the test injection of saline confirms appropriate placement of the needle, the stopcock is switched to the radionuclide syringe for administration of the radiopharmaceutical. A short delay before injecting the radiopharmaceutical is suggested to eliminate the tourniquet effect artifact. During the injection, passage of the saline or radiopharmaceutical through the veins over the wrist or foot can be observed and felt beneath the technologist's index finger. Once the radiopharmaceutical syringe is empty, the residual activ-ity within the stopcock and tubing is flushed with the remaining saline.

Other methods of radiopharmaceutical dose adminis-tration include oral, inhalation, and intrathecal routes. Intravenous administration has already been discussed. Oral delivery of radiopharmaceutical can be by mouth, indwelling nasogastric tube, or gastrostomy tube, depending on the procedure. If such an administration is required the patient is fed as tolerated. If delivery is by inhalation, such as for ventilation study, the patient is fit with an appropriate size mask and they will then practice breathing before actual administration of the radiopharmaceutical. Intrathecal administration for cerebrospinal fluid (CSF) studies requires sterile tech-nique and is always performed by a physician according to established protocols. A free flow of bloodless CSF is critical to a successful intrathecal administration.

Regardless of the method of administration, the dose administered must be recorded. Often this documenta-tion is an administered dose sticker that includes the initials of the technologist injecting, the time injected, the method of administration and the site of injection. This dose sticker is affixed to the exam requisition and is scanned into picture archiving and communications system (PACS) to remain a permanent part of the patient's record.

Calculation of a Pediatric Radiopharmaceutical Dose

The several methods proposed to calculate the amount of administered radioactivity for a specific study may be based on the child's weight and/or body surface area, estimation of organ volume, or a percentage of an adult dose, or it may even be a fixed dose. However, these methods often underestimate administered doses at the lower end of the scale or overestimate them at the upper end of the scale. A minimum amount of radioactivity is required for adequate imaging, even in the smallest child. Selection of a method or individual administered dose should be based on the principle of ALARA. Conversely, a maximum limit should be established. The method used for radiopharmaceutical administered dose deter-mination at many institutions is empirically derived. That is, the administered dose ranges are determined by experience based on several factors, including the patient's condition, the imaging technique desired (e.g., static versus dynamic imaging, and limited bone imaging versus SPECT imaging), the imaging equipment to be used, the radionuclide energy, the biological half-life of the radiopharmaceutical, and the percentage of the administered dose that localizes in the organ of interest.

The empirically determined radiopharmaceutical dose is primarily based on the interval for which most patients are able to remain still. When they are being fed, most children and even babies are able to remain still for as long as 5 minutes. Based on that assumption, the empiri-cal method estimates the radiopharmaceutical dose required to obtain a specific type of image at the appro-priate time interval after injection that can be acquired in 5 minutes for a specific imaging technique; that is, the use of magnification, choice of collimator, and the sen-sitivity of the camera. Based on the empirical method and experience, recommended radiopharmaceutical dose ranges for common radionuclide studies are provided in Table 23-2.

Some radiopharmaceutical package inserts contain information about the recommended administered dose to be used in children. Some do not, however, because many radiopharmaceuticals have not been tested specifi-cally for safety and efficacy in the pediatric population. This is because phase II and III clinical trials are costly and difficult to perform in the pediatric population. The U.S. Food and Drug Administration (FDA), in coopera-tion with its Radiopharmaceutical Drug Advisory Com-mittee and members of the Pediatric Nuclear Medicine Council of the Society of Nuclear Medicine, has worked to provide labeling information for pediatric radiophar-maceuticals and continues to do so. Most radiopharma-ceutical companies provide technical support services to give assistance in cases in which the package insert infor-mation is not available. These services maintain informa-tion derived from the literature on pediatric administered doses for their products to disseminate to their custom-ers. Other sources of information on recommended pediatric administered doses are the local commercial radiopharmacies.

TABLE 23-2	Pediatric Administered Doses			
Procedure	**Radiopharmaceutical**	**Administered Dose***	**Minimum**	**Maximum**
Brain SPECT perfusion	^{99m}Tc-HMPAO	285 µCi/kg	10 mCi	20 mCi
Cardiac shunt	^{99m}Tc-pertechnetate	5 mCi	5 mCi	5 mCi
Liver scintigraphy	^{99m}Tc–sulfur colloid	85 µCi/kg	2 mCi	6 mCi
Lung scintigraphy	^{99m}Tc-MAA	0.07 mCi/kg	0.4 mCi	2 mCi
Renogram	^{99m}Tc-DTPA	0.5 mCi/kg	1 mCi	10 mCi
	^{99m}Tc-MAG3	0.15 mCi/kg	0.5 mCi	2 mCi
Renal scintigraphy	^{99m}Tc-DMSA	0.05 mCi/kg	1.35 mCi	3 mCi
Bone scintigraphy	^{99m}Tc-diphosphonate	0.25 mCi/kg	2.7 mCi	15 mCi
PET bone scintigraphy	^{18}F-sodium fluoride	0.06 mCi/kg	0.5 mCi	10 mCi
Cystogram	^{99m}Tc-DTPA	Standard dose	1 mCi	1 mCi
Thyroid uptake/scintigraphy	^{123}I sodium iodide	4 µCi/kg	0.14 mCi	0.27 mCi
Thyroid scintigram	^{99m}Tc-pertechnetate	0.03 mCi/kg	0.27 mCi	2 mCi
Gallium scintigraphy	^{67}Ga-citrate	0.14 mCi/kg	3 mCi	10 mCi
MUGA study	^{99m}Tc–red blood cells	0.28 mCi/kg	5 mCi	20 mCi
Meckel scintigraphy	^{99m}Tc-pertechnetate	0.05 mCi/kg	2.0 mCi	5 mCi
Gastrointestinal bleeding	^{99m}Tc labelled RBC	0.14 mCi/kg	2 mCi	10 mCi
Gastroesophageal reflux	^{99m}Tc–sulfur colloid	Standard dose	0.54 mCi	0.54 mCi
Gastric emptying	^{99m}Tc–sulfur colloid	Standard dose	0.54 mCi	0.54 mCi
Hepatobiliary study	^{99m}Tc-mebrofenin	0.05 mCi/kg	0.8 mCi	5 mCi
MIBG scintigraphy	^{131}I-MIBG	0.14 mCi/kg	5 mCi	10 mCi
Testicular scintigraphy	^{99m}Tc-pertechnetate	0.05 mCi/kg	2.0 mCi	5 mCi
PET imaging	^{18}F-FDG	0.1 to 0.14 mCi/kg	1.0 mCi	10 mCi

DTPA, Diethylenetriamine pentaacetic acid; *FDG*, fluorodeoxyglucose; *HMPAO*, hexamethyl propyleneamine oxime; *HSA*, human serum albumin; *MAA*, microaggregated albumin; *MAG3*, mercaptoacetyl triglycine; *MIBG*, metaiodobenzylguanidine; *MUGA*, multiple gated acquisition.
*The nuclear medicine physician might double or increase the dose depending on the clinical situation, such as an uncooperative or retarded child or a critical condition, to expedite the study and optimize results.

Often the administered pediatric dose is weight-based as a multiplier of adult dose with a minimum and maximum range (see Table 23-2). A survey of North American pediatric nuclear medicine centers on their administered doses has shown variability in the administered dose of radiopharmaceutical.[80] In an attempt to standardize doses of radiopharmaceuticals, the European Association of Nuclear Medicine (EANM) published a pediatric dose card based on a baseline activity and the weight of the child (www.eanm.org/scientific_info/dosagecard/dosagecard.php). The calculation for administered activity in MBq is baseline activity × multiple depending on weight, with minimum of 40 MBq administered activity.[42] The EANM website has the dosage card for all common radiopharmaceuticals and recommended administered radiopharmaceutical doses in children.[47] However, the appropriateness of using international references must be determined for one's own country.

Preparing the Patient and the Camera

Given the differences of children in accepting new surroundings and clinical procedures, advance preparation of the room and equipment facilitates a smooth onset to the study. It is preferable to obtain as many images as possible with the gamma camera beneath the patient. This serves two purposes: (1) it is a frightening experience for the child to have the massive detector overhead, and (2) it is easier to monitor condition and vital signs without the detector obscuring the view of the child. In addition, older children are able to watch television, read a book, or be otherwise distracted. For anterior images the child can be placed prone on the imaging table. A small patient can be placed directly on top of the collimator for imaging.

Of paramount importance is appropriate positioning of the child within the gamma camera's field of view. The determination of abnormal radionuclide localization depends on comparison of one site with its contralateral side. This can readily be accomplished only if the patient's position is anatomical and symmetrical (Figure 23-4). If it is impossible to position the patient anatomically because of the clinical condition, both sides should be malpositioned identically and symmetrically to allow comparison. Anatomical positioning is even more important for SPECT imaging because a slight rotation can cause the appearance of increased or decreased activity on individual tomographic slices as an artifact of positioning. Current state-of-the-art SPECT software can correct some poor positioning rotational artifacts. When using the SPECT imaging table, it might be preferable to place the patient prone, because many children sleep in this manner and therefore are more comfortable in this position. It also may be advantageous to position the child feet first, rather than head first, in the gantry, so that the patient can look up from that position and see something other than the back of the gantry.

Of particular concern is the safety of the patient on the narrow SPECT imaging table. A patient safety restraint was developed that wraps around the child and the imaging table using Velcro strapping, thus securing the patient to the table to prevent falls (Figure 23-5) and ensure immobilization. The device does not attenuate, because it is made of vinyl and Velcro strapping.

CLINICAL APPLICATIONS

This section reviews the most commonly performed pediatric nuclear medicine procedures, with particular attention to technique. This is not meant to be a comprehensive review of all pediatric nuclear medicine procedures. For specific topics not included in this section, the reader should examine the current literature and the other chapters of this textbook related to specific imaging procedures.

Skeletal System

Bone scintigraphy is among the most common scintigraphic procedures performed in children. It requires particular attention to technical detail. The technologist should be familiar with the appearance of normal pediatric bone radiopharmaceutical localization and with skeletal anatomy so as to use appropriate positioning and to recognize artifacts.

Clinical indications for bone scintigraphy include infection, occult trauma, tumor localization, sports injuries, and orthopedic disorders such as avascular necrosis.[16] Additional indications include inflammation,

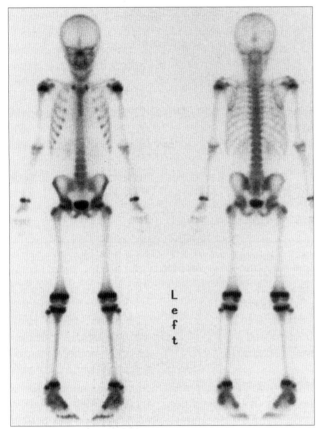

FIGURE 23-4 Symmetrical positioning for a whole-body bone scan allows comparison of one side with the other.

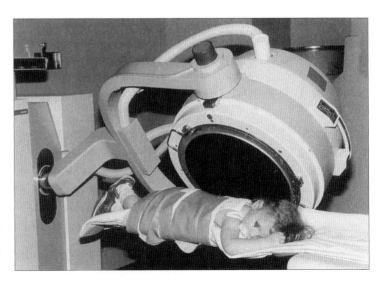

FIGURE 23-5 Patient restraining device is used as a safety belt during SPECT imaging. Note the patient's position, prone and with the feet toward the detector gantry; this position is comforting to some patients.

staging primary bone malignancy, evaluation of metastatic disease, nonaccidental injury, bone dysplasia, and evaluation for chronic regional pain syndromes. Finally, the bone scintigram has a valuable whole-body survey role in the case of a child who limps or refuses to bear weight, when the cause is not apparent on plain radiography. In these cases, a negative bone scintigram excludes significant pathology with a very high degree of confidence. Because the technique of bone scintigraphy requires a 3-hour delay between injection of the radiopharmaceutical and acquisition of the static images, the technologist has adequate time to assess the patient's ability to cooperate and to arrange for appropriate medication or sedation and monitoring, if necessary. The administration of medication or sedation should be given at an appropriate time before the scheduled imaging procedure to allow adequate time for the sedation to take effect. If SPECT imaging is to be done, the SPECT study should be obtained as soon as the patient has fallen asleep, if possible, to ensure adequate sedation throughout the SPECT acquisition. At times this is not possible, because the site of the abnormal localization is unknown and routine static images must be acquired first to identify the location.

For specific clinical indications, bone scintigraphy is performed in one to three phases. A one-phase bone scan consists of delayed static images acquired at 3 hours after injection. For a two-phase bone imaging procedure, an immediate extracellular (blood pool) whole-body image and or image of the area of interest is acquired within the first few minutes after injection, and delayed static images are acquired at 3 hours. The three-phase bone scan includes a dynamic acquisition of the area of interest begun immediately after injection, followed by blood pool images and routine static images at 3 hours after injection. Some pediatric nuclear medicine physicians no longer use a three-phase bone scan and feel that a two-phase scan with whole-body blood pool imaging and then delayed imaging is the optimum technique.[71]

Whole-body images allow the interpreter to survey the entire skeleton, which is helpful in recognizing patterns of distribution, malposition, and subtle asymmetrical localizations. Because, diseases in children are often systemic but can present with localized pain, a potential diagnosis of metastatic bone disease may be missed if the whole body is not surveyed. The distribution pattern often defines the disease process, such as in **child abuse,** in which diaphyseal localization in the extremities may be indicative of a shaken child.

A normal distribution pattern in the physes of the child is recognized.[3,22] The physes at the knees have greater activity than the physes at the ankles, which in turn have greater activity than the physes of the hips. The reverse is true in the upper extremities. The physes at the shoulder have greater activity than the physes at the wrists, which have greater activity than the physes

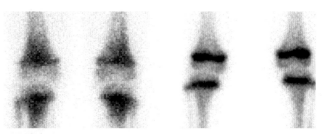

FIGURE 23-6 Symmetrical metaphyseal abnormality that can be seen in children with neuroblastoma, lymphoma, leukemia on *left image*, compared to normal metaphyseal appearance on *right image*.

at the elbows. Knowledge of these patterns allows differentiation of abnormalities, increased or decreased, at any given joint.[14] The differences in the various physes are altered if the images are obtained in the anterior or posterior position because of varying distances from the camera. However, the physes should always appear linear on good quality spot or whole-body images. Single spot images of the extremities do not allow detection of subtle differences in localization because exact positioning of the areas of interest is difficult to achieve. Patterns of subtle symmetrical metaphyseal abnormality that can occur with various tumors such as neuroblastoma, leukemia, and lymphoma can be missed when this pattern is not recognized (Figure 23-6).[15]

It should also be noted that recent bone or joint intervention will affect tracer distribution and confound interpretation, and for this reason bone scintigraphy following procedures such as joint aspiration and bone biopsy is to be avoided. The acquisition of 24-hour delayed images may be useful in certain cases, for example, where the distinction between cellulitis and osteomyelitis cannot be confidently made on the basis of the standard imaging protocol. It should be noted that although the background to lesion activity ratio is advantageous at 24 hours, the absolute count rate is low and image acquisition time needs to be extended accordingly. The use of side markers is also mandatory in pediatric bone scintigraphy.

In children, the affected limb in the majority of cases of reflex sympathetic dystrophy (RSD) shows decreased tracer activity, rather than increased, as is more commonly seen in the adult population. In RSD, the localization is dependent upon the stage of the process, and children complain earlier than adults. As in adult practice, the bone scintigram must be interpreted within the context of the other imaging investigations that have been obtained.

Careful attention should be paid to the statistics of the images acquired. When a whole-body imaging device is used, a minimum of 1 million counts per image is required. Both anterior and posterior whole-body images with the patient positioned anatomically and symmetrically are necessary for an adequate survey (Figure 23-7).

Patients younger than 5 years and older patients of short stature should have survey images done as spot films with magnification as necessary to provide sufficient detail. In addition to the whole-body survey images, spot images should be acquired for either time or counts so that an optimized image is obtained. Subsequent spot magnification of particular areas of interest should be acquired using sufficient time or count acquisition parameters individualized for the specific equipment. Limited one-phase bone scintigraphy is used in some facilities for follow-up examination, such as for Legg-Calvé-Perthes disease follow-up. Such a study consists of whole body view, spot views of the pelvis (anterior anatomic projection of the hips and posterior frog-leg lateral of the hips), plus pinhole anterior and/or frog-leg magnified views of the hips as well as SPECT. These magnified views should exclude the bladder and include only the acetabulum and hips to the level of the lesser trochanter (Figure 23-8).

For bone scintigraphy usually noncontrast, non-attenuation correction CT scan is performed of the area of interest using limited CT acquisition to the area of abnormality on the bone scintigram to minimize exposure to the patient. The parameters for acquisition of the CT study would be similar to those used for conventional stand-alone CT study. Dose modulation is applied to all CT acquisitions. Images are reconstructed and displayed in multiple formats for both fused and unfused images. All advanced processing that can be performed for conventional CT can be applied to CT images acquired on a multislice SPECT-CT hybrid device.

Infection. Bone scintigraphy is the most sensitive and specific imaging technique currently available for differentiating septic arthritis, cellulitis, and osteomyelitis.[41] Frequently x-ray examinations are completely normal in these disorders. Musculoskeletal infection is associated with pain and limitation of motion, and the patient usually but not always has an elevated erythrocyte sedimentation rate and frequently fever. In the neonatal population, however, the only clinical finding may be the lack of movement of an extremity. Early identification of septic arthritis or osteomyelitis is imperative to prevent bone or joint destruction and subsequent deformity. For example, an untreated septic arthritis of the hip of longer than 5 days' duration has a 50% probability

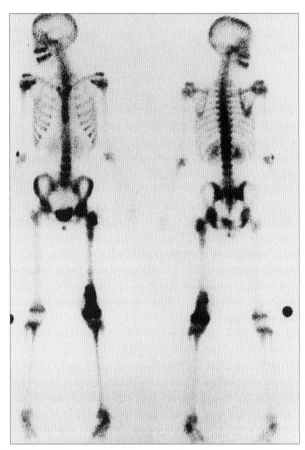

FIGURE 23-7 Whole-body images allowed recognition of abnormal localization of radionuclide in the scapula, which was not recognized on a limited bone scan performed at another institution.

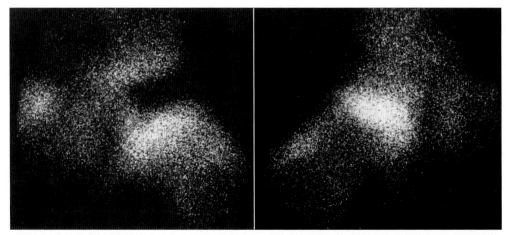

FIGURE 23-8 Pinhole views of the hips are acquired by positioning the hip in the center of the field of view and lowering the camera until the collimator is pressing on the patient's skin. The left hip demonstrates total avascularity of the epiphysis; the right hip is normal.

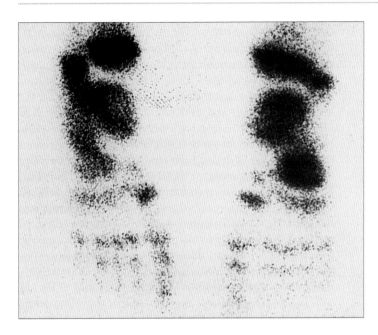

FIGURE 23-9 Electronically magnified image of both feet, which took 10 minutes of acquisition time and was required to visualize abnormal localization adequately.

of developing avascular necrosis of the proximal femoral epiphysis.[12]

The typical scintigraphic appearance of acute osteomyelitis is a well-defined focus of increased radionuclide localization, or "hot" lesion, seen on all three phases of the bone scan. The lesion is commonly in the metaphysis of the bone. On occasion, however, it presents as a photopenic, or cold lesion, when the vascular supply to the bone is compromised by surrounding tissue edema (compartment syndrome) or vascular thrombosis.[6] Detection and identification of ischemic osteomyelitis, which produces a cold area on the bone scan, warrant an emergency surgical drainage procedure to reduce the pressure in the tissues and enhance the return of blood flow. It should be noted that symptoms of infection should be present a minimum of 24 hours before performing bone scintigraphy to reduce the possibility of a false negative scintigram. It is therefore important to have all pertinent history as to onset of symptoms and prior treatment/procedures before undertaking to perform a bone study in a child.[25] Long-term intravenous antibiotic therapy may affect the scintigram.

Trauma. Because radionuclide scintigraphy has a high sensitivity for defining bone changes caused by trauma, it is an extremely useful tool for several disorders in the pediatric population. The normal bumps and bruises of childhood play do not produce abnormalities on bone scintigraphy. Significant or repeated trauma is required to produce perfusion and metabolic changes that are evident on bone scintigraphy. Several such conditions are well recognized, including occult fractures,[76] child abuse,[79] sports injuries,[62,66,67,85] and stress changes in the spine associated with spondylolysis.[33] Other conditions readily obvious on bone imaging and thought to be related to trauma are RSD[40] and myositis ossificans.[61] It

is important to note that all these disorders have a normal radiograph appearance in the early and sometimes even late stages.

A young child who is limping or refusing to walk but has a normal x-ray result will often demonstrate increased localization of radionuclide at a site of occult trauma. The lesion might be an occult undisplaced fracture or a microtrabecular bone injury. Frequent sites include the calcaneus, cuboid, patella, and metatarsal bones. Identification of abnormal radionuclide localization in the bones of the foot, particularly in a small child, requires magnification images to adequately distinguish the bone involved (Figure 23-9).

Correlative studies of bone scintigraphy versus x-ray survey examinations have documented that scintigraphy has a 27% greater sensitivity for recognizing bone trauma in child abuse.[79] Although radiographs provide better evidence of healed fractures and undisplaced hairline skull fractures, bone scintigraphy better demonstrates injuries of flat bones, such as the ribs, pelvis, and spine, and of soft-tissue injury. X-ray and bone scintigraphy, therefore, are used in a complementary manner to document evidence of child abuse. The technical quality of bone scintigraphy in child abuse is important, because most child abuse occurs in infants and children younger than 2 years. Their small bone structure requires high-resolution magnification imaging to define the appropriate information for interpretation.[2,22,47,86]

Organized competitive sports for children have become more popular in recent years. Because athletic activities require repeated practice of a particular motion or series of motions, a chronic and repetitive stress effect is exerted on the bones. This stress can produce focal metabolic changes that are evident on bone scintigraphy and that often are related to a particular type of sport. For example, teenagers who train as runners often develop shin splits or stress fractures of the tibia. Speed skaters, because of uneven stress on the feet as a result of the specific direction in which they race, may have a stress injury in one foot and not the other. Baseball pitchers demonstrate hypertrophy of the throwing arm. Frequently an athlete overlooks a specific trauma incident and is brought to the nuclear medicine department because of chronic and persistent bone pain. In many cases the information that the child participates in a particular sport frequently is either not conveyed or is not known by the referring physician. Often it is the nuclear medicine technologist who, when seeking a cause for the abnormal appearance on the bone scan, finally elicits the history of a specific sports trauma, which explains the scintigraphic findings.

Stress on the pars interarticularis of the vertebrae can cause spondylolysis, which can be evident on bone scintigraphy as a focal area of increased localization. The patient develops back pain without fever. It is common in weight lifters and football and basketball players. SPECT imaging is necessary in this disorder if the routine static images fail to demonstrate an abnormality or are equivocal.[19] SPECT imaging detects approximately one third more abnormalities than planar scintigraphic images. The addition of hybrid devices to perform SPECT-CT should also be considered. The CT would be performed as a limited noncontrast nonattentuation study through the area of scintigraphic abnormality or if no obvious lesion is seen scintigraphically, the fused imaging through the area of maximal pain may often detect unsuspected abnormality.[58] The addition of CT to the study is usually after the planar and SPECT imaging is reviewed with the patient still on the table. Radionuclide scintigraphy is much more sensitive than x-ray examinations in recognizing all the forms of sports trauma.

Hip Pain. Hip pain in the child may have a variety of causes, including toxic synovitis, septic arthritis, slipped capital femoral epiphysis,[75] and avascular necrosis of the femoral head.[16] Adequate imaging of the hip is achieved with the use of magnification techniques with a pinhole collimator,[63] SPECT, SPECT-CT, or a combination of these techniques. The technologist should position the pinhole collimator as close to the patient's normal hip as possible to include the entire area of interest. An anterior image is acquired for at least 100,000 counts. Subsequent images of the normal hip in the frog-leg lateral position and the painful hip in the anterior and frog-leg lateral positions are acquired for the same time as for the anterior image of the normal hip. The bladder must be emptied before imaging so that activity from a full bladder does not degrade the images by reducing the number of counts from the area of interest. If the child is unable to void, the bladder should be excluded from the image by using a lead shield.

Oncological Disorders. Children with oncological disorders benefit from bone scintigraphy for the diagnosis, staging, and assessment of disease response to therapy. These patients can also show a variety of focal abnormalities on bone scintigraphy that are unrelated to the neoplastic disease and that might be confusing in their interpretation. Children with oncological disorders may have osteoporosis from chemotherapy or poor nutrition; their bones are weaker; furthermore, they may be more susceptible to trauma or injury because of a physical handicap, such as an amputation and use of a prosthesis. Consequently, traumatic bone lesions frequently are detected on bone imaging performed for oncological reasons. Amputees can display abnormal radionuclide localization at the end of the stump or in the hemipelvis because of altered ambulation caused by a prosthetic device that induces uneven stress in the bone.[4] The use of crutches frequently causes increased radionuclide localization on the inner aspect of the proximal portion of the humeri. Conversely, diminished radionuclide localization, which appears as an asymmetry in the images, may be related to radiotherapy. It is important that the technologist who performs the bone scintigraphy procedure document such potential causes of abnormal localization to alert the nuclear medicine physician to allow for an appropriate interpretation of the abnormality.[37]

Bone SPECT Technique. As mentioned previously, SPECT bone scintigraphy is extremely valuable because of its greater sensitivity in detecting subtle localization abnormalities from occult metastases, occult trauma, or localized early infection. This is especially true in the examination of the spine. The anatomy of the spine is complex, x-ray changes appear late in the disease, and planar scintigraphy defines relatively gross abnormalities.

For studies of the hips and pelvis, artifacts caused by radionuclide accumulation in the bladder can be controlled by catheterization of the bladder with continuous drainage. The upper extremities in the field of view for chest SPECT are an additional problem, which can be controlled by strapping the arms above the head for studies of the thorax.

Data processing may be time-consuming in order to manipulate data from statistically poor frames as a result of limitation of the radionuclide administered dose or patient motion. Resolution recovery software, which is currently available, can improve image quality and may allow studies to be done with either decreased time or dose or a combination of the two. Standard protocols should not be used for data processing, because the information varies greatly from patient to patient. Computer systems that allow single-slice reconstruction with a variety of filters are helpful in determining the appropriate filter to be used for each individual patient. For SPECT images of the spine, quantification of abnormal localization of the radionuclide can be performed by

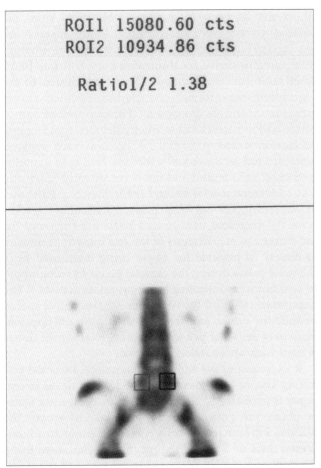

ROI1 15080.60 cts
ROI2 10934.86 cts

Ratio1/2 1.38

FIGURE 23-10 Quantitation of localization of radionuclide for bone SPECT imaging. Note the typical hot appearance of spondylolysis.

placing regions of interest over the abnormal area and the contralateral normal site to derive a ratio of activity (Figure 23-10).

Genitourinary System

Genitourinary procedures performed on pediatric patients include renography and renal scintigraphy, diuresis renography, direct radionuclide cystography (RNC), and scrotal scintigraphy. RNC and frequently renography require placement of a urinary bladder catheter to provide adequate drainage. It is useful for nuclear medicine technologists to develop the skill of bladder catheterization or for the nuclear medicine department to have an identified individual readily available to expedite the procedure and to prevent increased anxiety in the child by unnecessary delays in beginning the study. The technique of catheterization is described in the discussion on RNC.[81]

Renal Scintigraphy, Renography, and Diuresis Renography. Several disorders in childhood require imaging and function studies of the urinary tract, including infection, ureteropelvic or ureterovesical junction obstruction, **neonatal hydronephrosis** or hydroureteronephrosis, renal transplantation, renal vein thrombosis, and congenital anomalies in the neonate. Horseshoe kidneys, duplications, hypoplastic kidneys, and ectopic kidneys all can be diagnosed with radionuclide studies.[24]

A variety of radiopharmaceuticals have been developed for scintigraphic imaging and functional evaluation of the kidneys. ^{99m}Tc-mercaptoacetyltriglycine (^{99m}Tc-MAG3) has become the radiopharmaceutical of choice for imaging and functional analysis in pediatric genitourinary nuclear medicine.[70]

Cortical Scintigraphy. Renal cortical scintigraphy is performed using either ^{99m}Tc-glucoheptonate (^{99m}Tc-GH) or ^{99m}Tc-dimercaptosuccinic acid (^{99m}Tc-DMSA). The absorbed dose per millicurie is much less with ^{99m}Tc-GH; therefore higher activity angiographic images can be obtained. Significant bowel, liver, or collecting system localization have not been observed to interfere with the interpretation of the cortical regions of the kidneys when using magnification and oblique projections. However, ^{99m}Tc-DMSA has its advantages. Approximately 40% to 65% of the injected dose of ^{99m}Tc-DMSA binds to proximal convoluted tubule cells by 2 to 3 hours following intravenous injection. Hepatobiliary elimination only becomes significant in renal failure. Static imaging is performed at 3 hours postinjection, and for patients under 6 months of age, posterior and posterior oblique pinhole planar images of the kidneys are obtained using a high resolution collimator. For children over this age, posterior and posterior oblique planar images of the kidneys are obtained and are supplemented by SPECT. Regions of interest (ROIs) drawn around each kidney on the posterior image are used to calculate the differential renal function. ^{99m}Tc-DMSA is not seen within the renal medulla or collecting system, although in neonates and young infants, some tracer excretion may be seen within the urinary bladder. A differential function of the left kidney in the range of 45% to 57% is considered normal. Acute pyelonephritic defects are usually geographic, single, or multiple focal photopenic regions without associated volume loss, or as a generalized reduction in tracer activity in one or both kidneys. Such defects typically take 6 to 12 months or longer to resolve. For this reason, follow-up studies for detection of renal scarring in children with recurrent urinary tract infections should not be done within 3 months of a documented acute infection. Persisting wedge-shaped, ovoid, or flattened photopenic defects with associated volume loss imply cortical scarring. Coexisting acute pyelonephritis and scarring may only be reliably distinguished with follow-up studies. In the context of acute infection, a negative ^{99m}Tc-DMSA scan excludes kidneys that are at risk of scarring. The differential diagnosis of photopenic defects on the scan could be hydronephrosis or any space-occupying lesion such as a cyst, tumor, or abscess. It is often necessary to correlate scan findings with renal ultrasonography.

Renography. As a means of assessing renal clearance and excretion, dynamic radionuclide renography is commonly performed in the pediatric setting and, in general, the techniques are similar to those used in adult practice. The techniques used and interpretation of these renal studies are variable and still controversial. Common indications in children include the evaluation of renal tract dilatation, assessment of the efficacy of surgical intervention in cases of renal tract obstruction, assessment of a complex duplex kidney, and evaluation of the kidneys in cases of renal trauma and renal transplantation.

Renal clearance is radiopharmaceutical-dependent. ^{99m}Tc-diethylenetriamine pentaacetic acid (DTPA) is filtered at the glomerulus whereas ^{99m}Tc-MAG3 undergoes tubular extraction. ^{99m}Tc-MAG3 achieves greater renal clearance, resulting in a more favorable background to kidney activity ratio, and for this reason is the preferred radiopharmaceutical, especially in infants of less than 1 year of age, in whom glomerular filtration has not yet reached adult rates.

The child must be well hydrated before the examination is started. It is well-known that the state of hydration significantly affects the excretion of radiopharmaceuticals, particularly with diuretic stimulation.[20] Because of this, it is appropriate to control and monitor the patient's state of hydration for renography. Oral hydration to tolerance for at least 2 hours before the study should be encouraged. An alternative means of hydration is an intravenous administration of normal saline beginning at least 15 minutes before injection of the radiopharmaceutical and continuing through the remainder of the study.

Immediately before the beginning of the study, the patient should void. If the patient is unable to void on demand, the bladder should be catheterized to ensure adequate drainage during the study. Continuous bladder drainage reduces the absorbed radiation dose to the bladder and gonads and precludes patient movement caused by impending urination. If the catheter does not adequately empty the bladder, as observed on the persistence scope, urine should be aspirated using syringe suction.

Having voided, the child is positioned supine on the imaging table with the collimator directly beneath and is immobilized. Since both supine positioning and the presence of a full bladder can affect renal drainage. A postvoid image should be taken so that renal drainage may be assessed after the bladder has emptied. Similarly, a change of position, for example to the upright or prone position, following diuretic administration is essential to preclude apparent impairment of drainage due simply to supine positioning.

After the patient has voided, ^{99m}Tc-MAG3 (22 μCi/lb) is injected as a bolus with the patient positioned supine and the kidney region in the field of view of the gamma camera. Magnification is used as needed to adjust the image to include only the area from the xiphoid to the symphysis pubis. Static images are obtained at intervals for 20 minutes. Digital information is acquired to derive renal function curves. A rate of 15 or 20 sec/frame is acceptable. At the conclusion of the acquisition, background-subtracted time-activity curves are generated on the computer.[20] The choice of an appropriate background (ROI) is a hotly debated topic among nuclear medicine practitioners because each method described has a drawback[21]; the best course of action is to choose one method and use it consistently. Currently a circumferential ROI around the kidney for derivation of the renogram curve is preferred at many institutions.[28,78] Different background ROIs are preferred for the diuretic phase. Regions of interest must approximate as closely as possible the organ being monitored (e.g., the renal pelvis during the diuretic phase of renography) to be accurate in reflecting the appropriate activity.[44] The background ROI for the furosemide (Lasix) curve should exclude the ureter, and the ROI should closely approximate only the renal pelvis. A separate ROI for the ureter is used with hydroureteronephrosis.

If excretion of the radiopharmaceutical from the collecting system is delayed, furosemide[31,74] diuresis renography is performed.[65] If a urinary bladder catheter is not in place, the patient should be asked to empty the bladder. Furosemide diuresis is induced using an administered dose of 1 mg/kg. Acquisition is continued using the same parameters as the renogram phase of the study.

A variety of data analyses, in addition to the generation of time-activity curves for the whole kidney, can be performed. The percent differential renal function is the total counts from the renogram curve for each kidney minus background counts during the interval between 60 seconds and the initial appearance of radioactivity in the calyces. The time is best determined by viewing the computer images sequentially. The importance of the percent differential renal function in the presence of bilateral disease is questionable. Parenchymal transit time has been advocated as an effective means of differentiating obstruction from other causes of hydronephrosis.[84] Cortical renal function is derived from areas of interest over the kidney cortex as opposed to the entire kidney. The clearance half-life ($t_{1/2}$) response for the diuresis phase of the renogram is a simple quantitative calculation of the disappearance half-life. Unfortunately, the $t_{1/2}$ can be measured in at least eight ways,[21] and all produce different $t_{1/2}$ values for the same data. It is no wonder that the correlation of diuresis renography with surgical results and clinical outcomes has been variable. Although computer software programs are commercially available to calculate the $t_{1/2}$, the validity of these automatic programs may not be documented with outcomes.

Techniques such as measurement of the glomerular filtration rate (GFR) and effective renal plasma flow (ERPF) are performed occasionally; however, these techniques are time-consuming when performed using multiple blood samples and are considered technically unreliable in the young child when gamma camera techniques are used. Only relative estimates (±10% to 20%) are realistically derived even with meticulous techniques.

Radionuclide Cystography. Direct RNC for the detection of vesicoureteral reflux (VUR) is more advantageous than the conventional x-ray method because the absorbed radiation dose to the patient is reduced by a factor of at least 100,[23] various functional parameters relating to bladder function and reflux can be quantified, and the quantitative data have prognostic significance regarding the spontaneous cessation of reflux. This study may be performed for the assessment of VUR, either as an initial or a follow-up investigation in females. The presence of a low-lying or ectopic kidney poses a relative contraindication for direct RNC due to the inherent unreliability of detecting VUR in these cases, secondary to renal proximity to the bladder.

The techniques of direct and indirect RNC have evolved, beginning with the use of iodine-131 (^{131}I)-labeled x-ray contrast agents in early investigations by Winter[88] to an indirect method used by Dodge[27] in an attempt to eliminate catheterization. The indirect method depends on the rapid and complete clearance of the radionuclide through the kidneys after intravenous injection of the radiopharmaceutical. Imaging is then performed during and after voiding. A sudden increase in radioactivity in the upper tracts during and after voiding indicates reflux. The indirect method of RNC has reduced sensitivity when compared to the direct method, because VUR that occurs only during voiding is identified. Direct RNC allows quantification of the bladder volume at which VUR occurs,[60] measurement of the volume of VUR into the upper tracts,[87] determination of the drainage time of refluxed urine after voiding, and quantification of the residual urine volume. The direct radionuclide technique is more advantageous than the indirect method because it provides continuous monitoring during the filling, voiding, and postvoiding phases of bladder function, whereas the indirect technique examines the urinary tract only during voiding. The direct technique therefore is more sensitive in detecting VUR, because a significant percentage of VUR occurs during the filling phase at low bladder pressure and low bladder volume, which is not recognized by the indirect method. RNC is strongly recommended for follow-up studies to evaluate the efficacy of therapy for VUR.

When performing direct RNC, ^{99m}Tc-DTPA is instilled into the urinary bladder via a catheter placed using aseptic technique. There is no systemic tracer activity since absorption of ^{99m}Tc-DTPA from the urinary bladder is negligible. The administered dose is injected into the catheter tubing followed by an infusion of sterile normal saline under hydrostatic pressure. The infusion is terminated when either the calculated age-dependent maximum volume is reached or the child appears uncomfortable—whichever occurs first. Dynamic imaging with a general purpose collimator commences with bladder filling and terminates with the final micturition.

It is important to note that catheterization can be a simple and atraumatic experience if performed properly; however, it can also result in both physical and psychological trauma if the procedure is poorly performed by improperly trained or inexperienced personnel. The child should never be held down forcibly to accomplish catheterization. Rather, one person should assist the child in maintaining a frog-leg position and should maintain a conversation with the child during the procedure. Because the child cannot observe the procedure directly, it usually is a good practice to explain everything that is being done as it happens. This usually calms the patient, because it eliminates fear of the unknown. To accomplish catheterization, a Foley catheter is inserted into the bladder after aseptic preparation of the glans penis or perineum. The size of the catheter used depends on the sex and age of the child. A soft, size 8 French Foley catheter is used for girls up to 1 year of age. For girls between ages 1 and 3 years, a size 10 French Foley catheter is recommended, and for girls older than 3 years a size 12 French Foley catheter can be used. Generally, a catheter one size smaller is used in boys for each age group. Nonballoon catheters are not recommended, because patients tend to void around them and eject the catheter from the bladder. The use of stiff feeding tubes is not recommended because they are more hazardous, and perforation of the urethra or bladder can occur. The Foley balloon is expanded slowly and carefully, while the child's reaction is observed, to prevent injury in case of urethral or ureteral location of the balloon. Any sudden increase in the perception of pain should stop filling of the Foley balloon and an assessment of the catheter localization.

Whether the technologist performs the catheterization or not, the technique of direct RNC requires careful attention to multiple details to achieve an adequate study with clinically useful information. Because VUR is a dynamic process and may appear only fleetingly and in minimal amounts, technologists must constantly monitor the image to initiate the study at the appropriate time to document the reflux. Complete filling of the bladder is required for adequate performance of cystography, and a serious urge to void usually is associated with it, which can affect the patient's ability to cooperate.

Quantitative Data. In RNC, dynamic imaging commences with bladder filling and terminates with the final micturition. As part of the procedure, after catheterization, the bladder is emptied of residual urine, which is collected, measured, and recorded. The expected bladder capacity can be estimated based on the patient's age according to the formula developed by Berger and associates.[5] Normal bladder capacity in milliliters equals (age in years × 2) × 30.

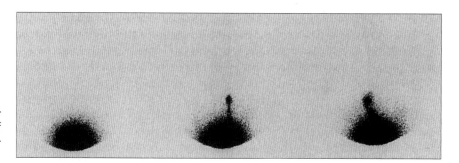

FIGURE 23-11 Posterior, left posterior oblique, and right posterior oblique images of the bladder and upper urinary tract, demonstrating vesicoureteral reflux on the right.

After 9 years of age, bladder capacities appear to vary from the formula. The formula is used only as rule of thumb, because capacities can also vary according to the health of the bladder. For example, smaller capacities have been documented after surgical procedures on the bladder or after recurrent infections.

A posterior and both posterior oblique images are obtained at a high-contrast setting with only the top of the bladder in the field of view. Only the top of the bladder should be included in the image; otherwise, the intense activity in the whole bladder will obscure recognition of small amounts of activity that may appear during reflux. Figure 23-11 demonstrates posterior and oblique views of the bladder and upper urinary tract demonstrating VUR. Using this technique, minimal amounts of VUR are adequately demonstrated. Dynamic Images are acquired at a rate of 5 seconds/frame. Rarely a fleeting minimal VUR occurs, which might not be demonstrated on permanent images. The technologist should note any other unusual occurrences to aid correct interpretation of the study. Then, a 2-minute posterior image is obtained, which includes the entire bladder and upper urinary tract. Total counts of the 2-minute image are recorded for use in calculating the residual volume. This image is acquired at a lower intensity setting to visualize any abnormalities of the bladder. The patient is then seated to void into a bedpan or a urinal, and the gamma camera is positioned against the patient's back. As the balloon of the catheter is deflated, the patient is encouraged to void. As the patient begins to void, the catheter should slide out of the bladder. Do not use suction to empty the Foley balloon, especially on boys since the balloon may wrinkle and obstruct the urethra. In such circumstance gently reinsert the catheter, refill it and allow it to drain slowly without suction. A voiding image is obtained as the patient empties the bladder. The same high-contrast setting as that used for the prevoid images is set for the voiding image to demonstrate the minimal reflux that can occur only during the higher pressures of voiding. Finally, a 2-minute postvoid image, including the bladder and the upper urinary tract, is obtained at a high-intensity setting. During data processing, ROIs may be drawn over the urinary bladder and kidneys to permit the generation of time-activity curves useful in study interpretation. An increase in tracer activity within the renal pelvis occurring during bladder filling, emptying, or both, and preferably shown on dynamic images as well as on time-activity curves derived from renal pelvic ROIs, implies VUR. It is described by the anatomical level to which it reaches, for example, ureter, renal pelvis, or parenchyma. The residual volume, total volume at maximum capacity, and the reflux bladder volume for each kidney can be determined according to formulas reported by Weiss and Conway.[82] It is important to remember that none of the calculated volumes is accurate if urine is lost during the procedure.

The addition of simultaneous recording of bladder pressures during direct RNC allows recognition of dysfunctional bladder abnormalities.[49] A physiological pressure transducer measures intravesical pressure through the drainage port of the Foley catheter. Using this method (the radionuclide cystometrogram), four pressure patterns have been characterized: normal, spastic-reflex, flaccid-paralytic, and uninhibited bladder contraction patterns. Patients with neurological bladder disorders have the spastic-reflex or flaccid-paralytic pattern. Children with voiding dysfunctions often have evidence of an uninhibited bladder contraction pattern.

Scrotal Scintigraphic Imaging. Scintigraphic imaging of a painful scrotum provides a useful screening study in determining the need for surgical exploration.[8,9] Torsion of the testis appears as a photopenic (cold) lesion because blood flow to the testicle is impaired by the torsion (Figure 23-12). Inflammatory lesions usually have increased activity in a painful scrotum. In general, ischemic lesions (torsion, abscess, tumor) are managed surgically, whereas hyperemic lesions (epididymitis, orchitis, torsion of the appendix testes) are managed nonsurgically.

Scintigraphy should be performed with a magnification technique such as converging or pinhole collimation. A lead apron shield is placed around and beneath the scrotum and over the thighs. U-shaped cutouts of an old lead apron are suitable for the variable sizes of the scrotum at different ages. The penis is gently taped upward on the abdomen with nonallergenic tape. ^{99m}Tc-pertechnetate is injected as a bolus to obtain a radionuclide angiogram of the scrotum so as to evaluate arterial perfusion. Angiographic images are obtained at 4 to 5 sec/image for 60 seconds. Static scintigraphy for a minimum of 1 million counts/view is obtained

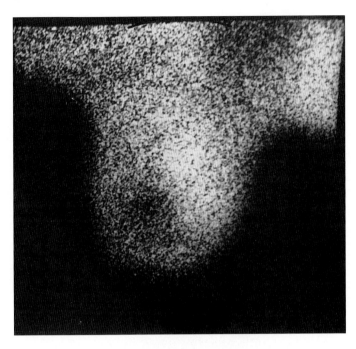

FIGURE 23-12 Magnified image of the scrotum demonstrates a photopenic (cold) lesion consistent with testicular torsion.

immediately after the angiogram and 10 minutes after injection. Finally, it is useful to obtain a static scan with a lead strip marker on the median raphe of the scrotum, because edema often distorts the size of the side of the scrotum involved, making comparison with the normal side difficult.

Although at one time, nuclear medicine was actively used for scrotal imaging, at this time, scrotal imaging is almost exclusively performed by medical ultrasonography techniques.

Gastrointestinal System

Radionuclide studies of the gastrointestinal tract in children have been a boon to pediatric gastroenterologists in the difficult diagnosis of such conditions as biliary atresia[50] and Meckel diverticulum.[68,69] Other conditions, such as **gastroesophageal reflux (GER)** and gastrointestinal (GI) bleeding, are investigated with radionuclide techniques. Technical considerations for the performance of these studies are different from those for the adult population, depending on the clinical condition in question.

Gastroesophageal Reflux. A common problem facing the pediatric practitioner is the infant or child who constantly "spits up" or vomits. Such findings may be a sign of GER. It is not unusual for a child to occasionally regurgitate after feedings, but frequent regurgitation can indicate a significant pathological cause. In addition to anatomical abnormalities such as esophageal stricture, tracheoesophageal fistula, and hiatal hernia, GER is associated with brain tumors, mental retardation, recurrent pneumonias, asthma, and sudden infant death syndrome (SIDS). Pediatricians are particularly concerned

about the relationship of GER to unexplained recurrent pneumonias.

Clinical Indications. GER studies can be used as a screening tool and as a confirmatory diagnostic tool. As a screening tool, radionuclide GER studies lack the ability to identify significant abnormalities of the swallowing mechanism, nasopharyngeal reflux, and significant anatomical abnormalities of the esophagus. Therefore it is recommended that in most circumstances, the x-ray esophagram be performed before the radionuclide GER study. If GER is present on the x-ray study, the radionuclide study is unnecessary. The radionuclide GER study is indicated if the x-ray study is normal, because the radionuclide procedure is a more sensitive technique, primarily because it examines the process of GER over a longer interval than is possible with the x-ray study. In addition, the clinician is interested in determining the frequency and magnitude of reflux. These factors help determine the necessity of surgical intervention, such as a Nissen fundoplication. The radionuclide study, therefore, assists in the determination of the severity of GER.

Factors Affecting Gastroesophageal Reflux. It is well documented that a number of factors increase the incidence of GER.

1. *Patient positioning.* GER occurs most frequently with the patient in the supine position.[64] The incidence of reflux in other positions, such as prone or decubitus, is significantly less. If reflux or vomiting occurs with the child in the supine position, the technologist must be prepared to turn the child's face to the side to prevent aspiration of the refluxed gastric contents. This is rare, but it can occur in child who is obtunded, has a neurological disorder, or is mentally challenged

unless preventive measures are taken. The vast majority of incidents of aspiration into the lungs occur during feeding and are caused by abnormal swallowing mechanisms.

2. *Volume.* A direct relationship exists between the volume of the stomach contents and GER. An over-distended stomach is more likely to exhibit GER. Minimal reflux, which can occur when the stomach is fullest at the initiation of the examination, might be less significant than what occurs later during the study.

3. *Consistency of stomach contents.* Liquids are more likely to reflux than solids. It is preferable to mix the radiopharmaceutical with the patient's normal meal. Milk or milk with cereal assumes a semisolid consistency in the stomach as the milk curdles with stomach acids. To ensure uniform mixing, the radiopharmaceutical is placed in the milk or formula and blended or shaken thoroughly before ingestion. A small amount of nonradioactive milk or formula is given lastly to wash radioactivity from the mouth and esophagus. If the child is a poor feeder, the radiopharmaceutical should be instilled as an initial bolus to ensure adequate count rates for imaging in the presence of small stomach volumes. If the radiopharmaceutical is instilled into the stomach via an orogastric or nasogastric tube, it is important to ensure that the tip of the tubing is in the fundus of the stomach. Frequently gastric tubes are inserted too far, often into the duodenum or even jejunum. This results in a failed study. Some nuclear medicine departments prefer to insert the gastric tubes themselves. Seldom is tubing longer than the first marker needed when a feeding tube is used. In addition, a small portion of the radiopharmaceutical dose can be instilled along with some saline to ensure that the tubing has been inserted into the stomach. If the child is crying lustily, the tubing is unlikely to be in the trachea. However, in a child who is obtunded, has a neurological disorder, or is mentally challenged, placement of the tubing may be difficult to assess without instillation of a small amount of radioisotope with the saline. The patient's formula or milk should not be used as the bolus in such circumstances.

4. *Abdominal pressure.* The adult technique for studying GER includes applying varying degrees of abdominal pressure with an abdominal band similar to a tourniquet. The GER appears dependent upon the varying degrees of applied abdominal pressure. Caution should be observed in attempting the same manipulation with a child, particularly with an infant, because the abdominal muscles play an important part in pediatric respiration. Abdominal venous return is also compromised by application of tourniquets around the abdomen.

5. *Aspiration of saliva.* Recent studies have demonstrated the normal aspiration of saliva in some

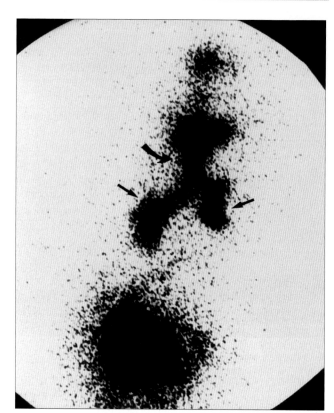

FIGURE 23-13 Salivagram image demonstrating activity in the trachea *(curved arrow)* and bronchi *(straight arrows).*

patients. For that reason, a "salivagram" can be performed before instilling radioactivity into the stomach or as a separate study. A drop of the radiopharmaceutical is placed on the patient's tongue, and the patient is monitored during the normal swallowing of saliva before the GER study is started. Data are acquired in the dynamic mode. Aspiration is readily recognized as activity in the trachea and bifurcation of the main bronchi (Figure 23-13). Time-activity curves are derived from ROIs over the lungs.[39]

Significance of Gastroesophageal Reflux. It is difficult to define the significance of GER. Taking into consideration all the influencing factors, it would seem that up to three episodes of GER during an examination, especially if they are minimal and occur at the beginning of the examination, would be of little clinical significance. Multiple episodes throughout the study of a large volume that reaches the level of the patient's mouth, particularly late in the study, would be significant because the contents can potentially be aspirated. Be that as it may, the potential for aspiration exists with any episode of GER, and findings should be correlated with the clinical situation, such as failure to thrive and multiple episodes of recurrent pneumonia.

Technical Considerations. The radionuclide technique for GER involves instillation of ^{99m}Tc–sulfur colloid into the stomach, along with a sufficient volume of nonradioactive liquid to fill the stomach. For the procedure, about 0.5 mCi (20 MBq) of ^{99m}Tc–sulfur colloid is instilled into the patient's stomach, either by ingestion orally or via an orogastric or a nasogastric tube, along with the infant's normal volume of formula, milk, juice, or glucose water. The patient should have fasted for a minimum of 2 hours before the procedure; at the time the radiopharmaceutical is given orally, the child usually accepts the radioactive feeding quickly. If the radionuclide is administered via orogastric or nasogastric tube, adequate placement of the tube in the fundus can be ensured by administering half the radiopharmaceutical and, if necessary, repositioning the tube before instillation of the remainder of the feeding and the radiopharmaceutical. The technologist should wear gloves and place absorbent disposable pads around the child's shoulders to protect the clothing and skin from contamination. If contamination occurs, the absorbent pad can be quickly removed even during the examination. The gastric tube is removed immediately after administration of the radionuclide and feeding.

Occasionally an examination is performed on a child who has a gastrostomy tube in place. In such instances, the tube should be clamped and its free end secured to the lower abdomen so that any residual radioactivity in the tube is not confused with reflux or aspirated activity on delayed images. The child is positioned supine on top of the gamma camera so both the stomach and thorax are in the field of view. A low-energy collimator is used, and magnification imaging may also be included, depending on the size of the child. A radioactive marker is placed at the level of the sternal notch and xiphoid. The patient is then fed and imaging begins simultaneously. Digital images are obtained using 64×64 matrix at 1 frame/15 sec for the 60-minute interval. After the 60-minute mark, 2-minute anterior and posterior images of the entire stomach and bowel are acquired to calculate the emptying percentage at 1 hour. In infants the gastric emptying rate at 1 hour varies considerably (10% to 90%), and standard values have not been defined.

Analysis of the data is performed by placing a ROI over the esophagus and a background region. A time-activity curve is generated from the background-subtracted esophageal area. Reflux episodes appear as spikes of increased activity above the background and may be categorized by the number of episodes occurring during one hour of imaging, for example, mild (<10 episodes), moderate (10 to 20 episodes), or severe (>20 episodes). Care must be taken to ensure that patient movement does not generate spurious spikes. The emptying percentage is calculated by placing the ROI over the stomach and the bowel for both the anterior and left lateral static images to obtain counts for each area. At a delayed interval of at least 3 hours, anterior and posterior images of the chest for 2 minutes are obtained, with markers at the shoulders and xiphoid, to seek any evidence of reflux aspiration. Aspiration appears as tracheal or lung activity on the 1- and 4-hour static thorax views.

It should be noted that contamination from vomit or regurgitation can mimic these appearances.

Gastric Emptying Study

The evaluation of children with chronic aspiration or GER constitutes a common indication for this examination, which is also performed in children with suspected or established motility disturbances, for example secondary to cystic fibrosis.

There is negligible systemic tracer absorption—only gastrointestinal tract activity should be seen. Age-dependent fasting is instituted before the examination. For infants, radiotracer is added to a small aliquot of infant formula, which is then fed to the child, followed by a volume of unlabeled formula equal to what the child normally takes. In older children who have already had dietary exposure to eggs, the tracer may be added to one egg before cooking, which the child will then eat as part of an egg meal. Radiolabeled feed or meal must be ingested as soon as possible after preparation, generally within 10 minutes; the time for ingestion should be recorded as well as whether the whole of the prepared feed or meal was ingested. For children with a gastrostomy tube, in order to prevent "dumping," a small volume (typically 20 ml) of unlabeled feed is initially introduced followed by the tracer dose in a small aliquot of feed and then an unlabeled volume of feed equal to what the patient normally takes. Anterior and posterior planar images with a field of view to include the distal esophagus, stomach, and small bowel are obtained immediately and at 15-minute intervals up to 90 minutes. Infants are held upright between images; older children are encouraged to walk. The patient is imaged in a supine position, carefully checked to ensure consistency. An ROI drawn around the stomach on both the anterior and posterior views allows a time-activity curve to be generated from the geometric mean of the counts. A follow-up study must always be performed in the same way as prior studies to permit a valid comparison of results. Patients may be retested on prokinetic medications to assess treatment efficacy. Our practice is to consider normal those studies where 50% or more of the gastric contents empties by 90 minutes postingestion, with a gastric emptying half-time of up to 90 minutes. Conversely, stomach activity residual of greater than 50% at 90 minutes or an emptying half-time greater than 90 minutes is considered evidence of delayed emptying. Institutional normal values should be established depending upon the constituents of the meal and the imaging technique that is followed.

Hepatobiliary Scintigraphy

The primary indication for hepatobiliary scintigraphy in the pediatric patient is differentiation of the various causes of neonatal jaundice. Indications for hepatobiliary scintigraphy include exclusion of biliary atresia, evaluation of suspected choledochal cyst, or postsurgical biliary leak. Patients with biliary atresia have hyperbilirubinemia and jaundice, which persists or increases in the neonatal period. Left untreated, biliary atresia is a lethal condition at an early age. It is often possible to differentiate an inflammatory liver disease (e.g., neonatal hepatitis) from obstructive biliary tract disease (e.g., biliary atresia) using a ^{99m}Tc-iminodiacetic acid (^{99m}Tc-IDA) derivative radiopharmaceutical. The ^{99m}Tc-IDA radiopharmaceuticals provide diagnostic images even in jaundiced patients with elevated direct serum bilirubin levels. A good hepatocyte extraction efficiency and short parenchymal transit time also are seen with these radiopharmaceuticals; ^{99m}Tc-mebrofenin is preferred because of its rapid clearance and limited renal excretion. Normal transit times have not been established for children but seem to be less than the normal $t_{1/2}$ for the adult.[34]

Other causes of neonatal jaundice, including neonatal hepatitis, usually are self-limiting conditions not associated with permanent interruption of the biliary drainage system. Differentiation of biliary atresia from other forms of obstruction or inflammatory disease is difficult based only on clinical laboratory tests and other radiological imaging tests such as ultrasonography. Invasive procedures such as percutaneous transhepatic cholangiography are difficult to perform in children and have associated risks.

The radiopharmaceuticals used for hepatobiliary imaging undergo the same hepatocyte uptake, transport, and excretion pathway as bilirubin. In evaluation of neonatal jaundice, phenobarbital can be used to activate hepatic excretory enzymes. A phenobarbital pretreatment of 5 mg/kg/day is divided into two equal doses 3 to 7 days before hepatobiliary imaging to increase the sensitivity of diagnosis to 90% or greater in distinguishing biliary atresia from other causes of jaundice.[50]

Oral intake is restricted for 2 hours before injection of the radiopharmaceutical. Administered radiopharmaceutical dose is weight based and is not dependent on bilirubin levels. Scintigraphy is begun immediately, with the patient in a supine position and with the appropriate magnification factor to obtain images that include only the xiphoid to the symphysis pubis within the field of view. Dynamic imaging is acquired for 45 to 60 minutes. Static images of the abdomen in the anterior/posterior and right/left lateral projection are obtained immediately thereafter. The key image is the left lateral projection. Any activity between the liver edge and the bladder within the abdomen anteriorly is evidence of GI activity, which excludes the diagnosis of biliary atresia. Depending on the magnification factor and the collimation, images are obtained for 2 minutes. Additional images are obtained at various intervals, typically 3, 6, and 24 hours, or until radioactivity is demonstrated in the GI tract.

SPECT may be helpful for diagnosis and may obviate the need for delayed imaging. If gallbladder filling is visualized, the patient is fed formula or a milk drink as a fatty meal while an additional dynamic sequence is obtained.

A normal neonatal study demonstrates radiopharmaceutical clearance from the blood pool by 5 minutes; the end point of the study is visualization of bowel activity, usually within 1 hour. The gallbladder and biliary tree are not typically visualized in the neonate. In a patient with biliary atresia, rapid radiopharmaceutical clearance from the blood pool is usually seen with lack of bowel activity by 24 hours. Delayed radiopharmaceutical clearance from the blood pool with delayed hepatic excretion into bowel implies neonatal hepatitis. In practice, however, bowel activity may be so delayed with severe hepatitis that it is effectively not visualized and in such cases biliary atresia cannot be excluded with certainty. Therefore the value of hepatobiliary scintigraphy lies in the exclusion of biliary atresia in cases where bowel activity is demonstrated, since in all other cases, the possibility of this diagnosis cannot be excluded.[55]

Nonobstructing choledochal cysts usually manifest as prolonged radiopharmaceutical retention at the site of a pericholecystic structure demonstrated by anatomical imaging. In cases of postsurgical biliary leak, progressive accumulation of either perihepatic or free abdominal radiopharmaceutical activity may be seen.

Meckel Diverticulum Imaging

The most common gastrointestinal congenital malformation is Meckel diverticulum, which occurs in approximately 1% to 3% of the population. Complications develop in about 25% of these individuals. Meckel diverticulum is the vestigial remnant of the omphalomesenteric duct and usually is found along the antimesenteric border of the distal ileum.[45] Meckel diverticula often contain gastric mucosa, which leads to complications such as peptic ulceration and hemorrhage from acid excretion. Such complications occur most frequently in children and young adults and require surgical correction.

Routine roentgenographic studies are usually considered of little value. Radionuclide imaging of Meckel diverticulum is based on the fact that ^{99m}Tc-pertechnetate concentrates in gastric mucosa via active transport by the mucous surface cells. Nearly 60% of all Meckel diverticula contain gastric mucosa and thus can be imaged. Radionuclide imaging has an accuracy of 90% to 98%, making it the optimum examination for identification of Meckel diverticulum. The clinical presentation varies. Meckel diverticulum is most often detected as an incidental finding at the time of surgery for other reasons. The patient may develop rectal bleeding as hematochezia (fresh blood tainting the stool), melena, or bright red, symptomless bleeding.

Radionuclide detection of Meckel diverticulum is technique dependent. False-positive results caused by migration of secreted ^{99m}Tc-pertechnetate from the stomach into the distal bowel have been reported. The following scintigraphic technique has been found to enhance the detectability of Meckel diverticulum.[17]

Radionuclide imaging should be performed before barium sulfate studies or colonoscopy of the bowel. Such procedures can stimulate radionuclide localization as a result of irritation of the mucosa and can cause false-positive interpretation. Barium sulfate attenuates photons and thus theoretically can mask localization of the radionuclide in the diverticulum, causing a false-negative interpretation. Another contraindication is having undergone a radiolabeled red blood cell scan within the preceding 24 hours, because there would be interference from background radiation. Because potassium perchlorate inhibits localization of pertechnetate in ectopic gastric mucosa, this drug should not be given before imaging. However, potassium perchlorate should be administered after the radionuclide study to reduce the radiation dose to the thyroid gland. The patient should fast for at least 2 hours before imaging to reduce secretion and migration of ^{99m}Tc-pertechnetate from the stomach into the bowel. Occasionally, in the presence of generalized bowel inflammation or irritable bowel, the radionuclide transit time throughout the bowel is rapid, resulting in difficult interpretation. The use of nasogastric suction to reduce transit of secreted nuclide may be helpful during a repeat examination. Premedications have also been used to enhance a Meckel study. Pretreatment with cimetidine is used because it inhibits secretion of pertechnetate from the cells into the lumen of the bowel. Pretreatment with ranitidine (1 mg/kg IV up to a maximum of 50 mg) administered as a slow infusion over 20 minutes is also used to reduce gastric mucosal secretion and increase mucosal radiopharmaceutical uptake. Because a Meckel diverticulum can be located close to the urinary bladder, the patient should void before and at intervals during the examination to prevent the ^{99m}Tc-pertechnetate excreted by the kidneys into the bladder from masking a small diverticulum located adjacent to the bladder.

For the procedure the patient is positioned supine. ^{99m}Tc-pertechnetate is administered intravenously, and imaging is begun immediately after injection. A two-phase dynamic study, to include the entire abdomen from the top of the diaphragm to the inferior extent of urinary bladder, should be acquired with the initial flow set at 5 sec/frame for 12 images followed by 1 minute/frame images acquired up to 15 minutes. Static views in the anterior/posterior and right/left lateral positions are acquired immediately thereafter. In children less than 2 years of age, static images of the thorax are also obtained to exclude ectopic gastric mucosa in a bronchopulmonary foregut malformation.

Ectopic gastric mucosa activity should appear at the same time as normal gastric mucosa and may occur

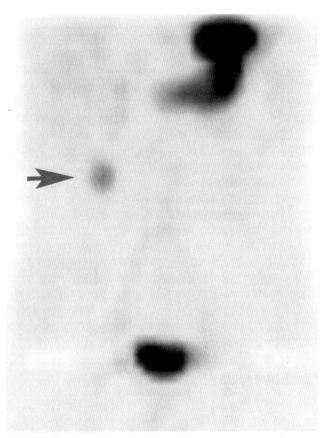

FIGURE 23-14 SPECT maximum intensity projection (MIP) image showing focal abnormal activity in the right mid abdomen in an area of ectopic gastric mucosa confirmed surgically to be a Meckel diverticulum *(arrow)*.

anywhere in the abdomen, although the right lower quadrant is the most common location (Figure 23-14). Ureteric or bladder activity may be confused for ectopic gastric mucosa but the latter should show activity first. With time, normal tracer activity will transit from the stomach lumen into the small bowel lumen but can be distinguished from ectopic gastric mucosa by its delayed appearance, movement, and lack of focality, tending to be more of an ill-defined, mildly increased region of radiopharmaceutical activity. With this technique, lateral, oblique, upright, and postvoid views, as well as SPECT, may be of use in localizing radiopharmaceutical activity. Giving the patient a drink of water may flush ureteric radiopharmaceutical activity into the bladder when there is doubt regarding the nature of a right lower quadrant focus of activity. Occasionally administration of a diuretic will be required to differentiate renal activity from the Meckel diverticulum. False-negative results are most commonly due to poor technique, with an imaging interval that is far too short, because it may occur from washout from an active bleeding site or it may be due to necrosis of an ulcerated focus of ectopic gastric mucosa. For this reason, in a child who presents with acute painless bleeding and is stabilized but has a normal exam, a repeat test after a short time interval such as 2 weeks can sometimes have a true positive result. So-called false-positive results may be caused by any inflammatory process, for example appendicitis, or a lesion containing ectopic gastric mucosa, such as a duplication cyst.

Scintigraphic Interpretation Criteria. Usually the Meckel diverticulum appears at the same time as the gastric mucosa at 10 to 20 minutes after injection. There might be a delayed appearance, but it rarely occurs after the 1-hour interval. The localization is usually prominent, rounded, and within a small focus. Most diverticula are found in the right lower quadrant of the abdomen, but they can be located anywhere in the abdomen and may be seen to move during the study. The activity should persist on multiple images during the study; however, the potential exists for emptying of the radioactive secretions from a Meckel lumen or dilution of the radioactivity by blood passing distally into the colon. This is a likely cause of the uncommonly reported false-negative studies. The diverticulum is generally intraabdominal and thus can be distinguished from activity in the retroperitoneal genitourinary tract, particularly on a lateral projection.[17]

Cardiovascular System

The most common radionuclide studies of the heart in children are those used to detect and quantify cardiac shunts, either left-to-right (through a septal defect or patent ductus arteriosus) or right-to-left. Surgically produced shunts also are frequently evaluated. All the techniques involve the use of a radiopharmaceutical such as ^{99m}Tc-pertechnetate or macroaggregated albumin (MAA) to document transit of the radionuclide through the cardiovascular system.[32] The major advantages of these techniques are their noninvasive nature, rapidity, and low radiation dose compared with alternative procedures such as cardiac catheterization and contrast angiography.

Left-to-right shunt quantification involves a rapid injection of a compact bolus of ^{99m}Tc-pertechnetate, preferably through the jugular vein, and digital acquisition of 0.5-second frames to document the transit through the cardiopulmonary circuit. Analog images are also acquired simultaneously. After acquisition the pulmonary time-activity curve is generated and analyzed via the gamma variate analysis to determine the pulmonary-to-systemic flow ratio (QP/QS ratio). This method provides precise quantification of left-to-right shunts with a pulmonary-to-systemic ratio of 1.2 to 3.0, as devised by Maltz and Treves.[51]

Right-to-left cardiac shunts are detected using ^{99m}Tc-MAA.[30] After injection of the radioactive particles, the distribution of activity between the systemic circulation and the lungs is determined. If no right-to-left shunt is present, more than 95% of the injected activity is trapped in the pulmonary vascular bed. Activity seen throughout the systemic circulation, including the kidneys, brain, and other organs, is evidence of a right-to-left shunt and

can be quantified by acquisition of whole-body images and placement of an ROI over the lungs and the rest of the body. The magnitude of the right-to-left shunt is calculated according to the following formula:

$$\text{Percentage right-to-left shunt} =$$
$$(\text{Total body count} - \text{Total lung count})/\text{Total body count}$$

The examination must be performed immediately after constitution of the radiopharmaceutical to avoid the possibility of radiopharmaceutical breakdown and increased counts from free pertechnetate in the kidneys or bladder.

ENDOCRINE

Neonatal Thyroid Scintigraphy

Neonatal thyroid scintigrams are indicated for neonates with elevated serum thyroid-stimulating hormone (TSH) that is detected on routine neonatal screening. After a dose of ^{99m}Tc-pertechnetate is injected, 1% to 2% is trapped but not organified by thyroid epithelial cells. Radioactivity is seen within the choroid plexus, salivary glands, thyroid gland, and gastric mucosa. The radiopharmaceutical undergoes urinary and intestinal excretion. Since the radiopharmaceutical is secreted into saliva, early imaging following intravenous injection is required, typically at 20 minutes, to avoid confusion between salivary pooling and ectopic thyroid tissue. The lower head, neck, and thorax are imaged with a parallel high-resolution collimator. Anterior and oblique views are obtained if the radioactivity appears in a normal suprasternal location. The examination is modified if the radioactivity localizes in an ectopic location. Anterior images are obtained, with and without markers at the suprasternal notch, and a lateral view with a chin marker is also obtained (Figure 23-15). Subsequently, higher quality images may be obtained with a pinhole collimator but without the use of markers—these images cannot be obtained with markers because of image distortion caused by the pinhole collimator. The role of markers is to permit differentiation of anatomical versus ectopic functioning thyroid tissue when present. Ectopic thyroid tissue often produces a hypothyroid state due to insufficient hormone production. Radioactivity in a normally-located gland associated with an elevated TSH indicates dyshormonogenesis. Absent thyroid radioactivity possibly reflects a nonfunctioning gland due to maternal auto-immune suppression due to transplacental antibody passage. A follow-up study is recommended at 4 to 6 months later.

MIBG Scintigraphy

Common uses for metaiodobenzylguanidine (MIBG) labeled with iodine-131 (^{131}I-MIBG) or iodine-123

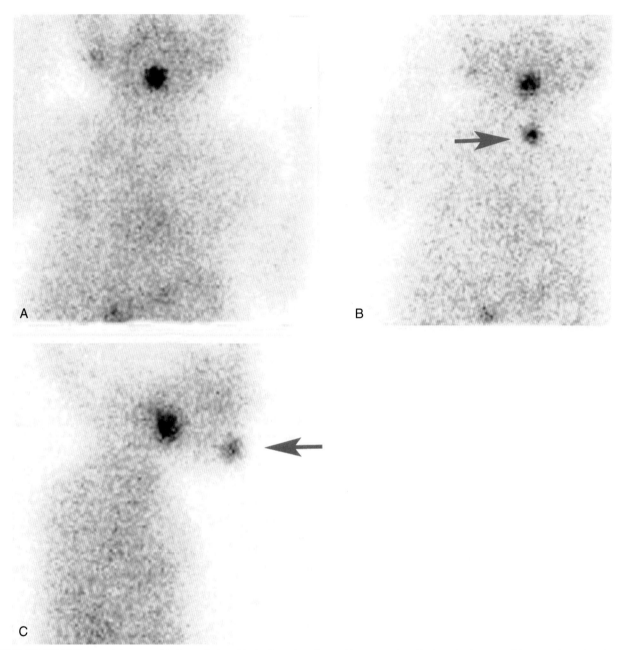

FIGURE 23-15 ^{99m}Tc thyroid scan with lingual thyroid. **A,** Anterior view without marker. **B,** Anterior image with sternal marker *(arrow).* Image **C,** Lateral view with chin marker *(arrow).*

(^{123}I-MIBG) is to confirm, stage, and monitor the post-treatment assessment of neuroectodermally-derived tumors such as neuroblastoma, pheochromocytoma, and ganglioneuroma.

MIBG is an analogue of noradrenaline with a specific active uptake mechanism believed to be responsible for uptake by tissues with sympathetic innervation including liver, spleen, myocardium, salivary glands, adrenal glands, and certain neuroendocrine tumors. Skeletal muscles, nasal mucosa, lungs, urinary tract, colon, gall-bladder and thyroid may also demonstrate accumulation of MIBG of variable intensity. No skeletal localization

should be seen. The extremities should demonstrate only slight muscular radioactivity and in these cases the bone may appear as a photon-deficient area.

Before the radiopharmaceutical injection, the patient's current therapy regimen must be checked to exclude agents known to interfere with MIBG imaging. The most common are β-adrenergic receptor agonist bronchodila-tors such as salbutamol. Many cardiac drugs such as calcium channel blockers, angiotensin-converting enzyme inhibitors and adrenergic receptor blockers also interfere with MIBG biodistribution, although such drugs are rarely found in a pediatric population. To provide thyroid blockade, an oral dose of potassium perchlorate is given one time immediately before the MIBG injection. The MIBG is injected slowly over 5 minutes, preferably into a peripheral vein rather than a central venous access device, since the radiopharmaceutical may persist within certain of these devices and may occasionally confound image interpretation. When possible, patients should be encouraged to drink copious fluids and to void frequently following the radiopharmaceutical injection. Imaging starts at 24 hours with whole body planar images ideally supplemented by spot views of the skull and torso. SPECT of the torso is recommended and additional 48-hour planar whole body images may also be obtained. When diagnostic hybrid imaging is available, the addition of a postcontrast enhanced diagnostic CT scan can be performed. This allows coregistration of the MIBG and anatomical imaging and should obviate the need for the patient to return for a separate diagnostic CT scan. It is our practice to try to perform these studies together where possible and when a CT scan would be required as well for response assessment as dictated by treatment protocols. In younger infants and children, this often requires sedation for the delayed 24 hour imaging and the CT scan. This can be specified at the time of scheduling of the examination when the nuclear medicine physician reviews the scheduled studies.

Primary tumor and metastases usually localize the MIBG. The degree of localization may be similar in benign and malignant tumors and maturation of neuroblastoma to ganglioneuroma may occur with no change in the localization intensity. Skeletal localization may be diffuse with the MIBG because of either cortical bone metastases, bone marrow infiltration, or both. False-negative images may occur in cases where lesions are smaller than the spatial resolution of the imaging system or where metastatic lesions are too close to the primary tumor to be recognized or too close to a site of physiological tracer localization to be differentiated. A small proportion (<6%) of neuroblastoma tumors are not MIBG-avid.[56] Additional information regarding MIBG imaging is located in Chapter 22.

PET Imaging

In adults, PET has become an indispensable imaging tool in clinical nuclear medicine. In combination with CT and magnetic resonance imaging (MRI), it is an established method in neurology, cardiology, infection imaging, and oncology. The pediatric indications in the fields of neurology (seizure disorders, brain tumors), cardiology, endocrinology, and infection are still limited; 2-deoxy-2-[^{18}F]fluoro-D-glucose (^{18}F-FDG) imaging in pediatrics is mainly performed to investigate oncological disorders. PET imaging is useful for differentiating benign and malignant masses, staging and restaging of malignancies, and monitoring response to therapy. It has proven useful in evaluating children with lymphoma, neuroblastoma, and primary bone and soft-tissue tumors.

Imaging Procedure. The same instructions are given to pediatric and adult patients.[26] The patient should fast for 4 to 6 hours before injection of the ^{18}F-FDG and refrain from strenuous exercise in the preceding 24 hours. Fasting for older children is not a difficulty, especially if the procedure is scheduled for the morning; however, cessation of feeding for infants and young children can be a problem. In infants and young children, an IV infusion of electrolytes is recommended. Water can be fed for all patients until 2 hours before the procedure.

An administered dosage of 0.1 to 0.2 mCi (4 to 5 MBq) of ^{18}F-FDG per kilogram of body weight is injected. Infants should be fed at 20 to 30 min after injection. To help eliminate metabolic brown fat radioactivity, pediatric patients are scheduled to arrive a minimum of 45 minutes before their expected injection time. This allows for any extra time that might be needed for the establishment of the IV site and for a delay to allow the patient to relax before the radiopharmaceutical is injected. The child should be kept quiet and in a warm and darkened room. The parents are allowed to be with the child during this time, with appropriate radiation protection precautions. Infants and children under the age of 3 years are sedated using intranasal or rectal midazolam. Sedation is used if necessary in older patients to prevent motion and to reduce anxiety. The urinary bladder is catheterized if structures in the pelvis are of importance for interpretation of the images or in cases of known bladder dysfunction. Furosemide may be given to enhance urinary excretion.

Imaging should begin at 60 minutes after injection. Transmission imaging is performed moving from head to feet, immediately followed by the emission images from feet to head with at least 3-minute acquisitions per bed position for PET-only systems.

For PET-CT systems, the CT component of the procedure should be performed with minimum exposure procedures.[29] For contrast-enhanced CT scans as part of the PET-CT protocol, the administered dose of nonionic contrast is weight-based: 2 ml/kg up to a maximum of 100 ml. The bolus is timed for portal venous opacification, with an injection duration of 50 seconds and image acquisition initiated at the end of the contrast infusion. Contrast is injected with a power injector, and a central venous line is not routinely used for the CT contrast injection, but an accessed central venous line can be used for the ^{18}F-FDG injection. If a peripheral line is established for ^{18}F-FDG and then IV contrast injection, the injection site should be remote from any anticipated disease localization. Both the PET and CT acquisitions are performed as craniocaudal acquisitions with the patient instructed to breath normally. The arms are usually positioned overhead unless the child is not able to hold this position.[29]

Clinical Applications

Lymphoma. Although lymphoma is the third most common type of cancer in childhood, the evaluation of PET in Hodgkin lymphoma in children is still limited. Similar to ^{67}Ga-citrate, FDG localization tends to be greater in higher-grade than in lower-grade lymphomas.[54] An overview of the literature with regard to the value of PET for initial staging of Hodgkin disease was published by Körholz and associates.[46] The main advantage of PET in diagnosing this disease is that PET is used as a whole-body imaging tool before and after therapy (Figures 23-16 and 23-17).

Primary Bone and Soft Tissue Tumors. In children, osteosarcoma and **Ewing sarcoma** are the two most frequently encountered primary malignancies of the bone. Routinely, MRI is used to define the local extent of the mass and soft-tissue involvement. Nuclear medicine methods have primarily been used to detect metastatic spread.

PET is a potentially useful clinical tool for the detection of Ewing sarcoma, metastases, therapy monitoring, and disease recurrence. In a comparison with whole-body MRI and skeletal scintigraphy, ^{18}F-FDG-PET showed the highest sensitivity in the detection of osseous metastases from primary bone tumors, followed by MRI and skeletal scintigraphy.[57] However, it was found that spiral CT was superior to ^{18}F-FDG-PET for the detection of pulmonary metastases from malignant tumors.[30] Therefore, for exclusion of lung metastases, ^{18}F-FDG-PET cannot be recommended at present. However, because of the high specificity of ^{18}F-FDG-PET, positive findings can be used to confirm abnormalities found on thoracic CT as being metastases. In soft-tissue sarcomas, ^{18}F-FDG-PET shows the ability to distinguish high-grade soft-tissue sarcoma from low-grade or benign tumors. Comparing the results of ^{18}F-FDG-PET, MRI, and CT in patients with soft-tissue sarcomas, ^{18}F-FDG-PET, as a one-step procedure, was confirmed to be the superior modality for the assessment of local and distant tumor recurrence and distant metastases (Figure 23-18).

Neuroblastoma. The primary diagnosis of **neuroblastoma** is usually based on MRI, CT, ^{123}I-MIBG, and bone scintigraphy. However, significant FDG localization was found in neuroblastoma lesions in most of the patients studied was found. When ^{18}F-FDG-PET was compared

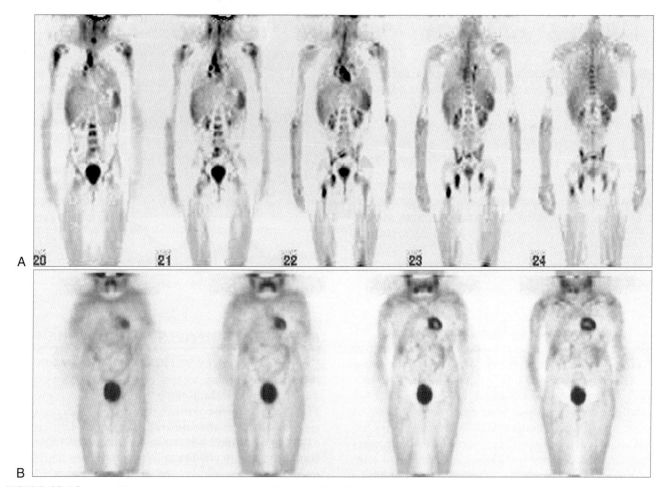

FIGURE 23-16 A, An ^{18}F-FDG PET scan of a 9-year-old boy, with widespread lymph node involvement of malignant lymphoma before chemotherapy. **B,** A follow-up scan after chemotherapy demonstrates complete remission.

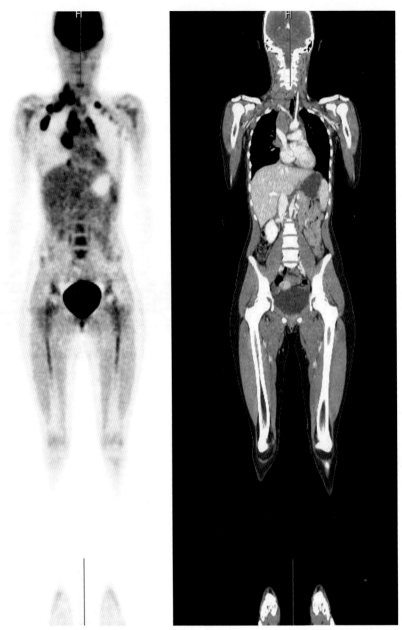

FIGURE 23-17 The ^{18}F-FDG PET coronal whole-body scan of 12-year-old with Hodgkin lymphoma stage III with extensive involvement of neck and mediastinum as well as disease below the diaphragm in the spleen.

with ^{123}I-MIBG localization imaging, a more intense ^{123}I-MIBG uptake before therapy could be seen, whereas ^{18}F-FDG-PET helped to define the posttherapeutic extent of ^{123}I-MIBG–negative neuroblastomas.[73] When ^{18}F-FDG-PET, bone scintigraphy, CT and/or MRI, urine catecholamine measurements, and bone marrow examinations were compared in children with high-risk neuroblastoma, it was found that after resection of the primary tumor and the absence of skull lesions, PET and bone marrow examinations were sufficient for monitoring neuroblastoma patients at high risk for progressive disease.

POTENTIAL PITFALLS IN PEDIATRIC PET

^{18}F-FDG-PET in children has some unique features of their normal appearance that are responsible for possible misinterpretation. In a number of studies, increased ^{18}F-FDG uptake in the normal thymus in children can be seen, mainly after chemotherapy (Figure 23-19). This has to be kept in mind when assessing the mediastinum in pediatric patients. In some cases, differentiation of normal thymic activity from tumor or inflammation in the anterior mediastinum may be difficult or even impossible, especially in lymphoma patients. A further source

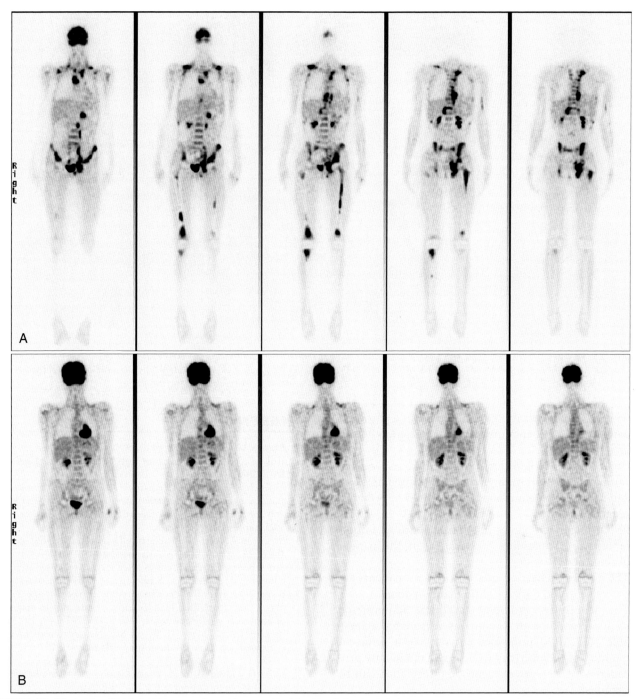

FIGURE 23-18 A, The ^{18}F-FDG PET scan of an 11-year-old girl with abdominal rhabdomyosarcoma before chemotherapy demonstrates multiple metastases. **B,** After chemotherapy, the patient is in complete remission.

of misinterpretation, especially in young patients, is physiologically increased ^{18}F-FDG activity in the myocardium, thyroid gland, GI tract, renal pelvis, and urinary bladder. In cases of radiopharmaceutical extravasation during injection, tracer accumulation in draining lymph nodes can simulate tumoral lymph node involvement. Other possible reasons for increased localization of ^{18}F-FDG are trauma, inflammatory foci, muscle and brown fat, and the normal ovary.

SUMMARY

- Pediatric procedures require special attention to nursing care, patient safety, immobilization techniques, instrumentation, and the technical requirements for specific procedures.
- High resolution is required using state-of-the-art instruments. Magnification collimators or zoomed images may be needed for some clinical procedures in order to obtain the highest resolution images.

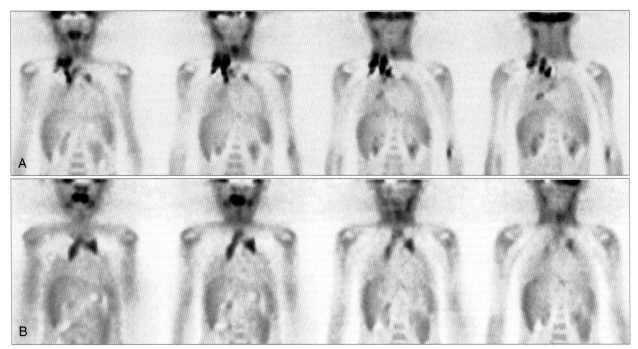

FIGURE 23-19 The ^{18}F-FDG PET scans of a 12-year-old boy with malignant lymphoma before chemotherapy **(A)** demonstrate multiple pathological lymph nodes in the thorax, and following chemotherapy **(B)** demonstrate increased normal ^{18}F-FDG uptake in the thymus.

- Pediatric immobilization techniques should allow the patient to be safe, comfortable, and motionless during imaging.
- Departments should have appropriate emergency equipment and procedures for pediatric patients.
- Appropriate guidelines must be followed in pediatric sedation.
- Pediatric patient–parent relationships are an important part of obtaining cooperation of the patient during the procedure.
- The preferred injection sites for pediatric patients are the veins in the dorsum of the hand or foot.
- The quantity of radiopharmaceutical administered should comply with "as low as reasonably achievable" (ALARA) principles but provide a sufficient quantity of radioactivity to ensure that a quality procedure with definitive diagnostic information can be obtained.
- Pediatric patients should be carefully positioned to provide body symmetry for comparison.
- Pediatric SPECT studies may require more acquisition time than adult SPECT procedures in order to obtain adequate image statistics.
- Most pediatric clinical indications for skeletal imaging require blood pool and delayed total body imaging.
- In renal imaging, the state of hydration will significantly affect the excretion of radiopharmaceuticals. Therefore oral hydration to tolerance is recommended for 2 hours before the study.
- Radionuclide studies of the gastrointestinal system should be performed before radiography studies with barium.

REFERENCES

1. Alessio AM, Kinahan PE, et al: Weight-based, low-dose pediatric whole-body PET/CT protocols, *J Nucl Med* 50(10):1570-1577, 2009.
2. American Academy on Pediatrics: Guideline for monitoring and management of pediatric patients during and after sedation for diagnostic and therapeutic procedures, *Pediatr Dent* 30(7 Suppl):143-159, 2008.
3. American Academy on Pediatrics: Diagnostic imaging of child abuse, *Pediatrics* 123(5):1430-1435, 2009.
4. Ami TB, et al: Stress fractures after surgery for osteosarcoma: scintigraphic assessment, *Radiology* 163:157-162, 1987.
5. Berger RM, et al: Bladder capacity (ounces) equals age (years) plus 2 predicts normal bladder capacity and aids in diagnosis of abnormal voiding patterns, *J Urol* 129:347-349, 1983.
6. Bressler EL, Conway JJ, Weiss SC: Neonatal osteomyelitis examined by bone scintigraphy, *Radiology* 152:685-688, 1984.
7. Bulas D, Goske M, et al. Image Gently: improving health literacy for parents about CT scans for children, *Pediatr Radiol* 39(2):112-116, 2009.
8. Chen DCP, Holder LE, Melloul M: Radionuclide scrotal imaging: further experience with 210 patients. I. Anatomy, pathophysiology, and methods, *J Nucl Med* 24:735-742, 1983.
9. Chen DCP, Holder LE, Melloul M: Radionuclide scrotal imaging: further experience with 210 patients. II. Results and discussion, *J Nucl Med* 24:841-853, 1983.
10. Cohen MD, Wood BP, Hodgman CH: The presence of parents with their children during imaging procedures, *Am J Roentgenol Radium Ther Nucl Med* 146:639-641, 1986.
11. Committee on Drugs (American Academy of Pediatrics): Guidelines for monitoring and management of pediatric patients during and after sedation for diagnostic and therapeutic procedures, *Pediatrics* 89:1110-1115, 1992.
12. Conway JJ: Avascular necrosis in septic arthritis of the hip (unpublished work).

13. Conway JJ: Communicating risk information in medical practice, *Radiographics* 12:207-214, 1992.
14. Conway JJ: *Musculoskeletal scintigraphy in children*, Audiovisual program CEL 6, New York, 1992, Society of Nuclear Medicine.
15. Conway JJ: Practical considerations in radionuclide imaging of pediatric patients. In Freeman LM, editor: *Freeman and Johnson's clinical radionuclide imaging*, ed 3, New York, 1984, Grune & Stratton.
16. Conway JJ: Radionuclide bone scintigraphy in pediatric orthopedics, *Pediatr Clin North Am* 33:1313-1334, 1986.
17. Conway JJ: Radionuclide diagnosis of Meckel's diverticulum, *Gastrointest Radiol* 5:209-213, 1980.
18. Conway JJ: Sedation, injection, and handling techniques in pediatric nuclear medicine. In James AE Jr, Wagner HN Jr, Cooke RE, editors: *Pediatric nuclear medicine*, Philadelphia, 1974, WB Saunders.
19. Conway JJ: *SPECT imaging in children: categorical course in nuclear radiology*, Weston, Va, 1989, American College of Radiology.
20. Conway JJ: The principles and technical aspects of diuresis renography, *J Nucl Med Technol* 17:208-214, 1989.
21. Conway JJ: "Well-tempered" diuresis renography: its historical development, physiological and technical pitfalls and standardized technique protocol, *Semin Nucl Med* 22:74-84, 1992.
22. Conway JJ, Collins M, et al: The role of bone scintigraphy in detecting child abuse, *Semin Nucl Med* 23(4):321-333, 1993.
23. Conway JJ, et al: Detection of vesicoureteral reflux with radionuclide cystography: a comparison study with roentgenographic cystography, *Am J Roentgenol Radium Ther Nucl Med* 115:720-727, 1972.
24. Conway JJ, Filmer RB: *Nuclear medicine in clinical pediatrics: kidney*, New York, 1975, Society of Nuclear Medicine.
25. Daldrup-Link HE, et al: Whole-body MR imaging for detection of bone metastases in children and young adults: comparison with skeletal scintigraphy and FDG PET, *Am J Roentgenol* 177:229-236, 2001.
26. Delbeke D, Coleman RE, et al: Procedure guideline for tumor imaging with 18F-FDG PET/CT 1.0, *J Nucl Med* 47(5):885-895, 2006.
27. Dodge EA: Vesicoureteral reflux: diagnosis with iodine-131 sodium orthoiodohippurate, *Lancet* 1:303-304, 1963.
28. Eskild-Jensen A, Gordon I, et al: Interpretation of the renogram: problems and pitfalls in hydronephrosis in children, *BJU Int* 94(6):887-892, 2004.
29. Fahey FH, et al: Dosimetry of pediatric PET/CT, *J Nucl Med* 50(9):1483-1491, 2009.
30. Franzius C, et al: FDG-PET for detection of pulmonary metastases from malignant primary bone tumors: comparison with spiral CT, *Ann Oncol* 12:479-486, 2001.
31. Furosemide (Lasix): In *Physician's desk reference (PDR)*, ed 43, Oradell, NJ, 1989, Medical Economics.
32. Gates GF, Orme HW, Dore EK: Cardiac shunt assessment in children with macroaggregated albumin technetium-99m, *Radiology* 112:649-653, 1974.
33. Gelfand MJ, Strife JL, Kereiakes JG: Radionuclide bone imaging in spondylolysis of the lumbar spine in children, *Radiology* 140:191-195, 1981.
34. Gilbert SA, Brown PH, Krishnamurthy GT: Quantitative nuclear hepatology, *J Nucl Med Technol* 15:38-47, 1987.
35. Goske MJ, Applegate KE, et al: The 'Image Gently' campaign: increasing CT radiation dose awareness through a national education and awareness program, *Pediatr Radiol* 38(3):265-269, 2008.
36. Goske MJ, Applegate KE, et al: The Image Gently campaign: working together to change practice, *AJR Am J Roentgenol* 190(2):273-274, 2008.
37. Hahn K, Fischer S, et al: *Atlas of bone scintigraphy in the developing paediatric skeleton: the normal skeleton, variants and pitfalls*, New York, 1995, Springer.
38. Hahn K, Pfluger T: Has PET become an important clinical tool in paediatric imaging? *Eur J Nucl Med Mol Imaging* 31:615-621, 2004.
39. Heyman S, Respondek M: Detection of pulmonary aspiration in children by radionuclide "salivagram," *J Nucl Med* 30:697-699, 1989.
40. Holder LE, Cole LA, Myerson MS: Reflex sympathetic dystrophy in the foot: clinical and scintigraphic criteria, *Radiology* 184:531-535, 1984.
41. Howie DW et al: The technetium phosphate bone scan in the diagnosis of osteomyelitis in childhood, *J Bone Joint Surg* 65:431-437, 1983.
42. Jacobs F, Thierens H, et al: Optimised tracer-dependent dosage cards to obtain weight-independent effective doses, *Eur J Nucl Med Mol Imaging* 32(5):581-588, 2005.
43. Keeter S et al: Sedation in pediatric CT: national survey of current practice, *Radiology* 175:745-752, 1990.
44. Koff SA, Binkovitz L, et al: Renal pelvis volume during diuresis in children with hydronephrosis: implications for diagnosing obstruction with diuretic renography, *J Urol* 174(1):303-307, 2005.
45. Kowalsky R, Falen S: *Radiopharmaceuticals in nuclear pharmacy and nuclear medicine*, Washington, DC, 2004, American Pharmacists Association.
46. Körholz D, et al: Importance of F18-fluorodeoxy-D-2-glucose positron emission tomography (FDG-PET) for staging and therapy control of Hodgkin's lymphoma in childhood and adolescence-consequences for the GPOH-HD 2003 protocol, *Onkologie* 26:489-493, 2003.
47. Lassmann M, Biassoni L, et al: The new EANM paediatric dosage card, *Eur J Nucl Med Mol Imaging* 34(5):796-798, 2007.
48. Ljung B, Andréasson S: Comparison of midazolam nasal spray to nasal drops for the sedation of children, *J Nucl Med Technol* 24:32-34, 1996.
49. Maizels M, et al: The cystometric nuclear cystogram, *J Urol* 121:203-205, 1979.
50. Majd M, Reba RC, Altman RP: Effect of phenobarbital on ^{99m}Tc-IDA scintigraphy in the evaluation of neonatal jaundice, *Semin Nucl Med* 9:194-204, 1981.
51. Maltz DL, Treves S: Quantitative radionuclide angiocardiography: determination of Qp: Qs in children, *Circulation* 47:1049-1056, 1973.
52. Mason KP: The pediatric sedation service: who is appropriate to sedate, which medications should I use, who should prescribe the drugs, how do I bill? *Pediatr Radiol* 38(Suppl 2):S218-224, 2008.
53. McKay RJ Jr: Diagnosis and treatment: risks of obtaining samples of venous blood in infants, *Pediatrics* 38:906-908, 1968.
54. Moog F, et al: Lymphoma: role of whole body 2-deoxy-2-[F-18]fluoro-D-glucose (FDG) PET in nodal staging, *Radiology* 203:795-800, 1997.
55. Nadel HR: Hepatobiliary scintigraphy in children, *Semin Nucl Med* 26(1):25-42, 1996.
56. Nadel HR: Nuclear oncology in children. In Freeman LM, editor: *Nuclear medicine annual*, New York, 1996, Raven Press, pp 143-193.
57. Nadel HR: Bone scan update, *Semin Nucl Med* 37(5):332-339, 2007.
58. Nadel HR: Pediatric bone scintigraphy update, *Semin Nucl Med* 40(1):31-40, 2010.
59. Nadel HR, Shulkin B: Pediatric positron emission tomography-computed tomography protocol considerations, *Semin Ultrasound CT MR* 29(4):271-276, 2008.

60. Nasrallah PF, et al: The quantitative nuclear cystogram: an aid in determining the spontaneous resolution of vesicoureteral reflux, *Urology* 12:645-658, 1978.

61. Orzel JA, Rudd TG: Heterotopic bone formation: clinical, laboratory, and imaging correlation, *J Nucl Med* 26:125-132, 1985.

62. Papanicolaou N, et al: Bone scintigraphy and radiography in young athletes with low back pain, *Am J Roentgenol Radium Ther Nucl Med* 145:1039-1044, 1985.

63. Paul DJ, et al: A better method of imaging the abnormal hips, *Radiology* 113:466-467, 1974.

64. Piepsez A, et al: Gastroesophageal scintiscanning in children, *J Nucl Med* 23:631-632, 1982.

65. Piepsz A, Tondeur M, et al. NORA: a simple and reliable parameter for estimating renal output with or without frusemide challenge, *Nucl Med Commun* 21(4):317-323, 2000.

66. Rosen PR, Micheli LJ, Treves S: Early scintigraphic diagnosis of bone stress and fractures in athletic adolescents, *Pediatrics* 70:11-15, 1982.

67. Roub LW, et al: Bone stress: a radionuclide imaging perspective, *Radiology* 132:431-438, 1979.

68. Sfakianakis GN, Conway JJ: Detection of ectopic gastric mucosa in Meckel's diverticulum and in other aberrations by scintigraphy. I. Pathophysiology and 10-year clinical experience, *J Nucl Med* 22:647-654, 1981.

69. Sfakianakis GN, Conway JJ: Detection of ectopic gastric mucosa in Meckel's diverticulum and in other aberrations by scintigraphy. II. Indications and methods: a 10-year experience, *J Nucl Med* 22:732-738, 1981.

70. Sfakianakis GN, Sfakianaki E, et al: A renal protocol for all ages and all indications: mercapto-acetyl-triglycine (MAG3) with simultaneous injection of furosemide (MAG3-F0): a 17-year experience, *Semin Nucl Med* 39(3):156-173, 2009.

71. Shalaby-Rana E, Majd M: (99m)Tc-MDP scintigraphic findings in children with leukemia: value of early and delayed whole-body imaging, *J Nucl Med* 42(6):878-883, 2001.

72. Shankar VR: Sedating children for radiological procedures: an intensivist's perspective, *Pediatr Radiol* 38(Suppl 2):S213-217, 2008.

73. Shulkin BL, et al: Neuroblastoma: positron emission tomography with 2-[fluorine-18]-fluoro-2-deoxy-D-glucose compared with metaiodobenzylguanidine scintigraphy, *Radiology* 199:743-750, 1996.

74. Shulkin BL, Mandell GA, et al: Procedure guideline for diuretic renography in children 3.0, *J Nucl Med Technol* 36(3):162-168, 2008.

75. Smergel EM, et al: Use of bone scintigraphy in the management of slipped capital femoral epiphysis (SCFE), *Clin Nucl Med* 12:349-353, 1987.

76. Starshak RJ, Simons GW, Sty JR: Occult fracture of the calcaneus: another toddler's fracture, *Pediatr Radiol* 14:37-40, 1984.

77. Strain JD, et al: Intravenously administered pentobarbital sodium for sedation in pediatric CT, *Radiology* 161:105-108, 1986.

78. Strauss BS, Blaufox MD: Estimation of residual urine and urine flow rates without urethral catheterization, *J Nucl Med* 11:81-84, 1970.

79. Sty JR, Starshak RJ: The role of bone scintigraphy in the evaluation of the suspected abused child, *Radiology* 146:369-375, 1983.

80. Treves ST, Davis RT, et al: Administered radiopharmaceutical doses in children: a survey of 13 pediatric hospitals in North America, *J Nucl Med* 49(6): 1024-1027, 2008.

81. Weiss S, Conway JJ: Radionuclide cystography, *J Nucl Med Technol* 15:66-74, 1987.

82. Weiss S, Conway JJ: The technique of direct radionuclide cystography, *Appl Radiol* 4:133-137, 1975.

83. Weiss SC, Conway JJ: An injection technique artifact, *J Nucl Med Technol* 12:10-12, 1984.

84. Whitfield HN, et al: The distinction between obstructive uropathy and nephropathy by radioisotope transit times, *Br J Urol* 39:433-436, 1978.

85. Wilcox JR, Moniot AL, Green JP: Bone scanning in the evaluation of exercise-related stress injuries, *Radiology* 123:699-703, 1977.

86. Williams G, Treves ST: A second radiographic skeletal survey for child abuse triggered by bone scintigraphy found positive after the initial survey was called negative, *Clin Nucl Med* 32(1):29-31, 2007.

87. Willi U, Treves S: Radionuclide voiding cystography, *Urol Radiol* 5:161-173, 1983.

88. Winter CC: A new test for vesicoureteral reflux: an external technique using radioisotopes, *J Urol* 81:105-111, 1959.

Radionuclides and Radiopharmaceutical Form Used in Clinical Nuclear Medicine

Radionuclide		Half-life	Radiopharmaceutical form or label	Nuclear medicine procedure
^{198}Au	β^- 0.962 max g 0.412 (95%)	2.69 days	Colloid	Therapy: synoviorthesis
^{11}C	β^+ 0.97 max (99%), annihilation photons (200%)	20.3 minutes	Acetate	Measurement of fatty acid that tracks the Krebs cycle. Used for prostate caner imaging and myocardial oxidative metabolism
			Choline	Measurement of cell membrane metabolism in oncologic applications
			Pittsburgh imaging compound B. (PIB)	Measurement of amyloid plaque
			Fatty acids (palmitate)	Measurement of myocardial fatty acid metabolism
^{14}C	β^- 0.156 max; no γ	5370 years	Urea	Determination of *Helicobacter pylori*
^{57}Co	EC 0.122 (87%)	270 days	Cyanocobalamin	Schilling test
			Cyanocobalamin with intrinsic factor	Schilling test
^{58}Co	EC (85%), β^+ 0.474 max (15%), annihilation photons 0.511 (30%), γ 0.810 (99%)	71 days	Cyanocobalamin	Schilling test
^{51}Cr	EC Vanadium x-rays 0.320 (9%)	27.8 days	Sodium chromate	Measurement of RBC volume
^{62}Cu	β^+ 2.91 max, annihilation photons (195%)	9.7 minutes	PTSM	Measurement of tumor or myocardial blood flow
			ATSM (diacetyl-bis[N^4-methyltiosemicabazone])	Measurement of hypoxia in tumor or myocardium
^{165}Dy	β^- 1.29 max g 0.095 (4%)	139 minutes	Ferric hydroxide	Therapy: synoviorthesis
^{169}Er	β^- 0.34 max	9.6 days	Colloid	Therapy: synoviorthesis (Europe)
^{18}F	β^+ 0.635 max (97%), annihilation photons (194%)	109 minutes	FDG	Measurement of myocardial metabolism (myocardial viability), brain metabolism, WBC activation, tumor glucose metabolism
			Fluorothymidine (FLT)	Measurement of cellular proliferation (DNA)
			Fluoromisonidazole (FMISO)	Measurement of hypoxia
			Fluoro-L-dopa (FDOPA)	Measurement of dopaminergic system integrity
			FTMA	Measurement of myocardial flow
			Sodium fluoride	Bone mineral imaging

Continued

Radionuclide		Half-life	Radiopharmaceutical form or label	Nuclear medicine procedure
^{67}Ga	EC γ 0.093 (40%), γ 0.184 (24%), γ 0.296 (22%), γ 0.388 (7%)	77.9 hours	Citrate	Imaging: inflammatory processes; soft-tissue tumor
			Imciromab pentetate	Monoclonal antibody for imaging; imaging myocardial necrosis
			Satumomab pendetide	Imaging metastatic disease of colorectal and ovarian cancer
^{123}I	EC Telurium x-rays 0.159 (83%)	13.3 hours	Fatty acids	Measurement of myocardial metabolism
			MIBG	Metabolism imaging: pheochromocytoma; neuroblastoma
			Sodium iodide	Measurement of sympathetic innervation thyroid imaging and uptake
^{125}I	EC Telurium x-rays 0.035 (7%)	60 days	Isothalamade	Measurement of GFR
			Human serum albumin (RISA)	Measurement of plasma volume
^{131}I	β⁻ max 0.606 (89.3%); 0.334 (7.4%); g 0.080 (2.6%), 0.364 (82%), 0.637 (7%), 0.723 (1.6%)	8.05 days	Iodide	Thyroid uptake therapy: thyroid
			Iodohippurate Iodomethylnorcholesteral (NP-59)	Renal imaging and function; imaging adrenal glands
			MIBG	Imaging pheochromocytomas and neuroblastomas
			Tositumomab	Therapy: non-Hodgkin's lymphoma
^{111}In	EC cadmium x-rays 0.173 (89%), 0.247 (94%)	2.81 days	Animyosin	Imaging to detect acute myocardial necrosis
			Capromab pendetide	Monoclonal antibody for imaging prostate
			Chloride	Labeling monoclonal antibodies and peptides; tumor and abscess imaging
			DTPA	Cisternography; gastric emptying
			Imciromab pentetate ibritumomab	Imaging to detect acute myocardial necrosis
			Tiuxetan iodothalamate	Imaging B-cell lymphoma
			Oxine	Labeling leukocytes and platelets
			DTPA	WBC migration study; imaging CSF
			Pentetreotide	Imaging neuroendocrine tumors
			Satumomab pendetide	Imaging metastatic disease from colon and ovarian cancer
^{81m}Kr	IT, no β⁺, Kr x-ray 0.190 (65%)	13 seconds	Gas	Pulmonary ventilation (not in United States)
^{13}N	β⁺ 1.20 max (100%), annihilation photons (200%)	9.96 minutes	Ammonia	Imaging to evaluate myocardial perfusion
^{15}O	β⁺ 1.73 max (99.9%), annihilation photons (200%)	2.03 minutes	Water	Perfusion imaging
^{32}P	β⁻ 1.71 max (100%)	14.3 days	Chromic phosphate	Therapy: malignant effusions, synoviorthesis
			Sodium phosphate	Therapy: polycythemia vera; bone pain
^{186}Re	β⁻ 1.00 max	140 days	Colloid	Therapy: synoviorthesis (Europe)
^{82}Rb	β⁺ 3.15 max (96%), annihilation photonsm (192%)	75 seconds	Rubidium cholide	Imaging evaluation of myocardial perfusion measurement of myocardial flow
^{153}Sm	β⁻ 0.80 max, Europium x-rays 0.070 (5.4%), 0.103 (28%)	47 hours	Lexidronan (EDTMP)	Palliative therapy: bone pain due to metastatic disease
^{89}Sr	β⁻ 1.46 max γ 0.91 (0.009%)	52 days	Chloride	Palliative therapy: bone pain due to metastatic disease
^{201}Tl	EC Hg x-rays 0.069 to 0.080 (94.4%); γ 0.167 (10%)	73.1 hours	Thallous chloride	Imaging: myocardial perfusion; parathyroid glands; tumors
^{133}Xe	β⁻ 0.364 max Cesium x-rays 0.080 (37%)	5.2 days	Gas	Imaging pulmonary ventilation

Radionuclide		Half-life	Radiopharmaceutical form or label	Nuclear medicine procedure
^{90}Y	β^- 2.27 max	64 hours	Ibritumomab tiuxetan	Therapy: B-cell non-Hodgkin's lymphoma
			Microspheres	Therapy: liver cancer
			Citrate silicate	Therapy: synoviorthesis (Europe)
^{99m}Tc	γ 0.140 (90%)	6.05 hours	Arcitumomab	Evaluation of colorectal cancer
			Apcitide	Thrombus imaging
			Albumin	Measurement of ventricular function
			Albumin colloid	Imaging RES
			Bicisate (ECD)	Imaging cerebral perfusion
			Denatured RBCs	Spleen imaging
			Depreotide	Imaging pulmonary masses
			DTPA	Renal imaging: glomerular filtration angiography: radioaerosol ventilation imaging; ventricular shunt study
			DMSA	Renal imaging: tubular function
			Disofenin (DISDA)	Imaging hepatobiliary
			Exametazine (HMPAO)	Imaging cerebral perfusion
			Tagged WBC	Imaging sites of infection (WBC labeling)
			Fanolesomab	Imaging infection (appendicitis)
			Glucoheptonate	Imaging: renal, brain
			Human serum albumin (HSA)	Lymphoscintigraphy
			Lidofenin (HIDA)	Hepatobiliary imaging
			Macroaggregated albumin (MAA)	Imaging pulmonary perfusion; LeVeen shunt study
			Mebrofenin	Hepatobiliary imaging
			Medronate (MDP)	Skeletal imaging
			Mercaptoacetyl-triglycerine mertiatide (MAG3)	Renal imaging: tubular secretion
			Nofetumomab merpentan (NR-LU-10)	Monoclonal antibody fragment (FAB) for imaging small cell lung cancer
			Oxidronate (HDP)	Skeletal imaging
			Pyrophosphate (PYP)	Imaging to detect acute myocardial necrosis
			RBCs	Imaging: GI bleeds, hemangioma; measurement of ventricular function
			Sestamibi (MIBI)	Imaging myocardial perfusion, breast, parathyroid; tumor viability study
			Sodium pertechnetate	Imaging: brain, thyroid, salivary glands ectopic gastric mucosa; testicular imaging; dacrocystography; cystography
			Sulfur colloid	Imaging: RES system, gastric emptying, GI bleed, bone marrow; LeVeen shunt study; cystography; lymphoscintigraphy; localization for ^{32}P chromic phosphate therapy; pulmonary aspiration study
			Teboroxime	Imaging myocardial perfusion
			Tetrofosmin	Imaging myocardial perfusion; tumor viability study

CSF, Cerebrospinal fluid; *DMSA,* dimercaptosuccinic acid; *DTPA,* diethylenetriamine-pentaacetic acide; *EC,* electron capture; *FDG,* fluorodeoxyglucose; *FTMA,* 4-[F-18]fluorotri-N-methylanilinium; *GFR,* glomerular filtration rate; *GI,* gastrointestinal; *IT,* isomeric transition; *MIBG,* meta-iodobenzylguanidine; *PTSM,* pyruvaldehyde bis(N4-methylthiosemicarbazone); *RBC,* red blood cell; *RES,* reticuloendothelial system; *WBC,* white blood cell.

Percentage Points and Chi-Square Distribution

$$F\left(\chi^2\right) = \int_0^{x^2} \frac{1}{2^{\frac{n}{2}}\Gamma\left(\frac{n}{2}\right)} x^{\frac{n-2}{2}} e^{\frac{-x}{2}} dx$$

F/N	.005	.010	.025	.050	.100	.250	.500	.750	.900	.950	.975	.990	.995
1	.0000393	.000157	.000982	.00393	.0158	.102	.455	1.32	2.71	3.84	5.02	6.63	7.88
2	.0100	.0201	.0506	.103	.211	.575	1.39	2.77	4.61	5.99	7.38	9.21	10.6
3	.0717	.115	.216	.352	.584	1.21	2.37	4.11	6.25	7.81	9.35	11.3	12.8
4	.207	.297	.484	.711	1.06	1.92	3.36	5.39	7.78	9.49	11.1	13.3	14.9
5	.412	.554	.831	1.15	1.61	2.67	4.35	6.63	9.24	11.1	12.8	15.1	16.7
6	.676	.872	1.24	1.64	2.20	3.45	5.35	7.84	10.6	12.6	14.4	16.8	18.5
7	.989	1.24	1.69	2.17	2.83	4.25	6.35	9.04	12.0	14.1	16.0	18.5	20.3
8	1.34	1.65	2.18	2.73	3.49	5.07	7.34	10.2	13.4	15.5	17.5	20.1	22.0
9	1.73	2.09	2.70	3.33	4.17	5.90	8.34	11.4	14.7	16.9	19.0	21.7	23.6
10	2.15	2.56	3.25	3.94	4.87	6.74	9.34	12.5	16.0	18.3	20.5	23.2	25.2
11	2.60	3.05	3.82	4.57	5.58	7.58	10.3	13.7	17.3	19.7	21.9	24.7	26.8
12	3.07	3.57	4.40	5.23	6.30	8.44	11.3	14.8	18.5	21.0	23.3	26.2	28.3
13	3.57	4.11	5.01	5.89	7.04	9.30	12.3	16.0	19.8	22.4	24.7	27.7	29.8
14	4.07	4.66	5.63	6.57	7.79	10.2	13.3	17.1	21.1	23.7	26.1	29.1	31.3
15	4.60	5.23	6.26	7.26	8.55	11.0	14.3	18.2	22.3	25.0	27.5	30.6	32.6
16	5.14	5.81	6.91	7.96	9.31	11.9	15.3	19.4	23.5	26.3	28.8	32.0	34.3
17	5.70	6.41	7.56	8.67	10.1	12.8	16.3	20.5	24.8	27.6	30.2	33.4	35.7
18	6.26	7.01	8.23	9.39	10.9	13.7	17.3	21.6	26.0	28.9	31.5	34.8	37.2
19	6.84	7.63	8.91	10.1	11.7	14.6	18.3	22.7	27.2	30.1	32.9	36.2	38.6
20	7.43	8.26	9.59	10.9	12.4	15.5	19.3	23.8	28.4	31.4	34.2	37.6	40.0
21	8.03	8.90	10.3	11.6	13.2	16.3	20.3	24.9	29.6	32.7	35.5	38.9	41.4
22	8.64	9.54	11.0	12.3	14.0	17.2	21.3	26.0	30.8	33.9	36.8	40.3	42.8
23	9.26	10.2	11.7	13.1	14.8	18.1	22.3	27.1	32.0	35.2	38.1	41.6	44.2
24	9.89	10.9	12.4	13.8	15.7	19.0	23.3	28.2	33.2	36.4	39.4	43.0	45.6
25	10.5	11.5	13.1	14.6	16.5	19.9	24.3	29.3	34.4	37.7	40.6	44.3	46.9
26	11.2	12.2	13.8	15.4	17.3	20.8	25.3	30.4	35.6	38.9	41.9	45.6	48.3
27	11.8	12.9	14.6	16.2	18.1	21.7	26.3	31.5	36.7	40.1	43.2	47.0	49.6
28	12.5	13.6	15.3	16.9	18.9	22.7	27.3	32.6	37.9	41.3	44.5	48.3	51.0
29	13.1	14.3	16.0	17.7	19.8	23.6	28.3	33.7	39.1	42.6	45.7	49.6	52.3
30	13.8	15.0	16.8	18.5	20.6	24.5	29.3	34.8	40.3	43.8	47.0	50.9	53.7

A number See *atomic mass.*

ablation (1) Separation or detachment. (2) Destruction, that is, by radiation.

abscess Localized collection of pus within tissue.

abscissa The *x*-, or horizontal, axis in a cartesian graph plot.

absolute activity calibration (well counter calibration) Well counter calibration is a historical term for a calibration more appropriately referred to as *absolute activity calibration.* Absolute activity calibration factors are used to convert pixel values into a measure of absolute activity per voxel.

absorption coefficient (α) Constant representing the fraction of ionizing radiation absorbed per centimeter thickness of absorbing material.

accelerator Device imparting high kinetic energy to a charged particle, causing it to undergo nuclear or particle reaction.

access time The time required for a computer to locate and retrieve information from a specified location. In the case of memory, this is related to the electronic speed of the address register and read/write circuits. In the case of disks, the access time is the sum of the time taken for the read/write head to locate a particular track plus the time required for information to rotate into the read/write position.

accumulator Register or data buffer used for temporary storage of data.

accuracy Refers to whether a given measurement or set of measurements reflects a true or exact value.

ACE Angiotensin-converting enzyme.

achalasia (1) Failure to relax; referring especially to pylorus, cardia, or any other sphincter muscles. (2) Obstruction of the terminal esophagus just proximal to the cardioesophageal junction.

acid Any chemical compound that can either donate a proton or accept a pair of electrons in a chemical reaction.

acidophilic (1) Stains easily with acid dyes. (2) Grows best in acid media.

acinus Smallest lobule of a gland; secretes the product of the gland.

acquisition Intake of data to the computer.

ACR American College of Radiology.

ACTH See *adrenocorticotropin.*

activation analysis Analytical procedure detecting and measuring trace quantities of elements after exposure to a flux of neutrons.

ADC See *analog-digital converters.*

A/D converter See *analog-digital converters.*

address Label, name, or number that designates a location where information is stored.

adduct An addition product, or complex, or one part of the same.

adenohypophysis Anterior lobe of the pituitary.

adenoma Epithelial tumor composed of glandular tissue.

adenosine An endogenously produced nucleoside that causes coronary and systemic vasodilation.

adenylate cyclase Enzyme found in the liver and muscle cell membranes.

adjuvant That which aids or assists.

adrenal cortex Outer portion of the adrenal gland; it produces cortisone.

adrenal medulla Central portion of the adrenal gland; it produces adrenalin.

adrenergic Relating to nerve fibers of the autonomic nervous system that liberate norepinephrine.

adrenocorticotropin (ACTH) Compound isolated from the anterior pituitary having a stimulating effect on the adrenal cortex.

aerosol Liquid particles suspended in a gas to be dispensed in a mist or spray.

afferent Carrying or conveying toward a center.

affinity (1) Attraction of a specific reactor substance for a ligand. (2) An inherent attraction for substances to undergo reactions with one another.

affinity chromatography Separation of compounds based on differences in their affinities for a given species.

agonist A drug capable of combining with receptors to initiate drug action.

akinesia Abnormal reduction of muscle movement.

ALARA U.S. Nuclear Regulatory Commission operating philosophy for maintaining occupational radiation exposures "as low as reasonably achievable."

albumin Class of simple proteins; found in most tissues.

alcohol Organic molecule containing the functional —OH group.

aldehyde Organic molecule containing the functional group:

$$\begin{array}{c} O \\ \| \\ -C-H \end{array}$$

aldosterone Sodium-retaining hormone of the adrenal cortex.

ALGOL (ALGOrithmic Language) High-level compiler language particularly well suited to arithmetic and string manipulations.

algorithm Prescribed set of well-defined rules or processes for the solution of a problem in a finite number of steps.

alimentary canal Food tract starting with the mouth and ending with the rectum and anus.

aliquot Specific measured amount of liquid.

alkane Hydrocarbon with a general formula of C_nH_{2n+2}.

alkene Hydrocarbon that has one double bond and a general formula of C_nH_{2n}.

alkyl Alkane with one hydrogen atom removed.

alkyne Hydrocarbon that contains a triple bond and a general formula of C_2H_{2n-2}.

alpha cells Cells in pancreatic islets containing large granules.

alpha decay Radioactive decay of radionuclides resulting in the emission of an alpha particle.

alpha particle (α) Nucleus of a helium atom emitted by certain radioisotopes upon disintegration.

ALU See *arithmetic unit.*

alveoli   Terminal air pockets in the lungs.

amelioration   Improvement of a disease.

amide   Organic molecule with the functional group:

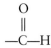

amine   Organic molecule containing the functional group —NH_2.

amino acid   Organic acid containing an NH_2 and a COOH group, thus having both basic and acidic properties.

aminophylline   A vasodilator and cardiac stimulant.

AMP   Adenosine monophosphate; nucleotide containing adenine, a pentose sugar, and one phosphoric acid; product of metabolism.

amphoteric   Having two opposite characteristics, especially having the capacity of reacting as either acid or base.

amplifier   A device used to linearly increase pulse size.

amplitude   The height of a waveform.

ampulla of Vater   Dilation of ducts from the liver and pancreas where they enter the small intestine.

AMU   See *atomic mass unit.*

amyloidosis   A disease characterized by extracellular accumulation of amyloid in various organs and tissues.

analog   (1) Representation of a parameter by a signal the magnitude of which voltage, current, or length is proportional to the parameter. (2) Structure with a similar function.

analog computer   A computer that parameterizes data in terms of the magnitude of the incoming signals.

analog-digital converter (ADC; A/D converter)   Electronic module used to convert an analog signal, such as a pulse height, into digital information recognizable by a computer.

anastomose   To unite an end to another end; to bridge two vessels with a section of a vessel.

androgenic hormone   Hormone stimulating male characteristics.

anemia   Deficiency of red blood cells.

aneurysm   Dilation of part of the wall of an artery.

Anger camera   Type of gamma ray scintillation camera, named for its inventor, Hal O. Anger.

angina   Chest pain usually due to insufficient oxygen supply to the heart.

angiography   X-ray photography of the blood vessels with use of a radiopaque substance.

angiotensin   Vasoconstrictor substance present in blood.

angstrom   A measurement of wavelength (10^{-8} cm).

anion   Negatively charged ion.

annihilation radiation   Reaction between a pair of particles resulting in their disintegration and the production of an equivalent amount of energy in the form of photons.

anode   A positively charged electrode that attracts electrons. In an x-ray tube of a CT, the anode accelerates electrons from the cathode to produce x-rays. The anode of a CT scanner has a rotating design to dissipate the heat produced because the beam must be on for many seconds.

anoxia   Deficiency of oxygen.

antecubital   Area in front of the elbow.

antibiotics   Drugs used to destroy bacteria; extracted from living organisms.

antibody   Substance capable of producing specific immunity to a bacterium or virus; found in the blood.

anticholinergic   Drugs blocking passage of impulses through the autonomic nerves.

anticoagulant   A substance that prevents the normal clotting of blood.

antigen   Molecule or particle capable of eliciting an immune response.

antineutrino   Neutral nuclear particle emitted in either positron decay or electron capture.

antiserum   Serum containing antibodies.

aorta   Large artery stemming from the left ventricle.

apatite   Crystalline phosphate of lime.

apex   The top of an organ.

aplasia   Failure of an organ to develop.

aplastic anemia   Anemia characterized by absence of red blood cell regeneration.

application program   Program that performs a task specific to a particular user's needs.

aqueous   Referring to anything dissolved in water.

arachnoid   Membrane covering the brain and spinal cord.

arene   Hydrocarbon compound that contains an aromatic portion.

arithmetic and logic unit (ALU)   See *arithmetic unit.*

arithmetic unit (AU)   Unit within the computer architecture that performs all mathematical and logical operations. Sometimes called *arithmetic and logic unit* (ALU).

aromatic compound   Chemical compound containing a ring system that has $(4n + 2)$ π electrons.

array processor   A specially devised high-speed computer that performs computations on image array elements in a parallel fashion.

Arrhenius concept   Concept stating that an acid is a compound that acts as a proton donor.

arrhythmia   Variation of the heartbeat.

arterial thrombus   Blood clot formed in an artery.

arthrography   Radiography after the introduction of opaque contrast material into a joint.

ASCII   Abbreviation for American Standard Code for Information Interchange, consisting of 128 seven-bit binary codes for uppercase and lowercase letters, numbers, punctuation, and special communication control characters.

ascites   An accumulation of serous fluid in the peritoneal cavity.

ascorbic acid   Vitamin C.

asepsis   Sterile state.

aseptic technique   Practice followed to prevent contact with or spread of microorganisms.

assembler   Programs that assemble symbolic programs into binary form.

assembly language   Commands for the minicomputer system written in symbolic or mnemonic form. Typically, three-letter abbreviations, called *mnemonics*, are used to represent each instruction, and each mnemonic can usually be equaled to one machine-code or binary instruction. An assembly language program is translated to binary code by an assembler.

asthma   A hyperreactive airway disease manifested as a chronic inflammatory disorder of airways of the lungs.

astrocytoma Central nervous system tumor composed of star-shaped cells.

ataxia Disorder of the neuromuscular system; lacking muscle coordination.

atherosclerosis Arterial hardening.

ATN Acute tubular necrosis.

atom Smallest unit of an element that can exist and still maintain the properties of the element.

atomic mass (A) Mass of a neutral atom usually expressed in atomic mass units.

atomic mass unit (AMU) Exactly one twelfth the mass of carbon 12; 1.661×10^{-24} g.

atomic number Number of protons in an atom, the symbol of which is Z.

atomic weight Average weight of the neutral atoms of an element.

ATP Adenosine triphosphate.

atrium Cavity of the heart receiving blood.

attenuation Any condition that results in a decrease of radiation intensity.

attenuation correction Compensation for the effects of radiation attenuation in computed tomography that may use mathematical estimate or measured transmission data.

Auger electrons Pronounced $\bar{o}$-'zhā. Electrons that participate in the production of x-rays.

AV block Impairment of the normal conduction between the atria and the ventricles.

avidity (1) Tendency of a specific reactor substance to hold its ligands. (2) The firmness of a combination of substances in reactions in terms of their dissociation.

AVN Avascular necrosis.

Avogadro's number Number of atoms in the gram atomic weight of a given element or the number of molecules in the gram molecular weight of a given substance: 6.022×10^{23} per gram mole.

axis of rotation In SPECT, an imaginary line passing through the center of the gantry about which the camera rotates.

axon The conducting portion of a nerve fiber.

background Detected disintegration events not emanating from the sample.

back-projection A computer manipulation of acquired image data back-projected into space.

backscattering Scattering of particulate radiation by more than 90 degrees.

bar phantom See *phantom*.

barn Area unit expressing the area of nuclear cross section; 1 barn = 10^{-24} cm^2.

Barrett esophagus Chronic peptic ulcer of the lower esophagus.

basal ganglia An aggregation of nerve cell bodies of the telencephalon.

base Any compound that either acts as a proton acceptor or an electron pair donor in a chemical process; the lower portion of the lung.

baseline Normal evaluation; evaluation before administration of a substance.

BASIC (Beginner's All-purpose Symbolic Instruction Code) High-level interactive, interpreter language for mathematical and string-variable manipulations.

batch mode Automatic computer mode that does not require specific programming instruction.

batch operation Computer operation that runs consecutively without operator intervention.

baud A unit of measurement of transmission speed; bits per second.

beam hardening An effective energy shift in the spectrum of an x-ray beam to more high energy photons due to the higher likelihood of the absorption of low energy x-rays.

becquerel (Bq) The Système Internationale unit of activity, equal to one disintegration per second, 1 Bq = 1 dps.

beta cells Pancreatic cells in the islets of Langerhans.

beta decay Radioactive decay of radionuclides resulting in the emission of beta particles.

beta (β^-) particle Electron whose point of origin is the nucleus; electron originating in the nucleus by way of decay of a neutron into a proton and electron (beta particle).

BGO Bismuth germinate; a PET scanner detection material.

biconcave Having two concave surfaces.

bifunctional chelates Complexing agent with two sites for complexation.

bifunctional drug Drug with ability to attack two types of symptoms or disease.

biliary atresia A congenital absence of bile ducts.

biliary system System including the liver serving both a digestive and an excretory function.

binary Pertaining to the number system with a radix of two.

binary code A code that uses two distinct characters, usually the numbers 0 and 1.

binary digit One of the symbols 1 or 0; called a *bit*.

binder See *specific reactor substance*.

binding constant The equilibrium constant for a reaction between an antibody or binding protein and its antigen or ligand.

binding energy Energy released when a chemical bond is formed; amount of stabilization energy holding a nucleon in the nucleus.

binding sites Sites on a protein where they bind to radionuclides.

bioassay Determination of chemical strength by tests of living tissues.

biochemical Referring to the chemistry of living organisms.

biochemical analogs Chemicals of the living system that resemble one another in function but not in structure.

bioeffects Effects on the biological system.

biological distribution Normal distribution of a substance within the living system.

biological half-life The elapsed time for the biological elimination of 50% of a material from the body.

biological matrix Basic materials of living systems.

biopsy Examination of tissue taken from the living body, usually without entirely removing the organ.

BIOS Basic input/output system.

biosynthesis Formation of a compound from other compounds by living organisms.

bisacodyl tablets   Drugs used as a laxative.

bismuth germinate (BGO)   A PET scanner detection material.

bit   An individual binary digit, either 1 or 0; acronym for *bi*nary digi*t*.

blank scan   A daily calibration of PET scanners using the transmission source to measure the count rate and uniformity of each detector with no attenuation material in the scanner. Blank scans are a reference for attenuation correction in addition to providing sinograms for visual evaluation of system uniformity.

bleomycin   An antibody substance having antineoplastic properties.

block   A group of bytes on a disk or magnetic tape used for data storage.

blood-brain barrier   A defense mechanism of the brain that prevents substances unnecessary for function from crossing into the brain.

blood pool   Vascular cavity.

body-contour orbits   A SPECT system that allows the orbit of the camera to be as close to the body as possible throughout the tomographic acquisition, thereby maximizing resolution.

bolus   Rounded mass or lump quantity; a concentrated radiopharmaceutical given intravenously.

bombardment   Exposure of a target to any ionizing radiation.

bootstrap program   Routine whose first instructions are sufficient to load the remainder of itself into memory from an input device and normally start a complex system of programs.

Bowman capsule   Sac at the end of uriniferous tubules in the kidneys.

bradycardia   Slow heartbeat.

Bragg curve   Curve showing specific ionization as a function of distance or energy.

bremsstrahlung x-rays   The German word for *braking radiation*. The mechanism that produces x-rays in a broad energy spectrum as the result of rapid deceleration of electrons that pass near the atomic nucleus. Also, photonic emissions caused by the slowing down of beta particles in matter.

bromination   Chemical addition of bromine to a compound.

bromocryptine   A dopamine receptor agonist.

bronchiectasis   Dilation of the small bronchial tubes.

bronchioles   Small bronchial tubes leading to air cells.

bronchus   Large passage carrying air within the lungs.

Brönsted-Lowry concept   Concept stating that an acid is a proton donor and a base is a proton acceptor in a chemical process.

brownian movement   Motion of minute particles suspended in liquid.

BSP   Body substance precautions.

BTU   British thermal unit; measurement of heat.

buffer   (1) Storage area used to temporarily hold information being transferred between two devices or between a device and memory; often a special register or a designated area of memory. (2) A solution of a weak acid and one of its salts that resists change in pH; usually used to maintain a constant pH for a reaction in solution.

buffer solution   A solution that has a specific pH value and is resistant to pH change by addition of acids or bases.

buffy coat   The grayish colored layer just above the red cells in a sample of blood, which is the white cell population in that sample of blood.

bug   An error in a program.

bullous   Referring to a bubble or a bladder.

bundle branch block   Interventricular block due to interruption of one of the two main branches of the bundle of His.

bus   A flat, flexible cable consisting of many transmission lines or wires; it interconnects computer system components to provide communication paths for addresses, data, and control information.

byproduct material   Radioactive material arising from controlled fission.

byte   A group of binary digits usually operated upon as a unit and usually 8 bits long. In ASCII code, one character occupies one byte of memory, and the maximum decimal integer that can be stored in an 8-bit byte is 255.

C   A computer programming language.

cache memory   A high-speed memory, usually part of the CPU.

CAD   Coronary artery disease.

calyx (*pl.* calyces)   Cuplike structure in the kidney that receives urine.

canaliculus   Small canal or channel.

cancer   A broad term used to describe genetic changes that result in the uncontrolled growth and spread of abnormal cells in the body; if left undetected, may become life-threatening, resulting in death.

carbohydrate   Compound consisting of carbon, hydrogen, and oxygen, such as sugars and starches.

carboxylic acids   Organic molecules with the functional group:

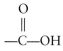

that have acidic properties because of this functional group.

carcinogen   Substance stimulating the formation of cancer.

carcinoma   Malignant tumor consisting of connective tissue enclosing epithelial cells.

cardiac cycle   One beat of the heart, which consists of systole, the period of ventricular contraction, and diastole, the period of ventricular relaxation.

cardiac ejection fraction (EF)   That fraction of the total volume of blood of the left ventricle ejected per contraction.

cardiac output   The quantity of blood ejected by the heart over a 1-minute interval.

cardiac reorientation   The generation of these standard sections (short axis, horizontal long axis, and vertical long axis) from the original transaxial images with the location of the left ventricular axis marked.

cardiomyopathy   Subacute or chronic disorder of the heart muscle.

carrier   Quantity of an element mixed with radioactive isotopes of that element to facilitate chemical operations.

carrier free Adjective describing a nuclide that is free of its stable isotopes.

carrier proteins Macroscopic amounts of nonlabeled proteins present with trace amounts of radiolabeled proteins.

cartesian coordinate system Utilization of numbers to locate a point in relation to two intersecting straight lines.

catabolism The breaking down within the body of complex chemical compounds into simpler ones.

cathode A negatively charged electrode that acts as a source of electrons. In an x-ray tube the cathode is the source of free electrons.

cathode ray tube (CRT) Electronic vacuum tube with a display screen where information is displayed.

cation Positively charged ion.

cauda equina End of the spinal cord containing the nerves that supply the rectal area.

CBG Cortisol-binding globulin.

CDC Centers for Disease Control and Prevention.

CEA Carcinoma embryonic antigen.

Celsius (1) Swedish astronomer and inventor. (2) Centigrade, the temperature scale in which there are 100 degrees between freezing and boiling water at sea level.

center of rotation (COR) Reference data used for correcting the slight misalignment of SPECT images taken from various projections.

central nervous system (CNS) That part of the nervous system containing the brain, spinal cord, and nerves.

central processing unit (CPU) Unit of a computing system that includes the circuits controlling the interpretation and execution of instructions—the computer proper, excluding I/O and other peripheral devices.

centrifuge (1) To rotate or spin at high speed for separation. (2) Instrument for rotating or spinning samples at high speed.

cerebral radionuclide angiogram, cerebral radioangiogram Rapid sequential scintiphotos of the blood vessels of the brain.

cerebrospinal fluid (CSF) Fluid found in the cavities of the brain, brain stem, spinal cord, and meninges.

Chagas disease South American trypanosomiasis.

character A single letter, numeral, or symbol used to represent information.

characteristic x-rays Monoenergetic x-rays that are produced by electrons dropping to a lower energy shell in the atom. These x-rays may result from ionization of the atom by a process that removes an inner shell electron such as a photoelectric interaction.

charged-particle accelerators Device used to electronically accelerate any charged particle. See also *cyclotron* and *electron accelerator*.

chart of nuclides The plotting of nuclides by their number of protons (vertical axis) and neutron number (horizontal axis).

chelate Ligand that has two or more potential bonding sites.

chemical equation Symbolic statement describing a process and showing the stoichiometric relationships among the individual species involved in the process.

chemical equilibrium State of lowest energy for a chemical system undergoing a chemical reaction.

chemical reaction Processes that result in chemical change of the participant molecules.

chemistry Study of matter and the changes that matter undergoes.

child abuse Any form of physical, emotional, or sexual maltreatment of children.

chi-square test A mathematical procedure applied to a series of observations to determine their amount of variability.

chloramine-T *N*-Chloro-4-methylbenzenesulfonamide sodium salt; an oxidizing agent used in radioiodination of proteins.

chlormerodrin Diuretic containing mercury.

cholecystitis Inflammation of the gallbladder.

cholecystokinin Hormone secreted by the small intestine; stimulates contraction of the gallbladder.

cholescintigraphy An imaging procedure to evaluate gallbladder function.

choroid plexus Membrane lining the ventricles of the brain, concerned with formation of cerebrospinal fluid.

chromatography Method of chemical analysis where the solution to be analyzed separates into component parts; some types are gel permeation chromatography, paper chromatography, and affinity chromatography.

cinematic display A dynamic sequence of images displayed in a continuous loop movie.

circumferential profile Normal boundaries or normal limits for each point in each profile are created based on statistical values amassed from a large number of normal subjects obtained from each angle on each slice for the purpose of determining perfusion defects in an image.

cistern Fluid reservoir; enclosed space.

CLIA 88 Clinical Laboratories Improvement Act of 1988.

clock A device within a computer system that keeps time, counts pulses, measures frequency, or generates periodic signals for synchronization.

closing capacity The volume of air in the lungs when closure begins.

cloud chamber Chamber where the paths of ionizing radiation can be observed.

COBOL (COmmercial and Business Oriented Language) A high-level incremental compiler language primarily suited to business applications.

cocktail A liquid scintillator.

code A system of symbols representing data or instructions executed by a computer.

coding The writing of instructions for a computer, using a system of symbols meaningful to a computer, an assembler, a compiler, or a language processor.

coefficient Constant by which a variable or other quantity is multiplied in an equation.

coefficient of variation A statistical measurement of the validity of serial observations on a changing parameter.

cohort labeling The labeling of blood cells all of the same age and therefore available only to the marrow precursors of a given cell type for a specific and limited length of time; it does not label cells already circulating.

coincidence counting A means of detecting radiation by two detectors placed in opposition to one another; an event is recorded only when seen by both detectors simultaneously.

coincidence lines Events recorded by detectors placed in opposition.

collagen Protein found in bone and cartilage.

collimator Shielding device used to limit the angle of entry of radiation.

colloid Molecules in a continuous medium that measure between 1 and 100 nm in diameter.

colonic transit The peristalsis mechanism to transport solid intake through the colon.

colorimetry Measurement of color.

colostomy Artificial opening in the colon.

column generator Column device using a parent radionuclide absorbed to a support in a column; the daughter radionuclide is usually obtained by elution of the column with a solution that interacts with the daughter but not with the parent.

command A word, mnemonic, or character that, by virtue of its syntax, is an input line that causes a computer system to perform a predefined operation.

competitive protein binding (CPB) Type of competitive binding radioassay in which the specific reactor substance is a native nonimmunological protein.

compile To produce a binary code program from a program written in source (symbolic) language, by selection of appropriate subroutines from a subroutine library, as directed by the instructions or other symbols of the source program; the linkage is supplied for combining the subroutines into a workable program, and the subroutines and linkage are translated into binary code.

compiler Program used to compile assembly code or source code.

complement A substance normally present in serum that is destructive to certain bacteria and other cells that have been sensitized by specific complement antibody.

complex ions The product resulting from the actions of neutral molecules with either a cation or an anion.

compliance The change in volume for a change in pressure.

compound Distinct substance formed by a union of two or more elements in definite proportions by weight.

Compton edge See *Compton scatter*.

Compton plateau See *Compton scatter*.

Compton scatter One process by which a photon loses energy through collisions with electrons.

computer Programmable electronic device that can store, retrieve, and process data.

computer program A plan or routine for solving a problem on a computer.

computer system A data processing system consisting of hardware devices, software programs, and documentation that describes the operation of the system.

concentration Strength of substance in a solution.

congener One of two or more things of the same kind.

congenital Existing at birth.

conjugate acid Remainder of a basic compound after it has either accepted a proton or donated an electron pair in a chemical process.

conjugate base Remainder of an acidic compound after it has either donated its acidic proton or accepted an electron pair in a chemical process.

constant A value that remains the same throughout a distinct operation.

contrast In scintigraphic imaging it is the measure of counts (or intensity) in the target (the object we are trying to image) compared with the intensity in a background region.

conversion electron Orbital electron that has been excited (ionized) by internal conversion of an excited atom.

coordinate covalent bond Covalent bond formed by two atoms in which one atom donates both electrons for the bond.

COPD Chronic obstructive pulmonary disease.

coronal plane Plane that takes its name from the coronal suture of the skull dividing the body into the front and back portions.

corticosterone Compound isolated from the adrenal cortex.

cortisol Adrenocortical hormone.

Coulomb's law Basic law of electrostatics, which states that:

$$F = \frac{q_1 q_2}{4\pi\varepsilon_0 r^2}$$

covalent bond Chemical bond formed by sharing a pair of electrons by two nuclei.

covalent compound Compound held together by covalent bonds.

CPB See *competitive protein binding*.

CPR Cardiopulmonary resuscitation.

CPU See *central processing unit*.

crash *Hardware crash* is the complete failure of a particular device, sometimes affecting the operation of an entire computer system; *software crash* is the complete failure of an operating system characterized by some failure in the system's protection mechanisms.

CRFS Comprehensive renal function study.

critical organ (1) Organ of interest. (2) Organ most affected by a technique.

cross-reactivity Reaction of a molecule with an immunoglobulin directed toward another substance.

CRT See *cathode ray tube*.

crystallography Study of the crystal structure of a molecule.

CSF See *cerebrospinal fluid*.

CT Computed tomography.

CT number See *Hounsfield unit*.

CU Control unit, a component of a computer's central processing unit.

curie Standard measure of rate of radioactive decay; based on the disintegration of 1 g of radium at 3.7×10^{-10} disintegrations per second.

cutie pie A type of ionization chamber.

cutoff frequency The frequency at which the filter magnitude drops below a certain value.

CVA Cerebrovascular accident.

cyanocobalamine Vitamin B_{12}.

cyclotron Device for accelerating charged particles to high energies using magnetic and oscillating electrostatic fields, causing the particle to move in a spiral path with increasing energy.

data   Facts, numbers, letters, and symbols; data are the basic elements of information that can be processed by a computer.

database   A computer's compilation of information.

daughter radionuclide   Decay product produced by a radionuclide. The element from which the daughter was produced is called the *parent*.

debusser   Device used to erase material from a computer or recording tape.

decay   Radioactive disintegration of a nucleus of an unstable nuclide.

decay constant   Decay rate of a radionuclide based on its half-life.

decay factor   Fraction of radionuclei that have decayed in a specified period, according to the following formula:

$$\lambda = 0.693/t_{1/2}$$

decay schemes   Diagram showing the decay mode or modes of a radionuclide.

dee   A component of a cyclotron in which particle acceleration takes place.

deiodinate   Removal of iodine from a compound.

delayed neutrons   Neutrons that are emitted in a radioactive process at an appreciable time after fission.

dementia   Mental deterioration from disease of the brain.

denaturation   Change in chemical and physical properties from the normal state, usually irreversible.

dendrite   One of the branching protoplasmic processes of the nerve cell.

densitometry   A method of determining bone mineral content from single or dual gamma ray or x-ray absorption measurements.

detector efficiency   The measure of the ability of a detector system to detect deposited energy and produce a response.

deuterons   Nucleus of a deuterium atom containing one proton and one neutron.

device   A hardware unit such as an I/O peripheral, magnetic tape drive, or line printer.

device control unit   A hardware unit that electronically supervises one or more of the same type of devices; it acts as a link between the computer and the I/O devices.

diabetes mellitus   Pathological condition with an absolute or relative insulin deficiency accompanied by elevated levels of glucose in the blood and urine.

diagnostic   (1) Referring to determination of the disease; analysis of symptoms. (2) Pertaining to the detection and isolation of a malfunction (hardware) or mistake (software).

dialysis   Process for separating crystalloids and colloids in solution by the difference in their rates of diffusion through a semipermeable membrane.

diastole   Relaxation and dilation of the heart.

diastolic pressure   The pressure in the heart during diastole.

diethylenetriamine pentaacetic acid (pentetic acid, DTPA)   Chelating agent that can be labeled with ^{99m}Tc and used for scintigraphy.

diffusion weighted imaging (DWI)   Diffusion imaging depends on the random motion of water molecules in tissue. Water diffusion characteristics can be displayed by using DWI where foci of bright intensity suggests restricted motion of water (ischemia or infarcted tissue) within that location,

digit   Character used to express one of the positive integers.

digital computer   Device that operates on discrete data, performing sequences or arithmetic and logical operations in these data.

digitalis   Cardiotonic agent from the *Digitalis* plant leaf.

dimer   A compound produced by the combination of two like molecules, in the strictest sense, without loss of atoms, usually by elimination of water or similar small molecule between the two, but often by simple covalent bonding.

diphosphonate   Organic phosphate compound that can be labeled with ^{99m}Tc and used for scintigraphy.

dipyridamole   A potent coronary vasodilator.

direct memory access (DMA)   Access to data in any location independent of sequential prohibitions.

directory   A file in the form of a table containing the names of and pointers to files on a mass storage volume.

DIS   Decay in storage.

discriminator   An electronic barrier used to eliminate low-amplitude noise pulses.

disintegration   General process of radioactive decay, usually measured per unit time; dps is disintegrations per second, and dpm, disintegrations per minute; dps is equal to counts per second (cps) divided by the efficiency of the detector; dpm is equal to counts per minute divided by the efficiency of the detector.

disk   Form of rotating memory consisting of a platter of aluminum coated with ferrous oxide that can be magnetized or read by a read/write head in proximity to the surface; most common form of bulk memory device.

display   A peripheral device used to represent data graphically; normally refers to some type of cathode ray tube system.

diuretic   Substance that promotes the secretion of urine.

diverticulum   Blind pouch; usually in the intestine.

DLIS   Digoxin-like immunoreactive substance.

DMA   See *direct memory access*.

DMSA   2,3-Dimercaptosuccinic acid; a chelating agent that can be labeled with ^{99m}Tc for renal imaging.

DNA   Deoxyribonucleic acid.

dopamine   An intermediate in tyrosine metabolism and the precursor of norepinephrine and epinephrine; it is present in the central nervous system.

DOS   Disk operating system.

dose   Amount of ionizing radiation absorbed by a specific area or volume or by the whole body.

dose calibrator   An ionization chamber designed to measure radionuclide doses.

dose response curve   The graphic relationship between counts bound and amount of standard added in a radioimmunoassay; a standard curve.

dosimetry   The accurate determination or calculation of dosage.

DOT   Department of Transportation.

DPA (dual photon absorptiometry)   A bone mineral content measurement technique using gamma or x-ray absorption with a dual energy photon-emitting source;

the dual photons allow for accurate correction of soft tissue interference.

DST   Dexamethasone suppression test.

DTPA   See *diethylenetriamine pentaacetic acid*.

DVT   Deep venous thrombosis.

dynode   One of several metal plates with a positive voltage that attracts and accelerates electrons within a photomultiplier tube. There are 8 to 14 dynodes in a photomultiplier tube, each multiplying the number of electrons by a factor of 3 to 6 times.

dysplasia   Abnormality of development.

dyspnea   Difficulty in breathing.

ECG   See *electrocardiogram*.

ECT   Emission computed tomography.

ED   End-diastole.

edema   Excess fluid in the body.

edetic acid (ethylenediaminetetraacetic acid, EDTA)   A chelating agent.

edge packing   An area of increased brightness around the edge of a scintillation camera image.

editor   Program to permit data or instructions to be manipulated and displayed. Most commonly used in the preparation of new programs or in the revision and correction of old programs.

EDTA   See *edetic acid*.

EEG   Electroencephalogram.

EF   See *cardiac ejection fraction*.

effective half-life   The elapsed time to eliminate a radioactive material from the body by a combination of biological elimination and radioactive decay, determined from physical and biological half-lives as:

$$1/t_e = 1/t_p + 1/t_b$$

EI   Excretion index.

ejection fraction   See *cardiac ejection fraction*.

EKG   See *electrocardiogram*.

elastic scattering   Scattering caused by elastic collisions between nuclei that result in a conversion of the system's kinetic energy.

electrocardiogram (ECG)   A graphic record of the electrical currents that traverse the heart and initiate its contraction.

electrochemical process   Chemical process involving oxidation and reduction of the reaction constituents.

electrolyte   Substance that forms ions when dissolved in water.

electrolytic reactions   Oxidation-reduction reactions.

electromagnetic radiation   Radiation as defined by wavelengths (e.g., heat waves, radio waves, infrared light, visible light, ultraviolet light, x-rays, gamma rays).

electrometer   Electrostatic instrument for measuring difference in potential.

electron   Elementary particle of an atom with a charge of -1 and a mass of 9.1×10^{-28} g.

electron accelerators   Machine used to accelerate electrons using potential differences.

electron capture   Method of radioactive decay in which the nucleus captures an orbital electron, which then interacts with a proton, effectively negating the proton and transmuting the nucleus to that of another element.

electron configuration   Refers to the space relationships of electrons in an atom.

electron microscope   Microscope that uses an electron beam to form an image on a fluorescent screen.

electron spin resonance (ESR)   Spectroscopic technique that determines structural features of a molecule based on electron resonance in a magnetic field.

electron volt (eV)   Kinetic energy gained by an electron passing through a potential difference of 1 V.

electronegativity   Tendency of a neutral atom to acquire electrons, measured relative to that of fluorine.

electronic collimation   Method to determine the positional location of radiation events without the use of physical collimators.

electronic structure   Structure of the orbital electrons in an atom that satisfies the quantum mechanical Schrödinger equation.

electrophoresis   Liquid paper chromatography carried out under the influence of an electric field.

element   Pure substance consisting of atoms of the same atomic number that cannot be decomposed by ordinary chemical means.

eluate   The material washed out of a chromatographic column.

elution   Separation by solvent extraction.

embolism   Matter that blocks a blood vessel.

emission computed tomography   See *single photon emission computed tomography*.

empiric, empirical   Referring to practical experience.

empirical formula   Chemical formula that reflects only the simplest molar ratio of the elements in the compounds, not the actual molar ratio.

EMS   Emergency medical system.

emulsion   (1) Mixture of two liquids, one suspended within another; colloid system. (2) Suspended mixture in which one of the components is gelatin-like.

end-diastolic volume   The quantity of blood in the ventricle at the end of diastole.

endocrine   Pertaining to a gland that secretes internally.

endocrine system   A group of organs and glands located throughout the body that secrete hormones that regulate bodily functions.

endocrinology   Study of hormonal secretion and of the endocrine glands.

endogenous   Originating or produced within the organism or its parts.

endogonic   Intake of energy.

endoscope   Tubular instrument carrying an illumination source, inserted into a body cavity to permit visual inspection.

endosteum   Membrane lining of a hollow bone.

endotoxin   Poison from dead bacterial cells; formed while cells are living.

energy levels   Quantum levels of an atom satisfying the Schrödinger equation that are allowed levels for electron location.

enterogastric reflux   Reflux of bile into the stomach.

enterogastric reflux index   The increase in ^{99m}Tc activity in the stomach area of interest divided by the decrease in ^{99m}Tc activity in the hepatobiliary tree, which indicates the activity in the stomach and hepatobiliary area at subsequent time intervals.

enzyme   Protein catalyzing specific transformation of material.

eosinophil (1) Cell stained readily by eosin. (2) White blood cell characterized by a two- or three-lobed nucleus and cytoplasms containing large granules.

EPA Environmental Protection Agency.

epidemiology Study of disease and its rate of occurrence, manner of spread, and prevalence.

epigastrium Space in the abdomen just below the ribs.

epiphysis (1) Portion of bone between the shaft and the cartilage. (2) Pineal gland.

epithelium Cells of skin and mucous membrane.

equal-time imaging A method of imaging where an area is selected with the ID marker, and an exposure is made until the ID in the region reaches a range of 2500 to 4000 counts. The time for this exposure is then used to obtain the other images.

equilibrium State of equality between two opposing substances.

equilibrium constant True constant that relates the concentration of products and reactants in a reversible chemical system where no further net change is occurring in those concentrations.

equivalent Weight of chemical species that contains either 1 mol of electrons and 1 mol of replaceable hydrogen, or combines with exactly 8 g of oxygen.

erg A unit of work in the gram-centimeter-second system equal to the amount of work of 1 dyne acting through the distance of 1 cm.

ergometer Instrument used for measuring energy expended.

ERPF Effective renal plasma flow.

error Any discrepancy between a computed, observed, or measured quantity and the specific value or condition.

erythrocyte Red blood cell.

erythrocytosis Increase in red blood cells from a known stimulant.

erythroid Reddish in color.

erythropoiesis Formation of erythrocytes.

ES End-systole.

esophageal transit The peristalsis mechanism to transport solid oral intake from the mouth to the stomach.

esters Organic compound formed by the action of an acid with an alcohol; contains the functional group:

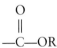

estradiol The most potent, naturally occurring estrogen in mammals.

estrogenic hormone Hormone producing female characteristics.

ether Organic compound containing a C–O–C linkage.

ethylenediaminetetraacetic acid (EDTA) See *edetic acid.*

etiology Study of the causes of disease.

Euler's number The base number (2.718) used in logarithmic calculations named after Leonhard Euler (1701-1783), a Swiss mathematician.

evagination The protrusion of some part or organ from its usual position.

Ewing sarcoma A type of bone cancer usually found in the shaft of large bones in children.

execute To perform an instruction or run a program on a computer.

exergonic Release of energy.

exogenous Originating or produced outside the subject of reference.

exponent In scientific notation, the exponent is the superscript next to the 10 that specifies how many places the decimal point in the number is to be shifted to the left (for negative exponents) or shifted to the right (for positive exponents).

exposure rate Rate of exposure to radioactivity usually measured in units of rad per hour.

extirpation Complete removal.

extractor Device that removes something; liquid that removes another substance with it.

extranuclear Referring to the space in an atom outside of the nucleus.

extravasation Escape of a fluid from a vessel into tissue.

extrinsic testing Scintillation camera uniformity testing done with the collimator in place.

Fab A fragment of an antibody.

families Sets of elements that have the same valence shell electron configurations.

fast neutron Neutron that has a minimum energy of 100 keV.

FDA The U.S. Food and Drug Administration.

FDG 2-Fluoro-2-deoxy-D-glucose.

ferrokinetics Study of iron within the body.

fibrinolysis Dissolution or splitting of fibrin.

file A logical collection of data that is treated as a unit, occupies one or more blocks on a mass storage volume, and has an associated file name and type.

film badge Photographic film shielded from light; worn by an individual to measure radiation exposure.

filter A computer algorithm applied to projections obtained from an imaging system to eliminate noise and artifacts.

filtered back-projection (reconstruction) A reconstruction algorithm to create axial slices from projection information.

filtration fraction The proportion of plasma that reaches the kidney and is filtered by the glomerulus.

fission Splitting of a nucleus accompanied by a release of energy and neutrons.

flat-field collimator See *collimator.*

flip angle A rotation of the magnetization vector that depends upon the strength and duration of the RF pulse

flood phantom See *phantom.*

flood-field uniformity The ability of a scintillation camera to depict a uniform distribution of activity as uniform.

fluid thioglycollate Medium that provides conditions for growth of aerobic and anaerobic bacteria; used in microbiological sterility testing of radiopharmaceuticals.

fluor A liquid scintillation medium.

fluorescence Emission of light by an activated chemical complex.

fluorodeoxyglucose 2-[^{18}F]-fluoro-2-deoxy-D-glucose (^{18}F-FDG); FDG.

focal spot The area on the anode of an x-ray tube where the electron beam strikes to produce x-rays.

folate Salt of folic acid.

follicle Sac or pouchlike depression; cavity.

follicle-stimulating hormone (FSH) Anterior pituitary hormone that stimulates follicle growth in the ovaries and spermatogenesis in the testes.

foramen magnum Large opening in the occipital bone between the cranial cavity and the vertebral canal.

foreshortening In phenomenon in planar scintigraphy when the kidney may appear smaller than its actual size if the long axis is not parallel to the surface of the crystal of the gamma camera.

FORTRAN (FORmula TRANslator) High-level compiler language for mathematical and scientific applications.

Fourier transform A mathematical process that converts matrix information into frequency space.

frame mode A method of computer data collection where x and y positional signals are stored in a single matrix.

free radicals Chemical complexes containing an unpaired electron.

frequency Number of cycles per unit time; normal unit is hertz, or cycles per second.

FSH See *follicle-stimulating hormone.*

F-test A statistical test of the null hypothesis.

FTI Free thyroxine index.

full width at half maximum (FWHM) A measurement of curve peak characteristics by comparing the curve width at half the peak height with the value at which the peak occurs. Used for a variety of applications, it is commonly used to express energy or spatial resolution. Results are expressed as a percentage:

$$\text{energy FWHM (\%)} = (DE/E) \times 100\%.$$

function An algorithm, accessible by name and contained in the system software, that performs commonly used operations; an example is the square root calculation function.

functional agents Radiopharmaceuticals that are rapidly taken up and excreted by the kidneys by a single, simple physiological mechanism such as ERPF or GFR.

functional group Portion of a molecule responsible for its specific chemical properties.

functional residual capacity The volume of air in the lungs at the end of a normal breath.

fundus Base of an organ.

fusion Nuclear process in which two discrete nuclei collide and join together, forming a larger nuclide.

FWHM See *full width at half maximum.*

g force Centrifugal force.

GABA Gamma-aminobutyric acid.

gallbladder ejection fraction (GBEF) The rate at which the gallbladder contracts.

gamma camera See *Anger camera.*

gamma decay See *gamma emission.*

gamma emission Nuclear process in which an excited nuclide de-excites by emission of a nuclear photon.

gamma globulin Globulins in plasma having the slowest mobility using electrophoresis in neutral or alkaline solutions.

gas-filled detector A container of gas with two electrodes, one positive (the anode) and one negative (the cathode) in which radiation is sensed by detecting the ionization of gas molecules produced by deposition of energy during passage of radiation through the gas-filled detector.

gastric emptying time The rate of gastric emptying, which is a complex process affected by the physical and chemical composition of the ingested meal, the intrinsic and extrinsic nervous innervation of the stomach, and circulating neuroendocrine transmitters.

gastrin Hormone stimulating secretion by the gastric glands.

gastroenteropathy Disease of the stomach and intestine.

gastroesophageal reflux Refers to the symptom complex of heartburn, regurgitation, and chest pain

gastroparesis A slight degree of stomach paralysis.

gate Electronic device capable of performing logic operations within a digital circuit. In nuclear medicine it implies a device that can provide a timing signal to the computer. This signal is usually associated with the QRS complex of the electrocardiograph.

gated acquisition The collecting of data in conjunction with a gate.

gauss Unit for measuring magnetic field strength; 10,000 gauss = 1 tesla.

Geiger-Mueller detector Ionization chamber measuring radiation in the region where the charge produced per ionizing event is independent of the number of primary ions produced by the initial ionizing event.

gel permeation chromatography Separation of compounds because of differences in their rates of permeation of a gel, especially useful for separation of large biomolecules such as proteins.

generator Device using a parent radionuclide to obtain its product, the daughter radionuclide, usually by addition of a solution that interacts only with the daughter.

genetic effects Dominant or recessive effects on progeny.

genitourinary tract Urinary system and the sex organs.

geometry A term used to denote the relationship of a radioactive source's position in terms of a detector's sensitive surface area.

GER Gastroesophageal reflux.

GFR Glomerular filtration rate.

GH, GHA, glucoheptonate A ^{99m}Tc-labeled carbohydrate used for imaging the renal cortex and collecting system, which may also be used for brain imaging.

globulin Simple protein found in serum and tissue.

glomerulus (*pl.* glomeruli) Small cluster of blood vessels or nerve fibers.

glucagon Pancreatic secretion that increases concentration of the blood sugars.

glucocorticoid Hormone secreted by the adrenal cortex, stimulating the conversion of proteins to carbohydrates.

glucoheptonate Chelating molecule that can bind ^{99m}Tc and be used as an imaging agent.

glucometer Instrument used to measure peripheral blood glucose levels.

glucose-6-phosphate (G-6-P) The form into which FDG is phosphorylated by the action of hexokinase and which cannot cross the cell membrane, therefore trapping ^{18}F within the cell.

glycogen Form in which carbohydrates are stored in animal tissue.

glycolysis The breaking down of glucose by a series of enzymatic steps in the cells' cytosol.

glycoprotein Protein and a carbohydrate that does not contain phosphoric acid, purine, or pyrimidine.

glycoside Compound formed between a sugar and another organic substance.

G-M detector See *Geiger-Mueller detector*.

gonad Ovary or testicle; the sex gland.

graafian follicle Ovarian follicle where the ovum matures.

gram atomic weight Weight in grams of 1 mol of an element.

gram molecular weight Weight in grams of 1 mol of a chemical compound.

granulocyte White blood cell.

granuloma Tumor or neoplasm consisting of newly formed tissue induced by the presence of a foreign body or of bacteria.

Graves disease Diffuse toxic goiter.

gray (Gy) A unit of absorbed dose equal to 1 joule per kilogram in any medium.

growth hormone (GH) Hormone secreted by the anterior pituitary; stimulates growth.

GSO Gadolinium orthosilicate; a PET scanner detection material.

GTT Glucose tolerance test.

half-life ($t_{1/2}$) A term used to describe the time elapsed until some physical quantity has decreased to half of its original value.

half-reaction Term used in an electrochemical reaction to describe either the oxidation process or the reduction process as a separate entity.

half-value layer (HVL) Thickness of absorbing material necessary to reduce the intensity of radiation by half; synonymous with half-thickness.

halide Compound containing a halogen.

halogens Family of chemical elements of similar electron structure (i.e., the valence shell is completely filled except for one electron)—fluorine, chlorine, bromine, iodine, and astatine.

HAMA Human antimouse antibodies.

hapten Molecule that cannot elicit immunoglobulin response by itself but can when bound to a larger carrier molecule.

hardware Physical equipment, such as mechanical, electrical, or electronic devices.

Hashimoto disease Infiltration of the thyroid gland with lymphocytes resulting in progressive destruction of the parenchyma and hypothyroidism.

haversian system System of canals in the bones where the blood vessels branch out.

HBV Hepatitis B virus.

HCFA Health Care Financing Administration.

HCG Human chorionic gonadotropin.

HD Hodgkin lymphoma.

HDP Hydroxymethylene diphosphonate, a ^{99m}Tc-labeled phosphate complex used in bone imaging.

heat-sensitive printer Type of printer that imprints characters on special sensitized paper by use of heat, without the use of an ink ribbon.

helium-3 (^{3}He) Isotope of helium with an atomic weight of three unified mass units.

hemangioma Tumor of blood vessels that is nonmalignant.

hematocrit Relative percentage of erythrocytes in whole blood.

hematology Study of blood and blood-forming organs.

hematopoietic system The blood system.

hemocytometer Instrument used to count blood cells.

hemoglobin Pigment of the blood that carries oxygen.

hemolysis Red blood cell destruction; escape of hemoglobin within the bloodstream.

hemorrhage Bleeding.

HEPA High-efficiency particulate air (filter).

heparin Mucopolysaccharide acid that occurs in tissues, mainly the liver; used in prevention and treatment of thrombosis, bacterial endocarditis, postoperative pulmonary embolism, repair of vascular injury, and to prevent clotting of blood.

hepatoblastoma Tumor of the liver.

hepatoma Tumor of the liver.

heptasulfide Technetium heptasulfide: ^{99m}Tc$_2$S$_7$; coprecipitates with colloidal sulfur particles stabilized with gelatin in ^{99m}Tc–sulfur colloid preparation.

hertz Basic unit of frequency; 1 hertz (Hz) = 1 cycle per second.

heterionic exchange Process of exchange of an ion native to bone for a labeled, bone-seeking ion.

hexadecimal Pertaining to the number system with a radix of 16.

hexane Alkane with the molecular formula C_6H_{14}.

hexokinase The first intracellular enzyme involved in glucose breakdown.

HIDA N,N-(2,6-dimethylphenyl) carbamolymethyl iminodiacetic acid; lidofenin; can be labeled with ^{99m}Tc and used as an imaging agent.

high-contrast resolution The ability to distinguish small objects and image details when there is a large difference between objects.

high-level language A programming language whose statements are translated into more than one machine language instruction; examples are BASIC and FORTRAN.

histochemical Referring to the deposit of chemical components in cells.

histogram A graph.

histology Study of the form and structure of tissues.

histopathology The science or study of diseased tissue.

HIV Human immunodeficiency virus.

HMO Health maintenance organization.

HMPAO Hexamethyl propylamineoxime.

homeostasis The state of equilibrium in the body with respect to various functions and to the chemical compositions of the fluids and tissues.

horizontal long axis Transverse sections of the heart in reoriented images.

hormone Chemical having a specific effect on the activity of a specific organ.

horseshoe kidney A congenital abnormality in which the bottoms of the two kidneys are joined.

Hounsfield unit A unit of measured value placed into the pixels of a CT image. The value represents a relative density to water, which has a value of zero on the Hounsfield scale, with densities lower than water having a negative number and densities higher than water having a positive value.

$$CT_{tissue} = (\mu_{tissue} - \mu_{water})/\mu_{water} \times 1000$$

HVL   See *half-value layer.*

hydrocarbon   Compound containing carbon and hydrogen exclusively.

hydrolysis   Processes of decomposition by the addition of water.

hydronephrosis   A term meaning the dilation of the renal pelvis and ureters.

hydroxide   The ion OH^-.

hydroxyapatite   Compound $Ca_{10}(PO_4)_6(OH)_2$; inorganic constituent of bone and teeth.

8-hydroxyquinoline (oxine)   Compound that can form a complex with indium and gallium and be used to label blood cells.

hygroscopic   Having an affinity for water.

hyperemia   Excess blood in an organ or part of the body.

hyperglycemia   Excessive sugar (glucose) in the blood.

hyperplasia   An increase in the number of cells in a tissue or organ, excluding tumor formation.

hypertension   Elevated blood pressure.

hyperthyroid   Overactive thyroid gland.

hypoglycemia   Not enough sugar (glucose) in the blood.

hypokinesia   Diminished motor function.

hypopituitarism   Insufficient secretion of the pituitary.

hypothalamus   Part of the forebrain below the cerebrum.

hypothyroid   Insufficient activity of the thyroid.

hypoxia   Abnormal reduction in oxygen in tissues.

ICANL   Intersocietal Commission on the Accreditation of Nuclear Medicine Laboratories.

ICRP   International Commission on Radiation Protection.

IDA   Iminodiacetic acid, a family of ^{99m}Tc-labeled radiopharmaceuticals used to evaluate the hepatobiliary system.

IF   See *intrinsic factor.*

ileal loop   A new bladder (neobladder) constructed from a portion of the small bowel (ileum) following the surgical removal of the patient's bladder.

ileostomy   A surgical opening into the ileum to allow for drainage of feces.

image matrix   The number of pixels used in an image acquisition.

iminodiacetic acid   Chelating group capable of binding technetium so that it can be attached to biologically active molecules, such as HIDA.

immobilization techniques   Methods used to prevent free movement of a patient during a procedure.

immunoactive   Immunity produced by stimulation of antibody-producing mechanisms.

immunoglobulin   Type of protein, isolated from the globulin fraction of serum having a characteristic shape and the ability to bind to molecules that are not endogenous to the species producing the immunoglobulin.

immunology   Study of resistance to disease or disease agents.

immunoreaction   Reaction taking place between an antigen and its antibody.

IMP   Iodoamphetamine.

incubate   To provide proper conditions for growth or a reaction to occur.

inelastic collision   Interaction between two particles resulting in a net loss of kinetic energy in the system.

infarct   Area deprived of its blood supply because of an obstruction.

infarction   The process formation of an infarct.

infiltration   The diffusion or accumulation of fluids in tissues where it is not normally located.

infundibular pulmonic stenosis   Obstruction in the outer passage from the right ventricle, restricting blood flow.

inhibition   Prevention or interference of a chemical reaction.

inhibitor   Substance preventing or interfering with a chemical reaction.

innominate vein   Vein receiving blood from the head and neck region.

inoculate   To protect against disease by injection of pathogenic microorganisms to stimulate production of antibodies.

inorganic   Branch of chemistry having to do with compounds and processes that do not involve carbon.

input   Transferal of data from auxiliary or external storage into the internal storage of a computer.

instruction   A coded command that tells the computer what to do and where to find the values it is to work with; symbolic instructions must be changed into machine instructions before they can be executed by the computer.

insulin   Hormone produced in cells of the pancreas essential for metabolism of carbohydrates.

interface   Connection between two systems, such as a scintillation camera and a computer.

internal conversion   Nuclear de-excitation process in which the radionuclide de-excites by transferring energy to an orbital electron.

interstices   Small gaps between tissues or structures.

intradermal   Through the skin.

intrathecal   Through the spinal cord.

intrinsic factor (IF)   Substance produced by the gastric mucosa and found in the terminal ileum that is necessary for absorption of vitamin B_{12}.

intrinsic testing   Scintillation camera uniformity testing with the collimator removed.

intussusception   The infolding of one segment of the intestine within another.

inulin   Polysaccharide that on hydrolysis yields levulose, which can be used to test kidney function.

inulin clearance test   Test of renal function.

inverse square law   The radiation intensity of any source decreases inversely as the square of the distance between the source and the detector.

in vitro   Outside a living organism.

in vivo   Within a living organism.

I/O (input/output) device   Computer device that either accepts input or prints out results.

iodination   Addition of iodine to a compound.

iodohippuran   Agent used for renal imaging.

ion   Atom or group of atoms with a net electronic charge.

ion exchange   Process involving reversible exchange of ions in a solution and in a solid.

ionic compound Compound held together by purely electrostatic forces.

ionic strength Half the sum of the terms obtained by multiplying the molarity of each ion by the square of its valence.

ionization Process of removing electrons from an atom to create an ion.

ionization chamber A gas-filled radiation detector.

IRMA Immunoradiometric assay.

irradiation Application of radiant energy for therapy or diagnosis.

ischemia Insufficient blood supply because of a spasm or constriction of the artery in an organ or part of the body.

ischemic damage Damage from a constriction of the blood vessel.

islets of Langerhans Pancreatic cells secreting insulin.

isobar Nuclides that have the same total number of neutrons and protons but are different elements.

isoelectric Having uniform electric potential; thus, no current is given off.

isomers Two compounds with the same molecular formulas and different structural formulas.

isometric transition Change in the extranuclear portion of an atom from a high-energy level to a lower energy level accompanied by the release of electromagnetic radiation.

isopleth Graph showing frequency of an event as a function of two variables.

isotones Nuclides having the same number of neutrons but a different number of protons.

isotonic Physiological; compatible with body tissues.

isotopes Nuclides of the same element with the same number of protons but different number of neutrons.

isotropic resolution The resolution obtained when the dimensions on the sides of a voxel are all equal.

iterative reconstruction An algorithm, or technique, that sequentially refines estimated pixel values and provides a more accurate reconstruction of the radiotracer's distribution in the body and significantly reduces streak artifacts.

ITLC Instant thin-layer chromatography.

ITP Idiopathic thrombocytopenia.

IUPAC International Union of Pure and Applied Chemistry.

joystick An electronic pointing device for computers.

kernel The image filter used in the CT reconstruction algorithm to calculate the sharpness of reconstructed image.

ketone Organic molecule with a carbon-oxygen double bond separating two alkyl portions:

$$\underset{(R—C—R)}{\overset{\displaystyle O \atop \displaystyle \|}{}}$$

kinetic energy That energy of a body due to its motion.

Kupffer cells Part of the reticuloendothelial system; star-shaped cells attached to the wall of the sinusoids of the liver.

kVp (kilovolt peak) The peak voltage that is applied between the cathode and anode of an x-ray tube.

lacuna Small hollow cavity.

lag phase The time on a gastric emptying curve during which no or little solid is evacuated.

LAL See *limulus amebocyte lysate*.

lambda (λ) Greek letter denoting the decay constant of radioactive species.

language Set of representations, conventions, and rules used to convey information.

Larmor equation Allows for the calculation of different precessional frequencies between fat and water for a given main magnetic field strength.

Larmor frequency The characteristic frequency at which the resonance of the nucleus is excited in magnetic resonance imaging.

law of constant composition If two (or more) elements combine chemically to form a compound, the relative weights of the constituent elements will always be in a constant proportion to each other.

law of definite proportions If two (or more) elements chemically combine to form a compound, the relative number of moles of each constituent element will be in a proportion of simple whole numbers with each other.

law of mass action The velocity of the chemical reaction is proportional to the masses of the reactants.

law of multiple proportions If two elements form more than one compound, the number of moles of one element in the first compound is proportional to the number of moles of the same element in the second compound.

law of reciprocal proportions Two chemical elements unite with a third element in proportions that are multiples of the union of the first two elements.

Le Chatelier principle A principle stating that if a system is initially at equilibrium and is forced away from equilibrium when a parameter is changed, the system will spontaneously return to a new equilibrium.

least squares curve fit The technique of visually estimating the best-fit straight line is fraught with inaccuracy and imprecision.

Legg-Calvé-Perthes disease Idiopathic osteonecrosis of the capital femoral head epiphysis.

lesion An area of damaged tissue either from disease or injury.

LET See *linear energy transfer*.

leukocyte White blood cell, either granular or nongranular.

leukopenia Less than the normal number of white blood cells.

leukotaxine Crystalline nitrogen substance appearing when tissue is injured.

Lewis concept A concept stating that an acid is an electron-pair acceptor and a base is an electron-pair donor.

LH Luteinizing hormone.

ligand (1) Molecule attached to a central atom using coordinate covalent bonds. (2) In radioimmunoassay, an antigen or small molecule that binds to a native carrier protein.

light pen A device resembling a pencil or stylus that is used to input information to a CRT display system.

limulus amebocyte lysate (LAL) In vitro test for pyrogens; it reacts with gram-negative bacterial endotoxins in nanogram or greater concentrations to form an opaque gel.

line of response   A path of an annihilation photon pair determined by the electronic collimation and coincidence detection.

line spread function   The profile of counts along a line running perpendicular to a line source.

linear attenuation coefficient   That quantity by which radiation is decreased per unit path length through matter.

linear energy transfer (LET)   Amount of energy lost by ionizing radiation by way of interaction with matter per centimeter of path length through the absorbing material.

linear regression   A calculation generally performed to show a linear relationship between two variables to predict some y variable based on measurement of some x variable.

lingula   Small tonguelike structure.

linker   A program that combines many relocatable object modules into an executable module; it satisfies global references and combines program sections.

lipid   Fat and fatlike substances.

lipophilic   Capable of dissolving, of being dissolved in, or of absorbing lipids.

lipophilicity   The degree to which a substance is lipophilic.

lipoproteins   Combination of a lipid and a protein.

liquid-drop model   Theoretical model of the nucleus that assumes a simple continuous nuclear potential and spheroid shape.

liquid scintillation counter   A system for detecting beta-emitting radionuclides using a liquid scintillator in which the radioactive source is dissolved.

list mode acquisition   A method of computer data collection where x and y positional signals are stored sequentially in memory in the form of a list.

listing   The printed copy generated by a line printer or terminal.

load   To store a program or data in memory; to mount a tape on a device such that the read point is at the beginning of the tape; to place a removable disk in a disk drive and start the drive.

location   An address in storage or memory where a unit of data or an instruction can be stored.

logarithm   Exponent of the power of a base that equals a given number.

logit   Mathematical relationship defined as ln $y/l - y$.

loop   A sequence of instructions executed repeatedly until a terminal condition prevails.

low-contrast resolution   The ability to distinguish small objects and image details when there is little density difference between objects.

low-pass filter   A filter used to remove noise by use of a cutoff frequency.

LSO   Lutetium oxyorthosilicate; a PET scanner detection material.

Lugol solution   An iodine solution.

lung quantification   Data obtained from lung images, usually perfusion images, to determine the function of different lobes and segments.

LV   Left ventricle.

LVEF   Left ventricular ejection fraction; see also *cardiac ejection fraction*.

lymphangiography   Radiography of the lymph channels.

lymphocyte   White blood cell with a single rounded nucleus.

lymphoma   Tumor composed of lymph node tissue.

lyophilize   To rapidly freeze and dehydrate a substance.

lysis   (1) Separation of adhesions binding different structures. (2) Destruction of a cell by a specific agent. (3) Abatement of disease symptoms.

LYSO   Lutetiumyttrium orthosilicate; a PET scanner detector material.

mA   Milliampere. A unit of electric current that describes the flow of charge per second.

MAA   Macroaggregated albumin.

Mab   Murine monoclonal antibody

machine code   See *object code*.

machine language   See *language*.

macro   (1) Directions for expanding abbreviated text; a boilerplate that generates a known set of instructions, data, or symbols; a macro is used to eliminate the need to write a set of instructions that are used repeatedly. (2) Prefix meaning huge or of large scale.

macroglobulin   Protein of high molecular weight.

macrophage   Large white blood cell; active in bacterial destruction.

MAG3   Mercaptoacetyl triglycine.

magnetic field   Field induced by moving electrical charges.

magnetic moment   Represents a vector indicating magnitude and direction, and describes the magnetic field characteristics of the nucleus.

magnetic quantum number   Quantum number (m, m_1, or M) that defines the orientation of an orbital in space.

magnetic tape   A plastic-base tape in which data is imprinted magnetically.

malabsorption   Inadequate absorption of nutrients in the gastrointestinal tract.

manometer   Device used to measure the pressure of liquids.

mass   Basic parameter of matter referring to the quantity of matter present. It is independent of the object's weight.

mass attenuation coefficient   The quotient of the linear attenuation coefficient divided by the density of the matter through which it passes.

mass defect   The difference in mass of an atom's constituent particles and its total mass.

matrix   A rectangular array of elements; any matrix can be considered an array.

maximum intensity projection (MIP)   A translucent 3D volume cinematic image.

maximum permissible dose (MPD)   Dose limitations, in rem, placed on each individual as specified by the Nuclear Regulatory Commission.

MDA   Minimum detectable amount.

MDP   Methylene diphosphonate, a ^{99m}Tc-labeled phosphate complex used in bone imaging.

mean   Average of two or more quantities.

Meckel diverticulum   Saclike pouch on the small intestine.

mediastinum   Space behind the breastbone containing the heart.

medulloblastoma   Tumor of the brain.

megakaryocyte   A cell found in the bone marrow developing into blood platelets.

magnetic resonance imaging (MRI)   Body imaging technique to observe chemical makeup of tissue using magnetic fields and radiofrequency electromagnetic waves.

MEK   Methyl ethyl ketone.

melanoma   Tumor characterized by dark pigmentation.

memory   Any form of data storage including main memory and mass storage in which data can be read and written; memory usually refers to the main memory.

mesenchyme   Primitive tissue of the embryo.

mesothelioma   A rare form of cancer that develops in the pleura, the lining of the chest, but can also occur in the peritoneum or the pericardium.

metabolism   Process for transforming foods into compounds used by the body.

metastable state   Excited state of a nucleus or atom that has a measurable lifetime; also known as an *isometric state*.

metastatic lesion   A lesion that is the result of the spread of disease.

metastasis   Spreading of a disease process from one part of the body to another.

metathesis   Chemical process in which two compounds exchange constituents.

MI   Myocardial infarction.

microbiological testing   Any test for bacteria, virus, or other microorganism.

microlysis   Destruction of a substance into microscopic size.

micrometer (µm)   One millionth of a meter; formerly *micron*.

microprocessor   A silicon chip containing many circuits.

microsphere   Round mass of a small size, visible only with a microscope.

microvilli   Projections of cell membranes greatly increasing the surface area of the cell.

migrating solvent   Chromatographic solvent; used to differentially carry the unknown solute to be separated.

MIP   See *maximum intensity projection*.

MIPS   Million instructions per second.

mitral stenosis   Deformity of the mitral valve of the heart.

mnemonic   Aiding the memory; use of an acronym or other pattern to aid the memory.

mobile phase   Phase in chromatography that differentially carries the unknown solutes.

modem   From *mo*dulate and *dem*odulate. A device used to transmit computer data over telephone lines.

modulation transfer function (MTF)   A curve depicting the image-to-object contrast ratio as a function of spatial frequency.

molal   Unit of concentration associated with molality equal to the number of moles of solute per kilogram of solvent.

molality   Unit of solution concentration defined as the number of moles of solute per weight (kg) of solvent.

molar   Concentration unit equal to number of moles of solute per liter of solution.

molarity   Measure of solution concentration defined as the number of moles of solute per volume (liter) of solution.

mole   See *gram molecular weight*.

molecular formula   Chemical formula that states the actual number of atoms of each constituent per molecule of the compound.

molecular imaging   Techniques that allow visualization of processing taking place at the molecular level.

molecular weight   Weight in unified mass units of one molecule of a particular chemical compound.

molecule   Basic unit of a chemical compound.

molybdate   Compound containing a MoO_4^{-2} group.

monatomic   One atom per molecule, usually referring to elements (e.g., the noble gases) in their native state.

monitor   The master control program that observes, supervises, controls, or verifies the operation of a computer system; the collection of routines that controls the operation of user and system programs, schedules, and operations; allocates resources; and performs I/O.

monoclonal antibodies   Immunoglobulins, chemically identical in structure, produced by a group of cells that are genetically identical.

monocyte   White blood cell having one rounded nucleus that increases in number during certain types of infections.

monoenergetic   Having a single energy.

morphological agents   Radiopharmaceuticals that are rapidly taken up by the kidney by complicated mechanisms that usually involve a complex interaction of the ERPF, GFR, tubular secretion, and tubular resorption.

morphology   Study of the structure of tissues.

motility   The power of spontaneous movement.

mouse   An electronic pointing device for computers.

MPD   See *maximum permissible dose*.

MPST   Mean platelet survival time.

MRI   See *magnetic resonance imaging*.

MTF   See *modulation transfer function*.

mucoid   (1) Mucuslike substance. (2) An animal-conjugated protein.

mucosal biopsy   Removal and examination of some of the tissue of the mucous membrane.

MUGA   See *multiple gated acquisition*.

multiformatter   A photographic system designed to produce images from a cathode ray tube in various positions and sizes.

multiple gated acquisition (MUGA)   Composite heart-imaging technique performed by synchronizing a patient's heartbeat by means of an electrocardiograph to a scintillation camera/computer.

murine   Pertaining to mice or rats.

myeloblast   A cell in the bone marrow that develops into a white blood cell.

myelofibrosis   Replacement of the bone marrow by fibrous tissue.

myeloid   (1) Referring to bone marrow. (2) Referring to the spinal cord. (3) Cell resembling a red bone marrow cell that did not originate in the bone marrow.

myocardial infarct   Heart muscle damage secondary to loss of its blood supply.

myocardial ischemia   Obstruction or constriction in the coronary arteries resulting in a deficiency of blood to the heart muscle.

myocardium   Heart muscle.

N See *neutron number.*

naperian logarithmic system Logarithmic system using the base *e*, which is a mathematical constant ($e = 2.71$).

nasogastric tube A tube that is inserted through a nostril and terminates in the stomach. It is used for feeding, to obtain specimens of gastric fluids, or to drain fluids from the stomach.

nasopharyngeal Referring to that part of the pharynx above the soft palate.

natural logarithm See *naperian logarithmic system.*

NCRP National Council on Radiation Protection and Measurement.

negatron Negative electron.

NEMA National Electrical Manufacturers Association.

neonate Newborn to 4-week-old infant.

neoplasia Condition characterized by new tumors or growths.

nephrology Study of the kidney.

nephron Part of the kidney that secretes urine.

nephrosis Degeneration of the kidney.

neurinoma Enlargement of a node or tumor on a peripheral nerve.

neuroblastoma Malignant tumors of the sympathetic nervous system and found most often in infants and children younger than 10 years.

neuroglia Nonnervous cellular elements of nervous tissue.

neurohormone Hormone stimulating the mechanism of the nerves.

neurohumeral Neural (autonomic) and humoral (circulating or hormonal); can refer to substances or transmission.

neurohypophysis Main part of the posterior pituitary (hypophysis cerebri).

neuron Principal functional unit of CNS.

neuropathology Study of nervous system diseases by examination of those tissues.

neutralization Chemical reaction in which an acid and a base react to form a salt and water.

neutrino Nuclear particle emitted during positron decay.

neutron Nuclear particle that is found in the nucleus, is electrically neutral, and has a mass of one mass unit.

neutron activation Nuclear process in which a nucleus absorbs a thermal neutron and de-excites by way of gamma-ray emission.

neutron flux Measure of neutron intensity defined as the number of neutrons passing through one square centimeter of area per second.

neutron number (N) Number of neutrons in a nucleus.

neutrophil White blood cell with three to five lobes connected by chromatin and cytoplasm containing five granules.

NHL Non-Hodgkin lymphoma.

nidus (1) Focus of infection. (2) Depression in the brain surface.

NIST National Institute of Standards and Technology. Formerly National Bureau of Standards (NBS).

NMR (nuclear magnetic resonance). See *magnetic resonance imaging (MRI).*

noble gas Any chemical element that has a completely filled valence-shell configuration in its neutral state—helium, neon, argon, krypton, xenon, and radon.

noise Extraneous interference in an electronic circuit of statistical manipulation.

nomogram Conversion scale.

nonpolar bond Chemical bond in which a pair of electrons is equally shared by two nuclei.

nonspecific binding (NSB) Binding of the radioligand to substances or surfaces other than the specific reactor substance.

normal Concentration unit defined as the number of equivalent weights of solute per liter of solution.

normality Method of expressing concentration defined as the number of equivalent weights of solute per volume of solution.

normalization A term used to mean that counts have been normalized.

normalization calibration Calibration method used to evaluate the differences in sensitivity of the crystals when compared to the detectors.

normalize A term used in association with computer-defined regions of interest to indicate that counts contained in the regions have been converted to the same size region.

NRC See *Nuclear Regulatory Commission.*

NSB See *nonspecific binding.*

nuclear charge Charge of the nucleus of an atom equal to the number of protons multiplied by the charge of a proton.

nuclear fission Nuclear process in which a nucleus splits into two pieces accompanied by neutron emission and energy release.

nuclear reactor Device that under controlled conditions is used for supporting a self-sustained nuclear reaction.

Nuclear Regulatory Commission (NRC) United States government agency regulating byproduct material.

nuclear stability Condition to describe a nucleus that is stable with respect to radioactive decay.

nucleons Any particle commonly contained in the nucleus of an atom.

nucleus (1) Portion of an atom containing the neutrons and the protons. (2) Spheric body that is the core of a cell. (3) Mass of gray matter in the central nervous system.

Nyquist frequency The highest frequency that can be represented in an image.

object code Relocatable machine language code.

obtund To dull or blunt, especially to blunt sensation or deaden pain.

occipital Referring to the back of the head or occiput.

Occupational Safety and Health Administration (OSHA) United States government agency regulating health standards in the workplace.

octal The number system with a radix of 8; for example, octal 100 is decimal 64.

OIH See *ortho-iodohippurate.*

oleic acid (octadecanoic acid) Straight-chained organic acid with the molecular formula $C_{18}H_{36}O_2$.

oncocytoma Granular cell adenoma of the parotid gland.

op code See *operation code.*

operand That which is affected, manipulated, or operated upon.

operating systems   Collection of programs, including a monitor or executive and system programs, that organizes a central processor and peripheral devices into a working unit for the development and execution of application programs.

operation code   Code used to start the operation of a program.

optic chiasma   The point of crossing of the fibers of the optic nerve.

orbital   Energy sublevels occupied by electrons in an atom.

ordered subset expectation maximization algorithm   See *OSEM.*

ordinate   The *y-*, or perpendicular, axis in a cartesian graph or plot.

organic chemistry   Branch of chemistry dealing with the study of compounds of carbon.

organic compounds   Any of the class of chemical compounds that contain carbon.

organomegaly   Abnormal enlargement of an organ.

ortho-**iodohippurate (OIH)**   Iodinated renal imaging agent.

OSEM   A reconstruction method used in SPECT and PET imaging that uses selected subsets of projection iteration data.

OSHA   See *Occupational Safety and Health Administration.*

osmoreceptor   Specialized sensory nerve ending that (1) gives rise to the sense of smell and (2) is stimulated by changes in osmotic pressures of the surrounding medium.

osseous   Composed of bone.

osteoblast   Immature bone-producing cell.

osteoclast   Large multinuclear cell associated with destruction of bone.

osteocyte   Cell lodged in flat oval cavities of the bone.

osteogenesis   Bone development.

osteomyelitis   Infection of the bone.

output   Information transferred from the internal storage of a computer to output devices or external storage.

ovary   Female reproductive gland.

oxidation   Process by which a substance loses electrons in an oxidation-reduction reaction.

oxidation-reduction   Chemical reaction in which electrons are transferred from one substance to another substance.

oxidizing agent   Substance in an oxidation-reduction reaction that causes another substance to lose electrons.

oxine   See *8-hydroxyquinoline.*

P wave   The first complex of the electrocardiogram representing depolarization of the atria.

Paget disease   Osteitis deformans.

PAH   *Para*-aminohippuric acid.

pair production   Photonic de-excitation process in which a photon disintegrates into an electron-positron pair, each of which gains an equal amount of kinetic energy.

pancreas   Large gland secreting enzymes into the intestines for digestion and manufacturing and secreting insulin.

papilla of Vater   Prominent tissue in the duodenum where the bile duct enters the intestine.

parathormone   Hormone secreted by the parathyroid gland.

parathyroid glands   Four small endocrine glands on the lateral lobe of the thyroid that control calcium and phosphorus metabolism.

parenchyma   Essential elements of an organ as distinguished from its framework.

parent radionuclide   Radionuclide that decays to a specific daughter nuclide either directly or as a member of a radioactive series.

parotid gland   Salivary gland.

PAS   *Para*-aminosalicylic acid.

Pascal   A computer programming language.

pathology   Study of disease based on examination of diseased tissue.

pathophysiology   Study of disordered function of organs.

Pauli exclusion principle   Two electrons in the same atom cannot have the exact same set of quantum numbers.

Pauling scale   A measure of electronegativity with fluorine arbitrarily assigned a value of 4.

PE   Pulmonary emboli

pediatric immobilization techniques   Techniques used to hold a patient still during imaging (e.g., wrapping, sandbagging, and sedation).

pedicle   Stemlike part of attaching structure.

PEG   Polyethylene glycol.

pellet   (1) A small pill. (2) A granule.

pentetic acid (diethylenetriamine pentaacetic acid, DTPA)   Chelating agent that can be labeled with ^{99m}Tc and used for scintigraphy.

peptide   Low molecular weight compound containing two or more amino acids.

peptide hormone   Hormones excreted by the pituitary, parathyroid, and pancreas.

percent trace binding   The amount of radioactivity bound by a specific reactor substance in a solution containing the substance of interest, divided by the amount of radioactivity bound by a solution where the substance of interest is undetectable, times 100.

perchlorate   Any chemical compound that contains the ClO_4 group.

perfusion   Passage of a fluid into an organ to thoroughly permeate it.

pericardium   Tissue sheath encasing the heart.

perineal region   Floor of the pelvis.

period   (1) In wave motion phenomena it is the time required to complete one cyclic motion, equalizing the reciprocal of the frequency. (2) Elements in a horizontal line on the periodic chart.

periodic table   A chart of the elements depicting the interrelationships among them based on their electronic configurations.

periosteal bone   Bone that develops directly from and beneath the periosteum.

periosteum   Thin tissue encasing bones that possesses bone-forming potential.

peripheral   (1) Near the surface, distant; distal, opposite of proximal. (2) Any device distinct from the central processor that can provide input or accept output from the computer.

peripheral blood   Blood that circulates in the vessels remote from the heart.

peripheral blood glucose   Glucose levels found in the peripheral blood vessels.

peripheral vessels   Blood vessels that are remote from the heart.

pernicious anemia   Anemia from lack of secretion by the gastric mucosa of intrinsic factor, which is important to blood formation.

pertechnetate   Any chemical compound containing the TcO_4 group.

PET   Positron emission tomography.

PGA   Pteroylglutamic (folic) acid.

pH   Measure of the hydrogen ion concentration in a solution; equals the negative logarithm of the hydrogen ion concentration.

pH meter   Device used to measure the pH of a solution based on the potential difference between the solution and a standard calomel electrode.

phagocyte   Cell that destroys bacteria or other foreign bodies.

phagocytize   To ingest cells or microorganisms by a cell (a phagocyte).

phagocytosis   Destruction of bacteria or other foreign bodies by phagocytes.

phantom   (1) Model of some part of the body in which radioactive material can be placed to simulate conditions in vivo. (2) A device that yields information concerning the performance of a medical imaging system.

pharmacokinetics   Study of the activity of drugs and medicines.

pharmacology   Study of drugs and medicine.

pharynx   Back of the nasal passages and mouth; the throat.

phase   The time relationship between two events.

phenols   Organic compounds with the functional group OH^- attached to an aromatic ring.

pheochromocytoma   A neuroendocrine tumor of the adrenal gland that causes hypersecretion of epinephrine and norepinephrine.

phosphor   Chemical compound that upon photonic absorption will de-excite slowly by emitting light.

phosphorylation   Chemical process in which a molecule acquires a PO_4^{-3} group.

phosphorylorate   The result from phosphorylation.

photocathode   Negative electrode of a photomultiplier tube.

photodisintegration   Disintegration event triggered by photonic interactions.

photoelectric effect   Process by which photons de-excite through absorption by electrons, resulting in ionization phenomena.

photomultiplication   Multiplication of the signal emitted by the interaction of a photon in a scintillation detector.

photomultiplier tube   An electronic tube that converts light photons to electric pulses.

photon   Discrete packet of electromagnetic energy.

photopeak   A peak or increase in a graphic representation of a radioactive spectrum characteristic of the radionuclide under study.

phrenic artery   Artery in the diaphragm.

phylogenetic, phylogenic   Referring to the developmental history of an organism or race.

physical half-life   The elapsed time to reach half of the original quantity of radioactivity by decay.

physiology   Study of the function of tissues or organs.

pipeline processing   Computer instructions carried out in an assembly-line fashion.

pipet (pipette)   (1) Device used to deliver a precise amount of a liquid. (2) The act of using such a device.

pitch   The ratio of table movement per revolution over the collimated slice thickness of one row of a multislice CT detector.

pituitary   Endocrine gland located at the base of the brain; regulates growth and secretions of other endocrine glands.

pixel   From *pic*ture *el*ement; a single image element.

placenta   Organ attaching the embryo to the uterus; the afterbirth.

placental barrier   Term used to describe the semipermeable barrier interposed between the maternal and fetal blood by the placental membrane.

Planck's constant 6.626186×10^{-27} erg-seconds.

planimetry   Measurement of plane surfaces.

plasma   Fluid of the blood not including the red and white blood cells.

plasmacrit   1.00—decimal hematocrit

platelet, blood platelet, thrombocyte   Small, colorless disks that aid in blood clotting found in circulating blood.

pledget   Cotton swab.

plethysmography   Measurement of changes in volume using a plethysmograph.

pleura   Membrane lining of the chest cavity and lungs.

pleural effusion   Fluid in the space that contains the lungs and the thoracic cavity.

PnAO   Propylene amine oxime, a ^{99m}Tc-labeled complex that crosses the blood-brain barrier and is used to image regional cerebral perfusion.

pneumonectomy   The surgical removal of a lung.

point spread function   The profile of counts along a line through a point source of radioactivity.

Poisson distribution   A statistical distribution of events.

polar covalent bond   Covalent bond formed by the unequal sharing of a pair of electrons between two atoms.

polar map   Concentric plot of cardiac short-axis slices from apex at the center to basal slices on the outside.

polarization   The development of differences in potential between two points in living tissues.

polyatomic ion   Ion composed of more than one atom.

polycythemia   Disease characterized by an overabundance of red blood cells.

polycythemia vera   Inherited disease characterized by increase of red blood cells and total blood volume accompanied by splenomegaly, leukocytosis, thrombocytosis, and bone marrow hyperactivity.

polymer   Compound formed of simpler molecules, usually of high molecular weight.

polymerization   Formation of a polymer.

polypeptide   Compound containing two or more amino acids linked by a peptide bond.

polyphosphate   Any molecule containing the $(PO_3)_n$ group.

pons   (1) Slip of tissue connecting two parts of an organ. (2) Part of the base of the brain.

popliteal fossa   Depression at the back of the knee.

porcine   From a pig.

porta hepatis   Part of the liver receiving the major blood vessels.

positron (β^+)   Transitory nuclear particle with a mass equal to that of an electron and a charge equal to that of a proton.

potentiometer   See *voltmeter*.

preamplifier   A device placed between a detector and an amplifier used to shape and increase pulse size.

precession   The combined effect of spinning and falling creates precession when a hydrogen nucleus is placed within a strong magnetic field. Precession follows a circular path around the magnetic field, and the precessional frequency is determined by the Larmor equation.

precipitate   Solid compound that is produced in a chemical reaction between two soluble compounds in a solution.

precision   Refers to the variations of individual measurements.

precordium   Upper abdominal region.

pressure   Force per unit area.

primary fluor   A liquid scintillator.

primordial   Formed early in the course of development.

principal quantum number (n or n_i)   Relative distance from the nucleus at which the electron will be found and also its relative energy.

processor   See *central processing unit*.

proerythroblast   Primitive erythrocyte.

progesterone   Hormone secreted by the ovaries.

program   Complete sequence of instructions and routines necessary to solve a problem.

program development   Process of writing, entering, translating, and debugging source programs.

projection   A point in space from several different angles.

prolactin   Hormone secreted by the anterior pituitary.

promonocyte   Intermediate cell between the monoblast and monocyte.

prompt neutrons   Neutrons from a fission event that are emitted immediately after or during the event.

proportional   Having the same or constant ratio

proportional counter   A gas-filled radiation detector.

proprioception   Process of receiving stimulation within the tissue.

prostaglandins   Substance causing strong contractions of smooth muscle and dilation of the vascular bed.

prostatic hypertrophy   Enlargement of the prostate because of an increase in the size of its cells.

protease   Enzyme that digests protein.

protein   High molecular weight compound of many amino acids linked by peptide bonds.

proteinuria   Protein in the urine.

prothrombin   Protein combining with other proteins to form thrombin, a clotting agent.

proton   Nuclear particle with a mass of one unified mass unit and a charge of $+1.6 \times 10^{-9}$ coulomb.

psi   Pounds per square inch; unit of pressure.

PTH   Parathyroid hormone; parathyrin.

PTHrP   Parathyroid horrmone–related peptide.

ptosis   Denotes a falling or downward displacement of an organ.

pulmonary   Referring to the lungs.

pulmonic stenosis   Obstruction from the right ventricle, restricting the outflow of blood.

pulse-height analysis   See *pulse-height analyzer*.

pulse-height analyzer (PHA)   Instrument that accepts input from a detector and categorizes the pulses on the basis of signal strength.

pulse-height window   See *window*.

pulse sequence   A series of radiofrequency waves; In MRI contrast it is controlled by pulse sequences.

PVC   Premature ventricular contraction.

pyelonephritis   Inflammation of the kidney and the pelvis of the kidney.

pylorus   Part of the stomach just before the duodenum.

pyogenic   Pus forming; bacterial.

pyrogen   Fever-inducing substance.

pyrophosphate   Chemical compound containing a $P_2O_7^{-4}$ group.

QA   See *quality assurance*.

QC   See *quality control*.

QF   See *quality factor*.

QMP   Quality management program.

QRS complex   The principal deflection in the electrocardiogram representing ventricular depolarization.

qualitative chemical analysis   Determination of the identity of each constituent in a chemical system.

quality assurance (QA)   Quality assurance; monitoring that follows a comprehensive plan with delineated quality, technical, operational, and clinical indicators.

quality control (QC)   The aggregate of activities as design analysis and inspection of defects to ensure adequate quality.

quality control serum   A serum sample that is analyzed many times to yield data about the statistical reproducibility of a radioassay.

quality factor (QF)   Linear energy transfer–dependent factor by which absorbed doses are to be multiplied to account for the varying effectiveness of different radiations.

quality management   Processes using statistical theories to eliminate variances in procedures.

quantitative chemical analysis   Branch of chemical analysis dealing with the determination of how much of a constituent there is in a chemical compound.

quantum mechanics   Branch of physics dealing with the mathematical description of the wave properties of atomic and nuclear particles.

quantum number   Value describing the location of an electron in the electron configuration of an atom.

quenching   (1) Action of a gas added to a Geiger-Mueller detector, allowing it to resolve. (2) An undesirable reduction of light output from a liquid scintillator.

R wave   A portion of the QRS electrocardiographic signal denoting ventricular contraction and relaxation.

rad   See *radiation absorbed dose*.

radial immunodiffusion   Immunochemical method used for the determination of serum concentrations of physiologically important substances.

radiation absorbed dose (rad)   Quantity of radiation that deposits 100 erg of energy per gram of absorbing material.

radiation dose   Quantity of radiation absorbed by some material.

radiation exposure Exposure to ionizing radiation.

radiation safety Methods of protecting workers and the general population from the deleterious effects of radiation.

radioactive decay The process undertaken by unstable nuclei in which a specific number of particles and a specific amount of energy are released. From radioactive decay, each radionuclide has its own "fingerprint" of characteristic radiation(s).

radiochemistry Study of the chemistry of radioactive elements.

radiochromatography Chromatography using NaI crystal for detection of substances labeled with a radioisotope.

radiocolloids Colloid of a solid in a liquid where the solid phase contains a radioisotope.

radiograph Image of the internal structure of objects by exposure of film to x-rays; roentgenogram.

radioimmunoassay (RIA) Assay by immunological procedures using radioactive antigens.

radioimmunotherapy A therapy that combines the killing efficiency of radiation with a monoclonal antibody engineered to target specific proteins expressed by a tumor cell.

radioligand A radioactive ligand.

radionuclide Unstable nucleus that transmutes by way of nuclear decay.

radionuclide cisternogram An imaging procedure used to evaluate the flow of cerebrospinal fluid or the status of a shunt.

radionuclidic purity Amount of total radioactive species in a sample that is the desired radionuclide.

radiopharmaceutical Radioactive drug used for therapy or diagnosis.

radiopharmacology Study of radioactive drugs and their therapeutic and diagnostic uses.

radiopharmacy Laboratory producing and dispensing solutions labeled with radioisotopes for therapeutic and diagnostic purposes.

radioreceptor Sensory nerve terminal stimulated by radiant energy.

radiosynoviorthesis (RSV) The destruction of synovitis in individual joints by an intra-articular injection of radiocolloid such as ^{32}P.

RAM (random access memory) Memory accessed in such a way that the next location from which data are obtained is not dependent on the location of the previously obtained data.

random count The counting of a false random event, which is when two atoms decay at nearly the same time or the photons from two different annihilation events are detected within the timing window.

random label A term that refers to the in vitro tagging of circulating cells of the peripheral blood with a radioisotope.

raphe A seam; the line of union of two contiguous and similar structures.

RAS Renal artery stenosis.

RAST Radioallergosorbent test.

rate meter Device, used in conjunction with a detector, that measures the rate of activity of a radioisotope; usually in units of counts per minute or counts per second.

RBE See *relative biological effectiveness.*

reaction Any process resulting in a net change to the constituents of the system.

reactor See *nuclear reactor.*

read-only input (ROI) Input only from the memory or from an internal source. (Contrast *region of interest [ROI].*)

read-only memory (ROM) Computer memory containing information that cannot be altered.

reagent Any chemical used in a process.

receptor Sensory nerve terminal responding to stimulation by transmission of impulses to the central nervous system.

rectilinear scanner An imaging device that passes over the area of interest in a rectilinear fashion.

red blood cell (RBC) Any blood cell containing hemoglobin.

redistribution A term used in nuclear cardiac imaging to describe the phenomenon when a once photon-deficient area gains activity over a period of time, e.g., thallium.

redox Abbreviation for an oxidation-reduction reaction.

reducing agent Substance that donates electrons in an oxidation-reduction reaction.

reduction In an oxidation-reducing reaction it is the process by which one substance gains electrons.

reflex A reaction or involuntary movement.

Regadenoson A vasodilator; a newer synthetic selective A2 adenosine receptor agonist, which is associated with bronchoconstriction.

region of interest (ROI) Portion of the data field that is to be studied. (Contrast *read-only input [ROI].*)

register A device capable of storing a specified amount of data such as a word. See also *accumulator.*

regression analysis See *linear regression.*

relative biological effectiveness (RBE) Ratio of the biological response derived from a particular radiation as compared with another radiation exposure.

relative renal function The determination of the degree to which one kidney (usually the diseased kidney) contributes to total renal function.

rem See *roentgen equivalent man.*

renal cortex Smooth outer layer of the kidney.

replacement reaction Chemical process in which an ion is replaced by another species in a compound.

resolution The ability of a counting or imaging system to accurately depict two separate events in space, time, or energy as separate.

resolving time The length of time taken by a detector to sense and process a nuclear event.

resonance When a system (or in MRI, a proton) oscillates with larger amplitude at different frequencies

resorption A loss of substance by lysis.

rest mass Mass that is not in motion.

reticuloendothelial cells Phagocytes.

RFQ Radiofrequency quadripole accelerator.

RIA See *radioimmunoassay.*

RISC Reduced instruction set computer.

RNA Ribonucleic acid; RNA, DNA, and proteins are the three major macromolecules that are essential for all forms of life. RNA, transfer RNA, and messenger RNA are involved in numerous processes associated with creating, coding, and processing genetic information.

RNC Radionuclide cystography.

ROC curve Receiver operating characteristic curve: a graphic representation of sensitivity and specificity.

ROCM Radiopaque contrast media.

roentgen (R) Quantity of x-radiation or gamma radiation per cubic centimeter of air that produces one electrostatic unit of charge.

roentgen equivalent man (rem) Unit of radiation dose defined as the product of rad and RBE.

ROI See *read-only input* and *region of interest*.

ROM See *read-only memory*.

rotation time The time required for one 360-degree rotation of the CT gantry.

rotor A cylinder within a CT x-ray tube that is attached to the rotating anode. The rotor is driven by rotating magnetic fields produced by the stator (wire-wrapped, torus-shaped device positioned on the outside of the x-ray tube).

RSO Radiation safety office(r).

run A single continuous execution of a program.

Rutherford scattering See *elastic scattering*.

RV Right ventricle.

RVG Radionuclide ventriculogram.

saccule Small sac or pouch.

sagittal (1) Plane or section parallel to the long axis of the body. (2) Arrowlike shape.

saline Sodium chloride in water.

saline solution, physiological Salt solution compatible with body tissues.

salivary glands Glands secreting saliva, connected to the mouth by ducts; the three glands are the parotids, submaxillaries, and sublinguals.

saturation analysis A type of competitive binding assay where the specific reactor substance–binding sites are all occupied (saturated) by ligand; RIA is a type of saturation analysis.

scaler An electronic pulse counter.

scanner configuration 2D, 3D Modes of image acquisition that determine image presentation.

Schilling test Test for primary pernicious anemia.

scientific notation A system of using signs or numbers to represent numbers of greater and lesser magnitudes.

scintigraphic agent Substance injected to produce images of internal organs; usually a radioactive solution.

scintigraphy Imaging the distribution of a radionuclide with scintillation detection.

scintillation Flash of light produced in a phosphor by radiation.

scintillation camera An imaging system based on the principles of scintillation detection and recording.

scintillation detector A type of detector that is based on the property of using certain crystals to emit light photons after deposition of energy in the crystal by ionizing radiation.

scleroderma (1) Thickening of the skin by swelling. (2) Thickening of the fibrous tissue.

scout scan An x-ray examination performed with the CT gantry in a fixed position to generate a planar image. The scout scan is used to define the body region to be imaged during the CT scan. This is sometimes referred to as a *topogram*.

secondary fluor (waveshifter) A liquid scintillator.

secretin Hormone-stimulating secretion of pancreatic juice and bile secreted by the duodenal mucous membrane.

secular equilibrium Parent-daughter radioisotope pair in which the parent has a much longer half-life than does the daughter radionuclide.

semiconductor Substance whose conductivity is enhanced by the addition of another substance or through the application of heat, light, or voltage.

senescent Growing old; characteristic of old age.

sensitivity (1) Pertains to the ability of a given test to determine what fraction or percentage of ill patients will have a positive test result. (2) Efficiency of a given detector system.

septal Referring to a wall or partition.

septum A wall or partition.

sequestration Destruction.

serous Referring to serum.

serum Liquid remaining after blood has clotted.

shells Energy levels in electronic configuration.

shielding Absorbing material used to attenuate ionizing radiation.

short axis Sagittal views of the heart in reoriented images.

shunt Bypass; an alternate course.

SI Serum iron; see also *specific ionization*.

sialography Salivary gland imaging.

SIDS Sudden infant death syndrome.

sievert (Sv) Unit for dose equivalent. For a quality factor (QF) = 1, one sievert is the dose equivalent of one gray (100 rad); 1 Sv = 100 rem.

signal-to-noise ratio A ratio describing the relationship between desired and unwanted information.

single photon absorptiometry (SPA) Bone mineral content measurement technique using gamma-ray or x-ray absorption with a single energy photon-emitting source.

single photon emission computed tomography (SPECT) An imaging technique associated with single gamma-ray–emitting radiopharmaceuticals obtained using a scintillation camera that moves around the patient to obtain images from multiple angles for tomographic image reconstruction.

sinogram A two-dimensional plot of SPECT or PET projection count profiles on the horizontal axis versus angle of the projection on the vertical axis.

sinusoid Beginning of the venous system in the spleen, liver, bone marrow, and so on that has an irregularly shaped, thin-walled space.

sinusoidal (1) Referring to a recess or cavity. (2) Referring to an abnormal channel that permits the escape of pus.

Sjögren syndrome An aggregate of signs and symptoms including dryness of mucous membranes, purpuric spots on the face, and bilateral parotid enlargement.

SNM Society of Nuclear Medicine.

SNR Signal-to-noise ratio.

software Collection of programs and routines associated with a computer.

software bootstrap A bootstrap activated by loading the instructions and specifying the appropriate load and start address.

sol Liquid colloid solution.

solid phase antibody An antibody chemically linked to a solid surface.

solitary pulmonary nodule (SPN)   A single nodule in the lung.

solute   Material dissolved into a solution.

solution   Physical system consisting of one or more substances dissolved in another substance.

solvent   Substance that acts as the dissolving agent in a solution.

solvent extraction   Use of a second solvent to preferentially dissolve a compound out of another solution.

somatostatin   A neuropeptide concentrated in numerous areas throughout the body (i.e., hypothalamus, cerebral cortex, brain stem, gastrointestinal tract, and pancreas).

sorption   Adsorption or absorption.

SPA   See *single photon absorptiometry*.

spallation   To chip or flake off.

specific activity   Unit pertaining to the disintegrations per gram of a radioisotope.

specific ionization (SI)   Linear rate of energy attenuation of ionizing radiation measured in terms of the number of ion pairs produced per unit distance traveled.

specificity   The ability of a given test to determine what fraction or percentage of well patients will have a negative test result. Ability of a substance to recognize and bind to only one other molecule.

specific reactor substance (SRS)   Material capable of specifically and reversibly reacting with another molecule.

SPECT   See *single photon emission computed tomography*.

spectrometer   Device measuring electromagnetic radiation characteristics in a spectrum.

spectrophotometry   Use of an instrument that measures light or color by photonic transmission.

spermatogenesis   Process of forming sperm.

sphincter   Muscle controlling a body opening.

spin-down   Based on quantum mechanics, it is when high-energy nuclei (e.g., H) align their magnetic moments in the antiparallel direction and are termed *spin-down nuclei*

spin-up   Based on quantum mechanics, it is when low-energy nuclei align their magnetic moments parallel to the external magnetic field and are termed *spin-up nuclei*.

splanchnic   Pertaining to the interior organs in any of the four great body cavities.

splenic hilum   Fissure where vessels and nerves enter the spleen.

SPN   Solitary pulmonary nodule.

spondylolysis   Breaking down or dissolution of the body of the vertebra.

SRS   See *specific reactor substance*.

SSKI   Saturated solution of potassium iodide.

SSTR   Somatostatin receptor.

stable electron configuration   Configuration of electrons about an atom in the atom's lowest energy state.

standard   A solution of pure substance of known concentration to which unknown substances may be compared.

standard deviation   The square root of the average of the squares of the deviation of the value of a set of measurements from each of the individual measurements.

stannous ion   Ion of tin in the +2 valence state.

stationary phase   Chromatographic phase that does not move with the solvent front.

steatorrhea   Excess fat in the feces.

stellate   Star shaped.

stenosis   A narrowing of a canal or vessel.

Stenson ducts   Canals that empty the parotid gland.

step and shoot   Movement of a SPECT system as it orbits the patient. The camera moves, stops, acquires an image, moves again, stops, and acquires another image.

steroid   Complex molecular structure containing four interlocking rings; three contain six carbon atoms each and the fourth contains five carbon atoms.

stoichiometry   Study of numeric interrelationships between chemical elements and compounds and the mathematical laws governing such relationships.

stoma   opening

storage   Device into which data can be entered and held and from which it can be retrieved.

stroke volume   The quantity of blood ejected by the heart in a single beat.

student *t*-test   A test of statistical significance of a deviation.

stunning   The term used to describe a decrease in subsequent radioiodine (^{131}I) uptake by residual thyroid and metastatic thyroid carcinoma following the administration of "scanning" doses of ^{131}I greater than 2 mCi.

subarachnoid   Below the membrane between the dura mater and the pia mater.

subarachnoid space   A space below the subarachnoid that contains cerebrospinal fluid.

subendocardial   Below the endocardium.

subphrenic   Below the diaphragm.

subprogram   A program or a sequence of instructions that can be called to perform the same task (although perhaps on different data) at different points in a program or in different programs.

sulcus   Any of the grooves or furrows on the surface of the brain.

supernatant, supernate   Liquid lying above or floating on a precipitated material.

survey meter   Meter that measures rate of radioactive exposure, usually in units of milliroentgens per hour.

SUV   Standard uptake value.

SVC   Superior vena cava.

synapse   The place where a nerve impulse is transmitted from one neuron to another.

synarthrosis   Immovable joint, where bones lock within one another.

synchronous   Performance of a sequence of operations controlled by an external clocking device; implies that no operation can take place until the previous operation is complete.

synchronous transfer   Sequenced computer program operated by an external clock that does not permit a step to proceed until the previous step is completed.

syncope   Fainting.

synovia   Transparent fluid found in joint cavities.

synovitis   Inflammation of joint-lining membrane.

Système Internationale (SI)   International system of units used to replace traditional units as a result of U.S. metrication laws PL 93-380 and PL 94-168.

systole   Contraction and expelling of blood from the heart.

systolic pressure   The pressure in the heart during systole.

T1   A weighted image in MRI that uses a short TE and short TR with a 90-degree pulse followed by a single 180-degree pulse.

T2   A weighted image in MRI that uses a long TR and long TE, which will maximize T2 contrast.

T_3   Triiodothyronine.

T_4   Tetraiodothyronine; thyroxine.

T wave   The next deflection in the electrocardiogram following the QRS complex; it represents ventricular repolarization.

tachycardia   Fast heart beat.

target   Object to be bombarded by ionizing radiation, usually in an accelerator or cyclotron.

TBG   See *thyroid-binding globulin.*

TBPA   Thyroxine-binding prealbumin.

tentorium   Fibrous tissue shelf separating the cerebrum from the cerebellum.

tesla   Unit for measuring magnetic field strength; 1 tesla = 10,000 gauss.

testosterone   Hormone produced by the testes, influencing the male characteristics.

tetrahedron   Molecular geometry in which the central atom is attached to four other atoms and the bond axes are directed along the diagonals of a cube.

tetralogy of Fallot   Birth defect involving deformities of the blood vessels and walls of the heart chamber.

thecal space   The space below the sheath covering the spinal cord.

therapeutic   Referring to the treatment of disease.

therapeutic window   Range of dosage of a pharmaceutical that produces a beneficial effect.

thermal neutrons   Neutrons with a maximum kinetic energy of 100 keV.

thermionic emission   Electrons freed from an atom by heat.

thermodynamics   Study of processes based on energy changes in the system.

thermoluminescent detector (TLD)   Type of crystal used to monitor radiation exposure by emitting light; used in a film badge or ring badge.

thiols   Family of organic compounds containing the functional group –SH.

thoracic cage   Chest cavity.

thrombin   Enzyme used as a clotting agent.

thrombocyte   See *platelet.*

thrombosis   Formation of a blood clot.

thyroid-binding globulin (TBG)   Serum protein that is the primary agent for transport for thyroid hormone.

thyroid gland   Endocrine gland that regulates metabolism.

thyrotropin (TSH)   Hormone stimulating the thyroid secreted by the anterior pituitary.

thyroxine   Hormone of the thyroid gland; 3,5,3,5-tetraiodothyronine.

tidal volume   The volume of air breathed out in a normal breath.

time constant   The speed of response of a rate meter.

titer   (1) Aliquot of titrant (solution of known concentration). (2) The quantity of a substance required to produce a reaction with a given amount of another substance.

Title 10 of the Code of the Federal Regulations, Part 20 (10 CFR, Part 20)   *United States Nuclear Regulatory Commission Rules and Regulations, Standards for Protection against Radiation;* Title 10 of the CFR pertains to atomic energy.

titration   Method of quantitative analysis in which one substance is volumetrically added to another substance with which it quantitatively reacts.

titrimetric procedures   Chemical laboratory procedure for quantitative analysis by addition of solution of a known concentration to a solution of unknown concentration.

TLD   See *thermoluminescent detector.*

tomograph   Any image representing three-dimensional information.

tomography   Process of recording a tomograph.

topogram   See *scout scan.*

torcula   Hollow, expanded area.

torsion   Twisting; in nuclear medicine this term is usually used to describe the twisting of the spermatic cord.

total count tube   A tube in an RIA to which an aliquot of labeled ligand only has been added to serve as a check on the delivery of that material.

total lung capacity   The volume of air in the lungs when as much air has been inhaled as possible.

TQM   Total quality management.

trabeculae   Fibrous tissue supporting the structure of an organ.

tracer study   Examination either in vivo or in vitro using a small amount of radionuclide-labeled substance to follow its path.

trackball   An electronic pointing device for a computer.

transcobalamin   Derivative of the cobalt-containing complex common to all members of the vitamin B_{12} group.

transferrin   Serum globulin binding and transporting iron.

transient equilibrium   Equilibrium reached by a parent-daughter radioisotope pair in which the half-life of the parent is longer than the half-life of the daughter.

transmission imaging   A study that is performed using an external source during acquisition for use in attenuation correction.

transmittance   The fraction of light that passes through photographic film.

transmutation   Nuclear process by which one element is changed into another element.

transudate   Term given to solvents and solutes that pass through a membrane.

transverse tomography   Transverse scanning of a cross section of an organ, done from multiple directions and then superimposed in a specific manner.

trauma   Injury; wound.

TRH   Thyrotropin-releasing hormone.

tritium   Isotope of hydrogen with a mass of three unified mass units, consisting of one proton and two neutrons.

true count   The counting of a pair of annihilation gamma rays striking the two detectors at the same time.

TSH   Thyroid-stimulating hormone. See *thyrotropin.*

turnkey   Computer system sold in a ready-to-use state.

Tyndall effect   Light reflected or dispersed by particles suspended in a gas or liquid.

tyrosine Amino acid present in proteins that are susceptible to radioiodination.

UIBC See *unsaturated iron-binding capacity.*

ultrasonic nebulizer Device used for dispersing liquids in a fine mist through the use of sound waves.

ultrasonography Use of sound waves to image an internal structure of the body.

uniformity correction Compensation for detector nonuniformity.

United States Pharmacopeia (USP) Official listing of all drugs and medications.

UNIX A computer operating system.

unsaturated iron-binding capacity (UIBC) Amount of serum transferrin that is not saturated with iron.

uptake probe A spectrometer system with a flat-field collimater; a major application is in thyroid uptake studies.

USP See *United States Pharmacopeia.*

vaccine Dead bacteria given to build specific immunity against disease.

valence electrons Electrons in the outermost energy level.

valence state Ionization state of an element in an ionic compound.

van der Waals bond Attraction between the charged portions of two molecules, known as dipoles.

variable The symbolic representation of a logical storage location that can contain a value that changes during a processing operation.

variance Degree of change.

vascular Referring to the vessels.

vascular bed Entire blood supply of an organ or structure.

vascular lesion Lesion that affects the vessels.

vasculature (1) Supply of vessels to a region. (2) Vascular system.

vasculitis Inflammation of a vessel.

vasoconstrictor Something that causes the constriction of blood vessels.

vasodilator Something that causes the dilation of blood vessels.

venipuncture Placement of a needle within a vein.

venography Radiography of the veins using a contrast medium; phlebography.

venous thrombi Blood clots within the veins.

ventilation Process of supplying air.

ventilation imaging The imaging procedure of the gas exchange mechanism in the lung, in which measurement of regional ventilation measurement of regional lung volumes, for closing volume, and for studying factors that influence the distribution of a single breath.

ventilation-perfusion ratio (V/Q) Comparison of functioning ventilatory space and perfused tissue within the lung; ratio of minute flow of air through alveoli to minute flow of blood through pulmonary capillaries.

ventricular Referring to a small cavity or chamber.

ventriculography Radiography of the ventricles of the brain.

vertical long axis Coronal images of the heart in the re-oriented images.

vesicoureteral reflux (VUR) Backward flow of urine through the bladder and into a ureter.

vitamin Organic compound necessary to maintain normal growth or function; found in some amounts in plants and animals.

volt Basic unit of electrical potential equal to one joule per coulomb.

voltmeter Device used to measure potential difference in electric circuits; potentiometer.

volume (1) Amount of space occupied in three dimensions. (2) A mass storage medium that can be treated as file-structured data storage.

volume dilution Dilution of a solution by addition of pure liquid solvent.

volume rendering Surface or MIP display of 3D tomographic data.

volumetric flask Flasks marked TC are calibrated "to contain" a specific volume, depending on the size of the flask, and allow volume measurement within noted accuracy limits.

voxel A three-dimensional picture element (pixel).

V/Q See *ventilation-perfusion ratio.*

VTE Venous thrombosis embolism.

VUR See *vesicoureteral reflux.*

wavelength Length per cycle in wave-motion mechanics.

well counter A thallium-activated sodium iodide crystal scintillation detector with a hole in the crystal to accommodate a sample vial.

white blood cell (WBC) Blood cell whose nucleus determines the type of cell: lymphocyte, monocyte, neutrophil, eosinophil, basophil.

whole gut transit The movement of solid material throughout the entire gastrointestinal tract.

window (1) Region of interest. (2) Limits of energy radiation accepted by a pulse-height analyzer.

wipe test Testing for removable contamination.

word Unit of data that may be stored in one addressable location (most microcomputers use 16-bit words).

WORM A type of optical disk drive; *w*rite *o*nce *r*ead *m*any.

x pulse In an Anger scintillation camera, those pulses emanating from the resistor/capacitor network positioned in a horizontal manner.

xerostomia Dryness of the mouth.

xiphisternum Inferior tip of the sternum.

x-ray Photonic radiation originating from electronic de-excitation.

x-ray diffraction Spectroscopic method for determining crystal structure by the interaction of x-rays with the atoms involved in the crystalline structure.

x-ray tube A vacuum tube that contains electrodes that produce electromagnetic energy in the x-ray portion of the spectrum.

y pulse In an Anger scintillation camera, those pulses emanating from the resistor/capacitor network positioned in a vertical manner.

Z number See *atomic number.*

z pulse In an Anger scintillation camera, it represents the sum of the *x* and *y* pulses.

zipper effect Overlap of two or more images.

Zollinger-Ellison syndrome Familial polyendocrine adenomatosis.

CHAPTER 1

1. b
2. c
3. c
4. a
5. d
6. c
7. b
8. a
9. d
10. a
11. b
12. d
13. c
14. b
15. d
16. c
17. b
18. c
19. a
20. b
21. c
22. b
23. c
24. b
25. c
26. b
27. c
28. b
29. b
30. c
31. a
32. b
33. b
34. a
35. d
36. c
37. b
38. d
39. d
40. b
41. b
42. c
43. c
44. c
45. b
46. c
47. a
48. d
49. b
50. a

Figure 2-7 courtesy Mallinckrodt, Inc., St Louis, Missouri.

Figure 3-9 courtesy Spectrum Dynamics LLC, Danville, California.

Figure 6-3 from Kowalsky RJ, Perry JR: *Radiopharmaceuticals in nuclear medicine practice*, Norwalk, Conn, 1987, Appleton & Lange.

Figures 6-4 and 6-19 courtesy GE Medical Systems-Americas, Milwaukee, Wisconsin.

Figure 7-8 from Ionizing radiation exposure of the population of the United States, *National Council on Radiation Protection Report No. 93*, Washington, DC, 1987, National Council on Radiation Protection.

Figure 7-9 from Nuclear Regulatory Commission Form 3, United States Nuclear Regulatory Commission, Washington, DC, 2010.

Figures 8-2, 8-3, 8-4, 8-6, 8-10, 8-13, 8-14, 8-17 through 8-22, 8-24 and 8-25 from Kowalczyk N, Donnett K: *Integrated patient care for the imaging professional*, St Louis, 1996, Mosby.

Figure 8-5 from Adler AM, Carlton RR: *Introduction to radiologic sciences and patient care*, ed 3, St Louis, 2003, Saunders.

Figures 8-7 and 8-23 modified from Potter PA, Perry AG: *Fundamentals of nursing: concepts, process, and practice*, ed 3, St Louis, 1994, Mosby.

Figures 8-8, 8-11, 8-15 and 8-19 from Ehrlich RA, Daly JA: *Patient care in radiography with an introduction to medical imaging*, ed 7, St Louis, 2009, Mosby.

Figure 8-9 from Ehrlich RA, McCloskey ED, Daly JA: *Patient care in radiography with an introduction to medical imaging*, ed 6, St Louis, 2004, Mosby.

Figures 10-7 and 10-18 courtesy General Electric Medical Systems, Waukesha, Wisconsin.

Figure 10-19 courtesy Henry Yeung, MD, Memorial Sloan Kettering Cancer Center, New York.

Figures 11-10 and 11-13 from Ballinger PW, Frank ED: *Merrill's atlas of radiographic positions and radiologic procedures*, ed 10, St Louis, 2003, Mosby.

Figure 11-23 Courtesy Jerry Payne, General Electric Medical Systems, Waukesha, Wisconsin.

Figure 14-1 from Agur AMR: *Grant's atlas of anatomy*, ed 9, Baltimore, 1991, Williams & Wilkins.

Figures 14-2, 14-4, and 14-5 from Anthony CP, Thibodeau GA: *Textbook of anatomy and physiology*, ed 10, St Louis, 1979, Mosby.

Figure 14-3 from Netter FH: *The CIBA collection—nervous system*, vol 1, West Caldwell, NJ, 1983, CIBA Pharmaceutical.

Figure 14-6 from Gilman S, Newman SW: *Manter and Gatz's essentials of clinical neuroanatomy and neurophysiology*, ed 7, Philadelphia, 1987, FA Davis.

Figures 15-1 and 15-2 from Thibodeau GA: *Anthony's textbook of anatomy and physiology*, ed 13, St Louis, 1990, Mosby.

Figure 15-14 from Becker DV, Hurley JR: Current status of radioiodine (^{131}I) treatment of hyperthyroidism. In Freeman L, Weissman HS, editors: *Nuclear medicine annual 1982*, New York, 1982, Raven Press.

Figure 15-19 redrawn from data reported by Melicow MM: One hundred cases of pheochromocytoma (107 tumors) at the Columbia-Presbyterian Medical Center, 1926-1976: a clinicopathological analysis, *Cancer* 40:1987-2004, 1977.

Figures 16-2 and 16-4 from Hammond EC: The effects of smoking, *Sci Am* 39:207, 1962. Copyright 1962 by Scientific American, Inc. All rights reserved.

Figures 16-7, 16-9, 16-10, 16-12, and 16-15 modified from and courtesy Missouri Baptist Medical Center, St Louis, Missouri.

Figures 16-13 and 16-14 courtesy Barnes-Jewish Hospital, St Louis, Missouri.

Figures 17-14 and 17-15 courtesy J. Machac, MD, Mount Sinai School of Medicine.

Figures 18-1, 18-19, and 18-30 from Thibodeau GA: *Anthony's textbook of anatomy and physiology*, ed 13, St Louis, 1990, Mosby.

Figure 18-31 from Hamilton WJ: *Textbook of human anatomy*, ed 2, St Louis, 1979, Mosby; courtesy Macmillan Press Ltd, Houndsmill Basingstoke, Hampshire, England.

Figure 19-20 from Henkin RE, Boles MA, Dillehay GL et al: *Nuclear medicine*, St Louis, 1996, Mosby.

Figure 20-1 from Anthony CP, Thibodeau GA: *Textbook of anatomy and physiology*, ed 10, St Louis, 1979, Mosby.

Figure 20-2 from Patton KT, Thibodeau GA: *Anatomy and physiology*, ed 7, St Louis, 2009, Elsevier.

Figures 20-4, 20-5, and 20-6 from Thibodeau GA: *Anthony's textbook of anatomy and physiology*, ed 13, St Louis, 1990, Mosby.

Figure 20-7 from Hamilton WJ: *Textbook of human anatomy*, ed 2, St Louis, 1979, Mosby; courtesy Macmillan Press Ltd, Houndsmill Basingstoke, Hampshire, England.

Figures 21-1 and 21-2 from Thibodeau GA, Patton KT: *Anatomy and physiology*, ed 5, St Louis, 2003, Mosby.

Page numbers followed by *f* indicate figures; *t*, tables; *b*, boxes.

713